Dietary Reference Intakes (DRIs): Recommended Intakes for Individuals, Elements
Food and Nutrition Board, Institute of Medicine, National Academies

Life Stage Group	Calcium (mg/d)	Chromium (μg/d)	Copper (μg/d)	Fluoride (mg/d)	Iodine (μg/d)	Iron (mg/d)	Magnesium (mg/d)	Manganese (mg/d)	Molybdenum (μg/d)	Phosphorus (mg/d)	Selenium (μg/d)	Zinc (mg/d)
Infants												
0-6 mo	210*	0.2*	200*	0.01*	110*	0.27*	30*	0.003*	2*	100*	15*	2*
7-12 mo	270*	5.5*	220*	0.5*	130*	11	75*	0.6*	3*	275*	20*	3
Children												
1-3 y	500*	11*	340	0.7*	90	7	80	1.2*	17	460	20	3
4-8 y	800*	15*	440	1*	90	10	130	1.5*	22	500	30	5
Males												
9-13 y	1300*	25*	700	2*	120	8	240	1.9*	34	1250	40	8
14-18 y	1300*	35*	890	3*	150	11	410	2.2*	43	1250	55	11
19-30 y	1000*	35*	900	4*	150	8	400	2.3*	45	700	55	11
31-50 y	1000*	35*	900	4*	150	8	420	2.3*	45	700	55	11
51-70 y	1200*	30*	900	4*	150	8	420	2.3*	45	700	55	11
>70 y	1200*	30*	900	4*	150	8	420	2.3*	45	700	55	11
Females												
9-13 y	1300*	21*	700	2*	120	8	240	1.6*	34	1250	40	8
14-18 y	1300*	24*	890	3*	150	15	360	1.6*	43	1250	55	9
19-30 y	1000*	25*	900	3*	150	18	310	1.8*	45	700	55	8
31-50 y	1000*	25*	900	3*	150	18	320	1.8*	45	700	55	8
51-70 y	1200*	20*	900	3*	150	8	320	1.8*	45	700	55	8
>70 y	1200*	20*	900	3*	150	8	320	1.8*	45	700	55	8
Pregnancy												
≤18 y	1300*	29*	1000	3*	220	27	400	2.0*	50	1250	60	13
19-30 y	1000*	30*	1000	3*	220	27	350	2.0*	50	700	60	11
31-50 y	1000*	30*	1000	3*	220	27	360	2.0*	50	700	60	11
Lactation												
≤18 y	1300*	44*	1300	3*	290	10	360	2.6*	50	1250	70	14
19-30 y	1000*	45*	1300	3*	290	9	310	2.6*	50	700	70	12
31-50 y	1000*	45*	1300	3*	290	9	320	2.6*	50	700	70	12

SOURCES: Dietary Reference Intakes for Calcium, Phosphorus, Magnesium, Vitamin D, and Fluoride (1997); Dietary Reference Intakes for Thiamin, Riboflavin, Niacin, Vitamin B6, Folate, Vitamin B12, Pantothenic Acid, Biotin, and Choline (1998); Dietary Reference Intakes for Vitamin C, Vitamin E, Selenium, and Carotenoids (2000); and Dietary Reference Intakes for Vitamin A, Vitamin K, Arsenic, Boron, Chromium, Copper, Iodine, Iron, Manganese, Molybdenum, Nickel, Silicon, Vanadium, and Zinc (2001). Copyright 2001 by the National Academy of Sciences. All rights reserved.

NOTE: This table presents Recommended Dietary Allowances (RDAs) in bold type and Adequate Intakes (AIs) in ordinary type followed by an asterisk (*). RDAs and AIs may both be used as goals for individual intake. RDAs are set to meet the needs of almost all (97 to 98 percent) individuals in a group. For healthy breastfed infants, the AI is the mean intake. The AI for other life stage and gender groups is believed to cover needs of all individuals in the group, but lack of data or uncertainty in the data prevent being able to specify with confidence the percentage of individuals covered by this intake.

Dietary Reference Intakes (DRIs): Tolerable Upper Intake Levels (UL[a]), Elements
Food and Nutrition Board, Institute of Medicine, National Academies

Life Stage Group	Arsenic[b]	Boron (mg/d)	Calcium (g/d)	Chromium	Copper (μg/d)	Fluoride (mg/d)	Iodine (μg/d)	Iron (mg/d)	Magnesium (mg/d)[c]	Manganese (mg/d)	Molybdenum (μg/d)	Nickel (mg/d)	Phosphorus (g/d)	Selenium (μg/d)	Silicon[d]	Vanadium (mg/d)[e]	Zinc (mg/d)
Infants																	
0-6 mo	ND[f]	ND	ND	ND	ND	0.7	ND	40	ND	ND	ND	ND	ND	45	ND	ND	4
7-12 mo	ND	ND	ND	ND	ND	0.9	ND	40	ND	ND	ND	ND	ND	60	ND	ND	5
Children																	
1-3 y	ND	3	2.5	ND	1000	1.3	200	40	65	2	300	0.2	3	90	ND	ND	7
4-8 y	ND	6	2.5	ND	3000	2.2	300	40	110	3	600	0.3	3	150	ND	ND	12
Males, Females																	
9-13 y	ND	11	2.5	ND	5000	10	600	40	350	6	1100	0.6	4	280	ND	ND	23
14-18 y	ND	17	2.5	ND	8000	10	900	45	350	9	1700	1.0	4	400	ND	ND	34
19-70 yr	ND	20	2.5	ND	10,000	10	1100	45	350	11	2000	1.0	4	400	ND	1.8	40
>70 y	ND	20	2.5	ND	10,000	10	1100	45	350	11	2000	1.0	3	400	ND	1.8	40
Pregnancy																	
<18 y	ND	17	2.5	ND	8000	10	900	45	350	9	1700	1.0	3.5	400	ND	ND	34
19-50 y	ND	20	2.5	ND	10,000	10	1100	45	350	11	2000	1.0	3.5	400	ND	ND	40
Lactation																	
<18 y	ND	17	2.5	ND	8000	10	900	45	350	9	1700	1.0	4	400	ND	ND	34
19-50 y	ND	20	2.5	ND	10,000	10	1100	45	350	11	2000	1.0	4	400	ND	ND	40

SOURCES: Dietary Reference Intakes for Calcium, Phosphorus, Magnesium, Vitamin D, and Fluoride (1997); Dietary Reference Intakes for Thiamin, Riboflavin, Niacin, Vitamin B6, Folate, Vitamin B12, Pantothenic Acid, Biotin, and Choline (1998); Dietary Reference Intakes for Vitamin C, Vitamin E, Selenium, and Carotenoids (2000); and Dietary Reference Intakes for Vitamin A, Vitamin K, Arsenic, Boron, Chromium, Copper, Iodine, Iron, Manganese, Molybdenum, Nickel, Silicon, Vanadium, and Zinc (2001). These reports may be accessed via www.nap.edu. Copyright 2001 by the National Academy of Sciences. All rights reserved.

[a] UL = The maximum level of daily nutrient intake that is likely to pose no risk of adverse effects. Unless otherwise specified, the UL represents total intake from food, water, and supplements. Due to lack of suitable data, ULs could not be established for arsenic, chromium, and silicon. In the absence of ULs, extra caution may be warranted in consuming levels above recommended intakes.

[b] Although the UL was not determined for arsenic, there is no justification for adding arsenic to food or supplements.

[c] The ULs for magnesium represent intake from a pharmacologic agent only and do not include intake from food and water.

[d] Although silicon has not been shown to cause adverse effects in humans, there is no justification for adding silicon to supplements.

[e] Although vanadium in food has not been shown to cause adverse effects in humans, there is no justification for adding vanadium to food and vanadium supplements should be used with caution. The UL is based on adverse effects in laboratory animals and this data could be used to set a UL for adults but not children and adolescents.

[f] ND = Not determinable due to lack of data of adverse effects in this age group and concern with regard to lack of ability to handle excess amounts. Source of intake should be from food only to prevent high levels of intake.

Foundations and Clinical Applications of

Nutrition

A Nursing Approach

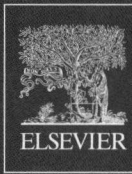

Third Edition

Foundations and Clinical Applications of

Nutrition

A Nursing Approach

Michele Grodner, EdD, CHES
Professor and Nutrition Coordinator
Department of Community Health
William Paterson University
Wayne, New Jersey

Sara Long, PhD, RD
Professor and Director, Didactic Program in Dietetics
Department of Animal Science, Food, and Nutrition
Southern Illinois University Carbondale
Carbondale, Illinois

Sandra DeYoung, EdD, RN
Associate Dean
College of Science and Health
William Paterson University
Wayne, New Jersey

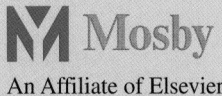
Mosby
An Affiliate of Elsevier

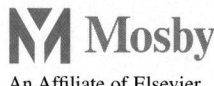

An Affiliate of Elsevier

11830 Westline Industrial Drive
St. Louis, Missouri 63146

FOUNDATIONS AND CLINICAL APPLICATIONS OF NUTRITION:
A NURSING APPROACH, THIRD EDITION   0-323-02009-7
Copyright © 2004, Mosby, Inc. All rights reserved.

NOTICE

Nutrition is an ever-changing field. Standard safety precautions must be followed, but as new research and clinical experience broaden our knowledge, changes in treatment and drug therapy may become necessary or appropriate. Readers are advised to check the most current product information provided by the manufacturer of each drug to be administered to verify the recommended dose, the method and duration of administration, and contraindications. It is the responsibility of the licensed prescriber, relying on experience and knowledge of the patient, to determine dosages and the best treatment for each individual patient. Neither the publisher nor the author assumes any liability for any injury and/or damage to persons or property arising from this publication.

Previous editions copyrighted 1996, 2000.

Library of Congress Cataloging-in-Publication Data
Grodner, Michele.
   Foundations and clinical applications of nutrition: a nursing approach / Michele
Grodner, Sara Long, Sandra DeYoung.—3rd ed.
      p. ; cm.
   Includes bibliographical references and index.
   ISBN 0-323-02009-7
   1. Diet therapy. 2. Nutrition. 3. Nursing.   I. Long, Sara. II. DeYoung, Sandra. III. Title.
   DNLM: 1. Diet Therapy—methods. 2. Nutrition. 3. Nursing Process. WB 400 G8735f2004
RM216.G946 2004
615.8'54—dc21   2003046490

Vice President and Publishing Director: Sally Schrefer
Senior Acquisitions Editor: Yvonne Alexopoulos
Senior Developmental Editor: Melissa K. Boyle
Publishing Services Manager: Catherine Jackson
Project Manager: Anne Gassett Konopka
Design Manager: Bill Drone
Cover Photos: PhotoDisc
Chapter Opening Photos: PhotoDisc

Printed in China

Last digit is the print number: 9 8 7 6 5 4 3 2

As our friend Claudio Pecori says:
"We're not here for a long time. . . we're here for a good time."

Michele Grodner

Sara Long

To my parents: examples of integrity, hard work, persistence, and love.

Sandra DeYoung

Contributors

Kem Louie, PhD, APRN, FAAN

Associate Professor
Department of Nursing
William Paterson University
Wayne, New Jersey
Nursing Approach boxes for Chapters 2, 9-11, 14-16, and 19
Cultural Considerations boxes for Chapters 1, 9-12, 14, and 17-21

Co-author Sandra DeYoung wrote *Nursing Approach* boxes for Chapters 3, 5, 6, 8, 13, and 20, as well as *Nursing Approach* boxes (revised by Kem Louie) for Chapters 1, 4, 7, 12, 17, 18, 21, and 22.

Marcia L. Nahikian-Nelms, PhD, RD, LD

Associate Professor
Director, Didactic Program in Dietetics
Southeast Missouri State University
Cape Girardeau, Missouri
Chapter 22: Nutrition in Cancer, AIDS, and Other Special Problems

Reviewers

Marianne Petrella Aloupis, RD, CNSD

Clinical Dietitian Specialist
Clinical Nutrition Support Services
Hospital of the University of Pennsylvania
Philadelphia, Pennsylvania

Ethan A. Bergman, PhD, RD, CD, FADA

Professor of Food Science and Nutrition
Department of Family and Consumer Sciences
Central Washington University
Ellensburg, Washington

Constance Locher Bussard, RD

Freelance Registered Dietitian
Springfield, Illinois

Barbara Cordell, PhD, RN, HNC, RMT

Director, ADN Program
Panola College
Carthage, Texas;
Private Practice, Holistic Nursing
Nacogdoches, Texas

Connie Breach Cranford, MS, RD, CSR

Renal Dietitian
Gambro Healthcare
Springfield, Illinois

Michele DeBiasse-Fortin, MS, RD, LDN, CNSD

Clinical Nutrition Manager/Nutrition Support Dietitian
Department of Food and Nutrition Services
Quincy Medical Center
Quincy, Massachusetts

Sandra P. Eardley, PhD, RD/LD

Assistant Professor (Emerita)
Department of Obstetrics & Gynecology
Southern Illinois University School of Medicine
Springfield, Illinois

Deena Elizalde, APRN, BC

Clinical Instructor
College of Nursing
Texas Woman's University, Houston Center
Houston, Texas

Dawn Goodholm, RD, LD/N

Clinical Nutrition Manager
Food and Nutrition Services
Brooks Rehabilitation Hospital
Jacksonville, Florida

Dorothy G. Herron, PhD, RN, CS
Assistant Professor, Adult Health Department
School of Nursing
University of Maryland
Baltimore, Maryland

Elizabeth Ann Kenyon, BS, RD, LMNT+
Consultant Dietitian and Dietitian for Diabetes Control Program
Panhandle Community Services
Gering, Nebraska;
Adjunct Faculty, Life Sciences
Western Nebraska Community College
Scottsbluff, Nebraska

Alice K. Lindeman, PhD, RD
Associate Professor
Department of Applied Health Sciences
Indiana University
Bloomington, Indiana

Sara A. Lopinski, MS, RD
Assistant Director
Food and Nutrition Services
St. John's Hospital
Springfield, Illinois

Debra L. McGinnis, MS, RD, LD
Clinical Dietitian, Department of Nutrition and Dietetics
Ohio State University Medical Center
Columbus, Ohio;
Adjunct Faculty, Department of Hospitality Management
Columbus State Community College
Columbus, Ohio

Ruth Novitt-Schumacher, RN, BSN, MSN
Instructor—Pediatrics
University of Illinois at Chicago
Chicago, Illinois

Anita K. Reed, MSN, RN
Instructor of Nursing
St. Elizabeth School of Nursing
Lafayette, Indiana

Sue G. Thacker, RN, C, PhD
Professor of Nursing
Wytheville Community College
Wytheville, Virginia

Martin M. Yadrick, MS, MBA, RD, FADA
Marketing Manager
Computrition, Inc.
Chatsworth, California

Preface

The process of achieving optimal health is a multidimensional endeavor. *Foundations and Clinical Applications of Nutrition: A Nursing Approach*, third edition, acknowledges this multidimensional approach by collaborating the worlds of nutrition and nursing. The role of nurses expands out of the medical clinic and into the community, thereby having a greater influence on the health promotion of individuals and communities. Consequently, the need for nurses to have a thorough background in both personal and clinical applications of nutrition becomes paramount. This nutrition text takes into account the personal nutrition needs of nurses to nourish themselves and their families and also their demanding professional responsibilities to implement and educate patients and clients (and their families) to follow prescribed medical nutrition therapy and to maintain or improve their health.

AUDIENCE

Nursing students are the primary audience for this book as they explore and apply nutrition and medical nutrition therapy. Secondary audiences include health education and health science students. Useful in a variety of healthcare settings, the text provides an excellent reference resource for nurses, nurse practitioners, and other healthcare professionals.

The book consists of four parts, which allows for adaptation for use within a one semester course. Similarly, Part I, *Wellness, Nutrition, and the Nursing Role;* Part II, *Nutrients, Food, and Health;* and Part III, *Health Promotion Through Nutrition and Nursing Practice* can be used for a basic one semester nutrition course, with Part IV, *Overview of Medical Nutrition Therapy,* then used as a future reference for medical nutrition therapy.

APPROACH

The perspective of this text tailors nutrition and medical nutrition therapy to the unique viewpoint of the nursing profession. Most other nutrition texts attempt to meet the needs of dietetic and nutrition majors in addition to nursing majors. Instead our focus is *the* nursing professional. This concentrated approach allows us to emphasize the skills applicable to nursing practice. Information needed by dietetic majors but not by nurses is omitted. We recognize that nurses do not prescribe or develop "diets" as medical nutrition therapy for patients. Instead, skills essential for nursing professionals are emphasized for implementation and education of patients and clients about prescribed dietary patterns.

FEATURES

Nursing Content Integrated with Nutrition. The unique role of nursing in the application of nutrition concepts provides a holistic perspective to patient care.

The Nursing Approach boxes in every chapter provide application of the nursing process and are written from a professional nursing perspective based on actual application to each content area.

Web Sites of Interest. Every chapter includes an average of three descriptions of web sites providing additional resources on chapter content. This use of the Internet provides a constantly updated "library" of information and incorporates computer skills.

Skill Application Support. Every chapter features **Applying Content Knowledge** or **Critical Thinking: Clinical Applications,** providing opportunities to apply information just learned in the chapter.

Life Span Health Promotion Explored in Three Chapters of Pregnancy, Lactation, and Infancy; Childhood and Adolescence; and Adulthood. Expanded coverage allows for more in-depth content of current issues affecting each life span category.

Life Span Approach. Age-related differences may affect dietary intake and nutrient utilization requiring modification of assessment and teaching strategies. Consequently, life span content is highlighted throughout the text as indicated by this special icon.

Cultural Sensitivity. Inclusion of ethnic food pyramids and **Cultural Considerations** boxes in every chapter highlights health and nutrition issues of specific ethnic groups. Students become sensitized and respectful of culturally defined food differences and are then able to approach, interview, and assess patients from diverse backgrounds. Appendix L presents cultural dietary patterns of different ethnic groups, allowing nurses to focus on the specific population with whom they work.

Food Allergy Issues. Awareness of food allergies and food intolerances is growing. This issue is explored with clear definitions and guidelines for recognizing and preventing food-related reactions, located within "Life Span Health Promotion: Childhood and Adolescence" (Chapter 12).

NEW Chapter 16: "Interactions: Complementary and Alternative Medicine, Dietary Supplements, and Medications." Complementary and alternative perspectives are challenging conventional medicine. This new chapter provides the integration of complementary and alternative medicine with traditional medicine. In addition, an expanded discussion of dietary supplements and medication interactions is provided. The chapter closes with consideration of the interaction occurring between medications and food, nutrients, and herbs.

REVISED Chapters on "Nutrition in Patient Care" and "Nutrition and Metabolic Stress." Reorganization of nutrition issues within these two chapters provides a more cohesive approach to information on patient care and the effects of metabolic stress on nutritional status.

UPDATED Chapters on "Nutrition for Diabetes Mellitus" and "Nutrition for Cardiovascular Diseases." Significant revisions of these chapters reflect the most current dietary recommendations for diabetes mellitus and cardiovascular diseases including user-friendly charts and teaching strategies.

Literacy Concerns. When appropriate, specific issues of literacy such as strategies for enhancing patient education for those with low literacy skills are presented in **Teaching Tool** boxes.

Contemporary Approach to Weight. The chapter on "Management of Body Composition" (Chapter 10) acknowledges that total fitness and wellness can be experienced by persons of all sizes and equips nurses to educate and support this approach.

Most Current Dietary Recommendations. The latest guidelines of the Dietary Reference Intakes (DRIs) and their rationales are included, providing students with tools to interpret ever-changing information, as well as the skills to make well-informed personal and professional decisions.

Incorporation of *Healthy People 2010.* The *Healthy People 2010* nutrition goals and objectives are incorporated where applicable, integrating personal nutrition goals with national objectives for communities. This framework clarifies how the nutritional status of our communities reflects individual nutritional health.

PEDAGOGY

Learning aids serve dual purposes throughout this text. Although primarily designed to support the understanding of concepts for the nursing student, the learning aids often represent means of educating patients and clients as well. Every chapter contains supportive features. For example, **Applying Content Knowledge** and **Critical Thinking/Clinical Applications** boxes provide readers the opportunity to apply knowledge learned in the chapters to real-life situations. **Web Sites of Interest** lists allow for further exploration of chapter concepts. Other supportive features that have been continued and strengthened include margin definitions of key terms, chapter summaries, and current references. Additional pedagogical features enhance the holistic, interdisciplinary approach to nutrition in nursing settings and provide contemporary critical thinking perspectives:

Teaching Tool boxes. Approaches to teaching clients about nutrient and medical nutrition therapy are incorporated within these boxes and within margin notes.

Health Debate boxes. Students are encouraged to develop their own opinions on controversial health issues.

Social Issue boxes. Ethical, social, and community concerns on local, national, and international levels are emphasized to reveal the various influences on health and wellness.

Myth boxes. Provide the basis for eliminating misconceptions about nutrition and health by clarifying the facts.

Cultural Considerations boxes. Highlight health and nutrition issues of specific ethnic groups to assist students as they approach, interview, and assess patients from diverse cultural backgrounds.

Toward a Positive Nutrition Lifestyle section. Features psychosocial strategies to support behavioral changes related to health for students and their clients (appears in Parts I, II, and III). This section recognizes the multidisciplinary skills needed to apply lifestyle changes for oneself and one's clients/patients.

Nursing Approach boxes. Demonstrate the continual application of the nursing process to each content area.

NEW Web Activities Icon. Placed at the end of various end-of-chapter pedagogy, refers readers to the *Student's Resource Online* for answers to questions posed, more case studies, and futher study.

Integrated Food Guide Pyramid. The Food Guide Pyramid is used throughout the text as an education guide for students and as a tool for teaching patients about dietary patterns. New to this edition are Food Guide Pyramids for Mexican and Puerto Rican dietary patterns, as well as the Healthy Eating Pyramid. The Food Guide Pyramid for Vegetarian Meal Planning is incorporated again in this new edition, and a Physical Activity Pyramid is also used to highlight the health benefits of physical activity.

SUPPLEMENTARY MATERIALS

An extensive ancillary package accompanies this text. Evolve Online Courseware for this third edition includes an **Instructor's Resource (CD-ROM and Online)** consisting of Chapter Objectives, Key Concepts, Chapter Outlines, Application Questions, Issues and Discussion Topics, Critical Thinking Activities, and Related Media, along with an extensive test bank (approximately 660 multiple-choice questions), an image collection (approximately 30 images from the text), and a comprehensive listing of all web sites found at the end of the chapters in the text. The **Student's Resource (Online)** includes Quick Review (with accompanying answers); Answers to *text* Applying Content Knowledge questions and Critical Thinking/Clinical Applications questions; one additional Applying Content Knowledge question (with accompanying answer); one additional Critical Thinking/Clinical Applications activity in Chapters 14-22 (with accompanying answer); matching questions (with accompanying answers); and WebLinks. The new version of *Mosby's NutriTrac Nutrition Analysis CD-ROM* is included with every copy of this text and features an expanded food database, greatly expanded activities database, Personal Profile screen, User Food Intake Record, Detailed Energy Expenditure log, Weight Management Planner, and a comprehensive nutritional evaluation.

ACKNOWLEDGMENTS

Our continued appreciation to the contributing authors who offered their unique perspectives on their areas of nutritional expertise to editions 1 and 2: Elaine H. Asp, PhD; Sharron Dalton, PhD, RD; Marcia L. Nahikian-Nelms, PhD, RD, LD; Marian L. Stone Neuhouser, PhD, RD; Ellen S. Parham, MSEd, PhD, RD, LPC; and Jaime S. Ruud, MS, RD. For this third edition, contributing author Marcia L. Nahikian-Nelms, PhD, RD, LD, has again ably authored Chapter 22, *"Nutrition in Cancer, AIDS, and Other Special Problems."* A new contributor, Kem Louie, PhD, APRN, FAAN, offers insight into the cultural aspects of client/patient care and to several of the Nursing Approach sections.

Our thanks to the reviewers who critiqued every aspect of nutrition fact and concept from Chapter 1 through Chapter 22. Reviewers' suggestions were incorporated, resulting in a strengthened third edition.

SPECIAL ACKNOWLEDGMENTS

This book continues its long and winding road from conception to this new third edition. As the book evolves, we again want to thank the supportive staff of Elsevier. We appreciate the guidance of Yvonne Alexopoulos, Senior Acquisitions Editor, who has gently nudged us to update features and to introduce new technology to support instructors as they enhance the learning experiences of their students. Our gratitude to Melissa Boyle, Senior Developmental Editor, for tracking the details, keeping us on task, and overseeing the manuscript during the adversity of our lives and of the publishing process. Thanks also to Anne Gassett, Project Manager, whose perceptive questions and editing skills allowed clarity of thought to reign and the production process to progress; and to Bill Drone, Design Manager.

In addition, we want to acknowledge the work of the Nursing Marketing Department for understanding what's special about our concept and for continuing to communicate this to our adopters.

Once again, thanks to our family and friends, who, by now, are used to having *the book* be an ongoing part of our lives, and view our sometimes late hours and "deadly deadlines" as part of our normal lives! Our journey has created personal bonds between us as we travel through our life spans together.

We continue to symbolize a collaboration of expertise in nutrition education, dietetics, and nursing. As we each become more sensitive to the multilayered responsibilities of nurses, we fine-tune our answers to the questions of "What do nurses need to know about nutrition?" and "How would they apply this knowledge to their patients and clients?" This edition reflects our ever-evolving responses to these questions.

Michele Grodner
Sara Long
Sandra DeYoung

Contents

Appendixes

Foundations and Clinical Applications of

Nutrition

A Nursing Approach

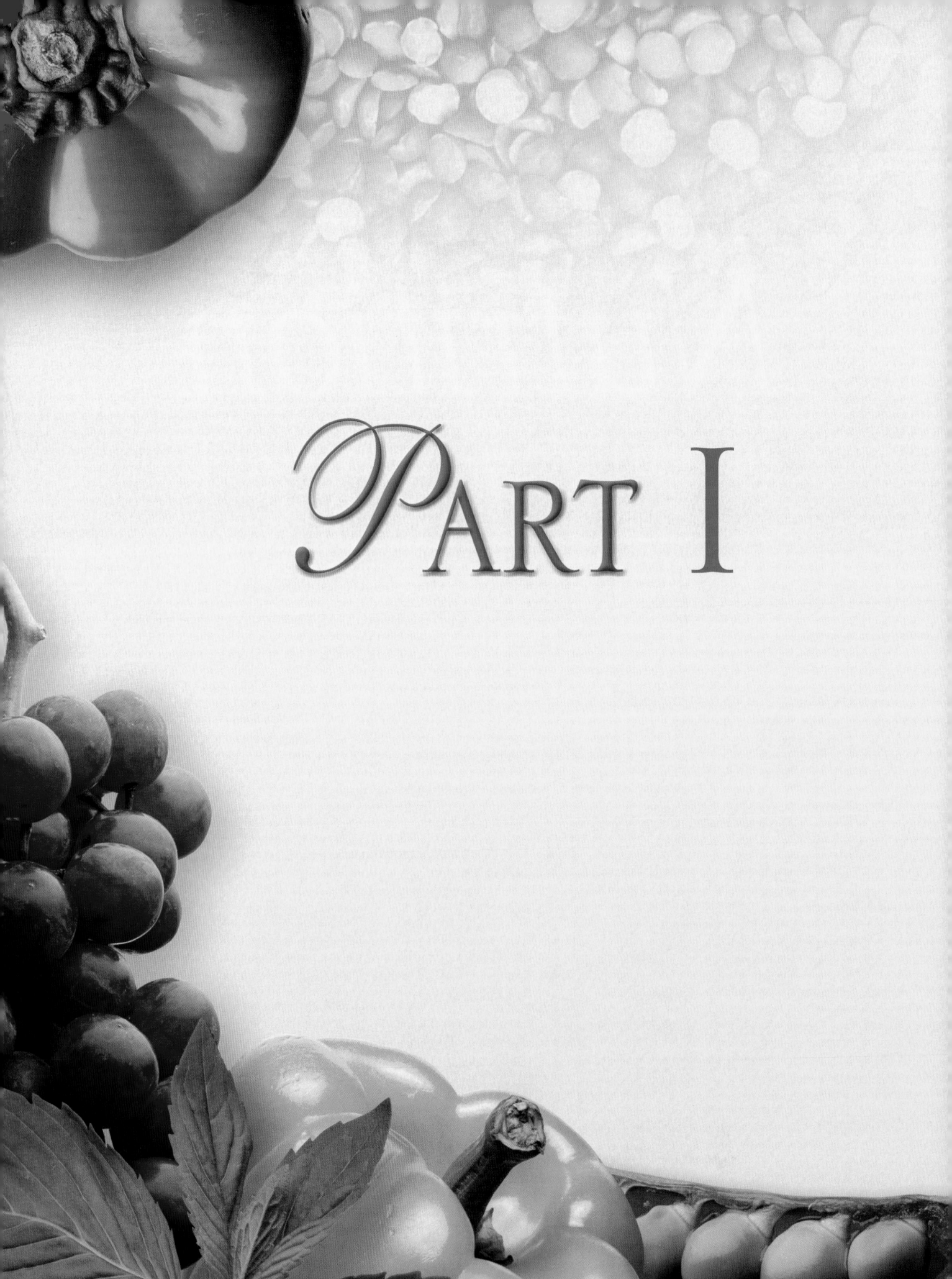

PART I

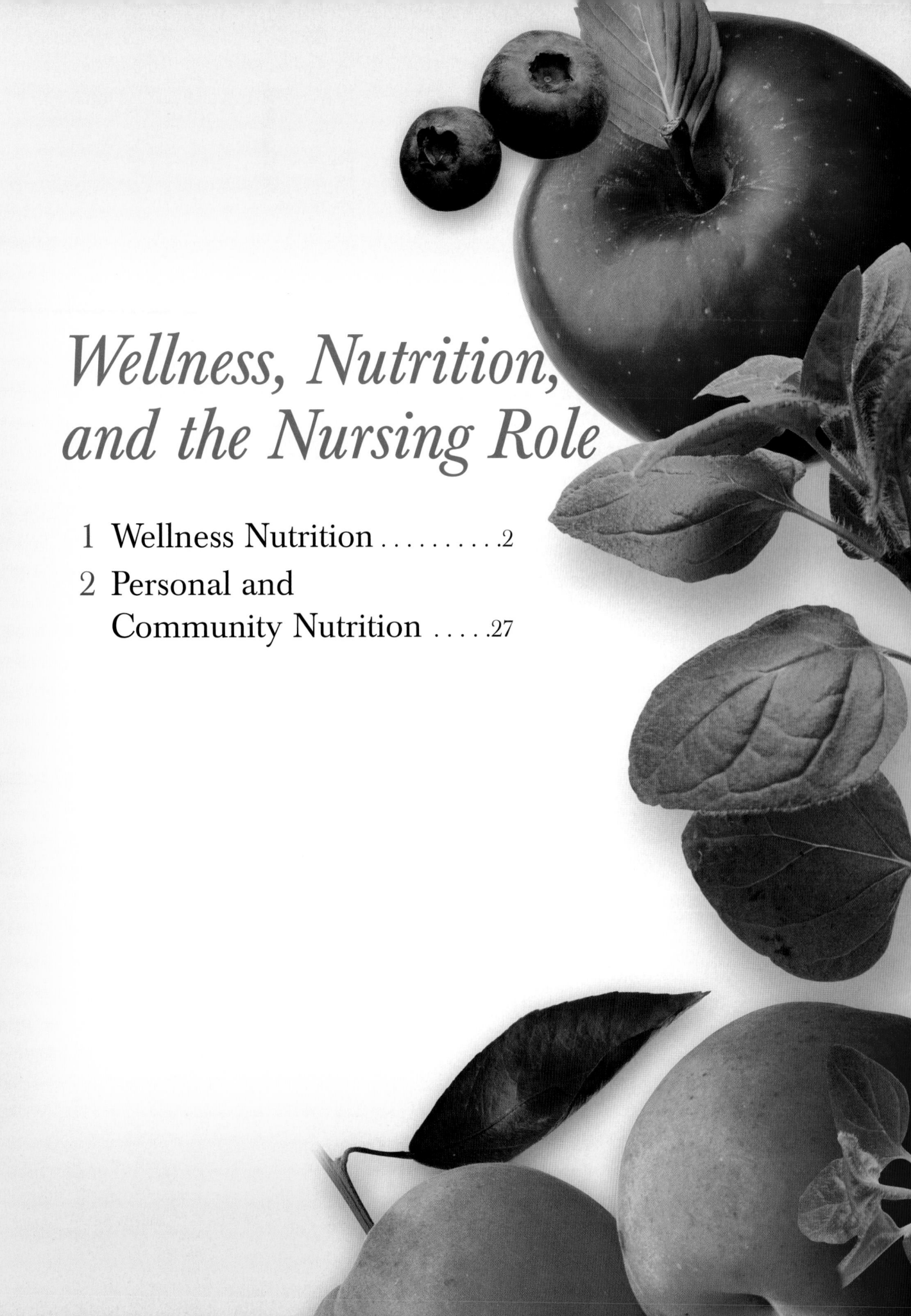

Wellness, Nutrition, and the Nursing Role

$\mathscr{C}$HAPTER 1

Wellness Nutrition

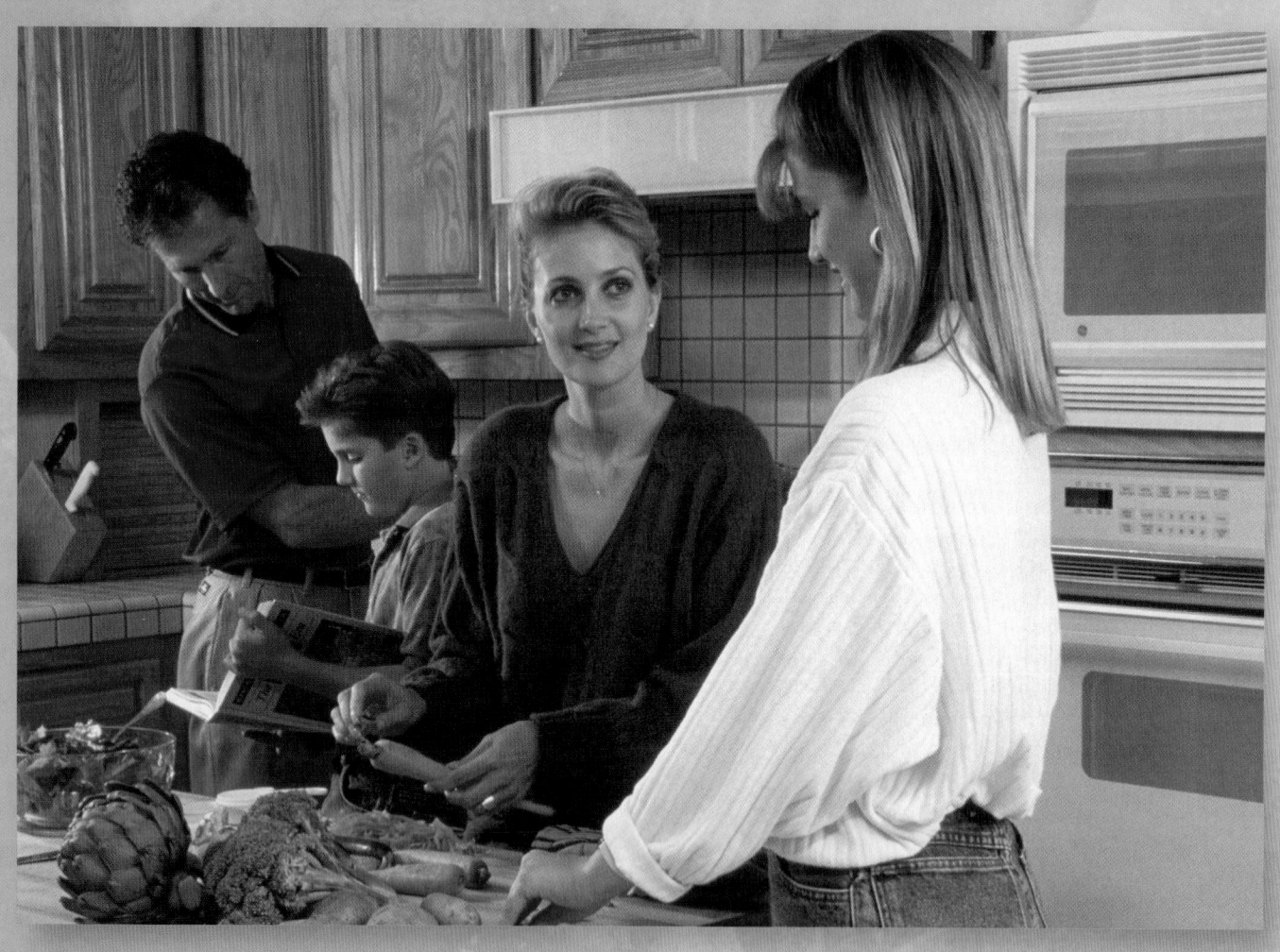

*Achieving wellness is a continuous,
never-ending journey.*

ROLE IN WELLNESS

Wellness is a lifestyle through which we continually strive to enhance our level of health. This text provides information, strategies, and techniques about food, nutrition, and health. These tools allow nurses and clients to achieve wellness through personal nutrition lifestyles.

Nutrition is a "hot topic" that generates interest easily; everyone seems to have opinions about what to eat and concerns about their own eating styles. The public is flooded with information and techniques related to health promotion through nutrition. This education of the public occurs in three different forms: formal, nonformal, and informal. *Formal education* is purposefully planned for implementation in a school setting. *Nonformal education* takes place through organized teaching and learning events in places such as hospitals, clinics, and community centers. *Informal education* encompasses a variety of educational experiences that occur through daily activities. These informal experiences may include watching television, reading newspapers and magazines, and conversing with other people.[1]

The most effective education results in behavior change. Nurses, through formal, nonformal, and informal educational interactions, can introduce knowledge and strategies for personal lifestyle choices that consider the social context of the patients' lives.[2] Formal education may be conducted by school nurses who teach health courses; topics can be approached through the health issues of the ethnic and cultural groups of the particular school's population. Nonformal education occurs when associations, such as the American Heart Association or hospital wellness programs, teach courses on risk-reducing lifestyle changes; these courses are usually open to the community. Informal education takes place when a nurse chats with a patient and his or her family, explaining the purpose of the dietary modifications recommended for the patient's particular disorder.

Never before have we had so much information about the effects of our personal behavior patterns on our level of health. Changing (or maintaining) our patterns of behaviors—and therefore our lifestyles—is the key to achieving wellness. Many social, community, and occupational forces affect our ability to change. Strategies and techniques ease our ability to modify our personal behaviors.

Modifying behaviors means changing lifestyles. Because this text is about food and nutrition, patterns of behaviors affecting the foods we choose to eat constitute our nutrition lifestyles. Our nutrition lifestyles won't all be the same. Some of us are caught in extremely hectic work, college, or sports schedules; we're lucky to find time to eat at all. Others find our families of origin still at the center of our eating patterns; our families, however, may not have adopted recent recommendations to decrease the risks of diet-related diseases. Many of us are part of new social settings on campus and need to adjust to rigid schedules and school cafeteria menus. Yet despite these variances, we have in common the ability to improve wellness through our nutrition lifestyles.

As healthcare professionals, we need to be concerned with our own nutritional patterns in addition to those of our clients. To reflect a health promotion perspective, individuals cared for by health professionals to maintain health are called *"clients."* Those who are ill or recuperating from illness are called *"patients."*

Enhancing personal health provides the stamina and well-being to fulfill the rigorous demands of nursing practice. A fundamental responsibility of nursing is client education. When teaching clients about nutritional wellness, nurses also function as role models for the positive effects of enhanced nutrition lifestyles.

DEFINITION OF HEALTH

In the past, health was defined as the absence of disease or illness. Modern medicine has conquered many life-threatening diseases, such as smallpox and polio. Public health measures of pasteurization and sanitation have reduced the risk of foodborne and environmental hazards. As concern about the physical status of the human body has lessened, we've been able to consider other aspects of the qualities of health.

One of the first expanded definitions of health was provided by the World Health Organization (WHO): "Health is a state of complete physical, mental, and social well-being and not merely the absence of disease and infirmity."[3] Although this definition addresses the concern that health is more than just the absence of disease, health is presented as a static concept that individuals achieve.

A more expanded definition of health was presented by Rene Dubos, biologist and philosopher, who wrote, "Health is a quality of life involving social, emotional, mental, spiritual, and biologic fitness on the part of the individual, which results from adaptations to the environment."[4] This view leads to our present understanding of health as a complex concept best represented by physical and psychologic dimensions. The dimensions include the following:

- *Physical health:* The efficiency of the body to function appropriately, to maintain immunity to disease, and to meet daily energy requirements.
- *Intellectual health:* The use of intellectual abilities to learn and to adapt to changes in one's environment.
- *Emotional health:* The capacity to easily express or suppress emotions appropriately.
- *Social health:* The ability to interact with people in an acceptable manner and to sustain relationships with family members, friends, and colleagues.
- *Spiritual health:* The cultural beliefs that give purpose to human existence. This belief may be found through faith in the teachings of organized religions, in an understanding of nature or science, or in an acceptance of the humanistic view of life.

Health is the merging and balancing of the five dimensions (i.e., physical, mental, emotional, social, and spiritual). This holistic view incorporates many aspects of human existence. Using this definition of health allows more individualized assessment of health status. As our health and the health of our clients are evaluated in relation to each dimension, some dimensions will be stronger than others (see the Teaching Tool box, "Dimensions of Health").

health
the merging and balancing of five physical and psychologic dimensions of health: physical, mental, emotional, social, and spiritual

Role of Nutrition

Nutrition is the study of nutrients and the processes by which they are used by the body. Nutrients are substances in foods required by the body for energy, growth, maintenance, and repair. Some nutrients are essential; they cannot be made by the human body and must be provided by foods.

nutrition
the study of essential nutrients and the processes by which nutrients are used by the body

nutrients
substances in foods required by the body for energy, growth, maintenance, and repair

TEACHING TOOL
Dimensions of Health

To broaden a patient's understanding of health, use the five dimensions of health. Describe the dimensions and then discuss with the patient each that pertains to his or her nutrition and health situation. By exploring aspects of health other than physical health, a person can then use all resources to restore the overall level of well-being.

WELLNESS THROUGH THE FIVE DIMENSIONS OF HEALTH

Physical health: Efficient body functioning
Intellectual health: Use of intellectual abilities
Emotional health: Ability to control emotions
Social health: Interactions and relationships with others
Spiritual health: Cultural beliefs about the purpose of life

Because the primary role of nutrients is to provide the building blocks for the efficient functioning and maintenance of the body, nutrition may appear to belong only within the physical health dimension. However, the effects of nutrients and their sources on the other health dimensions are far-reaching. Nutrition is the cornerstone of each health dimension.

Physical health is dependent on the quantity and quality of nutrients available to the body. The human body, from skeletal bones to minute amounts of hormones, is composed of nutrients in various combinations.

Intellectual health relies on a well-functioning brain and central nervous system. Nutritional imbalances can affect intellectual health, as occurs with iron deficiency anemia. Although milk is an excellent source of protein, calcium, and phosphorus, it provides a negligible amount of iron. Some young children drink so much milk that it affects their appetite for other foods such as meats, chicken, legumes, and leafy green vegetables, all of which are good sources of iron. As a result, iron deficiency may affect children with nutritional imbalances. The cognitive abilities of iron-deficient children may be affected, which could lead to possible learning problems.

Emotional health may be affected by poor eating habits, resulting in hypoglycemia or low blood glucose levels. Low blood glucose occurs normally in anyone who is physically hungry. When the body's need for food is ignored (e.g., when we miss meals because of poor planning or are too busy to eat), feelings of anxiety and confusion and trembling may occur. Emotions may be harder to control when we feel this way. Although blood glucose levels may affect our emotions, there are, of course, other factors that influence emotional health.

Social health situations often center around food-related occasions, ranging from holiday feasts to everyday meals. Nutritional status is sometimes affected by the quality of our relationships with family and friends. Are family meals an enjoyable experience or a tense ordeal? How might this affect a person's dietary intake?

Spiritual health often has ties to food. Several religions prohibit the consumption of specific foods. Many followers of Islam and Judaism adhere to the dietary laws of their religions. Both forbid consumption of pork-related products. Seventh Day Adventists follow an ovo-lacto vegetarian diet in which they consume only plant foods and dairy products and thus do not consume meat, fish, or poultry. In India cows are

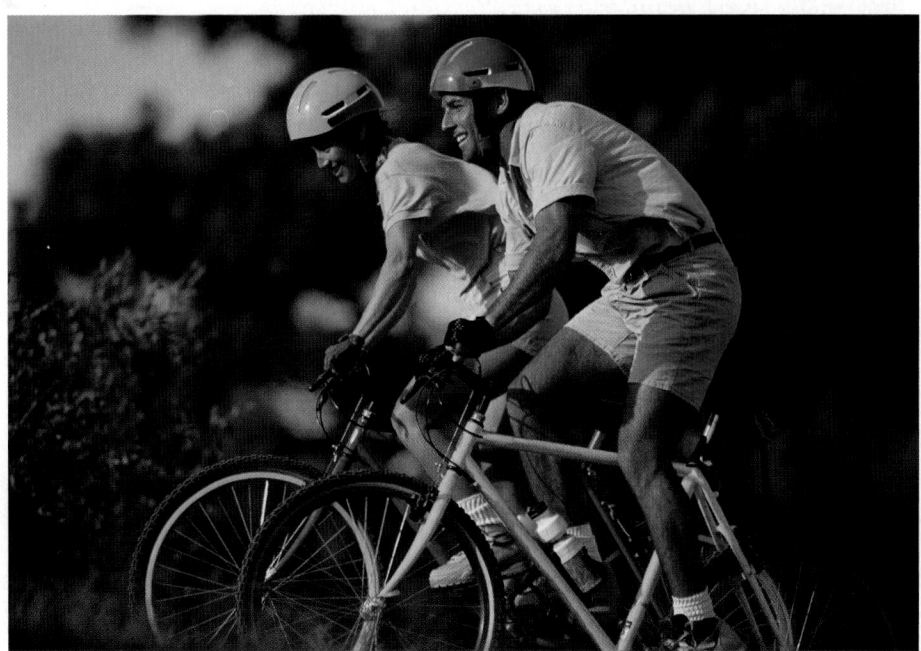

Physical health benefits from a good diet. (From PhotoDisc.)

viewed as sacred animals not eaten but instead revered as a source of sustenance (milk), fuel (burning of feces), power (as a work animal), and fertilizer (manure).

HEALTH PROMOTION

health promotion
strategies used to increase the level of health of individuals, families, groups, and communities

The goal of health promotion is to increase the level of health of individuals, families, groups, and communities. In community and occupational health settings, health promotion strategies implemented by nurses often focus on lifestyle changes that will lead to new, positive health behaviors. Development of positive behaviors may depend on knowledge, techniques, and community supports (see the Teaching Tool box, "Literacy and Health"):

1. *Knowledge:* Learning new information about the benefits or risks of health-related behaviors
2. *Techniques:* Applying new knowledge to everyday activities; developing ways to modify current lifestyles
3. *Community supports:* Availability of environmental or regulatory measures to support new health-promoting behaviors within a social context

Role of Nutrition

For more than 20 years, national health targets have been set. In 1979 the first initiative, the Surgeon General's report entitled *Healthy People,* laid out life-stage targets that continue to be tracked today. The second national prevention initiative,

---

TEACHING TOOL
Literacy and Health

Although health professionals take their high level of literacy for granted, many clients do not have command of basic literacy skills. About 25% of Americans are unable to understand written materials even at a basic literacy level, and another 25% have limited skills. In fact, low reading skills are associated with poor health and increased use of health services. The implications of these limitations are important because a nurse's efforts to educate clients to increase their knowledge and compliance may not be effective.

The most common form of media is print material. These materials are the least effective to reach the almost 50% of the adult population with limited reading skills. This highlights the need for the appropriate selection of client education materials for the level of readability to fit the client's reading ability. Ability may be lower than the stated years of education of clients and thereby compromise the measured readability of educational pamphlets.

We tend to assume that other forms of print and audio/visual media are more comprehensible to the public. This depends on several factors. If a poster is poorly designed and contains confusing graphics or too much technical information, the target audience may simply ignore the poster. If a video is too long, contains unfamiliar cultural habits, and is too specialized, the intended viewer may not comprehend the significant health messages embedded in the video.

Throughout this textbook, strategies are provided for working with low literacy clients, discussing the cultural connection, and evaluating and writing health education materials—all with the goal of enhancing health outcomes.

References: Bastable SB: Literacy in the adult patient population: Nurse As Educator: *Boston, 1997, Jones & Bartlett; Communicating with patients who have limited literacy skills.* Report of the National Work Group on literacy and health, *J Fam Pract 46:168, 1998; French KS, Larrabee JH: Relationships among educational material readability, client literacy, perceived beneficence, and perceived quality,* J Nurs Care Quality *13(6):68-82, 1999.*

Healthy People 2000, was a collaboration among the government, voluntary and professional health associations, businesses, and individuals under the direction of the secretary of Health and Human Services. The objectives focus on the decisions and policies that affect prevention efforts and create a standard from which to later assess the performance of meeting these goals.

The results of *Healthy People 2000* were used to develop the next set of national health targets, *Healthy People 2010 (HP2010).* This collaborative effort again welcomed the comments of thousands of health professionals. This document's intent is to have broad appeal and usefulness for policy makers ranging from the federal government down to state and local government initiatives. In addition, the interrelatedness of the health of communities and individuals is emphasized. The health status of an individual is dependent on the health supports of the community within which the individual lives.[5] This theme is also discussed in Chapter 2, Personal and Community Nutrition.

HP2010 is based on achievement of the following two paramount goals:

1. *Increase quality and years of healthy life.* This goal relates to life expectancy and the health-related quality-of-life concerns, which consider healthy days and years of healthy life of individuals by reduction of the risk factors of chronic disorders.
2. *Eliminate health disparities.* This pertains to the populations whose health status is affected by gender, race and ethnicity, education, and income.

The *HP2010* document is organized into 28 focus areas, each with its own objectives. Nutrition continues to be a priority for achievement of national goals, as evidenced by the inclusion of 18 nutrition-related objectives (Box 1-1). In addition, 13 other focus areas are impacted by or related to nutrition. Some of these focus areas include cancer, diabetes (particularly type 2 diabetes), food safety, and health communication.[5]

One nutrition objective is to have individuals reduce their daily intake of dietary fat to an average of 30% or less of total caloric intake.[5] To achieve this through health promotion strategies, health professionals need to know the relationship between fat consumption and the risk of developing coronary artery disease, certain cancers, and obesity; which foods are high in the kind of fats that affect health most; and effective ways to translate technical information to the public. Techniques include teaching clients how to shop for and cook foods that contain lower levels of fat. Community supports include health professionals recognizing supermarkets that stock low-fat food alternatives. Other community supports include restaurants that offer low-fat entrees, friends and family who provide social support, and media reports that publicize the relationship between dietary fat intake and coronary artery disease and cancer. Health professionals can make clients aware of these supports.

Data from analysis of *Healthy People 2000* reveal that a slight decrease in fat consumption occurred during the past 10 years, with the average fat intake now at about 33% of kcalorie intake.[5] However, increased education and continued application of strategies to reduce dietary fat intake are still necessary to reach the objective of a daily intake of dietary fat of 30% or less of total caloric intake. In a variety of healthcare and community settings, nurses may be asked to explain to their communities the purposes of priority health objectives.

Nutrition Monitoring

The nutritional status of the American population is monitored through several ongoing surveys. The National Nutrition Monitoring Act of 1990 provides for collaboration among government organizations that conduct national surveys of the nation's health and nutritional status. This collaboration supports the use of similar standards and research methods so the surveys' findings can be compared.

Box 1-1 *Healthy People 2010:* Nutrition and Weight Objectives

GOAL

Promote health and reduce chronic disease associated with diet and weight.

WEIGHT STATUS AND GROWTH OBJECTIVES

Healthy weight in adults: Increase the proportion of adults who are at a healthy weight from 42% to 60%.

Obesity in adults: Reduce the proportion of adults who are obese from 23% to 15%.

Overweight or obesity in children and adolescents: Reduce the proportion of children and adolescents who are overweight or obese from 11% to 5%.

Growth retardation in children: Reduce growth retardation among low-income children less than 5 years of age from 8% to 5%.

FOOD AND NUTRIENT CONSUMPTION OBJECTIVES

Fruit intake: Increase the proportion of persons who consume at least two daily servings of fruit from 28% to 75%.

Vegetable intake: Increase the proportion of persons who consume at least three daily servings of vegetables, with at least one third being dark green or orange vegetables, from 3% to 50%.

Grain product intake: Increase the proportion of persons who consume at least six daily servings of grain products, with at least three being whole grains, from 7% to 50%.

Saturated fat intake: Increase the proportion of persons who consume less than 10% of calories from saturated fat from 36% to 75%.

Total fat intake: Increase the proportions of persons who consume no more than 30% of calories from total fat from 33% to 75%.

Sodium intake: Increase the proportion of persons who consume 2400 mg or less of sodium daily from 21% to 65%.

Calcium intake: Increase the proportion of persons who meet dietary recommendations for calcium from 46% to 75%.

IRON DEFICIENCY AND ANEMIA OBJECTIVES

Iron deficiency in young children and in women of childbearing age: Reduce iron deficiency among young children and women of childbearing age.

Anemia in low-income pregnant women: Reduce anemia among low-income pregnant women in their third trimester from 29% to 20%.

Iron deficiency in pregnant women: Reduce iron deficiency among pregnant women.

SCHOOLS, WORKSITES, AND NUTRITION COUNSELING OBJECTIVES

Meals and snacks at school: Increase the proportion of children and adolescents aged 6 to 19 years whose intake of meals and snacks at school contributes to good overall dietary quality.

Worksite promotion of nutrition education and weight management: Increase the proportion of worksites that offer nutrition or weight management classes or counseling from 55% to 85%.

Nutrition counseling for medical conditions: Increase the proportion of physician office visits made by patients with a diagnosis of cardiovascular disease, diabetes, or hyperlipidemia that include counseling or education related to diet and nutrition from 42% to 75%.

FOOD SECURITY OBJECTIVE

Food security: Increase food security among U.S. households from 88% to 94% and reduce hunger in doing so.

From US Department of Health and Human Services, Public Health Service: Healthy people 2010, *ed 2, Washington, DC, 2000, US Government Printing Office; www.healthypeople.gov/.*

Two ongoing research projects that focus on nutritional status are the National Health and Nutrition Examination Survey (NHANES) and the National Food Consumption Surveys (NFCS). NHANES focuses on data from the dietary intake, medical history, biochemical evaluation, physical examinations, and measurements of American population groups who are carefully chosen to represent the total population. About every 10 years, the NFCS surveys subgroups of the American population to monitor nutrient intake. Records of food intake for 2 days are kept. These nutrient values are then compared with recommended dietary standards.

wellness
a lifestyle enhancing our level of health

lifestyle
a pattern of behaviors

DEFINITION OF WELLNESS

Wellness is a lifestyle (pattern of behaviors) that enhances each of the five dimensions of health. Individuals engaged in wellness lifestyles feel a sense of competency and achievement in their ability to modify their behaviors to increase or maintain positive levels of health.

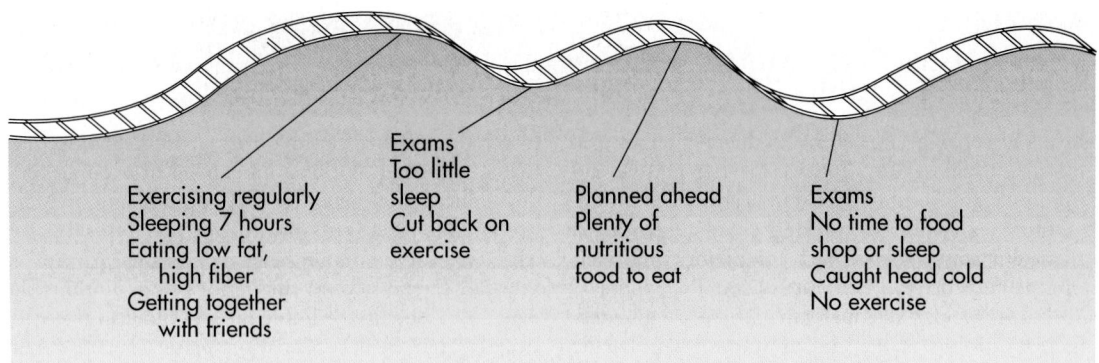

Exercising regularly
Sleeping 7 hours
Eating low fat,
   high fiber
Getting together
   with friends

Exams
Too little
sleep
Cut back on
exercise

Planned ahead
Plenty of
nutritious
food to eat

Exams
No time to food
shop or sleep
Caught head cold
No exercise

Figure 1-1 Wellness effort roller coaster. (From Rolin Graphics.)

Hectic contemporary schedules may seem to interfere with efforts to achieve wellness. The aim is to strive for wellness even if the path may seem more like a roller coaster than a smooth uphill climb (Figure 1-1). At times, clients may falter in their efforts, but the key is to renew positive behaviors as soon as possible.

Role of Nutrition

"Wellness nutrition" approaches food consumption as a positive way to nourish the body. This approach focuses on ways to organize our lives so we can more easily follow an eating pattern designed to enhance health status. Consuming a diet based on lower fat/higher fiber and moderate caloric consumption is then not a chore but rather an affirmation of our competency to care for ourselves. Conveying this approach to clients is a nursing challenge.

DISEASE PREVENTION THROUGH NUTRITION

Disease prevention is the recognition of a danger to health that could be reduced or alleviated through specific actions or changes in lifestyle behaviors. The hazard may be caused by disease, lifestyle or genetic factors, or an environmental threat. The three classifications of disease prevention are primary, secondary, and tertiary.[6] Disease prevention has strong ties to nutrition (see the Cultural Considerations box, "*Healthy People 2010* and Culturally Competent Care").

Primary prevention consists of activities to avert the initial development of a disease or poor health. A primary disease prevention approach is to eat a variety of foods to avert nutrient deficiencies. Adopting a low-fat, high-fiber eating style before diet-related health problems develop is a form of primary prevention.

Secondary prevention involves early detection to halt or reduce the effects of a disease or illness. Some diseases cannot be prevented, but early detection can minimize negative health effects. Secondary prevention strategies are useful to reduce the effects of chronic diet-related diseases. Controlling the intake of certain nutrients can decrease the severity of some disorders. Some individuals with high blood pressure (hypertension) are sodium sensitive, and simply reducing the amount of sodium consumed can decrease blood pressure levels and thus bring the disorder under control. Because hypertension is a risk factor for coronary artery disease, strokes, and renal disease, reduction of blood pressure through decreased sodium consumption is a secondary prevention strategy.

Tertiary prevention occurs after a disorder develops. The purpose is to minimize further complications or to assist in the restoration of health. These efforts may involve continued medical care. Often, learning more about the disorder is helpful for

disease prevention
the recognition of a danger to health that could be reduced or alleviated through specific actions or changes in lifestyle behaviors

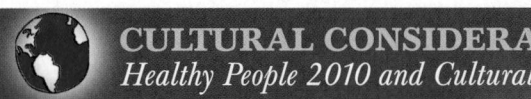

CULTURAL CONSIDERATIONS
Healthy People 2010 and Culturally Competent Care

Lifestyle and behavior are central to the maintenance of health and wellness. To influence lifestyle and behavior, health professionals need to take into account the values, attitudes, culture, and life circumstances of individuals. Changes in health status, particularly of minority populations, require professionals to take into account the increasing ethnic/cultural diversity of Americans. There are four recognized minority groups in the United States: Asian/Pacific Islanders, African Americans, Hispanic Americans, and Native Americans. Currently, it is estimated that one in five Americans belongs to a minority group. Minority populations are projected to grow to one third of the population by the year 2050.

HP2010 documents that the number of premature and excess deaths of ethnic minority populations far outweighs the majority groups. Research shows the factors that contribute to this are complex and involve multiple factors. Socioeconomic status among minority groups is generally lower than Caucasian majority groups. Socioeconomic status is measured by the combination of occupation, income, and educational attainment. A second major factor is the use of and access to healthcare programs by minorities. Many of the available health programs are not culturally relevant or sensitive to the minority populations they serve. There is a paucity of bilingual and bicultural health professionals, and health education materials are generally not culturally specific.

Application to Nursing: Diet and nutrition assessment is imperative to provide culturally competent care. Efforts to understand dietary patterns of clients need to go beyond relying on their membership in a defined group. For example, by learning the assimilative practices of an individual, nurses can assist dietitians in developing the most effective and culturally sensitive medical nutrition therapy recommendations. Together they can develop a treatment regimen that does not conflict with cultural food practices of the client.

patients and their families. Tertiary prevention frequently involves diet therapy. Direct treatments of many disorders have a dietary component. Some of these disorders include ulcers, diverticulitis, and coronary artery disease; they usually occur during the middle and older years of adulthood. Other disorders may affect food intake and the ability of the body to absorb nutrients. For example, chemotherapy for cancer may have the side effects of nausea and loss of appetite. Nutrition counseling during and after these treatments is necessary so patients are as well-nourished as possible to aid the healing process. The five dimensions of health can be an excellent teaching tool in promoting health and preventing diseases related to nutrition.

OVERVIEW OF NUTRIENTS WITHIN THE BODY

Which nutrients are the cornerstones of health and disease prevention? What do they do to make them so important? Why can't we just take a nutrient pill?

Nutrient Categories

Nutrients can be divided into the following six categories:

1. Carbohydrates
2. Proteins
3. Lipids (fats)
4. Vitamins
5. Minerals
6. Water

Nutrients may be either essential or nonessential, depending on whether the body can manufacture them. When the body requires a nutrient for growth or maintenance but lacks the ability to manufacture amounts sufficient to meet the body's needs, the nutrient is essential and must be supplied by the foods in our diet. Table 1-1 lists the essential nutrients needed in our diet. Other nutrients that the body can make on its own are called *nonessential*.

Table 1-1
Known Essential Nutrients

Nutrient	Source
Carbohydrates	Glucose
Lipids (fats)	Linoleic acid, linolenic acid
Protein	Amino acids: Histidine, isoleucine, leucine, lysine, methionine, phenylalanine, threonine, tryptophan, valine
Vitamins	Fat-soluble vitamins: A (retinol), D (cholecalciferol), E (tocopherol), K Water-soluble vitamins: Thiamine, riboflavin, niacin, pantothenic acid, biotin, B_6 (pyridoxine), B_{12} (cobalamin), folate, C (ascorbic acid)
Minerals	Major minerals: Calcium, phosphorus, sodium, potassium, sulfur, chlorine, magnesium Trace minerals: Chromium, cobalt, copper, fluorine, iodine, iron, manganese, selenium, zinc
Water	

The functions of essential nutrients in the body include aiding growth and repair of body tissues, regulating body processes, and providing energy. Some nutrients are diverse in their impact, whereas others have very specific functions.

Only carbohydrates, proteins, and lipids are nutrients that provide energy. Whereas carbohydrates primarily contribute only energy, proteins and lipids are also essential for the growth and repair of body tissues and are required for regulating body processes. Although vitamins and minerals cannot provide energy, they have indirect roles as catalysts for the body's use of nutrients for energy. Each vitamin serves a different specific function related to regulation of body processes. Minerals and water also regulate body processes and are required for tissue growth and maintenance.

FOOD, ENERGY, AND NUTRIENTS

Although the discussion to this point has focused on nutrients, we must remember that nutrients are found in foods. Because foods usually contain a mixture of nutrients, we often categorize a food based on the most predominate nutrient found in the food. A bagel is a carbohydrate food and contains mostly complex carbohydrates, although it also contains protein, water, small amounts of vitamins and minerals, and an even smaller amount of lipids or fat[7] (Figure 1-2).

The gold mine of nutrients found in whole foods is one of the reasons why taking a nutrient-specific pill will not provide for all the necessities of the human body.

Energy

Let's consider the energy-containing nutrients of carbohydrates, protein, and lipids. These contain energy because they are organic. Being organic means they are composed of a structure that consists of hydrogen, oxygen, and carbon. Living or once-living things, including plants and animals, produce organic compounds.

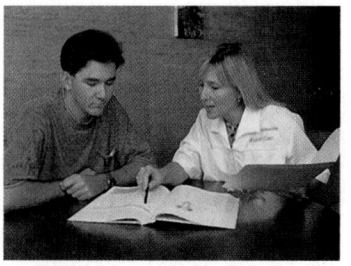

Nutrition is an integral part of healthcare education. (From Joanne Scott/Tracy McCalla.)

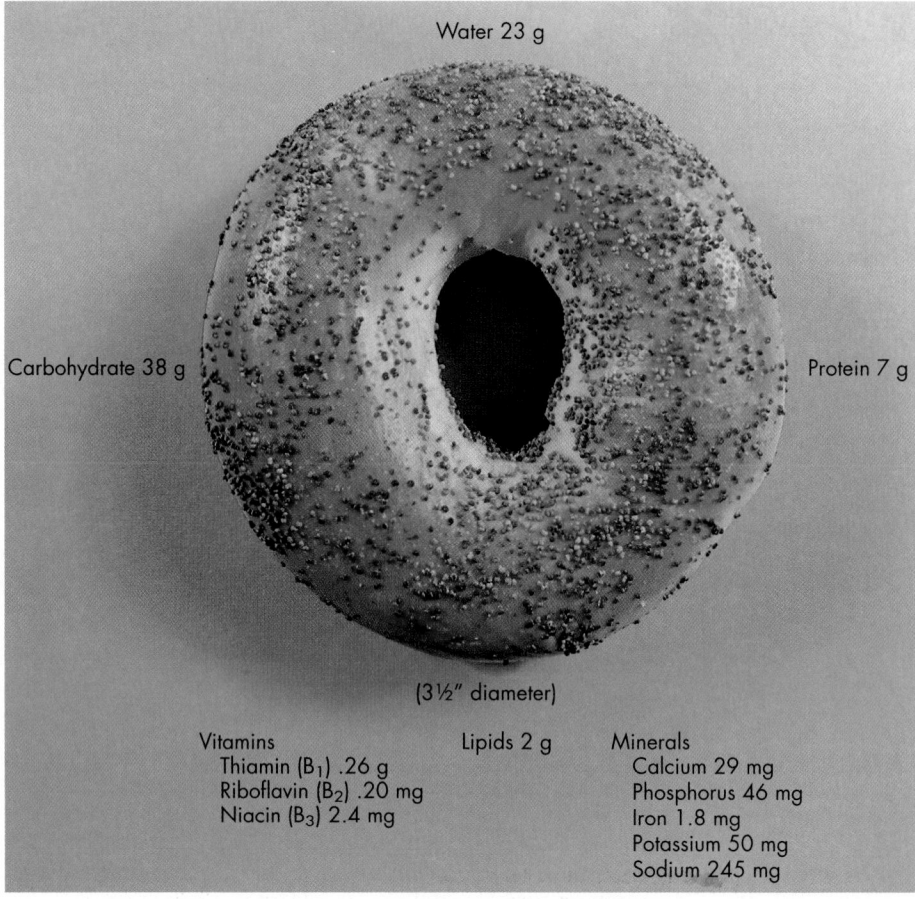

Water 23 g

Carbohydrate 38 g

Protein 7 g

(3½" diameter)

Vitamins
  Thiamin (B₁) .26 g
  Riboflavin (B₂) .20 mg
  Niacin (B₃) 2.4 mg

Lipids 2 g

Minerals
  Calcium 29 mg
  Phosphorus 46 mg
  Iron 1.8 mg
  Potassium 50 mg
  Sodium 245 mg

Figure 1-2 Most foods contain a mixture of nutrients. (From Joanne Scott/Tracy McCalla. Data from *Nutrient Data Laboratory*, www.nal.usda.gov/fnic/foodcomp/.)

The carbon-containing structure identifies these nutrients as being organic. When these nutrients are oxidized (burned in the body), energy is released and available for use by the cells. Although vitamins are also organic, they do not provide energy for the human body. Only carbohydrates, proteins, and lipids are energy-yielding nutrients.

The energy released from food is measured in kilocalories (thousands of calories) or calories. Technically, a calorie is the amount of heat necessary to raise the temperature of a gram of water by 1° C (0.8° F). When someone asks how much energy is in an 8-oz. glass of skim milk, the correct response is 90,000 calories or 90 kilocalories. For numeric simplicity, we commonly refer to the *"calories"* in a food rather than use the correct term of *kilocalories*. To assure accuracy, the term *kilocalories* will be used throughout this text, abbreviated as "kcalories" or "kcal."

Energy-yielding nutrients provide different amounts of energy (Table 1-2). Carbohydrates and protein each provide 4 kcalories per gram. Lipids contain more than twice as much energy and provide 9 kcalories per gram. The kcalorie content of a specific food—for example, a bagel—is based on the amount of carbohydrate, lipid, and protein energy contained in the food (Figure 1-3). When we consume energy-yielding foods, we usually ingest other nutrients as well, including vitamins, minerals, and water.

Another energy-yielding substance is alcohol. Alcohol provides 7 kcalories per gram. Although alcohol provides energy, it is not considered a nutrient because the body does not need it. In fact, the body treats it as a toxin. Breaking down or metabolizing alcohol is not only stressful to the body but also uses essential nutrients that could be better used to nourish the body. Some studies suggest that moderate

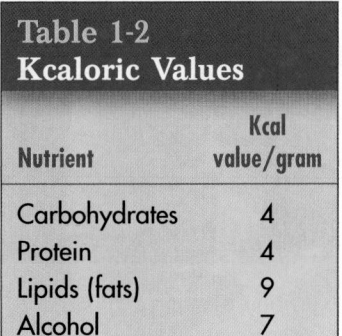

Table 1-2 Kcaloric Values	
Nutrient	**Kcal value/gram**
Carbohydrates	4
Protein	4
Lipids (fats)	9
Alcohol	7

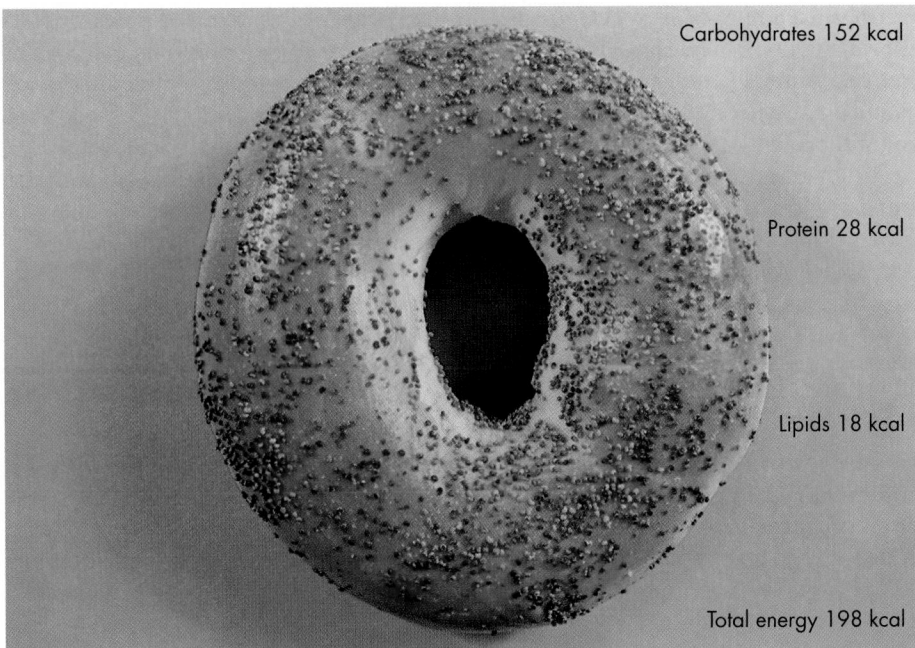

Carbohydrates 152 kcal

Protein 28 kcal

Lipids 18 kcal

Total energy 198 kcal

Figure 1-3 A food's kcalorie content is based on the energy-yielding nutrients it contains. (From Joanne Scott/Tracy McCalla. Data from *Nutrient Data Laboratory,* www.nal.usda.gov/fnic/foodcomp/.)

consumption of alcohol-containing beverages such as red wine may be protective for heart disease. The beneficial components are most likely phytochemicals, nonnutritive plant substances found in the ingredients (such as red grapes) used to produce the alcoholic beverages.

Although protein, lipids, and carbohydrates provide energy, they—along with the other three nutrient categories of vitamins, minerals, and water—have other important functions. A brief introduction to each nutrient category follows.

Carbohydrates

Carbohydrates are a major source of fuel. They consist of simple carbohydrates, often called sugars, and complex carbohydrates that include starch and most fiber. Simple carbohydrates are found in foods such as white sugar, fruits, and milk. Complex carbohydrates are found in cereals, grains, pastas, fruits, and vegetables. All, except fiber, are broken down to units of glucose, which is one of the simple carbohydrates. Glucose provides the most efficient form of energy for the body, particularly for muscles and the brain.

Most fiber cannot be broken down by the human digestive system; therefore, it provides little, if any, energy. However, consuming fiber is necessary for good health. Dietary fiber provides several beneficial effects on the digestive and absorptive systems of the body. These effects range from preventing constipation to possibly reducing the risk of colon cancer and heart disease.

Proteins

Proteins, in addition to providing energy, perform an extensive range of functions in the body. Some of these functions include roles in the structure of bones, muscles, enzymes, hormones, blood, the immune system, and cell membranes. The linking of amino acids in various combinations forms proteins. Twenty amino acids are required to create all the necessary proteins to maintain life. The body forms some amino acids whereas others, called *essential amino acids,* must be consumed in foods. The nine essential amino acids are found in animal and plant sources. Animal sources include meat, fish, poultry, and some dairy products such as milk and cheeses. Plant sources include grains, legumes (peas and beans that contain protein), seeds, nuts, and many vegetables (albeit in small amounts).

Although protein is important nutritionally, eating too much of it can be a problem. Eating substantially more than the recommended amounts of protein does not produce superhumans. Instead, our physical systems can become overworked. Excess protein is broken down to amino acids. The amino acids are then used for energy or broken down further in metabolic processes and either are stored as body fat or excreted through the kidneys in urine.

Lipids (Fats)

Fats are the densest form of energy available in foods and as stored energy in our bodies. Fats, or lipids, serve other purposes, such as functioning as a component of all cell structures, having a role in the production of hormones, and providing padding to protect body organs. Essential fatty acids and the fat-soluble vitamins A, D, E, and K are found in food lipids. It is the fats in certain foods that make them taste so appealing.

Lipids are divided into three categories: triglycerides, phospholipids, and sterols. Triglycerides are called *saturated, monounsaturated,* or *polyunsaturated fats* based on the types of fatty acids they contain. Fatty acids are carbon chains of varying lengths and degrees of hydrogen saturation. The most common phospholipid is lecithin; among sterols, we hear most about cholesterol. Although we consume lecithin and cholesterol in food, our bodies manufacture them as well.

Fats and cholesterol are often in the news. Saturated fats or triglycerides found in some fat-containing foods and dietary cholesterol are associated with increased blood lipid levels. Elevated blood lipid levels, whether formed by our bodies or consumed in dietary sources, are a risk factor for the development of coronary artery disease. Saturated fats, and to a certain extent polyunsaturated fats, have also been associated with increased risk for certain cancers. Coronary artery disease and cancer are serious public health diseases that affect millions of North Americans. Consequently, medical and health professionals emphasize the need to reduce intake of foods that contain fats and cholesterol.

Vitamins

Vitamins are compounds that indirectly assist other nutrients through the complete processes of digestion, absorption, metabolism, and excretion. Thirteen vitamins are needed by the body, and each has a specific function. As noted earlier, vitamins provide no energy but instead assist in the release of energy from carbohydrates, lipids, and proteins.

Vitamins are divided into two classes based on their solubility (i.e., ability to dissolve) in water. The water-soluble vitamins include the B vitamins (thiamin, niacin, riboflavin, folate, cobalamin [B_{12}], pyridoxine [B_6], pantothenic acid, biotin) and vitamin C. The fat-soluble vitamins, which dissolve in fats, are vitamins A, D, E, and K.

Vitamins are found in many foods; fruits and vegetables are particularly good sources. Because some foods are better sources of specific vitamins, eating a variety of foods is the best way to consume sufficient amounts.

Minerals

Minerals serve structural purposes (e.g., bones and teeth) in the body and are found in body fluids. Minerals in body fluids affect the nature of the fluids, which in turn influence muscle function and the central nervous system. Sixteen essential minerals are divided into two categories: major minerals and trace minerals. Although this distinction is based on the quantity of minerals required by the body, each is equally important.

Minerals are plentiful in fruits, vegetables, dairy products, meats, and legumes. Although minerals are indestructible, some may be lost through food processing. For example, when whole-wheat flour is processed or refined to white flour, minerals such as phosphorus and potassium are lost and not replaced.

Water

Water is a major part of every tissue in the body. We can live only a few days without water. Water functions as a fluid in which substances can be broken down and reformed for use by the body. As a constituent of blood, water also provides a means of transportation for nutrients to and from cells.

Many of us probably do not drink enough water or liquids to best meet the needs of our bodies. We should consume the equivalent of about 8 to 10 cups of water a day from foods and beverages. Awareness of the value of water consumption is growing as bottled water companies heavily advertise their products to the public. Bottled waters have become a fashionable alternative to other beverages. These products seem to offer convenience and status against which tap water cannot compete. Although more money may be spent on bottled water than is necessary, the health benefits are still achieved. Unflavored, plain water, whether purchased bottled or from public water supplies, provides the best value; waters fortified with vitamins, minerals, and herbs are not necessary.

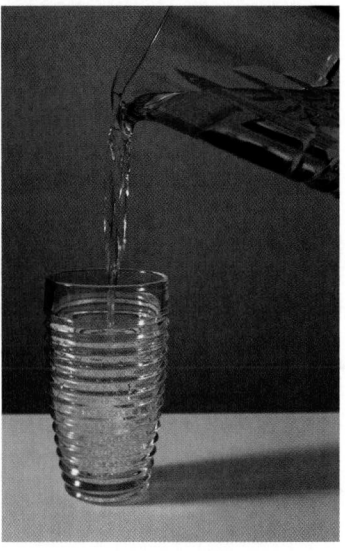

The need for water is more urgent than the need for any other nutrient. (From PhotoDisc.)

DIETARY STANDARDS

Simply knowing which nutrients are essential to life is not sufficient. We need to know how much of each nutrient to consume to be assured of basic good health. Similarly, eating foods without awareness of their nutrient value does not assure an adequate intake of nutrients. Dietary standards provide a bridge between knowledge of essential nutrients and food consumption. They also provide a guide of adequate nutrient intake levels against which to compare the nutrient values of foods consumed.

dietary standards
a guide to adequate nutrient intake levels against which to compare the nutrient values of foods consumed

Dietary Reference Intakes

In the United States past dietary standards were based on providing nutrients in amounts that would prevent nutritional deficiency diseases. New perspectives of nutrient needs, availability of nutrients, food components, and dietary supplements have emerged. A new set of nutrient standards, Dietary Reference Intakes (DRIs), combines the classic concerns of deficiency diseases that were the original focus of nutrient recommendations with the contemporary interest to reduce the risk of chronic diet-related diseases such as coronary artery disease, cancer, and osteoporosis.[8,9] The DRIs are also applicable to various individuals and population groups.

Responsibility for these new dietary standards lies with the Standing Committee on the Scientific Evaluation of Dietary Reference Intakes of the Food and Nutrition Board, Institute of Medicine, and National Academy of Sciences, along with the participation of Health Canada. The DRIs are now the nutrient recommendations for the United States and Canada.

The DRIs are based on (1) reviewing the available scientific data about specific nutrient use; (2) assessing the function of these nutrients to reduce the risk of chronic and other diseases and conditions such as coronary artery disease and cancer; and (3) evaluating current data on nutrient consumption levels among U.S. and Canadian populations.[8,9]

Dietary Reference Intakes (DRIs)
dietary standards including Estimated Average Requirement (EAR), Recommended Dietary Allowance (RDA), Adequate Intake (AI), and Tolerable Upper Intake Level (UL)

Estimated Average Requirement (EAR)
the amount of a nutrient needed to meet the basic requirements of half the individuals in a specific group; the basis for setting the RDAs

Recommended Dietary Allowance (RDA)
the level of nutrient intake sufficient to meet the needs of almost all healthy individuals of a life-stage and gender group

Adequate Intake (AI)
the approximate level of an average nutrient intake determined by observation of or experimentation with a particular group or population that appears to maintain good health

Tolerable Upper Intake Level (UL)
the level of nutrient intake that should not be exceeded to prevent adverse health risks

Lingo of Dietary Reference Intakes

The DRIs comprise the Estimated Average Requirement (EAR), Recommended Dietary Allowance (RDA), Adequate Intake (AI), and Tolerable Upper Intake Level (UL).

Estimated Average Requirement (EAR) is the amount of a nutrient needed to meet the basic requirements of half the individuals in a specific group that represents the needs of a population. The EAR considers issues of deficiency and physiologic functions. Public health nutrition researchers and policymakers primarily use the EARs to determine the basis for setting the RDAs.

Recommended Dietary Allowance (RDA) is the level of nutrient intake that is sufficient to meet the needs of almost all healthy individuals of a life-stage and gender group. The aim is to supply an adequate nutrient intake to decrease the risk of chronic disease. The RDA is based on EARs for that nutrient plus an additional amount to provide for the particular need of each group. Some nutrients do not have an RDA but an Adequate Intake (AI) level.

Adequate Intake (AI) is the approximate level of an average nutrient intake determined by observation of or experimentation with a particular group or population that appears to maintain good health. The AI is used when there are not sufficient data to set an RDA.

Tolerable Upper Intake Level (UL) is the level of nutrient intake that should not be exceeded to prevent adverse health risks. This amount includes total consumption from foods, fortified foods, and supplements. The UL is not a recommended level of intake but a safety boundary of total consumption. ULs exist only for nutrients of which adverse risks are known.

The DRIs are designed to meet the needs of most healthy individuals. Individuals generally use the RDAs and AIs when assessing their nutrient intakes. Those with special nutritional needs, such as those suffering from disease, injury, or other medical conditions, may have nutrient needs that are higher than the DRIs.

Use of Dietary Reference Intakes

The DRIs are widely used throughout the U.S. food systems. Uses include the following:

- Planning meals for large groups, such as the military
- Creating dietary standards for governmental food assistance programs such as the Special Supplemental Food Program for Women, Infants and Children (WIC) and Food Stamp programs
- Interpreting food consumption information on individuals and populations. Although originally intended only for analysis of the diets of large groups of people, DRIs can be used for individuals if compared with an average intake over a period of time. The intake of a single day does not have to meet the recommended levels. A comparison with the DRIs does not determine nutritional status but is only one of several measurements used to assess nutritional status.
- Meeting national nutrition goals such as those listed in *HP2010*
- Developing new food products, such as imitation products, that duplicate the nutrient values of the original

However, the DRI standards are not the basis of the nutrient information that appears on food and supplement products. The Daily Value (DV) is used for nutrition labeling and is based on dietary standards from 1968—when nutrition labeling was first implemented. When the current food labeling standards were revised in 1994, the Food and Drug Administration (FDA) did not update the nutrient values. (See Chapter 2 for a detailed discussion of food labeling.)

Additional Standards

The Median Heights and Weights and Recommended Energy Intake standard presents the average heights and weights of Americans. The energy intake recommendations are an average of the need for each category. A margin of safety is not added to avoid recommending potentially excessive intakes of energy; consuming too much energy may be a primary cause of obesity, a major public health issue.

Standards Around the World

Other countries have developed dietary standards based on energy needs, food supply, or environmental factors that affect their populations. In addition, organizations such as the Food and Agriculture Organization of the United Nations, along with the WHO, have developed dietary standards that meet the practical needs of healthy adults worldwide.

Why aren't nutrient recommendations the same for every country or population? After all, the needs of the human body must be the same around the world. The difference lies in the definitions and purposes of nutrient recommendations.

Standards may be designed to provide the basic amount of a nutrient to prevent deficiency symptoms or to supply sufficient amounts for basic good health. These amounts may differ substantially based on the nature of the nutrient, such as whether it is stored in the body. In addition, health professionals of a nation or organization may interpret the same scientific data differently, arriving at various recommended amounts.

Whether a standard is set to provide for only basic nutrient needs may depend on the availability of food. In the United States, where access to food is easy and the supply plentiful, the setting of nutrient recommendations higher than minimum levels is reasonable; most citizens have access to foods to meet those levels. In parts of the world where the food supply is more limited, the immediate goal is to supply as many individuals as possible with basic needs to prevent deficiencies.

Some values differ from the U.S. standards based on the most common sources of nutrients worldwide. For example, most of the world relies heavily on plant protein sources, whereas North Americans use mainly animal sources. Recommended protein levels reflect this difference.

Ultimately, all standards are simply guidelines. Even when set at a specific amount, standards represent a range of the requirement of the nutrient. Individual needs may vary, so consuming enough food to meet the basic amounts should be each person's nutritional goal.

ADEQUATE EATING PATTERNS

Knowing the DRIs makes nutrition seem simple. Just eat enough of the DRI nutrients and good health seems assured. However, we don't eat nutrients; we eat foods. For an eating pattern to be considered adequate, the foods we eat must provide all the essential nutrients plus fiber and energy. An adequate eating pattern takes into account assortment, balance, and nutrient density.

Assortment addresses the value of eating a variety of foods from every food group. Eating the same foods every day may be convenient but may not serve health and nutrient needs. The limited selection of foods may not contain sufficient amounts of essential nutrients and dietary fiber or may be high in some nutrients, such as fat, and low in others, such as vitamin A. As shown in Figure 1-4, eating a ham and cheese sandwich every day may seem like a quick lunchtime solution, but an assortment of selections over a 5-day period provides a daily average of fewer calories, less fat, less cholesterol, and less sodium. A good strategy is to adopt a habit of selecting different foods for lunch or, at the least, rotating food choices throughout the week.

An eating pattern exhibiting *balance* will provide foods from all food groups in quantities so essential nutrients are consumed in proportion to each other; thus there is a balance among the levels of nutrients eaten. The Food Guide Pyramid represents this concept by taking into account different food groups and number of servings. Balance also ensures that energy plus nutrient needs will equal the intake of energy and nutrients to satisfy adequacy (Figure 1-5).

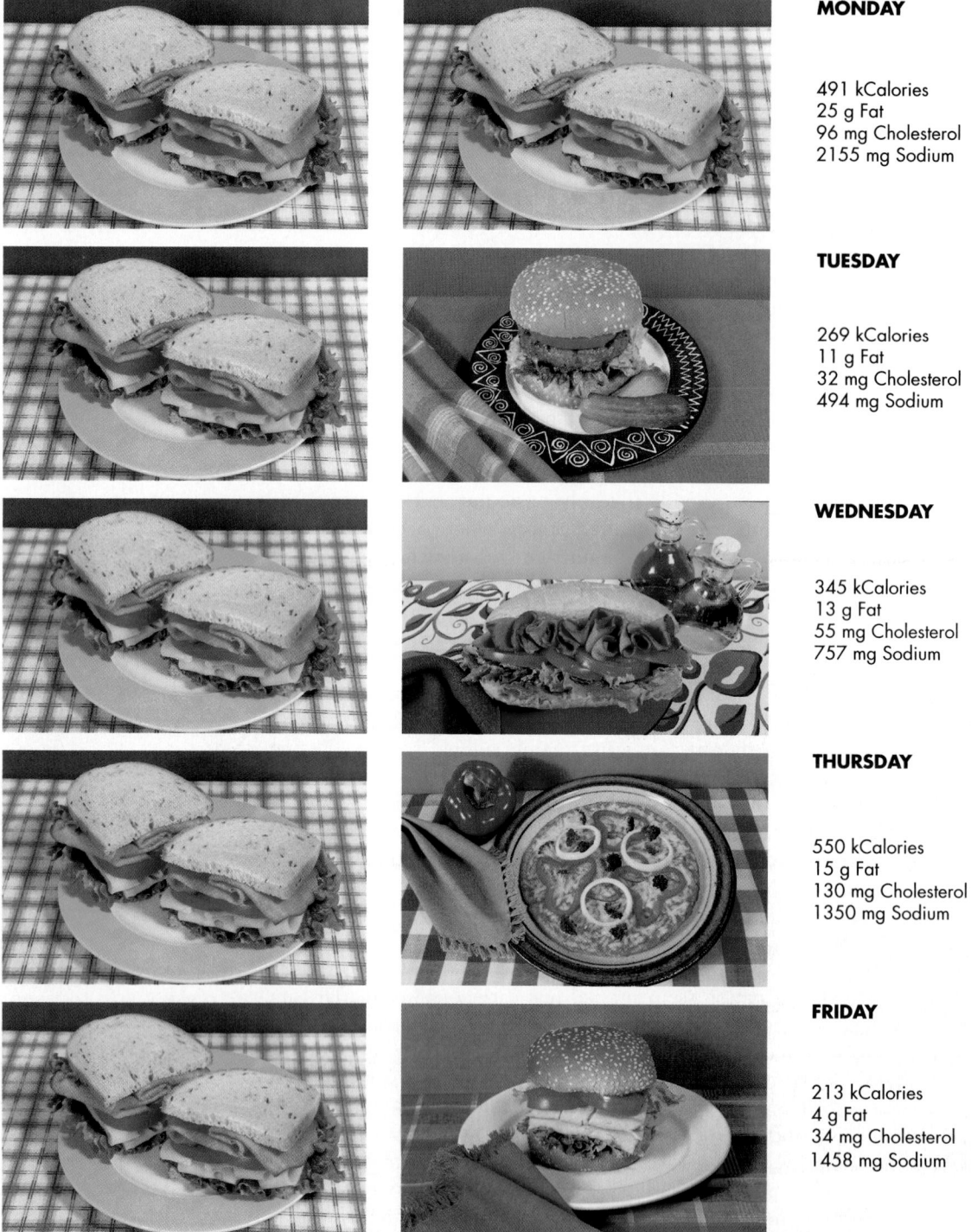

MONDAY

491 kCalories
25 g Fat
96 mg Cholesterol
2155 mg Sodium

TUESDAY

269 kCalories
11 g Fat
32 mg Cholesterol
494 mg Sodium

WEDNESDAY

345 kCalories
13 g Fat
55 mg Cholesterol
757 mg Sodium

THURSDAY

550 kCalories
15 g Fat
130 mg Cholesterol
1350 mg Sodium

FRIDAY

213 kCalories
4 g Fat
34 mg Cholesterol
1458 mg Sodium

Figure 1-4 An adequate eating pattern incorporates an assortment of foods. Eating a ham and cheese sandwich every day may seem like a quick lunchtime solution, but an assortment of foods over a 5-day period provides a daily average of fewer calories. (From Joanne Scott/Tracy McCalla. Data from *Nutrient Data Laboratory,* www.nal.usda.gov/fnic/foodcomp/.)

Nutrient density assigns value to a food based on a comparison of its nutrient content with the kcalories the food contains. The more nutrients and the fewer kcalories a food provides, the higher its nutrient density. Figure 1-6 demonstrates that a 12-oz glass of orange juice contains many more nutrients than a 12-oz soda that contains empty kcalories. The orange juice is nutrient dense compared with

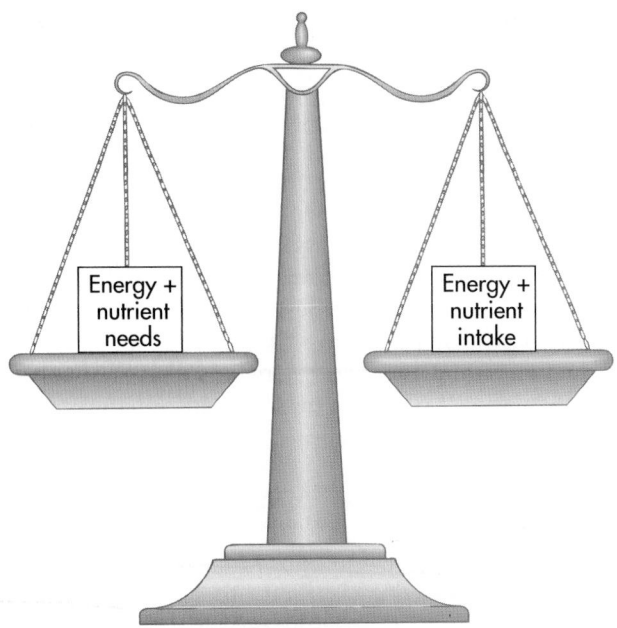

Figure 1-5 A balance of nutrients in the diet helps ensure adequacy. (From Rolin Graphics.)

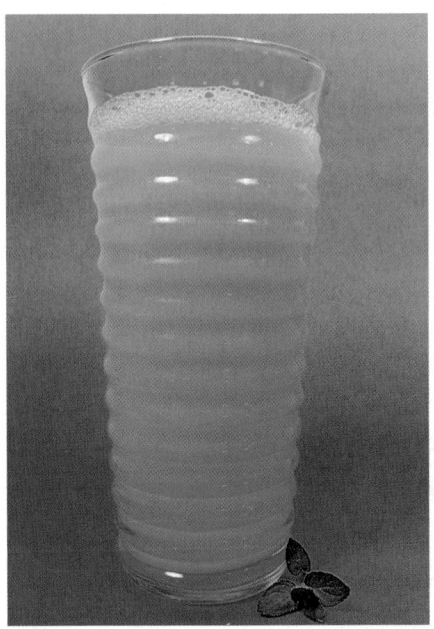

Orange juice: 12 oz, 120 kcal
Nutrients:
Phosphorus	63 mg
Potassium	744 mg
Iron	.75 mg
Sodium	3 mg
Calcium	40 mg
Vitamin A	75 re
Thiamin (B$_1$)	.33 mg
Riboflavin (B$_2$)	.15 mg
Niacin	1.5 mg
Vitamin C	186 mg

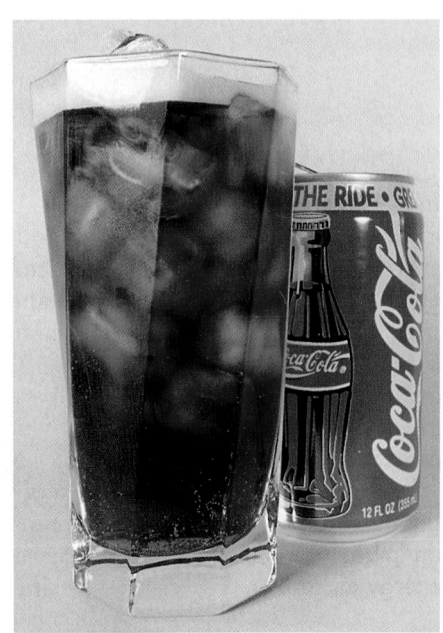

Soda: 12 oz, 160 kcal
Nutrients:
Phosphorus	52 mg
Potassium	7 mg
Iron	.2 mg
Sodium	18 mg

Figure 1-6 The more nutrients and the fewer kcalories a food provides, the higher its nutrient density. (From Joanne Scott/Tracy McCalla. Data from *Nutrient Data Laboratory,* www.nal.usda.gov/fnic/foodcomp/.)

the soda. Although both may quench a thirst and taste sweet, the orange juice supplies so much more for similar kcalories.

NUTRITIONAL ASSESSMENT

Nutritional assessment is the process of determining nutritional status. The assessment may reveal nutrient deficiencies or excesses. A deficiency may be either a primary nutrient deficiency caused by an inadequate intake of a nutrient or a

No single food contains all the nutrients essential for optimum health. An adequate eating pattern incorporates an assortment of foods.

secondary nutrient deficiency caused by the body's inefficient use of the nutrient once it is absorbed.

There are two levels of nutritional assessment. One level evaluates dietary intake of the foods we eat to determine the quantities of nutrients consumed as compared with the DRI standard. The other level evaluates dietary intake but also considers how the body uses the nutrients for growth and maintenance of health. Several methods of evaluation may be used. Although registered dietitians and nutritionists perform in-depth nutritional assessment, nurses as members of a health team approach require an awareness of this process as well. Nurses may conduct simple nutritional assessments to provide patient/client information that can be used by nutrition professionals.

A brief introduction to nutritional assessment follows. Chapter 14 contains a detailed nursing orientation for comprehensive nutritional assessment to be used as a basis for medical nutritional therapy.

Assessment of Dietary Intake

The DRIs offer guidelines for safe and appropriate levels of nutrients to be consumed by individuals or provided in the food supply. If a person's intake does not meet DRI levels, however, the diet is not necessarily deficient because the DRIs do not reflect the use of nutrients by individual bodies, nor do they take into account overconsumption of specific nutrients, health problems, or environmental influences. Therefore, when evaluating nutritional status, a healthcare worker may note whether a client's dietary intake meets the DRI standard but should not base the evaluation solely on a comparison with the DRIs. A complete nutritional assessment is necessary to evaluate a person's nutritional status.

Estimates of food consumption are often used to determine the nutritional status of individuals and populations. Sometimes if the dietary intake is imbalanced, undernutrition, overnutrition, or malnutrition may be diagnosed.

Undernutrition is the underconsumption of energy or nutrients based on RDA and DRI values. This means either not eating enough food to take in all the essential nutrients or eating enough food for energy but choosing foods that lack certain nutrients. In the United States some women do not consume enough of the vitamin folate, although the rest of their nutrient intake is adequate.

Overnutrition is consumption of too many nutrients and too much energy compared with DRI levels. North Americans generally overconsume saturated fats, which is a risk factor for the development of heart disease.

Malnutrition is a condition that results from an imbalanced nutrient and/or energy intake. Malnutrition is both undernutrition *and* overnutrition—undernutrition of too few nutrients or energy intake and overnutrition of excess nutrient or energy consumption. An obese man who consumes an excessive amount of kcalories is malnourished because his intake is out of balance. His intake does not equal his energy output. A nutrient overdose is malnutrition. In contrast, a college student who constantly diets for slimness or sports, consuming below the DRI for nutrients and energy, is also malnourished.

✿ Portraits of Malnutrition

As discussed earlier, not all who are malnourished resemble famine victims. The effects of long-term famines represent extreme forms of malnutrition (see Chapter 6). Lesser degrees of malnutrition are all around us. Consider the nutritional status of hospital patients, older adults, and chronic alcohol users.

For hospital patients, the nature of an illness, combined with medications, may affect appetite and the absorption of nutrients. The effects of malnutrition may be caused by the illness rather than by improper nutrient intake. Clinical nurses are trained to detect hospital malnutrition in acute care settings.

Nutritional assessment determines nutritional status. The assessment techniques include two levels:

1. The quality or range of nutrients consumed
2. The body's use of nutrients for growth and maintenance of health

undernutrition
the underconsumption of energy or nutrients based on RDA and DRI values

overnutrition
consumption of too many nutrients and too much energy compared with DRI levels

malnutrition
an imbalanced nutrient and/or energy intake

Older adults may be at risk for malnutrition. They may be unable to afford fresh fruits and vegetables or may be unable to get to the supermarket regularly because of transportation difficulties. Dental and other health problems may make chewing or digesting foods difficult. Social factors may affect appetite as well. Cooking for one and eating alone are not appealing and may affect food intake. Home health nurses must be alert to the social and economic factors that contribute to malnutrition in older adults.

Individuals who consume alcohol excessively and who may still be functional (e.g., able to work or attend school) are often malnourished because alcohol replaces nutrient-dense foods; alcohol affects the gastrointestinal tract and so impairs absorption of nutrients. The health needs of chronic alcohol abusers may be noticed by nurses in community and occupational health centers.

It is hard to imagine malnutrition happening close to home, especially when we shop in supermarkets that overflow with food products. Although hidden malnutrition among hospital patients, older adults, and chronic alcohol users is not as severe, it affects their health and productivity.

Diet Evaluation

Ways to gather data on the food a person eats may include the use of the 24-hour recall, usual food intake, a food record, a food frequency checklist, or a diet history. The 24-hour recall is a report on what an individual ate during the previous 24 hours. The information is usually gathered in a personal interview or by telephone. Usual food intake may be obtained by asking what the person usually eats at a typical meal or snack. This helps to develop an eating pattern. The individual who measures and records the amounts and kinds of food and beverages consumed during a certain time period creates a food record. Maintaining a food record is somewhat time consuming because the individual needs to keep careful notes on intake and to use measuring utensils to provide accuracy. A food frequency checklist records how often a person eats a specific type of food. This helps to focus on groups of foods that are either deficient or excessive. A diet history is an approximate representation of a person's eating habits over a long period. The data are gathered through interviews or questionnaires. None of these methods is totally accurate. They depend on good memories and recording skills and accurate measurements. Currently, these methods are the most convenient ways to collect data on dietary intake. When possible, it may be helpful to use multiple methods to double check the accuracy of information collected.

Once the data are collected, they can be analyzed through several computer dietary analysis programs and compared with the DRI for the individual. When this analysis is performed on a representative group of individuals of the larger population, estimates based on the dietary intake analysis can be made of the nutritional status of the population.

Assessment of Nutritional Status

Assessing nutritional status uses several methods of evaluation. Each method provides different data by which to assess nutritional status. See Chapter 14 for specific instructions for implementing these methods.

Because the methods for assessing nutritional status involve dietary, clinical, and biochemical analyses, collaboration by a multidisciplinary health team is usually required. In addition to dietary evaluations conducted by dietitians, methods may include the following:

- A *clinical examination performed by a primary health provider, nurse, or dietitian to note outward signs of nutritional health.* This includes physical examination through observation of the eyes, mucous membranes, skin, hair, mouth, teeth, and tongue. Clinical observations are limited in value because overt symptoms of nutrient deficiencies would not become apparent until late stages of deficiencies. In addition, some of the symptoms observed could be caused by conditions other than dietary deficiencies. Therefore a client's medical history from medical records or through direct interview and a social history are also important data to consider.

- *Biochemical analysis of samples of body tissues, such as blood or urine tests, to assess how the body uses nutrients.* If the blood level of a nutrient is low, it could mean the dietary intake was low, the nutrient was consumed but was poorly absorbed, or the individual has a higher than average requirement for the nutrient. Iron is a nutrient assessed through blood levels. Urine analysis can reveal the efficiency with which our bodies use glucose and protein and excrete other nutrients. Although a primary healthcare provider, nurse, or technician would draw the actual tissue samples, a dietitian would complete the nutritional analysis and interpret the results.

- *Anthropometric measurements, such as measuring the height, weight, and limb circumference of an individual and comparing those dimensions with national standards, to determine healthy growth patterns.* Body composition may also be used to determine percentages of lean body mass and body fat levels. In addition to height, weight, and limb circumference, various techniques are often used to assess body fat composition. These may include skin fold measurements, waist-to-hip ratios, densitometry, and bioelectric impedance analysis. Skill gained through careful practice is necessary to minimize the margin of error in taking body measurements. Before an assessment of this kind of data is completed, a family history should be conducted. Heredity plays a role in the growth patterns and final height and weights we achieve.

Through consideration of data from clinical, biochemical, and anthropometric measurements, the nutritional status of individuals can be determined. As with dietary assessment, if these analyses are performed on enough individuals who are representative of the total population, the nutritional status of nations can be estimated.

Nurses who provide maintenance healthcare to nonhospitalized clients may implement a limited form of dietary evaluation as a screening procedure. For example, community and home health nurses who may not have access to computer analysis when conferring with clients can compare the results of the 24-hour recall or food record to the recommended servings of the Food Guide Pyramid (see Figure 2-2) or, if the client receives medical nutritional therapy, to a prescribed diet. Clients can then use this form of quick assessment to periodically check the status of their intake. This quick assessment does not, however, provide the same indepth analysis as the comprehensive nutritional assessment performed by a dietitian who works with a multidisciplinary health team.

The Nutrition Specialist

Who is the nutrition specialist—the dietitian or the nutritionist? The answer is *both*. The difference is in the type of training and credentialing completed after majoring in foods and nutrition on the college or university level. Among health professionals, there has always been a concern that individuals may present themselves as nutritionists based on self-study (a personal interest in nutrition) or from completion of nonaccredited programs. Most states have established licensing for health specialists in nutrition. To be qualified requires years of a specially designed course of study. This is because the ramifications of medical nutrition therapy are crucial to recovery from illness and because lifestyle counseling concerning the optimum dietary intake for healthy individuals requires years of a specially designed course of study. Other states defer to the registering process developed by the American Dietetic Association (ADA) that confers the registered dietitian, or "RD," credentials. Nutrition professionals who are not registered dietitians should

medical nutrition therapy
the use of specific nutrition services to treat an illness, injury, or condition

have graduate degrees in nutrition from accredited university or college nutrition programs.

A registered dietitian (RD) is a professional trained in normal and clinical nutrition, food science, and food service management who is credentialed by the Commission on Dietetic Registration of the ADA. Credentialing is based on completing a bachelor of science degree from an accredited program, receiving clinical and administrative training, and passing a national registration examination. Continuing education is mandatory for continued registration. RDs may also have advanced training in specialized areas of medical nutritional therapy.

A nutritionist is a professional who has earned graduate degrees of master of science (MS), doctorate of education (EdD), or doctorate of philosophy (PhD) in foods and nutrition. In 43 states, dietitian/nutritionist is a legally defined and licensed or certified title. Meeting strict requirements allows for the use of designated titles. These may include certified dietitian nutritionist (CDN) or licensed dietitian (LD). These professionals may also be RDs. Within some states, it may be illegal to practice dietetics, such as medical nutrition therapy, without a license.[10]

Similar to nurses, dietitians and nutritionists practice in a variety of healthcare settings. Clinical dietitians and nutritionists focus on the therapeutic needs of individuals and their families in institutional settings such as hospitals, long-term care facilities, and rehabilitation centers. Others work in community-based practice settings as community nutritionists, dietitians, and educators; they may concentrate on health promotion and disease prevention in addition to therapeutic issues. Public health nutritionists attend to diet-related health issues of the larger community to include state, national, and international nutrition concerns. Dietitians may also work in the food industry conducting research or marketing for the food industry and for pharmaceutical companies.

registered dietitian (RD)
a professional trained in foods and the management of diets (dietetics) who is credentialed by the Commission on Dietetic Registration of the American Dietetic Association; credentialing is based on completing a bachelor of science degree from an approved program, receiving clinical and administrative training, and passing a registration examination

nutritionist
a professional who has completed a master or doctorate degree in foods and nutrition

Toward a Positive Nutrition Lifestyle: Self-Efficacy

Achieving wellness is an ongoing process. We all experience times when meeting our personal dietary goals is easy and other times when it seems as if we will never regain a sense of control over our nutrition lifestyles. These "ups and downs" are all part of the process of achieving wellness.

To support our pathway toward achieving wellness, this section in each chapter will feature psychosocial strategies to enhance positive self-efficacy. *Self-efficacy* is our perception of our ability to have power over our lives and behaviors. Positive self-efficacy means believing that personal behaviors can be changed and one has control over one's life. Negative self-efficacy refers to feeling as if one is powerless, with little control over circumstances. A sense of positive self-efficacy is essential to attain and then maintain nutrition lifestyles for optimum health. These strategies may be applicable in our own life situations and are useful for our clients as they, too, strive for enhanced self-efficacy.

Summary

Health is the merging and balancing of physical, intellectual, emotional, social, and spiritual dimensions. Nutrition, the study of essential nutrients and the ways they are used by the body, is a cornerstone of each health dimension. To improve health and nutrition, health promotion strategies can be implemented. These strategies often rely on knowledge, techniques, and community supports to initiate and maintain lifestyle behaviors to enhance health. Wellness is a lifestyle through which the five dimensions of health are further enhanced. "Wellness nutrition" approaches food consumption as a positive way to nourish the body.

The essential nutrients obtained from foods are divided into six categories: carbohydrates, proteins, fats, vitamins, minerals, and water. These nutrients aid growth and repair of body tissues, regulate body processes, and provide energy. Some nutrients are diverse in their impact, whereas others have specific functions. This chapter explores how the recommended daily levels of essential nutrients are determined. To prevent nutrient deficiencies and decrease the risk of the development of chronic disorders, dietary standards have been developed to provide guidelines about sufficient nutrient intakes. The DRIs are the standards for the United States and Canada.

Nutritional assessment determines nutritional status and nutrient deficiency in individuals. The techniques include two levels of assessment: evaluation of the quality of nutrients consumed and the body's use of nutrients for growth and maintenance of health.

THE NURSING APPROACH
Holistic Assessment and Nutrition: The Nursing Process

The nursing process is a systematic method of planning and providing care. The goal of the nursing process is to identify a client's healthcare status, identify actual or potential health problems, establish plans to meet the identified needs, and deliver specific nursing implementations. To achieve this goal, the nursing process components logically follow in sequence from assessing, diagnosing, planning, implementing, and evaluating.

The nursing process can be applied to patients' nutritional needs as it can to all human needs. This section, The Nursing Approach, in most chapters includes assessment, planning, implementation, and evaluation of some aspect of nutritional or medical nutritional therapy needs. In other chapters, only a portion of the nursing process is addressed, such as critical thinking, assessment, or diagnosis. Nursing diagnoses, when given, are usually based on the North American Nursing Diagnosis Association (NANDA) diagnosis, such as "Nutrition, altered: less than body requirements," "Knowledge deficit," or "Fluid volume deficit."

The following are possible NANDA (1999) diagnoses related to nutrition:
- Body image disturbance
- Breastfeeding, effective
- Breastfeeding, ineffective
- Breastfeeding, interrupted
- Constipation, risk for
- Diarrhea
- Fluid volume, deficit
- Fluid volume, deficit, risk for
- Fluid volume, excess
- Fluid volume, imbalance, risk for
- Growth, risk for altered
- Growth and development, altered
- Infant feeding pattern, ineffective
- Knowledge deficit
- Nutrition, altered, less than body requirements
- Nutrition, altered, more than body requirement
- Nutrition, altered, risk for more than body requirements
- Self-care deficit: feeding

The nurse, whether hospital or clinic staff nurse, home health nurse, occupational health nurse, nurse practitioner, or school nurse, is in a unique position regarding an individual's nutritional needs. Although the nurse may not be as knowledgeable as the dietitian regarding nutrition, it is the nurse who does a holistic assessment of each patient and who diagnoses strengths and weaknesses in nutritional lifestyle. It is through

THE NURSING APPROACH–cont'd
Holistic Assessment and Nutrition: The Nursing Process

this systematic assessment that the nurse can also begin to identify factors that affect nutritional status, such as cultural beliefs, socioeconomic status, physiologic changes, and social circumstances. Implementations may follow in the form of reinforcement, education, consultation with the primary health provider, or referral to a dietitian.

The nurse who has a thorough knowledge of basic nutrition will appreciate the importance of dietary intake in maintaining health and in recovery from disease or injury.

Reference: NANDA International (2002). NANDA Nursing Diagnoses: Definitions and Classification, 2003-2004, *Philadelphia: NANDA.*

APPLYING CONTENT KNOWLEDGE

Health promotion strategies often involve lifestyle changes. Bob needs to reduce his dietary fat intake because he is at risk for coronary artery disease. He lives in a suburban community and takes a train into New York City where he works. Although it is only a half-mile to the train station, he usually drives his car there to save time. Breakfast is often coffee, with a midmorning break that consists of a Danish and more coffee; lunch is obtained from street vendors who sell hot dogs and sausage sandwiches; dinner is usually eaten with his family but often features meat and potatoes, his favorites. Because he leaves early in the morning and returns tired in the evening, he says he doesn't know how to change his behaviors.

Using the strategies of knowledge, techniques, and community supports, describe the education care plan that could be developed with Bob.

(See *Student Resource Online* for answer.)

Web Sites of Interest

American Dietetic Association
www.eatright.org
As the Web site of the American Dietetic Association (ADA) and the ADA National Center of Nutrition and Dietetics, this site is a wealth of information on nutrition, health, and wellness. Career and member information is available as well as referrals to registered dietitians in the United States.

Healthy People
www.healthypeople.gov
The official Web site of *HP2010* provides the basis for development of new objectives and the progress toward achieving goals.

National Academy Press of the National Academy of Sciences
www.nap.edu/readingroom
The National Academy of Sciences is a nonprofit organization that through its Institute of Medicine formulates dietary standards such as the RDAs and the DRIs. This site provides online publications and a bookstore.

Nutrient Data Laboratory
www.nal.usda.gov/fnic/foodcomp/
This U.S. Department of Agriculture Web site includes information on the nutrient content of foods consumed in the United States. About 6000 items

are included, and these form the basis of nutrient information for government surveys and research studies.

Nutrition Navigator
navigator.tufts.edu
Developed by Tufts University School of Nutrition Science and Policy, this site is the first online rating and review guide of sources and quality of nutrition information on the Internet.

References

1. Thomas PR, ed: *Improving America's diet and health: from recommendations to action,* Washington, DC, 1991, National Academy Press.
2. Burns CM: Toward *Healthy People 2000:* the role of the nurse practitioner and health promotion, *J Am Acad Nurse Pract* 6(1):29, 1994.
3. World Health Organization: "Constitution of the World Health Organization," *Chronicles of the World Health Organization*, Geneva, Switzerland, 1947; www.who.int/aboutwho/en/definition.html.
4. Dubos R: *So human the animal*, New York, 1968, Scribners.
5. US Department of Health and Human Services, Public Health Service: *Healthy People 2010,* ed 2, Washington, DC, 2000, US Government Printing Office; www.healthypeople.gov/.
6. Simons-Mortons B, Greene WH, Gottlieb NH: *Introduction to health education and health promotion,* ed 2, Prospect Heights, Ill, 1995, Waveland Press.
7. Pennington J: *Bowes & Church's food values of portions commonly used,* ed 17, Philadelphia, 1997, Lippincott-Raven.
8. Standing Committee on the Scientific Evaluation of Dietary Reference Intakes, Food and Nutrition Board, Institute of Medicine: *Dietary reference intakes: applications in dietary assessment,* Washington, DC, 2000, National Academy Press.
9. Standing Committee on the Scientific Evaluation of Dietary Reference Intakes, Institute of Medicine: *Dietary reference intakes: calcium, phosphorus, magnesium, vitamin D, and fluoride,* Washington, DC, 1998, National Academy Press.
10. Klausner A: Deciphering the alphabet soup of nutrition advice, *Environmental Nutrition,* July 1998.

CHAPTER 2

Personal and Community Nutrition

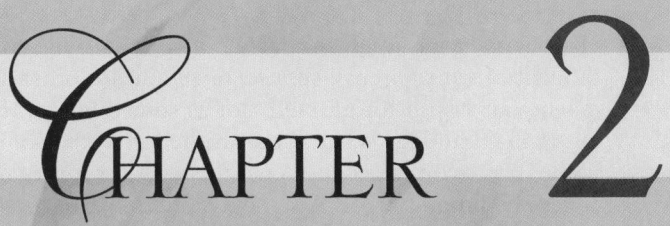

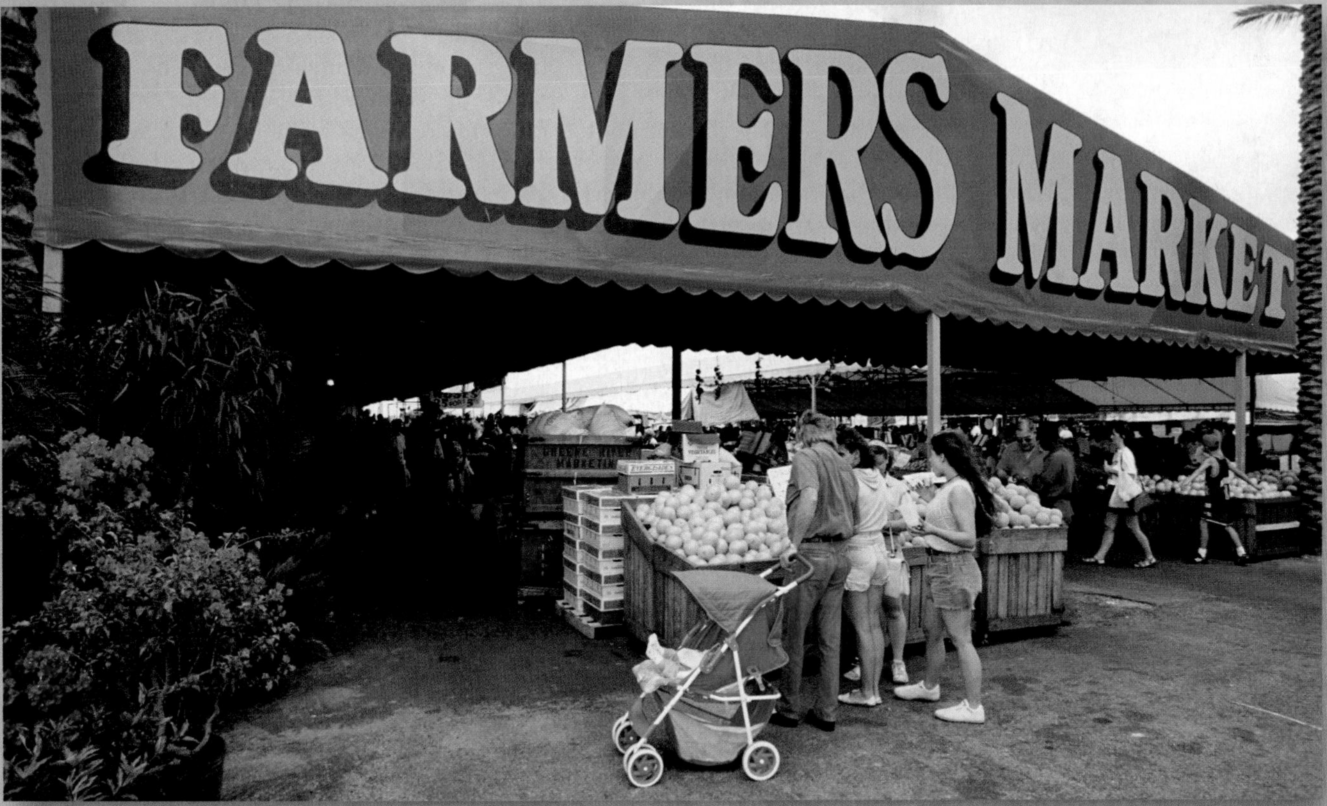

. . . A person's food behavior is influenced by personal factors as well as community issues affecting food availability, consumption and expenditure trends, consumer information, and food safety.

Have you ever thought about who is responsible for your health? Perhaps you thought of your parents, spouse, or significant other. Or possibly you have always taken your health for granted, not as something to actively work toward improving or maintaining. What about the health of the community in which you live or work? Have you ever considered the health status of the residents of your town or college community?

As stated in *Healthy People 2010*:

> Over the years, it has become clear that individual health is closely linked to community health—the health of the community and environment in which individuals live, work, and play. Likewise, community health is profoundly affected by the collective beliefs, attitudes, and behaviors of everyone who lives in the community.[1]

We must take responsibility for our personal health and the health of our communities-at-large. This chapter considers strategies to improve our health by taking charge of our personal nutrition and becoming aware of the nutrition issues of our communities.

ROLE IN WELLNESS

As presented in Chapter 1, wellness is a lifestyle through which we continually strive to enhance our level of health. Health is the merging and balancing of physical, intellectual, emotional, social, and spiritual dimensions. Considering these dimensions in relation to personal and community nutrition broadens our understanding. The physical health dimension is represented by the food guides presented in this chapter. By following the recommendations of the food guides, we may reduce the risk of diet-related diseases. Consumer decisions about food purchases and application of food safety recommendations depend on reasoning abilities that reflect the intellectual health dimension. The emotional health dimension may affect the ability to be flexible when adopting suggested guideline changes. If we (or our clients) have problems doing so, will we view ourselves as "failures"? Social health dimension is tested as we (and our clients) interact with family and friends when we attempt to follow the guidelines. Can we be role models for others without being perceived as threats? Many religions stress personal responsibility for caring for one's body, which embodies the spiritual dimension of health. Part of that responsibility includes the foods we choose to eat.

The decisions individuals make about the food they eat determine their health and wellness. Health professionals frequently give advice about appropriate foods for clients to consume. Therefore it is important for nurses in institutional and community settings to understand how personal factors and community issues that affect food availability, consumption and expenditure trends, consumer information, and food safety can influence a person's food behavior. Effects of these personal and community factors on consumers' food decisions are some of the major topics of this chapter.

PERSONAL NUTRITION

As adults, each of us is ultimately responsible for the quality of our dietary intake. Although external forces may affect our everyday food choices, we can decide to have the internal self-awareness to consciously modify those forces. To be accountable for our nutritional status and health may require adjustment of some personal goals to allow time to work on achieving a wellness lifestyle.

Food Selection

Our food preferences, food choice, and food liking affect the foods we select to eat. Although these terms reflect similar food-related behaviors, they are different.[2]

Food preferences are those foods we choose to eat when all foods are available at the same time and in the same quantity. Factors affecting preferences include genetic determinants and environmental effects. Genetic factors include inborn desires for sweet and salty flavors. One study of taste receptors notes that because of genetic taste markers, some people experience the taste of vegetables such as broccoli and brussels sprouts as bitter and therefore avoid such foods, whereas other people find this flavor enjoyable.[3] Consumption of cruciferous vegetables, such as broccoli and brussels sprouts, may be associated with a decreased risk of developing certain cancers.[3] If some people avoid them because of perceived bitter taste, will they be more at risk for cancers?

Environmental effects are learned preferences that are the result of cultural and socioeconomic influences. We often adjust our choices to those we are around. Because we are around our families the most, their influence is the most significant factor in the choices we make; therefore the dietary patterns we experience as children affect us throughout our lives[4] (see the Cultural Considerations box, "Hispanic Food Shopping Habits"). In fact, even the food a mother eats prenatally affects the preferences of her child in the future.[5]

food preferences
the foods we choose to eat when all foods are available at the same time and in the same quantity

CULTURAL CONSIDERATIONS
Hispanic Food Shopping Habits

Hispanic Americans are the largest minority group in the United States, with 35.3 million people based on the U.S. Census Bureau data for 2000. Hispanic Americans are not a homogenous group because they come from a variety of countries such as Mexico, Puerto Rico, Dominican Republic, and Latin American countries. Nonetheless, Hispanics share many common concerns and needs.

In 2001 the Food Marketing Institute (FMI) conducted a study that consisted of 1200 telephone interviews with Hispanic grocery shoppers. Of the respondents, 1000 were from the top 10 Hispanic markets in the United States and 200 were from Puerto Rico. The institute's findings highlight the need to understand how we are alike and how we differ as a nation of food shoppers.

Hispanic shoppers decide where to shop based on the availability of fresh, high-quality fruits and vegetables; polite and pleasant staff; sanitary and orderly store appearance; low prices; and superior meats and poultry. Because many Hispanic shoppers do not use prepared "ready-to-serve" products, but instead cook from scratch every day, the freshness of ingredients is important. Of the respondents, 85% report preparing traditional Hispanic meals. Shoppers also prefer Hispanic elements, such as the following, in the supermarkets where they shop:
- Availability of Hispanic products
- Bilingual store signs
- Bilingual employees who understand Hispanic products
- Advertisements in Hispanic and Spanish-language media
- Advertising that addresses family needs

Although supermarkets are the most visited, many Hispanic shoppers also go to independent bakeries and butcher shops more often than the typical American shopper. Shopping trips are often organized around a shopping list and with consideration of advertised specials and store price comparisons.

An important fact to note is that Hispanic shoppers usually do not shop alone but consider grocery shopping as a family function. More than half of Hispanics shop with another adult from their household. This may also reflect that mealtimes are an important part of family life for Hispanic Americans—who rarely eat their main meal out in restaurants. This tends to change as more income is earned. In addition, younger Hispanic adults tend to eat out more often than older Hispanic adults.

The report notes that the level of acculturation (adaptation to the culture of the dominant group) of Hispanic Americans may significantly affect the use of the supermarket. As acculturation increases, the value of Hispanic-specific features of grocery shopping will probably lessen and shopping strategies may be more similar to those of other Americans.

Application to nursing: When assisting Hispanic American clients, assumptions cannot be made simply based on a client's surname or use of language because different levels of acculturation may affect food choice and preparation. When dietary recommendations are given, strategies for shopping and preparing foods can be discussed within the information presented by the Food Marketing Institute. Where does the client shop? With whom do they shop? Are meals prepared from scratch? Who cooks meals for the family? Should other members of the household be present when dietary recommendations are explained? Sensitivity to all aspects of a client's life enhances the path to wellness.

Reference: Food Marketing Institute: US Hispanics: insights into grocery shopping preferences and attitudes, 2002, *Washington, DC, 2002, Food Marketing Institute.*

An indirect influence on food preferences is the media, particularly television. Television advertising is a potent force that influences the foods we prefer and buy. Programs spread messages as to food and lifestyle preferences of different socioeconomic groups. A TV show about a working class family presents images of food intake associated with those of a lower socioeconomic status—dinner might be hot dogs and beans. In another TV show, an upper socioeconomic family might sit down to a meal of baked salmon and salad. Each unintentionally sends messages about appropriate food intake for individuals belonging to each socioeconomic group.

Health promotion issues are tied to food preferences. If recommendations call for changes in foods whose preference is rooted in genetic determinants, the motivation for change needs to be different than if the food preference is environmentally learned. New preferences can be learned; genetic preferences are more difficult to change.

food choice
the specific foods that are convenient to choose when we are actually ready to eat

Food choice concerns the specific foods that are convenient to choose when we are actually ready to eat; rarely are all our preferred foods available at the same time to satisfy our preferences. Food choices are restricted by convenience. With hectic lifestyles, we tend to avoid foods that take long to prepare. Instead, we often repeatedly choose foods that are easy to prepare and eat, regardless of their nutritional value. Cost is also a factor. We sometimes weigh cost benefits against time benefits. If a food costs more but saves time, we may choose it. We may decide that a food item, even if nutrient dense, costs too much money for the benefits received. Again, nutritional value may not be a prime concern that affects food choice.

food liking
foods we really like to eat

Food liking considers which foods we really like to eat. We may want to eat foods that enhance our health, but we like to eat chocolate layer cake, for example. We constantly weigh all the factors of preference, choice, and liking when we select the foods we eat. Ultimately, these three types of food behaviors greatly affect individual nutritional status.[2]

It is the small steps we take that eventually lead to cumulative change. As we study different aspects of food and nutrition, we will present suggestions that will move us and our clients toward significant change. These suggestions will lead to the formation of new personal food habits.

✿ COMMUNITY NUTRITION

The nutritional status of our communities is a reflection of our individual nutritional health. Perhaps the most significant factor affecting the nutritional status of communities is economics. Having sufficient funds to purchase adequate food supplies is a necessity. Public health nutrition efforts to prevent nutrient deficiencies include the U.S. government's food stamp program. This program provides individuals and families below certain income levels with coupons to purchase nutritious foods. Another such effort is the Special Supplemental Food Program for Women, Infants, and Children (WIC). The WIC program provides medical care, nutrition counseling, and supplemental foods to women who are pregnant or breastfeeding and to infants and children up to the age of 5 who are at nutritional risk. Both programs have a significant impact on improving the nutritional status of those who participate. Additional government programs are discussed in Chapters 12 and 13.

Another level of public health nutrition is aimed at the nutrient excesses of our dietary intake. In the late 1970s, a new era in nutrition recommendations began in the United States. Rather than focusing on nutrient deficiencies as a cause of poor health, health professionals began to notice that the cause of an increasing amount of chronic illness was possibly tied to excessive intake of certain nutrients such as saturated fats, cholesterol, sodium, and sugars.[6] As knowledge of diet-related diseases (e.g., heart disease, hypertension, cancer, diabetes, osteoporosis, obesity) has increased, several sets of dietary recommendations from different government agencies and voluntary health and scientific associations have been released to address this issue.

Each set of recommendations serves a different purpose. For example, recommendations from the American Heart Association focus on lifestyle and dietary factors that affect risk factors of coronary artery disease, whereas those of the American Cancer Society center on issues related to cancer development. Despite differences in the focus of the recommendations, consensus has developed on the guidelines for maintaining general good health.[7,8] These recommendations are incorporated into our national goals. All recommendations suggest a reduced intake of saturated fat, total fat, cholesterol, sodium, sugar, and excessive kcalories and an increased intake of fiber, complex carbohydrates, fruits, and vegetables. These goals form the basis of health promotion efforts to implement primary, secondary, and tertiary prevention strategies. Education at the community level to reach as many individuals and families as possible has been a challenge for health professionals.

Dietary Guidelines for Americans

In response to the dietary recommendations, the U.S. Department of Agriculture (USDA) and U.S. Department of Health and Human Services (USDHHS) developed in 1977 the *Dietary Guidelines for Americans*. These guidelines, most recently revised in 2000, contain general suggestions regarding food selection for healthy Americans more than 2 years of age (Figure 2-1). The 10 recommendations are divided into 3 clusters of ABC: **A**im for fitness, **B**uild a healthy base, and **C**hoose sensibly.[9]

Lifestyle Applications

Your clients and patients would certainly like to follow the *Dietary Guidelines for Americans,* but how should they do this? Their busy schedules barely allow time for any food at all. Have them consider the following suggestions (see also Box 2-1):

- In the morning, choose dry cereals and bread products (e.g., English muffins) that contain whole grains and alternate or mix these with less-fiber favorites. If no time can be found for breakfast, stock up on portable juices and portable fruit, such as apples or bananas, that can be eaten on the way to class or work. Bring fruit in backpacks or briefcases for a quick snack.
- Be creative with vending machine selections. Choose lower-fat and lower-sugar selections such as raisins, bagel chips, pretzels (rub off excess salt), popcorn, and even some plain cookies or crackers. Some vending machines stock small cans of tuna fish, yogurts, and fruits. Contact the staff responsible for filling the vending machines to request healthier selections.
- If lunch and dinner are on the run and fast-food drive-throughs are the only option, select lower-fat items such as grilled chicken sandwiches or plain hamburgers without the sauce. Don't have French fries or milkshakes (unless they are low fat) every time but instead alternate with salads and low-fat milk, juice, or water.
- Perhaps lunch and dinner are in a college or employee cafeteria. Try to select turkey, chicken (without skin), fish, and lean beef dishes. Include whole grain bread, a grain (rice or pasta), several vegetables, and salad. Try fruit for dessert; it is good with frozen low-fat yogurt, if available.
- Maybe your clients don't really eat "meals" but eat snacks throughout the day. This is called *grazing.* It is possible to graze and follow the *Dietary Guidelines for Americans* by choosing wholesome foods instead of candy bars and soda. High-quality grazing foods that are often available include bagels (with a little cream cheese), yogurt, fruits, pretzels, pizza (but not daily because of the high-fat content of cheese), and dry cereals with milk.

LEADING CAUSES OF DEATH IN THE UNITED STATES, NOTED FROM MOST COMMON TO LEAST COMMON

1. Heart disease
2. Cancers
3. Stroke (cerebrovascular diseases)
4. Chronic lower respiratory diseases
5. Accidents
6. Diabetes mellitus
7. Pneumonia and influenza
8. Alzheimer's disease
9. Kidney disorders
10. Blood infections (septicemia)
11. Suicide
12. Chronic liver disease and cirrhosis
13. High blood pressure (hypertension)
14. Lung inflammation (pneumonitis)
15. Homicides

From Minino AM, Smith BL: Deaths: Preliminary data for 2000, *National Vital Statistics Report* 49(12), October 9, 2001.

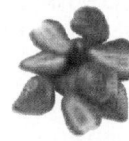
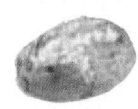
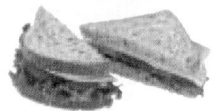
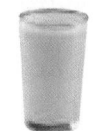
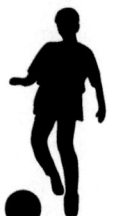
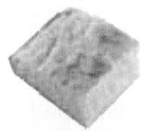
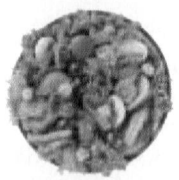
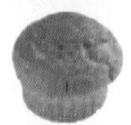
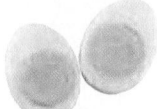

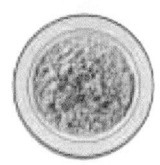
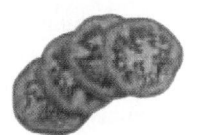
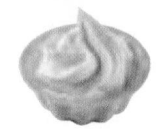
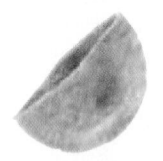
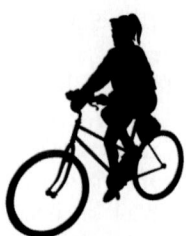
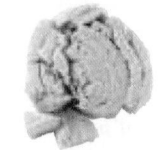
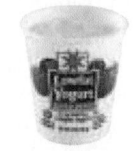
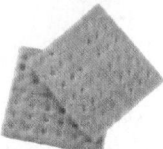

DIETARY GUIDELINES FOR AMERICANS

AIM FOR FITNESS...

▲ Aim for a healthy weight.

▲ Be physically active each day.

BUILD A HEALTHY BASE...

■ Let the Pyramid guide your food choices.

■ Choose a variety of grains daily, especially whole grains.

■ Choose a variety of fruits and vegetables daily.

■ Keep food safe to eat.

CHOOSE SENSIBLY...

● Choose a diet that is low in saturated fat and cholesterol and moderate in total fat.

● Choose beverages and foods to moderate your intake of sugars.

● Choose and prepare foods with less salt.

● If you drink alcoholic beverages, do so in moderation.

...for good health

Figure 2-1 The recommendations made by the current version of *Dietary Guidelines for Americans.* (From US Department of Agriculture, US Department of Health and Human Services: *Nutrition and your health: dietary guidelines for Americans,* ed 5, Home and Garden Bulletin 232, Washington, DC, 2000, USDA; www.usda.gov/cnpp.)

Box 2-1 Implementing Dietary Guidelines: Easier Said Than Done

As most of us become familiar with the *Dietary Guidelines for Americans* recommendations and the Food Pyramid, we probably reflect on the different food choices available to us and what changes we could most easily implement. But many low-income and unemployed individuals and families don't have the luxury of deciding among a variety of available foods. Instead, their problem is one of food insecurity.

Food insecurity is the limited access to safe, nutritious food and may be measured as a marker of undernutrition among persons who are also poor and isolated from mainstream society. Retarded growth and iron deficiency along with food insecurity may lead to health disparities because of income, race, and ethnicity. The available financial resources of these households may not be able to stretch far enough to provide sufficient quantities of high-quality foods. A recurring strain for these families is to provide enough food for their children and themselves; sometimes they may all experience hunger.

In this context, the definition of hunger is not just the physiologic need for food. Instead, a social definition of hunger is the inability to access enough food to feel nourished and satisfied.

Although government programs like Food Stamps and WIC and private nonprofit food banks do fill hunger gaps, they are often insufficient to provide enough food for all of those in need. When clients struggle to adopt new dietary guidelines, keep in mind the range of food choices easily available.

From US Department of Health and Human Services, Public Health Service: Healthy People 2010, *ed 2, Washington, DC, 2000, US Government Printing Office; www.health.gov/healthypeople.*

Next time your clients are food shopping or grabbing a snack or meal, encourage them to stop a moment and consider the best choices available.

FOOD GUIDES

When we are armed with the latest nutrient recommendations, we can easily apply this knowledge to the way we eat every day. Because we think about what *food* to eat rather than what *nutrients* we need, these nutrient recommendations are most useful when translated into real food. To help us do this, food guides have been developed.

The Food Guide Pyramid

The Food Guide Pyramid (Figure 2-2) is designed to help us follow most of the *Dietary Guidelines for Americans*.[10] Developed by the USDA, it is a guide to the amounts and kinds of foods we should eat daily to maintain health and to reduce the risk of developing diet-related diseases.

As an outline of what to eat, the Food Guide Pyramid presents the following five major food groups:

1. Bread, cereal, rice, and pasta group (6 to 11 servings/day)
2. Vegetable group (3 to 5 servings/day)
3. Fruit group (2 to 4 servings/day)
4. Milk, yogurt, and cheese group (2 to 3 servings/day)
5. Meat, poultry, fish, dry beans, eggs, and nuts group (2 to 3 servings/day)

The small tip of the Pyramid is for fats, oils, and sweets. There is no serving number suggested for this category because these should be consumed in small quantities only.

Each food group is visually displayed to represent the number of servings we should eat daily; the number is a range of servings. This range takes into account our different energy needs and personal food preferences. Everyone should eat at least the minimum number of servings for each group. By doing so, we consume an adequate quantity of essential nutrients.

The Pyramid allows us to choose between foods that contain different levels of fats (lipids), fiber, and sodium. To use the Pyramid as a guide for choosing a low-fat, high-fiber meal pattern, we also need to understand the effect of food preparation on the fat and fiber content of meals. By arming ourselves with more information about the foods we choose and how we prepare them, we can develop an optimum meal pattern. This textbook provides this information in the chapters that discuss fats, carbohydrates, and sodium (a mineral). The Health Debate box, "Controversy Brewing," also provides information about an alternative pyramid, the "Healthy Eating Pyramid."

Life span nutrition concerns are reflected by two variations of the original Food Guide Pyramid—The Food Guide Pyramid for Children (see Figure 12-2) and Tufts Food Guide Pyramid for Older Adults (go to: www.nutrition.tufts.edu) address the different nutrient emphasis suggested for these two age groups.

Alternative and ethnic food pyramids are also available that provide specific food selections that conform to the general Pyramid categories. These recognize that traditional dietary patterns of other cultures also offer opportunities to decrease the risk of diet-related disorders. The Asian, Mediterranean, and Latin American Diet Pyramids are accessible from the Oldways Preservation & Exchange Trust Web site located at www.oldwayspt.org. These pyramids differ from the Food Guide Pyramid in the number of servings of animal foods, legumes, nuts, and seeds.[11] Vegetarian and soul food pyramids have been created as well. Other countries and commonwealths have food guides that reflect their national food supply, food consumption patterns, and nutritional status. Examples of the food guides for Mexico and Puerto Rico are shown in Figure 2-3. Although the shapes of the guides may differ from the U.S. Food Pyramid, all recommend similar distributions of food category servings.[12] Ethnic food guides may be useful when caring for clients from other countries.

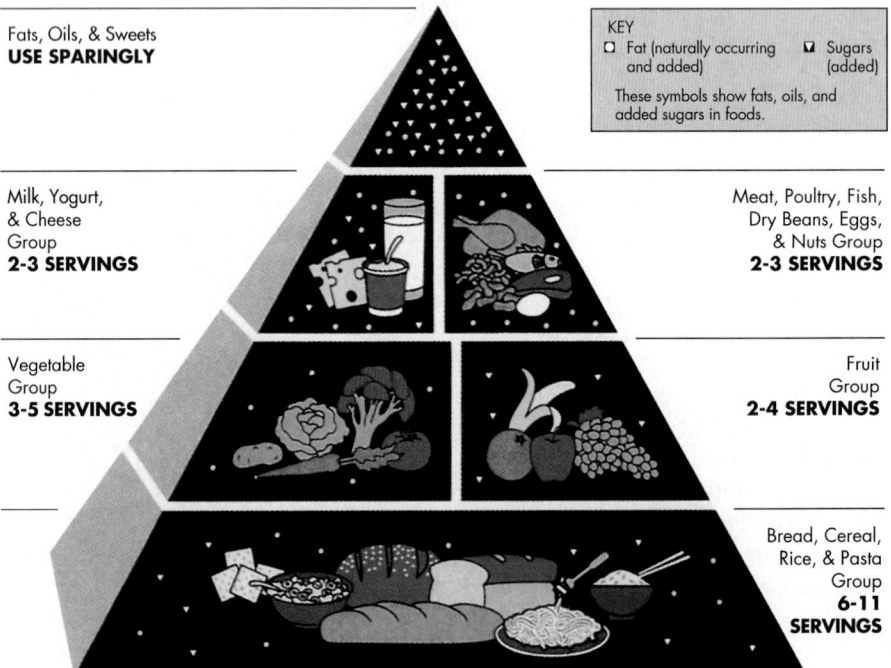

Figure 2-2 The Food Guide Pyramid: a guide to daily food choices. (From US Department of Agriculture Center for Nutrition Policy and Promotion: *The Food Pyramid*, Home and Garden Bulletin 249, Washington, DC, 1992, revised 1996, US Government Printing Office; www.usda.gov/fcs/cnpp.htm.)

*A*lthough the Food Guide Pyramid has been around for a number of years, not all health professionals view its recommendations as the most sound to improve and maintain health. Some cite the increasing incidence of diet-related disorders such as type 2 diabetes, obesity and Syndrome X. (Syndrome X, or metabolic syndrome, is a group of heart disease risk factors of abdominal obesity, glucose intolerance, high blood pressure, and abnormal blood lipid levels.) Increases of diet-related disorders may indicate the traditional Pyramid does not meet our health goals because the prevention and treatment of these three conditions have dietary components. Perhaps the Pyramid is not being followed correctly. If it is being followed, the emphasis of the Pyramid on complex carbohydrates from grains and the use of animal-derived foods as the focus of two categories (dairy and protein sources) as the foundation of our dietary intake does not provide the expected health benefits. Another factor may be that the Pyramid does not distinguish between refined and unrefined grain products. Health benefits are lost that could be derived from unrefined complex carbohydrate grain products, such as whole wheat bread.

One of the first alternative pyramids to address these concerns was developed by Dr. Walter Willett, chairperson of the Department of Nutrition at the Harvard School of Public Health. Based on accumulated scientific research, this pyramid—the Healthy Eating Pyramid—changes the focus of food selection and distinguishes between whole and refined grain foods as well as highlights plant sources of protein, such as nuts and legumes, that contain healthful plant oils (see the "Healthy Eating Pyramid" below). Animal-derived foods are pushed high up on the Healthy Eating Pyramid to reflect that they are foods that should only be consumed occasionally. For example, red meat is to be used sparingly or infrequently. Fish, poultry, and eggs are to be consumed zero to two times a day. This is different from the traditional Pyramid, which groups animal and plant sources of protein together (meat, poultry, fish, dry beans, eggs, and nuts) with suggested servings of two to three times a day without distinguishing between the nutrient content of these foods. In addition, the Healthy Eating Pyramid includes recommendations for daily exercise and weight control.

Will this additional pyramid prove to be more beneficial? Would you follow it?

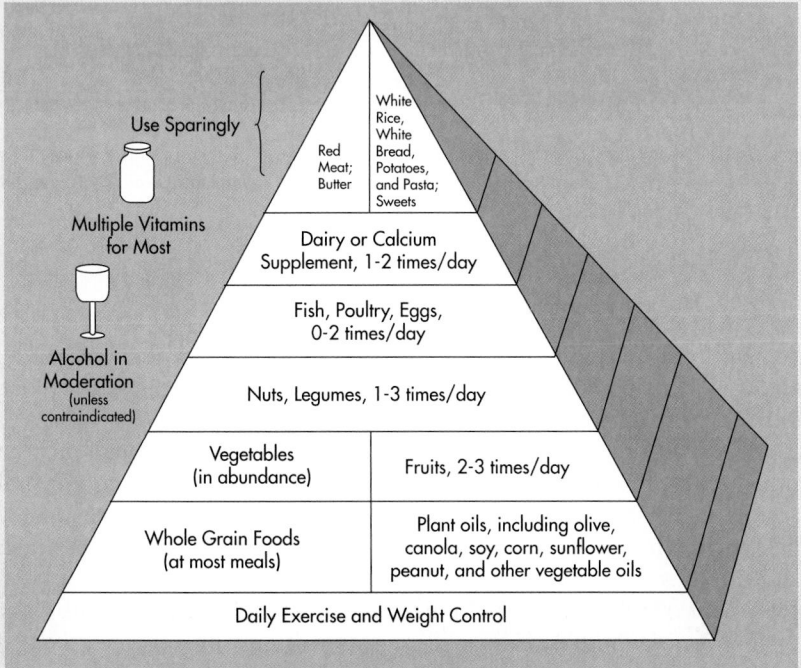

Healthy Eating Pyramid. (Reprinted with the permission of Simon & Schuster. Source: EAT, DRINK, AND BE HEALTHY by Dr. Walter C. Willett, Copyright © 2001 by President and Fellows of Harvard College.)

Reference: Willett W: Eat, drink, and be healthy, *New York, 2001, Simon & Schuster.*

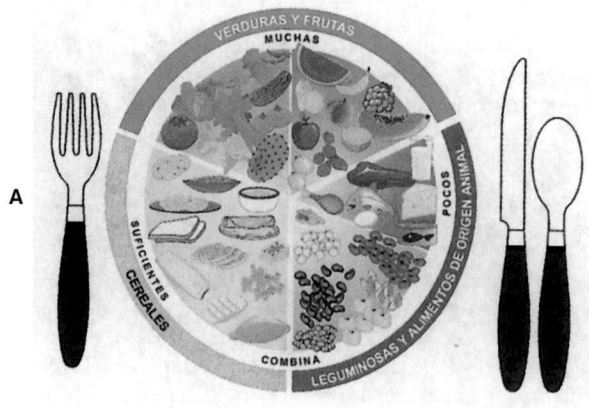

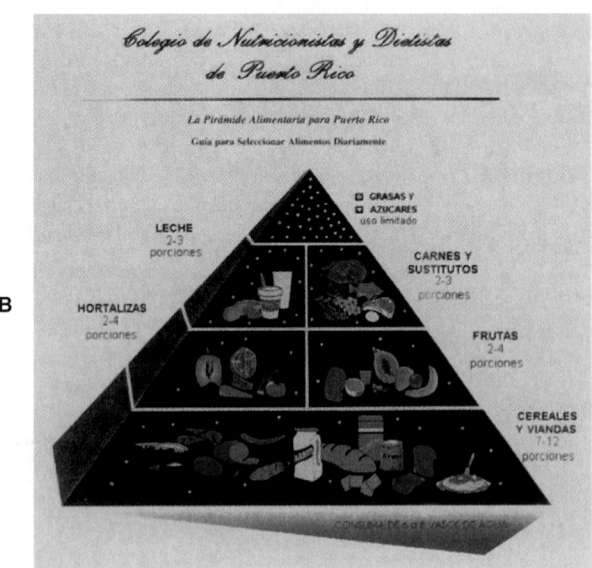

Figure 2-3 International food guides. **A,** Mexico. **B,** Puerto Rico. (From Painter J, Rah J-H, Lee Y-K: Comparison of international food guide pictorial presentations, *J Am Dietetic Assoc* 102(4):483, Apr 2002.)

5 a Day Program

Perhaps you have noticed banners and brochures in your local supermarket that proclaim "5 a Day—for Better Health" and other posters that advise increased consumption of fruits and vegetables (Figure 2-4). These banners are part of the national "5 a Day—for Better Health" program. This program represents the first government and private industry partnership to improve health and is a collaborative effort of the National Cancer Institute, the National Institutes of Health, and the Produce for Better Health Foundation, a nonprofit consumer education foundation funded by the fruit and vegetable industry.[13]

The purpose of the program is to increase the number of Americans who consume at least five servings of fruits and vegetables a day. By doing so, the goals of the *Dietary Guidelines for Americans, Healthy People 2010,* and other dietary recommendations may be achieved.

Research shows that 28% of Americans consume only two fruits and only 3% consume three servings of vegetables a day.[1] Consequently, most Americans do not meet the recommended five servings of fruits and vegetables a day, although this amount is the minimum number recommended by the Food Guide Pyramid. By

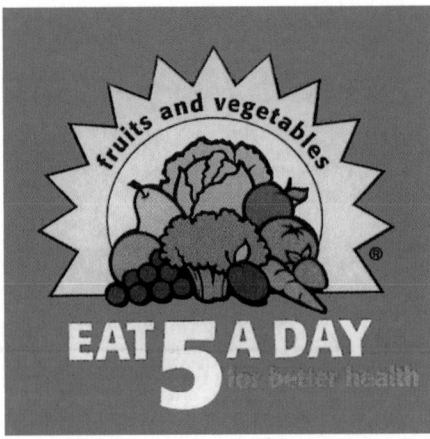

Figure 2-4 "5 a Day" logo. (From Produce for Better Health Foundation, 2002, Newark, Del.)

focusing on only fruits and vegetables, this guide becomes an easy way to decrease intake of fats because fruits and vegetables are naturally low in fat. With five servings of fruits and vegetables each day, increased consumption of fiber, vitamin C, and beta-carotene will also occur. These nutrients, in addition to their functions as essential nutrients, are recognized as having the potential to reduce the risk of developing heart disease and certain cancers. In addition, fruits and vegetables are excellent sources of antioxidants and phytochemicals for which potential health benefits are continually being uncovered.

Although it may be difficult to determine the percentage of daily dietary fat consumed, it is easy to count the number of servings of fruits and vegetables. If more fruits and vegetables are eaten everyday, appetites for high-fat foods will decrease (see sample menu in margin).

Exchange Lists

The food guides refer to eating a number of servings of specific foods daily. But what is a serving size? A resource for serving sizes is the *Exchange Lists for Meal Planning,* published by the American Dietetic Association and the American Diabetes Association[14] (see Appendix B).

Foods are divided into different groups or lists: carbohydrates, meat and meat substitutes, and fats. Each list or exchange contains sizes of servings for foods of that category; each serving size provides a similar amount of carbohydrate, protein, fat, and kcalories. The carbohydrate group is subdivided into lists of starch, fruit, milk, other carbohydrates, and vegetables. The meat and meat substitute group is sorted by fat content (Table 2-1).

The exchange lists were first developed for use by persons with diabetes. A dietitian can create both an appropriate dietary program that prescribes the number of kcalories and units of each exchange category to be consumed daily as well as a plan for when foods should be eaten. By using the exchange lists, an individual can choose favorite foods from each list while controlling the amount and kind of carbohydrates consumed throughout the day.

Guidelines for individuals with diabetes, published by the American Dietetic Association, de-emphasize prescribed calculated kcaloric diets that only use the exchange lists.[15] The focus is now on adapting dietary intake to meet individual metabolic nutrition and lifestyle requirements (see Chapter 19).

The exchange lists encourage variety and help to control kcalories and grams of carbohydrates, protein, and fats. As a tool for dietary instruction, these lists have

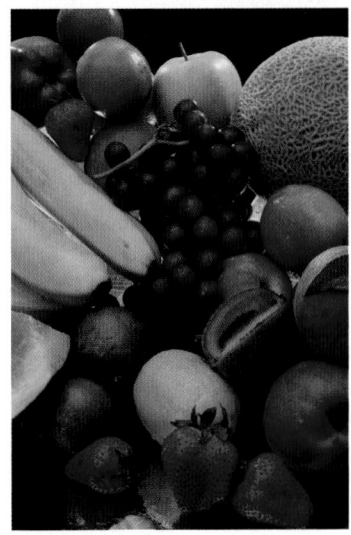

Choose fruits and vegetables each day to reduce the risk of diet-related diseases. (From PhotoDisc.)

SAMPLE MENU TO ACHIEVE "5 A DAY"

Breakfast: orange juice **(1)**, oatmeal, toast, coffee with milk

Snack: orange or apple **(2)**

Lunch: turkey sandwich with lettuce and tomato **(3)**, skim milk

Snack: popcorn and ice tea

Dinner: lemon pepper catfish, baked potato **(4)**, broccoli **(5)**, tossed green salad **(6)**, French bread with butter or margarine, skim milk

Table 2-1
Exchange Group Nutrient Value

The following table shows the amount of nutrients in one serving from each list.

Groups/Lists	Carbohydrate (g)	Protein (g)	Fat (g)	Calories
Carbohydrate Group				
Starch	15	3	0-1	80
Fruit	15	—	—	60
Milk				
Fat-free	12	8	0-3	90
Reduced-fat	12	8	5	120
Whole	12	8	8	150
Other carbohydrates	15	varies	varies	varies
Vegetables	5	2	—	25
Meat and Meat Substitute Group				
Very lean	—	7	0-1	35
Lean	—	7	3	55
Medium-fat	—	7	5	75
High-fat	—	7	8	100
Fat Group	—	—	5	45

From American Diabetes Association and American Dietetic Association: Exchange lists for meal planning, (revised), Alexandria, Va, 1995, American Dietetic Association.

been adapted to meet the needs of weight reduction programs and medical nutrition therapy planning. The Food Pyramid also uses the concept of units of servings by recommending a range of servings for each food category. A difference is that the Food Pyramid categorizes groups of foods based on the nutrients they contain whereas the exchange lists categorize groups by proportion of carbohydrate, protein, and fat.

Criteria for Future Recommendations

Although the current recommendations are expected to provide sound advice for a while, other organizations may issue their own guidelines in the future. Which guidelines should we follow? Should we change our eating habits and revise client dietary recommendations for each new study? Or, to avoid confusion, should new recommendations just be ignored?

Criteria to evaluate future dietary guidelines and recommendations follow:

- *Consider the source of the nutrition advice.* Are the recommendations from a federal government agency? If so, the work of these agencies is usually reviewed by health and nutrition professionals before release to the public. If the advice is from a private nonprofit group, is the group nationally recognized? A number of well-respected organizations are devoted to prevention and treatment of specific diseases, such as the American Heart Association, American Cancer Society, and American Diabetes Association. In addition, there are professional associations, including the American Dietetic Association and the Society for Nutrition Education, that specialize in the relationship of nutrition and health. (See Appendix C for a complete listing of organizations.)
- *Assess the comprehensiveness of the recommendations.* Do the recommendations address only one health problem? If so, is that a health problem that

Box 2-2 **Types of Research**	
Experimental Study	Consists of an experimental group receiving treatment (or dietary change) and a control group receiving no treatment (or dietary change); differences, if any, are then analyzed; may use animals or human subjects. Also called *clinical* or *laboratory study*.
Case Study	Analyzes an individual case of a disease or health difference to determine how factors may influence health; a naturalistic study because no manipulation of dietary intake or behaviors occurs.
Epidemiologic Study	Studies populations; tracks the occurrence of health or disease processes among populations; may use historical data, surveys, and/or medical records to determine possible factors influencing the health of a group of people.

affects your clients? Would following these recommendations have any negative effects? Would a category of nutrients be underconsumed? Recommendations that address several health issues are usually more complete and provide an increased level of prevention.

- *Evaluate the basis of the recommendations.* How were the recommendations determined? The current recommendations are based on many research studies on the relationships between diet and diseases. If new recommendations are issued, are they based on the results of new studies? If so, how many and what kinds of studies (Box 2-2)? Collecting this type of information means more than just listening to a 2-minute radio announcement or a 5-minute TV report. Some newspapers contain in-depth evaluations of research; others just skim the surface. It may be necessary to read the original study in the library or to discuss the recommendations.
- *Estimate the ease of application.* Can the recommendations be easily adopted? Are they presented in terms of foods (easier to apply) or nutrients (harder to apply)? Is a degree in nutrition needed to understand the recommendations?

CONSUMER FOOD DECISION-MAKING*

Community supports can have an impact on the quality of personal nutrition. Most important are the consumer decisions made daily when buying food to be prepared in the home or when eating out.

Food Selection Patterns

Food selection patterns may be estimated through assessment of government data gathered through national surveys and programs. One approach is to evaluate information based on the Healthy Eating Index. Developed by the USDA's Center for Policy and Promotion, the Healthy Eating Index measures the dietary quality of an individual's food intake based on the extent to which the intake follows the *Dietary Guidelines for Americans* and the Food Guide Pyramid. Factors considered

---

*Elaine H. Asp, PhD, contributed this section for the first and second editions of this text.

in this assessment are total fat intake, saturated fat, cholesterol, sodium, and the range of foods consumed.[16]

According to research, those with higher index scores, that is more healthful dietary intakes, have higher levels of nutrition knowledge and have achieved higher education levels. Consequently, the data reveals that higher socioeconomic characteristics are related to a greater understanding of nutrition and the effects of healthy diets in reducing the risks of diet-related disorders.[16] This difference may reflect access to resources (e.g., time and financial means) that support preparation and consumption of foods that follow the dietary guidelines.

Nonetheless, most Americans attain an average index score of 64, which is significantly below the optimum index score of 100. As a nation, we need to improve our nutrient intake. An aspect of doing so must take into account our beliefs and attitudes toward our dietary intake. A recent study using national data reveals that only 23% of the surveyed population are interested in improving their intake while 37% are not interested in doing so and 40% believe their intake does not need to change. Most view healthy eating as too complicated. In addition, the majority views snacking as an unhealthy practice, and as a result, the majority chooses snacks that are also unhealthy.[17]

Application to nursing: When working with clients, we can be aware of their attitudes toward nutrition and dietary change. Although changing dietary intake is a prime strategy to reduce the risk of diet-related chronic disorders, many Americans are not interested in changing their eating behaviors. In addition, the belief that snacking is unhealthy is unfortunate. Snacks do not have to be high fat, high sodium, or calorie-laden. Consuming additional fruits, vegetables, and whole grain foods is often best accomplished through wisely selected additional "mini-meals" or snacks. We may need to educate or remind clients about the nutritional benefits of dietary change as a disease prevention strategy, and we should definitely emphasize the positive value of snacking on wholesome foods. Providing clients with simple techniques for changing food selection habits is crucial.

Food Consumption Trends

Food consumption trends reflect the food decisions Americans have made in the past. Tracking these trends is the responsibility of the USDA. Following changes in consumption trends across the years for specific foods reveals information about food substitutions, including food prices or technologic changes that bring new types of food products to the marketplace. Food consumption trends now show that, generally, Americans eat more food in larger portions with additional snacks, which results in a greater caloric intake than in the past.[18]

Implications of Food Consumption Trends

Food consumption trends have an impact on the nutritional status of the U.S. population. Consumption of fruits and vegetables is increasing and is ideal to reduce risk factors associated with diet-related chronic diseases.[18] Generally, however, many of us need to learn how to prepare the wider variety of vegetables now available in the supermarkets so they taste and look good and are safe to eat. Teaching how to prepare foods is an adjunct goal of nutrition education. Programs such as 5 a Day that provide point-of-purchase preparation techniques and recipes should prove effective. Additionally, the popularity of TV cooking shows, such as those broadcast on the Food Network, increase our knowledge base. Some shows such as *Emeril Live*—through its use of theme programs such as "firehouse" cooking and "tailgate" parties—have become popular with some men who have not previously been interested in food preparation.

Similarly, because of increased consumption of cereals and grains,[18] we need new ways to prepare different kinds and forms of grains, such as wheat, rice, buckwheat, and corn, in the forms of pastas, couscous, and tortillas to meet the dietary recommendations of 6 to 11 servings a day. For the best nutrient value, grains and cereals should be consumed as whole grains, when possible, not refined. Breakfast cereals can be a way to become accustomed to whole grains. These products have qualities in demand by today's consumers; they are convenient, may contain fiber, are good sources of nutrients, and are low in calories.

Animal sources of protein—meat, poultry, and fish—are increasing.[18] In recent years, within the meat, poultry, and fish category, beef and egg consumption decreased while poultry and fish consumption increased. More fish is being consumed because of increased availability of fresh and frozen fish due to the development of refrigerated and frozen storage techniques.

The cooking method of meat, poultry, and fish determines the final dietary fat content. The message to reduce dietary fat and cholesterol intake has affected how we consume and prepare animal protein. Health benefits are greatest when we choose low-fat cooking methods. Some popular ethnic cuisines extend meat, poultry, or fish by combining protein sources with cereals, grains, vegetables, and sauces.

Dairy product trends reflect dietary recommendations to consume products lower in fat. The consumption of whole milk with high amounts of fat is decreasing while the consumption of low-fat and nonfat milk and other dairy products is increasing because of the wide array of new products in the marketplace. Consumption of yogurt and other fermented dairy products with live cultures continues to rise because of their health benefits.

Caloric sweetener consumption continues to increase.[18] Consumption of cane and beet sugars has decreased, but corn and noncaloric sweetener consumption has increased. These changes occurred because the technologies associated with producing corn sweeteners from cornstarch and manufacturing noncaloric sweeteners reduced their costs, allowing them to compete economically with cane and beet sugars. Sweetener and beverage consumption trends affect the nutritional status depending on whether the type of sweetener or beverage chosen increases or decreases intake of energy and other nutrients. Other issues of sweeteners are discussed in Chapter 4.

Although these trends reflect per capita consumption patterns based on the total population, it is our individual food choices that have the greatest influence on our personal level of wellness.

Effective Food Buying Styles

This chapter is full of information about consumer decisions, but how is it to be applied? How do you and your clients become better shoppers? The first step is to tailor a shopping style to one's particular situation. Consider the following to formulate the most effective approach to food shopping:

- *Food budget*: A food budget should take into account the funds needed to keep a moderate amount of food in the home and the money spent on meals away from home.
- *Consumer diversity*: Buying food for a single young adult is different from buying for a family. Lifestyles of household members affect the number and types of meals served and the kinds and amounts of food served.
- *Dietary preferences*: We all have food preferences based on ethnicity, habits, chronic illness, or ethical views such as vegetarianism. Each preference affects food-buying selections.
- *Shopping frequency*: Each household works best with a shopping plan— perhaps weekly, every 2 weeks, or on the way home from school or work when things are needed.
- *Location and types of food stores*: Different types of food stores provide a range of services and products. Conventional supermarkets, superstores, super centers, and super warehouse stores are valuable for fresh produce,

perishables, and basic grocery items; wholesale clubs and limited assortment warehouse stores are good for bulk foods at low prices; specialty stores offer unique foods at high prices; and convenience stores "save the day."

CONSUMER INFORMATION AND WELLNESS

The more information consumers have about the food they eat, the better they can choose foods that contribute to wellness. Nutrition education is necessary for consumers to use the additional information appropriately.

Food Labeling

Food labels are the best way for consumers to see how individual foods fit their nutritional needs. The function of food labels is twofold. The first function is to assist consumers to select foods with the most health-providing qualities (Box 2-3). The second is to motivate food companies to enhance the nutritional value of food products because labels reveal ingredient and nutrient content.[19]

Food labeling for processed foods in the United States is based on standards established under authority of the 1990 Nutrition Labeling and Education Act. Although nutrition labeling is mandatory for most processed products, it is voluntary for fresh meat, poultry, fish, milk, eggs, and produce. An example of the label for processed foods is shown in Figure 2-5.

The "Nutrition Facts" panel must list the quantities of energy (kcalories), fat, and the following other specific nutrients in a serving:

- Total food energy
- Food energy from fat
- Total fat
- Saturated fat
- Cholesterol
- Sodium
- Total carbohydrates
- Dietary fiber
- Sugars
- Protein
- Vitamins A and C

Box 2-3 New Labeling Definitions for Organic Foods

To continue to make food labels consumer-friendly, the National Organic Program division of the USDA has created new levels of certification for foods that contain organically grown ingredients. These regulations will help defuse consumer confusion about organic products.

A product label may display the following:

"100% ORGANIC"

All ingredients meet or exceed USDA specifications for organic foods, which bans the use of synthetic pesticides, herbicides, chemical fertilizers, antibiotics, and hormones.

"ORGANIC"

At least 95% of ingredients meet or exceed USDA specifications for organic foods.

"MADE WITH ORGANIC INGREDIENTS"

At least 70% of ingredients meet or exceed USDA specifications for organic foods.

If less than 70% of ingredients are organic, but one or more ingredients are organic, the specific organic ingredients can be identified as organic but only in the small type on the ingredient panel.

From National Organic Program, US Department of Agriculture: Labeling packaged products under the national organic standards, *August 1, 2002; www.ams.usda.gov/nop/LabelingTable073102.pdf.*

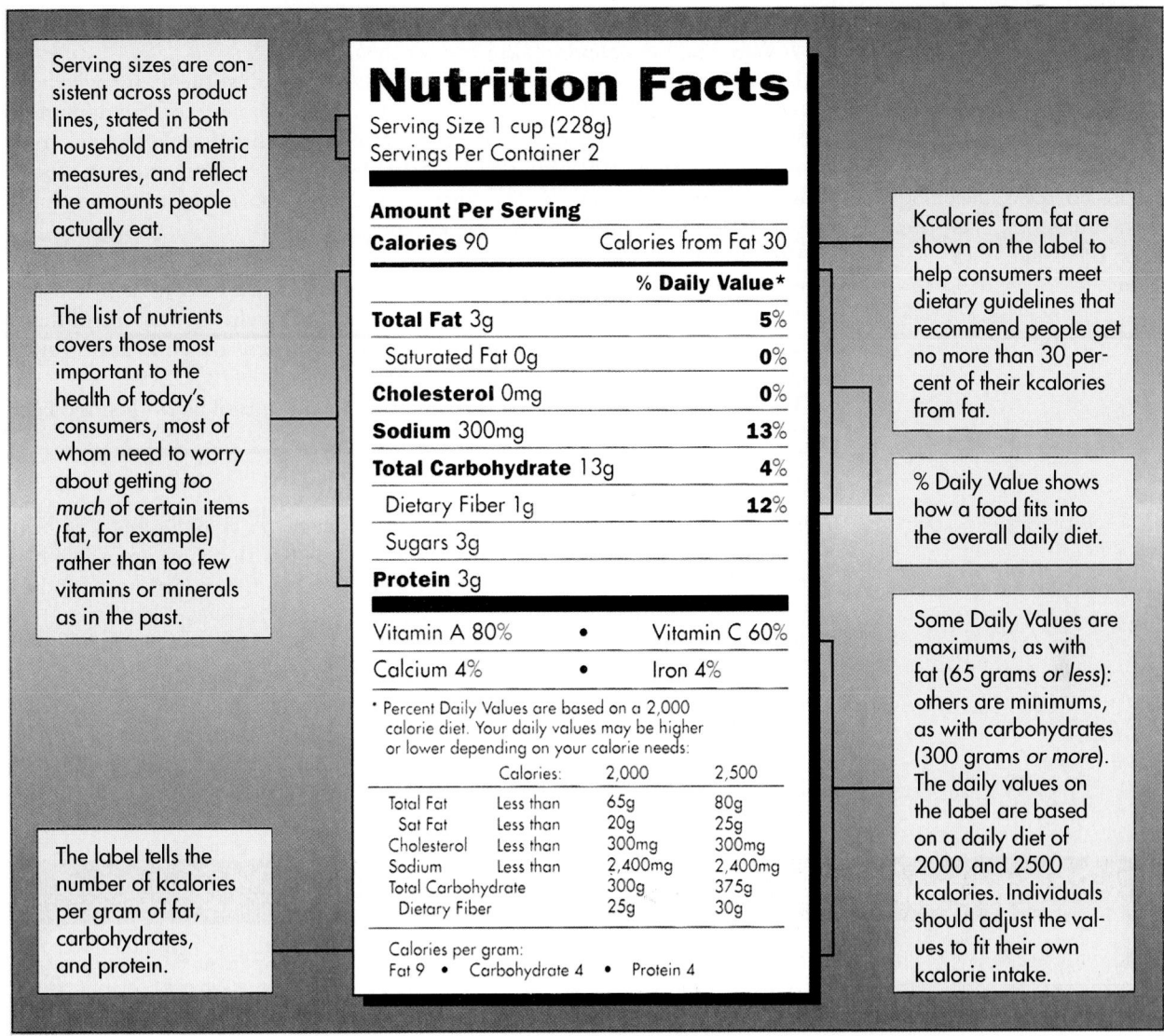

Serving sizes are consistent across product lines, stated in both household and metric measures, and reflect the amounts people actually eat.

The list of nutrients covers those most important to the health of today's consumers, most of whom need to worry about getting *too much* of certain items (fat, for example) rather than too few vitamins or minerals as in the past.

The label tells the number of kcalories per gram of fat, carbohydrates, and protein.

Kcalories from fat are shown on the label to help consumers meet dietary guidelines that recommend people get no more than 30 percent of their kcalories from fat.

% Daily Value shows how a food fits into the overall daily diet.

Some Daily Values are maximums, as with fat (65 grams *or less*): others are minimums, as with carbohydrates (300 grams *or more*). The daily values on the label are based on a daily diet of 2000 and 2500 kcalories. Individuals should adjust the values to fit their own kcalorie intake.

Nutrition Facts

Serving Size 1 cup (228g)
Servings Per Container 2

Amount Per Serving

Calories 90   Calories from Fat 30

% **Daily Value***

Total Fat 3g	5%
Saturated Fat 0g	0%
Cholesterol 0mg	0%
Sodium 300mg	13%
Total Carbohydrate 13g	4%
Dietary Fiber 1g	12%
Sugars 3g	
Protein 3g	

Vitamin A 80%	•	Vitamin C 60%
Calcium 4%	•	Iron 4%

* Percent Daily Values are based on a 2,000 calorie diet. Your daily values may be higher or lower depending on your calorie needs:

		Calories:	2,000	2,500
Total Fat	Less than		65g	80g
Sat Fat	Less than		20g	25g
Cholesterol	Less than		300mg	300mg
Sodium	Less than		2,400mg	2,400mg
Total Carbohydrate			300g	375g
Dietary Fiber			25g	30g

Calories per gram:
Fat 9 • Carbohydrate 4 • Protein 4

Figure 2-5 An example of the food label format that currently is mandatory in the United States. (From Food and Drug Administration, Washington, DC.)

- Calcium
- Iron

The percent of Daily Values (DVs) information, based on a 2000-kcalorie diet, is intended to show consumers how much of a day's ideal intake of a particular nutrient they are eating. DVs for selected nutrients and food components based on a 2500-calorie diet are also given at the bottom of the label. DVs are based on either of two sets of reference values: Reference Daily Intakes or Daily Reference Values, depending on the nutrient or food component. These reference values are used primarily by food and nutrition professionals, whereas consumers use the DVs.

Reference Daily Intakes set standards for protein, vitamin, and mineral intake based on the current U.S. Recommended Daily Allowances (U.S. RDAs). The U.S. RDAs were created specifically for nutrition labeling and are set on the highest RDAs determined by the 1968 set of values of any nutrient (except for calcium and phosphorus, which were set at 1 g each) for any sex and age category, except for pregnancy and lactation. Reference Daily Intakes are the basis for the standards of the federal programs that provide nutritional support. The four sets of Reference Daily Intakes values categorized by age and physiologic state are as follows: adults

Daily Values (DVs)
a system for food labeling composed of two sets of reference values: Reference Daily Intakes and Daily Reference Values

Reference Daily Intakes
a set of daily nutrient values for protein, vitamins, and minerals based on allowances of the 1968 RDAs

Daily Reference Values
a set of daily nutrient and food constituent values for which there are no RDAs, including carbohydrates, fat, fiber, cholesterol, potassium, and sodium

and children 4 years of age and older; children 1 to 4 years old; infants 1 year old or younger; and pregnant or lactating women.

Daily Reference Values are for nutrients and food constituents for which there are no RDAs, including carbohydrates, fat, fiber, cholesterol, potassium, and sodium. Daily Reference Values have been developed because these food components are important to health, as recognized by current recommendations for minimum or maximum intakes. The fiber recommendation is a minimum value and the cholesterol recommendation is a maximum value.

Uniform definitions for food descriptors, such as light, low fat, and others for nutrient content claims, are now clearly defined and must be consistently used for all foods (Box 2-4). This information helps consumers who try to control their intakes of specific nutrients and food components. Similarly, the content of fruit beverages as juices is also defined by government regulations (Box 2-5).

To help clients evaluate food labels, see the Teaching Tool box, "Just the Facts."

Health Claims

Health claims relating a nutrient or food component to risk of a disease or health-related condition now appear on food labels. Only health claims approved by the FDA may be on the label. This information helps consumers select those foods that can keep them healthy and well.

So far, the health claims allowed include a relationship between the following:[19,20]

- a diet with enough calcium and a lower risk of osteoporosis
- a diet low in total fat and a reduced risk of some cancers
- a diet low in saturated fat and cholesterol and a reduced risk of coronary heart disease

---

Box 2-4 Food Descriptors

FREE

Contains only a tiny or insignificant amount of fat, cholesterol, sodium, sugar, and/or calories. For example, a "fat-free" product will contain less than 0.5 grams of fat per serving.

LOW

"Low" in fat, saturated fat, cholesterol, sodium, and/or calories; can be eaten fairly often without exceeding dietary guidelines. So "low in fat" means no more than 3 grams of fat per serving.

LEAN

Contains less than 10 grams of fat, 4 grams of saturated fat, and 95 mg of cholesterol per serving. "Lean" is not as lean as "low." "Lean" and "extra lean" are USDA terms for use on meat and poultry products.

EXTRA LEAN

Contains less than 5 grams of fat, 2 grams of saturated fat, and 95 mg of cholesterol per serving. Although "extra leaner" is leaner than "lean," it is still not as lean as "low."

REDUCED, LESS, FEWER

Contains 25% less of a nutrient or calories. For example, hot dogs might be labeled "25% less fat than our regular hot dogs."

LIGHT/LITE

Contains one third fewer calories or one half the fat of the original. "Light in sodium" means a product with one half the usual sodium.

MORE

Contains at least 10% more of the daily value of a vitamin, mineral, or fiber than the usual single serving.

GOOD SOURCE OF . . .

Contains 10% to 19% of the daily value for a particular vitamin, mineral, or fiber in a single serving.

From Food and Drug Administration, Center for Food Safety and Applied Nutrition: A food labeling guide: Appendix A, *September 1994 (revised 1999); www.cfsan.fda.gov/ ~ dms/flg-69.htm.*

TEACHING TOOL
Just the Facts—Using Labels to Teach Nutrition Literacy

Healthcare providers view nutrition as a basic component of health education and refer patients to nutritionists for nutrition education. Nurses are in the position to reinforce nutrition concepts first presented by nutritionists. Although physicians may be viewed as the experts on health, patients who have low literacy skills tend to use their social network of family and friends for health and nutrition information. Consequently, for interventions to be successful, members of social networks should be included. The approach should be visual, interactive, and culturally appropriate. This lesson on label comprehension fits these three criteria.

Clients should be presented with three boxes of cereal or Nutrition Facts labels from three cereal products. Choose products that are different. For example, include a heavily presweetened cereal, a lightly sweetened cereal, and one with no added sweeteners. Ask the following questions:

- *Which has the most kcalories per serving?* This may be affected by weight, volume of the cereal (popped with air), and the density of added ingredients like raisins.
- *Which has the largest serving size?* Servings sizes are the same by weight for all products in a food category.
- *Which contains the most dietary fat?* Fat is not an issue with cereals, except for granola.
- *Which contains the most sodium?* Some cereals contain about 300 mg, which is high for sodium-sensitive clients.
- *Which contains the most added sugars?* Added sugars can range from none to 13 grams per serving.
- *How many calories come from sugars?* Multiply the number of grams of sugars by 4 kcalories. By dividing this number by the total kcalories per serving and multiplying the decimal by 100, you can determine the percentage of sugar content.
- *Which contains the most fiber?* Fiber content can range from none to about 5 grams per serving.

As your study of nutrition continues, you may add other questions and be able to relate client responses to preventive heath issues of diet-related diseases or to address specific dietary needs of a patient's medical nutrition therapy.

Information on literacy from Macario E et al.: Factors influencing nutrition education for patients with low literacy skills, J Am Dietetic Assoc 98:559, 1998; Teaching Tool (use of cereal boxes) created by Michele Grodner; Photograph by Joanne Scott/Tracy McCalla.

- a diet rich in fiber-containing grain products, fruits, and vegetables and a reduced risk of some cancers
- a diet rich in fiber-containing grain products, fruits, and vegetables, and a reduced risk of coronary heart disease
- a diet low in sodium and a reduced risk of high blood pressure
- a diet rich in fruits and vegetables and a reduced risk of some cancers (Box 2-5)
- folic acid and a decreased risk of neural tube defect-affected pregnancy
- dietary sugar alcohols and a reduced risk of dental caries
- soluble fiber from certain foods, such as whole oats and psyllium seed husk, as part of a diet low in saturated fat and cholesterol and a reduced risk of heart disease

Food labeling legislation also covers dietary supplements. The Dietary Supplement Health and Education Act of 1994 (DSHEA) requires the FDA to prove that a dietary supplement is unsafe or adulterated or has false or misleading labeling. The act does not allow claims about diagnosis, treatment, or prevention of disease but does allow claims of certain benefits that must be truthful. A standard statement is required on the label by the FDA[21] (see Chapter 16).

Interested in getting the latest information and updates related to nutrition, food labeling, and dietary supplements and other announcements from the FDA? Log on at www.cfsan.fda.gov/~dms/infonet.html to subscribe to the free FDA-DSFL (Dietary Supplement/Food Labeling) electronic newsletter.

Box 2-5 Not All Juices Are Created Equal

If you don't want to concentrate all your strength on choosing a juice, the information below will help make the choice easier:

100% PURE OR 100% JUICE

Guarantees only 100% fruit juice, complete with all its nutrients. If this label is missing, it's not all juice.

"COCKTAIL," "PUNCH," "DRINK," "BEVERAGE"

Terms used to signify diluted juice cotaining less than 100% juice, often with added sweeteners.

FRESH SQUEEZED JUICE

Squeezed from fresh fruit. It is not pasteurized and is usually located in the produce or dairy section of the grocery store.

FROM CONCENTRATE

Water is removed from whole juice to make concentrate; then water is added back to reconstitute to 100% juice or to diluted juice (e.g., lemonade).

NOT FROM CONCENTRATE

Juice that has never been concentrated.

FRESH FROZEN

Freshly squeezed, packaged, and frozen without pasteurization or further processing. It is usually sold in plastic bottles in the frozen food section of the grocery store and is ready to drink after thawing.

JUICE ON UNREFRIGERATED SHELVES

Shelf-stable product usually found with canned and bottled juices on unrefrigerated shelves of the store. It is pasteurized juice, or diluted juice, often from concentrate, packaged in sterilized containers.

CANNED JUICE

Heated and sealed in cans to provide extended shelf life of more than 1 year.

From Lewis C: Not all juices are created equal, Publication No. (FDA) 99-2324, FDA Consumer, September-October 1998 (revised May 1999); vm.cfsan.fda.gov/ ~ dms/fdjuice.html.

FOOD SAFETY

Food safety is influenced by community decisions and personal behaviors. We expect the larger community, such as government agencies, to supervise the production and preparation of food products to ensure the safety of the foods we purchase. But once we as consumers purchase food products, we are responsible for the proper handling of foods to prevent foodborne illness.

These concerns apply equally in the nursing setting. Our clients are also consumers. Our recommendations regarding nutritional intake are "translated" by our clients when they become consumers. As we advise about nutrition concerns, public and personal food safety is an issue.

The knowledge, attitudes, perceptions, and concerns that consumers have about food safety affect the food decisions they make. There is enormous concern from consumers and the food industry that the U.S. food supply be safe. To have a safe food supply, it is essential that each sector of the food chain (producers, manufacturers, wholesalers, food stores, food service outlets, and consumers) follow correct food-handling procedures. Such procedures, called Hazard Analysis Critical Control Points (HACCP) programs, have been or are being developed for the various segments of the food system to improve food quality.

Consumers are periodically surveyed regarding their confidence in the safety of the food supply and in their ability to select safe food products. In 2000 results showed that consumers were satisfied with food labels and the food safety consumer alerts that the FDA provides. Consumers are not aware, however, of the advocacy role of the FDA regarding food safety initiatives.[22] Regardless of government actions and manufacturing procedures concerning safe food preparation, responsibility ultimately is on the individual consumer who prepares food at home.

Risk Analysis and Food Safety

Setting risk standards involves determining a balance between risk and benefit for those who produce and consume foods. Risks to human health and to the environment are balanced against the economic benefits sustained by the use of insecticides, fungicides, and rodenticides. However, like the other approaches used to set risk standards, risk-benefit estimates for foods are limited by the unavailability of reliable quantitative data to use in the analysis.

Biotechnology: Consumer Risk or Benefit?

No, biotechnology does not mean that the androids are coming. Instead, the most recent form of food biotechnology is the controlled modification of the genetic structure of foods at the molecular level to improve nutrient content, increase crop or animal yield, inhibit spoilage, and otherwise enhance desirable characteristics of food products.

Traditional biotechnologic efforts resulted in random mutations from cross-breeding of plants or animals. These changes seem to have shown little risk to consumers or the environment. However, the new molecular biotechnology raises concerns by some consumers and scientists although risks are decreased compared with traditional biotechnology.

A recent example of biotechnology involves the transfer of a bacterium gene to corn and cotton plants that allows the plants to create pesticides as part of their natural growth cycle. The created pesticides are harmful only to insects that prey on those plants and are harmless to humans and other insects and animals. Consequently, fewer pesticides can be used while maintaining or increasing crops.[23]

Currently, genetically engineered crops are commonly used for feeds for animals. More than half of soybean and a quarter of corn crops are genetically altered forms. This means that the poultry and meats we consume most likely were raised on these crops.

To ensure safety, food that has been transformed with genes should be tested to determine whether toxic substances have been unwittingly produced or whether the food produces a protein that may elicit an allergic reaction in susceptive individuals. Routine testing determines whether the modified product now contains an allergen not previously detected. The FDA or Environmental Protection Agency (EPA) should regulate this testing.[23]

Additional questions need to be considered as other food products are genetically modified. Will such changes increase supply and availability, thereby lowering the price of nutritious foods? An example is the increased milk yield from cows treated with bovine somatotropin (BST). Another change is the use in cheese making of pure chymosin enzyme from molecular biotechnology rather than the more expensive rennet from calves' stomachs. The FDA has approved both of these products of biotechnology.[24]

How would lower prices affect the farmers who grow the crops or whose cows produce the milk? If these genetic manipulations keep prices high by producing "status" perfect quality produce, who gains? Or are these scientific developments simply a continuation of the food biotechnology time line started when milk was first pasteurized to destroy bacteria? There are no clear answers at this time.

Food Safety and Manufactured Products

Once produce is grown and ready to be eaten or processed into multi-ingredient products, other issues of food safety arise. Food safety approaches consider *risk* as keeping substances out of the food supply and *benefits* as enhancing the shelf life and maintaining the nutrition quality of food products. This was the basis of the original Delaney Clause that addresses food additives and other detailed government regulations. In 1996 the Food Quality Protection Act was passed, which replaced the zero tolerance for cancer-causing agents in foods of the *Delaney Clause* by reforming federal standards for pesticide residues in foods with a standard of "reasonable certainty of no harm."

Additives considered safe and already in use when the food safety acts first went into effect are on a Generally Recognized As Safe (GRAS) list; new additives are added as their safety is established. However, in the years since the establishment of the original GRAS list, methods of analysis have become more sensitive and can detect lower and lower levels of these substances, thus calling into question the safety of additives on the original list. As a result, a comprehensive review of the list and all chemicals added to food is conducted periodically by the Federation of American Societies for Experimental Biology (FASEB).

intentional (direct) food additives
substances purposely added during manufacturing to food products

incidental (indirect) food additives
substances that inadvertently contaminate processed foods

Additives used for their functional properties in foods during processing, that is, to improve food quality in some way, are called intentional (direct) food additives, and those that inadvertently become a part of a food at some time as it passes through the food system are called incidental or (indirect) food additives. Direct additives are used to improve, maintain, and stabilize food quality; to increase availability across the country and lengthen storage time; to increase convenience; to decrease waste; and to stabilize or increase nutrient content. Table 2-2 lists selected intentional GRAS food additives. Indirect additives include pesticide and herbicide residues, animal drugs, processing aids, and packaging constituents that migrate from the package into the food. Regardless of their source, indirect additives seem to be of greatest concern to consumers.

Foodborne Illness

From the practical standpoint of keeping people well, consumers and professionals must acknowledge the importance of microbiologic contaminants; both groups need to work together to help prevent foodborne illness. In addition to the discomfort, these illnesses cause greater economic costs in terms of lost time at work and productivity than most people can imagine. Unfortunately, the incidence of foodborne illness in the United States is increasing, according to the federal Centers for Disease Control and Prevention (CDC), which keeps statistical data on these illnesses. Because many cases of foodborne illness are not reported, federal agencies must rely on estimates to define the size of the problem. The FDA estimates an annual incidence of 25 to 81 million cases of foodborne illness. Foodborne illness is estimated to cost almost $10 billion annually.

Food can become contaminated with bacteria, molds, parasites, and viruses during production, processing, transporting, storage, and retailing. It can become contaminated in the home. Although the entire food distribution system may contribute to foodborne illness, improper handling of food in the home is a commonly overlooked source of contamination and growth of illness-causing microorganisms. The severity of foodborne illness varies with the microorganism, the susceptibility of the person, and the amount of bacteria or enterotoxin ingested. Information about sources, symptoms, and special control recommendations for common bacterial infections and intoxications are identified in Box 2-6.

As the palates of Americans become more accustomed to exotic sensations, the Japanese meal of sushi—raw fish with vinegared rice—is ordered more often in the growing number of Japanese restaurants. However, the fish must be served fresh and free of parasites; Anisakidae nematode parasites can be a problem when eating raw fish. Sushi is not a dish to prepare at home. It is safest when prepared by specially trained chefs. Licensing of sushi chefs is not mandatory in the United States; therefore sushi chefs are not required to meet the strict standards of licensed chefs. As a precaution, persons with reduced immune system disorders or liver disorder, and other at-risk persons, should consider avoiding raw and undercooked fish and animal foods such as sushi and sashimi (raw fish

Table 2-2
Intentional Food Additives

Type of Additive	Purpose
Processing Aids	
Anticaking agents	Prevent particles from collecting together in clumps (e.g., keep salt free flowing)
Conditioners	Make dough less sticky and easy to handle
Dough strengtheners	Help dough to withstand mechanical action of automatic processing
Drying agents	Absorb moisture to keep packaged products from becoming soggy or lumpy
Emulsifiers	Prevent oil separation in salad dressings
Enzymes	Speed up reactions that otherwise would be very slow
Firming agents	Stabilize and prevent flow of a dough
Flour treatments	Modify response of flour to mixing, as in making a dough
Leavening agents	Make baked products rise and become light (e.g., yeast baking powder, soda)
Lubricants	Ingredients such as fat in a dough that help keep it pliable and moldable
Propellants	Gases used to make sprays from fluids (e.g., oil spray for coating pans)
Solvents	Fluids in which particles of another compound dissolve (e.g., water is solvent for sugar)
Stabilizers	Used to keep fat globules small in ice cream or air bubbles small in whipped cream
Texturizers	Contribute to texture in some way (e.g., crunchy)
Thickening agents	Increase thickness (viscosity) of liquids
Preservatives	
Acidulants	Acids that prevent growth of microorganisms in food
Antimicrobials	Control growth of microorganisms in food
Antioxidants	Help prevent or slow down development of off-flavors and odors of fat-containing foods
Curing and pickling agents	Control microbial growth in meat, pickles, and sauerkraut
Fumigants	Chemical control of pests and/or deterioration; usually leave residues in the food
Oxidizing and reducing agents	Influence interactions in food systems that cause deterioration
Appearance and Flavor Enhancers	
Clarifying agents	Combine with and precipitate or disperse compounds that prevent liquids from being clear
Color	Natural or synthetic compounds added to improve the color of food
Flavor enhancers	Improve flavor by strengthening flavors in a product
Flavoring agents	Added to foods to improve flavor or for special effects
Nonnutritive sweeteners	Noncaloric compounds usually with high intensity of sweetness
Nutritive sweeteners	Sweeteners that supply calories

only).[25] Regardless, these foods should not be an everyday treat but can be enjoyed safely in moderation.

What could be more wholesome and healthful than fresh cider straight from the cider mill? Unfortunately, a number of people who sipped cider at an apple farm in Massachusetts learned otherwise when they fell victim to a pathogenic type of *Escherichia coli (E. coli)* bacteria and experienced gastrointestinal distress. It seems that apples used for cider are often those that have fallen to the ground and have

Box 2-6 Foodborne Illness: Ten Least-Wanted Foodborne Pathogens*

The U.S. Public Health Service has identified the following microorganisms as the biggest culprits of foodborne illness, either because of the severity of the sickness or the number of cases of illness they cause. Beware of these pathogens: *Fight BAC!*

CAMPYLOBACTER

This is the most common cause of diarrhea in the United States. **Sources:** Raw and undercooked meat and poultry, raw milk, untreated water.

CLOSTRIDIUM BOTULINUM

This organism produces a toxin that causes botulism, a life threatening illness that can prevent the breathing muscles from moving air in and out of the lungs. **Sources:** Home-prepared foods, herbal oils; honey should not be fed to children less than 12 months old.

E. COLI O157:H7

This bacterium can produce a deadly toxin and causes approximately 73,000 cases of foodborne illness each year in the United States. **Sources:** Meat, especially undercooked or raw hamburger; produce; raw milk.

LISTERIA MONOCYTOGENES

This causes listeriosis, a serious disease for pregnant women, newborns, and adults with weakened immune systems. **Sources:** Soil, water. It has been found in dairy products including soft cheeses and in raw and undercooked meat, poultry, seafood, and produce.

NOROVIRUS

This virus is the leading cause of diarrhea in the United States. Any food can be contaminated with norovirus if handled by someone who is infected with this virus.

SALMONELLA

This is the most common cause of foodborne deaths and is responsible for millions of cases of foodborne illness a year. **Sources:** Raw and undercooked eggs, undercooked poultry and meat, dairy products, seafood, fruits, vegetables.

STAPHYLOCOCCUS AUREUS

This bacterium produces a toxin that causes vomiting shortly after ingesting. **Sources:** Cooked foods high in protein, such as cooked ham, salads, bakery products, dairy products.

SHIGELLA

This causes an estimated 300,000 cases per year of diarrhea illnesses. Poor hygiene causes *Shigella* to be easily passed from person to person. **Sources:** Salads, milk and dairy products, unclean water.

TOXOPLASMA GONDII

This parasite causes toxoplasmosis, a severe disease that can produce central nervous system disorders, particularly mental retardation and visual impairment in children. Pregnant women and people with weakened immune systems are at higher risk. **Sources:** Meat, primarily pork.

VIBRIO VULNIFICUS

This causes gastroenteritis or a syndrome called *primary septicemia*. People with liver diseases are especially at high risk. **Sources:** Raw or undercooked seafood.

From Partnership for Food Safety Education; www.fightbac.org/10least.cfm.
*For more information on these and other foodborne pathogens, check out the "Bad Bug Book" at http://vm.cfsan.fda.gov/~mow/intro.html.

As of November 1998, all packaged juices that have not been pasteurized or treated to prevent the growth of illness-causing microbes must have warning labels stating the following:

WARNING: This product has not been pasteurized and, therefore, may contain harmful bacteria that can cause serious illness in children, the elderly, and persons with weakened immune systems.

blemishes. The problem is those apples may come in contact with animal feces and manure fertilizer; unless the apples are washed well or the cider is pasteurized or preserved with sodium benzoate, this contamination can lead to illness.[26,27] Unpasteurized apple juice has, on occasion, still been problematic as noted by the case of a 3-year-old who was hospitalized for almost a month as a result of consuming unpasteurized apple juice contaminated with *E. coli* 0157:H7, which has caused death and illness in those who have consumed undercooked hamburger.[28]

Some types of *E. coli* are normally found in the human intestinal system; they are responsible for producing vitamins B_{12} and K and for limiting the growth of other undesirable bacteria. But we have few defenses against the pathogenic *E. coli* 0157:H7. This form of *E. coli* was found in a batch of meat distributed to restaurants in the northwest United States in 1993. When the cooks at a fast-food restaurant chain undercooked hamburgers containing this *E. coli* organism, 4 children died and about 500 people became ill. The bacteria attacked the intestinal walls, which allowed the effects to then spread to other parts of the body, particularly the kidneys. Cooking the meat to a "well-done" stage with no trace of redness would have destroyed the *E. coli* bacteria.[29] As a result of this outbreak, the USDA now recommends that ground beef and venison be cooked to a minimum internal temperature of 160° F (71° C) and poultry to 180° F (82° C) in restaurants and in the home.[29] *E. coli* 0157:H7 is also thought to have been responsible for illnesses from raw milk, dry cured salami, lettuce, produce from manure-fertilized gardens, potatoes, radish sprouts, alfalfa sprouts, yogurt, sandwiches, and water.[27] The CDC estimates that at least 20,000 cases of *E.coli*-related foodborne illnesses occur each year.[28]

Preparing food for parties also requires adherence to food safety principles. Appropriate temperatures must be maintained to keep hot foods hot and cold foods cold. But other factors may also cause illness. In a 1996 party in upstate New York, 30 people became ill with diarrhea after consuming food that was inadvertently contaminated by water infected with *Plesiomonas shigelloides* and *Salmonella* serotype Hartford. The catered food was prepared with well water that was incidentally contaminated with pathogens from runoff surface water from nearby farmlands and for which inadequate water-treatment was implemented.[30] Untreated drinking water is often the cause of *P. shigelloides* infections, as is eating uncooked shellfish or travel to developing countries. *Salmonella* serotype Hartford is tied to fecal contamination, such as from animals. Symptoms for both bacteria are similar, occur within 12 to 48 hours of exposure, and include bloody or mucuos diarrhea, cramps, vomiting, or fever.

Food Preparation Strategies

Although government inspection programs should guard against foodborne illnesses, we must adhere to safe food handling procedures in the home and follow food safety guidelines when we eat away from home as an aspect of personal responsibility for our nutrition. Here are some recommendations from Fight Bac!, a public-private coalition of The Partnership for Food Safety Education that informs the public about food safety strategies[31] (Figure 2-6):

- To ensure sanitary food handling in the home, make sure food preparer's hands are clean, clean equipment is used, and a clean surrounding is maintained, including cutting boards and countertops.

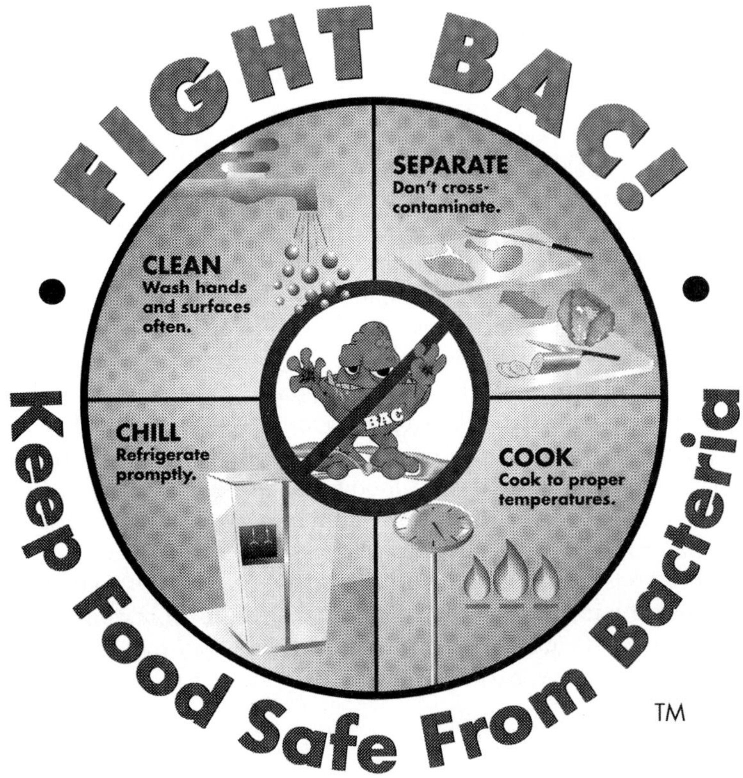

FOODBORNE ILLNESS HOTLINES

Center for Food Safety and Applied Nutrition Outreach and Information Center: (888) SAFE FOOD

FDA Foodborne Illness Reporting Emergency Line: (301) 443-1240

FDA Medical Products Reporting Medwatch Line: (800) FDA-1088 (This group monitors adverse reactions to medical products [medicines, special nutritional products such as dietary supplements, infant formula, medical foods].)

USDA Meat and Poultry Food Safety Hotline: (800) 535-4555

Figure 2-6 Fight Bac! This logo represents the public-private coalition of The Partnership for Food Safety Education to inform the public about food safety strategies. (From Partnership for Food Safety Education, Washington, DC.)

- Wash hands with soap and hot water before preparing and cooking foods.
- Wash cutting boards, utensils, and countertops that come in contact with uncooked meats, poultry, or fish with hot soapy water and a disinfectant.
- Do not place cooked foods on unwashed surfaces where uncooked foods have been prepared because the cooked foods will become contaminated with the microorganisms on these surfaces. Cooking destroys bacteria, but bacteria from uncooked foods on unwashed surfaces can reinfect any cooked food placed on them.
- Keep foods either colder than 40° F (4° C) or hotter than 140° F (60° C). The "danger zone" for rapid growth of microorganisms is a temperature inside this range. Foods can easily fall into this zone at a picnic or a potluck meal.
- Refrigerate cooked foods *immediately* after meals or after they are cooked. DO NOT cool to room temperature and then refrigerate.
- Boil all home-canned vegetables, meats, poultry, and fish for 10 minutes before tasting.
- Discard or boil marinades used with uncooked meats, poultry, and fish after marination is completed; bacteria are not destroyed until heated.
- Cook all meat (160° F), poultry (180° F), shellfish, and fish to the well-done stage.
- Do not eat or taste any uncooked foods containing raw eggs, including cookie and cake batters. They could contain *Salmonella*.
- NEVER use a recipe that calls for raw eggs and is not cooked or baked after addition of the eggs. When making homemade ice cream, cook the eggs by making soft custard; do not use raw eggs in the mixture to be frozen.
- Microwave cooking can be tricky and dangerous. NEVER store defrosted and/or partially cooked meats and poultry. Cook them completely to the well-done stage first, and then eat or refrigerate.
- When food shopping, choose perishable foods (those from the refrigerator or freezer cases) last and get them home as soon as possible. Don't leave them sitting in the car while doing other errands.
- Never buy or use foods in a bulging can, cracked jar, or bulging lid. Damage to containers may have allowed botulism to develop. Don't taste to determine if spoiled; this toxin is extremely dangerous.

Additional common food safety mistakes include the following:

- Thawing on countertop
- Cooling leftovers on the counter
- Marinating at room temperature
- Delaying refrigeration of restaurant "doggie bags"
- Tasting stirring spoon
- Consuming hide-and-seek Easter eggs[32]
- Buying foods with expired use dates

We tend to be casual about food preparation. After all, we eat all the time. However, sometimes being too relaxed allows for these bacterial and viral contaminations to occur. In our homes, we must implement basic food safety procedures when preparing and storing foods; in food retail markets and food service facilities, we count on the expertise and supervision of public health officers to enforce regulations that provide for safe food availability.

As nurses we must recognize our role in providing safe foods to patients. When handling foods for patients, care must be taken to prevent contamination by using the techniques of food handlers, such as hand washing before serving meals or assisting patients with their meals.

Food Preservation to Control Foodborne Illness

Through the years, many methods have been developed and used to preserve food for future use by controlling decomposition and microbial growth that could lead to foodborne illness. Besides drying and dehydrating, which limit moisture in the food, methods developed include canning, refrigerating and freezing, pasteurizing, curing and smoking, modified atmosphere packaging, aseptic packaging, and irradiating foods. In canning, heat is used to destroy microorganisms; in pickling, salt, acid (vinegar), and usually heat control microbial growth; and in jellies and jams, sugar is the preservative. Refrigerating and freezing limit the growth of microorganisms by the use of cold temperatures. Pasteurizing uses heat to destroy pathogenic organisms in milk and other undesirable ones in other foods. The use of various salts and smoke cure and preserve meat, poultry, and fish. Modified atmosphere packaging provides an atmosphere of various gases within the package that helps control microbial growth to preserve the food. Aseptic packaging preserves food and prevents contamination by placing food products that are sterilized separately from the packaging into sterilized containers, which are immediately sealed.

Irradiation is a food preservation technology beginning to be used not only to control the microorganisms causing foodborne illness but also to increase international and domestic food trade. By decreasing economic losses caused by food spoilage, insects, sprouting, parasites, microorganisms associated with foodborne disease, and changes associated with ripening, irradiated products can be shipped farther and still remain safe to eat.[33] Irradiation involves exposure of food to gamma irradiation using cobalt-60 or cesium-137 or to an electron beam from electron accelerators.[17,27] The machine sources may be the least controversial of the sources of radiation because they are independent of nuclear energy, so there is no radioactive waste. Extensive testing has shown that irradiated foods are wholesome, do not become radioactive, and provide consumers with a reduced risk of foods contaminated with microorganisms that cause foodborne illness.[34,35]

Worldwide, at least one food is now approved for irradiation in 40 countries.[35] In the United States irradiated foods were first produced commercially in 1992,[34] although food irradiation has been researched, evaluated, and tested for more than 50 years.[35] The foods most often irradiated are spices and dried vegetable seasonings. With the banning or potential banning of fumigants now used for these foods and for fresh fruits and vegetables, dried fruits, tree nuts, and cocoa beans, it is anticipated that irradiation will increase. The use of irradiation for poultry products is a specific example of efforts to control *salmonellosis* and *campylobacteriosis*.[33]

Irradiated whole foods (as opposed to foods containing irradiated ingredients) in the United States must be labeled as "Treated with Radiation" or "Treated by Irradiation" and must display the international symbol for irradiated foods, radura[34,35] (Figure 2-7).

As health professionals, we can assist other food and nutrition professionals to educate our clients as consumers about the value of this technology as safeguarding our food supply in the marketplace and in our homes.

TOWARD A POSITIVE NUTRITION LIFESTYLE: LOCUS OF CONTROL

Do things just happen to you? Does it seem as if school, family, or society affect what you do without your input? Or do you feel that you have control over what takes place? Do you have a life plan (or weekly plan) that you follow? Locus of control is the perception of one's ability to control life events and experiences. Having an internal locus of control means feeling as if you can influence the forces with which you come into contact. You have an inner sense of your ability to guide life events. An external locus of control is defined as the perception of not being able to control what happens to you and that outside forces have power over what you experience.

Let's apply these concepts to your style of making food choices when shopping. In particular, consider the nutritional implications of locus of control. If you have an internal locus of control, you may develop a basic plan of the types of nutritious

irradiation
a procedure by which food is exposed to radiation that destroys microorganisms, insect growth, and parasites that could spoil food or cause illness

Figure 2-7 The "radura" symbol must be carried by all foods that have been treated with radiation, although it need not be carried by processed foods that include irradiated ingredients.

locus of control
the perception of one's ability to control life events and experiences

foods to be purchased during a shopping trip. You may make a few unplanned purchases, but they would be limited in number. You feel in control of your choices. Having an external locus of control means that you might start out with a shopping list, but you are probably easily swayed by in-store promotions, coupons, and even colorful packaging to select products not on your list. You often buy more than needed because so much "looked good."

Awareness of our type of locus of control allows us to develop strategies to improve our food decisions. Individuals with an internal locus of control tend to develop their own approaches for changing food-related behaviors; those with an external locus of control may need a structured program or group support to provide guidance to modify their food behaviors.

SUMMARY

This chapter considers factors of personal and community nutrition. Food preferences, food choices, and food liking greatly influence the foods we choose and so affect our overall nutritional status. As knowledge of the relationship between diet and disease increases, public health approaches to diet-related disease prevention have been formulated to encourage us to select foods not just for their nutrient and energy content but for their primary disease prevention value as well. Food guides have been created to implement the dietary recommendations on a daily basis. These guides address the concerns of nutrient adequacy and primary disease prevention. The Food Guide Pyramid and 5 a Day program are easy to follow to improve our nutritional intake. Food consumption trends in the United States are an indication of changes in the American diet. These trends for fruits and vegetables; cereals and grains; meat, poultry, and fish; dairy products; and sweeteners reflect the availability and food choices of per capita consumption. This information helps us translate nutrients into food categories and attend to consumer needs and issues when advising clients or patients.

Providing health professionals and consumers with more information about foods through food labels increases the probability that decisions made and advice given about which foods to eat will be based on nutrition as well as on taste, thus contributing to health and wellness. Food safety is of concern because of its potential to eliminate or at least substantially decrease foodborne illness as more is learned about the various causes of this illness. Knowledge of how bacteria, molds, parasites, and viruses can be problems in the food supply helps us understand how to control these problems to stay well.

THE NURSING APPROACH
Dietary Teaching: The Nursing Process

One of the main nursing roles in health education includes teaching individuals and groups. Clients have a variety of learning needs. The goal of learning is to change behavior. The learning session needs to be related to the assessment and to the identified goals.

Factors that contribute to learning include the person's ability to comprehend English, literacy, motivation, readiness, involvement, relevance of the topic, and environment. Obviously, if the person does not speak or understand English, it is important to obtain an interpreter.

Some learning principles include (1) developing appropriate teaching materials that are age specific (e.g., children, older adults), (2) providing information that clients can relate to and covering what is known before proceeding to what is unknown, (3) pacing the learning session, (4) providing teaching aids and materials (e.g., visual handouts), (5) using layperson's terms, and (6) providing feedback and praise when needed.

THE NURSING APPROACH–cont'd
Dietary Teaching: The Nursing Process

There are a variety of teaching methods that the nurse can implement, such as explanation, discussion, demonstration, group discussion, and role-playing.

An important component is the evaluation of the planned teaching session. The evaluation should include the timing, teaching methods, amount of information, and whether the client or group actually mastered the information provided by the nurse. Evaluation methods can include direct observation, written tests, questions, demonstrations, and self-reports.

Following is an example of how the nursing process could be used.

ASSESSMENT

Objective Data

Knowledge of the following:
- Dietary Reference Intakes (DRIs)
- Height/weight/energy intake recommendations
- Protein/fat/carbohydrate ratios
- Food Guide Pyramid
- Dietary contributions to prevention of chronic diseases
- Food safety issues
- Ability to pay for food
- Access to government food programs

Subjective Data

- Food preferences, choices, and likes based on culture, religion, and other variables
- Interest in changing dietary patterns
- Motivation to make needed changes

NURSING DIAGNOSIS

From the list of possible nursing diagnoses identified in Chapter 1, the assessment data may reveal a nutritional problem, which can be formulated into many different nursing diagnoses. For example, a nursing diagnosis of "Nutrition, Altered, less than body requirements" may be related to a lack of knowledge about the Food Guide Pyramid as evidenced by a insufficient take of fruit and vegetables.

PLANNING

Goals are identified for individuals or groups based on the diagnosis. Goals need to be short term, long term, and measurable. For example, for Glenn, who follows a kosher diet, goals could include the following:

Short-term goal:

Glenn will increase daily intake of fruits and vegetables to five servings daily.

Long-term goal:

Glenn will not experience constipation.

A short-term goal for a group of clients in a senior citizens center might be, "The members will demonstrate understanding of the importance of fiber intake." A long-term goal would be, "The members will not experience symptoms of constipation."

IMPLEMENTATION

Specific nursing activities or interventions are selected with each of the goals. Interventions should reinforce positive behaviors or alter the causes of problems. These interventions might include the following:

Short-term implementations:

1. Teach Glenn about the importance of eating fruits and vegetables.
2. Explain the Food Guide Pyramid, keeping in mind any food restrictions in a kosher diet.

Continued

THE NURSING APPROACH–cont'd
Dietary Teaching: The Nursing Process

3. Discuss the health risks of inadequate fruit and vegetables.
4. Assist the client in selecting appropriate foods from a list of choices, depending on his food preferences.

Long-term implementations:

1. Glenn will keep a food diary and include the recommended amounts of fruits and vegetables.
2. Glenn will continue to exercise by walking and drinking water along with his balanced meals.

EVALUATION

Each goal should be evaluated for how well the desired outcomes were met. Evaluation approaches that can be used for dietary teaching include the following:

- Questions and answers
- Short verbal quiz
- A word game such as a crossword puzzle or word search
- Selection of appropriate food choices

Evaluation of a follow-up food record for a week's intake

APPLYING CONTENT KNOWLEDGE

Jenny is again visiting her primary healthcare provider for a "stomach virus." She has been seen several times for the same problem over the past few months. When conducting the intake interview, you wonder if she could have a recurring foodborne illness. What are three assessment questions you might ask her?

Web Sites of Interest

Dietary Guidelines for Americans
www.nal.usda.gov/fnic/dga
Provides links to the basis of each of the Dietary Guidelines.

Food Guide Pyramid
www.nal.usda.gov/fnic/Fpyr/pyramid.html
Features an interactive Food Guide Pyramid that provides information on related topics.

National Center for Food Safety and Technology (NCFST)
www.iit.edu/~ncfs/
Consortium of industry, government, and academia that works toward the assurance of a safe and high-quality food supply; considers the issues that develop from new food technologies.

NutriBase
www.nutribase.com
Provides online nutrient database of 19,344 food items including 3160 menu items from 71 restaurants; also offers a weight-loss calculator, a calorie requirements calculator, "desirable" weight and body fat content charts, a directory of food and supplement makers, a healthy food substitutions list, a food and cooking glossary, and toll-free telephone numbers for food makers.

The Partnership for Food Safety Education
www.fightbac.org
Private-public partnership that educates the public about food safety strategies through multiple media approaches.

U.S. Food and Drug Administration (FDA)
www.fda.gov
As the home page of the FDA, provides links to all the areas serviced and supervised by this federal consumer protection agency.

References

1. US Department of Health and Human Services, Public Health Service: *Healthy People 2010,* ed 2, Washington, DC, 2000, US Government Printing Office; www.health.gov/healthypeople.
2. Logue AW: *The psychology of eating and drinking: an introduction,* ed 2, New York, 1992, Freeman.
3. Drewrowski A, Henderson SA, Barratt-Fornell A: Genetic taste markers and food preferences, *Drug Metab Dispos* 29(4 pt2):535, Apr 2001.
4. Birch LL, Fisher JA: The role of experience in the development of children's eating behavior. In Capaldi ED, ed: *Why we eat what we eat: the psychology of eating,* Washington, DC, 1996, American Psychological Association.
5. Mennella JA, Beauchamp GK: The early development of human flavor preferences. In Capaldi ED, ed.: *Why we eat what we eat: the psychology of eating,* Washington, DC, 1996, American Psychological Association.
6. Senate Select Committee on Nutrition and Human Needs: *Dietary goals for the United States,* ed 2, Washington, DC, 1977, US Government Printing Office.
7. American Heart Association: *An eating plan for healthy Americans,* Dallas, 2000, The Association; www.americanheart.org; Krauss RM et al.: AHA Dietary Guidelines, Revision 2000: a statement for healthcare professionals from the Nutrition Committee of the American Heart Association, *Circulation* 2000:2296.
8. American Cancer Society: *Nutrition for risk reduction,* January 2001; www.cancer.org/eprise/main/docroot/PED/content/PED_3_2X_Recommendations?sitearea=PED.
9. US Department of Agriculture, US Department of Health and Human Services: *Nutrition and your health: dietary guidelines for Americans,* ed 5, Home and Garden Bulletin 232, Washington, DC, 2000, USDA; www.usda.gov/cnpp.
10. US Department of Agriculture Center for Nutrition Policy and Promotions: *The Food Pyramid,* Home and Garden Bulletin 249, Washington, DC, 1992, revised 1996, US Government Printing Office; www.usda.gov/fcs/cnpp.htm.
11. Mediterranean Diet Pyramid, Latin American Diet Pyramid, Asian Diet Pyramid, Cambridge, Mass, 2002, Oldways Preservation & Exchange Trust; www.oldwayspt.org.
12. Painter J, Rah J-H, Lee Y-K: Comparison of international food guide pictorial presentations, *J Am Dietetic Assoc* 102(4):483, Apr 2002.
13. National Cancer Institute/National Institutes of Health: *5 a Day for better health: a baseline study of Americans' fruit and vegetable consumption,* Rockville, Md, 1992, The Institute.
14. American Diabetes Association, American Dietetic Association: *Exchange lists for meal planning (revised),* Alexandria, Va, 1995, American Dietetic Association.
15. American Diabetes Association position statement: Evidence-based nutrition principles and recommendations for the treatment and prevention of diabetes and related complications, *J Am Dietetic Assoc* 102(1):109, 2002.
16. US Department of Agriculture Center for Nutrition Policy and Promotion: *The Healthy Eating Index, 1994-1996,* Washington, DC, 1998, US Government Printing Office; www.usda.govnews/releases/1998/05/0209.
17. Dinkins JM: Beliefs and attitudes of Americans toward their diet, *Family economics and nutrition review* 13(1):98, 2001.
18. Putnam JJ, Allshouse JE: *Food consumption, prices, and expenditures, 1970-97,* Statistical Bulletin No. 965, Washington, DC, 1999, Economic Research Service, USDA, 1999.
19. Kurtzweill P: Food label close-up, *FDA Consumer* 28(3):15, 1994 (revised 1998); www.fda.gov/fdac/reprints/closeup.html.
20. Food and Drug Administration: *FDA talk paper,* February 17, 1998; www.cfsan.fda.gov/label.html.
21. Food and Drug Administration: *Food and nutrition news,* Spring 1997.
22. US Department of Health and Human Services: Customer satisfaction results for the Food and Drug Administration remain constant, *HHS News,* December 22, 2000; www.fda.gov/bbs/topics/NEWS/NEW00746.html.
23. Center for Science in the Public Interest: Genetically engineered foods: are they safe? *Nutrition Action Health Letter* 28(9):1,3, November 2001.
24. Food and Drug Administration: *Report on the FDA review of the safety of recombinant bovine somatotropin recombinant,* February 10, 1999.

25. Food and Drug Administration /Center for Food Safety and Applied Nutrition: *Food safety A to Z reference guide,* September 2001.

26. Besser RE et al.: An outbreak of diarrhea and hemolytic uremic syndrome from *Escerichia coli* 0157:H7 in fresh-pressed apple cider, *J Am Med Assoc* May 5, 1993.

27. Food and Drug Administration: *FDA Consumer,* September-October 1998 (revised 1999); www.vm.cfsan.fda.gov.

28. Lewis C: Critical controls for juice safety, *FDA Consumer,* September-October 1998 (revised 1999), www.vm.cfsan.fda.gov.

29. Buchanan RL, Doyle MP: Foodborne disease significance of *Escherichia coli* 0157:H7 and other enterohemorrhagic *E. coli, Food Technology* 51(10):69, 1994.

30. *Plesiomonas shigelloides* and *Salmonella* serotype Hartford infestations associated with a contaminated water supply—Livingston County, New York, 1996, *MMWR* 396, May 22, 1998.

31. Partnership for Food Safety Education: *Fight bac!;* www.fightbac.org.

32. Anon. Washington News, *Food Technology* 50(9):37, 1996.

33. Loaharanu P: Cost/benefit aspects of food irradiation, *Food Technology* 48(1):1, 1994.

34. Olson DG: Irradiation of food: scientific status summary, *Food Technology* 52(1):56, 1998.

35. American Dietetic Association: Food irradiation: position of the American Dietetic Association, *J Am Dietetic Assoc* 00(100):246, 2000.

PART II

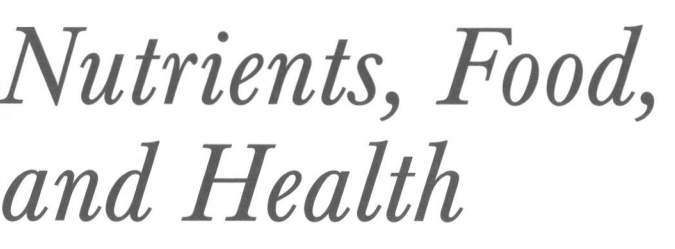

Nutrients, Food, and Health

CHAPTER 3

Digestion, Absorption, and Metabolism

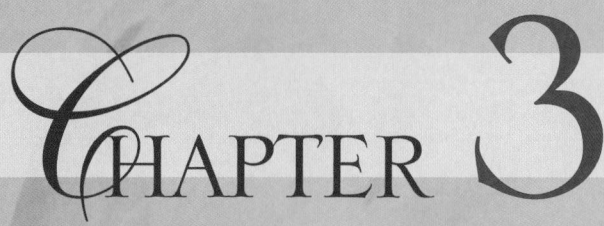

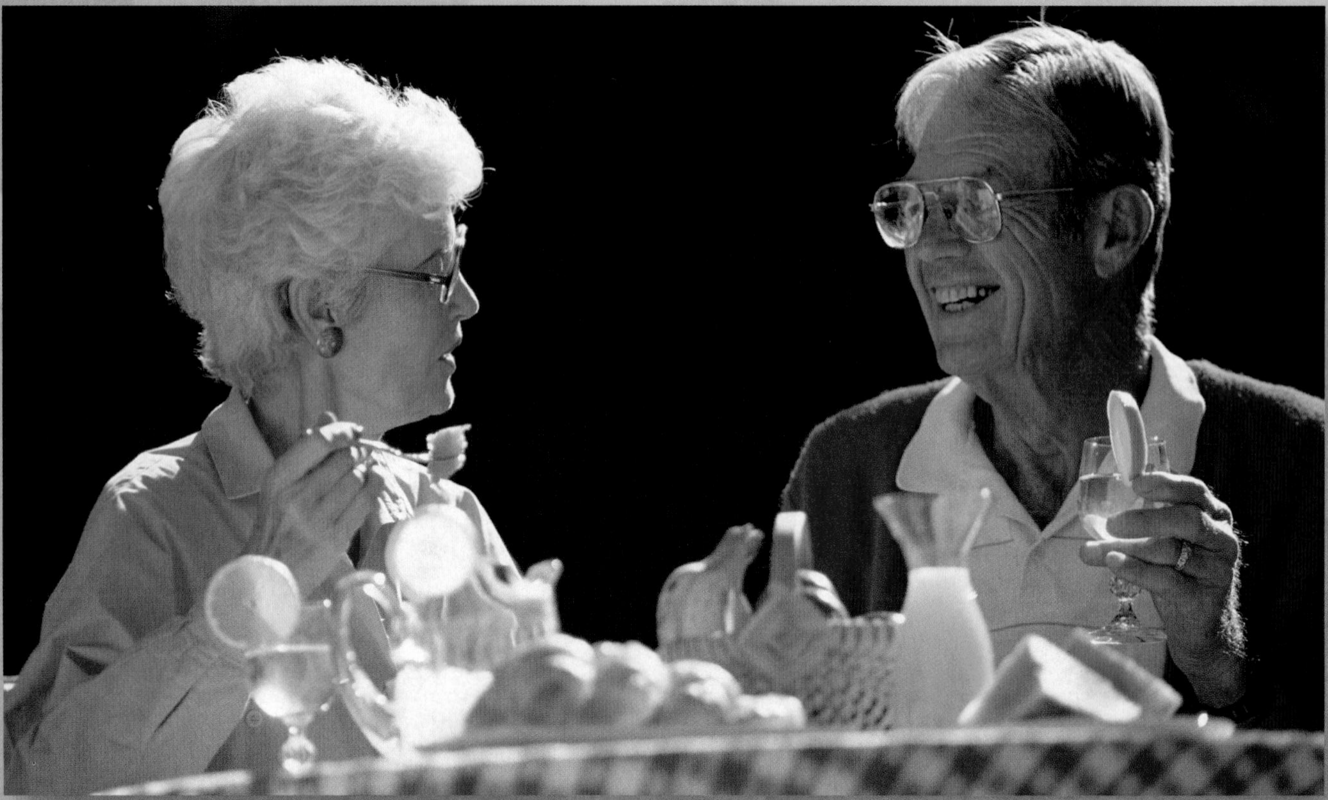

The digestive system, responsible for processing foods, is itself dependent on our nutrient intake for its maintenance.

ROLE IN WELLNESS

Gulping down breakfast on the way to class or work, skipping lunch, and then eating dinner late may not seem to affect the health status of adults. However, if this kind of eating pattern becomes routine, not only does it begin to affect health status but it also characterizes an individual's lifestyle.

The body's health is based on the nutrients available to support growth, maintenance, and energy needs. Inadequate nutritional intake can affect the body's ability to use the foods consumed. The digestive system, responsible for processing foods, depends on nutrient intake for its maintenance. Although the body is resilient, we stress our physical limits when we adopt habits that do not support optimal health. A primary way to decrease the risk of future disease and achieve wellness is to use lifestyle choices that support positive health behaviors.

Physical health begins with the gastrointestinal (GI) tract as the first stop to maintain body functioning; unless nutrients in foods are digested and absorbed, life cannot continue. The decision and follow through to change lifestyle behaviors to positively improve health in relation to digestive disorders are aspects of intellectual health. Several disorders of the GI tract are tied to one's emotional state and the ability to handle stress; emotional health effects of lifestyle behaviors may cause constipation, diarrhea, and heartburn. Reducing the causes of intestinal gas guards against socially embarrassing moments. Again, our food choices and styles of eating may affect the level of flatus experienced. Negativity associated with body smells is defined by society and thus affects our social dimension of health. Respecting the sanctity of the human body, thereby acknowledging our spiritual dimension, may include one's willingness to follow dietary and lifestyle changes to enhance the functioning of the GI tract (see the Cultural Considerations box, "Wholeness of Body, Mind, and Self").

This chapter presents a brief orientation to the processes of digestion, absorption, and metabolism. These processes work together to provide all body cells with energy and nutrients.

DIGESTION

The main organs of the digestion system (Figure 3-1 and Box 3-1) form the gastrointestinal (GI) tract, or alimentary canal, which creates an open tube that runs from the mouth to the anus. Everything we eat is processed through the GI tract.

gastrointestinal (GI) tract
the main organs of the digestive system that form a tube that runs from the mouth to the anus

CULTURAL CONSIDERATIONS
Wholeness of Body, Mind, and Self

This text's presentation of digestion and absorption is based on Western perspectives. To most Westerners, body organs tend to be viewed separately from mind and spiritual influences. In contrast, Ayurveda, traditional Indian medicine, meaning "the science of life," is based on living a balanced life. Consequently, Ayurveda treats physical disorders as the body (organs) or life being out of balance. Treatment works to bring balance or harmony back to the life of the individual. The wholeness of life is represented by body *(shira)*, mind *(manas)*, and self *(atman)*. All three require attention to achieve and maintain health. Because each component is important, Ayurveda is a holistic approach that recognizes the interdependent roles of body, mind, and self. A person is viewed as a combination of three forces or humors that are called "doshas."

Each person is a different combination of these forces, which are "vata," "pitta," and "kapha." *Vata* is a force similar to air, *pitta* a force similar to fire, and *kapha* a force like mucus and water. Health occurs when these *doshas* are in balance; otherwise disease occurs. If *pitta* is too strong, fever, ulcers, and liver disorders may occur. An individual would need to strengthen the other *doshas* through (1) changes in behaviors and food choices, (2) use of natural medicines, and (3) yoga and meditation to decrease *pitta* and regain balance.

Application to nursing: This concept may assist clients to understand that their illnesses may be affected by other components of their lives. Sometimes illnesses force us to confront factors that may influence our ability to maintain health or to achieve balance in our lives.

Reference: Nakamura RM: Health in America: a multicultural perspective, *Boston, 1999, Allyn and Bacon.*

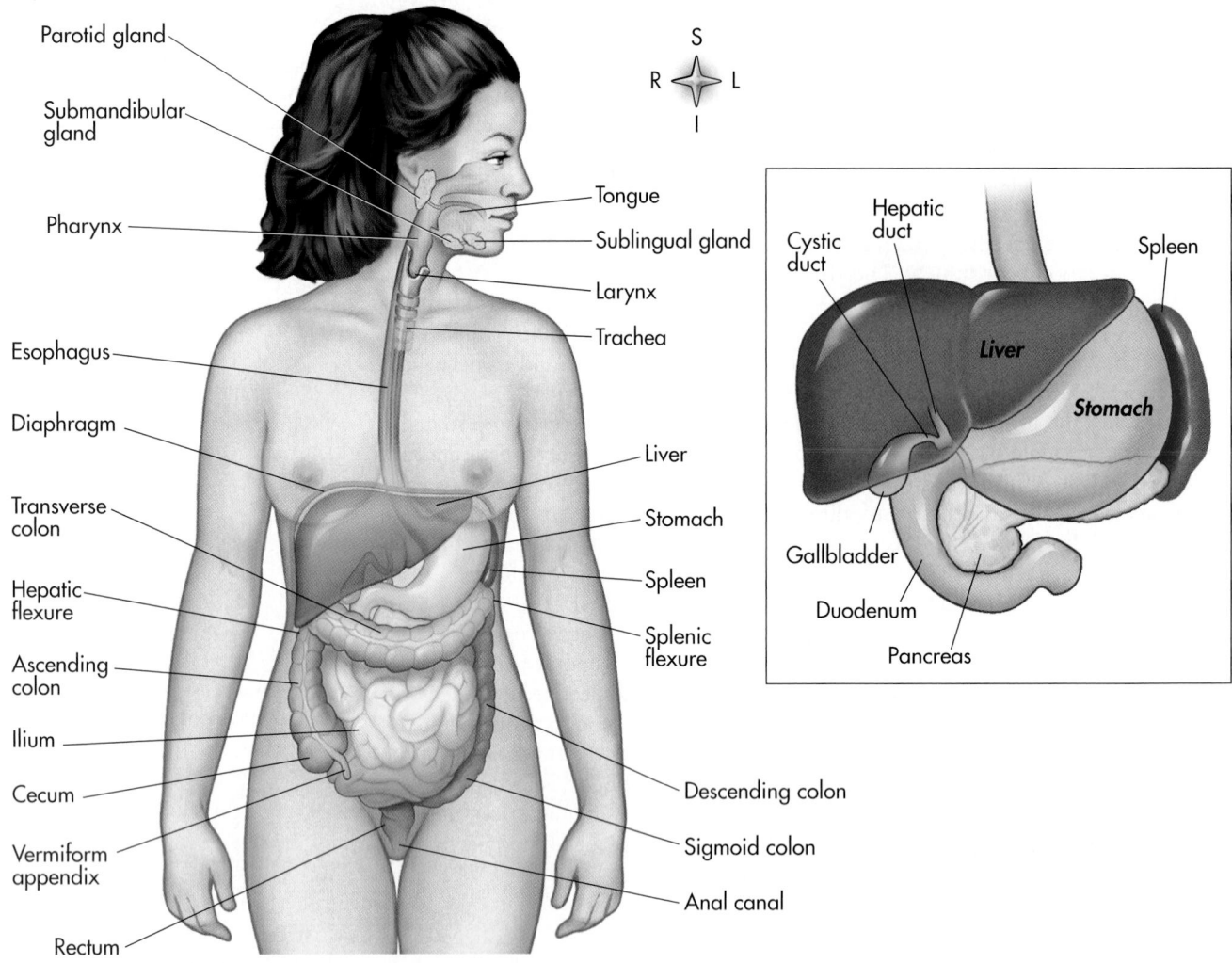

Figure 3-1 Digestive system. (From Thibodeau GA, Patton KT: *Anatomy and physiology,* ed 5, St Louis, 2003, Mosby.)

Box 3-1 Digestive System Organs

SEGMENTS OF THE DIGESTIVE TRACT	ACCESSORY ORGANS
Mouth	Salivary glands
Oropharynx	Parotid gland
Esophagus	Submandibular gland
Stomach	Sublingual gland
Small intestine	Tongue
Duodenum	Teeth
Jejunum	Liver
Ileum	Gallbladder
Large intestine	Pancreas
Cecum	Vermiform appendix
Colon	
Ascending colon	
Transverse colon	
Descending colon	
Sigmoid colon	
Rectum	
Anal canal	

The **digestive system** prepares ingested nutrients for **digestion** and absorption and protects against consumed microorganisms and toxic substances.[1] To achieve these functions, a series of processes occur. These processes of ingestion, digestion, absorption, and elimination depend on the motility or movement of the GI wall and the secretions of digestive juices and enzymes.[2]

🎋 The Mouth

Are you hungry? Thinking about your favorite food? Is your mouth watering? Our mouths really do "water" when we think about or begin to eat foods. However, it is not actually water we sense but a thin mucouslike fluid, called **saliva**. Saliva is the term for the secretions of the three salivary glands of the mouth. As **exocrine glands**, each set of salivary glands produces a different type of secretion that is released into the mouth. The parotid glands create watery saliva that supplies enzymes; the submandibular glands produce mucus and enzyme components; and the sublingual glands, the smallest, create a mucous type of saliva. A reflex mechanism controls these secretions.

Food in the mouth stimulates chemical and mechanical digestion. **Chemical digestion** occurs through the action of saliva that not only moistens the foods we chew but also contains amylase, an enzyme that begins the digestive process of starches.

Another digestive process that occurs in the mouth, **mechanical digestion**, depends on teeth. Teeth rhythmically tear and pulverize food. The enamel that covers teeth is the hardest substance in the body and therefore protects teeth from the harsh effects of chewing. The tongue assists with mechanical digestion by guiding food into chewing positions and then leading the pulverized food into the esophagus. Another function of the tongue is that of taste. More than 2000 taste buds are responsible for our sensations of sweet, bitter, sour, and salty when tasting foods (Figure 3-2).

As toddlers, we have the highest number of taste buds and a higher degree of taste sensitivity, so bland foods are more appealing. The number of taste buds declines as we grow older, which explains why older adults have diminished taste

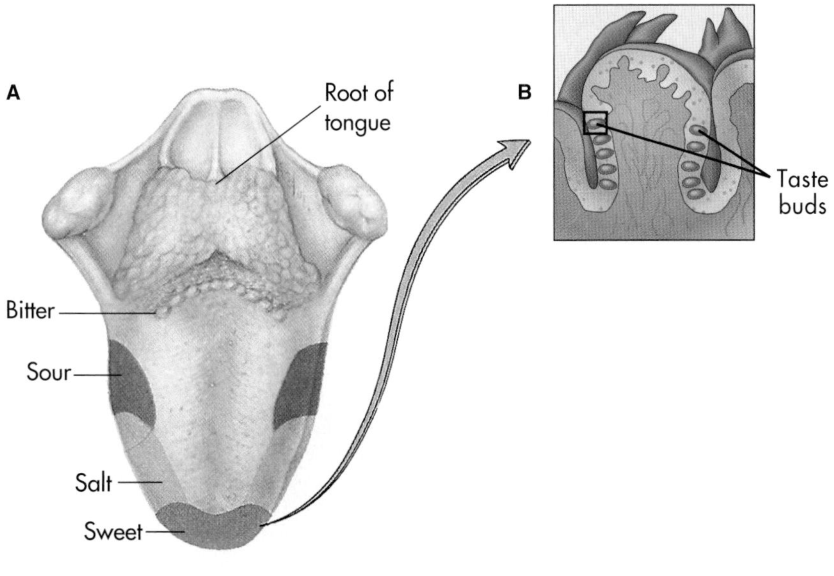

digestive system
a series of organs that functions to prepare ingested nutrients for digestion and absorption

digestion
the process through which foods are broken down into smaller and smaller units to prepare nutrients for absorption

saliva
the secretions of the salivary glands of the mouth

exocrine glands
glands that secrete chemicals into ducts that release into a cavity or to the surface of the body, such as salivary glands (mouth) and the liver (gallbladder)

chemical digestion
the chemical altering effects of digestive secretions, gastric juices, and enzymes on food substance composition

mechanical digestion
the crushing and twisting effects of teeth and peristalsis that divide foods into smaller pieces

Figure 3-2 A, Areas of sensations of sweet, bitter, sour, and salty. **B,** A detailed site of a taste bud. (**A** from Marsha J. Dohrmann. In Thibodeau GA, Patton KT: *Anatomy and physiology,* ed 2, St Louis, 1993, Mosby. **B** from Network Graphics. In Thibodeau GA, Patton KT: *Anatomy and physiology,* ed 4, St Louis, 1999, Mosby.)

sensitivity. Older adults may need to be encouraged to avoid the use of too much salt, particularly if they have hypertension or cardiac disorders.[2]

Our sense of smell works along with our taste bud sensations. These two combined senses actually account for the perception (and enjoyment) of the flavors of different foods. Our positive or negative response to specific foods based on our sensory perception affects our food choices.[3]

Portions of the pulverized or masticated food get formed into the shape of a ball called a **bolus.** The tongue effortlessly forms the bolus, which is then swallowed and passed by the epiglottis into the esophagus within about 5 to 7 seconds. The epiglottis is a flap of tissue that closes over the trachea to prevent the bolus from entering the lungs.

The Esophagus

The esophagus is a muscular tube through which the bolus travels from the mouth to the stomach. The process begins at the top of the esophagus when **peristalsis,** the involuntary movements of circular and longitudinal muscles, begins and draws the bolus further into the GI tract. This mechanical action further breaks down the size of foodstuff and increases exposure to digestive secretions. Muscular actions depend on the four layers of tissues that form the tube of the GI tract (Figure 3-3). The **mucosa** is composed of mucous membrane and forms the inside layer. Under the mucosa is the **submucosa,** which is a layer of connective tissue. Digestion depends on the blood vessels and nerves of the submucosa to regulate digestion. Surrounding the submucosa is a thick layer of muscle tissue called the **muscularis.** The outermost layer of the GI wall is made of serous membrane called **serosa,** which is actually the visceral layer of the peritoneum that lines the abdominal pelvic cavity and covers organs.[2]

The coordination of these layers provides the varied movements required for digestion. Essentially, muscular action controls the movement of the food mass through the GI tract. Churning action within a segment of the GI tract allows secretions to mix with food mass. Circular muscles surround the GI tube. Rhythmic contractions of these muscles cause wavelike motions of peristalsis that move food downward. Longitudinal muscles run parallel along the GI tube. The combined effect of the circular and longitudinal muscles causes **segmentation** as a forward and

bolus
a masticated lump or ball of food ready to be swallowed

peristalsis
the rhythmic contractions of muscles causing wavelike motions that move food down the GI tract

mucosa
the inside GI muscle tissue layer composed of mucous membrane

submucosa
a layer of connective muscle tissue under the mucosa

muscularis
a thick layer of muscle tissue surrounding the submucosa

serosa
the outermost layer of the GI wall; made of serous membrane

segmentation
the forward and backward muscular action that assists in controlling food mass movement through the GI tract

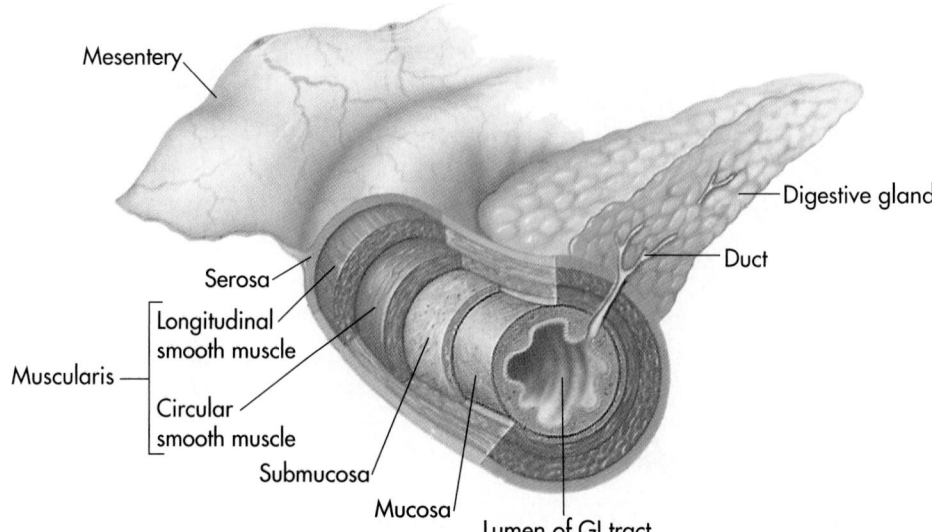

Figure 3-3 Muscle layers of the GI tract. (From Christy Krames. In Thibodeau GA, Patton KT: *Anatomy and physiology,* ed 2, St Louis, 1993, Mosby.)

backward movement. Sphincter muscles are stronger circular muscles that act as valves to control the movement of the food mass in a forward direction. In effect, sphincter muscles prevent reflux by forming an opening when relaxed and closing completely when contracted.

At the bottom of the esophagus, the cardiac sphincter controls the movement of the bolus from the esophagus into the stomach. It also prevents the acidic contents of the stomach from moving upward back through the esophagus.

The Stomach

The bolus enters the fundus, the upper portion of the stomach that connects with the esophagus. The other divisions of the stomach include the body, or center portion, and the pylorus, the lower portion. The stomach wall contains gastric mucosa that contains gastric pits. At the base of the pits are the gastric glands whose chief cells create gastric juice, a mucous fluid that contains digestive enzymes, and parietal cells, which secrete stomach acid called *hydrochloric acid.*

Gastric secretions occur in three phases: cephalic, gastric, and intestinal.[2] The cephalic phase is called the "psychic phase" because mental factors can stimulate gastrin, a hormone. In the gastric phase, gastrin increases the release of gastric juices when the stomach is distended by food. The third phase is the intestinal phase in which the gastric secretions change as chyme passes through to the duodenum. Gastric secretions are inhibited by exocrine and nervous reflexes of gastric inhibitory peptides, secretin, and cholecystokinin (CCK) (also called *pancreozymin*), a hormone secreted by intestinal mucosa.

Some gastric juices provide acidity in the stomach to assist the effective function of certain enzymes. As agents of chemical digestion, enzymes are specific in action, working only on individual classes of nutrients and changing substances from one form to a simpler form. Enzymes are "organic catalysts" formed from protein structures; they function at specific pHs and are continually created and destroyed. Specific enzymes are required for energy release and digestion.

Hormones, which regulate the release of gastric juices and enzymes, act as messengers between organs to cause the release of needed secretions. In digestion, hormones affect the secretions from the stomach, intestines, and gallbladder. These secretions may slow or speed digestion and affect the pH levels of gastric juice. Overall, the mechanical and chemical actions work together to complete the process of digestion.

Gastric motility, or movement of food mass through the stomach, requires 2 to 6 hours. The churning and mixing of the food mass with gastric juices creates a semiliquid mixture called chyme. When chyme enters the pylorus section of the stomach, it causes distention and the release of the hormone gastrin. Gastrin sends a message that hydrochloric acid (HCl) is needed to continue the breakdown of chyme. As HCl is released from the stomach lining, thick mucus is also secreted to protect the stomach walls from the harsh HCl.

Every 20 seconds, chyme is released into the duodenum, the upper portion of the small intestine; this action is controlled by the hormonal and nervous system mechanism of enterogastric reflex. This consists of duodenal receptors in the mucosa that are sensitive to the presence of acid and distention. The impulses over sensory and motor fiber in the vagus nerve cause a reflex restriction of gastric peristalsis. For example, the gastric inhibitory peptide released in response to fats in the duodenum decreases peristalsis of stomach muscles and slows chyme passage. This results in decreased motility, and the stomach empties more slowly when a person eats a high-fat diet.

The combined action of mechanical digestion (the strong muscular movements of peristalsis) and chemical digestion (the effects of the gastric juices) works to prepare nutrients for the process. Chyme is kept in the stomach by the actions of the pyloric sphincter, which slowly releases it into the duodenum.

FROM THE PLATE TO THE CELL: FOOD TRANSIT TIMES

Chewing and swallowing:	Depends on texture and quantity
Esophagus:	5-7 seconds
Stomach:	2-6 hours
Small intestine:	About 5 hours
Large intestine:	9-16 hours
TOTAL:	16-27 hours ingestion to elimination

gastrin
a hormone secreted by stomach mucosa that increases the release of gastric juices

cholecystokinin (CCK)
a hormone secreted by the small intestine that initiates pancreatic exocrine secretions, acts against gastrin, and activates the gallbladder to release bile

chyme
a semiliquid mixture of food mass

Functions of the stomach include the following:

- Holding food for partial digestion
- Producing gastric juice
- Providing muscular action, which, combined with gastric juice, mixes and tears food into smaller pieces
- Secreting the intrinsic factor for vitamin B_{12} absorption
- Releasing gastrin
- Assisting in the destruction, through its acidity of secretions, of pathogenic bacteria that may have inadvertently been consumed[2]

The Small Intestine

The chyme entering the duodenum soon moves through to the jejunum and ileum of the small intestine. During intestinal motility, because of peristalsis and segmentation, it takes about 5 hours for chyme to pass through the small intestine. Segmentation in the duodenum and upper jejunum mixes chyme with digestive juices from the pancreas, liver, and intestinal mucosa. Peristalsis is controlled by intrinsic stretch reflexes and initiated by CCK, the hormone secreted by intestinal mucosa.

In the small intestine, the nutrients in chyme are completely prepared for absorption. The small intestine is the major organ of digestion, and the final stages of the digestive process occur here. Because it is also the site of almost all of the absorption of nutrients, the intestinal lining must be able to accommodate the actions of both digestion and absorption. The intestinal walls are covered with a thin layer of mucus that protects the walls from digestive juices. The walls are also adapted to enhance the absorption process. Fingerlike projections called **villi** greatly increase the amount of mucosal layer available for the absorption of nutrients (Figure 3-4).

villi
fingerlike projections on the walls of the small intestine that increase the mucosal surface area

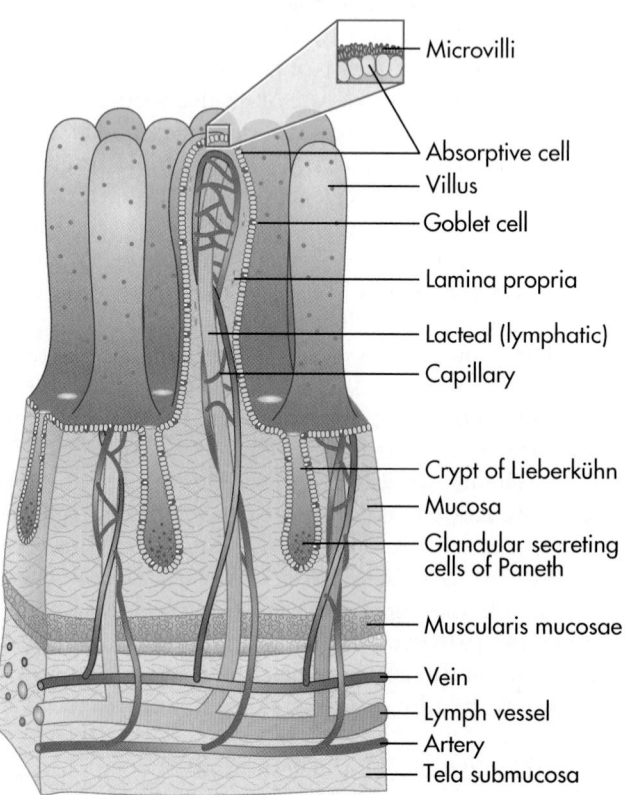

Figure 3-4 Structure of the intestinal wall. The circular folds, villi, and microvilli multiply the surface area and enhance absorption. (From Mahan LK, Escott-Stump S: *Krause's food, nutrition, and diet therapy*, ed 10, Philadelphia, 2000, WB Saunders.)

On the villi are hairlike projections called *microvilli*. These also enhance absorption by their structure and movements.

As chyme enters the small intestine, **hormones** begin sending messages that regulate the release of digestive juices to continue the process of chyme digestion. Some hormones are provided by the small intestine; several are released by other organs into the small intestine. These secretions include enzymes from the small intestines, bile produced in the liver, and digestive juices from the pancreas.

One of the first hormones released by the small intestine is **secretin**. This hormone causes the pancreas to send bicarbonate to the small intestine to reduce the acidic content of the chyme. As the acidic level decreases, other pancreatic juices enter and begin their work. Another hormone secreted by the small intestine is cholecystokinin (CCK), or pancreozymin; it functions to initiate pancreatic exocrine secretions; act against gastrin by inhibiting gastric HCl secretion; and activate the gallbladder to contract, causing bile to be released into the duodenum.

Bile, secreted by the liver and stored in the gallbladder, is released to emulsify fats, which aids in the digestion of lipids. The emulsification creates more surface area that allows lipid enzymes to digest fats to their component parts. The liver always secretes bile. CCK and secretin spur the gallbladder to release bile for the digestion of fats. In addition, the small intestine produces enzymes to assist in the digestive process. Although much of the chyme is absorbed, the rest—which usually consists of fiber, minerals, and water—passes through the next sphincter (ileocecal valve) and into the large intestine (ascending colon).

The Large Intestine

The large intestine consists of the cecum, colon, and rectum. The cecum is a blind pocket; therefore the mass bypasses it and enters the ascending colon, which leads into the transverse colon that runs across the abdomen over the small intestine to the descending colon. The descending colon extends down the left of the abdomen into the sigmoid colon and leads into the descending colon, on to the rectum, and into the anal canal. Finally, any remaining mass passes out through the anus. The journey through the large intestine takes about 9 to 16 hours.

In the large intestine or colon, final absorption of any available nutrients, usually water and some minerals, occurs. Bacteria residing in the large intestine produce several vitamins, which are then absorbed. Water is withdrawn from the fibrous mass, forming solidified feces. Mucous glands in the intestinal wall create mucus that lubricates and covers feces as it forms. Again, peristalsis continues to move substances through the GI tract, resulting in the excretion of feces from the colon through the anus, the last sphincter muscle of the GI tract.

The movement of the food mass through the GI tract is controlled to enhance digestion and absorption. During passage through the GI tract, more than 95% of the carbohydrates, fats, and proteins ingested are absorbed. Some minerals, vitamins, and trace elements may be less absorbed.[1]

Table 3-1 summarizes the primary mechanisms of the digestive system. Details of carbohydrate, protein, and lipid digestion follow in specific chapters.

ABSORPTION

Although the food mass has possibly spent several hours in the tube of the GI tract, it is not yet actually inside the body until its nutrient components are absorbed. **Absorption** is the process by which substances pass through the intestinal mucosa into the blood or lymph. Transport processes provide the means for nutrients to actually pass through the wall of the small intestine. These include passive diffusion and osmosis, facilitated diffusion, energy-dependent active transport, and engulfing pinocytosis (Figure 3-5). Passive diffusion occurs when pressure is greater on one side of the membrane and the substance then moves from the area of

hormones
substances that act as messengers between organs to cause the release of needed secretions

secretin
a hormone secreted by the small intestine that causes the pancreas to release bicarbonate to the small intestine

bile
a substance that emulsifies fats to aid the digestion of lipids; produced by the liver and stored in the gallbladder

absorption
the process by which substances pass through the intestinal mucosa into the blood or lymph

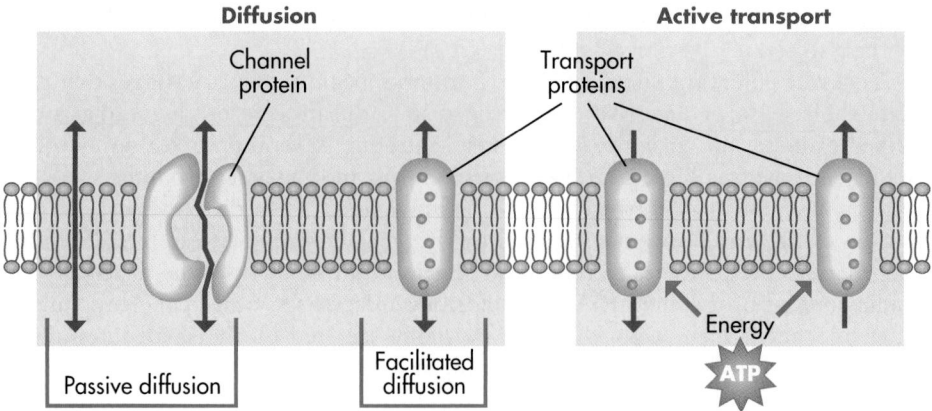

Figure 3-5 Methods of absorption. *Passive diffusion*, the movement of molecules from a region of high concentration to low concentration; *facilitated diffusion*, the movement of molecules by a carrier protein across the cell membrane from a region of high to low concentration; *active transport*, the movement of molecules and ions by means of a carrier protein against fluid pressures that require expenditure of cellular energy. (From Mahan LK, Escott-Stump S: *Krause's food, nutrition, and diet therapy*, ed 10, Philadelphia, 2000, WB Saunders.)

Table 3-1
Digestive Processes

Mechanism	Description
Ingestion	Process of taking food into the mouth, starting it on its journey through the digestive tract
Digestion	A group of processes that break complex nutrients into simpler ones, thus facilitating their absorption; *mechanical digestion* physically breaks large chunks into small bits; *chemical digestion* breaks molecules apart
Motility	Movement by the muscular components of the digestive tube, including processes of mechanical digestion; examples include *peristalsis* and *segmentation*
Secretion	Release of digestive juices (containing enzymes, acids, bases, mucus, bile, or other products that facilitate digestion); some digestive organs also secrete endocrine hormones that regulate digestion or metabolism of nutrients
Absorption	Movement of digested nutrients through the GI mucosa and into the internal environment
Elimination	Excretion of the residues of the digestive process (feces) from the rectum, through the anus; defecation

Reference: Thibodeau GA, Patton KT: Anatomy and physiology, ed 4, St Louis, 1999, Mosby.

greater pressure to less pressure, allowing molecules to travel through capillaries. Facilitated diffusion takes place when, despite positive pressure flow, molecules may be unable to pass through membrane pores unless aided. Specific integral membrane protein supports the movement by bringing the larger nutrient molecules through the capillary membrane.

Energy-dependent active transport happens when fluid pressures work against the passage of nutrients. As an active process, energy is required. This energy is supplied by the cell and a "pumping" mechanism, which are assisted by a special membrane protein carrier. Engulfing pinocytosis takes place when a substance, either fluid or nutrient, contacts the villi membrane, which then surrounds the substance and creates a vacuole that encompasses the substance. Passing through the cell cytoplasm, the substance is then released into the circulatory system.[4] The amounts of vitamins and minerals absorbed depend on the body's storage levels and immediate need for these nutrients. Nutrients such as fats, carbohydrates, and protein are easily absorbed regardless of the level of need. The structure of the small intestine, the site of almost all nutrient absorption, allows for efficient absorption to occur. The microvilli are sensitive to the exact nutrient needs of the body. Their wavelike motions, caused by peristalsis, result in the most exposure of the nutrient-laden chyme to the absorbing cells. This exposure allows needed nutrients to leave the GI tract and pass through the microvilli cells. At this point, the nutrients are truly "inside" the body.

Various factors may affect absorption of nutrients. Combinations of naturally occurring substances such as fiber or binders may move nutrients through the GI tract too quickly for optimum absorption to occur. Individual nutrient absorption and other issues of bioavailability are addressed in other chapters. The relationship between food and drug absorption is also an important issue of medical treatment. Ingesting medications with food may decrease the absorption rate of the medication and may also interfere with the absorption of other nutrients contained in the food consumed. This issue is explored in depth in Chapter 16.

Once "inside" the body, the nutrients enter the circulatory systems of the bloodstream or lymphatic system. The general circulatory or blood system receives absorbed protein, carbohydrates, small parts of broken down fats, and most vitamins and minerals. This system transports these nutrients throughout the body. The lymphatic system, a secondary circulatory system, receives large lipids and fat-soluble vitamins. The nutrients traveling in the lymphatic system are deposited into the bloodstream near the heart. All nutrients then circulate throughout the body in the blood, providing for the nutrient requirements of cells.

Soon after entering the bloodstream, nutrients pass by the liver. This allows the liver to have "first choice" of the available nutrients. The liver is a powerhouse organ that provides a wide variety of services and substances; thus its nutrient needs are a priority. From there, the bloodstream's journey of nutrients continues to the heart to also give it a prime nutrient selection. The journey then continues through the circulatory system to all cells. Some nutrients end up in nutrient storage sites of the body. These sites include the bones, liver, and kidneys. Other nutrients, if not discarded or used by cells, are filtered out of the blood by the kidneys to be reabsorbed or excreted in urine.

Elimination

The expulsion of feces or body waste products is called *defecation*. When the rectum is distended because of waste accumulation, the reflex to defecate occurs. The residue may include substances, such as cellulose and other dietary fibers and connective tissue from meat collagen, that are unable to be digested by human enzymes. Undigested fats may combine with dietary minerals, such as calcium and magnesium, and form residue. Additional residue may include water, bacteria, pigments, and mucus. Figure 3-6 summarizes the functions of the digestive system, and the Teaching Tool provides suggestions for client and patient teaching.

Digestive Process across the Life Span

Over the course of the life span, the main and accessory organs of digestion develop and change. The immature GI tract, particularly the intestinal mucosa of young infants, may allow intact proteins to be absorbed without complete

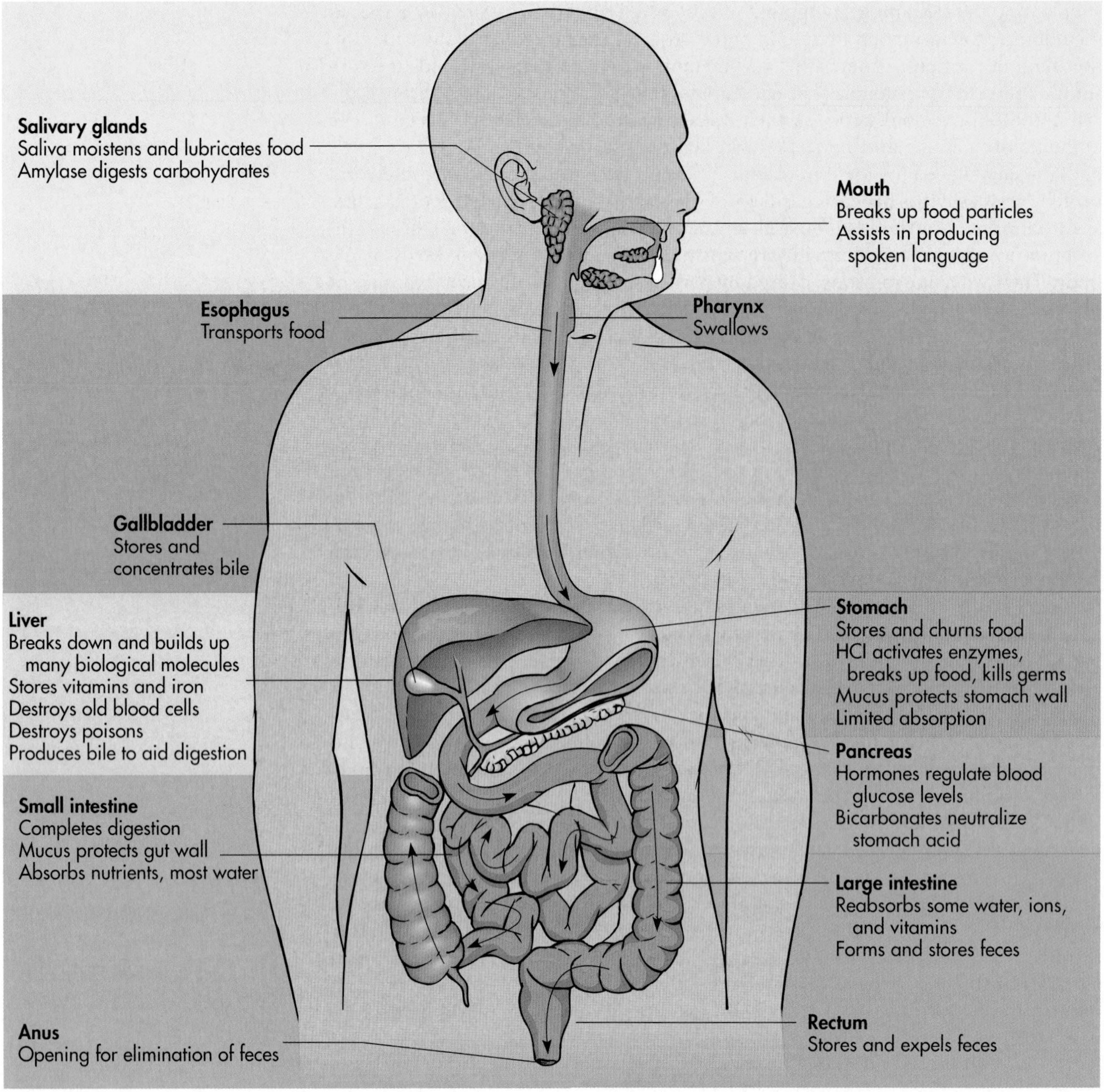

Salivary glands
Saliva moistens and lubricates food
Amylase digests carbohydrates

Mouth
Breaks up food particles
Assists in producing
   spoken language

Esophagus
Transports food

Pharynx
Swallows

Gallbladder
Stores and
concentrates bile

Stomach
Stores and churns food
HCl activates enzymes,
   breaks up food, kills germs
Mucus protects stomach wall
Limited absorption

Liver
Breaks down and builds up
   many biological molecules
Stores vitamins and iron
Destroys old blood cells
Destroys poisons
Produces bile to aid digestion

Pancreas
Hormones regulate blood
   glucose levels
Bicarbonates neutralize
   stomach acid

Small intestine
Completes digestion
Mucus protects gut wall
Absorbs nutrients, most water

Large intestine
Reabsorbs some water, ions,
   and vitamins
Forms and stores feces

Anus
Opening for elimination of feces

Rectum
Stores and expels feces

Figure 3-6 Summary of digestive organ functions. (From Rolin Graphics.)

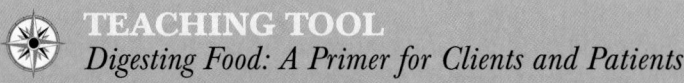

TEACHING TOOL
Digesting Food: A Primer for Clients and Patients

As healthcare professionals, we may assume that our clients understand the way the body works as easily as we do. More than likely, however, their knowledge is limited, and even if they studied digestion years ago in a health education class, they may have forgotten or replaced facts with misinformation.

When working with clients for health promotion or with patients recovering from GI disorders, consider using the summary of digestive organ functions (see Figure 3-6) as a teaching tool. By visually reviewing the digestive organs and processes, clients and patients can have a clearer concept of the purposes of dietary recommendations and may therefore find compliance easier.

digestion occurring. This incomplete digestion may result in an allergic response by the immune system and is part of the reason to delay the introduction of solid foods (e.g., cereals) until the GI tract has matured sufficiently. Another age-related condition is lactose intolerance in which the body ceases to produce lactase, the enzyme that breaks down the milk carbohydrate of lactose. For some people, this occurs once the primary growth need for nutrients contained in milk is met. For others, this may not occur until adulthood or not at all (see Chapter 4). Older adults sometimes experience lactose intolerance as the secretion of enzymes, such as lactase, decreases as part of the aging process. Conditions of the middle years include gallbladder disease and peptic ulcers (sores that may occur on the epithelial surfaces of the stomach or small intestine). Older years may be marked by problems of constipation and diverticulosis. These conditions may be associated with age-related reduced peristalsis and decreased physical activity, and may be worsened by a lifelong history of chronic low dietary fiber consumption.[2] Other issues related to aging are discussed in later chapters, particularly in Chapter 13.

METABOLISM

It is hard to imagine that a lunch consisting of tuna on rye bread will actually end up being part of the cells of the body. Fortunately, the human body is able to transform the nutrients of the sandwich into substances usable by cells. Metabolism is a set of processes through which absorbed nutrients are used by the body for energy and to form and maintain body structures and functions. The two main processes of metabolism involve catabolism and anabolism. Catabolism is the breakdown of food components into smaller molecular particles, which causes the release of energy as heat and chemical energy.[2] Anabolism is the process of synthesis from which substances are formed, such as new bone or muscle tissue. Both processes happen within cells at the same time.

When nutrients finally reach individual cells, they may be chemically changed through anabolism to help form new cell structures or to create new substances such as hormones and enzymes. Some vitamins and minerals assist in the use of other nutrients within the cell. They act as catalysts or coenzymes to initiate and support the transformation and use of carbohydrates, proteins, and lipids. Other nutrients may be used as energy to continue life-supporting processes. These processes include the energy needed to support deoxyribonucleic acid (DNA) reproduction and create proteins and other molecules, nerve impulses, and muscle contractions. Some energy is stored in a ready-to-use state. Specific metabolic functions of individual nutrients are discussed in later chapters (Chapters 4 to 8).

Waste products from metabolism are discarded by the cells and wind up circulating in the blood. They are then excreted through the lungs, kidneys, or large intestine. The lungs release excess water and carbon dioxide. The kidneys filter and excrete metabolic waste and excess vitamins and minerals but reabsorb nutrients that the body needs to retain. Waste products may also be discarded through the large intestine in feces.

Fortunately, we do not have to consciously control these processes. Our responsibility is to provide an adequate selection of nutrients through the foods we choose to eat and to eat those foods in a way that enhances the functioning of the GI tract.

metabolism
a set of processes through which absorbed nutrients are used by the body for energy and to form and maintain body structures and functions

Metabolism across the Life Span

Metabolic changes are most noticeable later in life as the amount of food energy required decreases in relation to lowered metabolic rates. Nutrient needs, however, remain constant. Our challenge as we (and our clients) enter the middle years and beyond is to meet nutrient needs while maintaining or reducing our kcaloric needs to equal actual metabolic use. Recognition of this change can forestall the unexpected weight gain that appears to accompany aging in the United States.

OVERCOMING BARRIERS

Some of our lifestyle behaviors affect the functioning and health of our GI tracts and therefore influence our nutritional status (see the Social Issue box, "Hunger Vs. Appetite Vs. Time"). Some common GI tract health problems are caused by the everyday decisions that we make but that can be changed. Prevention suggestions and treatment strategies for some common GI tract health problems follow.

SOCIAL ISSUE
Hunger Vs. Appetite Vs. Time?

---

*O*ur daily schedules often determine our responses to hunger. Ever notice how differently you eat during the week compared with the weekend? The weekday mosaic of classes, studying, work, and possibly sports training makes fitting in time to get to the campus cafeteria a Herculean feat. Or, if you prepare your own meals, time must be set aside for buying and cooking foods. Weekends may be more leisurely without classes or work, or perhaps we find time for socializing.

Yet somehow we manage. Although fewer meals may be eaten during the week, we are not any less hungry nor are energy needs lower. Sometimes, chaotic schedules may be accommodated by telling ourselves we are not really hungry or we just do not have time to eat.

How can we do that? Isn't hunger a physiologic need for energy and nutrients? Can we just think ourselves through the hunger sensation? To understand this process, we need to explore the feeding regulating mechanism of the body.

Our sense of hunger and satiety is governed by the hypothalamus, a small portion of the brain. Its purpose is to maintain homeostasis (a state of balance) through regulation of food intake through a feeding (hunger) center and a satiety center. The response of the hypothalamus, which initiates the hunger sensation, is thought to be related either to low blood glucose levels or to the lack of chyme in the stomach.

When we eat, blood glucose levels rise and chyme is once again in the stomach. The hypothalamus responds by providing a feeling of satiety or satisfaction, and we stop eating.

When we "feel" hungry, we are recognizing the internal stimuli of hunger. Perhaps our stomach seems to be rumbling or "empty" or we are "starving." These sensations are tied to physical events in our bodies. When we act on this, we eat. However, we can also choose to ignore these signals. This means we cognitively override the sensation and do not respond. There are physical mechanisms to cope with the lack of new energy sources, but it is still stressful to our bodies.

External stimuli also affect our desire or appetite for eating. Referred to as *environmental cues*, these include the smell and sight of food, which may artificially increase our hunger. Simply seeing a food commercial on television or talking about food can excite the feeding center even if the stomach is not actually "empty." We also associate eating with specific social settings and time of day, regardless of our physical need for food. How can a birthday be celebrated without a cake? Religious holidays are often associated with special foods or meals. Throughout our elementary school experience, we ate lunch when we were scheduled, not necessarily when we were hungry.

All those years of eating by schedules and events have led us to adapt by overriding our cognitive cues about our real sense of hunger. Now, when personal schedules are more individualized, we may find that the external stimuli supporting our appropriate intake of food are gone; we must develop our own cues to ensure optimal nutritional intakes.

Compiled from Logue AW: The psychology of eating and drinking: an introduction, *ed 2, New York, 1991, Freeman; and Mahan LK, Escott-Stump S:* Krause's food, nutrition, and diet therapy, *ed 10, Philadelphia, 2000, WB Saunders.*

Heartburn

Heartburn, fortunately, has nothing to do with the health of the heart. Instead, it is a burning sensation felt in the esophagus when food that has already been passed to the stomach refluxes or passes back up through the cardiac sphincter into the esophagus. The esophagus is not lined with acid-resistant mucus, as is the stomach, so the acidic mixture of food burns the walls of the esophagus and causes pain. Heartburn, or **gastroesophageal reflux (GER)**, is a common experience. Depending on the frequency and severity of heartburn, including symptoms such as asthma, chronic cough, and other ear, nose, and throat ailments, a diagnosis of either gastroesophageal reflux disease (GERD) or laryngopharyngeal reflux (LPR) (in which reflux affects the larynx or pharynx) may occur. See Chapter 17 for a detailed discussion of GERD.

Prevention and treatment strategies attempt to reduce the amount of pressure in the stomach so that the cardiac sphincter is not opened by excess pressure from stomach contents. A primary approach is to avoid overeating, so that the stomach can easily accommodate its contents. Other strategies include avoiding the following[5,6]:

- *Constipation.* Straining to defecate affects the contents of the stomach by creating additional pressure.
- *Lying down shortly after eating.* Resting or sleeping with a full stomach may push contents against the cardiac sphincter. Wait several hours after a meal before lying flat or keep head and shoulders elevated when reclining.
- *High-fat meals.* Slow emptying of the stomach from eating high-fat food increases the chance of reflux.
- *Tight clothing.* Wearing restrictive clothing around the waist and midriff affects the functioning of the stomach and may increase stomach pressure.
- *"Eating on the run."* Eating meals while under stress or trying to do other activities at the same time may cause food to not be chewed enough. Big clumps of foods in the stomach force the stomach muscles to react strongly, which may cause reflux (see the Health Debate box, "Are Advertisers Leading Us Astray?").
- *Certain foods and drinks.* Consuming chocolate, alcohol, peppermints, spearmints, or liqueurs and possibly caffeine, tomatoes, and citrus fruits and juices may irritate and cause heartburn.
- *Some medications.* Taking certain medications regularly may initiate heartburn. If heartburn often occurs when taking birth control pills, antihistamines, tranquilizers (e.g., diazepam [Valium]), or any drug taken often, check with the primary care provider. Heartburn could be caused by these medications.

If these strategies do not help and heartburn remains, consult a primary care provider. Chronic heartburn or GER may result in **esophagitis** or may be caused by **hiatal hernia**, which requires medical intervention.

✸ Vomiting

Although vomiting is not usually related to lifestyle behaviors, it is a common digestive disorder worthy of review. **Vomiting** is reverse peristalsis. Instead of food moving down the GI tract, the peristalsis muscles move the contents of the stomach back through the esophagus and forcefully out the mouth. It is an involuntary muscular action that we cannot easily control. Often it is painful; the contents of the stomach already consist of a mixture of food and acidic gastric juices that burns the unprotected esophagus.

Vomiting is a way of the body protecting itself. Perhaps an intruding virus or toxin has entered the GI tract; vomiting removes the offending substance. Mixed messages regarding the body's sense of equilibrium during air or sea travel can result in motion sickness, of which vomiting may be a symptom. Dehydration is a concern when vomiting is continuous. Vomiting causes a loss of fluid and elec-

gastroesophageal reflux (GER)
return of gastric contents into the esophagus that results in a severe burning sensation under the sternum; commonly called *heartburn*

HEARTBURN CAN BE REDUCED BY AVOIDING THE FOLLOWING:
Alcohol
Caffeine
Chocolate
Citrus fruits
Citrus juice
High-fat food
Liquor
Peppermint
Spearmint
Tomatoes

esophagitis
inflammation of the lower esophagus

hiatal hernia
herniation of a portion of the stomach into the chest through the esophageal hiatus of the diaphragm

vomiting
reverse peristalsis

HEALTH DEBATE
Are Advertisers Leading Us Astray?

A TV commercial begins with a man and his adult daughter shopping in a gourmet deli. The daughter displays a spicy sausage she has just selected for their dinner; he protests that it will upset his stomach and cause him bad heartburn. Allaying his fears, she presents him with an over-the-counter (OTC) drug product that will prevent his painful symptoms if taken in advance. Everyone is happy!

What's wrong with this picture? Advertisers paint a false picture of the appropriate use of OTC histamine receptor antagonists such as Tagamet, Axid, Zantac, and Pepcid. These drugs were originally developed to treat peptic ulcers. Because it is now known that most ulcers are caused by the bacterium *Helicobactor pylori* and can be cured with antibiotics, pharmaceutical companies whose sales of histamine receptor antagonist drugs would diminish are attempting to expand the use of these medications to other somewhat related conditions. In lower doses, these drugs can relieve heartburn symptoms but cannot treat the cause of the discomfort. By promoting the use of these drugs to alleviate symptoms caused by hard to digest foods or overeating, underlying conditions such as gastroesophageal reflux (GER) and esophagitis, for which heartburn is a symptom, may be overlooked. Although immediate reflux discomfort may be eased, the dosage in these OTC drugs is not high enough to prevent damage to the esophagus. Rather than emphasizing lifestyle and dietary changes, this approach encourages abuse of medication and disregard for dietary common sense.

Should these drugs be advertised as a premeal cure-all for heartburn, or should OTC advertisements be restricted?

Compiled from USP DI-Volume II advice for the patient: drug information in lay language, *ed 17, Rockville, Maryland, 1997, US Pharmacopeail Convention, Inc; and Gower T: Heartburn: everything you need to know to tame the fire within, Health 11(4):100, 1997.*

trolytes, such as magnesium, potassium, and sodium, which stresses the functioning of the body. Infants are at particular risk for dehydration because their bodies consist mostly of fluids.[5] A primary healthcare provider should be consulted to determine the cause of vomiting and to recommend treatment.

Also at medical risk are individuals who vomit as a way to control their weight and suffer from eating disorders such as anorexia nervosa and bulimia. Repetitive self-induced vomiting can injure the esophagus and wear away the enamel of teeth.[7] Anyone practicing this self-destructive behavior should consult a primary care provider or mental health professional as soon as possible (see Chapter 12).

Intestinal Gas

flatus
intestinal gas

Annoying, embarrassing, and offensive are all terms that come to mind when intestinal gas, or flatus, is the subject. Actually, everyone's body produces and releases gas from the lower intestinal tract. Most gas leaves the GI tract without our awareness because it is odorless. Sometimes if the gas passes through too quickly, it is quite noticeable!

Bacteria in the large intestine may cause gas formation when specific indigestible carbohydrates ferment. These may include some of the carbohydrates found in legumes (dried beans) such as soybeans and black beans. Another cause may be lactose intolerance, the inability to break down lactose, the carbohydrate in milk. The lactose then begins to ferment, causing gas buildup, bloating, and diarrhea (see Chapter 4). The longer any undigested substances linger in the large intestine, the more likely it is that fermentation will occur, leading to gas formation. This may result from constipation that slows the passage of chyme through the GI tract. Another factor contributing to flatulence may be eating so quickly that food is swallowed in large clumps, which thereby requires more time to sufficiently process the chyme before it is excreted.[5, 6]

Generally, however, intestinal gas can probably be decreased through some simple changes of food-related behaviors. Here are some suggestions:

- If making dietary changes to increase fiber intake, gradually add more fibrous foods such as legumes to allow the system to adjust.
- Notice the effects of drinking milk. Drink fluid milk in small quantities over several weeks, working up to an 8-oz glass. Note at what level gas may develop. If a problem occurs, consider eating other milk-related products such as yogurt, cheese, or lactose-reduced milk.
- Increase fluid intake and consume sufficient amounts of fiber to prevent constipation.
- Take the time to consider which foods may be problematic. Each person's cause of flatulence may be different.
- Eat slower and chew foods more thoroughly.

Constipation

There is no clear definition of constipation. It is usually considered as difficulty and discomfort associated with defecation. Individuals may interpret these terms differently and may vary in their natural urge to defecate. Not everyone needs to pass a bowel movement daily. Normal functioning ranges from once a day to every 3 days. Generally, constipation is recognized as straining to pass hard, dry stools.[5,6,8]

The causes of constipation are usually related to lifestyle behaviors that can easily be changed. The following strategies address these behaviors:

- *Choose foods that are high in fiber, particularly insoluble fiber such as wheat bran.* Whole grain breads, fruits, and vegetables are important foods to consume. Fiber provides bulk that softens the stool and makes elimination easier.
- *Listen to body signals and follow a schedule that allows time for a bowel movement to occur.* Ignoring the natural urge to defecate causes feces to remain in the colon longer. This allows more water to be withdrawn, resulting in harder, drier feces.
- *Exercise regularly.* Lack of exercise can lead to a loss of tone in the muscles of the lower GI tract.
- *Drink enough liquids.* Fluid intake should be approximately 8 to 10 cups a day. Most of us need to consciously remember to drink water or other liquids to fulfill this need.
- *Relax.* Stress tightens muscles throughout the body and may inhibit proper bowel functioning.
- *Consume regular meals.* The body works best with an intake of nutrients and fiber throughout the day.

Constipation caused by lifestyle behaviors should respond to these strategies. If using these strategies does not relieve constipation, consult a primary care provider to rule out more serious disorders (see the Health Debate box, "Laxative Use: By Prescription Only?").

✺ Diarrhea

Diarrhea is the passing of loose, watery bowel movements that result when the contents of the GI tract move through too quickly to allow water to be absorbed in the large intestine. Diarrhea may be caused by bacterial or viral infections (e.g., stomach virus or intestinal flu), lactose intolerance, spoiled foods, or even stress.[2,5] An occasional bout is not a problem. However, if diarrhea continues, too much

constipation
straining to pass hard, dry stools; slow movement of feces through colon

diarrhea
frequent passing of loose, watery bowel movements

HEALTH DEBATE
Laxative Use: By Prescription Only?

Over-the-counter (OTC) drugs can be purchased without a prescription. This allows individuals the opportunity for self-care for minor health discomforts. Some OTC drugs, when misused, allow individuals to often inappropriately self-medicate. Laxatives as an OTC are among those drugs that may be misused.

Laxatives stimulate the colon by increasing peristalsis or causing water to be pulled into the colon to increase and soften the bulk of feces. Those that increase peristalsis are stimulant cathartics (e.g., Ex-Lax, Correctol), chemicals that have a pharmacologic effect by irritating intestinal mucosa to action. Laxatives that increase the bulk of feces are called *bulk-forming* (e.g., Naturacil, FiberCon, Metamucil); the water that is absorbed by the high-fiber laxative increases and softens feces, which facilitates elimination.

Both actions of laxatives replicate what fibrous foods and sufficient fluids do. Consider that prunes and prune juice naturally contain dihydroxyphenyl isatin, a chemical that initiates peristalsis, and wheat bran is especially effective for softening stool consistency. Consuming 20 to 35 g of dietary fiber daily from fruits, vegetables, and whole grains plus an adequate fluid intake most often alleviates the need for laxatives.

Although the action of laxatives seems harmless, the long-term effects are not. The following issues should be considered regarding laxative use:

- Regular use of laxatives to relieve constipation prevents underlying health problems from being diagnosed. Serious health disorders such as blockages from tumors or colon cancer might be masked by misuse of laxatives.
- Laxative use can become a habit. The muscles of the lower GI tract become addicted to or dependent on the pharmacologic effect of laxatives. Eventually after weeks and months of laxative use, the muscles are unable to respond on their own to contract with enough force for elimination to occur. They require the stimulation from cathartic laxatives to initiate bowel movements.
- Laxatives are too easily abused. Use of laxatives is not a weight-loss technique. Some individuals who are obsessed with their body weight have misconceptions about laxatives. They believe that by taking laxatives after eating, the food just eaten will leave the body without being absorbed and so will not cause weight gain. This is not the case. Most of the caloric value of food is still absorbed, but what is lost are vitamins and minerals, particularly calcium. These nutrients need to be in the digestive system longer to be absorbed. Often, laxative abuse is a symptom of anorexia nervosa or bulimia. The abuse may consist of taking laxatives several times during the course of a day. The physical effects of the laxative drugs may cause additional health problems. Addiction to laxatives requires medical assistance as soon as possible.

Most cases of constipation can be resolved by lifestyle changes as suggested in this chapter. By relying on a drug to alleviate a health problem, we are not taking responsibility for maintaining our own health.

Primary care providers may recommend the use of laxatives to relieve constipation that results from drug interactions, therapeutic dietary restrictions, or specific medical conditions. Most use of laxatives, however, is self-prescribed.

If laxatives are often misused, should they be available as an OTC drug or only by prescription? What do you think?

Compiled from Mahan LK, Escott-Stump S: Krause's food, nutrition, and diet therapy, ed 10, Philadelphia, 2000, WB Saunders; and Payne WA, Hahn DB: Understanding your health, ed 6, New York, 2000, McGraw-Hill.

fluid and electrolytes may be lost and dehydration is possible. Efforts should be made to drink enough fluids to replace those lost. This is particularly a concern for infants and older adults who are most at risk for dehydration; their fluid levels are delicately maintained. Infants cannot easily communicate their thirst, and a greater proportion of their bodies consists of fluid; the excessive loss of fluid has serious consequences of electrolyte imbalance and a distorted ability to maintain body temperature and functions.

Among older adults, the ability to detect thirst may be diminished; disorientation, sometimes assigned to senility, may actually be a sign of dehydration that, if not diagnosed, may further deteriorate health. Because it is a symptom of illness, diarrhea that lasts more than 2 days should be discussed with a primary care provider to uncover the actual cause.

TOWARD A POSITIVE NUTRITION LIFESTYLE: CONTRACTING

Have you ever made a bet? Contracting is similar to making a bet with a friend; only the object of the bet is a health behavior. A contract is a specific agreement with yourself or between you and a friend, spouse, or other relative. The agreement represents your willingness to attempt to change a health-related behavior. The advantage to contracting is that the goal or behavior change is clearly defined and observable. You also decide on a specific period within which to achieve the goal. As with a bet, you determine a reward or penalty for not completing the contract. (Yes, contracts with oneself are much easier to break.) By practicing a new health-related behavior for a specific period, the expectation is that the change will be permanent.

A contract with yourself might be to drink eight glasses of water a day for a week to relieve constipation. The change to increase fluid intake is a behavior you can directly control and observe. Although the aim is to alleviate constipation, which may not be a behavior you can consciously change, its risk factors can be reduced. At the end of the week, your reward could be to see a movie with a friend, whereas the penalty might be to clean out your messy bedroom closet.

Perhaps you have noticed that you regularly work through lunch and eat at your desk. The result is that heartburn has become a regular discomfort, and a discussion of remedies is often the topic of work breaks. A co-worker complains that she seems unable to break her habit of buying a high-calorie Danish pastry with her coffee each morning. You could contract with her that for the next 2 weeks you will eat lunch away from your desk, either in the employee cafeteria or at a local restaurant. She contracts with you that she will buy fruit instead of a Danish pastry for her morning snack. If you both complete the contracts, a reward could be to lunch together at a special restaurant. If only one person completes a contract, the penalty could be for the "loser" to pack a brown bag lunch for a week for the "winner."

Contracting is applicable to many aspects of contemporary lifestyles and is limited only by our imagination.

SUMMARY

The processes of digestion, absorption, and metabolism work together to provide all body cells with energy and nutrients. Within the digestive system, all foods are digested. The organs forming the GI tract include the mouth, esophagus, stomach, small intestine, and large intestine or colon. Peristalsis, segmentation, and the action of sphincter muscles regulate the movement of foodstuff through one organ to the next. Other structures support the digestive system, including the teeth, tongue, salivary glands, liver, gallbladder, and pancreas. They assist with mechanical digestion (chewing) and chemical digestion (producing or storing secretions).

The main site of nutrient digestion and absorption is the small intestine. Once absorbed, nutrients are truly "inside" the body. Nutrients then enter the circulatory system of the bloodstream or lymphatic system and become available to all cells. When the nutrients reach the cells, they may be metabolized. The metabolic changes allow the nutrients to fulfill many cell functions.

Some common GI tract health problems are caused by lifestyle behaviors that can be changed. Prevention suggestions and treatment strategies for heartburn, intestinal gas, and constipation consider the effect of lifestyle behaviors. Although vomiting and diarrhea are not usually related to lifestyle, each has an impact on the functioning of the GI tract.

THE NURSING APPROACH
Using Your Skills in Informal Situations

As a student nurse—and ultimately a licensed nurse—you may often be approached by patients and their families, neighbors, friends, and your own family for advice on common health problems. As your nursing judgment grows, you will gain confidence in distinguishing situations where general health advice can be given apart from situations that require referral to another healthcare professional.

The GI health problems discussed in this chapter are the kinds of problems about which people feel comfortable seeking the advice of a nurse. For example, someone may ask which over-the-counter (OTC) remedy you recommend for heartburn. Although you may suggest one or two products, this is a good opportunity for you also to engage in some health teaching about the prevention of heartburn.

Media advertisements try to "sell" people on the idea of taking OTC heartburn prevention medication before meals that tend to cause them distress. Often, if people would eat more sensibly and avoid foods that cause them to have heartburn, they wouldn't need the medication. They should be discouraged from relying on the "quick fix" offered by a pill.

It's amazing how, even in a social situation, people you don't know well confide personal information just because you are a nurse. A good example of this is the problem of constipation. Some people will describe the details of their malady and a long history of their home remedies. You might wish you didn't know such intimate information about people you associate with socially. However, in some situations you can give brief but helpful information about dietary solutions to the problem or make arrangements to talk to the person in more detail at a more suitable time.

It doesn't always take a lot of time to give valuable advice about health and wellness, and it can make a big difference in the life of the questioner.

APPLYING CONTENT KNOWLEDGE

James, a senior at the local university, is completing his internship at the rock radio station while continuing to work at his part-time job. Without any time to spare, he has been eating meals whenever he can, often from fast-food restaurants. These meals are usually gobbled quickly in his car. Lately, though, he is feeling stressed and is experiencing heartburn. List three lifestyle behaviors that James could change to possibly reduce heartburn.

Web Sites of Interest

American College of Gastroenterology

www.acg.gi.org

The American College of Gastroenterology is an organization that focuses solely on the study and medical treatment of disorders of the GI tract. This Web site provides extensive information for consumers and health professionals and is a particularly good site for the latest information on GERD.

American Dental Association

www.ada.org/index.html

This official site of the American Dental Association presents a wealth of knowledge related to maintaining the health of our teeth and mouths through up-to-date news items and search tools.

American Medical Association

www.ama-assn.org

As the official site of the American Medical Association, this site supplies information on the organization along with press releases, journal articles, and valuable links to related topics.

Health Care Information Resources

www-hsl.mcmaster.ca/tomflem/top.html

This site provides links to general health information through numerous sites on specific illnesses, wellness, professional U.S. and Canadian health associations, alternative medicine, and more.

References

1. Klein S, Cohn SM, Alpers DH: The alimentary tract in nutrition. In Shils ME et al, eds.: *Modern nutrition in health and disease,* ed 9, Philadelphia, 1999, Williams & Wilkins.
2. Thibodeau GA, Patton KT: *Anatomy and physiology,* ed 4, St Louis, 1999, Mosby.
3. Logue AW: *The psychology of eating and drinking: an introduction,* ed 2, New York, 1991, Freeman.
4. Williams SR: *Nutrition and diet therapy,* ed 8, St Louis, 1997, Mosby.
5. Mahan LK, Escott-Stump S: *Krause's food, nutrition, and diet therapy,* ed 10, Philadelphia, 2000, WB Saunders.
6. Wellness Letter Berkeley, ed: *The new wellness encyclopedia,* Boston, 1995, Houghton Mifflin.
7. Garner DM, Garfinkel PE: *Handbook for treatment for eating disorders,* ed 2, New York, 1997, Guilford Press.
8. Food and Nutrition Board, National Research Council: *Diet and health: implications for reducing chronic disease risk,* Washington, DC, 1989, National Academy Press.

CHAPTER 4

Carbohydrates

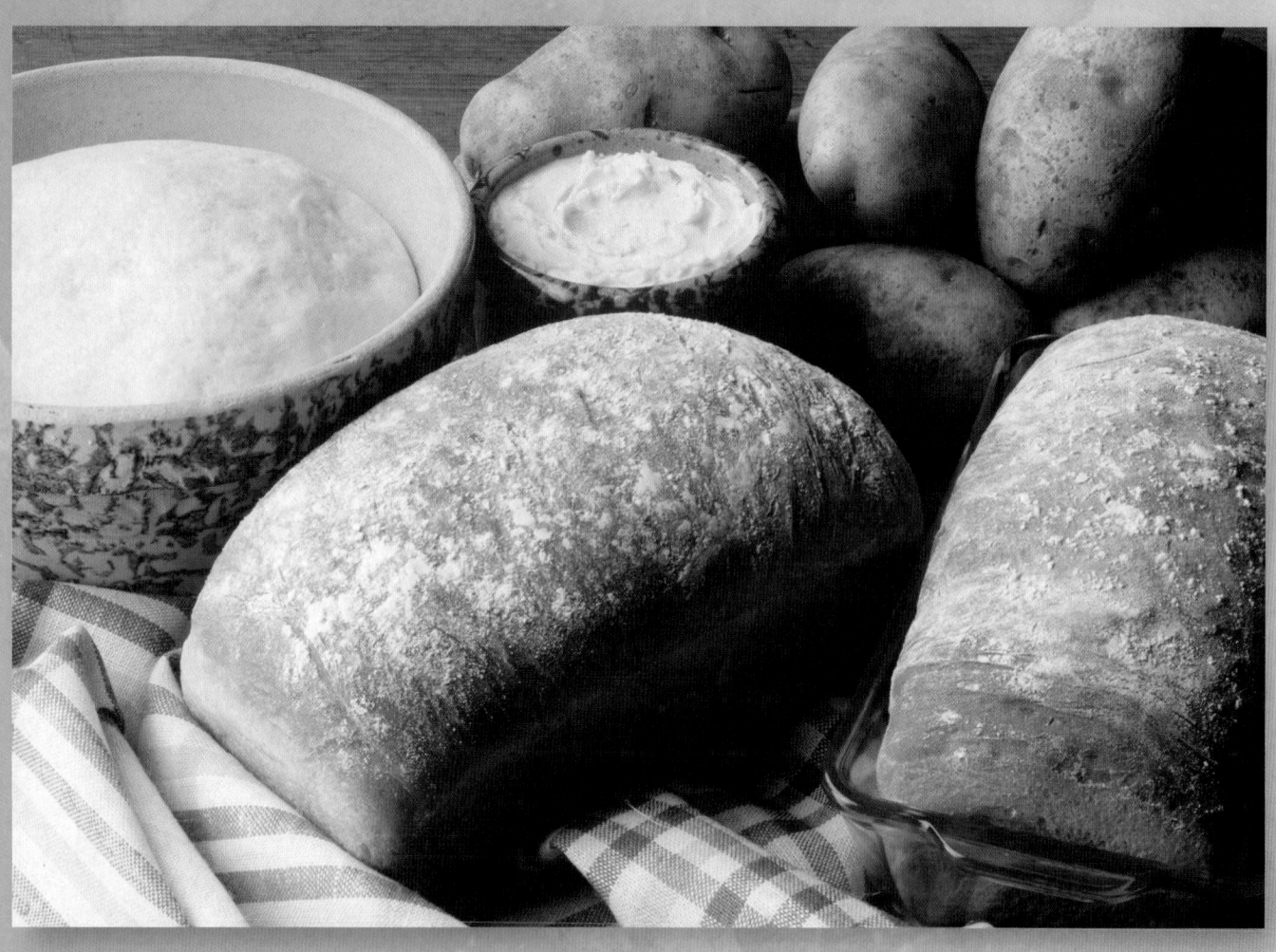

All carbohydrates are organic compounds composed of carbon, hydrogen, and oxygen in the form of simple carbohydrates or sugars.

ROLE IN WELLNESS

Nature has provided us with an excellent source of energy—carbohydrates. Found primarily in plants, carbohydrates are a convenient and economical source of calories for people throughout the world. Carbohydrates include simple carbohydrates, such as glucose and sucrose, and complex carbohydrates, which include starch and dietary fiber. Each type of carbohydrate serves a distinct role in nourishing the body.

In addition to serving as an energy source, some carbohydrates are also used as sweetening agents. When carbohydrate sweeteners are found naturally in foods, such as in fruits, they are also accompanied by essential nutrients. The sweetness makes eating nutrient-dense foods even more enjoyable. Some carbohydrates also supply dietary fiber.

The energy value of carbohydrates was discovered in 1844.[1] The recognition that increasing our consumption of carbohydrates provides preventive health benefits is more recent. Increased levels of complex carbohydrates appear to reduce the risk factors associated with chronic diet-related disorders such as heart disease, diabetes, and some cancers.[2] The Acceptable Macronutrient Distribution Range (AMDR) for carbohydrate is 45% to 65% of kcaloric intake per day as primarily complex carbohydrates.[2] *Healthy People 2010* concurs, recommending that we meet the dietary guideline's minimum average daily goals of at least five servings of vegetables (including legumes) and fruits and at least six servings of grain products.[3] This advice is reflected in the Food Guide Pyramid. The five to six servings of fruits and vegetables and six to eleven servings of bread, cereal, rice, and pasta provide adequate amounts of complex carbohydrates (Figure 4-1).

Considering carbohydrates through the health dimensions provides perspective on their role in wellness. The physical health dimension depends on our ability to provide our bodies with enough carbohydrate kcalories for energy and enough complex carbohydrates and fiber consumption for optimum body functioning.

carbohydrates
organic compounds composed of carbon, hydrogen, and oxygen

Acceptable Macronutrient Distribution Range (AMDR)
intake range for an energy source associated with reduced chronic disease risk while supplying adequate essential nutrients

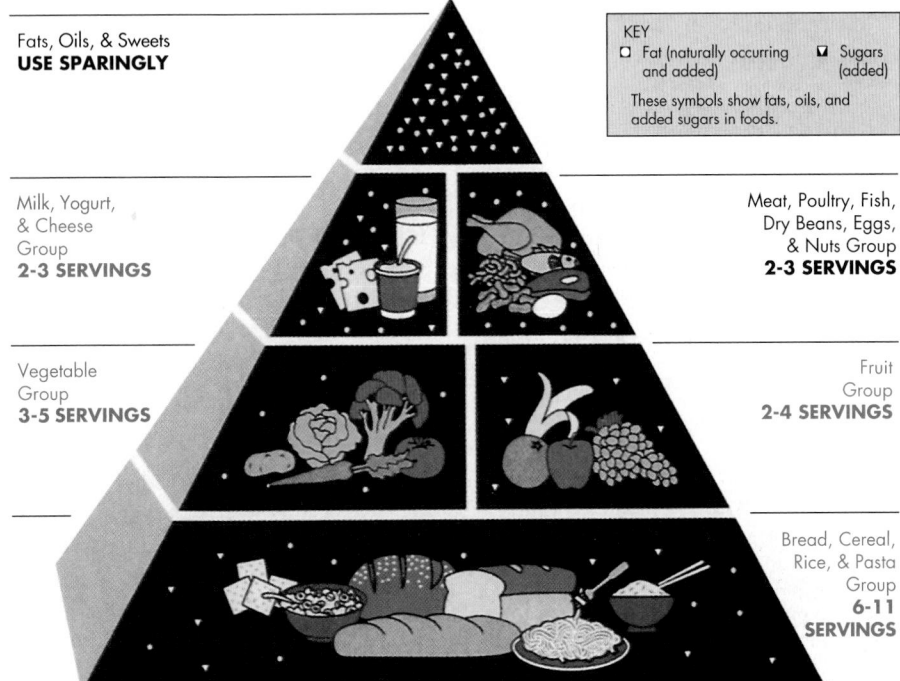

Figure 4-1 The Food Guide Pyramid, highlighting sources of complex carbohydrates. (From US Department of Agriculture: *USDA human nutrition information*, Pub No 249, Washington, DC, 1992, US Government Printing Office.)

Issues related to the role of carbohydrates are often in the headlines. Our ability to process research findings and decide the level of impact on our food choices reflects our level of intellectual, or reasoning, health dimension. For some of us, emotional health may depend on the ability to distinguish hypoglycemic (low blood glucose) symptoms. If we are aware of our personal response to normal hypoglycemia, can we then distinguish real emotional issues from those caused by hypoglycemia? The social dimension of health may also be tested. Social groups can support change or make changes more difficult to achieve. Will you or your client feel comfortable snacking on a banana (a good fiber source) while chocolate bars are unwrapped? The spiritual health dimension has ties to carbohydrates because several religions view bread, a carbohydrate, as the "staff of life."

FOOD SOURCES

The carbohydrates we consume are primarily from plant sources. As plants grow, they capture energy from the sun and chemically store it as carbohydrates. This process, called *photosynthesis,* depends on water from the earth, carbon dioxide from the atmosphere, and chlorophyll in the plant leaves to form carbohydrates.

All carbohydrates are organic compounds composed of carbon, hydrogen, and oxygen in the form of simple carbohydrates or sugars. When linked together, these simple sugars form three sizes of carbohydrates: monosaccharides, disaccharides, and polysaccharides (Figure 4-2).

Monosaccharides are composed of a single carbohydrate unit. Glucose, fructose, and galactose are monosaccharides.

Disaccharides consist of two single carbohydrates bound together. Sucrose, maltose, and lactose are disaccharides.

simple carbohydrates
monosaccharides and disaccharides

monosaccharides
a sugar composed of a single carbohydrate unit; glucose, fructose, and galactose are monosaccharides
disaccharides

a sugar formed by two single carbohydrate units bound together; sucrose, maltose, and lactose are disaccharides

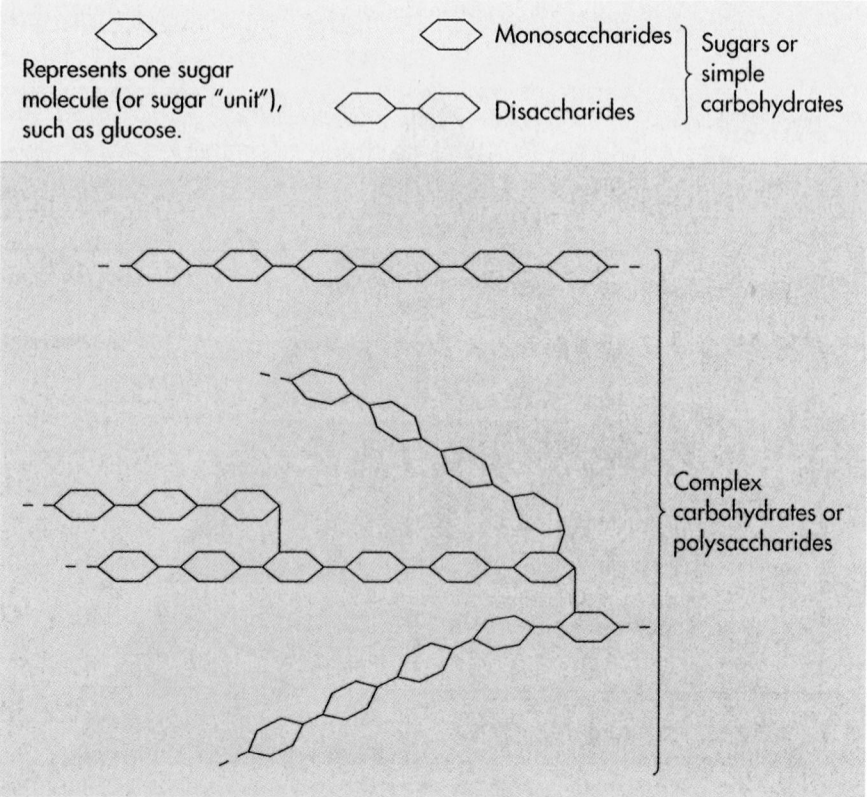

Figure 4-2 Structure of monosaccharides, disaccharides, and polysaccharides. (From Pagecrafters; in Guthrie HA, Picciano MF: *Human nutrition,* New York, 1995, McGraw-Hill.)

Table 4-1
Dietary Carbohydrates

Carbohydrate Type	Common Names	Naturally Occurring Food Sources
Simple		
Monosaccharides		
Glucose	Blood sugar	Fruits, sweeteners
Fructose	Fruit sugar	Fruits, honey, syrups, vegetables
Galactose	—	Part of lactose, found in milk
Disaccharides		
Sucrose (glucose + fructose)	Table sugar	Sugar cane, sugar beets, fruits, vegetables
Lactose (glucose + galactose)	Milk sugar	Milk and milk products
Maltose (glucose + glucose)	Malt sugar	Germinating grains
Complex		
Polysaccharides		
Starches (strings of glucose)	Complex carbohydrates	Grains, legumes, potatoes
Fiber (strings of monosaccharides, usually glucose)	Roughage	Legumes, whole grains, fruits, vegetables

Polysaccharides consist of many units of monosaccharides joined together. Starch and fiber are food sources of polysaccharides, whereas glycogen is a storage form in the liver and muscles.

The three sizes of carbohydrates are divided into two classifications: *simple carbohydrates* (monosaccharides and disaccharides) and *complex carbohydrates* (polysaccharides) (Table 4-1). Both are valuable sources of carbohydrate energy. There are differences, however, between the health values of simple and complex carbohydrates found in the foods we consume. Although simple carbohydrates primarily provide energy in the form of glucose, fructose, and galactose, complex carbohydrates may also provide fiber in addition to glucose.

polysaccharides
a carbohydrate consisting of many units of monosaccharides joined together; starch and fiber are food sources, and glycogen is a storage form in the liver and muscles

CARBOHYDRATE AS A NUTRIENT WITHIN THE BODY

Function

Carbohydrates provide energy, fiber, and naturally occurring sweeteners (sucrose and fructose). Energy is the only real nutrient function of carbohydrates; the roles of fiber and carbohydrate sweeteners are discussed later in this chapter. Carbohydrates supply energy in the most efficient form for use by our bodies. If enough carbohydrate is provided to meet the energy needs of the body, protein can be spared or saved to use for specific protein functions. This service of carbohydrates is called the *protein-sparing effect*.

When adequate amounts of carbohydrates are available, both carbohydrates and small amounts of fats are used for energy. When there are not enough carbohydrates available, fat is metabolized, which results in the formation of ketones, intermediate products of fat metabolism. The body without distress easily disposes of low levels of ketones. If carbohydrate levels continue to be insufficient to meet energy demands, increased levels of ketones overwhelm the physiologic system and ketoacidosis develops; ketoacidosis affects the pH balance of the body, which can be lethal if uncontrolled. Although lipids and proteins can, if necessary, provide energy for most bodily needs, the brain and nerve tissues function best on glucose from carbohydrates.

Digestion and Absorption

Our food sources of carbohydrates tend to be disaccharides (sugars) and polysaccharides (starches). The gastrointestinal (GI) tract has the role of digesting carbohydrates into monosaccharides for easy absorption. The digestive process begins in the mouth. Mechanical digestion breaks food into smaller pieces and mixes the carbohydrate-containing food with saliva that contains amylase, called *ptyalin*. This begins the hydrolysis of starch into the simpler carbohydrate intermediary forms of dextrin and maltose. In the small intestine, intestinal enzymes and specific pancreatic amylase work on starch intermediary products to continue the breakdown to monosaccharides.

Enzymes specific for disaccharides (lactase for lactose, sucrase for sucrose, maltase for maltose) are secreted by the small intestine's brush border cells, which then hydrolyze disaccharides into monosaccharides. (For more information, see the Cultural Considerations box, "The Missing Enzyme," and the Teaching Tool box, "Lacking Lactose? No Problem!") After an active absorption process (i.e., one that requires energy input), absorptive cells in the small intestine take up these monosaccharides. Once glucose, fructose, and galactose enter the villi, the portal blood circulatory system transports them to the liver. The liver removes fructose and galactose and converts them to glucose. This glucose may be used immediately for energy or for glycogen formation, a storage form of carbohydrate that provides an always-ready source of energy. Figure 4-3 summarizes carbohydrate digestion.

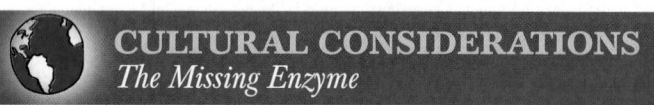

CULTURAL CONSIDERATIONS
The Missing Enzyme

Many adults throughout the world are unable to easily digest the lactose found in milk. Approximately 75% of the adult world population and 25% of the U.S. population are lactose maldigesters. This condition, lactose intolerance, occurs when the body does not produce enough lactase, a digestive enzyme that breaks lactose into glucose and galactose. When the lactose sits in the large intestine, bacteria begin to ferment the undigested lactose, causing diarrhea, bloating, and increased gas formation.

Lactase deficiency may be the result of a primary or secondary cause. Primary lactose intolerance is caused by a genetic factor that limits the ability to produce lactase. Although small amounts of lactose can often be tolerated, the level of lactase produced cannot be enhanced. The condition is common among Asian/Pacific Islanders (Asian Americans), Africans (African Americans), Hispanics (Hispanic Americans), Latinos, and Native Americans. In the United States the prevalence of lactose intolerance caused by maldigestion or low lactose levels is about 62% to 100% in Native Americans, 90% in Asian/Pacific Islanders, 80% in African Americans, 53% in Hispanic Americans, and 15% in Caucasians.

One explanation for primary lactose intolerance is that the ability to digest milk is age-related. Consider that the milk of mammals, including humans, was intended for the young to consume during periods of major growth. The ability to digest milk may diminish because the biologic need is lessened as maturity is reached. Older adults may also develop lactose intolerance as the aging process diminishes the production of some digestive enzymes such as lactase.

Sometimes secondary lactose intolerance occurs when a chronic gastrointestinal illness affects the intestinal tract, reducing the amount of lactase produced (see Chapter 17). Even a bout of an intestinal virus or flu can cause temporary lactose intolerance. Most of these individuals recover and are again able to digest lactose.

Application to nursing: Health professionals can guide clients to determine what amounts of lactose-containing foods can be tolerated despite low lactase levels. Fine tuning eating styles may require the assistance of a registered dietitian (RD) to assure adequate consumption of calcium-containing foods.

Compiled from McBean LD, Miller GD: *Allaying fears and fallacies about lactose intolerance*, J Am Dietetic Assoc 98:671, 1998; Suarez FL, Savaiano DA: *Diet, genetics and lactose intolerance*, Food Technol 51:74, 1997; *National Institutes of Health:* Lactose intolerance, *National Institutes of Health Pub No 94-2751, Washington, DC, 1994, National Digestive Diseases Information Clearinghouse.*

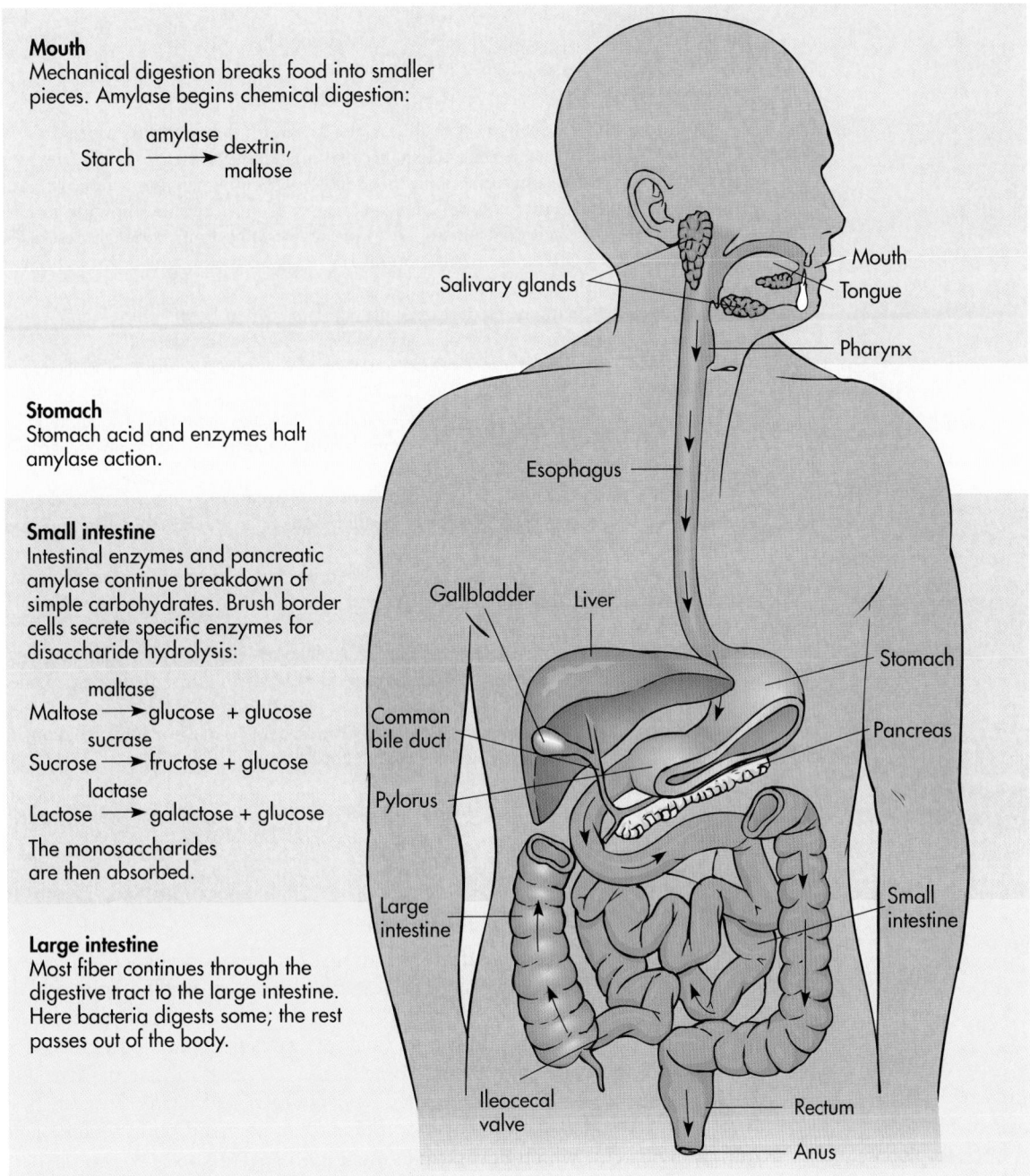

Mouth
Mechanical digestion breaks food into smaller pieces. Amylase begins chemical digestion:

$$\text{Starch} \xrightarrow{\text{amylase}} \text{dextrin, maltose}$$

Stomach
Stomach acid and enzymes halt amylase action.

Small intestine
Intestinal enzymes and pancreatic amylase continue breakdown of simple carbohydrates. Brush border cells secrete specific enzymes for disaccharide hydrolysis:

$$\text{Maltose} \xrightarrow{\text{maltase}} \text{glucose + glucose}$$
$$\text{Sucrose} \xrightarrow{\text{sucrase}} \text{fructose + glucose}$$
$$\text{Lactose} \xrightarrow{\text{lactase}} \text{galactose + glucose}$$

The monosaccharides are then absorbed.

Large intestine
Most fiber continues through the digestive tract to the large intestine. Here bacteria digests some; the rest passes out of the body.

Salivary glands — Mouth — Tongue — Pharynx — Esophagus — Gallbladder — Liver — Common bile duct — Pylorus — Large intestine — Ileocecal valve — Stomach — Pancreas — Small intestine — Rectum — Anus

Figure 4-3 Summary of carbohydrate digestion and absorption. (From Rolin Graphics.)

Glycogen: Storing Carbohydrates

Glycogen is carbohydrate energy stored in the liver and in muscles. The amount held in the muscles of an adult is 150 grams (600 kcalories); 90 grams (360 kcalories) are stored in the liver. Retrieved as needed for energy, glycogen is quickly broken down by enzymes to produce a surge of energy. The process of converting glucose to glycogen is glycogenesis.

Glycogen levels can be significantly increased through physical training and dietary manipulations (see Chapter 9). It is still considered a relatively limited source of energy compared with the amounts of energy stored in body fat.

glycogen
carbohydrate energy stored in the liver and in muscles

glycogenesis
the process of converting glucose to glycogen

Lactose intolerance is not an illness and should not undermine a person's sense of wellness. To assure that clients receive an adequate supply of nutrients usually consumed in lactose-containing dairy products—especially calcium, riboflavin, and vitamin D—without the use of supplements, consider suggesting the following to clients:

- Experiment with different portion sizes of lactose-containing foods to determine individual levels of tolerance; small amounts up to 1/2 cup consumed throughout the day can often be tolerated.
- Use over-the-counter lactase-enzyme tablets when consuming dairy products (presently available as Lactaid, Lactrase, Dairy Ease, and others).
- If available, purchase lactose-reduced dairy products such as fluid milk, ice cream, and soft cheeses.
- Consume foods high in nutrients found in lactose-containing foods; high-calcium foods include broccoli, eggs, kale, spinach, tofu, shrimp, canned salmon, sardines with bones, and calcium-fortified orange juice.
- Consume hard cheeses (in moderate amounts because of fat content) that contain lower lactose levels such as Swiss, cheddar, Muenster, Parmesan, Monterey, and provolone.
- Avoid softer cheeses (or experiment to learn level of tolerance), including ricotta, cottage cheese, mozzarella, Neufchâtel, and cream cheese (see Appendix L for lactose content of foods).
- Test tolerance of different brands of yogurt; lactose levels may vary according to processing variations. Generally, lactase bacteria in yogurt culture hydrolyzes some of the lactose.
- Consider supplementation if these dietary modifications are not achieved; consult with a nutritionist for an appropriate supplement.

Data from Nelson JK et al.: Mayo Clinic diet manual, *ed 7, St Louis, 1994, Mosby.*

Metabolism

A primary aspect of carbohydrate metabolism is the maintenance of blood glucose homeostasis at a level between 70 to 120 mg/dl. Sources of blood glucose, the most common sugar in the blood, may be from carbohydrate and noncarbohydrate sources. Dietary starches and simple carbohydrates provide blood glucose after digestion and absorption; glycogen stored in the liver and muscle tissue is converted back to glucose in a process called glycogenolysis. Intermediate carbohydrate metabolites are also a source of blood glucose. The metabolites include lactic acid and pyruvic acid, which occur when muscle glycogen is used for energy.

Noncarbohydrates can also provide blood glucose. Gluconeogenesis is the process of producing glucose from fat and protein. It is not as efficient as using carbohydrate directly for glucose. As fat is metabolized into fatty acids and glycerol (see Chapter 5), the smaller glycerol portion can be converted by the liver into glycogen, which is then available for glucose needs through glycogenolysis. Protein, which is composed of numerous combinations of amino acids, may also be a source of glucose. Some of these amino acids are glucogenic; if they are not used for protein structures, they can be metabolized to form glucose.

Blood glucose is a source of energy to all cells. Glucose may be used immediately as energy or converted to glycogen or fat; both conversions provide energy for the future. Although glycogen can be converted back to glucose, the conversion of glucose to fat is irreversible. Glucose cannot be formed again but is stored as fat and, if needed, is metabolized later as fat, although its original source was carbohydrate.

Glucose is essential for brain function and cell formation, particularly during pregnancy and growth. Because the body can form glucose through gluconeogenesis

glycogenolysis
the process of converting glycogen back to glucose

gluconeogenesis
the process of producing glucose from fat and protein

from protein and fat, glucose technically is not an essential nutrient. Gluconeogenesis can provide some glucose but not enough to meet essential needs if dietary carbohydrate is insufficient. To compensate (as previously discussed), **ketone bodies** can be used for energy. Ketone bodies are created when fatty acids are broken down for energy when sufficient carbohydrates are unavailable; this process of fat metabolism, however, is incomplete. If dietary carbohydrate continues to be insufficient, a buildup of ketones results, causing ketosis.

ketone bodies
a breakdown product of fatty acid catabolism

Blood Glucose Regulation

Metabolism of glucose and regulation of blood glucose levels are controlled by a sophisticated hormonal system. **Insulin**, a hormone produced by the beta cells of the islets of Langerhans, functions to lower blood glucose levels. It does this by enhancing the conversion of excess glucose to glycogen through glycogenesis or to fat stored in adipose tissue. Insulin also eases the absorption of glucose into the cells so that the use of glucose as energy is increased.

insulin
a hormone produced by the pancreas that regulates blood glucose levels

Whereas insulin functions to lower blood glucose levels, other hormones raise glucose levels. The pancreas produces two hormones with this function, glucagon and somatostatin. **Glucagon** stimulates conversion of liver glycogen to glucose, assisting the regulation of glucose levels during the night; **somatostatin,** secreted from the hypothalamus and pancreas, inhibits the functions of insulin and glucagon. Several adrenal gland hormones also have a role in raising blood glucose levels. Epinephrine enhances the fast conversion of liver glycogen to glucose. Steroid hormones function against insulin and promote glucose formation from protein. Produced by the pituitary gland, growth hormone and adrenocorticotropic hormone (ACTH) function as insulin inhibitors. The thyroid hormone thyroxine affects blood glucose levels by enhancing intestinal absorption of glucose and releasing epinephrine.

glucagon
a pancreatic hormone that releases glycogen from the liver

somatostatin
a hormone produced by the pancreas and hypothalamus that inhibits insulin and glucagon

SIMPLE CARBOHYDRATES

Monosaccharides

Glucose, often called *blood sugar,* is the form of carbohydrate most easily used by the body. It is the simple carbohydrate that circulates in the blood and is the main source of energy for the central nervous system and brain. Glucose is rapidly absorbed into the bloodstream from the intestine, but it needs insulin to be taken into the cells where energy is released.

Fructose is the sweetest of the sugars. Although fruits and honey contain a mixture of sugars, including sucrose, fructose provides the characteristic taste of fruits and honey. After absorption from the small intestine, fructose circulates in the bloodstream. When it passes through to the liver, liver cells rearrange fructose into glucose.

Galactose is rarely found in nature by itself but is part of the disaccharide lactose, the sugar found in milk. Absorbed like fructose, galactose is converted to glucose by the liver.

Disaccharides

Sucrose is formed from the pairing of units of glucose and fructose. We know it as *table sugar.* Sugar cane and sugar beets are two sources of sucrose, and it is found naturally in fruits. Because it contains fructose, sucrose is quite sweet. Sucrose has a special place in our history of food consumption and is further explored in the section titled "Sugar—A Special Disaccharide."

Maltose is created when two units of glucose are linked. It is available when cereal grains are about to germinate and the plant starch is broken down into maltose. The majority of maltose in human nutrition is created from the breakdown of starch in the small intestine. Maltose is of particular value in the production of beer and other malt beverages. When maltose ferments, alcohol is formed.

Lactose is composed of glucose and galactose. It is sometimes called *milk sugar* because it is the primary carbohydrate in milk.

Sugar–A Special Disaccharide

The term *sugar* is a word with many meanings. Sugar may refer to the simple carbohydrates (monosaccharides and disaccharides). Sucrose, the disaccharide naturally found in many fruits, is also called sugar. White table sugar refers to sucrose extracted from sugar cane and sugar beets. Sugar may also be an umbrella term used to cover numerous kcaloric-sweetening agents used in our food production system, although U.S. commercial law defines sugar as "sucrose." There is a distinction between how the term *sugar* is used on a label versus its use by a biologist, chemist, or nutritionist. Often, blood glucose levels are called *blood sugar levels*. It is important that we, as health professionals, be aware that our clinical use of the term may confuse clients. Concerns about sugar focus on the following three issues: (1) sources in the food supply, (2) consumption levels, and (3) health effects.

Sources in the Food Supply.   Sugar in our food supply may include the following nutritive sweeteners: refined white sugar, brown sugar, dextrose, crystalline fructose, high fructose corn syrup (HFCS), glucose, corn sweeteners, lactose, concentrated fruit juice, honey, maple syrup, molasses, and reduced energy polyols or sugar alcohols (e.g., sorbitol, mannitol, xylitol)[4] (Table 4-2). All forms of sugar are chemically similar; each provides kcalories and most do not contain any other nutrients. Blackstrap molasses does contain iron, but other more nutrient-dense sources of iron are easily available. Honey, which seems less processed than other sweeteners, provides only a trace of minerals and therefore is as nonnutritious as any other sweetener.

The Food and Drug Administration (FDA) categorizes some sweeteners as Generally Recognized as Safe (GRAS) ingredients and others as food additives (see Chapter 2). For food additives, an acceptable daily intake (ADI) is determined as the amount that a person can safely consume daily over one's life without risk. Table 4-2 lists descriptions, regulatory status, and energy amounts provided by sweeteners.

Consumption Levels.   Our national intake of refined white sugar has declined, whereas consumption of HFCS has greatly increased since the 1970s. In the 1970s, a process was perfected in which HFCS, a very sweet-tasting syrup, can be made from corn syrup. HFCS is less expensive to produce than refined sugar and is also sweeter. Used extensively in food manufacturing, it has replaced refined white sugar in many products, such as soft drinks.

Health Effects.   The health concerns regarding sugar consumption include nutrient displacement, dental caries, and the related issues of obesity and diabetes.

Does it matter to our bodies what the source of the sweet taste is? That depends. A major health concern is nutrient displacement. Displacement occurs when whole foods, which are minimally processed, are not eaten and are replaced by foods containing added sugars. If we eat candy and soda instead of a sandwich and juice for lunch, we lose a number of important nutrients (Figure 4-4).

Foods and drinks with added sugars often contain empty kcalories that provide few nutrients. Because all forms of sugar are chemically similar, the sucrose in fruits is actually the same as the sucrose in a cream-filled doughnut. The difference, however, is that naturally occurring vitamins, minerals, and fiber available in the fruit are not available in the doughnut. The doughnut's empty kcalories can replace kcalories from other foods that might contain a natural sweetener and also provide vitamins, minerals, protein, complex carbohydrates, and fiber. Consumption of excessively sugared food does not support wellness goals because it probably replaces other more nutrient-dense foods.

Dental caries are related to eating concentrated sweets and sticky carbohydrates. Sugar supports the growth of bacteria, which promotes the formation of

Table 4-2
Nutritive and Nonnutritive Sweeteners

Descriptions, other names, regulatory status, and amount of energy provided by nutritive and nonnutritive sweeteners

Sweetener	Kcal/g	Regulatory Status	Other Names	Description
Sucrose	4	GRAS[b]	Granulated: coarse, regular, fine; powdered; confectioner's; brown; turbinado, demerara; liquid: molasses	Sweetens; enhances flavor; tenderizes, allows browning, and enhances appearance in baking; adds characteristic flavor with unrefined sugar.
Fructose	4	GRAS	High fructose corn syrups: 42%, 55%, 90% fructose; crystalline fructose: 99% fructose	Sweetens; functions like sucrose in baking. Some persons experience a laxative response from a load of fructose (greater than or equal to 20 g). May produce lower glycemic response than sucrose.
Polyols-monosaccharide				
Sorbitol	2.6	GRAS (label must warn about a laxative effect)	Same as chemical name	50% to 70% as sweet as sucrose. Some persons may experience a laxative effect from a load of sorbitol (greater than or equal to 50 g).
Mannitol	1.6	Permitted for use on an interim basis (label must warn about a laxative effect)	Same as chemical name	50% to 70% as sweet as sucrose. Some persons may experience a laxative effect from a load of mannitol (greater than or equal to 20 g).
Xylitol	2.4	GRAS	Same as chemical name	As sweet as sucrose.
Saccharin	0	Permitted for use on interim basis (label must contain cancer warning and amount of saccharin in the product)	Sweet 'n Low	200% to 700% sweeter than sucrose. Noncariogenic and produces no glycemic response. Synergizes the sweetening power of nutritive and nonnutritive sweeteners. Sweetening power is not reduced with heating.
Aspartame	4[a]	Approved as a general-purpose sweetener	Nutrasweet, Equal	160% to 220% sweeter than sucrose. Noncariogenic and produces limited glycemic response. New forms can increase its sweetening power in cooking and baking.
Acesulfame K	0	Approved for use as a tabletop sweetener and as an additive in a variety of desserts, confections, and alcoholic beverages	Sunette[c]	200% sweeter than sucrose. Noncariogenic and produces no glycemic response. Sweetening power is not reduced with heating. Can synergize the sweetening power of other nutritive and nonnutritive sweeteners.
Sucralose	0	Approved for use as a tabletop sweetener, and as an additive in a variety of desserts, confections, and nonalcoholic beverages	Splenda[d]	600% sweeter than sucrose. Noncariogenic and produces no glycemic response. Sweetening power is not reduced with heating.

From Position of the American Dietetic Association: Use of nutritive and nonnutritive sweeteners, J Am Dietetic Assoc 98:580, 1998.
[a]Provides limited energy to products because of its sweetening power.
[b]GRAS = Generally Recognized As Safe by the US Food and Drug Administration.
[c]Hoechst Food Ingredients, Edison, NJ.
[d]McNeil Specialty Products Company, New Brunswick, NJ.

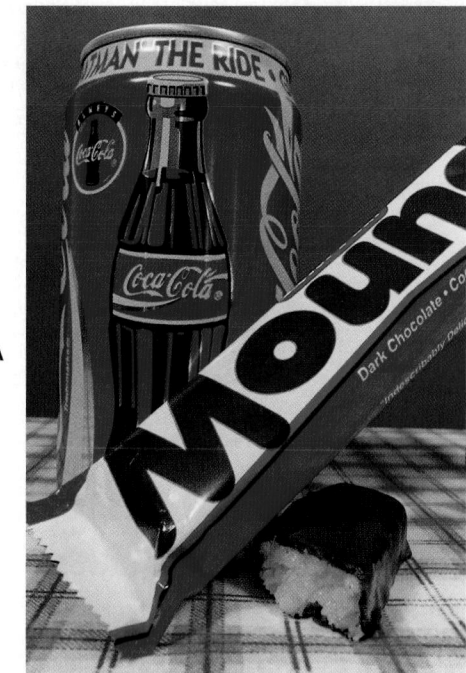
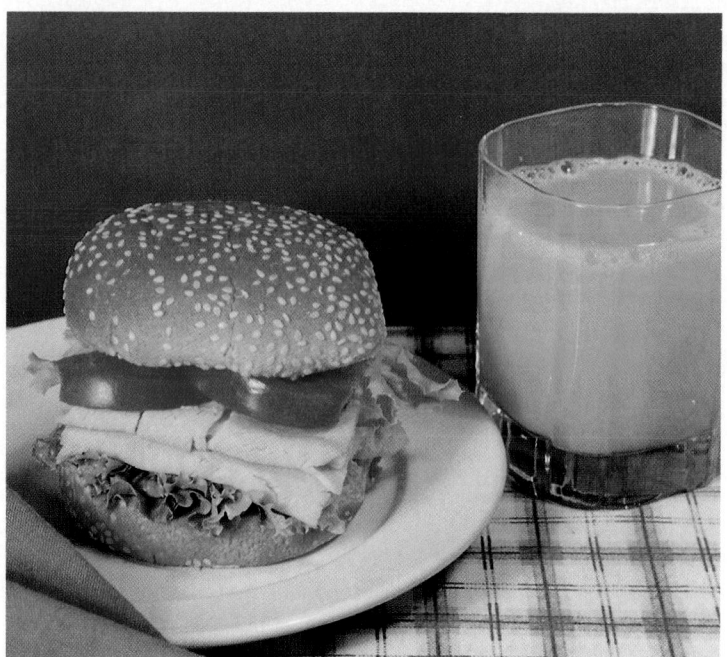

Figure 4-4 Consuming products with added sugars (**A**) can displace more nutrient-dense foods (**B**). (From Joanne Scott/Tracy McCalla.)

plaque. Plaque leads to tooth decay. Ways to decrease the development of caries are to eat sweets at the end of meals—rather than between meals—and to monitor the quantity and frequency of sugar intake. Sticky, sugary foods are more cariogenic than sweet liquids. Optimal dental hygiene reduces plaque formation and promotes dental health.

A misconception is that obesity is caused by high sugar intake only. In fact, obesity may be caused by an excess intake of kcalories from any of the energy nutrients, which is then stored as body fat. Many sugared foods are also high in fat. Because fat is the most energy-dense nutrient, fat intake may be more of a risk factor for obesity than sugar intake.

There is no confirmed relationship between the level of sugar intake and increased risk of developing type 2 diabetes mellitus.[2] Persons with diabetes are counseled to restrict their intake of concentrated sweets to assist the regulation of insulin needs once the disorder is confirmed. However, consumption of sweets does not cause the disorder. These issues become complicated because obesity is a risk factor for type 2 diabetes mellitus. Health concerns related to obesity and type 2 diabetes mellitus are explored in Chapters 10 and 19.

A myth that sugar consumption by children produces hyperactivity or disorders such as attention-deficit hyperactivity disorders (ADHD) continues to be perpetuated. Controlled research studies have consistently failed to support this assertion.[4] More than likely, excessively active behavior is related to the occasions at which sugared foods such as cake and candy are ingested. If children regularly consume excessive amounts of refined sugar, their overall dietary intake may be nutritionally deficient, possibly resulting in altered behaviors.

So how much sugar is acceptable? Moderate amounts are alright when our diets are low in fat and high in fiber. The *Dietary Guidelines for Americans* suggests consuming sugars in moderation (see Chapter 2). The DRI report on carbohydrates suggests that added sugars be kept to 25% or less of energy intake on a daily basis. Less added sugar intake assures a dietary intake that is adequate in complex carbohydrates.[2] By following recommendations to increase consumption of fruits and vegetables to at least five servings a day and complex carbohydrates to six servings a day, we can reduce our intake of simple sugars.

Other Sweeteners

Other available sweeteners are sugar alcohols (polyols) and alternative sweeteners. **Sugar alcohols**, also called sugar replacers to avoid confusion with noncarbohydrate alcohol, are nutritive sweeteners because they provide 2 to 3 kcalories per gram but less than the 4 kcalories per gram of carbohydrates. They occur naturally in fruits and berries. Sorbitol, mannitol, and xylitol are the most commonly used sugar alcohols. **Alternative sweeteners** are nonnutritive substances produced to be sweet-tasting; however, they provide no nutrients and few, if any, kcalories. For food production purposes, sugar alcohols are synthesized rather than derived from natural sources.[4] Aspartame and saccharin are commonly used alternative sweeteners.

Sugar alcohols have several advantages when replacing sugar. They are less cariogenic than sucrose. In contrast to carbohydrate sugars, sugar alcohols do not encourage the growth of bacteria in the mouth that leads to tooth decay. In fact, xylitol may actually prevent cavity formation and be protective when used in chewing gum. Although chemically related to carbohydrates, sugar alcohols are absorbed more slowly and incompletely than carbohydrates. The longer absorption time leads to a slower rise in blood glucose levels or reduced glycemic response. Persons with diabetes may be able to consume moderate amounts of these sweeteners and still control their blood glucose levels.

A disadvantage of sugar alcohols is that if large quantities are consumed, they may ferment in the intestinal tract because of their slower absorption rate. This fermentation may cause gas and diarrhea. The incomplete absorption results in a lower caloric value per gram, and thus less energy is available. Therefore the sugar alcohols are called *reduced-energy* or *low-energy sweeteners*.[4]

Alternative sweeteners, also called *artificial sweeteners*, are manufactured to be used as sweetening agents in food products. Their function is to replace naturally sweet kcaloric substances such as sugar, honey, and other sucrose-containing substances. Alternative sweeteners most commonly used in the United States and approved by the FDA are aspartame, saccharin, acesulfame potassium (K), and sucralose. Often, a combination of alternative sweeteners is used that results in an increased sweet sensation.[4]

Aspartame is formed by the bonding of the amino acids phenylalanine and aspartic acid. When consumed, aspartame is digested and absorbed as two separate amino acids. Although aspartame contains the same kcalories as sucrose, much less aspartame is needed to get the same sweet taste because it is 180 to 200 times sweeter than sucrose. This provides so few kcalories that aspartame can be considered a nonkcaloric sweetener. Approved in 1981 and used in a wide variety of products such as soft drinks, cereals, chewing gum, frozen snacks, and puddings, aspartame is consumed in more than 100 countries. In 1996, aspartame was approved as a general purpose sweetener for all foods and beverages.

Several studies have shown aspartame to be safe, yet some individuals have reported side effects thought attributable to aspartame consumption. These included allergic reactions such as rashes; edema of the lips, tongue, and throat; and respiratory difficulties.[5] However, within controlled settings, these reactions were not replicated; this means that aspartame consumption was not responsible for the allergic reactions.[6,7] The Internet has been used by some individuals to spread false information about aspartame, linking its consumption to disorders that range from multiple sclerosis to brain tumors to arthritis. Logically, one substance would not cause an array of serious disorders. Investigation of the authors of the e-mails revealed noncredible sources, and therefore the FDA maintains its approval of aspartame.[8]

Individuals with the genetic disorder **phenylketonuria (PKU)** should not consume aspartame because their bodies cannot break down excess phenylalanine,

sugar alcohols
nutritive sweeteners related to carbohydrates that provide 2-3 kcalories per gram; sorbitol, mannitol, and xylitol are sugar alcohols, also called sugar replacers.

alternative sweeteners
nonnutritive sweeteners (or artificial sweeteners) synthetically produced to be sweet-tasting but do not provide nutrients and few, if any, kcalories; aspartame, saccharin, acesulfame K, and sucralose are alternative sweeteners

aspartame
a nonnutritive sweetener formed by the bonding of the amino acids phenylalanine and aspartic acid

phenylketonuria (PKU)
a genetic disorder in which the body cannot break down excess phenylalanine

which results in a buildup that causes medical problems. All products containing aspartame have a warning label to alert individuals with PKU. This warning should apply to pregnant women as well. Because the fetus would be exposed to excess phenylalanine before the presence of PKU could be determined, the safest approach is to restrict consumption of aspartame during pregnancy.

The general adult population (for a 132-lb person) is advised to keep daily aspartame consumption at or below 50 milligrams per kilogram body weight (the equivalent of 83 packets of Equal, an aspartame product) or 14 12-oz cans of aspartame-sweetened soda.[4] Aspartame, when added to products, is most often listed by its original brand name of Nutrasweet.

saccharin
a nonnutritive sweetener

Saccharin has had a stormy history since it was accidentally discovered more than 100 years ago.[8] The storm began when some animal studies indicated an association between excessive saccharin consumption and the development of bladder cancer.[8] In 1977 the FDA proposed a ban of saccharin. Many Americans were upset that the only available nonkcaloric sweetener was to be banned. The public outcry was so great that Congress, in an unusual move, created a moratorium to prevent the ban. In addition, Congress passed legislation requiring all products that contain saccharin to clearly state a warning that the consumption of saccharin may be hazardous to health.

The danger from saccharin is probably minimal. The risk of bladder cancer does not appear to apply to humans because no noticeable increase of bladder cancer has occurred. In addition, an association between cancers and saccharin is not supported by studies of individuals with diabetes who tend to consume high amounts of saccharin.[4] Consequently, the moriatorium is no longer in effect as the FDA is not pursuing the ban on saccharin. Saccharin is now considered an interim food additive to be used in cosmetics, pharmaceuticals, and foods and beverages.[4] For food products, the amount of saccharin contained must be identified on the product label. Restrictions include that beverages may contain no more than 12 mg/oz or less than 30 mg per food serving.[9]

Compared with other alternative sweeteners, saccharin has a bitter aftertaste. To mask this, it is often used in combination with other alternative sweeteners. Saccharin is still valuable because it is extremely sweet—300 to 700 times as sweet as sucrose.[9]

acesulfame K
a synthetically produced non-nutritive sweetener

Acesulfame K received FDA approval in 1988. Synthetically produced, it tastes 200 times sweeter than sucrose, but it is not digestible by the human body and therefore provides no kcalories. Acesulfame K is approved for use in a variety of products, from chewing gum to nondairy creamers, but so far its use has been limited. One advantage of this product over aspartame is that it can be used for baking. Heat does not affect its sweetening ability, whereas heat destroys the sweet taste of aspartame.[8] Persons who must severely limit potassium intake because of medical nutritional therapy for renal disorders should consult a registered dietitian about acceptable levels of acesulfame K.

sucralose
a nonnutritive sweetener, suitable for cooking, that provides no energy

Sucralose (trichlorogalactosucrose) was approved by the FDA in April 1998 for use in desserts, candies, nonalcoholic beverages, and as a tabletop sweetener. Made from chemically altered sucrose, sucralose provides no energy but is 600 times sweeter than sucrose. Because the body poorly absorbs it, sucralose passes through the digestive tract and is excreted in urine. An advantage of sucralose is that it can be used in baking and cooking.[4]

Other artificial sweeteners are awaiting approval. Cyclamate, a sweetener used in Canada, appeared in the United States for only a 20-year period until it was banned in 1970.[8] At that time the FDA determined that cyclamate consumption caused bladder cancer in animals. Although reevaluation of the data revealed that the risk to humans is minimal, the ban is still in effect. It is, however, being appealed.[4] Stevia is created from the leaves of a South American shrub. Although it is used as a sweetener, it cannot be sold as such because it does not have FDA approval as a food additive. Sufficient evidence of safety has not been submitted to meet U.S. standards. Nonetheless, stevia can be sold as a dietary supplement based on the dietary supplement legislation of 1994.[8] Because it is used in very small quantities and has no caloric value, individuals with diabetes may use stevia as another sweetener alternative.

Sweet Decisions

Should you consume foods with real sugar or artificial sugar? Which is the best? Which is the worst? There are no clear answers, but here is a way to decide. A concept used with food safety issues is a benefits-risks analysis. Does the benefit of consuming a substance outweigh the risk? This analysis can be applied to the decision of whether to consume artificial sweeteners.

Benefits of consuming artificial sweeteners include experiencing a sweet taste with lower kcalories and less cariogenic effect than sucrose. Many people believe these sweeteners are an important part of their weight reduction effort. For most, though, the saved kcalories are often replaced by consuming other kcaloric foods, thereby undermining their weight-loss efforts.[10] However, within a formal multidiscipline weight-control program, aspartame-sweetened foods and beverages supported long-term weight-loss maintenance among obese women.[11] In other words, individuals who successfully lose weight and maintain that weight loss do not depend solely on alternative sweeteners. Instead, changes in exercise and food selection behaviors are the basis of the weight change.

Risks associated with the use of alternative sweeteners may involve safety concerns. This is a difficult issue to sort. Because sucrose in the form of white table sugar has been used for thousands of years, we essentially have a large-scale study of its safety for humans. In contrast, alternative sweeteners have existed only for a century or less. Because alternative sweeteners are not naturally formed in plants or animals, their safety must be determined through research studies.

The research process is difficult. Rather than using humans as test subjects, researchers use animals. The test animals are given extremely large doses of the artificial sweeteners and are followed by researchers for several generations of their species. If the physiology of the animals is affected, particularly in regard to cancerous tumors, the substance may be regarded as too dangerous for consumption by humans. The difficulty is that the extremely large doses given to the animals does not replicate the amounts that would be typically consumed by humans. Concerns raised include whether the substance caused the tumor or whether the excessive quantity interfered with normal cell function. Also, how many animals need to be affected for a substance to be considered dangerous and in what animal generation of the experiment? Attention should also be paid to who funds such studies. If the company manufacturing the substance pays for the research, does that affect the interpretation of the results? These are difficult questions with which health scientists and FDA officials grapple.

This is an area, however, in which we can make a personal decision whether to consume products that contain alternative sweeteners. Based on our analysis of the benefits and risks, we can decide if our wellness goals are better met by consuming a moderate amount of sucrose or a reasonable intake of alternative sweetened products.

COMPLEX CARBOHYDRATES: POLYSACCHARIDES

Polysaccharides are many units of monosaccharides held together by different kinds of chemical bonds. These types of bonds affect the ability of the body to digest polysaccharides and therefore account for the classification of polysaccharides as complex carbohydrates.

complex carbohydrates
polysaccharides of starch and fiber

Starch

All starchy foods are plant foods. Starch is the storage form of plant carbohydrate. The strings of glucose that form starch are broken down by the digestive tract to provide glucose. Food sources of starch include grains, legumes, and some vegetables and fruits. Grains are the best source of starch. Grains provide more carbohydrates than any other food category.[2] Grains are consumed in many forms and include wheat, oats, barley, rice, corn, and rye. The overall health value of processed grain products differs based on their sugar, fat, and fiber content.

Breads, bagels, breakfast cereals, pasta, pancakes, grits, oatmeal, and other cooked cereals provide high-quality complex carbohydrates. These grain products may also contain fiber if made with whole grains. Depending on the spreads and toppings served, they may also be low in fat. Main dish items such as pizza, rice casseroles, and pasta mixtures create another category of complex carbohydrate foods. Other foods such as crackers, cakes, pies, cookies, and pastries also provide carbohydrates but often contain considerable amounts of added sugar and fats; they should be eaten in moderation.

Legumes (beans and peas) are another significant source of complex carbohydrates. They are low in fat and are also an excellent source of fiber, iron, and protein. Available dried, canned, or frozen, beans can be easily incorporated into commonly eaten foods.

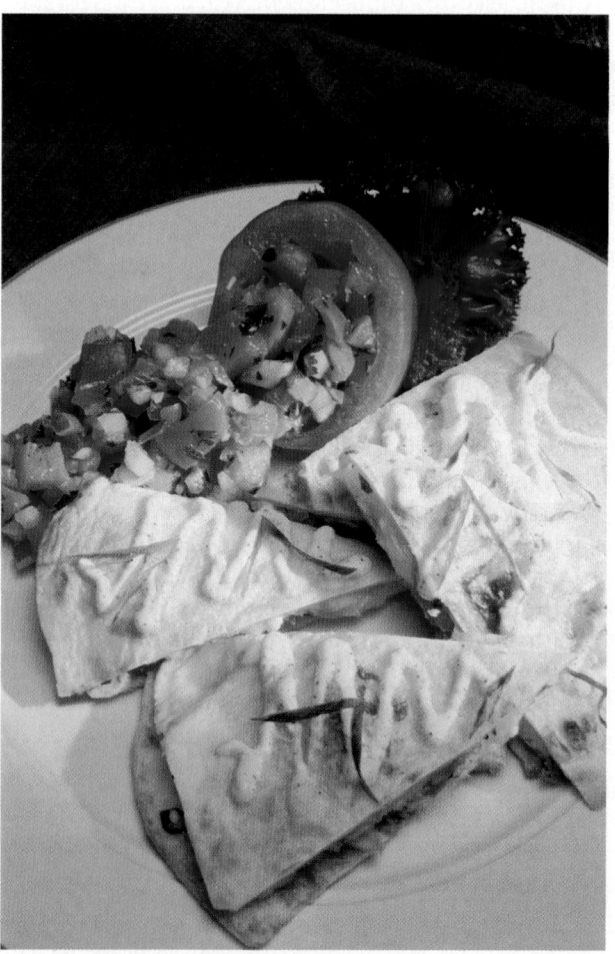

Ethnic cuisines can provide a source of complex carbohydrates and variety in one's diet. (From PhotoDisc.)

Multicultural influences have expanded our exposure to inexpensive and versatile legumes. Mexican foods feature kidney beans as an ingredient of taco fillings and chili. Puerto Rican and Caribbean meals highlight rice and beans in savory sauces. Hearty Italian-style soups often depend on white and kidney beans combined with pasta. An African influence is reflected in dishes that combine black-eyed peas with meats or green vegetables. Hummus, a chickpea paste dip of Middle Eastern heritage, is often served with pita bread or vegetables.

Among vegetable sources of starch, potatoes lead the way. We consume potatoes in so many ways that we sometimes forget their humble "roots." As a root vegetable, the potato is a powerhouse of complex carbohydrates, fiber, vitamins, and even some protein. Unfortunately, some of the ways we prepare potatoes undo their positive health benefits. Most potatoes are processed into products loaded with fat and sodium. Nutritionally, potato chips have little in common with baked potatoes. The best health value is to eat potatoes in the least-processed form. Instead of French fries, choose a baked potato or prepare mashed potatoes with skim milk and a small amount of margarine.

Other starchy root vegetables include parsnips, sweet potatoes, and yams. Sweet potatoes and yams provide the same nutrients as white potatoes plus significant amounts of beta-carotene. Carrots and some varieties of squash such as acorn and butternut also provide starch and beta-carotene. Beta-carotene, a substance the body can convert into vitamin A, may have a protective effect against some forms of cancer.

Fiber

Fiber, like starch, also consists of strings of simple sugars. Unlike starch, however, human digestive enzymes cannot break down fiber. Dietary fiber consists of substances in plant foods including carbohydrates and lignin that, for the most part, cannot be digested by humans.[2] We do not produce digestive juices strong enough to break down the bonds that hold the simple carbohydrates of most plant fibers, so fiber "passes through" our bodies without providing kcalories or nutrients. Its texture provides bulk that thickens chyme and eases the work of the gastrointestinal (GI) muscles that regulate movement of the food mass.

Although human digestive juices cannot digest fiber, micro flora that normally reside in the colon use fiber as a medium for microbial fermentation, resulting in the synthesis of vitamins and the formation of short chain fatty acids (SCFA). The bacteria that reside in the colon synthesize several vitamins, including vitamin K, biotin, B_{12}, folate, and thiamin. Only vitamin K and biotin can be absorbed in sufficient amounts from the colon to be significant; the other vitamins are absorbed from the small intestine so that the synthesized vitamins are not bioavailable.[12] The SCFA that are produced can be absorbed and used for energy by the mucosa of the colon, thereby maintaining the health of the colon epithelial cells.[12] The effects of SCFA also increase fecal matter bulk.

Dietary fiber actually refers to several kinds of carbohydrate substances from different plant sources; all serve similar functions in the human body. Dietary fibers are divided into two categories based on their solubility in fluids. Soluble dietary fibers, which dissolve in fluids, include pectin, mucilage, psyllium seed husk, guar gum, and other related gums. Soluble fiber thickens substances. Insoluble dietary fibers do not dissolve in fluids and therefore provide structure and protection for plants. Some insoluble dietary fibers are cellulose and hemicellulose. Lignin, considered a dietary fiber, is composed of chains of alcohol rather than carbohydrate.

Foods are sometimes classified based on the predominate type of fiber they contain. Oatmeal is a good source of soluble fiber because oat bran, part of the whole oatmeal grain, is particularly high in soluble fiber. But the whole grain is a good source of insoluble fiber as well. Although Table 4-3 specifically lists foods con-

dietary fiber
carbohydrates (polysaccharides) and lignin in plant foods that cannot be digested by humans

soluble dietary fibers
dietary fibers that dissolve in fluids

insoluble dietary fibers
dietary fibers that do not dissolve in fluids

Table 4-3
Dietary Fibers and Food Sources

Fibers	Food Sources
Insoluble	
Cellulose Hemicellulose Lignin	Whole grains, brown rice, buckwheat groats, whole wheat flour, whole wheat pasta, oatmeal, unrefined cereals, vegetables, wheat bran, seeds, popcorn, nuts, peanut butter, leafy green vegetables such as broccoli
Soluble	
Pectin Mucilage Guar and other gums	Kidney beans, split peas, lentils, chick peas (garbanzo beans), navy beans, soybeans, apples, pears, bananas, grapes, citrus fruits (oranges and grapefruits), oat bran, oatmeal, barley, corn, carrots, white potatoes

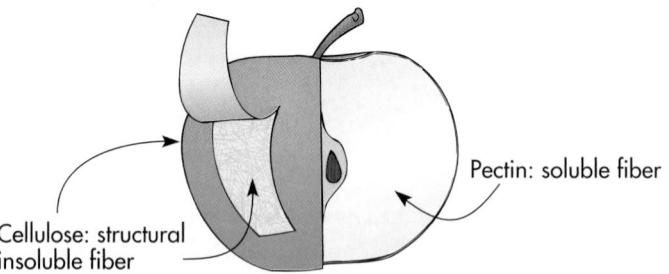

Pectin: soluble fiber

Cellulose: structural insoluble fiber

Figure 4-5 In an apple, insoluble fiber (cellulose) inside and in the skin provides structure, and soluble fiber (pectin) inside adds substance.

taining soluble and insoluble dietary fiber, many fiber-rich foods contain some of each kind of fiber. For example, an apple is a source of the soluble dietary fiber pectin, which is part of the inside "stuff" of the apple. An apple also provides cellulose, an insoluble dietary fiber that forms the structure of the apple and gives it its characteristic shape (Figure 4-5). Popcorn is another source of insoluble dietary fiber that has been with us for a long time (see the Cultural Considerations box, "The 'Pop' Heard Through the Centuries").

Health Effects

All the health benefits of fiber improve the physical functioning of the human body. The benefits are not directly nutritional but instead allow the body to function at a more efficient level. Each of the following disorders listed may develop because of genetic predisposition, environmental factors, or lifestyle behaviors. However, the risk of developing these disorders seems to increase when consumption of dietary fiber is low. Because eating sufficient fiber appears to be a preventive factor, we consider the benefits of fiber on primary disease prevention. Primary prevention aims to avert the initial development of a disorder or health problem. The risk of developing obesity, constipation, hemorrhoids, diverticular disease, and colon cancer may be decreased by regularly consuming sufficient amounts of fiber.

Obesity.   Eating high-fiber foods seems to make weight control easier. The volume of fibrous foods makes us feel fuller, so less food is consumed. Often, fibrous foods replace those that are higher in fat and kcalories. Regularly eating foods high in fiber and low in fat may reduce or prevent obesity.

Constipation.   Fiber, particularly insoluble fiber such as wheat bran and whole grains, prevents the dry, hard stools of constipation (see Chapter 3). A sufficient

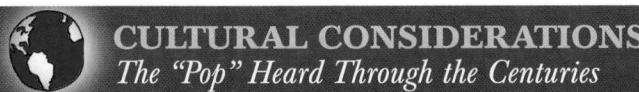

CULTURAL CONSIDERATIONS
The "Pop" Heard Through the Centuries

Next time you're at the movies digging into a giant tub of popcorn, be sure to appreciate one of the tastier contributions of Native Americans to our food supply. Five thousand years ago, popping corn was first created over an open fire. The delectable popcorn added variety to ways to prepare corn, a mainstay of the Native American diet. Gifts of popcorn necklaces and popcorn beer were made by the Indians of the Caribbean in the 1500s, and the Aztecs used popcorn in religious ceremonies. And what would Thanksgiving have been without some popped corn—compliments of the Wampanoag tribe?

Popcorn most likely originated in Mexico, but it was also grown in India, Sumatra, and China years before Columbus "discovered" America. Biblical stories of "corn" in Egypt were not entirely true. The term *corn* meant the most commonly used grain of a region. In Scotland and Ireland, corn referred to oats; in England, corn was wheat. In the Americas, the common corn was maize and the two terms, *corn* and *maize*, became synonymous.

Today, special varieties of corn have been developed for their "popping" characteristics. When heated, water in the corn kernel creates steam. This steam, unable to escape through the heavy skin of the kernel, causes an explosion that exposes the white starchy center. Fortunately, the skin remains attached to the starch, which makes popcorn an excellent source of dietary fiber.

Although all popcorn provides dietary fiber, some of the ways it is prepared negate this health benefit. Popcorn laden with butter and covered with salt is not a healthful snack. Nor is a batch popped with the aid of oil, even if vegetable oil is used. Microwaveable packets of popcorn are equally deceiving because they contain oil and other additives. We also may easily be mislead into eating more than we should because each bag contains four servings, which most of us devour single-handedly.

Instead, return to the native style—fresh air-popped corn. Air-popping appliances and microwave containers eliminate the need for oil. Better toppings include sodium-reduced salt, garlic powder, or Cajun spices. While devouring your wholesome snack, remember to acknowledge the inventiveness of Native Americans.

Compiled from Early popcorn history, *Chicago*, 1996, *Popcorn Institute*; Elkort M: The secret life of food, *Los Angeles*, 1991, Jeremy P. Tarcher.

fiber intake assures larger, softer stools that are easier to eliminate. Less straining during elimination also reduces the risk of developing hemorrhoids (enlarged veins in the anus) and diverticular disease.

Diverticular Disease. Diverticular disease is a disorder that primarily afflicts people in their 50s and 60s. Some 30% of Americans over the age of 50 are estimated to have the disorder.[13] It begins, however, earlier in life because of a consistently low intake of dietary fiber.

Diverticular disease affects the large intestine. Pockets (diverticula) develop on the outside walls of the intestine, as shown in Figure 4-6. Low-fiber diets may create increased internal pressure from segmentation muscles attempting to move the food mass because the bulk of fiber is not available. This pressure may then weaken intestinal muscles. Weakened muscles are more at risk for the formation of diverticula. If feces get caught in the pockets, bacteria may develop, multiply, and cause serious and painful inflammation (diverticulitis). Medical treatment and nutritional therapy are necessary and are discussed in Chapter 17.

Colon Cancer. Eating enough dietary fiber may also reduce the risk of developing colon cancer. Two risk factors for colon cancer related to fiber intake are a high dietary fat intake and exposure to carcinogenic substances in the GI tract.[14] The higher our fat intake, the more at risk we are for colon cancer. By eating more fiber, we tend to eat less fat. Fiber foods tend to replace foods that are high in fat. Because foods containing fiber are bulkier, they seem to fill the stomach quicker, providing satiety sooner and with less kcalories than foods containing fat. Fiber-containing foods such as fruits and vegetables may contain other substances that may be protective for the colon.

Consumption of sufficient fiber also speeds the movement of substances through the GI tract, potentially reducing exposure of the colon to potential carcinogens.[2,14] In particular, the longer feces sit in the large intestine or colon, the greater the chance for carcinogenic substances to form and affect the colon. A direct mecha-

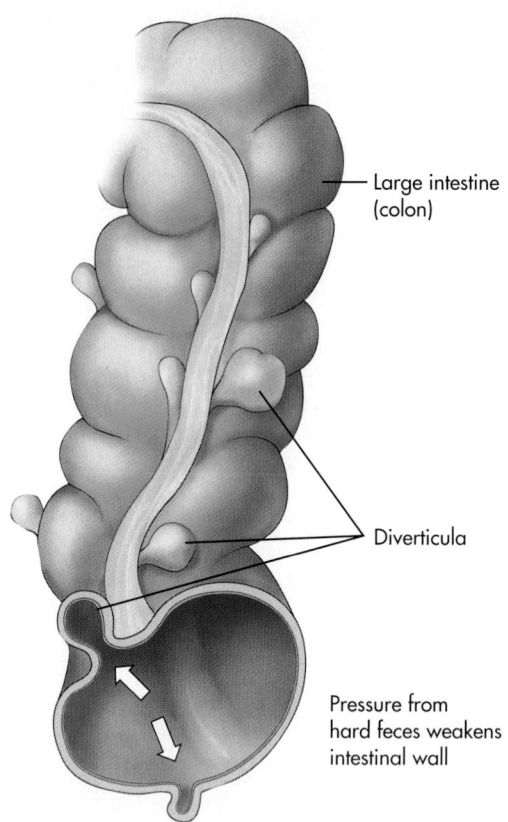

Figure 4-6 Diverticulosis in the colon. A low-fiber diet may increase the risk for this disorder.

nism of dietary fiber occurs when dietary fiber absorbs potential carcinogens that then leave the body in feces. Wheat bran has been shown to provide this benefit.[15]

Ongoing laboratory research has led to speculation that the SCFA (also called *volatile fatty acids*) produced by the fermentation of fiber in the colon may have a role in protecting colon cells from cancer and may inhibit cholesterol synthesis. These roles, although still being explored, may reveal further physiologic benefits of dietary fiber.[12]

Heart Disease.   Two heart disease risk factors are high blood cholesterol and increased lipid levels (see Chapter 5 for recommended levels). Increasing dietary fiber consumption can lower blood cholesterol and lipid levels in two ways: (1) fiber foods replace higher fat foods, particularly those containing dietary cholesterol and saturated fats; and (2) soluble fiber such as pectin (citrus fruits and apples), guar gum (legumes), and oat gum (oat bran) binds lipids and cholesterol as they move through the intestinal tract.[16] Because fiber is not digested, neither are the bound lipids and cholesterol, which make less cholesterol and lipids available to the bloodstream.

Diabetes Control.   Dietary fiber intake may help persons with diabetes to stabilize blood glucose levels. Diabetes mellitus affects the body's ability to regulate blood glucose levels. When fiber is consumed, particularly soluble fiber, glucose may be absorbed more slowly. The slower absorption rate of glucose may keep blood glucose within acceptable levels.[16]

Consuming increased amounts of dietary fiber may seem to decrease the risk for developing certain diseases; however, reduced risk may not be caused by the increased dietary fiber but by other dietary changes. By eating more foods that contain fiber, we may reduce our intake of high-fat foods. It may be the lower fat intake that reduces the risk, not the higher dietary fiber intake.

When the recommended increase of dietary fiber intake is fulfilled by fiber-containing foods, there tend to be few health risks. Problems may develop when fiber supplements or other forms of processed or purified fiber, such as oat or wheat bran, are consumed in large quantities. When used as a supplement, excessive quantities of purified fiber can overwhelm the GI tract and lead to blockages in the small intestine and colon.[16] This is a serious medical condition that fortunately is a rare occurrence.

Bioavailability of minerals may be lowered by the presence of fiber-containing foods. Some fibers and substances in whole grains, such as phytates and oxalates, may bind minerals, making them unable to be absorbed. However, higher fiber dietary patterns tend to also be higher in mineral content; therefore absorption of minerals remains adequate.[16]

As fiber passes through the GI tract it provides several health-promoting services that are still being discovered. Some foods that contain fiber also contain an assortment of essential nutrients. That is why it is best to get fiber from real foods rather than from supplements.

Because some benefits do vary between soluble and insoluble fiber, should daily intakes of each kind of fiber be calculated? Not at all. Increase total dietary fiber to recommended levels slowly by gradually substituting whole grain foods, fresh fruits, and vegetables for some lower fiber foods (see the Teaching Tool box, "What's Your Fiber Score Today?"). This allows the body to adjust to the additional fiber, reducing the possible formation of intestinal gas.

 TEACHING TOOL
What's Your Fiber Score Today?

Although the foods below are particularly good sources of dietary fiber, many other foods—all fruits and vegetables—contain smaller amounts that add up by the day's end. Does your typical intake meet the recommended levels of about 20 to 38 grams per day?

ABOUT 2 g/SERVING	ABOUT 3 g/SERVING	ABOUT 4 g OR MORE/SERVING
Apricot	Apple with skin	Baked beans
Banana	Corn	Bran cereals
Blueberries	Orange	Kidney beans
Broccoli	Pear	Lentils
Cantaloupe	Peas	Navy beans
Carrot	Potato with skin	Whole wheat spaghetti
Cauliflower	Raisins	
Grapefruit	Shredded wheat cereal	
Oatmeal	Strawberries	
Peach		
Pineapple		
Rye crisp		
Whole wheat bread		
Whole wheat cereals		

Data from Pennington JAT: Bowes & Church's food values of portions commonly used, *ed 17, Philadelphia, 1997, Lippincott-Raven.*

Food Sources and Issues

Although dietary fiber is not absorbed and does not serve a nutrient function in the body, the effects of fiber are important for optimum health.

An Adequate Intake (AI) of dietary fiber is about 20 to 38 grams per day, depending on age and gender.[2,16] Most Americans consume much lower levels of fiber; adults often average only 14 to 15 grams of fiber per day, whereas children and young adults average 12 grams.[17] This is because of several factors. First, many Americans do not consume enough fruits and vegetables on a daily basis. Somehow, high protein and dietary fat intakes have pushed fruits and vegetables out of our meal patterns. Also, possibly the most significant factor is that most Americans regularly eat foods made with refined grains from which dietary fiber has been removed. Consumption of legumes and high-fiber cereal foods provides considerably more fiber.

Unrefined Vs. Refined Grains

unrefined grains
grains prepared for consumption containing all edible portions of kernels

whole grain products
food items made using unrefined grains

refined grains
grains that contain only some of the edible kernel

Unrefined grains are prepared for consumption containing their original components. These grains are really seeds or kernels that include all the nutrients necessary to support plant growth and are segmented inside the kernel to be used when needed. Whole grain products refer to food items made using all the edible portions of kernels.

In contrast, refined grains have been taken apart. Only portions of the edible kernel are included in refined grain products. Although both unrefined and refined grain products are good sources of complex carbohydrates, other nutritional qualities of the whole grain are lost when grains are refined. Grains most often refined are wheat, rice, oats, corn, and rye.

To better understand how the nutrients are lost, consider the wheat kernel shown in Figure 4-7. The kernel consists of three nutrient-containing components. The outer layer, bran, is an excellent source of cellulose dietary fiber and also contains magnesium, riboflavin, niacin, thiamin, vitamin B_6, and some protein.

The germ found in the base of the kernel contains a wealth of nutrients to support the sprouting of the plant. Some of these include thiamin, riboflavin, vitamin B_6, vitamin E, zinc, protein, and wheat oil (polyunsaturated vegetable oil).

The endosperm, the largest component of the kernel, contains starch, the prime energy source for the sprouting plant. It also contains protein and riboflavin but much smaller amounts of niacin, thiamin, and B_6.

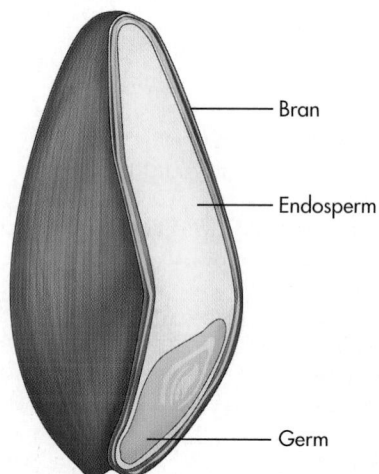

— Bran

— Endosperm

— Germ

Figure 4-7 Inside a wheat kernel.

When flour is refined, the bran and germ are removed; the bran affects the physical lightness of the flour, and the oil in the germ may become rancid, reducing the shelf life of the flour. Only the starchy endosperm is used to mill refined flour. Because flour is the mainstay of grain products, the loss of nutrients to the population is significant. In the 1940s it was determined that deficiencies of thiamin, riboflavin, niacin, and iron occurred because of the refining process. To counteract this loss, those four nutrients were added back to flour. Now, flour with these specific nutrient additives is called *enriched flour.*

Enrichment is the replacement of nutrients to the level that was present before processing. Although the four lost nutrients are replaced, other vitamins, minerals, and fiber originally in whole wheat are not. Zinc, magnesium, vitamin E, and dietary fiber are not returned to the refined white flour. Consequently, any product made with enriched white flour is still nutritionally inferior to whole wheat flour (see the Health Debate box, "If Dietary Fiber Is So Important, Should Grain Products Be Allowed to Be Refined?").

The preference for refined complex carbohydrates may be changing. The health benefits of dietary fiber have been so newsworthy and the focus of such intensive advertising that consumer perception of fiber has evolved from a negative selling point to a positive one.[18] Twenty years ago, if products claimed to be high in fiber or made from whole grains, sales would decline. Today, high-fiber food items are among the better sellers in categories such as cereals and breads[18] (see the Cultural Considerations box, "Cereals Around the World").

enrichment
returning nutrients lost because of processing to their original levels

OVERCOMING BARRIERS

As we eat throughout the day, our bodies respond to the available glucose and easily adjust to provide glucose during the hours between food intake. For some of us, however, these regulating mechanisms malfunction. When this happens, the effect of food consumption on blood glucose levels needs to be considered to avoid sudden rises and falls in blood glucose levels. The two conditions most related to

---

HEALTH DEBATE
If Dietary Fiber Is So Important, Should Grain Products Be Allowed to Be Refined?

This chapter highlights the health benefits of eating the recommended levels of fiber. Also emphasized are nutrition losses that occur when fruits, vegetables, and grains are processed or refined. The process of refining can lead to the extensive loss of fiber and various nutrients. Although some nutrients are replaced, some, such as dietary fiber, are not.

If health benefits of dietary fiber and nutrients are so valuable, should there be government regulations to restrict or prohibit the removal of valuable nutrients and dietary fiber? Several of the diseases associated with low-fiber intake are chronic diseases. Treating these long-term diseases places a burden on the entire U.S. healthcare system.

Is it fair for all of us to bear the financial burden for those not consuming the most healthful form of foods available? Should there be a law against the processing of whole grains? Should white flour production be restricted? Or is the availability of white (or wheat) and whole wheat products sufficient? Is it our "freedom of choice" to be able to select among different food products although some are more beneficial to health than others?

What do you think?

carbohydrate metabolism are hypoglycemia and diabetes mellitus. These conditions are introduced here; nutritional therapy for diabetes mellitus is detailed in Chapter 19.

Hypoglycemia

hypoglycemia
blood glucose levels that are below normal values

Hypoglycemia, or low blood glucose level, is a symptom of an underlying disorder; it is not a disease. We may all experience hypoglycemia when we haven't eaten for a few hours and begin to feel hungry. If we don't eat, our bodies switch to an alternative source of energy. This causes the release of epinephrine and glucagon, which act to make the liver glycogen release glucose to be available for energy. For some individuals, the transition to this energy source or the experience of hypoglycemia may be uncomfortable, causing rapid heartbeat, sweating, weakness, anxiety, and hunger.

If these symptoms occur regularly, even when an individual eats well, a primary healthcare provider should be consulted. The underlying cause of hypoglycemia needs to be determined. Some health problems for which hypoglycemia may be a symptom are over-production of insulin by the pancreas, which excessively lowers blood glucose levels, and intestinal malabsorption of glucose or insufficient glucose storage (glycogen) in the liver.

Other disorders may have symptoms similar to hypoglycemia. A tumor on the adrenal gland may cause excessive amounts of epinephrine to be released, or a circulatory problem may affect blood flow to the brain, thus causing the confusion, headaches, and other symptoms often associated with hypoglycemia.[14]

Symptoms similar to chronic hypoglycemia may also occur when patterns of food intake are erratic or when we simply don't eat enough. True hypoglycemia is rare.[14] If hypoglycemia is suspected, dietary intake patterns are analyzed. Is the day's food intake full of concentrated sweets and sodas? This would cause an excessive release of insulin that could then lead to a low blood glucose response. That is not true hypoglycemia. Instead, a mix of carbohydrate and protein foods should be eaten throughout the day and hypoglycemic symptoms will probably decrease. However, if the best efforts at diet control do not eliminate hypoglycemic episodes, medical advice should be sought.

hyperglycemia
elevated blood glucose levels (>120 mg/dl)

Diabetes Mellitus

diabetes mellitus
a disorder of carbohydrate metabolism characterized by hyperglycemia caused by insulin that is either defective or deficient

Whereas hypoglycemia involves low blood sugar, diabetes is concerned with very high blood glucose levels, or hyperglycemia. Diabetes mellitus (DM) is a disorder of carbohydrate metabolism characterized by hyperglycemia caused by insulin that is either ineffective or deficient. The impact of diabetes is that the energy supply of glucose keeps circulating in the bloodstream; it is not available in sufficient quantities to support the energy needs of the cells.

There are several types of diabetes: type 1, type 2, and gestational.

Type 1 Diabetes Mellitus

In type 1 diabetes mellitus (DM), the pancreas produces insufficient amounts of insulin. Insulin must be provided through daily insulin injections to control blood glucose levels. Type 1 DM tends to occur early in life, caused by viral or autoimmune destruction of the area of the pancreas responsible for insulin production; genetic factors may also be associated with type 1 DM. This disorder is not risk related. We cannot prevent or develop type 1 DM by our dietary intake or lifestyle behaviors. When the disorder occurs, lifelong treatment depends on dietary intake that balances food intake with insulin injection and on lifestyle behaviors to reduce the complications of type 1 DM. Individuals with type 1 DM are at more risk for heart disease, kidney disorders, and retinal damage.

type 1 diabetes mellitus (DM) a form of diabetes mellitus in which the pancreas produces no insulin at all

Type 2 Diabetes Mellitus

In type 2 diabetes mellitus (DM), the pancreas produces some insulin, but it is ineffective and unable to meet the needs of the body. Risk is related to genetic, environmental, and lifestyle factors. The risk of developing type 2 DM increases with family history, age, weight, and caloric intake. Type 2 DM is associated with advancing age, being overweight, and consuming excess kcalories. If family members have type 2 DM, adopting preventive lifestyle behaviors as young adults can reduce the risk of developing this disorder later in life. Preventive lifestyle behaviors include exercising regularly and eating a moderately kcaloric, high-fiber, low-fat diet to avoid weight gain, as we grow older. Both of these behaviors also work to treat type 2 DM as well.

type 2 diabetes mellitus (DM) a form of diabetes mellitus in which the pancreas produces some insulin that is defective and unable to serve the complete needs of the body

As a nation we are becoming more concerned as the prevalence of type 2 DM is increasing rapidly—even among children and young adults. Health professionals are recognizing prediabetic disorders, and efforts to begin prevention earlier are becoming public health goals. A recent panel of experts from the American Diabetes Association and the U.S. Department of Health and Human Services recommends screening adults younger than 45 if they are seriously overweight and have one or more of the following risk factors:

- Family history of diabetes
- Low high-density lipoprotein (HDL) cholesterol and high triglycerides
- High blood pressure
- History of gestational diabetes or gave birth to an infant that weighed more than 9 lbs
- Minority group heritage (e.g., African Americans, Native Americans, Hispanic Americans, and Asian/Pacific Islanders are at increased risk for type 2 diabetes)[19]

Gestational Diabetes Mellitus

Gestational diabetes mellitus (GDM) may occur during pregnancy when blood glucose levels remain abnormally high. This form of diabetes may affect the health and development of the fetus as well as the health of the mother. Although it seems as if the pregnancy triggers the diabetic response in some women, studies show that some women who develop gestational diabetes tend to develop type 2 DM later in life. Many exhibit several of the risks factors of type 2 DM before pregnancy and thus are predisposed to develop diabetes.[20] To limit the negative impacts of GDM, which if not controlled may lead to pregnancy-induced hypertension, premature birth, large fetus size, congenital abnormalities, future obesity and diabetes in the infant, and other birth complications, routine screening for diabetes is part of quality prenatal care.[21]

gestational diabetes mellitus (GDM) a form of diabetes occurring most commonly after the 20th week of gestation

Dietary modifications are an important part of controlling diabetes. This is accomplished through individually developed dietary prescriptions based on metabolic nutrition and lifestyle requirements. Basic changes include reduced intake of simple sugars such as white table sugar and syrups. These are replaced by more complex carbohydrates and a balanced intake of nutrients, particularly carbohydrates, throughout the day. To make implementation of the treatment plan easier, registered dietitians (RD) use the *Exchange Lists* to assist clients with diabetes with meal planning. The *Exchange Lists* (see Appendix B) was first developed for diabetic meal planning but has become a basic tool for almost all food guides and dietary recommendations.[22] Another system to control diabetes, carbohydrate counting, has recently been introduced. This system allows the client to keep track of carbohydrate intake during the course of the day. Chapter 19 provides more details on this approach.

Overall management of GDM takes into account the physical, psychosocial, and educational requirements. Whereas an RD has primary responsibility for developing and teaching the individualized dietary prescription, nurses reinforce these dietary modifications and also teach the skills of blood glucose monitoring, insulin therapy, and exercise. Health professionals can develop a supportive relationship with clients by consideration of cultural orientation and learning styles.[23]

TOWARD A POSITIVE NUTRITION LIFESTYLE: TAILORING

Consider what a tailor does. A tailor takes a bolt of cloth and by cutting, shaping, and sewing, fits a garment to the exact measurements of a person. Tailoring as a behavior-change technique takes a health recommendation and by "cutting," "shaping," and "sewing," fits the recommendation to the limitations or requirements of our individual lifestyles.

Strong recommendations to increase our fiber intake are made in this chapter. Ideally, fiber intake should be about 20 to 38 grams a day. The most efficient means of intake would be to replace all refined grain products with whole grain products. But is that possible considering contemporary lifestyles? Often we are not able to control available food choices, and thus we have difficulty changing our behavior to implement this type of recommendation. By tailoring the recommendation or goal to our individual lifestyles, we can succeed. Here's some "tailoring" in practice:

- Overwhelmed by the thought of eating only whole grain foods? Decide to eat more whole grain products for breakfast and dinner, which are eaten at home when control is easier.
- No time to cook vegetables? Prepare or order salads and keep fresh fruits of any kind handy.
- Needing to add fiber to your diet? When possible, choose fiber-rich foods for lunch. Be realistic, however, because foods available at the cafeteria or coffee shop are limited.
- Attending a family holiday dinner or special event or going on vacation? Enjoy what's served. Then resume a regular fiber-rich dietary pattern when back at work or school.

Although the goal is to increase fiber intake, the objective is to fit positive dietary choices and habits to the shape of our nutrition lifestyles.

SUMMARY

Carbohydrates are composed of carbon, hydrogen, and oxygen. There are three sizes of carbohydrates: monosaccharides (glucose, fructose, and galactose), disaccharides (sucrose, maltose, and lactose), and polysaccharides (starch and dietary fiber). These three sizes are divided into the two categories of simple carbohydrates (monosaccharides and disaccharides) and complex carbohydrates (polysaccharides).

Primarily found in plant foods, carbohydrates are an abundant food source of energy and dietary fiber. Glucose is the carbohydrate form through which energy circulates in the bloodstream. Blood glucose levels are naturally regulated through hormonal systems that aim to keep the body in balance. Hypoglycemia and diabetes mellitus may occur when these systems cannot regulate glucose within normal levels. In contrast to glucose, dietary fiber does not provide energy. Although dietary fiber is a carbohydrate, it is not digestible by humans. The health benefits of consuming sufficient quantities of dietary fiber, however, are significant.

The best food energy sources of carbohydrates are grains, legumes, and starchy root vegetables. Dietary fiber is available in many foods such as fruits, vegetables, and whole grain products. Dietary fiber and other nutrients are often lost when foods, particularly grains, are processed.

The most recent dietary guidelines recommend the increased consumption of complex carbohydrates. The Food Pyramid suggests 6 to 11 servings of grains and 5 to 9 servings of fruits and vegetables. The intent is to reduce our fat intake by increasing intake of starch and dietary fiber. By following these guidelines, our risk of developing diet-related diseases will be decreased.

THE NURSING APPROACH
Fiber Case Study

Debbie, age 25, visits a nurse practitioner's (NP) office for a physical examination before starting a new job. When collecting the health history, the NP finds that Debbie has complaints of occasional constipation. The NP recognizes that constipation generally becomes worse with age, therefore the NP would like to correct Debbie's problem early. Further data are needed and are collected by means of interviewing Debbie.

ASSESSMENT

Subjective
- Small, hard stool
- Difficulty defecating every few weeks
- Fiber intake minimal; prefers white bread and low-fiber cereals and vegetables
- Fluid intake of 4 to 6 glasses per day
- Noticeable change in usual bowel habits

NURSING DIAGNOSIS
- Altered health maintenance, related to lack of knowledge, as evidenced by inadequate fiber intake
- Risk for constipation as evidenced by inadequate fiber intake

PLANNING

The NP sets the following goals with Debbie:
1. Increase fiber-rich foods by three servings per day (e.g., prunes, apples, broccoli, peas, bran cereal, kidney beans).
2. Increase fluid intake to 6 to 8 glasses per day (e.g., warm or hot beverages, fruit juices).

IMPLEMENTATION
1. Explain the importance of fiber.
2. Provide written information on types and sources of fiber.
3. Explore food likes and preferences to determine high-fiber foods acceptable to Debbie.
4. Encourage Debbie to add one serving of fiber per day every 2 weeks until three servings per day have been added to daily intake.
5. Encourage Debbie to add 2 glasses of fluids (e.g., water, fruit juices) to her intake each day.
6. Discuss ways in which #4 and #5 can be done in light of her lifestyle.

EVALUATION

Have Debbie contact the NP in 1 month to see if the goals of increased fiber and fluid intake have been met and whether she experiences the absence of constipation.

APPLYING CONTENT KNOWLEDGE

You are at a restaurant having lunch with friends. After a friend hears you order a sandwich on whole wheat bread, the friend comments, "Whole wheat bread, white bread, what's the big deal? They're all complex carbohydrates." How would you respond?

Web Sites of Interest

American Diabetes Association
www.diabetes.org
The official site of the American Diabetes Association provides a wealth of information for health professionals and the public ranging from Internet resources to research updates to volunteer opportunities for members.

The Grains Nutrition Information Center
www.wheatfoods.org
This site, sponsored by the Wheat Council, provides nutrition and food preparation information and resources on ways to incorporate more grains into the American diet for better health.

USA Rice Federation
www.usarice.com
Sponsored by the USA Rice Federation, a national industry association of rice producers, millers, and related businesses, this site offers information about rice production, research, and environmental issues. The Rice Cafe presents a wide variety of recipes for consumers.

References

1. Dolan JP, Adams-Smith WN: *Health and society: a documentary history of medicine,* New York, 1978, The Seabury Press.
2. Institute of Medicine, Food and Nutrition Board: *Dietary reference intakes for energy, carbohydrate, fiber, fat, fatty acids, cholesterol, protein, and amino acids,* Washington, DC, 2002, National Academy Press.
3. US Department of Health and Human Services, Public Health Service: *Healthy People 2010,* ed 2, Washington, DC, 2000, US Government Printing Office; www.health.gov/healthypeople.
4. American Dietetic Association: Position of the American Dietetic Association: use of nutritive and nonnutritive sweeteners, *J Am Dietetic Assoc* 98:580, 1998.
5. US Department of Health and Human Services: *Health hazard evaluation: summary of adverse reactions attributed to aspartame,* Washington, DC, 1995, U.S. Government Printing Office.
6. Garriga M, Berkebile C, Metcalfe D: A combined single-blind, double-blind, placebo-controlled study to determine the reproducibility of hypersensitivity reactions to aspartame, *J Allergy Clin Immunol* 87:821, 1991.
7. Geha R et al.: Aspartame is no more likely than placebo to cause urticaria/angioedema: results of a multicenter, randomized, double-blind, placebo-controlled crossover study, *J Allergy Clin Immunol* 92:513, 1993.
8. Henkel J: Sugar substitutes: Americans opt for sweetness and lite, *FDA Consumer,* Nov-Dec 1999; www.cfsan.fda.gov/dms/fdsugar.html.
9. Food and Drug Administration: *Code of federal regulations: food and drugs,* Apr 1, 1996: Parts 10 to 199, Washington, DC, The Office of the Federal Register.
10. Chen LA, Parham ES: College students' use of high-intensity sweeteners is not consistently associated with sugar consumption, *J Am Dietetic Assoc* 91:686, 1991.

11. Blackburn G et al.: The effect of aspartame as part of a multidisciplinary weight-control program on short- and long-term control of body weight, *Am J Clin Nutr* 65:409, 1997.

12. Klein S, Cohn SM, Alpers DH: The alimentary tract in nutrition: a tutorial. In Shils ME et al., eds.: *Modern nutrition in health and disease,* ed 9, Philadelphia, 1999, Williams & Wilkins.

13. Simmang CL, Shires FT: Diverticular disease of the colon. In Feldman M, Sleisenger MH, Scharschmidt BF, eds.: *Gastrointestinal and liver disease,* ed 6, Philadelphia, 1998, WB Saunders.

14. Levin RJ: Carbohydrates. In Shils ME et al., eds.: *Modern nutrition in health and disease,* ed 9, Philadelphia, 1999, Williams & Wilkins.

15. Ferguson LR, Harris PJ: Studies on the role of specific dietary fibres in protection against colorectal cancer, *Nutat Res* 350(1):173, 1996.

16. American Dietetic Association: Position of the American Dietetic Association: health implications of dietary fiber, *J Am Dietetic Assoc* 97:1157, 1997.

17. Jenkins DJA, Wolever TMS, Jenkins AL: Fiber and other dietary factors affecting nutrient absorption and metabolism. In Shils ME et al., eds.: *Modern nutrition in health and disease,* ed 9, Philadelphia, 1999, Williams & Wilkins.

18. Nicklas TA et al.: Dietary fiber intake of children and young adults: the Bogalusa Heart Study, *J Am Diet Assoc* 95(2):209, 1995.

19. US Department of Health and Human Services: HHS, ADA warn Americans of "pre-diabetes," encourage people to take healthy steps to reduce risks, *HHS News,* Mar 27, 2002; www.hhs.gov/news/press/2002pres/20020327.html.

20. McMahan MJ, Ananth CV, Liston RM: Gestational diabetes mellitus: risk factors, obstetric complications and infant outcomes, *J Reprod Med* 43(4):372, Apr 1998.

21. Hod M, Meizner I: Diabetes in pregnancy, *Ann 1st Super Sanita* 33(3):317, 1997.

22. American Diabetes Association, American Dietetic Association: *Exchange lists for meal planning,* Alexandria, Va, 1995, American Dietetic Association.

23. Jones MW, Stone LC: Management of the woman with gestational diabetes mellitus, *J Perinat Neonatal Nurs* 11(4):13, Mar 1998.

CHAPTER 5

Fats

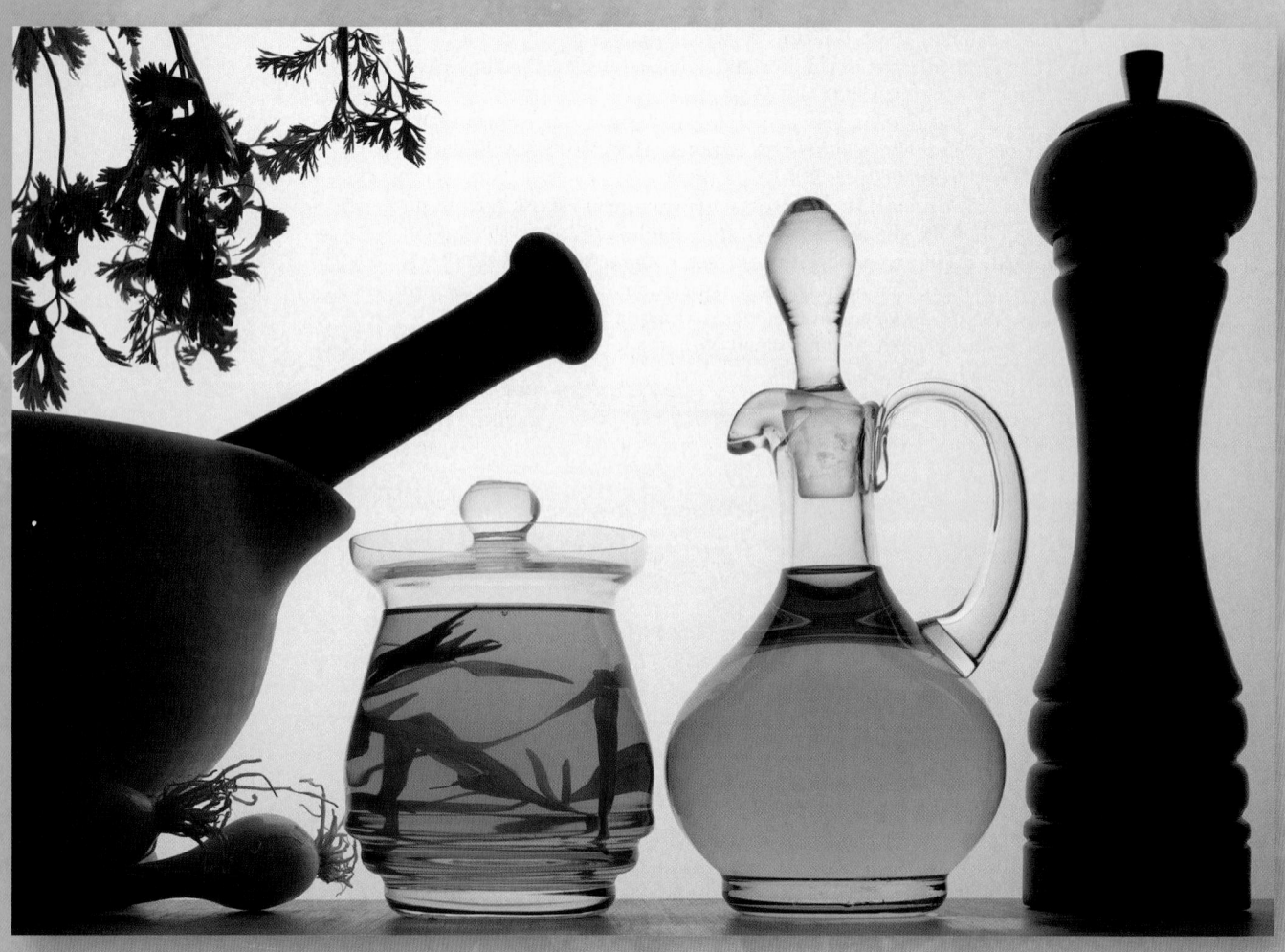

The term fats actually refers to the chemical group called lipids. Lipids are divided into three classifications: fats (or triglycerides) and the fat-related substances of phospholipids and sterols.

✿ ROLE IN WELLNESS

Some people fear fat. We may have friends who have so-called "fat attacks." These attacks are reported to be both the craving for tasty, fatty foods and the worrying about the way fat appears on the body. However, fat is not always an enemy. Fat is valuable and necessary to health. It is important to learn about fat in food, what the fat we eat does in our bodies, and how it can be both helpful and harmful to our health. Individual preference for fat is developed either in infancy or early childhood; innate preferences for sweet taste are observed at birth.[1] Thus children learn to prefer tastes, flavors, and textures that are associated with foods that are rich in fat, sweet, or both. Aging may be associated with increasing acceptance of bitter tastes and consumption of more fruits, vegetables, and whole grains.[1] Nonetheless, decreasing fat consumption takes time and effort, perhaps because of food selection habits, symbolic meaning associated with certain foods, and sensory values of fats in foods.

The five dimensions of health provide ways to think about the effects of changing dietary fat consumption. Physical health is maintained by consuming dietary fats that are necessary for essential fatty acids, for energy, and for fat-soluble vitamins. Excessive intake of fats, though, may increase the risk of obesity and diet-related diseases. The intellectual health dimension encompasses the skills necessary to assess the type of dietary fat modification most appropriate for our clients' and our own health needs. How we emotionally approach nutritional lifestyle changes for our clients and ourselves affects success, which reflects the emotional health dimension. Can these emotions be expressed, or are changes simply disregarded because they make us feel uncomfortable? The social dimension is tested as change is initiated. Are relationships of family and friends based on sharing high-fat meals? Can you or your clients refuse to take part in social situations without jeopardizing relationships or making others feel defensive? Can food preparation suggestions to lower the fat content be made without seeming overly critical? Some religions maintain that taking care of one's body is necessary to achieve spiritual goals. Adopting a healthier fat intake supports these spiritual health dimension goals.

Fat actually refers to the chemical group called *lipids*. Lipids are divided into three classifications: fats (or triglycerides) and the fat-related substances of phospholipids and sterols. Triglycerides are the largest class of lipids and may be in the form of fats (somewhat solid) or oils (liquids). About 95% of the lipids in foods and in our bodies are in the triglyceride form of fat. The other two lipid classifications are the fat-related substances of phospholipids and sterols. Lecithin is the best-known phospholipid; cholesterol is the best-known sterol. All are organic, composed of carbon, hydrogen, and oxygen; and cannot dissolve in water.

FUNCTIONS

The functions of lipids may be divided into two categories: (1) the characteristics of lipids in foods and (2) the physiologic health of our bodies.

Food Functions

Source of Energy

Fat is the densest form of stored energy in both food and in our bodies. This means that gram for gram, food fat—in the form of triglycerides—can produce more than twice the energy in kcalories as carbohydrate or protein. For example, a gram of nearly pure fat (9 kcal), such as butter, provides more than twice the kcalories as a gram of nearly pure carbohydrate (4 kcal), such as sugar, or a gram of nearly pure protein (4 kcal), such as dried, lean fish.

Sharron Dalton, PhD, RD, contributed this chapter in the first and second editions of this text.

Palatability

Fat makes food smell and taste good. Deep-fat fried potatoes outrank all other vegetable choices among North Americans. Whether it's bread with butter (or margarine), salad with dressing, or desserts with cream, fat makes these foods taste pleasant for many people. For patients who are anorectic because of illness, strategically adding small amounts of fats to meals may increase their nutrient intake.

Satiety and Satiation

Fat helps prevent hunger between meals. Fat slows down digestion because of the hormones released in response to its presence in the gastrointestinal (GI) tract, causing us to feel full and satisfied; we call this feeling *satiety*. *Satiation* is another, different aspect of fat consumption that occurs during, not after, eating. In contrast to satiety, satiation tends to increase our desire to eat additional fatty foods, not less. The effect of fat on satiation is likely to be more important than its effect on satiety and may lead to overeating.[2] A situation that often occurs with the last slice of pizza provides a good example: You want it, you eat it, and half an hour later, you feel too full.

Food Processing

Certain qualities of lipids, besides their nutritional purposes, make them a valuable resource for the processing of foods. The use of processed hydrogenated fats helps keep the fat in food products from turning rancid. Lecithin, a phospholipid, has an extensive role as an **emulsifier**. These functions, which will be described in more detail, also increase our overall intake of lipids by allowing its use in numerous processed foods.

Nutrient Source

Some fats contain or transport the fat-soluble nutrients of vitamins A, D, E, and K and the essential fatty acids of linoleic and linolenic fatty acids.

These essential fatty acids (EFAs), components of fat triglycerides, are necessary materials for making compounds, such as prostaglandins, that regulate many body functions, including blood pressure, blood clotting through platelet aggregation, gastric acid secretions, and muscle secretions. The overall strength of cell membranes depends on EFAs. Overt deficiency symptoms of EFAs include skin lesions and scaliness (eczema) caused by increased permeability, which leads to membrane breakdown throughout the body (Figure 5-1). Inflammation of epithelial tissue and increased susceptibility to infections throughout the body are also possible.

emulsifier
a substance that works by being soluble in water and fat at the same time

essential fatty acids (EFAs)
polyunsaturated fatty acids that cannot be made in the body and must be consumed in the diet

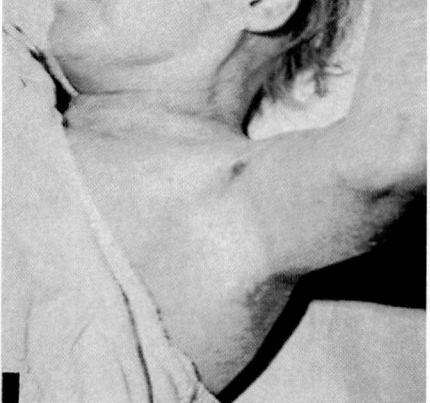

Figure 5-1 A, Essential fatty acid deficiency. Patients receiving fat-free parenteral nutrition have developed biochemical abnormalities and skin lesions as shown here. **B,** Resolution in same patient after 2 weeks of treatment. (Courtesy Dr. M.C. Riella; from McLaren DS: *A colour atlas and text of diet-related disorders,* ed 2, London, 1992, Mosby-Year Book Europe Limited. By permission of Mosby International Ltd.)

Because the minimum amount of EFA required is contained in only about 2 teaspoons of polyunsaturated vegetable oil, deficiencies of EFAs were thought to be rare. However, deficiencies have been noted in (1) older patients with peripheral vascular disease (a potential complication of diabetes mellitus); (2) patients with fat malabsorption, such as cystic fibrosis; and (3) patients receiving treatment for protein malnutrition with low-fat, high-protein diets. Individuals recovering from serious accidents and burns are also at risk.[3] It is possible that individuals who strive to achieve extremely low dietary fat intake could develop EFA deficiencies.

Physiologic Functions

Stored Energy

Body fat cells contain nearly pure fat, also in the form of triglycerides. This means a pound of adipose tissue, the storage depot of body fat, could produce about 3500 kcalories as energy. Because glucose stored in our bodies as glycogen is stored with water, carbohydrate is a bulkier form of stored energy than body fat. Adipose tissue provides important fuel during illness or times of food restriction and is a major energy source for muscle work.

Organ Protection

Stored fat safely cushions and protects body organs during bumpy activities, such as participating in impact aerobics or riding a toboggan.

Temperature Regulator

The fat layer just under our skin serves as insulation to regulate body temperature by minimizing the loss of heat.

Insulation

A substance composed largely of fatty tissue, called *myelin*, covers nerve cells. This covering provides electrical insulation that allows for transmission of nerve impulses.

adipose tissue
stored form of fat (mainly triglycerides) in the body

Functions of Phospholipids and Sterols

So far, we have discussed the major roles of triglycerides. Phospholipids are also important as a part of all cell membrane structure and serve as emulsifiers to keep fats dispersed in body fluids.

Lecithins are the main phospholipids. Lecithin is a constituent of lipoproteins—carriers or transporters of lipids—including fats and cholesterol in the body. This characteristic has earned lecithin a reputation for carrying fat and cholesterol away from plaque deposits in the arteries. Although lecithin does play a role in transporting fat and cholesterol, supplementary lecithin from sources outside of the body does not help make the body's transportation system more efficient. Instead, dietary lecithin is simply digested and used by the body as any other lipid.

As a lipid group, sterols are critical components of complex regulatory compounds in our bodies and provide basic material to make bile, vitamin D, sex hormones, and cells in brain and nerve tissue. Cholesterol in particular is a vital part of all cell membranes and nerve tissues and serves as a building block for hormones. When exposed to ultraviolet light, a cholesterol substance in our skin can be converted to vitamin D by the kidneys and liver. The liver synthesizes cholesterol to make bile, the emulsifying substance necessary to absorb dietary lipids.

STRUCTURE AND SOURCES OF LIPIDS

Fats: Saturated and Unsaturated

triglycerides
the largest class of lipids found in food and body fat; composed of three fatty acids and one glycerol molecule

Triglycerides are compounds consisting of three fatty acids and one glycerol molecule (Figure 5-2). The glycerol portion is derived from carbohydrate, but it is a small part compared with the fatty acids that may be alike or different from each other. Fatty acids can be made of long or short chains of carbon atoms. Each carbon atom has four bonding sites or imaginary arms where it can attach to other atoms. To form a carbon chain, one site on each side of the carbon bonds to a neighboring carbon, as if one arm on each side were outstretched to form a chain. Because these atoms have four arms, the two extra arms each attach to a hydrogen atom, which makes the chain saturated with hydrogen.

If a hydrogen atom is removed from two neighbor carbons, freeing the extra arm on each, the carbons are bonded to each other at two sites. The two arms on the same side both clasp the two arms of the neighboring carbon, forming a double bond. We call this an *unsaturated carbon chain* because there is a possibility that hydrogen could come along and saturate the chain by breaking one set of clasped arms and attaching to them. In foods, this is sometimes done artificially through the process of hydrogenation, which forces hydrogen atoms to break a double bond and attach to the carbons, creating a saturated fat (Figure 5-3). Hydrogenation is discussed in the section on processed fats.

hydrogenation
breaking a double bond on a fatty acid carbon chain and saturating it with hydrogen

All natural fats are mixtures of different types of fatty acids. Most plant oils contain some saturated fatty acids, and animal fats contain amounts of polyunsaturated fats (Figure 5-4). The predominant type of fat in a food determines its category.

saturated fatty acid
a fatty acid with carbon chains completely saturated or filled with hydrogen

A saturated fatty acid has a single-bonded carbon chain that is fully saturated because hydrogen atoms are attached to all available bonding sites. Palmitic acid (16 carbons atoms) (Figure 5-5, *A*), a saturated fatty acid, is contained in meats, butterfat, shortening, and vegetable oils. Other saturated fatty acids include stearic (18 carbon atoms), myristic (14 carbon atoms), and lauric (12 carbon atoms).[2] Ad-

Three fatty acids join to glycerol in a condensation reaction to form a triglyceride.

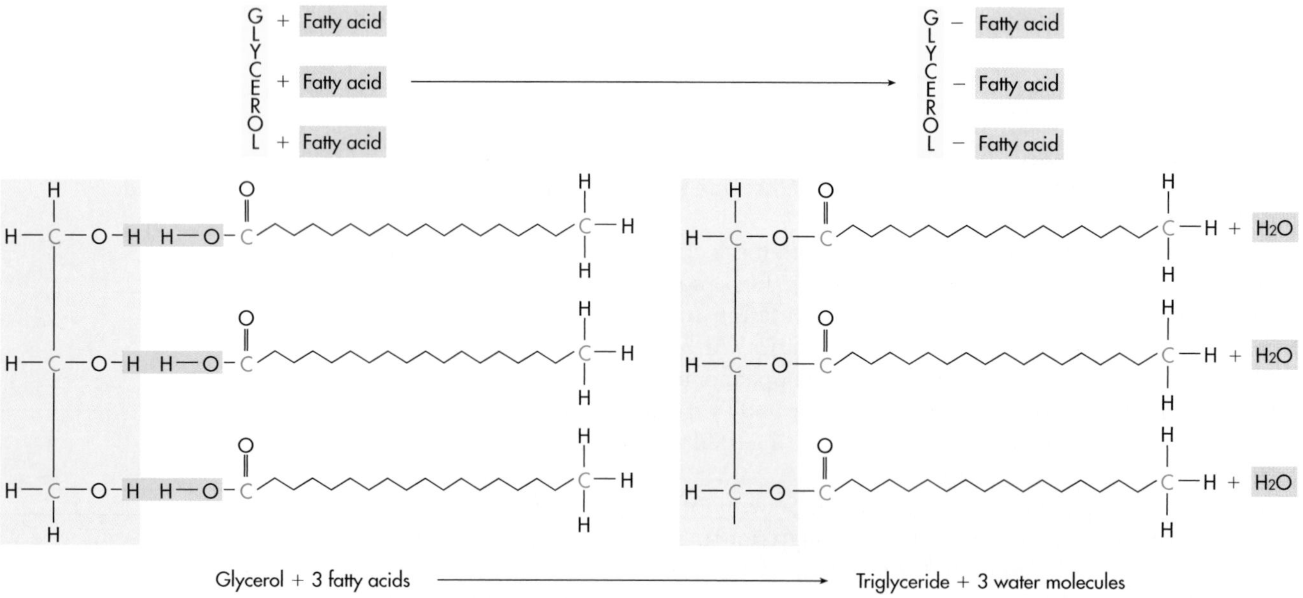

Glycerol + 3 fatty acids ⟶ Triglyceride + 3 water molecules

A bond is formed with the O of the glycerol and the C of the last acid of the fatty acid because of the removal of water from the glycerol and fatty acids.

Three fatty acids attached to a glycerol form a triglyceride. Water is released. Triglycerides often contain different kinds of fatty acids.

Figure 5-2 Formation and structure of a triglyceride.

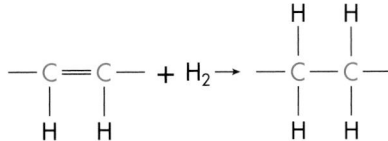

Figure 5-3 Process of hydrogenation.

ditional food sources of saturated fatty acids are primarily animal, including beef, poultry, pork, lamb, luncheon meats, egg yolks, and dairy products (milk, butter, and cheeses); the only major plant sources are palm and coconut oils (often called *tropical oils*) and cocoa butter.

Unsaturated fatty acids have one or more unsaturated double bonds along the carbon chain. If a carbon chain has only one unsaturated double bond, it is a **monounsaturated fatty acid.** Oleic acid (Figure 5-5, *B*) is the main monounsaturated fatty acid in foods. Dietary sources include olive oil, peanuts (peanut butter and peanut oil), and canola oil.

If a carbon chain has two or more unsaturated double bonds, it is a **polyunsaturated fatty acid (PUFA).** Food sources include vegetable oils (corn, safflower, wheat germ, canola, sesame, and sunflower), fish, and margarine.

monounsaturated fatty acid
a fatty acid containing a carbon chain with one unsaturated double bond

polyunsaturated fatty acid (PUFA)
a fatty acid containing two or more double bonds on the carbon chain

Dietary fat	Cholesterol (mg/tbsp)	Percent breakdown of fatty acid content (normalized to 100%)
Canola oil	0	6 · 22 · 10 · 62
Safflower oil	0	10 · 77 · Trace · 13
Sunflower oil	0	11 · 69 · 20
Corn oil	0	13 · 61 · 1 · 25
Olive oil	0	14 · 8 · 1 · 77
Soybean oil	0	15 · 54 · 7 · 24
Margarine	0	17 · 32 · 2 · 49
Peanut oil	0	18 · 33 · 49
Vegetable shortening	0	28 · 26 · 2 · 44
Palm kernel oil	0	49 · 9 · 37
Coconut oil	0	81 · 2 · 11
Palm oil	0	87 · 2 · 6
Lard	12	41 · 11 · 1 · 47
Beef fat	14	52 · 3 · 1 · 44
Butter fat	33	66 · 2 · 2 · 30

Legend:
- Saturated fat
- Linoleic acid ⎤
- Alpha-linoleic acid ⎦ Polyunsaturated fat
- Monounsaturated fat

Figure 5-4 Comparison of dietary fats in terms of cholesterol, saturated fat, and the most common unsaturated fats.

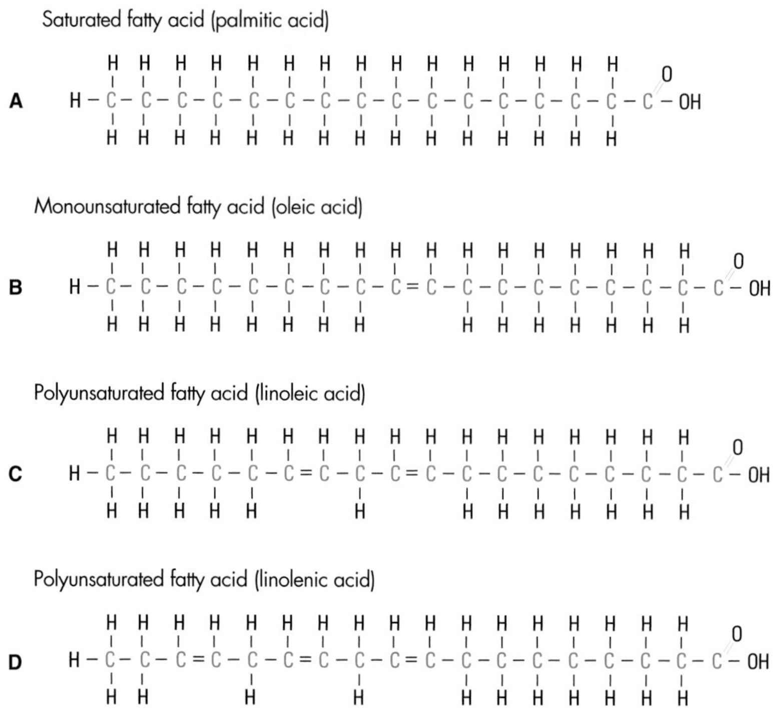

Saturated fatty acid (palmitic acid)

A $H-C-C-C-C-C-C-C-C-C-C-C-C-C-C-C-C-OH$ (with O double bond)

Monounsaturated fatty acid (oleic acid)

B $H-C-C-C-C-C-C-C-C=C-C-C-C-C-C-C-C-C-OH$ (with O double bond)

Polyunsaturated fatty acid (linoleic acid)

C $H-C-C-C-C-C=C-C-C=C-C-C-C-C-C-C-C-OH$ (with O double bond)

Polyunsaturated fatty acid (linolenic acid)

D $H-C-C-C=C-C-C=C-C-C=C-C-C-C-C-C-C-C-OH$ (with O double bond)

Figure 5-5 Examples of fatty acids found in foods. Foods with these fatty acids include **A,** Animal-derived foods (beef, poultry, lamb, pork, eggs, dairy, tropical oils); **B,** Olive oil, peanuts (butter and oil), canola oil; **C,** Vegetable oils (margarine and salad dressings), some animal fats, prepared foods; **D,** Fatty fish (bluefish, tuna, salmon, etc.), fish, canola oil.

PUFAs are categorized by the location of the unsaturation in the molecular structure of the fatty acid. Two categories of polyunsaturated fatty acids, omega-6 and omega-3, contain two fatty acids (linoleic and linolenic) that our bodies cannot manufacture; these acids are EFAs and must be provided by dietary intake. The characteristic that distinguishes them from other PUFAs is the position of the first double bond in relation to the end of the carbon chain. The first double bond is at the sixth carbon from the omega end of the chain in linoleic acid (Figure 5-5, *C*), the main member of the omega-6 family. The first double bond is at the third carbon atom from the omega end in linolenic acid (Figure 5-5, *D*), the main member of the omega-3 family.

Americans consume an abundance of linoleic acid from consumption of large amounts of vegetable oils, such as margarine and salad dressing, and large amounts of prepared foods. Another source of linoleic acid may be animal foods; for example, although poultry fat is predominately saturated, it also contains some PUFA, including linoleic acid.

In contrast, American consumption of linolenic acid is not abundant at all. Linolenic acid is associated with fish consumption because that is how it was first recognized as important in health. A low incidence of heart disease among the native people of Greenland and Alaska, in spite of a very high-fat diet, was traced to the oils in deep-water fish, the staple in their diet.[4] One of the main omega-3 fatty acids in fish is eicosapentaenoic acid (EPA), which is derived from linolenic acid. Fish are more efficient in this conversion of fatty acids than humans. Omega-3 fatty acids appear to lower the risk of heart disease by reducing the blood clotting process; clots can cause blockages in the arteries if plaques exist. Although consuming extra omega-3 fatty acids is likely to have little effect on blood cholesterol levels, it may reduce the risk of clots that may cause a myocardial infarction (heart attack) and possible sudden death.[5] According to prospective studies, reduced risk of coronary artery disease (CAD), because of higher consumption of fish or omega-3 fatty acids, appears applicable to men and women.[5,6]

linoleic acid
an essential polyunsaturated fatty acid with the first double bond located at the sixth carbon atom from the omega end

linolenic acid
an essential polyunsaturated fatty acid with the first double bond located at the third carbon atom from the omega end

eicosapentaenoic acid (EPA)
the main omega-3 fatty acid in fish

Table 5-1
Food Sources of Omega-3 Fatty Acids

Food	% of Lipid as Omega-3	
Oils		**Grams/Oz***
Menhaden	23	6.9
Salmon	22	6.6
Cod liver	20	6.0
Canola	10	3.0
Soybean	7	2.1
Butterfat	2	0.6
Corn	1	0.3
Fish		**Grams/4 Oz**
Cod	42	0.3
Shrimp	38	0.5
Tuna	30	2.3
Pink salmon	29	1.0
King crab	20	0.6
Mackerel	17	1.8-2.6
Herring	6	1.0-2.0

*1 oz = 2 tbsp; 1 oz provides 246 kcal.

Certain fish provide more omega-3 fatty acids than others. Good sources include tuna, salmon, bluefish, halibut, sardines, and lake trout. Table 5-1 lists additional sources. Eating fish twice a week or using canola oil, another source of linolenic acid, should provide an adequate balance between sources of omega-6 and omega-3 fatty acids, although the best balance is still unknown.

Native people of Greenland and Alaska consume 4 to 5 grams of EPAs daily,[4] about the amount in 1.5 to 3 lbs of certain deep-water fish. Because it is unlikely that most Americans will consume this quantity of fish, fish oil supplements of these fatty acids are manufactured. However, questions about proper dosages, safety, and side effects are still being researched. Symptoms that may potentially occur from high intakes of omega-3 fatty acids include infections, increased bleeding time, and diabetes.[7] For now, the best approach is to increase consumption of foods containing these potentially important fatty acids, unless a healthcare professional prescribes fish oil supplements indicating dose levels.

Phospholipids

Phospholipids are similar to triglycerides except they have only two fatty acids; the third spot contains a phosphate group. The body manufactures phospholipids, found in every cell, therefore they are not essential nutrients. Lecithin, the main phospholipid, contains two fatty acids, with the third spot filled by a molecule of choline plus phosphorus (Figure 5-6). In the body, lecithin's function as an emulsifier is to work by being soluble in water and fat at the same time.

Lecithin from soybeans is used in food processing to perform an emulsification role. Lecithin, naturally found in egg yolks, is the versatile ingredient in mayonnaise that prevents separation of vinegar and oil. Lecithin is also used in manufacturing chocolates to keep the cocoa butter and other ingredients combined and in cakes and other bakery products to maintain freshness.

phospholipids
lipid compounds that form part of cell walls and act as a fat emulsifier

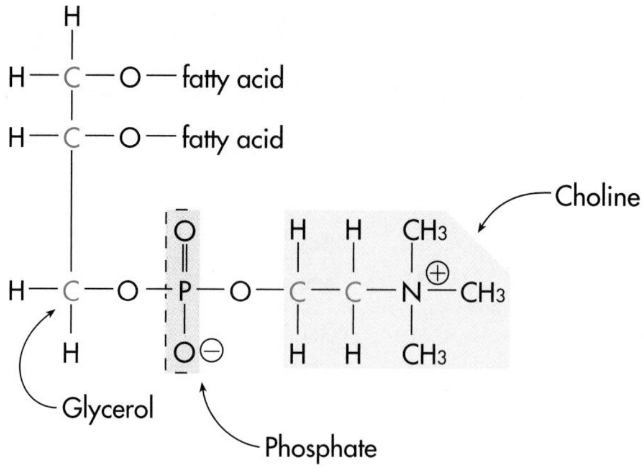

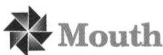

Figure 5-6 A phospholipid: lecithin.

Sterols

sterols
fatlike class of lipids that serve vital functions in the body

Sterol structures, including cholesterol, are carbon rings intermeshed with side chains of carbon, hydrogen, and oxygen, which make them more complex than triglycerides (Figure 5-7). Like phospholipids, sterols are synthesized by the body and are not essential nutrients. For example, if dietary cholesterol is not consumed, the liver will produce the amount required for body functions.

Generally, dietary cholesterol accounts for about 25% of the cholesterol in the body. The rest, which is made in the liver, seems to be produced in relation to how much is needed. The only food sources of cholesterol are animal and include beef, pork (bacon), chicken, luncheon meats, eggs, fish, and dairy products (milk, butter, and cheeses); plant foods do not contain cholesterol.

FATS AS A NUTRIENT WITHIN THE BODY

Digestion

Mouth

The mouth's only digestive process is mechanical, as teeth masticate fatty foods. Although the tongue produces a fat-splitting enzyme (lingual lipase), this enzyme is most important during infancy for digestion of long-chain fatty acids found in milk, but it is not significant for adult fat digestion.

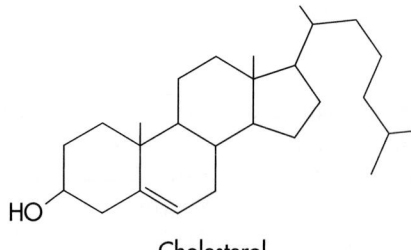

Cholesterol

Figure 5-7 A sterol: cholesterol. Foods with cholesterol include animal-derived foods such as beef, pork, chicken, bacon, luncheon meats, eggs, fish, and dairy products.

Stomach

Mechanical digestion continues through the strong actions of peristalsis. Fat-splitting enzymes such as gastric lipase hydrolyze some fatty acids from triglycerides.

Small Intestine

Fats entering the duodenum initiate the release of cholecystokinin (CCK) hormone from the duodenum walls. CCK, as described in Chapter 3, then sparks the gallbladder to release bile into the small intestine. The bile emulsifies fats to facilitate digestion. Mechanical digestion through muscular action allows for increased exposure of the emulsified fat globules to pancreatic lipase. This enzyme is the primary digestive enzyme that breaks triglycerides into fatty acids, monoglycerides, and glycerol molecules. Note that fats may not be completely broken down. Some may also pass through without being digested or absorbed. Figure 5-8 summarizes digestion of triglycerides.

Absorption

Fatty acids, monoglycerides, and cholesterol are assisted by bile salts in moving from the lumen to the villi for absorption. Micelles, created by bile salts encircling lipids, aid diffusion through the membrane wall. When through the membrane wall, fatty acids and glycerol combine back into triglycerides. These triglycerides are incorporated into chylomicrons, containing fats and cholesterol coated with protein, to allow travel through the lymph system to the blood circulatory system toward the hepatic portal system and the liver. Some glycerol and any short- and medium-chain fatty acids are absorbed directly into the blood capillaries leading to the portal vein and liver.

At the cell membranes, the triglycerides in the chylomicrons are broken down into fatty acids and glycerol with assistance from an enzyme called *lipoprotein lipase*. Muscle cells, adipose cells, and other cells in the vicinity take up most of the fatty acids released by the breakdown of chylomicrons. Cells can use the absorbed fatty acids immediately as fuel, or they can reform them into triglycerides to be stored as reserve energy supplies.

Metabolism

Lipid metabolism consists of several processes. Catabolism (breakdown) of lipids for energy involves the hydrolysis of triglycerides into two-carbon units that become part of acetyl coenzyme A (acetyl CoA). The acetyl CoA then enters the series of reactions called the TCA cycle, eventually leading to the oxidation of the carbon and hydrogen atoms derived from fatty acids (or carbohydrates or amino acids) to carbon dioxide and water with the release of energy as adenosine triphosphate (ATP). If fat catabolizes quickly because of a lack of carbohydrate for energy, the liver cells form intermediate products called *ketone bodies*. These ketone bodies accumulate in the blood, causing a condition called ketosis.

Anabolism (synthesis) of lipids, or lipogenesis, results in the formation of triglycerides, phospholipids, cholesterol, and prostaglandins for use throughout the body. Triglycerides and phosphates form from fatty acids and glycerol or from excess glucose or amino acids. Extra carbon, hydrogen, and oxygen from any source can be converted to and stored as triglycerides in adipose tissues, so we can gain fat from foods other than fat.

Lipid metabolism is regulated mainly by insulin, growth hormone, adrenocorticotropic hormone (ACTH), and glucocorticoids.

---

chylomicrons
the first lipoproteins formed after absorption of lipids from food

Triglycerides are composed of long chains of fatty acids. To aid fat digestion in those patients with malabsorption, synthetically manufactured medium-chain triglycerides (MCTs) may be incorporated into a patient's dietary intake. MCTs should not be used to completely replace dietary fats because they do not contain EFAs.

acetyl coenzyme A (acetyl CoA)
important intermediate byproduct in metabolism formed from the breakdown of glucose, fatty acids, and certain amino acids

TCA cycle
cellular reactions that liberate energy from fragments of carbohydrates, fats, and protein; also called the *tricarboxylic acid cycle* or *Krebs cycle*

ketosis
a condition in which the absence of plasma glucose results in partial oxidation of fatty acids and the formation of excessive amounts of ketones

lipogenesis
anabolism (synthesis) of lipids

adrenocorticotropic hormone (ACTH)
an adrenal cortex hormone that stimulates secretion of more hormones

glucocorticoid
an adrenal cortex hormone that affects food metabolism

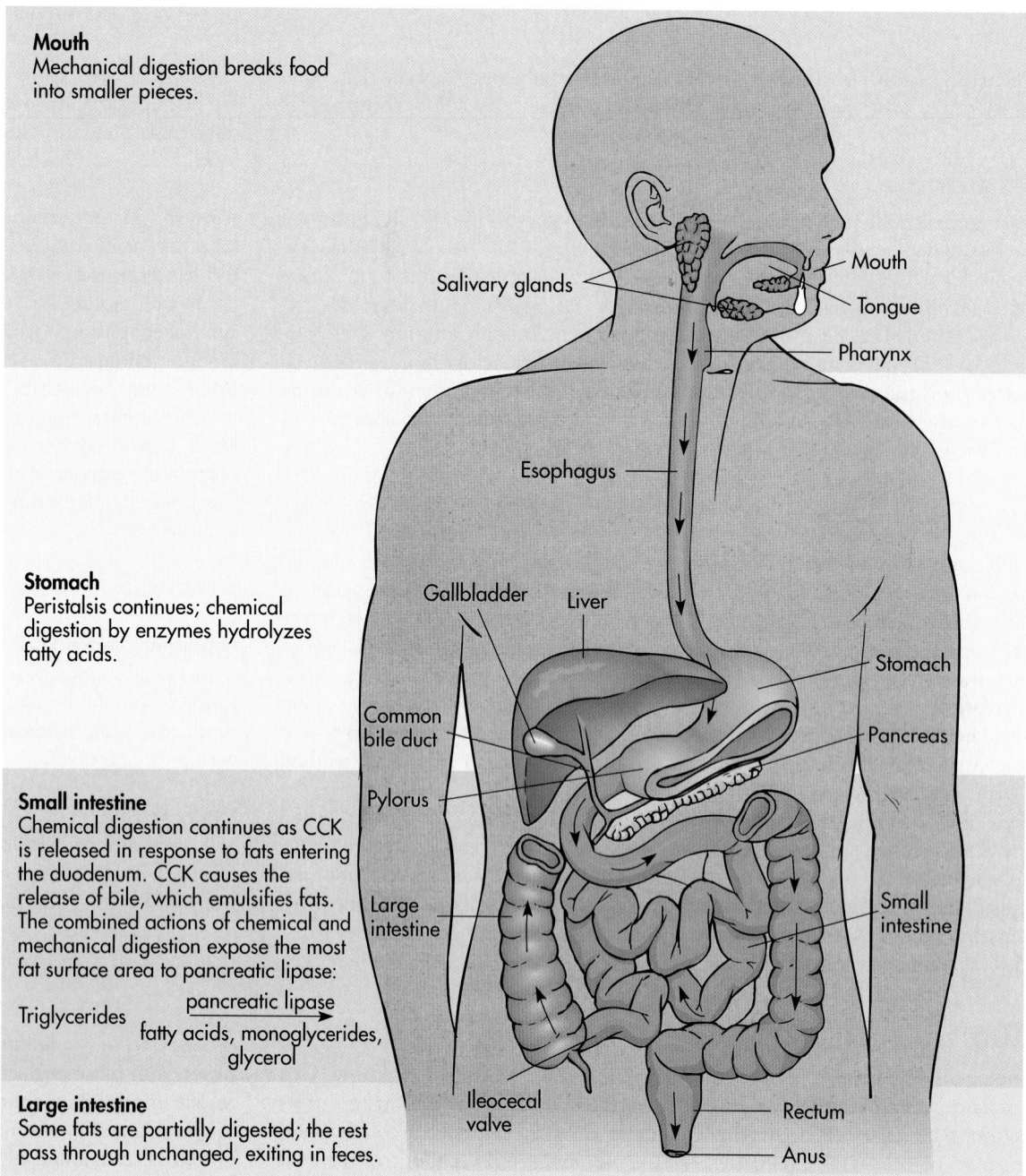

Mouth
Mechanical digestion breaks food into smaller pieces.

Stomach
Peristalsis continues; chemical digestion by enzymes hydrolyzes fatty acids.

Small intestine
Chemical digestion continues as CCK is released in response to fats entering the duodenum. CCK causes the release of bile, which emulsifies fats. The combined actions of chemical and mechanical digestion expose the most fat surface area to pancreatic lipase:

$$\text{Triglycerides} \xrightarrow{\text{pancreatic lipase}} \text{fatty acids, monoglycerides, glycerol}$$

Large intestine
Some fats are partially digested; the rest pass through unchanged, exiting in feces.

Salivary glands — Mouth — Tongue — Pharynx — Esophagus — Gallbladder — Liver — Stomach — Common bile duct — Pancreas — Pylorus — Large intestine — Small intestine — Ileocecal valve — Rectum — Anus

Figure 5-8 Summary of fat digestion and absorption. (From Rolin Graphics.)

FAT INTAKE AND ISSUES

Awareness of the fat content of foods is steadily growing. Whether we are consuming a sophisticated gourmet feast or chowing down hot dogs and hamburgers at a summer barbecue, the fat levels of our meals may be of interest. Concerns about fat in our diets center around health issues of excessive intake of energy, excessive fat intake that replaces other nutrients, and the relationship between dietary fat intake and the development of chronic diet-related diseases. Some lipids consumed in foods are essential to our bodies to achieve wellness.

Fat Content of Foods

High-fat foods are always high-calorie foods. This is because fats are the most concentrated source of food energy, supplying 9 kcalories per gram; carbohydrates and proteins supply 4 kcalories per gram. Because most foods contain a mixture of nutrients, we can identify the fat content of food by the number of fat grams in a serving or the percent of Daily Value of recommended fat intake in a serving. Nutritional labels on packaged food contain this information.

 The Dietary Reference Intakes, based on Acceptable Macronutrient Distribution Ranges (AMDRs), recommend that we eat 20% to 35% of our kcaloric intakes from fats, with 10% or less of kcalories from saturated fats.[8] Based on the daily values, total fat intake for an average daily kcaloric intake of 2000 to 2500 kcalories should range from about 40 to 97 grams or less (400 to 875 kcalories or less). Saturated fat should be 25 to 20 grams or less (225 to 180 kcalories or less). Children less than 5 years of age require at least 20% of kcalories as fat. A greater restriction may compromise growth or the ability to properly process cholesterol as an adult.[9]

There is growing evidence that diets with fat levels of 18% to 22% may have undesirable effects including lower HDL levels and higher triglyceride levels.[10] The evidence does not support reducing fat much below 26% kcalories as fat—not a problem for most Americans, who have a long way to go toward lower fat diets. In fact, although only about one third of adult Americans have reached 30% of total energy as fat,[11] the majority believe they are avoiding or limiting high-fat foods.[12] One reason may be because high-fat foods have both potent sensory qualities and high-energy density; overeating is then often more passive than active. Another reason is that people who eat a lot of high-fat foods are unsure whether their diets are high in fat because home cooking has fallen sharply; the cook no longer knows exactly what goes into each dish. Also, portion sizes at restaurants are often twice the size of that recommended for good health by the Food Guide Pyramid. Then there is the "less fat, more carbs" message that has been incorrectly translated into sweet, kcalorie-dense, low-fiber carbohydrate foods, so the low-fat diet has become a high-calorie, processed-carbohydrate diet. It is also likely that people are misled by labels of "reduced fat" foods and thus actually *increase* the total intake of such foods. The individual foods we eat daily may have a higher or lower fat content, but overall we should generally average 25% to 30% of kcaloric fat intake from all the foods we eat each day (see the Teaching Tool: "Calculating Your Daily Fat Intake").

TEACHING TOOL
Calculating Your Daily Fat Intake

*H*ere's how to calculate your daily grams of fat:

1. Use the Recommended Energy Intake chart in Chapter 9 to determine your appropriate energy needs for the day. Multiply that number of kcalories by 0.25 for 25% fat intake or by 0.30 for 30% fat intake.
2. Divide that number by 9, because each gram of fat has 9 kcalories. For example, if you consume 1800 kcal a day and want to get 25% of those kcalories from fat: $0.25 \times 1800 = 450$. Then divide 450 by 9 to get 50 grams of fat. Energy needs for the day _____ kcal $\times$ 0.30 = _____ kcal fat intake/day. _____ kcal fat intake a day $\div$ 9 kcal = _____ grams of fat/day.
3. Next, check food labels and/or use food composition tables (see Appendix A) for the grams of fat per food serving. You then can compare the sum of the fat grams consumed with the recommended levels for your particular energy needs.

How do we measure the fat in foods without labels, such as fresh foods, home-cooked recipes, and restaurant items? One way is to classify foods into groups according to fat content. The Food Guide Pyramid illustrates the density of fat in different food groups by the concentration of symbols for fat in each section (Figure 5-9). There are few fat symbols in the bottom sections for bread and cereal, fruits, and vegetables, and many more in the three top sections for dairy foods; meat, fish, and nuts; and added fats. Of course there are some exceptions to these guidelines. Half an avocado contains 15 grams of fat and 150 kcalories, about 90% fat. Six medium shrimp contain 2 grams of fat and 150 kcalories, less than 2% fat. Grams of fat, saturated fat, and cholesterol in examples from different food groups are listed in Tables 5-2 and 5-3.

Detecting Dietary Fat

Some fats are visible; others are invisible. Visible fat is fairly easy to find and control; just cut off the white fat on the outside of a steak and measure the butter or sour cream on the baked potato. Invisible fat is harder to measure. Fat in milk, cheese, and yogurt is nearly impossible to see, but many people learn to taste the difference between whole and low-fat dairy products. In addition, dairy foods are all labeled so fat content is known. Some foods give other clues that they contain fat. Press a napkin on a slice of pizza, a Danish pastry, or an egg roll. Look for oil around the edge of stir-fried Chinese food.

Be aware of general characteristics that signal the level of fat in foods. Some cooking methods, such as deep-frying, add fat. The way a prepared food is usually eaten may also increase fat intake, such as spreading butter or oil on bread rather than just dipping it in soup. Whether eating in or dining out, the amount of food regularly selected from high-fat animal sources such as meat and cheese compared

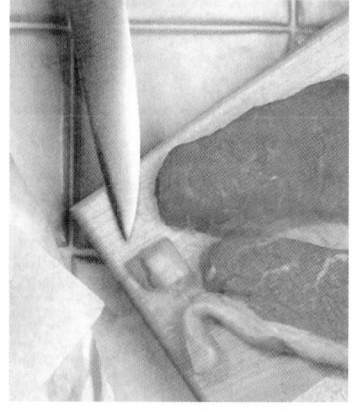

Trim meat before cooking to reduce fat intake. (From National Cancer Institute, Bethesda, Md.)

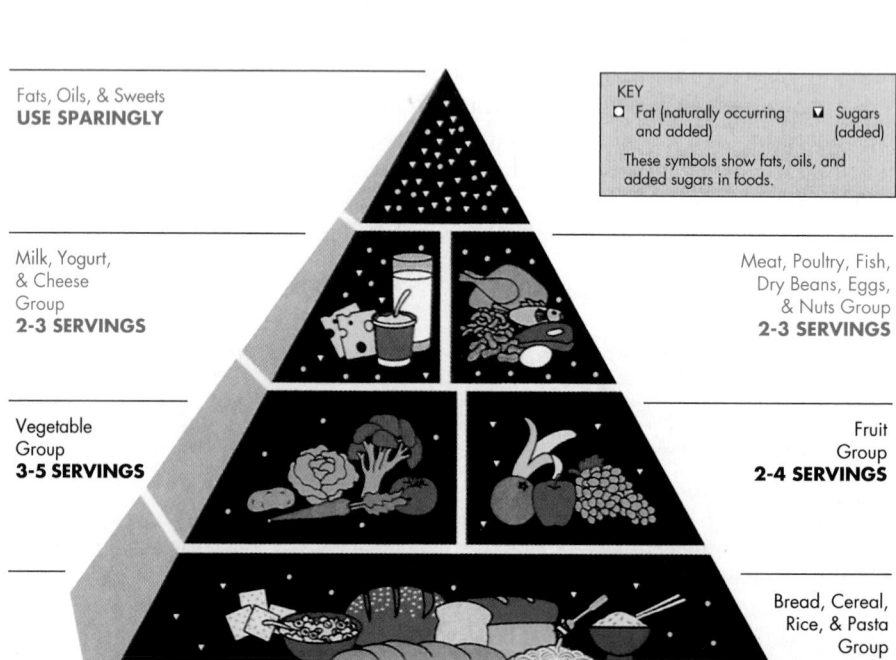

Figure 5-9 The Food Guide Pyramid, highlighting major sources of fat. Note that the fat symbol also appears in the Vegetable and Bread, Cereal, Rice, and Pasta groups; be alert to fat hiding in individual items in these food groups. For example, an avocado contains about 30 grams of fat. (From US Department of Agriculture: The Food Guide Pyramid, *Human Nutrition Information Pub No 249,* Washington, DC, Revised 1996, US Government Printing Office.)

with the amount of food consumed from low-fat grains, vegetables, and fruit affects total dietary fat consumption levels.

Government and consumer groups have encouraged restaurants and institutional food service operations to offer identifiable low-fat, low-calorie food choices. These choices allow clients to meet health promotion goals while maintaining social interactions. Encourage clients to identify healthy menu choices when eating away from home.

Table 5-2
Fat in Food Servings

Food	Serving Size	Fat Content
Butter/Margarine	1 Tbs	11 g
Salad dressing	1 Tbs	7 g
Mayonnaise	1 Tbs	11 g
Cream cheese	1 Tbs	10 g
Carrots	½ cup	trace
Broccoli	½ cup	trace
Potato, baked	1	trace
French fries	10	8 g
Apple	1	trace
Orange	1	trace
Banana	1	trace
Fruit juice	1 cup	trace
Rice or pasta	½ cup	trace
Bagel	1	trace
Muffin	1 medium	6 g
Danish pastry	1 medium	13 g
Skim milk	1 cup	trace
Low-fat milk	1 cup	5 g
Whole milk	1 cup	8 g
American cheese	2 oz	18 g
Cheddar cheese	1½ oz	14 g
Frozen yogurt	½ cup	2 g
Ice milk	⅓ cup	3 g
Ice cream	⅓ cup	7 g
Lean beef	3 oz	6 g
Poultry	3 oz	6 g
Fish	3 oz	6 g
Ground beef	3 oz	16 g
Bologna (2 slices)	1 oz	16 g
Egg	1	5 g
Nuts (⅓ cup)	1 oz	22 g

Table 5-3
Cholesterol Content of Selected Foods*

Food	Amount	Cholesterol (mg)
Milk, nonfat/skim	1 cup	4
Mayonnaise	1 Tbsp	8
Cottage cheese, lowfat/2%	½ cup	10
Milk, lowfat/2%	1 cup	18
Cream cheese	1 oz	28
Hot dog†	1	29
Ice cream, 10% fat	½ cup	30
Cheddar cheese	1 oz	30
Butter	1 Tbsp	31
Milk, whole	1 cup	33
Clams, fish fillets, oysters	3 oz	50-60
Beef,† pork,† poultry	3 oz	70-85
Shrimp	3 oz	166
Egg yolk†	1	213
Beef liver	3 oz	410

*In ascending order.
†Leading contributors of cholesterol to U.S. diet.

The cuisines of China and Italy are based on rice, pasta, and bread. When prepared with small amounts of fat and eaten with little fatty meat and plenty of vegetables, these cultural food patterns are excellent examples of healthful diets. Yet, when Chinese and Italian foods are prepared to please the American palate, large amounts of fat are used in cooking the food, and portion sizes are larger than usual for specific ethnic tradition (see the Cultural Considerations box, "Choosing Lower Fat Ethnic Dishes").

Fast, But High-Fat, Foods

Contemporary lifestyles sometimes leave little room for meal planning and preparation. Often we may find ourselves heading for the nearest fast-food restaurant or snack bar as we dash off to school or work. What impact do these meals have on our nutritional status? A positive trend among fast-food chains is the use of less saturated fat in fried potatoes and the addition of items such as salads and skim milk to the menu. On the negative side, between 40% and 50% of fast-food kcalories come from fat, far higher than the recommended 30%.

When we study the major food contributors of fat in the American diet, hamburgers, cheeseburgers, meat loaf, and hot dogs top the list. Whole milk beverages including shakes are next, followed by cheese and salad dressings. Doughnuts, cookies, and cake tie with fried potatoes.[13] It is no surprise that the majority of fat in the American diet happens to appear in menu favorites served in fast-food restaurants (Box 5-1). In addition, the majority of fat in these foods tends to be saturated, with hamburgers and cheeseburgers leading the pack.

One may wonder why some foods that are fast to fix, such as apples, oranges, and bananas, are not considered fast foods, nor are they sold in fast-food restaurants. The answer probably has to do with the fact that fat lends a seductive flavor to fast-food favorites (see the Teaching Tool: "But Fast Foods Are So Convenient . . .").

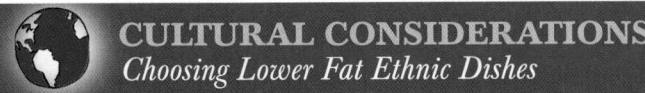

CULTURAL CONSIDERATIONS
Choosing Lower Fat Ethnic Dishes

*P*erhaps you've grown up eating rice and beans, home-made lasagna, or Chinese takeout. Regardless of who prepares the food, Americans are consuming more international foods than ever before. We have a smorgasbord of ethnic foods from which to choose. Chinese, Indian, Mexican, and Greek dishes have become commonplace.

We may assume that because these foods are different and exotic, they are healthier for us. After all, aren't hamburgers and hot dogs—all-American favorites—the worst offenders for our health? However, although some ethnic dishes are lower in fat and higher in dietary fibers, other ethnic delights aren't much better than traditional all-American favorites.

The Chinese foods eaten in America would be considered far too rich (and high in fat) by the Chinese; they are reserved for banquets and even then are eaten in moderation. To enhance the healthfulness of prepared Chinese foods, avoid fried dishes, especially egg rolls, and make rice the centerpiece of your meal. Top the rice with moderate portions of entrees of chicken or seafood mixed with vegetables.

Italian dishes of pasta and gravy (i.e., tomato sauce) are healthful but become problematic when teamed with sausage, meatballs, fried breaded meats, and layers of cheeses or when tomato sauce is replaced by a cream Alfredo sauce. Each adds substantial amounts of saturated fats. Be aware of portion sizes and focus on large portions of pasta served with smaller servings of the high-fat foods.

Mexican and Latino foods are sometimes made with lard, a heavily saturated animal fat, and with fatty portions of pork. These negatives, however, are somewhat offset by the generous (and delicious) use of beans, rice, and soft tortillas made from corn or wheat. When possible, avoid or reduce the use of lard; vegetable oils are a good substitute. Generally the less fat used, the healthier the entree. For example, a taco made with a soft tortilla contains less fat than one made with a hard fried tortilla. And be sure to pile on lots of lettuce, tomatoes, and salsa!

Application to nursing: Become familiar with the exotic tastes of international cuisines. By doing so, you'll be able to assist clients in understanding the fat content of their ethnic favorites. Just remember that the palatability of fat is a worldwide phenomenon, so choose wisely.

Box 5-1 Ballparks and Healthy Food: An Unlikely Combination?

*A*cross the country, American major league ballparks provide hungry and thirsty fans with a wide selection of food choices. But can healthy guidelines still be followed? Here's a sample of the results of an American Dietetic Association (ADA) survey of food selections found at America's 28 ballparks:

AVAILABLE AT ALL PARKS

Hot dogs, peanuts, nachos, ice cream, popcorn, pretzels, sodas, and beer

AVAILABLE AT MOST PARKS

Pizza, bottled water, hamburgers, French fries, grilled or baked chicken sandwiches, a variety of sausages, frozen yogurt, cotton candy and other candies

AVAILABLE AT EIGHT OR FEWER PARKS

Fresh fruit, fresh vegetables, salads, milk (whole only), garden or vegetable burgers

SOME REGIONAL AND ETHNIC SELECTIONS

- Ahi tuna sandwiches at the San Francisco Giants' 3Com Park
- California roll (a type of sushi) at the California Angels' Anaheim Stadium
- Biscotti (Italian cookie) and pierogies at the Cleveland Indians' Jacob's Field
- Carrot juice and herbal teas at the Oakland A's Coliseum
- Arepas (South American cornmeal crepes with cheese), rice and beans, and plantains at the Florida Marlins' Pro-Player Stadium

The ADA advises it is best to have a nutrition plan before getting to the stadium. That way choosing pizza or a hamburger won't be an impulse selection but rather part of an overall eating plan for the day. So enjoy the game!

Reference: Take me out to the buffet, *Press Release, Chicago, June 11, 1997, American Dietetic Association; www.eatright.org/press061197.html.*

How can fat intake be lowered? First, start early to include children and the whole family in buying food, preparing it, and having low-fat foods on hand. Many people prefer fast food because they don't have fresh or partly prepared foods ready to cook. Teaching children cooking skills from simple recipes, videos, and friends has been shown to establish low-fat food preferences early. Studies

TEACHING TOOL
But Fast Foods Are So Convenient . . .

*O*ur advice to clients needs to be realistic, which means accepting the fact that most people occasionally eat at fast-food restaurants. Rather than attempting to dissuade them from going at all, give clients the following tools for helping to make lower-fat selections.

Advice about reducing fat intake sounds good when we have the time to prepare wholesome meals. If you are one of the harried millions rushing between school, work, and extracurricular activities, cooking advice sounds like a foreign language. Here are reality-based fast-food restaurant strategies for reducing fat intake while eating quickly.

- Avoid deep-fried fish and chicken sandwiches. Although fish and chicken are lower in fat and cholesterol than beef, when they are breaded and fried, more fat is soaked up than in a hamburger.
- Choose grilled chicken sandwiches and, if possible, remove the high-fat sauces.
- Always order a side salad or top sandwiches with lettuce and tomato.
- Try the junior size of the specialty sandwiches. This is true particularly for lunch; we don't need to eat half our daily intake of calories in one meal.
- Order quarter-pound hamburgers plain, without cheese or bacon. Enough fat calories will be saved to occasionally order fries—a small portion, of course!
- Order a plain baked potato as a side dish. Top with a small amount of butter or just eat it plain with a bit of salt and pepper.
- Salad bars can be deceiving. Fat lurks in salad dressing, mayonnaise-based cole slaw, and potato and macaroni salads. Go heavy on the lettuce, carrots and other sliced vegetables, beans, and fruits. Put salad dressing in a small pile. Dip your fork into the dressing, then into the salad. This gives you the same taste but less fat.

Eat quickly, but smartly.

---

show that people are more likely to adopt low-fat diets if eating partners or families do the same.[14]

Second, most major secondary and tertiary healthcare settings have an active dietetic department, often geared to pediatrics and family practice. Programs offered may include healthy cooking classes for children and their parents or nutrition and wellness classes. Providing lists of such programs is a valuable resource for clients.

Third, never say never. It is okay to include some high-fat foods in food plans because they taste good. If a mixture of low-fat and high-fat foods is eaten, preferences for both are developed; this automatically controls overdoing the fatty foods. The Teaching Tool that discusses fast foods is packed with other strategies for fast-food, low-fat eating patterns.

Preserving Fats in Foods

Processed Fats and Oils: Hydrogenated and Emulsified

A problem with unsaturated fats in foods is that oxygen attacks the unsaturated double bonds (oxidation), causing damage that makes them rancid; rancid fats have an odor and bad flavor and may cause illness. One way to reduce vulnerability to oxidation is to artificially saturate the fatty acids by adding hydrogen at the double bonds. This process of *hydrogenation* makes the fat solid and more stable, which provides cooking benefits. When vegetable oil, which is polyunsaturated, is completely hydrogenated, it becomes a white, waxy or plasticlike substance called *vegetable shortening*. Because it is saturated with hydrogens, the body processes it as if it were a saturated fat. The ingredient list on a product label can truthfully state that the product contains more unsaturated liquid oil although it is mixed with the partially hydrogenated fat. Partially hydrogenated fats are used in a variety of food products.

Sometimes the solution to one problem causes another problem. Although it stabilizes fat, hydrogenation changes the structure of some of the fatty acids, from *cis* fatty acids to *trans* fatty acids (Figure 5-10). Most fatty acids in natural foods are in the cis form, but margarine and vegetable shortening contain high concentrations of trans fatty acids (trans-fats). Some margarines are now processed to contain no trans fatty acids. Often manufacturers will note if their margarine products are free of trans fatty acids. Controversy over the impact of trans-fats in relation to cancer vulnerability and elevated blood cholesterol levels has confused the public.

Before completely deciding butter is better, consider that although some margarines are fairly high in trans-fats, they usually have less than many commercially made foods such as French fries, potato chips, and bakery products made from partially hydrogenated vegetable oils. Some margarines are now offered as "transfree." On the other hand, of the 34% of kcalories consumed as fat by Americans, only 3% to 4% of total kcalories come from trans-fats.[15]

Nonetheless, trans-fat consumption appears to increase risk for CAD. Risk is increased because the trans-fat raises the blood cholesterol component (low-density lipoproteins [LDLs]), which delivers cholesterol throughout the body, and while doing so, may contribute to plaque formation in arteries. Trans-fat also decreases the blood cholesterol component (high-density lipoproteins [HDLs]) that removes excess and used cholesterol from the body. Maintaining higher levels of this component decreases risk of CAD. Considering these effects on blood cholesterol, consumption of trans-fat should be limited.[15,16] Listing trans fatty acid content on nutrition labels is currently optional. Consumer groups such as the Center for Science in the Public Interest (CSPI) advocate for trans-fat content listing to be mandatory.[17]

Because trans-fat content is not required on the nutrition facts panel of food labels, look for saturated fat instead. Although saturated fat does not not have the same effect as trans-fat, generally foods that contain less saturated fat have less trans-fat. "Partially hydrogenated fat" as an ingredient is another clue that

cis fatty acids
cis indicates the configuration of the double bond of fatty acids in a natural oil

trans fatty acids (trans-fats)
fatty acids with unusual double-bond structures caused by hydrogenated unsaturated oils

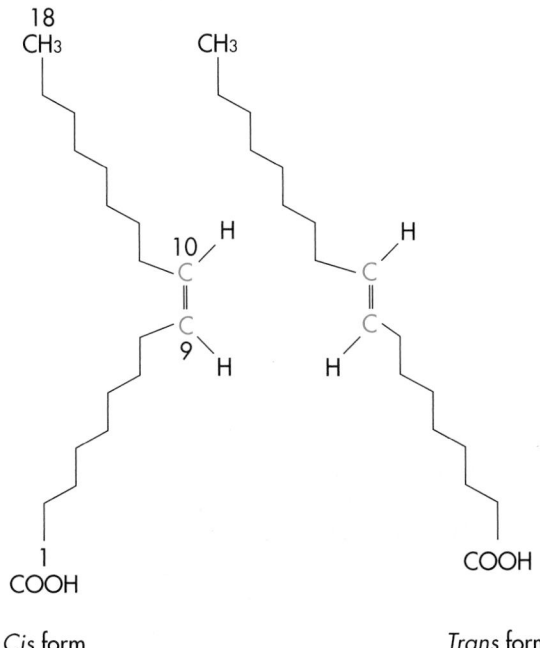

Cis form   *Trans* form

Figure 5-10 Cis bond to trans bond.

trans-fat is present in the product. When possible, trans-fat should be replaced by a monounsaturated fat such as canola oil. Guidelines currently suggest as a priority to reduce overall food fat to 30% of total kcalories; less fat means less trans-fats as well. This means eating less margarine, French fries, potato chips, cakes, and cookies, as well as less fried chicken, fried fish, fatty meat, and ice cream.

Antioxidants

Another way to preserve polyunsaturated fats without hydrogenation is through the use of antioxidant additives. These substances block oxidation, or the breakdown of double bonds by oxygen. Food manufacturers can use either natural or synthetic forms of antioxidants. Natural sources include vitamin E (tocopherol) and vitamin C (ascorbic acid). Their use not only helps to preserve foods but also adds essential vitamins. Synthetic forms consist of the food additives of butylated hydroxyanisole (BHA) and butylated hydroxytoluene (BHT). These forms are used in packaging as well to help prevent the oxidation of the foods.

Food Cholesterol Vs. Blood Cholesterol

Cholesterol is a waxy substance found in all tissues in humans and other animals, thus all foods from animal sources, such as meat, eggs, fish, poultry, and dairy products, contain cholesterol. The highest sources of cholesterol are egg yolks and organ meats (liver and kidney). No plant-derived food contains cholesterol, not even avocado or peanut butter, which are very high in fat. People often misunderstand this because they confuse food (dietary) cholesterol with blood cholesterol.

A high level of cholesterol in the blood is a risk factor for CAD. To understand blood cholesterol levels, the role of lipoproteins—specialized transporting compounds—needs clarification. Lipoproteins are compounds that contain a mix of lipids—including triglycerides, fatty acids, phospholipids, cholesterol, and small amounts of other steroids and fat-soluble vitamins—that are covered with a protein outer layer (Figure 5-11). The outer layer of protein allows the compound to move through a watery substance, such as blood. Lipoproteins transport fats in the circulatory system.

The amount of fat and protein determines the density or weight of the lipoprotein. The more fat and lipid substances, the lower the density (or lighter) the compound. Four forms of these compounds are most important for understanding the route of cholesterol in the body; they are chylomicrons, very low-density lipoproteins, low-density lipoproteins, and high-density lipoproteins.

Chylomicrons transport absorbed fats from the intestinal wall to the liver cells. Fats are then used for synthesis of lipoproteins. **Very low-density lipoproteins (VLDLs)**

very low-density lipoproteins (VLDLs) lipoproteins that carry fats and cholesterol to body cells and are made of the largest proportions of cholesterol

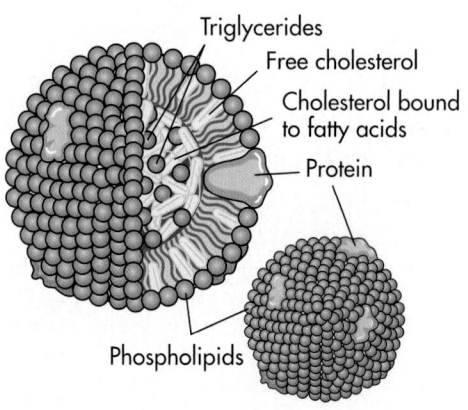

Figure 5-11 Lipoprotein.

leave the liver cells full of fats and lipid components to transfer newly made (endogenous) triglycerides to the cells. Low-density lipoproteins (LDLs) form from VLDLs as density is reduced as fats and lipids are released on their journey through the body. LDLs carry cholesterol throughout the body to tissue cells for various functions. In contrast to the delivery functions of the first three lipoproteins, high-density lipoproteins (HDLs) are formed within cells to remove cholesterol from the cell, bringing it to the liver for disposal.

A total blood cholesterol reading reflects the level of cholesterol contained in LDL and HDL. To get a clearer assessment of cholesterol activity in the body, the individual levels of LDL and HDL are valuable. The risk of CAD associated with blood cholesterol levels is presented in Table 5-4. LDL levels reflect the amount of cholesterol brought to cells that have the potential to be dropped off along the way to clog vessels and arteries, contributing to plaque formation. As this happens, HDLs remove cholesterol from the circulatory system. Removal of cholesterol is a positive action that reduces CAD risk.

Health guidelines generally recommend a dietary cholesterol intake of 300 mg or less per day. However if LDL cholesterol is elevated, dietary cholesterol intake should be less than 200 mg.[18] Table 5-3 lists the cholesterol content of selected foods. However, the major culprit that raises blood cholesterol is not dietary food cholesterol but too much *food fat* (dietary triglycerides), particularly saturated fats; food cholesterol alone makes a minor difference for most people. Too much food cholesterol becomes a problem when it is eaten in conjunction with very high-fat diets. Sometimes, this extra cholesterol in the blood may be dropped off, staying in the vessels and arteries. It is a factor involved in plaque buildup, called atherosclerosis, or CAD (Figure 5-12).

One reason for the confusion is the way food is cooked and eaten. Eggs, for example, are high in cholesterol and are often cooked and served with high-fat bacon or sausage. The combined meal of eggs and bacon then gets a bad reputation for raising blood cholesterol. The fact is that the large amount of fat in bacon and sausage is more likely to raise blood cholesterol than the food cholesterol in eggs. Shrimp are high in cholesterol but low in fat. That is, low in fat if the shrimp are steamed or broiled, not encased in a deep fat fried coating. Of course, moderation is recommended when eating eggs or shrimp.

Another source of confusion is that cooking oils made from corn, safflower, and soybeans are often labeled as cholesterol free (see the Myth box, "No-Cholesterol Potato Chips Must Mean Fat Free!"). Of course they are cholesterol free; only foods from animals contain cholesterol. Yet vegetable oils are virtually 100% food fat, and large amounts of dietary fat can also raise blood cholesterol.

In addition to the amount of fat, another characteristic of food fat that causes it to affect blood cholesterol differently is whether the fat is saturated or unsaturated;

low-density lipoproteins (LDLs)
lipoproteins that carry fats and cholesterol to body cells and are made of large proportions of cholesterol

high-density lipoproteins (HDLs)
lipoproteins that carry fats and cholesterol from body cells to the liver and are made of large proportions of proteins

plaque
deposits of fatty substances, including cholesterol, that attach to arterial walls

atherosclerosis
accumulation of plaques that result in blockage in the arteries

We usually classify beef and chocolate as cholesterol-raising foods. Stearic acid is a major long-chain saturated fatty acid in beef fat and cocoa butter (the fat that gives chocolate its appealing mouth feel). Stearic acid does not seem to raise blood cholesterol levels by itself, but because of other fatty acids in the beef and chocolate that do raise blood cholesterol, the entire food is assigned to the cholesterol-raising category. Although growers are trying to manipulate animal feed, we can do little to alter the mixture of fatty acids in beef fat. However, we might seek chocolate products that are not made with added saturated fatty acids such as butterfat, coconut, and hydrogenated fats.

Table 5-4
Blood Cholesterol Levels

Risk Classification	Total Cholesterol	LDL-Cholesterol
Desirable	<200 mg/dl	<130 mg/dl
Borderline-high	200-239 mg/dl	130-159 mg/dl
High	≥240 mg/dl	≥160 mg/dl

Modified from National Cholesterol Education Program: ATP III guidelines at-a-glance quick desk reference, NIH Pub No 01-3305, Washington, DC, 2001, US Department of Health and Human Services; Public Health Services; National Institutes of Health; National Heart, Lung, and Blood Institute.

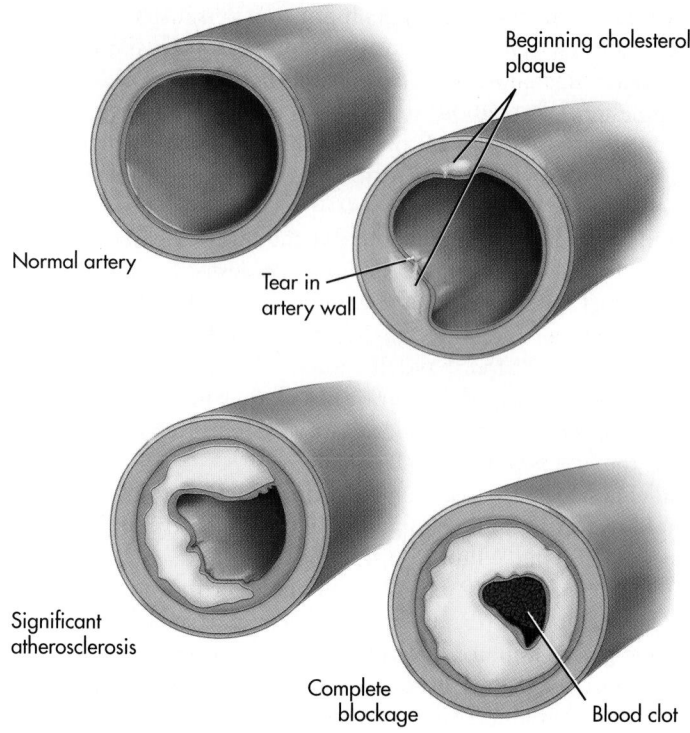

Figure 5-12 Development of atherosclerosis.

⭐ **MYTH**
No-Cholesterol Potato Chips Must Mean Fat Free!

*H*ave you ever noticed how some food packages proclaim the contents are cholesterol free? Often, this gives us the impression the products are reformulated to be healthier than their old version. We might then be tempted to buy the products. But are they really cholesterol free?

Many of us still associate dietary cholesterol with being our only lipid concern in foods. Fats tend to have a greater impact on health than dietary cholesterol. To be a savvy consumer, read ingredient labels and be aware of some finer points of fat education.

- Hydrogenated vegetable oils—corn, soybean, and cottonseed—contain transfatty acids and cholesterol-forming saturated fats often used to prepare potato and corn chips.
- Tropical oils of palm, palm kernel, and coconut are the only naturally saturated fat plant source. Found in many food products, they should be consumed only occasionally. (Popcorn popped in tropical oils came under fire; many movie theater chains now offer air-popped popcorn in addition to traditionally prepared popcorn.)
- Margarines are cholesterol free if made from vegetable oils but still contain the same number of calories as butter; both are about 100% lipid. Margarines, however, contain unsaturated fatty acids. Note that the level of hydrogenation used to form the margarine affects the amount of trans and saturated fatty acids contained. Use label information to select the least saturated product.
- Advise clients to check the labels of foods regularly eaten; a cholesterol-free product might not be as healthy as it seems.

that is, whether the fat contains mostly saturated or unsaturated fatty acids. Saturated fatty acids generally raise blood cholesterol by providing the liver with the best building blocks for making cholesterol.

A simple guideline followed by many people is that blood cholesterol is *raised* by eating solid saturated fats and *lowered* by unsaturated and monounsaturated liquid fats. However, this rule is oversimplified for two reasons. First, food fats are a mixture of the three types. Second, although saturated fatty acids as a group raise cholesterol, some individual ones do not. Therefore, although we classify food fats as cholesterol raising (butter/saturated) and cholesterol lowering (corn oil/PUFA and olive oil/monounsaturated), these guidelines are based on the proportion of specific fatty acids in each food and how much each individual fatty acid affects blood cholesterol. Total fat intake can also influence blood cholesterol levels regardless of the source. Table 5-2 and Figure 5-4 clear up some confusion over the finer points of fat.

Researchers have studied individual fatty acids as well as combinations regarding their effects on blood cholesterol[10] and other mechanisms including cancer.[19] We discuss these effects in the section titled "Fats as a Nutrient Within the Body."

Synthetic Fats and Fat Replacers

Many people dream about eating brownies and ice cream that are magically stripped of fat but still richly satisfying in taste and texture. Although surveys show that sugar substitutes have not reduced the amount of sugar we consume, optimists hope fat substitutes will reduce fat in our diets. Scientists are working to develop reduced-fat or fat-free substances that replace fat yet retain the taste and mouth-feel of fat in foods.[20]

Fat replacers, as they are called, are generally classified two ways: already existing in nature or synthesized in the laboratory. The naturally occurring ones do not change chemically and thus require less rigorous testing before the Food and Drug Administration (FDA) allows them to be used in foods. Heating and then blending protein from milk or eggs in a process called *microparticulation* produces one type of fat replacer. Simplesse is an example. Food applications include ice cream, frozen yogurt, and salad dressings—but not baked or deep-fried foods.

Carrageenan, a carbohydrate extracted from seaweed, has been used for centuries to thicken foods. Added to lean ground beef, carrageenan yields moist, juicy cooked meat with the texture of higher-fat beef. Similar gumlike products from oats, corn, and potatoes are under development and would provide lower kcalorie fatlike properties in food.

Salatrim, which stands for *short- and long-chain triglyceride molecules,* is made in the laboratory and provides sensory qualities with reduced energy content (5 kcal/g vs. 9 kcal/g). Olestra is a fat replacer made in the laboratory that binds fatty acids in a nontraditional way to sugar so that enzymes in the digestive tract are not able to break away the fatty acids. Olestra resembles standard fats and oils in many ways, including the ability to withstand frying and baking at high temperatures. Several characteristics of Olestra are attractive to manufacturers and consumers, including the sensory properties of taste and texture, the no-kcalorie value because of the body's inability to digest it, and the reduced absorption of fat and cholesterol from the intestine. Potato chips cooked in Olestra have 75 kcal/oz—half that of regular chips. Because of its swift passage through the gut and attraction of fat-soluble nutrients such as vitamins and carotenoids, the FDA requires product labels of foods containing Olestra to read in part, "Olestra may cause abdominal cramping and loose stools. Olestra inhibits the absorption of some vitamins and other nutrients."

As the story of fat replacers continues to unfold, we need to study their effect on people's food choices. Will we be misled into thinking that low- or no-fat foods automatically are low kcalorie? Many fat-reduced foods will increase the amounts of other ingredients, such as carbohydrates, and do not result in low-kcalorie items.

To what degree will products containing fat replacers stimulate mechanisms to compensate for reduction in fat? Some studies suggest that incorporating reduced-fat products into the diet results in total fat reduction.[21] Yet, diets reduced in fat may not result in a reduction of total kcalories.[20] Thus fat-free foods help some people consume fewer kcalories overall; other times people eat a fat-free food at one meal, then make up the kcalories by eating more at the next. What about appetite guiding what we eat? If mouth-feel is maintained in reduced-fat foods, we may not distinguish between high- and reduced-fat foods. Then there is the "bargain" appeal. In studies in which people did not know which chips were regular and which were Olestra, they ate similar amounts of each. When they did know, they ate significantly more Olestra chips, thus mistakenly thinking they got two for the "fat price" of one.

One of the objectives of *Healthy People 2000* was to "increase to at least 5000 brand items the availability of processed food products that are reduced in fat and saturated fat."[22] By 1992, 8 years ahead of schedule, more than 5600 reduced-fat products were available.[23] Consequently, because this objective has been met, other objectives are included in *Healthy People 2010 (HP2010)* (see Table 1-1).

Although fat replacers are widely available, the most prudent and health-promoting approach is for products to be reformulated or developed without the use of fat replacers so products contain lower-fat ingredients but still taste good. Research studies suggest that eating a low-fat diet can lead to a decrease in the preference for fat.[12] Is it possible that fat replacers could undermine this healthful change? Nutritionists and scientists undoubtedly will continue to seek answers to make our fat-free brownie and ice cream dreams come true—without side effects.

OVERCOMING BARRIERS

Health concerns about our dietary fat intake fall into several categories: energy intake, reduced intake of other nutrients because of dietary fat consumption, and the relationship between dietary fat intake and diet-related diseases.

Energy Intake

Foods containing significant amounts of dietary fat will naturally provide more kcalories than other lower-fat foods. Although high-fat treats are fine occasionally, indulging too often or not even realizing which foods are fat-laden can result in consumption of too many kcalories. These kcalories may end up stored as body fat in adipose tissues.

Fat is even more efficient at being stored than are carbohydrate and protein, which means that we may gain more body fat from eating fat kcalories than eating the same number of carbohydrate kcalories. The evidence for this comes from studying people who eat low-fat, high-calorie diets, as discussed earlier. A likely explanation for this is that the energy cost to convert dietary fat to body fat requires only 3% of the kcalories consumed,whereas carbohydrate requires 23% of the energy consumed to be converted to body fat. Both fat storage and fat oxidation differ from those of carbohydrates and fat.

In striking contrast to the closely regulated balance between intake and use of carbohydrate and protein, the fat oxidation rates in some people are low in response to high-fat diets. This may lead to weight gain.[24] But can we say dietary fat determines body fat? In short-term studies, low-fat diets result in modest reduction in body weight; but long-term studies show diets within the range of 18% to 40% fat kcalories have little effect on body fatness.[25] Our average kcalorie daily intake increased by 300 kcalories between 1980 and 1993, to 2700 for men and 1800 for women. Fat increased 2.8 g (about 1/2 teaspoon for men and about 6 g [about 1 tsp] for women).[26,27] The increase in overall kcalories explains why the percent of fat as kcalories dropped from 37% to 33% although we actually ate more fat.

Diets high in fat are not the primary cause for the high prevalence of excess body fat in our society, nor is the reduction in dietary fat the sole solution to the problem. We have an "all-food-all-the-time" lifestyle coupled with an aversion to physical activity. Overeating and underactivity are likely reasons for the steady increase in overweight and obese Americans. Another reason may be the ability to be aware of internal cues of hunger. Consider if we mistake fatigue as a cue of hunger. Consumption of food becomes a way to relieve tiredness, which of course does not work. Still, for many individuals struggling with moderate or even excessive weight, awareness of their dietary fat intake sources can make a difference. By gradually reducing fat intake—without increasing carbohydrate intake—energy intake decreases and weight maintenance becomes easier to achieve.

Extreme Dietary Fat Restrictions

Dietary intake of fat can also get too low. Although general population recommendations are for fat consumption to be 30% or less of our kcalorie intake, Dr. Dean Ornish developed a regimen to reverse CAD that is based on a dietary fat intake of 10% or less of kcaloric intake. The Ornish program has been successful in reducing cardiac risk factors, slowing the advance of CAD, and supporting continuation of lifestyle behaviors such as dietary modifications, regular exercise, and relaxation techniques.[28] However, an intake this low, based on a primarily vegetarian dietary pattern, may be difficult for most Americans to maintain. Adequate intake of EFAs must also be provided. There is also concern that a low-fat, high-carbohydrate diet may lower HDL cholesterol and raise triglycerides.[29]

Our health warnings about fat intake can also be taken too seriously and interpreted too intensely, creating health hazards throughout the life span. Infants and young children depend on dietary fats and cholesterol for the formation of brain and nerve tissue and to provide adequate kcalories for growth. Cases of failure to thrive have been reported when parents restricted the intake of dietary fats of their infants.[30] Dietary fats should not be restricted for children less than 2 years of age.[9] After that, a prudent diet with recommended levels of fats can be followed.[9]

Persons afflicted with the eating disorder of anorexia nervosa envision their bodies as being fat and, although they are emaciated, they often focus on their dietary fat consumption. They may reduce dietary fat intake to dangerously low levels through the erroneous belief that fat consumption at *any* kcaloric level would make them fat.

Among older adults, fear of dietary fat and cholesterol may cause malnutrition. Some older adults have become so focused on the potential negative effects of cholesterol on the health of their hearts that their food intake is overly restrictive of all nutrients. Although our dietary fat and cholesterol intake impacts the course of CAD, it is most potent during the early and middle years of adulthood, rather than in the later years of life.

Reduced Intake of Other Nutrients

Even if dietary fat consumption does not result in weight gain, foods high in fat tend not to contain much dietary fiber and may be low in other nutrients. Not consuming enough dietary fiber, as noted in Chapter 4, is a risk factor for several chronic conditions. The seductive nature of foods containing fats may lead us to crave these foods and neglect others. The best guarantee toward achieving the goal of nutritional wellness is to consume a balanced intake of nutrients, based on recommended guidelines, through consumption of at least five to seven servings of naturally low-fat fruits and vegetables per day.

Dietary Fat Intake and Diet-Related Diseases

The presence in the American diet of too much fat is directly related to several chronic diseases such as CAD and certain types of cancer. High-fat diets are indirectly related to type 2 diabetes mellitus and hypertension. Health guidelines to prevent and treat these diseases call for less dietary fat than the average American eats. The *HP2010* daily recommendations are to eat a total fat intake of 30% or less of kcalories, saturated fatty acid less than 10% of kcalories, and less than 300 mg of cholesterol. [31] Surveys indicate that Americans daily actually eat 33% to 34% of kcalories as total fat, 11% to 12% as saturated fat, and about 370 mg of cholesterol.[27] Consider how this affects our risk for these diet-related diseases.

Coronary Artery Disease

The relationship between CAD and dietary fat intake, particularly of saturated fats, seems strong. Based on the effects of saturated fat and cholesterol intake on blood cholesterol levels, a high-fat diet is a risk factor for the development of CAD.

Compared with recommended guidelines (see Table 5-4), more than 50% of Americans have high or borderline high blood cholesterol levels.[18] Although a downward trend in blood cholesterol levels is evident, according to National Health and Nutrition Examination Survey III (NHANES III) data collected between 1978 and 1991, an elevated blood cholesterol count is considered a signal for risk of CAD and a potential heart attack, especially when the ratio of LDL to HDL is high.[18] We also have good evidence that eating a lot of saturated fat is related to high blood cholesterol and, conversely, eating mostly monounsaturated and polyunsaturated fats is related to low blood cholesterol and low rate of heart disease deaths. Consequently, new recommendations have been released from the National Cholesterol Education Program, Adult Treatment Panel III report. This report focused on Therapeutic Lifestyle Change (TLC) recommendations for those most at risk for CAD. Although the general recommendations are to keep saturated fat intake to 10% or less of daily kcaloric intake, the TLC recommends 7% or less; instead of 300 mg of dietary cholesterol a day, the TLC recommends less than 200 mg.[18] Yet, what exactly is the connection between saturated fat and heart disease?

The suggested steps in the theory linking saturated fat to heart disease go like this:

1. Large amounts of saturated fat produce more LDL to circulate in the blood.
2. The cholesterol carried in the LDL is more likely to be attacked by oxygen, which in turn attracts big scavenger cells called macrophages.
3. The macrophages consume the oxidized material that accumulates in a modified form, called *foam cells*.
4. The foam cells cluster under the lining of the artery wall, forming bulges that cause fatty streaks, which is the first event in plaque formation.
5. The foam cells produce chemicals that further damage the artery wall and cause changes that produce artery-clogging plaque.

Saturated fat started this entire process by requiring too many LDL buses to carry it around. To reduce the amount of LDL, we should eat less saturated fat. If we eat more saturated fat than we need, the gradual buildup of plaque as atherosclerosis is likely to follow. In addition, some people seem to be more disposed than others to this series of events that lead to atherosclerosis.

An active area of research is whether the oxidation of LDLs can be inhibited or retarded by antioxidants, particularly those derived from diet. Vitamin E, beta-carotene, and vitamin C are antioxidants in fruits and vegetables. Because the optimal amount to prevent oxidative damage is unknown and there is evidence that high doses of some antioxidants, particular carotenoids, may be harmful, the safest source is fruits and vegetables rather than supplements. The same goes for reducing homocysteine in the blood. Homocysteine is a compound linked to increased

macrophages
cells that are able to surround, engulf, and digest microorganisms and cellular debris; big scavenger cells

risk of CAD and stroke. High homocysteine levels may be related to low folate and vitamins B_6 and B_{12}. Fruits, vegetables, and low-fat animal products are safe sources of these nutrients.

There is growing evidence that genetic factors may determine who will—and who won't—benefit from dietary changes designed to lower cholesterol. Geneticists have claimed discovery of a gene that could account for the characteristics of what is called an *atherogenic profile*, which describes an estimated 30% of the U.S. population. These characteristics include upper-body obesity, low concentration of HDL, and a preponderance of LDL fatty compounds in the blood.[32] This finding suggests that some people may indeed be predisposed to atherosclerosis and heart disease.

Because we cannot control our heredity, prevention is the main goal for everyone, regardless of genes, to lower the risk factors for atherosclerosis and heart disease that are within our control. High blood cholesterol, especially LDL cholesterol, is one risk factor affected by diet, mainly by reducing total fat intake and particularly saturated fatty acids. Blood cholesterol level is just one of several risk factors. Other widely known risk factors are tobacco, sedentary lifestyle, stress, overweight, alcohol, and hypertension (see the Cultural Considerations box, "Disproving the 'Hispanic Paradox'"). Experts stress the importance of reducing each risk factor to prevent or reduce the symptoms of heart disease.

Cancer

Since the 1960s, a connection between consumption of dietary fat and the development of various cancers was thought to exist. This assumption was based on international comparison studies, which produced incomplete findings because important factors related to cancer initiation were not considered. New, more carefully designed studies suggest that the relationship between dietary fat intake and cancer development is weak or nonexistent.

Within the past decade, prospective large-scale studies have investigated the relationship between dietary fat intake and the development of cancers of the breast,

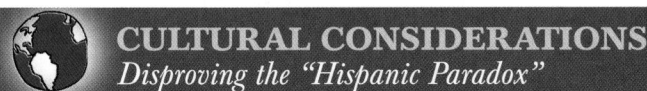

CULTURAL CONSIDERATIONS
Disproving the "Hispanic Paradox"

Health professionals have been confused for years by the commonly called "Hispanic paradox." The paradox refers to epidemiologic reports that Mexican Americans are less likely to die from cardiovascular disease (which includes hypertension, coronary artery disease, and stroke) than Caucasian Americans. This appears as a paradox because Mexican Americans have high rates of obesity and diabetes, which are risk factors for heart disease. Consequently, Mexican Americans should be at greater risk for heart disease-related death as compared with the total population. A new study appears to begin to disprove this paradox.

Instead of relying on population reports such as census records, this study followed, for more than an average of 13 years, U.S.-born Mexican Americans, Mexico-born Mexican Americans, and non-Hispanic Caucasians between the ages of 50 and 64 who participated in the San Antonio Heart Study. Findings revealed that the risk of dying from cardiovascular disease for U.S.-born Mexican Americans was 1.7 times the risk for non-Hispanic Caucasians and 1.9 times greater from coronary heart disease. For Mexico-born Mexican Americans, the risk was 1.5 times more than non-Hispanic Caucasians.

Application to nursing: These results imply the risk is *greater* for Hispanics—not lower as implied by the Hispanic paradox. Because this is only one study, more research is necessary to confirm these findings. It is possible, because previous studies analyzed death certificates, that the most accurate cause of death may not have been listed or the ethnicity identification may not have been correctly recorded on the death certificates. Nonetheless, this new study confirms the current wisdom that identifies obesity and diabetes as significant risk factors for cardiovascular disease regardless of ethnicity. Considering that Hispanics are the largest and fastest growing minority group in the United States—and within that group, Mexican Americans are the largest subgroup—attention to reducing risk factors is the most reasonable course of action.

Reference: American Heart Association: Mexican Americans more likely to die of heart disease than Caucasians, Meeting Report and Press Release, American Heart Association, Apr 25, 2002; www.americanheart.org.

colon, and prostate. Most recently, larger prospective case-controlled studies such as the 20-year-old Nurses' Health Study, which follows thousands of participating nurses, reveal that there appears to be no relationship between breast cancer and dietary fat consumption.[33] A stronger risk factor for breast cancer, based on human and animal studies, is consistent consumption of too many calories from any food source. For colon cancer, there may be an association between consumption of significant amounts of red meats and colon cancer development. This may be caused by specific fats in meats or the carcinogenic substances formed when meats are cooked at high temperatures. Again, a stronger relationship exists between consuming too many calories compared with energy expenditure (exercise) as a risk factor for colon cancer. Other ways to decrease colon cancer risk include exercising regularly, not smoking, and consuming adequate amounts of the B vitamin folic acid. In the case of prostate cancer, not much research has been conducted, but based on international comparisons, genetic factors—rather than diet—appear stronger. The different rates of prostate cancer when individuals switch, for example, from an Asian dietary pattern (low in fat) to a Western pattern (higher in animal fat) still supports genetic factors but does show the influence of animal fat or meat-related effects on cancer rates.[33,34]

More research is needed to accurately determine the association between dietary fat intake and cancer. Recommendations for heart healthy dietary fat intake (increase PUFA and monounsaturated fats) should not affect cancer risk but will decrease the risk of heart disease.[33]

Type 2 Diabetes Mellitus and Hypertension

Type 2 diabetes mellitus (DM) and hypertension are indirectly related to dietary fat intake. Both of these disorders may stress the circulatory system; a high dietary fat intake may further limit the functioning of the circulatory system through the potential development of atherosclerosis. In addition, these disorders are managed better when weight moderation is achieved; dietary fat reduction may enhance this process. Medical nutritional therapy for these disorders is detailed in Chapters 19, 20, and 22.

TOWARD A POSITIVE NUTRITION LIFESTYLE: GRADUAL REDUCTION

It's the subject of TV situation comedies. One member of the family becomes a health food fanatic, serving blades of grass, sprouts, and weird mixtures of soybeans, nuts, and who knows what. And what is the immediate response of the sit-com family? Disgust and rebellion, of course.

As we make recommendations to our clients to reduce their fat intake (and perhaps for ourselves and our families, too), consider that often the most effective way to achieve permanent change is through gradual reduction. That's the mistake made by the TV character: too many changes made too quickly.

An action plan for gradual reduction of dietary fat intake could include the following:

1. For 1 week, record all food and beverages consumed.
2. Based on reading this chapter, assess which foods are likely to be high in fat. Particularly note if one high-fat food item, such as whole milk, is consumed often or if a certain meal or snack regularly includes fatty foods. Perhaps scrambled eggs and bacon are eaten almost every morning for breakfast, and an afternoon coffee break always includes either a sweet Danish pastry or a huge, buttery muffin.
3. The next week, choose one item and either reduce consumption or replace it with a lower-fat substitute. Instead of whole milk, use 2% or 1% fat milk or replace the coffee break treat with an English muffin with a bit of butter or margarine and jelly.

4. The following week, select another food item or meal and make a simple substitution.

This process can continue with small changes—gradual reductions—resulting in major reductions in dietary fat intake.

SUMMARY

Lipids are organic and are composed of carbon, hydrogen, and oxygen. They include fats and fat-related substances divided into three classifications. About 95% of the lipids in foods and in our bodies are in the form of fat as triglycerides, the largest class of lipids. The other two lipid classifications are the fat-related substances of phospholipids and sterols. Lecithin is the best-known phospholipid; cholesterol is the best-known sterol.

The functions of lipids fall into two categories: their food value and their physiologic purposes in the body. Food value functions take into consideration that fat is the densest form of stored energy in both food and in our bodies. Foods containing fat smell and taste good and provide satiety. Fat-soluble nutrients—vitamins A, D, E, K, and linoleic and linolenic fatty acids, the EFAs—are available through foods. Physiologic functions of stored fat include providing a backup energy supply, cushioning body organs, and serving to regulate body temperature.

Phospholipids are part of body cell membrane structure and serve as emulsifiers. Cholesterol, a sterol, has a role in the formation of bile, vitamin D, sex hormones, and cells in brain and nerve tissue.

Triglycerides are compounds made of three fatty acids and one glycerol molecule. The fatty acids may be saturated, monounsaturated, or polyunsaturated depending on their number of double bonds. Phospholipids are similar to triglycerides except they have only two fatty acids; the third spot contains a phosphate group. Sterol structures, including cholesterol, are carbon rings intermeshed with side chains of carbon, hydrogen, and oxygen. All three types of lipids can be manufactured in our bodies. The only exceptions are two fatty acids, linolenic and linoleic fatty acids, found in triglycerides; these cannot be formed by the body and are essential nutrients.

Digestion of lipids occurs mainly in the small intestine; absorption depends on the transportation of lipids through the lymph and blood circulatory systems. Lipids travel through the body in lipoprotein packages containing triglycerides, protein, phospholipids, and cholesterol. Lipoproteins differ according to the proportions or ratio of these ingredients. Very low-density lipoproteins (VLDLs), low-density lipoproteins (LDLs), and high-density lipoproteins (HDLs) are found in the blood. Because they contain cholesterol, the levels of LDLs and HDLs may serve as medical markers of one of the risks of CAD.

Health concerns about our dietary fat intake fall into several categories, including appropriate energy intake, reduced intake of other nutrients because of excessive dietary fat consumption, and the relationship between dietary fat intake and diet-related diseases.

THE NURSING APPROACH
Critical Thinking: The Nursing Process

Nurses must use critical thinking as part of their nursing role. You cannot carry out the nursing process accurately and intelligently without using critical thinking. What are the critical thinking skills in nursing? They incorporate the ability to identify missing data and misconceptions and the ability to identify assumptions and cause-effect relationships. Also included is the skill of seeing patterns, clusters, and inconsistencies of information and the skill of prioritizing and planning action in a logical way.

Continued

THE NURSING APPROACH–cont'd
Critical Thinking: The Nursing Process

Bring your critical thinking skills to bear on the following situations and questions and, if necessary, refer to this chapter to find clues to the answers.

1. A patient tells you she has lowered fat intake in her diet by switching from beef to chicken. What else would you have to ask this patient before accepting her conclusion that she has lowered fat intake?
2. A friend complains that, although he eats a lot, he is always starving between meals. What might account for this?
3. A man who has heart disease tells you he has clogged arteries in his heart. He says if he can reduce his cholesterol intake, he knows he can get the problem under control. Is he correct? Why or why not?
4. A mother states she wants to teach her 6-year-old daughter to eat a fat-controlled diet so she will have good eating habits in adulthood. Is her premise valid?
5. A teenager thinks just drinking skim milk instead of whole milk is adequate fat control for her age. Is this a true assumption?
6. Is it possible to eat fats containing only high-density lipoproteins?
7. Is reducing sugar and carbohydrates in your diet the most efficient way to reduce kcalories?
8. The wife of a patient with diabetes tells you she has adhered to cooking a low-fat diet for her husband by trimming external fat from meat and serving skim milk. What other assessments would you have to make to decide if her husband's fat intake is appropriate?

APPLYING CONTENT KNOWLEDGE

Disease prevention for chronic diet-related diseases depends on changes in lifestyle behaviors. Consider the lifestyle behaviors John could adopt based on his personal history. John is a 20-year-old Caucasian man. His brother and father both have high cholesterol levels and histories of CAD in their families. Although John's cholesterol level is average for his age, what three disease prevention strategies could he pursue? Would these strategies be primary, secondary, or tertiary?

Web Sites of Interest

Center for Science in the Public Interest
www.cspinet.org
The Center for Science in the Public Interest (CSPI) is a nonprofit advocacy and educational organization that is dedicated to promoting health by increasing the nutritional quality and safety of the American food supply through legislative, regulatory, and judicial means. The CSPI's *Nutrition Action Healthletter* has focused public attention on health and safety issues of foods, alcohol, and food-production environmental concerns.

Drive Thru Diet
www.bgsm.edu/nutrition/FFMainF.htm
Sponsored by the Bowman Gray School of Medicine, Wake Forest University, this site lets the user select healthier fast-food meals by providing nutrient content of menu items from seven fast-food restaurants. Information on items containing the lowest fat, cholesterol, calorie, and sodium is available, along with the ability to determine the nutrient content of a whole meal.

Eating Well On-Line
www.eatingwell.com
This online version of *Eating Well Magazine* presents articles and recipes on nutrition, food, and low-fat cooking. It is a good resource for those learning how to lower their dietary fat intake.

References

1. Drewrowski A: Sensory control of energy density at different lifestages, *Proc Nutr Soc* 59(2):239, 2000.
2. Blundell JE et al.: The fat paradox: fat-induced satiety signals versus high fat overconsumption, *Int J Obesity* 19:832, 1995.
3. James PJH, Kubow S: Lipids, sterols and their metabolites. In Shils ME, Olson JA, Shike M, eds.: *Modern nutrition in health and disease,* ed 9, Philadelphia, 1999, Lea & Febiger.
4. Harris WS: Fish oils and plasma lipid and lipoprotein metabolism in humans: a critical review, *J Lipid Res* 30:785, 1989.
5. Albert CM et al.: Blood levels of long-chain omega-3 fatty acids and risk of sudden death, *J Am Med Assoc* 346(15):1113, 2002.
6. Hu FB et al.: Fish and omega-3 fatty acid intake and risk of coronary heart disease in women, *J Am Med Assoc* 287(14):1815, 2002.
7. Drevon CA: Marine oils and their effects, *Nutr Rev* 50:38, 1992.
8. Institute of Medicine Food and Nutrition Board: *Dietary reference intakes for energy, carbohydrate, fiber, fat, fatty acids, cholesterol, protein, and amino acids,* Washington, DC, 2002, National Academy Press.
9. American Academy of Pediatrics, Committee on Nutrition: Statement on cholesterol, *Pediatrics* 101:141, 1998.
10. Knopp RH et al.: Long-term cholesterol-lowering effects of 4 fat-restricted diets in hypercholesterolemic and combined hyperlipidemic men, *J Am Med Assoc* 278:1509, 1997.
11. Enns CW, Goldman JD, Cook A: Trends in food and nutrient intakes by adults: NFCS 1977-78. CSFII 1989-91, and SCFII 1994-95, *Fam Econ Nutr Rev* 10:2, 1997.
12. Greene GW, Rossi SR: Stages of change for reducing dietary fat intake over 18 months, *J Am Dietetic Assoc* 98:529, 1998.
13. Subar AF et al.: Dietary sources of nutrients among US adults, 1989 to 1991, *J Am Dietetic Assoc* 98:537, 1998.
14. Barnard N, Akhtar A, Nicholson A: Factors that facilitate compliance to lower fat intake, *Arch Fam Med* 4:153, 1995.
15. Byers T: Hardened fats, hardened arteries? *N Engl J Med* 333:1544, 1997.
16. Lichtenstein AH: Trans fatty acids, plasma lipid levels, and risk of developing cardiovascular disease: a statement for health care professions from the American Heart Association, *Circulation* 95:2588, 1997.
17. CSPI Newsroom: *Dangerous "trans fat" present in foods, absent on labels,* July 26, 2002, Center for Science in the Public Interest; www.cspinet.org/new/200207261.html.
18. Van Horn L, Ernst N: A summary of the science supporting the new National Cholesterol Education Program dietary recommendations: what dietitians should know, *J Am Dietetic Assoc* 101(10):1148, 2001.
19. Dwyer JT: Human studies on the effects of fatty acids on cancer: summary, gaps, and future research, *Am J Clin Nutr* 66(suppl):1581S, 1997.
20. Position of the American Dietetic Association: Fat replacers, *J Am Dietetic Assoc* 98:463, 1998.
21. Kennedy E, Bowman S: Assessment of the effect of fat-modified foods on diet quality in adults, 19 to 50 years, using data from the Continuing Survey of Food Intake by Individuals, *J Am Dietetic Assoc* 101:455, 2001.

22. US Department of Health and Human Services, Public Health Service: *Healthy People 2000: midcourse review and 1995 revisions,* Washington, DC, 1995, US Government Printing Office.
23. Dornblaser L: New product news, *Prepared Foods* 4:37, 1996.
24. Ravussin E, Swinburn BA: Pathophysiology of obesity, *Lancet* 340:404, 1992.
25. Willett WC: Is dietary fat a major determinant of body fat? *Am J Clin Nutr* 67(suppl):556S, 1998.
26. Centers for Disease Control and Prevention: Daily dietary fat and total food-energy intakes: Third National Health and Nutrition Examination Survey, Phase 1, 1988-1991, *MMWR* 43:116, 1994.
27. Ernst ND et al.: Cardiovascular health risks related to overweight, *J Am Dietetic Assoc* 97(suppl):S47, 1997.
28. Billings JH: Maintenance of behavior changes in cardiorespiratory risk reduction: a clinical perspective from the Ornish Program for reversing coronary heart disease. *Health Psychol* 19(1 Suppl):70, 2000.
29. Katan MB, Grundy SM, Willett WC: Beyond low-fat diets, *N Eng J Med* 337:563, 1997.
30. Pugliese MT et al.: Parental health beliefs as a cause of failure to thrive, *Pediatrics* 80(2):175, Aug 1987.
31. US Department of Health and Human Services, Public Health Service: *Healthy People 2010,* ed 2, Washington, DC, 2000, US Government Printing Office; www.health.gov/healthypeople.
32. Nishina PM: Linkage of atherogenic lipoprotein phenotype to the low density lipoprotein receptor locus on the short arm of chromosome 19, *Proceedings of the National Academy of Sciences, USA* 89:708, 1992.
33. Willet W: *Eat, drink, and be healthy,* New York, 2001, Simon & Schuster.
34. Moyad MA: Dietary fat reduction to reduce prostate cancer risk: controlled enthusiasm, learning a lesson from breast cancers, and the big picture, *Urology* 59(4 Suppl 1):51, 2002.

CHAPTER 6

Protein

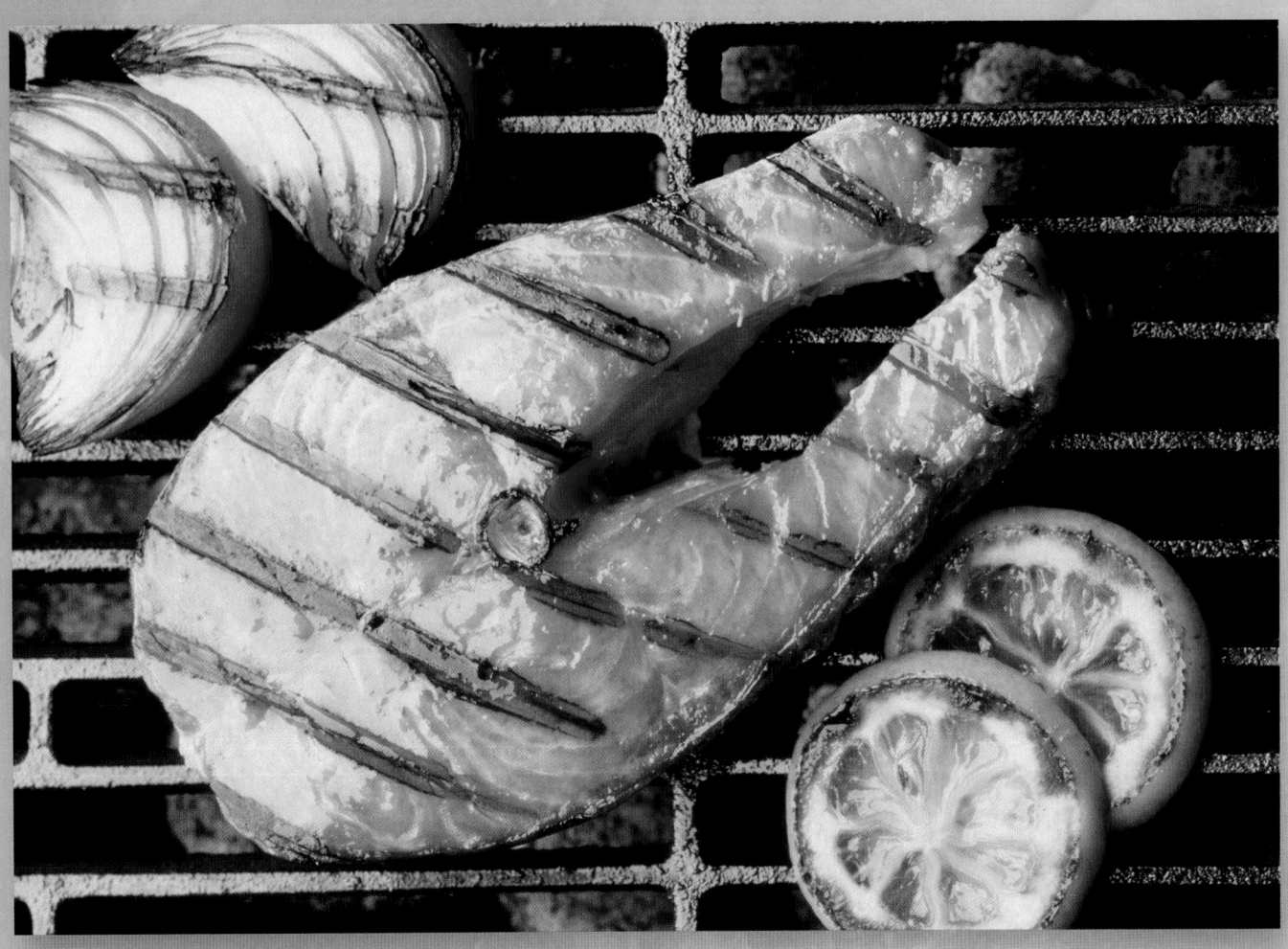

Protein in food is our only source of amino acids, which are absolutely necessary to make the thousands of proteins that form every aspect of the human body.

ROLE IN WELLNESS

"A chicken in every pot!" was a political motto used during the past century. At that time, being able to afford animal protein on a daily basis was the mark of a high standard of living and an assurance of good health. Today the motto might be, "Rice and beans for all of us!" We now know that there are many sources of protein available in our food supply. Some offer advantages over others by being lower in fat and higher in other nutrients such as complex carbohydrates and fiber.

Protein in food is our only source of amino acids, which are absolutely necessary to make the thousands of proteins that form every aspect of the human body. No wonder protein, which is plentiful in our food supply, has gained the status of a super nutrient for Americans. A common but inaccurate belief is that we expect that the more protein we eat, the stronger our immune system will be, the less we will weigh, and the more muscles we will develop.

Although proteins formed by our bodies do have a role in those functions, the amounts we consume are often greater than we need. Awareness of protein sources and portion sizes is important as we work toward achieving health promotion goals to decrease our risk of diet-related diseases (Figure 6-1).

The five dimensions of health provide ways to think about the effects of protein consumption. Our overall physical health and well-being depend on our eating enough essential amino acids for body protein synthesis. The ability to comprehend and apply new approaches to protein consumption by adapting to different protein sources (e.g., legumes and grains) and reducing portion sizes depends on our intellectual health capacity to implement change. Protein is a super-status food for some Americans; favorite sources may provide emotional health security. Clients needing to make dietary changes, such as changing to lower fat sources of protein (e.g., cutting back on sausages), may need our advice on coping strategies. As we and our clients follow different eating patterns, such as practicing vegetarianism or reducing consumption of animal protein, family and social dynamics may be affected when one member changes and thereby tests our level of social health.

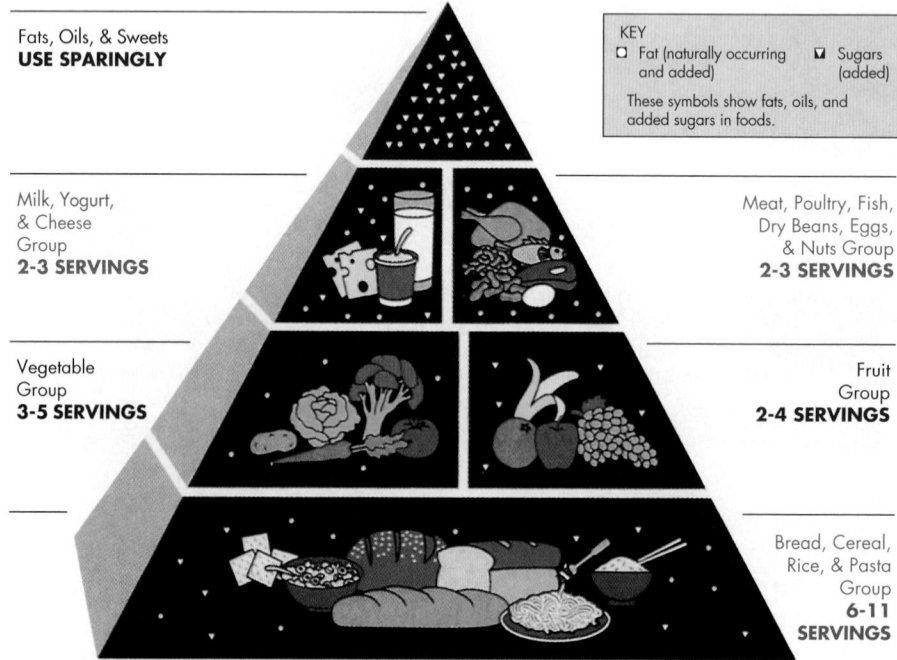

Figure 6-1 The Food Guide Pyramid, highlighting major sources of protein. (From US Department of Agriculture: *Food Guide Pyramid*, Human Nutrition Information Pub No 249, Washington, DC, 1992, revised 1996, US Government Printing Office.)

Religious and spiritual beliefs lead individuals to nourish their bodies through a nonharming philosophy that views humans as being civilized enough to nourish their bodies without taking life.

STRUCTURE OF PROTEIN

Proteins are formed by the linking of many smaller molecules of amino acids. Amino acids, like glucose, are organic compounds made of carbon, hydrogen, and oxygen. However, amino acids also contain nitrogen, which clearly distinguishes protein from other nutrients.

There are 20 amino acids from which all the proteins that are required by plants and animals are made. The human body is able to manufacture some of the amino acids for its own protein-building function, however nine amino acids cannot be made by the cells of the body. Therefore these essential amino acids (EAAs) must be eaten in food, digested, absorbed, and then brought to cells by circulating blood. The remaining 11 are nonessential amino acids (NEAAs) (Box 6-1). The liver can create NEAAs as long as structural components, including nitrogen, from other amino acids are available to use for NEAA formation.

Each cell constructs or synthesizes the proteins it needs. To build proteins, the cell must have access to all 20 amino acids. This available supply of amino acids is in the metabolic amino acid pool. The amino acid pool is a collection of amino acids that is constantly resupplied with EAAs (from dietary intake) and NEAAs (synthesized in the liver). The pool allows the cell to build proteins easily.

Protein Composition

The functions of proteins are closely related to their structures. The complex composition of proteins is best understood through four structural levels: primary, secondary, tertiary, and quaternary[1] (Figure 6-2).

The primary structure of protein composition is determined by the number, assortment, and sequence of amino acids in polypeptide chains. Amino acids are linked together by peptide bonds to form a practically unlimited number of proteins. The peptide bond occurs at the point at which the carboxyl group of one amino acid is bound to the amino group of another amino acid (Figure 6-3).

The 20 amino acids form chains that may contain any combination or assortment of amino acids. This allows for thousands of different proteins to be formed. Two proteins may contain the same assortment and number of amino acids yet still have different functions because of the sequencing or order of the amino acids.

proteins
organic compounds formed from chains of amino acids

amino acids
organic compounds containing carbon, hydrogen, oxygen, and nitrogen

essential amino acids (EAAs)
amino acids that cannot be manufactured by the human body

nonessential amino acids (NEAA)
amino acids manufactured by the human body

amino acid pool
the assortment of amino acids available to cells

Box 6-1 Amino Acids

ESSENTIAL AMINO ACIDS	NONESSENTIAL AMINO ACIDS
histidine	alanine
isoleucine	arginine
leucine	aspartic acid
lysine	cysteine
methionine	cystine
phenylalanine	glutamic acid
threonine	glutamine
tryptophan	glycine
valine	proline
	serine
	tyrosine

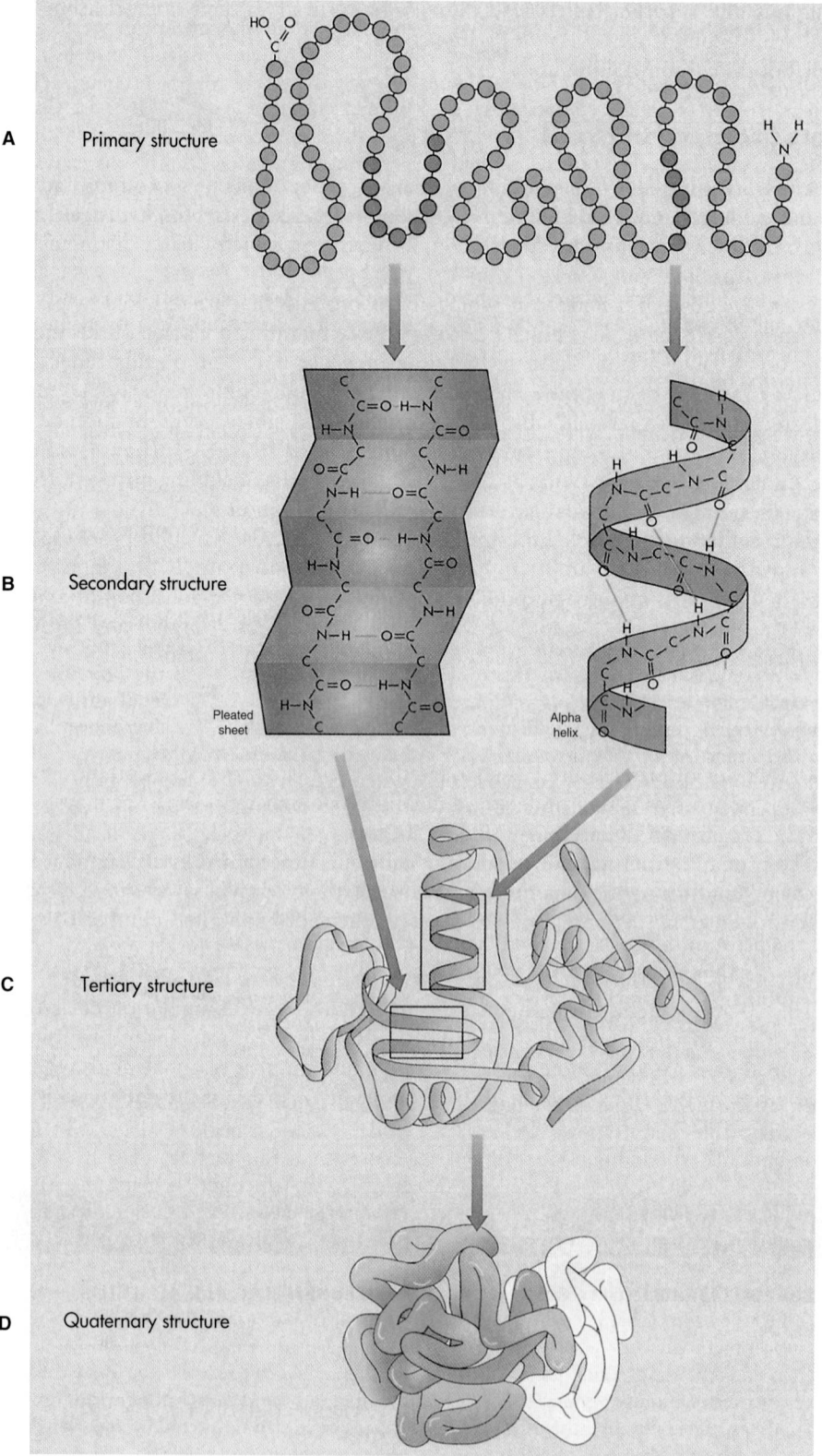

Figure 6-2 Structural levels of protein. **A,** Primary structure: determined by number, kind, and sequence of amino acids in the chain; **B,** secondary structure: hydrogen bonds stabilize folds of helical spirals; **C,** tertiary structure: globular shape maintained by strong intramolecular bonding and by stabilizing hydrogen bonds; **D,** quaternary structure: results from bonding between more than one polypeptide unit. (Bill Ober; In Thibodeau GA, Patton KT: *Anatomy and physiology,* ed 4, St Louis, 1999, Mosby.)

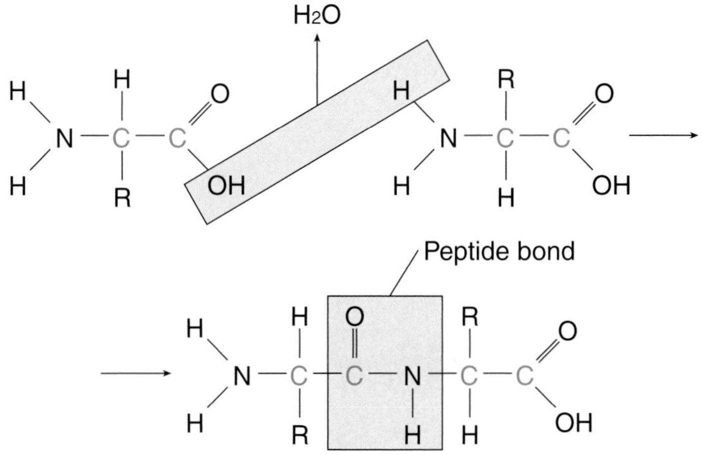

Figure 6-3 Peptide bonds.

The secondary structure level of proteins affects the shape of the chain of amino acids; they may be straight, folded, or coiled. The tertiary structure results when the polypeptide chain is so coiled that the loops of the coil touch, forming strong bonds within the chain itself. The quaternary structural level is proteins containing more than one polypeptide chain.

If the structure of a protein changes, the protein may not be able to perform its original function. The shape may be changed by heat (cooking), ultraviolet light (exposure to sunlight), acids (vinegar), alcohol, and mechanical action. When the shape of a protein is affected (e.g., a folded chain unfolding), the protein has been denatured and has been physically changed.

An example of denaturing a food protein is the change that occurs when the white of an uncooked egg (a clear liquid) is beaten. The clear liquid turns white, foamy, and stiff. The protein in the egg has been denatured; however, it is still a valuable source of amino acids. The amino acids are not affected; only the shape of the chain has been changed.

Inside the body, denaturing of proteins is controlled by mechanisms that keep the internal body environment from getting too basic or too acidic. Either extreme can lead to the denaturation of vital proteins within the body. Body temperature also affects the protein structure of the body. High fevers can become lethal when protein structures within the body become denatured. When body proteins are denatured, they cannot perform their original functions.

Although uncontrolled denaturation can be dangerous, it is helpful for digestion. Denaturing changes the three-dimensional structure of a protein, providing more surface area on which digestive juices act to release the amino acids of the food proteins.

denatured
a change in the shape of protein structures caused by heat, light, acids, alcohol, or mechanical actions

PROTEIN AS A NUTRIENT WITHIN THE BODY

The proteins we consume in foods are not the same proteins used by our bodies. Actually, the only nutrient role protein in foods serves is to provide amino acids, the building blocks of all proteins.

Digestion and Absorption

Because of the complex structure of proteins, a number of protein enzymes, or proteases, produced by the stomach and pancreas are required to hydrolyze proteins into smaller and smaller peptides until individual amino acids are ready for absorption (Figure 6-4).

proteases
protein enzymes

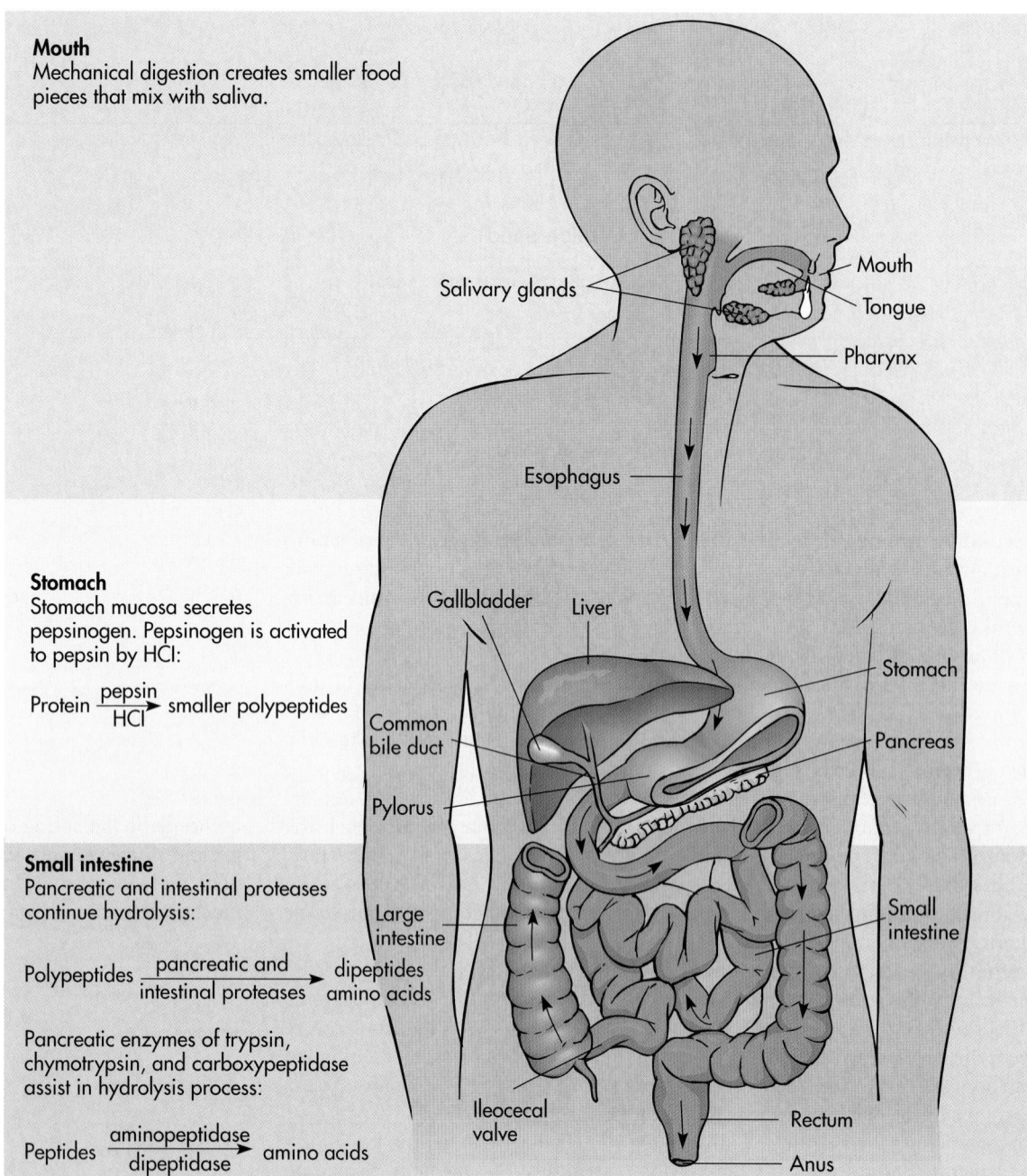

Mouth
Mechanical digestion creates smaller food pieces that mix with saliva.

Salivary glands

Mouth
Tongue
Pharynx

Esophagus

Stomach
Stomach mucosa secretes pepsinogen. Pepsinogen is activated to pepsin by HCl:

$$\text{Protein} \xrightarrow[\text{HCl}]{\text{pepsin}} \text{smaller polypeptides}$$

Gallbladder   Liver

Stomach

Common bile duct

Pancreas

Pylorus

Small intestine
Pancreatic and intestinal proteases continue hydrolysis:

$$\text{Polypeptides} \xrightarrow[\text{intestinal proteases}]{\text{pancreatic and}} \begin{array}{c}\text{dipeptides}\\\text{amino acids}\end{array}$$

Pancreatic enzymes of trypsin, chymotrypsin, and carboxypeptidase assist in hydrolysis process:

$$\text{Peptides} \xrightarrow[\text{dipeptidase}]{\text{aminopeptidase}} \text{amino acids}$$

Large intestine

Small intestine

Ileocecal valve

Rectum

Anus

Figure 6-4 Summary of protein digestion and absorption. (From Rolin Graphics.)

Mouth

Only mechanical digestion of protein occurs in the mouth. Mastication breaks protein-containing food into smaller pieces that mix with saliva passing through to the stomach.

Stomach

pepsinogen
the inactive form of pepsin

pepsin
a gastric protease

Pepsinogen, an inactive form of the gastric protease pepsin, is secreted by the stomach mucosa. Pepsin becomes activated when it mixes with hydrochloric acid (HCl), also produced by stomach secretions. Pepsin then begins the process of protein hydrolysis, breaking the bonds linking the amino acids of the protein peptide bonds. The result is smaller-sized polypeptides, rather than single amino acids or dipeptides. The polypeptides pass through to the small intestine for further hydrolysis.

Rennin, an important gastric protease, is only produced during infancy. It functions with calcium to thicken or coagulate the milk protein casein; this slows the movement of milk nutrients from the stomach, allowing additional digestion time.[2]

Small Intestine

In the small intestine, pancreatic and intestinal proteases continue the hydrolysis of polypeptides. As these smaller peptides touch the intestinal walls, peptidases are released, which complete the hydrolyses of protein into absorbable units of individual amino acids and dipeptides.

The primary pancreatic enzyme is **trypsin**. It is first secreted as trypsinogen, an inactive form. The intestinal hormone enteropeptidase activates trypsinogen into trypsin, which continues the hydrolysis of polypeptides. Two other pancreatic enzymes assist in the hydrolysis process; **chymotrypsin** hydrolyzes polypeptides into dipeptides, and **carboxypeptidase** breaks polypeptides and dipeptides into amino acids. Two intestinal peptidases are **aminopeptidase**, which releases free amino acids from the amino end of short-chain peptides, and **dipeptidase**, which completes the hydrolysis of proteins to amino acids.

Absorption of amino acids occurs through the intestinal walls by means of competitive active transport that requires vitamin B_6 (pyridoxine) as a carrier. Because amino acids are water soluble, they easily pass into the bloodstream.

Metabolism

To understand the importance of protein metabolism in the growth and maintenance of the body, consider that most protein functions are a result of protein anabolism (synthesis) in cells. Hormones have a major role in the regulation of protein metabolism. Anabolism is enhanced by the effect of growth hormone (from the pituitary gland) and the male hormone testosterone. Hormones affecting the catabolism (break down) of proteins are the glucocorticoids that are enhanced by adrenocorticotropic hormone (ACTH); these hormones are secreted from the adrenal cortex. This process releases proteins in the cells to break down to amino acids and then the amino acids travel in the bloodstream, contributing to an available pool of amino acids (Figure 6-5).

trypsin
the primary pancreatic protease

chymotrypsin
a pancreatic protease that hydrolyzes polypeptides into dipeptides

carboxypeptidase
a pancreatic protease that hydrolyzes polypeptides and dipeptides into amino acids

aminopeptidase
an intestinal peptidase that releases free amino acids from the amino end of short-chain peptides

dipeptidase
an intestinal peptidase that completes the hydrolysis of proteins to amino acids

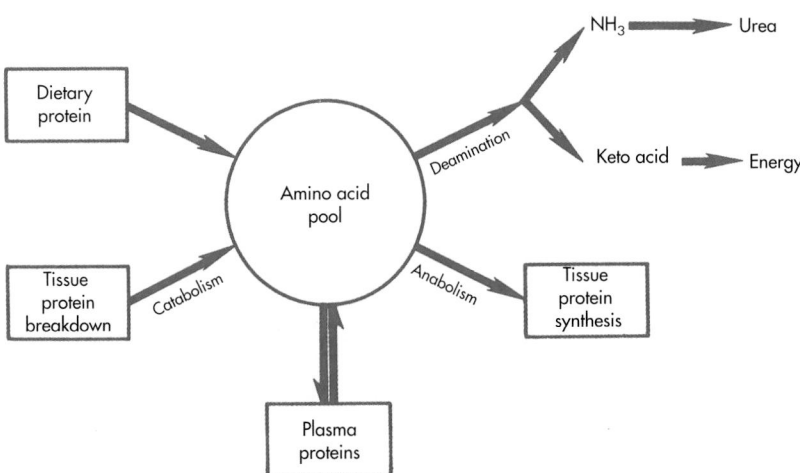

Figure 6-5 The body's equilibrium depends on a balance between the rates of protein breakdown (catabolism) and protein synthesis (anabolism). (Modified from Williams SR: *Essentials of nutrition and diet therapy*, ed 7, St Louis, 1999, Mosby.)

deamination
a process through which an amino acid group breaks off from an amino acid molecule, resulting in molecules of ammonia and keto acid

urea
product of ammonia conversion produced during deamination

The liver cells begin the process of catabolism through deamination. Deamination results in an amino acid (NH_2) group breaking off from an amino acid molecule, resulting in one molecule each of ammonia (NH_3) and a keto acid. Liver cells convert most of the ammonia to urea, which is later excreted in urine. The keto acid may enter the TCA cycle to be used for energy or, through gluconeogenesis and lipogenesis, be converted to glucose and fat[1] (see Figure 6-5).

Protein Excess

An excessive intake of protein results in increased deamination by the liver. The increased deamination may result in high levels of keto acids, possibly putting the body into a state of ketosis. The increased urea is excreted by the kidneys. Because the liver and kidneys are both involved with the deamination process, the increased stress on the organs could initiate underlying disorder of these organs. Because there are no definitive benefits of excessive protein intake, the general recommendation is to consume no more than twice the Recommended Dietary Allowance (RDA) for protein.

In fact, the source of excess protein may be a health concern. Animal-derived protein sources such as meats may also be high in saturated fat and cholesterol. This may increase the risk of coronary artery disease (CAD) and some cancers. The relationship between protein intake and osteoporosis has also been considered. When protein intake is high, there is a slight increase of calcium excretion from the body, but calcium absorption is not affected. Studies have yielded mixed results about this effect on the risk of osteoporosis. Because osteoporosis is multifactorial, this specific relationship is difficult to determine. Recommendations to consume moderate amounts of protein and to meet the new Dietary Reference Intake (DRI) levels for calcium are the best dietary approaches to decrease risk of CAD and cancer (see Chapter 8 for an in-depth discussion of osteoporosis).

Nitrogen Balance

nitrogen-balance studies
measurement of the amount of nitrogen entering the body compared with the amount excreted

Nitrogen-balance studies are used to determine the protein requirements of the body throughout the life cycle and to assign value to the protein quality of foods to determine their biologic value.[2] Because nitrogen (N) is a primary component of protein, the body's use of protein can be determined by comparing the amount of nitrogen entering the body in food protein with the nitrogen lost from the body in feces and urine.

Nitrogen lost or excreted from the body may be endogenous nitrogen (from catabolism of body protein), metabolic nitrogen (from intestinal cells), or exogenous nitrogen (from dietary proteins). Nitrogen in feces may be metabolic and exogenous (from cells and dietary proteins) and in urine may be endogenous (catabolism of body protein) and exogenous (from dietary proteins).

An individual is in nitrogen equilibrium or zero nitrogen balance if the amount of nitrogen consumed in foods equals the amount excreted. This occurs in normal, healthy adults when nitrogen in food protein entering (input) the body equals the nitrogen leaving the body (output). Because adults are no longer growing, the nitrogen that enters the body is not needed to build new tissue but is used simply to maintain the body.

Positive nitrogen balance occurs when more nitrogen is retained in the body than excreted. The nitrogen is used to form new cells for growth or healing. This occurs in growing children and in pregnant women who require additional nitrogen (and protein) for the growth of the fetus. Individuals recovering from illness or injury may be in positive nitrogen balance as the body heals. Negative nitrogen balance happens when more nitrogen is excreted from the body than is retained from dietary protein sources. This occurs when there is a breakdown of proteins within the body, such as in muscles and organs. Negative nitrogen balance may be caused by aging, physical illness, extreme stress, starvation, surgery, or eating disorders.

FUNCTIONS

Proteins created in our bodies perform numerous functions, including the following:
- Growth and maintenance
- Creation of communicators and catalysts
- Immune system response
- Fluid and electrolyte regulation
- Acid-base balance
- Transportation

Growth and Maintenance

Each body cell contains proteins. All growth depends on a sufficient supply of amino acids. The amino acids are needed to make the proteins required to support muscle, tissue, bone formation, and the cells themselves.

Maintaining our bodies also requires a constant supply of amino acids. There is a continual turnover of body cells, which are composed of protein. The cells break down and must immediately be replaced. Each replacement cell requires the formation of additional protein.

Also needed for growth and maintenance is the protein collagen, found throughout the body. Collagen forms connective tissues such as ligaments and tendons and acts as a glue to keep the walls of the arteries intact. In addition, collagen has a role in bone and tooth formation by forming the framework structure that is then filled with minerals such as calcium and phosphorus. Synthesis of scar tissue also depends on collagen. Other structures such as hair, nails, and skin are composed of similar protein substances.

Creation of Communicators and Catalysts

Many vital substances produced by our bodies are formed of protein. Some hormones are proteins. Hormones act as communicators to alert different parts of the body to changes or to regulate functions of organs. Insulin, a hormone that directs cells to take in glucose, is a protein. Enzymes are also proteins. Enzymes are catalysts that enable chemical reactions or biologic changes to occur within the body. Each enzyme has a specific target; consequently, numerous enzymes are continually formed.

Blood clotting depends on protein substances as well. Twelve blood clotting factors must be in place for blood to clot when injury has occurred; several of the factors, such as fibrogen, are composed of protein.

Immune System Response

The defense system of our bodies depends on proteins produced in response to foreign virus and bacteria that invade our bodies. The proteins, or antibodies, are specific to each intruder. If sufficient levels of amino acids are not available to form these antibodies, we may have difficulties maintaining our health. Our overall immunologic response—our resistance to disease—depends on proteins formed within our bodies.

Fluid and Electrolyte Regulation

Water is balanced among three compartments in the body: intravascular (within veins and arteries), intracellular (inside cells), and interstitial (between cells). Proteins and minerals attract water, creating osmotic pressure. As proteins circulate through our bodies, they maintain body fluid and electrolyte balance by keeping water appropriately divided among the three compartments.

Acid-Base Balance

Some reactions occurring within the body lead to the release of acidic substances; others cause basic matter to enter the fluids of the body. Blood proteins can buffer the effects of fluids to maintain a safe acidic level in body fluids. The ability of protein to regulate the balance between the acidic and base characteristics of fluids is called the *buffering effect* of protein. Because the chemical structure of amino acids combines an acid (the carboxyl group [COOH]) and base (amine), an amino acid can function either as an acid or base depending on the pH of its medium. This is why the buffering effect of blood proteins is possible. This function is crucial to protect all proteins in the body. If fluids become either too acidic or too basic, the shape of proteins is altered or denatured. Denatured proteins are not able to perform their usual functions.

Many of the constituents of blood are protein based, and if protein functions are affected, the result can be lethal. Therefore proteins maintain a delicate pH level to assure the proper functioning of all body systems (Box 6-2).

Transportation

Throughout our bodies, proteins are able to transport nutrients and other vital substances. For individual cells, proteins act as pumps, assisting the movement of nutrients in and out of cells. Many nutrients, including lipids, minerals, vitamins, and electrolytes, are carried in the blood by proteins such as lipoproteins. This allows the nutrients to be available to all parts of the body. Hemoglobin, a special carrier composed of protein, transports oxygen in blood. Oxygen is stored in our muscles in another protein carrier, myoglobin. These protein carriers, hemoglobin and myoglobin, are essential for a well-functioning body.

FOOD SOURCES

Quality of Protein Foods

complete protein
proteins containing all nine essential amino acids

The proteins in foods are categorized by the EAAs they contain. Complete protein contains all nine EAAs in sufficient quantities that best support growth and maintenance of our bodies. Animal-derived foods, including meat, poultry, fish, eggs,

---

Box 6-2 Genetic Disorders

Phenylketonuria (PKU) is a genetic disorder with a protein link. This disorder is characterized by the inability to use or break down excess phenylalanine, an essential amino acid. The excess phenylalanine circulating inside the body can cause various health problems. Infants with this disorder consume low-phenylalanine formulas whereas children and adults follow a limited protein diet to control the intake of phenylalanine.

Another genetic protein disorder is sickle cell disease, which affects the shape of red blood cells. Because of abnormalities of the hemoglobin molecule, the red blood cell is curved or sickle shaped rather than round. The sickle shape can cause these blood cells to clog small blood vessels. This can be painful, may cause damage to internal organs such as the kidneys and heart, and may lead to frequent infections throughout the body. Early screening, followed by long-term penicillin treatment, can prevent secondary infections.

Having the sickle cell disease trait is not the same as having the disease itself. Both parents have to have the trait for a child to be at risk. Even then, there is only a 25% chance of developing the disorder. Sickle cell disease may occur in any ethnic group, but it is more common among Africans and African Americans; some states screen all infants to determine susceptibility.

From Phenylketonuria: screening and management, NIH Consensus Statement, *17(3):1, October 16-18, 2000;* Facts about sickle cell anemia, *National Institutes of Health Pub No 96-4057; www.nhlbi.nih.gov/health/public/blood/sickle/sca_fact.pdf.*

and most dairy products, contain complete protein. (A notable exception is gelatin, which is incomplete.) Soybeans are the only plant sources providing all nine essential amino acids. Foods that contribute the best balance of EAAs and the best assortment of NEAAs for protein synthesis and are easily digestible are **high-quality protein** foods. The two highest quality protein foods are eggs and human milk. The egg is of high quality because it contains all the necessary nutrients to support life. Human breast milk is the perfect food; its nutrient profile is ideal for human growth.

Incomplete protein lacks one or more of the nine essential amino acids. These proteins will not provide a sufficient supply of amino acids and will not support life (Box 6-3). Many plant foods contain considerable amounts of incomplete proteins. Some of the better sources are grains and legumes.

The EAAs that incomplete proteins lack are called **limiting amino acids**. The limiting amino acid reduces the value of the protein contained in the food. Unless the limiting amino acid is consumed in other foods, the amino acid pools inside the cells would be missing some of the essential amino acids. Protein production within the cell would be affected, and fewer proteins could be formed. Consequently, limiting amino acids reduces the number of proteins that can be made by our bodies. Generally, we consume a sufficient mix of complete and incomplete proteins, therefore this is not a health problem. Only those who adopt a dietary pattern restricting certain types of protein foods are at risk for an imbalanced intake.

high-quality protein
a food containing the best balance and assortment of essential and nonessential amino acids for protein synthesis

incomplete protein
proteins lacking one or more of the essential amino acids

limiting amino acid
the essential amino acid or amino acids that incomplete proteins lack

---

Box 6-3 Sources of Complete and Incomplete Proteins

FOODS CONTAINING COMPLETE PROTEINS

Fish
Shellfish
Chicken
Turkey
Duck*
Beef*
Lamb*
Pork*
Eggs*
Soybeans (tofu)
Cheese
  Hard cheeses
    Cheddar
    Muenster
    Swiss
  Soft cheeses
    Cottage cheese†
    Ricotta†
Milk†
Ice milk/reduced-fat ice cream
Yogurt†
Frozen yogurt

FOODS CONTAINING INCOMPLETE PROTEINS

Cereals
  Ready-to-eat
  Oatmeal
  Wheatena
Grains
  Wheat
  Rice
  Corn
  Oats/oatmeal
  Barley
  Spaghetti/pasta
  Bagels
  Bread
Legumes
  Black-eyed peas
  Lentils
  Beans
  Peanuts/peanut butter
  Chickpeas
  Split peas
Broccoli
Potatoes
Green peas
Leafy green vegetables

---

*Possible high-fat source of protein.
†Protein in skim, 2%, and whole milk products.

Complementary Proteins

By eating different kinds of plant foods throughout the day, the total protein intake will equal that of complete proteins found in animal-related products. The advantages to complementing proteins are that plant foods cost less and tend to contain less fat; consuming less dietary fat is a prevention strategy for several chronic diet-related diseases.

A balance of amino acids is required throughout the day for protein synthesis. A sufficient assortment of EAAs is provided without planning if both animal and plant protein foods are eaten. If animal foods are not eaten, more care is required to assure that limiting amino acids are consumed. Combinations of plant foods that provide all the EAAs are grains (e.g., wheat or rice) with legumes (e.g., kidney beans or chickpeas) and grains or legumes with small amounts of animal protein from dairy, meat, poultry, or fish (Box 6-4).

Measures of Food Protein Quality

Many foods contain protein; however, the value of specific foods as protein sources varies. Perhaps the protein contained is incomplete or is difficult to digest (bound tightly to fiber). If food proteins are not digested, the amino acids can't be absorbed to nourish our bodies.

Several methods are used to analyze the quality of proteins in food, including biologic value, amino acid score, and protein efficiency ratio. Biologic value measures how much nitrogen from a protein food is retained by the body after digestion, absorption, and excretion. This measurement of nitrogen balance reveals how available the protein of that food is to the human body. An egg has the highest reference protein score of 100; all of the egg protein can be used. It has become a standard against which all other food proteins are judged. Fish has a score of 75 to 90, and corn, which contains protein but also has lower amino acid ratios, has a score of 40.[2]

Amino acid score is a simple measure of the amino acid composition of a food as compared with a reference protein. The score is based on the limiting amino acid of the food. Digestibility of the protein is not considered.

A third method for assessing protein quality is protein efficiency ratio (PER). Using this method, rats are fed a set amount of protein and then, based on weight gain, the physiologic value of the food protein consumed is determined.[2]

$$PER = \frac{Weight\ gain}{Protein\ intake}$$

biologic value
a method to determine the quality of food protein by measuring the amount of nitrogen kept in the body after digestion, absorption, and excretion

amino acid score
a simple measure of an amino acid composition of a food as compared with a reference protein; based on the limiting amino acid

protein efficiency ratio (PER)
a method to determine the quality of food protein by comparing weight gain to protein intake

---

Box 6-4 Food Combinations that Provide Complete Proteins

GRAINS + LEGUMES = COMPLETE PROTEIN

Peanut butter sandwich
Tacos with refried beans
Rice and beans
Split pea soup with croutons
Falafel (chickpea balls) on pita bread
Lentil soup with rye bread
Baked beans with bread

GRAINS OR LEGUMES + ANIMAL PROTEIN (SMALL AMOUNT) = COMPLETE PROTEIN

Chili with beans and cornbread
Ready-to-eat cereal with skim milk
Cheese sandwich
Pasta with cheese
Rice pudding
French toast
Pancakes (made with milk and/or eggs)
Tuna casserole

Protein RDA

The RDA for protein provides for sufficient intake of the EAAs and enough total protein to provide the amino groups needed to build new NEAAs. Other factors that affect the RDA for protein are age, gender, physiologic state, and sources of protein.[3]

Age affects protein requirements because when growth occurs, such as during childhood, a greater percentage of dietary intake of protein is needed compared with adulthood. Growth results in additional muscle and tissues, all of which require the amino acids contained in dietary protein. Theoretically, older adults may require lower levels of protein because muscle mass is reduced as we age; protein use may also be affected by variables of decreased physical activity, illness, and chronic use of medications. However, few studies exist to confirm a lower requirement, so the protein RDA for adults age 50 and more is the same as for younger adults.[3] Gender differences also affect protein needs. Men tend to have more lean body mass or muscle than women. Lean body mass requires more protein for maintenance (see the Health Debate box, "Amino Acid Supplements").

Certain physiologic states, such as pregnancy and lactation, require different amounts of nutrients. Pregnant women should consume additional protein to meet the needs of the growing fetus as well as those of their own bodies. RDA recommendations for protein are 20% higher (from 50 grams to 60 grams) for pregnant women. Lactation, the production of breast milk, also requires consumption

lactation
the production of breast milk

HEALTH DEBATE
Amino Acid Supplements

Bodybuilders focus on muscles, muscles, muscles! Unfortunately, many believe that because protein loss occurs during strength and endurance exercise and muscles are composed of protein, excessive amounts of protein must be eaten. However, just a moderate increase of dietary protein is indicated. Because most Americans eat significantly higher amounts of protein than the RDA, this additional need is most likely consumed. In any event, simply eating extra protein does not build muscles. It is only by working a muscle, when adequate protein is present in the diet, that will cause it to develop and strengthen.

There is also a mistaken belief that certain NEAAs, such as arginine and ornithine, should be taken as supplements. The perception is that they have special abilities to enhance muscle development. However, studies show that amino acids taken as supplements are ineffective for increasing lean body mass.

When ingested, these supplements are treated as any other protein source of amino acids. Too much of any one may prevent absorption—and result in a deficiency—of another because they compete for the same absorption sites.

Once a supplement is absorbed, the liver views any protein supplement as a source of amino acids. The supplemental amino acids will not necessarily be directed to muscle development. They may just be converted to other NEAAs. Or, if too much protein or too few kcalories are consumed, amino acids will be used for energy immediately or stored as body fat.

Some bodybuilders also use drugs illegally to pump up muscles. These drugs, such as anabolic steroids, produce dangerous emotional and physical side effects. Amino acid supplements that are perceived to build muscles, although ineffective, are less dangerous than steroids. Should this misperception continue to be fostered as a safer option? Should bodybuilders use drugs at all? What do you think?

Compiled from Armsey TD, Green GA: Nutrition supplements: science vs hype, The Physician and Sportsmedicine 25(6), 1997; Christensen HN: Amino and nutrition: A two-step absorptive process, Nutrition Reviews 51(4):95, 1993; and Williams M: Erogenic and ergolytic substances, Medicine and Science in Sports and Exercise 24(9X supplement): S344-348, 1992.

of additional protein. Breast milk contains high quality protein that is formed from amino acids provided by the woman. The protein RDA for lactation is even higher than during pregnancy (from 50 grams to 65 grams). Special circumstances of serious physical illness, wound healing, fevers (increased metabolic rate), or unusual stress may also increase protein needs.

The type of food sources also affects the amount of protein needed. In the United States most of the protein eaten is complete protein from animal sources. These sources are considered when the RDA for protein is set. Other countries rely on more plant sources of incomplete proteins, so worldwide recommendations, such as those of the World Health Organization, differ from the U.S. guidelines.

The RDA for protein is 0.8 g/kg (or 2.2 lb). For an average adult man, the RDA is 58 to 63 grams; for an average adult woman, the RDA is 46 to 50 grams (see the DRI table inside the front cover). Recent research suggests that recommended levels for athletes are 1.0 to 1.5 g/kg body weight. Because most Americans eat more protein than recommended, even athletes tend to easily meet protein recommendations.[4] Determine your recommended protein intake using the formula in the Teaching Tool box, "Calculating Your Recommended Protein Intake."

The Acceptable Macronutrient Distribution Ranges (AMDRs) suggests that protein consumption range between 10% to 35% of energy intake. Depending on the percentage of protein energy consumed, consumption of energy from carbohydrates and lipids should be adjusted accordingly.[3]

VEGETARIANISM

vegan dietary pattern
a food plan consisting of only plant foods

lacto-vegetarian dietary pattern
a food plan consisting of only plant foods plus dairy products

ovo-lacto vegetarian dietary pattern
a food plan consisting of only plant foods plus dairy products and eggs

Vegetarian dietary patterns have long been a part of human history. Instead of animal protein sources, vegetarian dietary patterns focus on plant proteins to provide EAAs. The vegan dietary pattern consists of plant foods including grains, legumes, fruits, vegetables, seeds, and nuts; no animal-related products are eaten. The lacto-vegetarian dietary pattern includes all the foods of the vegan plus dairy products such as milk, cheese, yogurt, and butter. The ovo-lacto vegetarian dietary pattern incorporates eggs into the lacto-vegetarian assortment of foods.

The Benefits of Vegetarianism

Vegetarian dietary patterns may be followed to achieve health, spiritual, economic, and/or environmental benefits. When well-planned, vegetarian dietary patterns result in health benefits that are similar to those of a low-fat, high-fiber diet and consist of reduced risk of obesity, CAD, type 2 diabetes mellitus, hypertension, gastrointestinal disorders, and certain cancers such as lung and colorectal cancers.[5]

Because animal foods are our primary source of saturated fat and only source of cholesterol, plant-based vegetarian dietary patterns tend to be lower in total fat and cholesterol. This reduced intake, combined with the high fiber content of plant

TEACHING TOOL
Calculating Your Recommended Protein Intake

To determine your personal protein recommendation, compute the following:

1. Divide your body weight by 2.2 to determine your weight in kilograms (kg).
2. Weight in lbs ÷ 2.2 = weight in kg. Here is an example:

$$140 \div 2.2 = 63.6 \text{ kg}$$

3. Multiply the kilogram weight by 0.8 g/kg to determine your protein RDA (i.e., weight in kg × 0.8 g/kg = g of protein/RDA). Here is an example:

$$63.6 \text{ kg} \times 0.8 \text{ g/kg} = 50.9 \text{ g protein/RDA}$$

foods, often results in lower blood cholesterol levels. In addition, the body weight of individuals following vegetarian dietary patterns is generally lower. This also reduces the risk of developing hypertension and diabetes.

The spiritual rationale for some individuals who are vegetarians is based on the belief in nonharming. Several religions, including Hinduism and Seventh-Day Adventists, see the consumption of animal flesh as being unhealthy or polluting to the body. Other vegetarians do not follow a formal religion but believe strongly in the protection of animal rights and are opposed to the slaughter of animals for human consumption.

The economic approach addresses the belief that animal-related products cost more than plant protein foods, not only financially but in terms of costs to our natural environment as well. Livestock and other domesticated animals are inefficient producers of protein. Although protein foods from cattle and chicken are of high quality, many pounds of grains are used by these animals to produce one pound of edible food. Some people maintain that by eating from lower on the food chain— that is, eating more plant foods—there will be less waste and limited environmental impact on our natural resources.

The Drawbacks of Vegetarianism

The vegetarian dietary pattern has several drawbacks. The most critical affects vegans. The vegan dietary pattern can provide all the essential nutrients except vitamins D and B_{12}.

Most dietary vitamin D is consumed through milk fortified with the vitamin. Because vegans do not consume any dairy products, this source of vitamin D is diminished. However, vitamin D is available through synthesis during exposure of the skin to direct sunlight. This source was thought to be adequate for adults and children, but recent reports reveal that rickets, the vitamin D deficiency disorder, has been diagnosed among some infants and young children of vegetarian African American Muslims.[6] The children were well-fed, but dietary sources of vitamin D were negligible. Even maternal breast milk may be low in vitamin D if not consumed in dietary form. It is possible that the combination of dressing young children in heavy clothing (restricting exposure of the skin to the sun) and darker skin pigmentation (which also reduces vitamin D synthesis) places some children at risk for vitamin D deficiency.

Reliable sources of vitamin B_{12} are all animal-related. By excluding animal-derived foods, including milk, sources of B_{12} are simply not available. Even ovo-lacto vegetarians may have low levels of vitamin B_{12}. Symptoms of vitamin B_{12} deficiency take years to appear and may cause permanent damage to the central nervous system. Individuals who restrict their intake or exclude animal foods should take B_{12} supplements or consume foods fortified with vitamin B_{12} such as fortified soy milk to insure adequate intake.[5]

Other nutrients in which vegans could be deficient are iron and zinc, minerals usually consumed in meat, fish, and poultry. Calcium levels may also be low if dairy products are excluded; few plants are good sources of calcium. These nutrients are available in a well-planned vegan diet of whole foods. Nonetheless, care must be taken to consume sufficient amounts of calcium during pregnancy and growth periods; supplements will be necessary. If the vegan dietary pattern is poorly implemented and depends on refined and processed foods, nutrients may be lacking.

Another drawback pertains to the dimension of social health. Social health is the ability to interact with people in an acceptable manner and to sustain relationships with family members, friends, and colleagues. Those following a vegetarian dietary pattern often find themselves rationalizing their behaviors to others. It can sometimes be tricky to do so without alienating others—especially while they are in the midst of a steak dinner. Perhaps the simplest approach is to emphasize the health benefits gained by adopting a vegetarian dietary pattern.

To ensure that a vegetarian dietary pattern is healthful necessitates learning about protein complementing and new ways of preparing meatless dishes. Simply replacing meat with a lot of cheese won't result in any health benefits. In fact, the fat content of a cheese dish is probably higher than a lean meat dish. The most helpful approach is to read vegetarian cookbooks that not only provide recipes but also include vegetarian nutrition information. Figure 6-6 presents the Food Guide Pyramid for Vegetarian Meal Planning, which is a valuable guide to assure adequate nutritional status.

Contemporary Vegetarianism

Other terms have evolved to describe semi-vegetarian dietary patterns. In addition to the foods consumed by ovo-lacto vegetarians, *pesco-vegetarians* consume small amounts of fish. Eating limited quantities of chicken is a *pollo-vegetarian dietary pattern*. These titles do not reflect the original ideals of vegetarianism. Instead, they are representative of new contemporary dietary patterns evolving in response to current health issues. These health issues center around the risk of developing one or more of the chronic diet-related diseases: CAD, cancer, type 2 diabetes mellitus, and hypertension. Risk is reduced as dietary fat intake is lowered. A major source of fat in our diets is our consumption of animal protein foods. Reducing levels of this category of dietary fat lowers risk for chronic diet-related diseases. By doing so, the health promotion goals of *Healthy People 2010* recommendations may be achieved.

DIETARY PATTERNS OF PROTEIN

So what should we eat for protein? No longer do we need to be confined to a meat and potatoes mentality when it comes to protein. The healthiest approach is to eat mixed sources of protein—animal and plant sources (see the Cultural Considerations box, "Rituals for Animal-derived Protein," for a discussion of the religious

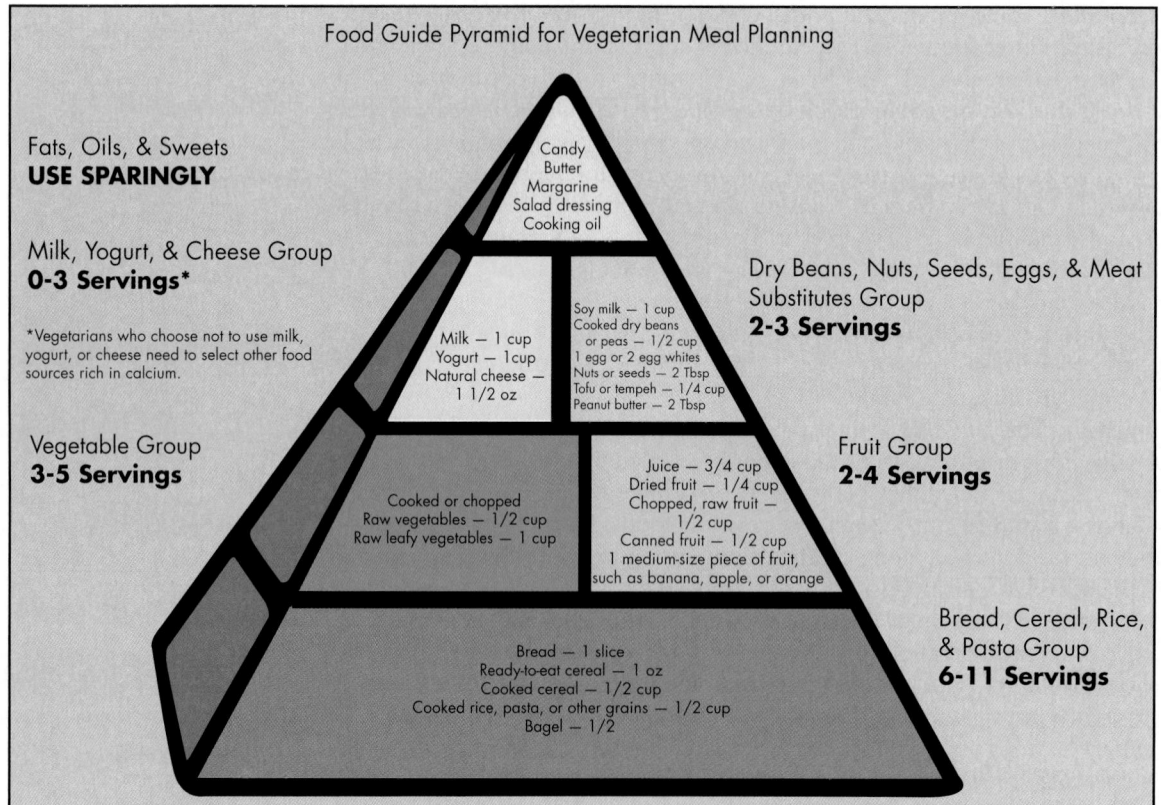

Figure 6-6 Food Guide Pyramid for Vegetarian Meal Planning. (From National Center for Nutrition and Dietetics. The American Dietetic Association: Based on the USDA Food Guide Pyramid. © ADAF 1997. Reprodution of this pyramid is permitted for educational purposes. Reproduction for sales purposes is not permitted.)

$\mathcal{M}$ost religions identify foods with specific holidays and rules regarding consumption. Two predominantly Western religions, Judaism and Islam, have rules regarding the daily preparation and consumption of foods; most of these directions focus on consumption of animal-derived protein foods.

KASHRUT, JEWISH DIETARY LAWS

The rules of *kashrut* were presented in the Torah, or bible of the Jewish people. *Kosher* means "fit" and is the concept referring to the Jewish dietary laws. Although most of the rules can be explained on the basis of physical health benefits, the foundation and observance of the restrictions is because of spiritual health rather than physical. By observing the kosher dietary laws, one is respecting God, oneself, and other Jews. There are about eight laws regarding consumption of animal-derived protein. They are briefly described below.

1. Only certain animals may be eaten. Only mammals with cloven hooves that chew the cud may be eaten and its milk consumed; this allows cattle, deer, goats, and sheep to be consumed but not pigs. Birds must also meet specific criteria; acceptable birds (and their eggs) include chickens, ducks, geese, and turkey. In addition, fish must have fins and scales to be consumed; therefore all shellfish, eel, and catfish are not permitted. Acceptable foods are viewed as coming from "clean" animals and unacceptable foods are viewed as "unclean."

2. Animals must be slaughtered in a specific manner that is quick and painless and that causes most blood to drain from the carcass.

3. Slaughtered animals must be free of any bruises or diseases to be consumed.

4. Only certain parts of permitted animals may be consumed. Animal blood from any animal and layers of solid fat may not be consumed.

5. Meat must be prepared for consumption in specific procedures. Blood must be completely drained and cuts of meat must avoid certain nerves and animal parts. Specially trained "kosher" butchers prepare animals foods according to kashrut.

6. Meat and dairy are not consumed together. Consequently, separate cooking utensils, plates, and utensils are maintained for meat consumption and dairy consumption. Some foods are considered neither meat nor dairy and may be eaten with either category. These foods are called *pareve*.

7. Products from unclean animals may not be consumed. The exception is honey. Although bees may not be consumed, honey is acceptable.

8. Foods are examined for insects and worms that may not be consumed but may be on vegetables, fruits, and grains.

To ensure that these rules are followed, food preparation is supervised by rabbis (spiritual teachers), after which the product may then display special logos to that effect. Most often it is a "K" that appears on product packaging (see examples at bottom of page).

HALAL, ISLAMIC DIETARY LAWS

The Islamic rules of *halal* or permitted foods, presented in the Koran (bible of Islam), consider food consumption as an aspect of worship. Consequently, eating is viewed as a way to keep one's body healthy. Food should not be consumed excessively and is to be shared with others. All food is permitted unless specifically prohibited. Specific rules concerning foods that may not be consumed include the following:

- Swine (pigs) and birds of prey may not be consumed.
- Animals that are not slaughtered according to specific Muslim procedures may not be consumed. These are similar to those of Jewish laws that regard the exact means of slaughter and blood drainage.
- Alcoholic beverages and drugs that affect consciousness, unless required for medicinal purposes, may not be consumed. Coffee and tea, because they contain the stimulant caffeine, are discouraged.
- Foods that are produced according to Islamic dietary laws sometimes bear the symbols approved by the Islamic Food and Nutrition Council of America (see examples directly below).

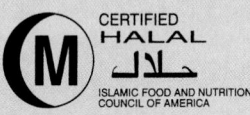 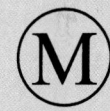

Application to nursing: In nursing practice, it is valuable to be knowledgeable and thereby respectful of the possible dietary restrictions of clients. Assistance can then be given as to the best dietary pattern to assure wholesome nutrient intakes and the alternative medications or treatment available. For example, because observant Jews and Muslims do not consume pigs or products derived from pigs, the source of insulin (usually from pigs) may be problematic for patients with diabetes.

Reference: Kittler PG, Sucher KP: Food and culture in America: a nutrition handbook, *ed 3, Belmont, Calif, 2002, West/Wadsworth.*

Ⓤ Union of Orthodox Jewish Congregations, New York, New York

Ⓚ O.K. (Organized Kashrut) Laboratories, Brooklyn, New York

K/M/H (K.V.H.) Kashrut Commission of the Vaad Horabanim (Rabbinical Council) of New England, Boston, Massachusetts

△K Rabbi J.H. Ralbag, New York, New York

  Kosher Supervision Service, Hackensack, New Jersey

Ⓚ Kosher Overseers Association of America, Beverly Hills, California

Ⓥ Vaad Hoeir of St. Louis, St. Louis, Missouri

aspects of protein consumption). The mix provides an excellent assortment of EAAs plus sufficient building block materials for constructing NEAAs. By eating fewer animal protein foods, dietary fat intake is reduced. By eating more plant protein foods, dietary fiber is increased.

Restructuring the Dinner Plate

If asked to plan a balanced meal, what would the plate look like? Perhaps animal protein (meat, fish, or poultry), vegetables (broccoli, potato, and a salad), and a grain (bread). But how much room on the plate would each portion be?

Before reading this chapter, a person's plate would most likely look like that in Figure 6-7. Notice how meat is the centerpiece that takes up the most space on the plate. Is this large portion of chicken necessary? Not at all.

A 6-oz serving of chicken provides about 53 grams of protein. Add to that amount the protein in the bread (3 g), potato (4 g), broccoli (2 g), salad (1 g), and skim milk (8 g), and the total protein intake from one meal alone is 71 grams. Because we eat protein throughout the day, no one meal needs to provide all our protein. Instead, the balance of the meal needs to be restructured. Because each component of the meal contains protein, whether from animal or plant sources, portion quantities can shift and still provide plenty of protein. An adequate serving of meat is about the size of a deck of cards or the size of your palm. Notice in Figure 6-8 how the chicken, reduced to 3 oz, is no longer the focus of the plate. Each item occupies a more equal space on the plate. The protein total is still high at 48 grams.

By spreading protein intake throughout the food groups, the objectives of the Food Guide Pyramid are met. The first plate (see Figure 6-7) provides the following:

- 1 serving of grains
- 3 servings of vegetables
- 0 servings of fruit
- 1 serving of dairy
- 2 servings from the meat/beans/eggs group

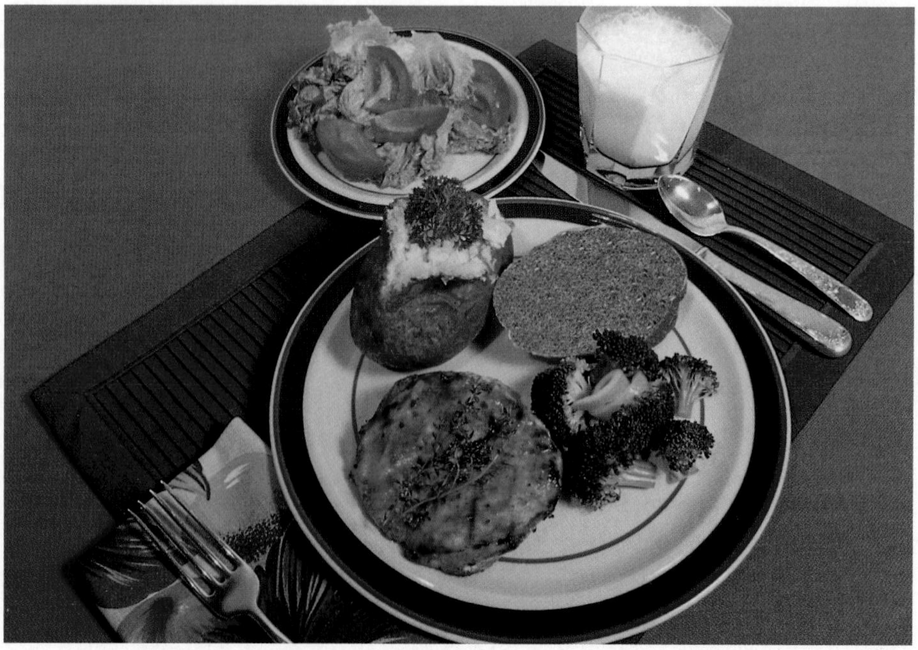

> Use the concept of the deck of cards and the restructured meal to visually display to clients appropriate animal-protein portion sizes.

Figure 6-7 A balanced meal. (From Joanne Scott/Tracy McCalla.)

The second plate (see Figure 6-8) provides the following:
- 2 servings of grains
- 4 servings of vegetables
- 1 serving of fruit
- 1 serving of dairy
- 1 serving of protein

The new plate provides more complex carbohydrates from grains, fruits, and vegetables while still providing sufficient amounts of protein.

OVERCOMING BARRIERS

Malnutrition

Malnutrition, the imbalance of nutrient intake, encompasses conditions that range from over-consumption of nutrients to extreme under-consumption. This discussion concerns the conditions related to under-consumption of nutrients. Under-consumption can result in nutrient deficiencies that range from marginal to severe starvation. Marginal deficiencies occur when lower than recommended levels of nutrients are regularly consumed. Although obvious signs of specific nutrient deficiencies may not be visible, the level of wellness and ability to function at an optimum level are compromised. As the other nutrient categories of vitamins and minerals are studied, specific symptoms of deficiencies will be explored.

Starvation has become a catch-all term. Although we may say "I'm starving" when we've missed a meal, our starvation in no way compares with that experienced by those who truly do not have access to sufficient quantities of high-quality food. The technical term for starvation is protein-energy malnutrition (PEM). PEM is an umbrella term for malnutrition caused by the lack of protein, energy, or both. PEM affects populations around the world. This form of malnutrition is responsible for about half of the 10.9 million child deaths per year. Of children with PEM, 70% are found in Asia, 26% in Africa, and 4% in Latin America and

malnutrition
an imbalanced nutrient and/or energy intake

protein-energy malnutrition (PEM)
malnutrition caused by the lack of protein, energy, or both

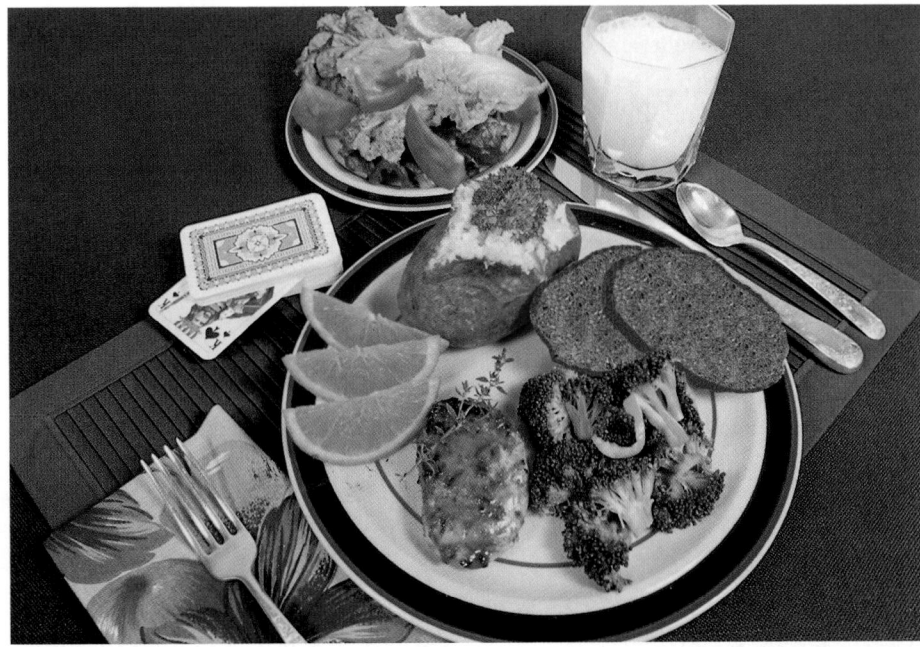

Figure 6-8 A restructured meal. (From Joanne Scott/Tracy McCalla.)

the Caribbean Islands.[7] In young children, PEM can cause permanent disabilities because most brain growth occurs during the early years of life. Extreme PEM results in the conditions of marasmus and kwashiorkor (Figure 6-9). These disorders can be fatal because of decreased resistance to infections; the body, lacking protein, is unable to create sufficient quantities of antibodies to support the immune system.

marasmus
malnutrition caused by a lack of energy (kcalorie) intake

Marasmus is malnutrition caused by a lack of sufficient energy (kcalorie) intake. An individual with marasmus is extremely thin; skin seems to hang on the skeletal bones. Fat stores that normally fill out the skin have been used for energy to maintain minimum body functioning. Muscle mass is also reduced, having also been used for energy, and nutrients are not available to rebuild it. If the condition continues, damage may occur to major organs such as the heart, lungs, and kidneys. Marasmic children will not grow. If the condition occurs between 6 and 18 months of age, the time during which the most brain development occurs, permanent brain damage may result.

kwashiorkor
malnutrition caused by a lack of protein while consuming adequate energy

In contrast to marasmus, the symptoms of kwashiorkor give the appearance of more than sufficient fat stores in the stomach and face. Kwashiorkor is malnutrition caused by a lack of protein while consuming adequate energy. The swollen belly and full cheeks of kwashiorkor are caused by edema (water retention). Edema occurs because protein levels in the body are so low that protein is not available to maintain adequate water balance in the cells and fluid accumulates unevenly. When adequate nutrition is provided, the fluid is no longer retained. Instead of a full belly and round cheeks, the loss of fat stores becomes apparent and the skin hangs loosely, similar to marasmus. An individual with kwashiorkor is apathetic and experiences muscle weakness and poor growth.

Without sufficient protein, lipids produced by the liver are unable to leave and thus accumulate there. The liver becomes fatty and unable to function well. Even hair quality is affected because protein is the main constituent of hair. Curly hair becomes straight, hair falls out easily, and the pigmentation changes.

The definition of kwashiorkor is evolving. Kwashiorkor was identified as a disorder that develops when very young children are switched from breast milk to solid foods. Although they are consuming enough kcalories, it seems that their protein intake is too low for the needs of their growing bodies.[8] Based on these observations, kwashiorkor is defined as malnutrition caused by protein deficiency although adequate energy is consumed.

This definition, however, does not explain why other children and adults in the same community develop marasmus instead of kwashiorkor. As researchers continue to study the disorder, they have noticed similarities between the locations where kwashiorkor is prevalent and where exposure to dietary aflatoxin occurs. They have also noted that that the symptoms of kwashiorkor are similar to those of aflatoxin poisoning. Aflatoxin is a mold that develops when grains are stored under poor conditions of heat and humidity. Eating grains affected by aflatoxin can affect liver function, even leading to liver cancer.[9]

The liver produces NEAAs, without which protein synthesis throughout the body is limited. If liver function is reduced, as with aflatoxin poisoning, production of protein-related structures and substances is decreased. Compared with healthier children and adults, it appears that when malnourished children consume aflatoxin-tainted grains, their weakened immune systems are not able to fight off the effects of aflatoxin. Aflatoxin also induces immunosuppression, creating a cumulative effect that may lead to the development of kwashiorkor.[9]

Malnutrition Factors

Malnutrition is often caused by several factors that affect food availability. Although poverty tends to be a dominant influence, other forces also affect the development of malnutrition. These include biologic, social, economic, and environmental factors (Box 6-5).

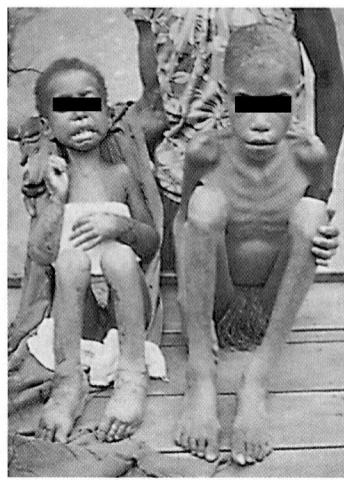

Figure 6-9 Children suffering from kwashiorkor (*left*) and marasmus (*right*) as a result of inadequate energy intake. (Courtesy Professor R. Hendricksen. In McLaren DS: *A colour atlas and text of diet-related disorders*, ed 2, London, 1992, Mosby-Year Book Europe Limited. By permission of Mosby International Ltd.)

Box 6-5 ✸ Malnutrition Factors

BIOLOGIC FACTORS

- Maternal malnutrition before or during pregnancy and/or lactation
- Infections that may affect nutrient absorption
- Chronic diarrhea as both a cause and effect of malnutrition
- Toxins such as aflatoxin
- Lack of food, particularly protein

SOCIAL FACTORS

- Ignorance of nutrient needs of children, resulting in inappropriate weaning foods
- Child abuse and neglect
- Eating disorders, particularly anorexia nervosa
- Drug abuse affecting the ability to care for oneself appropriately
- Social isolation of older adults, leading to an inability to purchase and prepare adequate quantities of food

- Alcoholism (kcalories from alcohol replace consumption of nutrient-dense foods)
- Wars/civil strife disrupting normal social and food production systems

ECONOMIC FACTORS

- Poverty and socioeconomic status
- Unemployment
- Under-education
- Political strife affecting distribution of wealth and land ownership

ENVIRONMENTAL FACTORS

- Polluted water, reducing food production and directly impacting the health of populations
- Famine caused by droughts or crop failures
- Improper farming techniques

Biologic factors affect the ability of the body to use nutrients. Economic effects encompass the ability to purchase food and also consider the structure of a country's economy and access to employment. Environmental factors directly affect the availability of food as related to crop production and food safety. Lack of education, social isolation, and the rippling effects of underemployment seem to be malnutrition factors throughout the world, regardless of the overall wealth of nations. Health and economic support systems provided throughout the life cycle may prevent the development of factors affecting food availability.

Groups at Risk in North America

Most people in North America are well-nourished, although growing numbers of homeless individuals living in shelters or other temporary sites are at risk for varying levels of malnutrition.[10] Without access to cooking facilities or the funds to purchase adequate quantities of foods, these individuals are at nutritional risk. In response to this crisis, food pantries and soup kitchens have been established by nonprofit and charitable groups to distribute food and meals (see the Social Issue box, "Hunger All Around: How to Help"). Also at risk are the working poor, whose incomes barely cover the basic expenses of housing, utilities, and health care and leave little for food purchases.

✸ Older adults are also at risk. Although their nutritional concerns will be covered in depth in Chapter 13, consider that the physical and financial limitations of older adults may reduce their ability to purchase and prepare wholesome meals. When these issues are also compounded by social isolation, the situation of older adults becomes serious.

Hospital patients and those with chronic illnesses such as acquired immunodeficiency syndrome (AIDS) and cancer are also at risk for PEM, even while under medical care. Depending on their illness, 25% of hospital patients may experience treatable malnutrition.[11] This is called *hospital malnutrition* or iatrogenic malnutrition. This condition may be caused by not consuming enough food, side effects from an illness, prolonged liquid diet (as a result of extended diagnostic testing), or medications that reduce the body's ability to absorb nutrients. An extended hospital stay may also increase the risk of poor nutritional status.[11] Weight loss associated with an extended hospital stay may be attributed to the illness rather than

iatrogenic
inadvertently caused by treatment or diagnostic procedures

to lack of nutrients. The patient seems sicker but is actually malnourished and not absorbing the nutrients needed to heal and recover.

Primary care providers, nurses, and dietitians all play a collaborative role in preventing, identifying, and treating hospital malnutrition. Astute nursing assessment may uncover early signs of malnutrition or factors predisposing a patient to it. Some patients may enter the hospital already malnourished. Dietitians work not only with individual patients but also with the healthcare industry to develop new products and technologies designed to either prevent or reduce the incidents of PEM among hospital patients.[12] Clinical guidelines, coupled with nutrition support teams, can enhance nutritional adequacy.[12]

Chronic Hunger

chronic hunger
a continual experience of undernutrition

Although famines and wars affect the nutritional status of people throughout the world, the population of North America has not experienced these extremes of deprivation. Instead, chronic hunger, defined as a continual experience of undernutrition (not enough food to eat), has become the norm for a subset of our population. This subset is growing as the economies of North America tighten, causing government food and welfare programs to be unable to provide an appropriate safety net to prevent and alleviate chronic hunger. Instead, more individuals and families are faced with a consistent lack of opportunities to improve their standard of living and most importantly, their health.

TOWARD A POSITIVE NUTRITION LIFESTYLE: CHAINING

Chaining refers to the linking together of two behaviors. If two actions consistently occur together, they often become linked or tied to each other. They become one behavior and a habit. Many of us already practice chaining; unfortunately, the results often have a negative impact on our dietary intake patterns. Frequently eating potato chips while studying can link these two actions—eating chips and studying. The chain requires that whenever studying takes place, chips need to be eaten. Chaining, however, can also be used to improve nutritional status.

Consider these chains:

- When you eat a sandwich, eat a fruit too. Instead of linking chips and a sandwich (or hoagie, grinder, or sub), this links a sandwich with a fruit.
- Have a glass of skim milk with the midday meal regularly to increase calcium intake. Skim milk becomes chained to lunch.
- At home, weigh portions of meat, fish, and poultry. Compare the size of an appropriate portion to the size of a deck of cards. Are they similar in size? Weigh portions regularly and consciously compare sizes. Animal protein portion sizes will be linked to the deck of cards and portion control can be achieved without weighing.

These are just a few chains related to protein consumption. Chaining can be applied to other nutrition and wellness situations of our clients as well.

SUMMARY

Proteins consist of chains of amino acids. Amino acids are organic compounds made of carbon, hydrogen, oxygen, and nitrogen. There are 20 amino acids from which all proteins are made. The body can manufacture some, but not all, of the amino acids. EAAs cannot be made by the body; these nine amino acids are needed from food. The other 11 NEAAs can be created by the liver. All are available to the cells through the amino acid pool to allow proteins to be synthesized.

The proteins in foods are categorized by the EAAs they contain. Complete proteins contain all nine essential amino acids, whereas incomplete proteins lack one or more of the essential amino acids.

The proteins in foods are not the same as those used by our bodies. During digestion, food protein is broken down to amino acids. Once absorbed, the amino acids circulate in the blood to build new proteins. The new proteins are used to perform numerous functions, including growth and maintenance, creation of essential substances, immune system response, fluid regulation, acid-base balance, and transportation of nutrients and other substances in the body. Malnutrition resulting in PEM, marasmus, and kwashiorkor is a worldwide concern.

THE NURSING APPROACH
Protein Case Study

Roy, a 69-year-old homeless man, comes to a neighborhood mobile van health clinic with a leg ulcer that he says he has had for several months and that continues to get larger. He is obviously poorly nourished. He says he eats what he can find on the street and sometimes goes to the city food center for a hot meal. The nurse cleans Roy's leg ulcer, and the physician orders laboratory tests.

Continued

THE NURSING APPROACH–cont'd
Protein Case Study

ASSESSMENT

Subjective
- Minimal intake of meat, eggs, or other protein foods
- Fatigue

Objective-
- Height 6'2"
- Weight 140 lb.
- Muscle atrophy in extremities bilaterally
- Decreased muscle strength
- Poor skin turgor
- Hair is dull and thin
- Slight ankle edema bilaterally
- Left lower leg ulcer 4 cm in diameter, Stage II
- Laboratory test results:
  - Total serum protein 5.4 (norm 6.6-7.9 Gm/dl)
  - Serum albumin 3.1 (norm 3.3-4.5 Gm/dl)
  - Serum transferrin 200 (norm 220-400 ug/dl)
  - Other laboratory tests are normal or close to normal

NURSING DIAGNOSIS

1. Altered nutrition, less than body requirements, of protein related to lack of food availability, evidenced by delayed healing of lower left leg ulcer and underweight status
2. Skin integrity impaired as evidenced by leg ulcer

PLANNING

Specific realistic goals and outcomes for Roy include the following:
1. Roy will express understanding of the importance of protein and the variety of food sources of protein.
2. His leg ulcer will heal within 2 months.
3. He will gain 4 lbs. in 2 months.

IMPLEMENTATION

1. Discuss with Roy protein and dietary sources of protein.
2. Supply Roy with cans of high-protein and vitamin supplements at each clinic visit.
3. Apply wet-to-dry dressing and antibiotic ointment to leg ulcers during clinic visits twice a week.
4. Encourage Roy to move into a homeless shelter affiliated with the clinic until the leg ulcer heals.
5. Encourage Roy to eat at least one meal per day in the shelter.

EVALUATION

Each goal should be evaluated to see if the outcome has been fully or partially met as evidenced by the following:
- After four clinic visits, client describes high-protein sources have been eaten each day
- Decrease the diameter of leg ulcer in 1 month to 2 cm and healing in 2 months
- Weight gain of at least 2 lb. in 1 month and 4 lb. in 2 months

APPLYING CONTENT KNOWLEDGE

Karen and her husband, Roger, want to reduce their intake of fat and increase their fiber intake. Both grew up in families that prided themselves as being the "meat and potatoes" type. Suggest three strategies they could adopt to restructure their dinner plates.

Web Sites of Interest

Healthfinder

www.healthfinder.gov

This U.S. government Web site links to consumer health and human services information through online publications, clearinghouses, databases, government agencies, and nonprofit organizations. It also includes a list/serv for immediate notification of new health research highlights and resources.

PKU: Information Sheet

www.modimes.org/HealthLibrary/334_607.htm

This information sheet is provided by the March of Dimes and contains facts about the prevention of PKU symptoms, facts about PKU during pregnancy, and current research findings.

The Sickle Cell Information Center

www.emory.edu/PEDS/SICKLE/

This site provides education, counseling, research updates, and international resources about sickle cell anemia for patients and health professionals.

The Vegetarian Resource Group

www.vrg.org/

This site is a comprehensive guide to vegetarian information, cookbooks, journals, and related links.

References

1. Thibodeau GA, Patton KT: *Anatomy and physiology*, ed 4, St Louis, 1999, Mosby.
2. Matthews DE: Proteins and amino acids. In Shils ME et al., eds.: *Modern nutrition in health and disease*, ed 9, Philadelphia, 1999, Williams & Wilkins.
3. Institute of Medicine Food and Nutrition Board: *Dietary Reference Intakes for energy, carbohydrate, fiber, fat, fatty acids, cholesterol, protein, and amino acids*, Washington, DC, 2002, National Academy Press.
4. Nutrition and Athletic Performance—position paper of the American Dietetic Association, Dietitians of Canada, and the American College of Sports Medicine, *J Am Dietetic Assoc* 100:1543, 2000.
5. Messina VK, Burke KI: Position of the American Dietetic Association: vegetarian diets, *J Am Dietetic Assoc* 97(11):1317, 1997.
6. Tortorella K: Rickets: a relic shows up again, *New York Times* 13:1, March 12, 1995.
7. *Nutrition: alleviating protein-energy malnutrition*, World Health Organization, March 13, 2002; www.who.int/nut/pem.htm.
8. Solomons NW, Molina S, Bluw J: Weanling diarrhea: a case report, *Nutr Rev* 48(5):212, 1990.
9. Hendricksen RG: Of sick turkeys, kwashiorkor, malaria, perinatal mortality, heroin addicts and food poisoning: research on the influence of aflatoxins on child health in the tropics, *Ann Trop Med Parasitol* 91(7):787, 1997.
10. Wolgamuth JC et al.: Wasting malnutrition and inadequate nutrient intakes identified in a multiethnic homeless population, *J Am Dietetic Assoc* 92(7):834, 1992.
11. Allison SP: The management of malnutrition in hospital, *Proc Nutr Soc* 55(3):855, 1996.
12. Pennington CR: Disease-associated malnutrition in the year 2000, *Postgrad Med J* 74(868):65, 1998.

CHAPTER 7

Vitamins

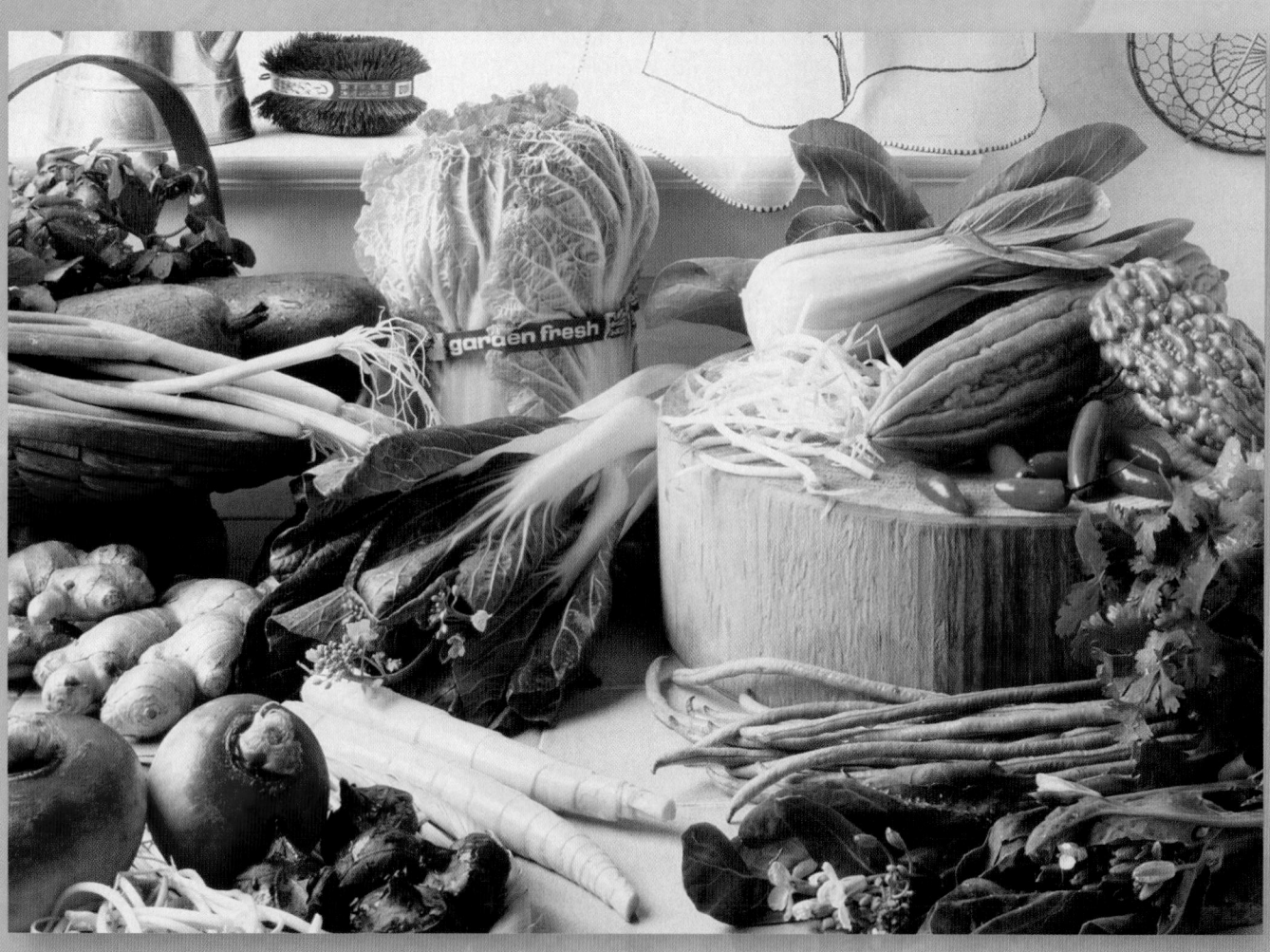

*Vitamins are organic molecules that
are required in very small amounts.*

ROLE IN WELLNESS

Vitamins seem to have a magical aura. Take enough and you'll have more energy and be healthier, smarter, and even better looking. If only it were so easy. Although vitamins are essential for life, they are only one of many factors required for wellness.

Knowledge of the existence of vitamins is recent; the discovery of vitamins slowly evolved, beginning in the early part of the twentieth century. The focus of research was to discover the amounts of vitamins needed to prevent deficiency symptoms and diseases that undermine the health and well-being of populations throughout the world.

The scientific view of vitamins, however, is in flux. Additional effects of vitamin use are surfacing as more is learned about the functions of vitamins as antioxidants and hormonelike substances. Some vitamins and related substances such as carotenoids may reduce the risk of developing certain chronic diseases. Information is emerging that points to relationships between consuming foods high in vitamins and a lower incidence of developing diseases.

The Dietary Reference Intakes (DRI) consider the concern of providing nutrient requirements necessary to prevent deficiencies and toxicity from overdoses and accounting for the value of nutrient intake as a means of reducing disease risk.[1] Recommendations within the DRI documents include the use of fortified foods or supplements for particular nutrients, such as folic acid for women of childbearing age to ensure proper neural tube formation of the fetus during pregnancy.

Vitamins are organic molecules required in very small amounts. Each vitamin performs a specific metabolic function. Vitamins, except for vitamin D, are not synthesized by our bodies and thus are essential nutrients that must be provided through dietary intake. Vitamin D is the only vitamin created by the human body.

Vitamins are vital to life and therefore to the five dimensions of health. Vitamins are essential nutrients without which the body cannot continue functioning within the physical dimension. Recommendations to eat five fruits and vegetables per day throughout the life span are made to reduce the risk of diet-related diseases in the future. Intellectual skills are used to envision future benefits that accrue from food choices today. Deficiencies of several B vitamins can produce irritability, confusion, and paranoia thereby affecting the emotional health dimension. Older adults may be at risk for deficiencies because of their inability to get to the store to buy fruits and vegetables; the physical health of older adults may depend on their social health in relation to neighbors who may provide assistance with shopping needs. Sometimes following religious teachings may jeopardize health, as noted by the development of rickets, the vitamin D deficiency disorder, among some African American children of families following the dietary and dress customs of the Islamic faith. Spiritual health is interdependent upon the other dimensions of health.

As vitamins are discussed, note that some are referred to by specific names or by letters and numbers. Each vitamin has a history that affects how we refer to it today. In 1929 Henrik Dam in Copenhagen, Denmark, discovered vitamin K. It was the only substance able to halt a hemorrhagic disease in which blood does not coagulate. Dam named the vitamin *K* for the Danish word *koagulation*. In another case, several B vitamins were isolated into the same test tube labeled B, and we therefore have vitamins numbered B_1, B_2, and B_3. In the 1970s the science community decreed that all vitamins should be called by their formal biochemical titles. The public and many health professionals still refer to the simpler letter and number names for vitamins. Both the formal and informal names are used in this chapter.

This chapter will list vitamin DRI. Because DRI is an umbrella term that includes Recommended Dietary Allowance (RDA), Adequate Intake (AI), and Tolerable Upper Intake Level (UL), applicable standards will be identified. Because there are different RDA and AI based on age, gender, and physiologic need, only those for men and women ages 19 to 30 are included for each vitamin, unless spe-

vitamins
essential organic molecules needed in very small amounts for cellular metabolism

DRI = Dietary Reference Intakes

RDA = Recommended Dietary Allowance

AI = Adequate Intake

UL = Tolerable Upper Intake Level

cial circumstances surrounding the need for a vitamin warrant discussion. The DRI tables are located inside the front cover of this book.

A primary deficiency of a vitamin occurs when the vitamin is not consumed in sufficient amounts to meet physiologic needs. A secondary deficiency develops when absorption is impaired or excess excretion occurs, limiting bioavailability. Most deficiencies are detected through clinical and biochemical assessment; specific diagnostic and laboratory procedures are beyond the scope of this text and are available elsewhere.[2]

Although vitamin deficiencies are no longer common among Americans, subgroups are at risk. Because of their increased needs, pregnant women are often at risk for marginal deficiencies of essential vitamins. Older adults may also be at risk because of decreased absorptive ability and limited economic and physical resources for food availability. Poverty is an overwhelming factor that affects the nutritional status of children and adults. Chronic alcohol and drug abuse not only alters psychologic and mental capacities but also limits the body's ability to absorb and use essential vitamins.

Health professionals can also take into account other special circumstances that may initiate vitamin deficiencies. Individuals dealing with long-term chronic disorders that affect the total body response, such as acquired immunodeficiency syndrome (AIDS) or liver or kidney disorders, have special vitamin concerns because the metabolic processes of the body may be compromised by these disorders and by the medications prescribed. Deficiencies have recently been documented that were possibly caused by the effects of cancer treatment, use of multiple alternative therapies, and lifestyle behaviors. These deficiencies were at first misdiagnosed because vitamin deficiencies were no longer thought to occur.[3-5]

Toxicities of vitamins rarely occur naturally from food consumption. Instead, inappropriate use of supplements may be toxic to our bodies. Vitamins have been studied for their physiologic effect or basic need for health maintenance. The recommended levels reflect this knowledge. Use of vitamin supplements at megadose levels is equivalent to a pharmacologic effect, with potential druglike physical responses. Some vitamins have UL; for others, a megadose (i.e., 10 times the RDA for a specific nutrient) of a vitamin is considered the highest amount of the nutrient that will not cause adverse health effects. Because most vitamins have not been studied to determine function and safety at these megadose levels, extensive use without guidance can be problematic.

VITAMIN CATEGORIES

Vitamins are divided into two categories based on their solubility in solutions. *Water-soluble vitamins* dissolve or disperse in water; they are the B complex vitamins (thiamine, riboflavin, niacin, pyridoxine, folate, vitamin B_{12}, biotin, and pantothenic acid), choline, and vitamin C. *Fat-soluble vitamins* dissolve in fatty tissues or substances; they are vitamins A, D, E, and K.

Solubility characteristics affect how vitamins are absorbed and transported in the body. Water-soluble vitamins are easily absorbed in the small intestine, and then pass into the bloodstream for circulation throughout the body. Fat-soluble vitamins follow the more complicated route of other fat-containing substances; bile is required for absorption from the small intestine. Fat malabsorption problems may also lead to potential deficiencies of fat-soluble vitamins.

The water solubility of the B vitamins and vitamin C allows for minimal storage of any excess vitamin consumed; tissues may be saturated with these vitamins, but they usually are not stored. Deficiencies can develop quickly—within weeks—therefore we need to consume these vitamins on a daily basis. Excesses are generally not toxic and are simply excreted in urine. However, damage may result if vitamin levels are chronically high because of supplementation.

If we consume more than the daily requirement of a fat-soluble vitamin, our bodies store the excess rather than excrete it. The DRI for fat-soluble vitamins take into account this storage capacity. Although storage is expected in organs such as the liver and spleen, other fatty tissues in the body can also retain excessive amounts of fat-soluble vitamins. Overloading the storage capabilities can be toxic and produce illness; toxicity rarely comes from excessive dietary intake but rather from improper use of vitamin supplements.

FOOD SOURCES

Vitamins are in almost all foods, yet no one food group is a good source of all vitamins. Fresh fruits and vegetables are particularly rich sources. Others include legumes, whole grains, and animal foods of meat, fish, poultry, eggs, and dairy products. Even the almost pure fats of vegetable oils and butter provide vitamins E and A, respectively. Although this does not mean we should consume these products for their vitamin content, it does mean we have a wide range of foods to choose from for our vitamin nutrition.

It is always best to consume vitamins from food sources. Although synthetic forms of vitamins will perform vitamin functions, there may be other factors in foods

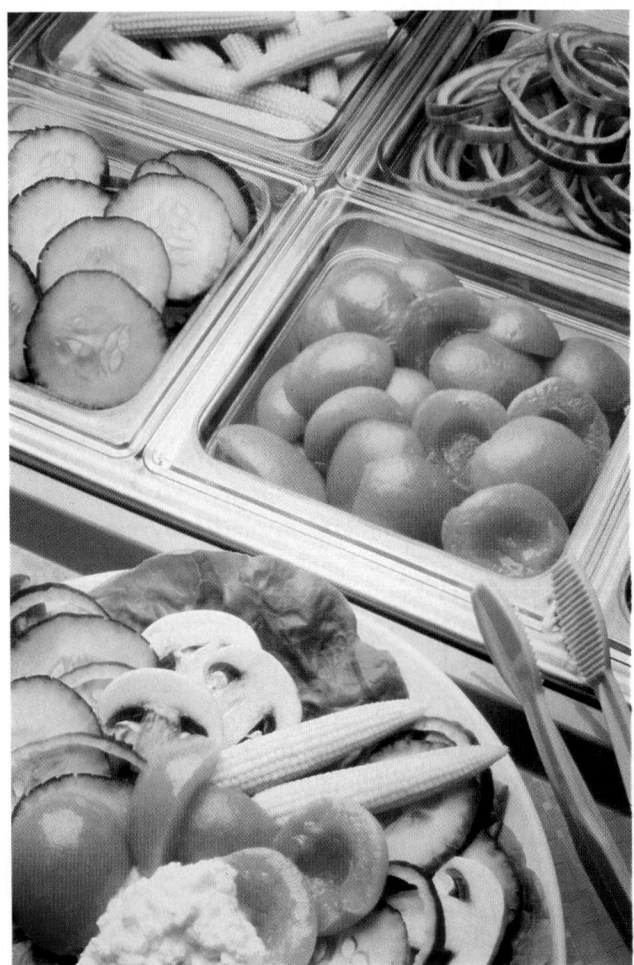

Although vitamins are in almost all foods, fruits and vegetables are especially rich sources. (From PhotoDisc.)

Box 7-1 Phytochemicals and Functional Foods: The Value of Food

Nutrition tends to focus on the nutrients required for the health and well-being of the human body. Other food components exist that may have other health benefits but do not qualify as "a nutrient."

Phytochemicals are nonnutritive substances in plant-based foods that appear to have disease-fighting properties. The health-promoting value of these substances is best obtained by eating a diverse assortment of vegetables, fruits, legumes, grains, and seeds. Green tea, soy, and licorice also contain phytochemicals with healthful qualities. *Functional foods* are foods that provide health benefits beyond the nutrients they contain. Phytochemicals and functional foods are of great interest because they may assist in the prevention or treatment of chronic diseases such as diabetes, coronary artery disease, cancer, and hypertension. Even incidence of osteoporosis, arthritis, and neural tube defects may be reduced by adequate consumption of these substances. Onions and garlic not only taste good but contain allylic sulfides—phytochemicals—that

enhance immune function, enhance excretion of cancer-inducing substances, decrease blood cholesterol levels, and reduce spread of tumor cells—quite a long list of benefits for foods that taste so good. Tomatoes provide lycopene, which appears to have the ability to halt cancer cells from spreading. Consequently, consumption of cooked tomatoes has been related to a decreased risk of certain cancers. Soy contains isoflavones, which also decrease blood cholesterol levels and flavonoids that may reduce menopausal symptoms. A number of products already use soy-derived ingredients and others are in development. Consumers can gain health benefits while consuming familiar foods that have added soy ingredients (see also the Health Debate box in Chapter 22).

Perhaps a significant means for disease prevention has always been available for us: consumption of adequate amounts of fruits and vegetables (at least five a day) along with less-processed grains and legumes, possibly topped off with a few cups of green tea.

Compiled from Position of The American Dietetic Association: Functional foods, J Am Dietetic Assoc 99:1278, 1999; *Review: The road to enhancing the food supply,* Food Insight, *May/June:1,4, 1998.*

---

phytochemical
nonnutritive substance in plant-based foods that appears to have disease-fighting properties

that provide benefits. For instance, broccoli and other cruciferous vegetables contain a wide variety of chemicals including sulforaphane, a phytochemical (Box 7-1). Sulforaphane appears to block the growth of tumors in animals.[6]

WATER-SOLUBLE VITAMINS

Thiamine (B₁)

For centuries, a mysterious disease afflicted people of all ages and status throughout Asia. The disease so wasted muscles that sufferers trying to stand would cry out, "Beri, beri," meaning, "I can't! I can't!" in Thai. This phrase, beriberi, became the name of a serious disease resulting from thiamine deficiency. In the 1890s it was discovered that beriberi resulted from consumption of hulled (white) rice, and that unhulled (brown) rice prevented or cured this disease. Later, researchers found that thiamine in the hulls of whole grains prevents or cures beriberi.

beriberi
a severe chronic deficiency of thiamine characterized by muscle weakness and pain, anorexia, mental disorientation, and tachycardia

Function

The main function of thiamine is to serve as a coenzyme in energy metabolism; it also has a role in nerve functioning related to muscle actions.

coenzyme
a substance that activates an enzyme

Recommended Intake and Sources

The RDA for thiamine is 1.2 mg for men and 1.1 mg for women. The amount of thiamine required increases as the metabolic rate rises. Those engaged in rigorous physical activity burn more energy, so they require more thiamine.

Lean pork, whole or enriched grains and flours, legumes, seeds, and nuts are good sources of thiamine. As a water-soluble vitamin, some thiamine can be lost in food processing or when foods are cooked at home.[2] Thiamine may be leaked into cooking fluid or destroyed by heat. Generally, however, most of us consume sufficient amounts of thiamine.

DRI = Dietary Reference Intakes

RDA = Recommended Dietary Allowance

AI = Adequate Intake Tolerable

UL = Upper Intake Level

Deficiency

Thiamine deficiency alters the nervous, muscular, gastrointestinal (GI), and cardiovascular systems.[7] In beriberi, a severe, chronic deficiency results, characterized by ataxia (muscle weakness and loss of coordination), pain, anorexia, mental disorientation, and tachycardia (rapid beating of the heart). Wet beriberi manifests with edema, affecting cardiac function by weakening the heart muscle and vascular system. Dry beriberi affects the nervous system, producing paralysis and extreme muscle wasting. Marginal deficiencies may occur, producing psychologic disturbances, recurrent headaches, extreme tiredness, and irritability.[7]

Beriberi still occurs in areas of the world, such as Asia, where the staple food is highly polished rice, which is low in thiamine. The practice of repeatedly washing the milled rice results in further loss of thiamine. Very high intakes of raw fish can also produce beriberi. Raw fish naturally contains an enzyme, thiaminase, that destroys thiamine. This does not affect those of us who occasionally enjoy sushi or sashimi, Japanese specialties of raw fish.

In the United States enrichment of refined flour has virtually eliminated thiamine deficiency. However, persons who are chronic alcohol users may develop thiamine deficiency because of decreased food intake and reduced intestinal absorption coupled with an additional need for thiamine by the liver to detoxify alcohol (see the Cultural Considerations box, "Cuban Crisis").

A severe deficiency of thiamine may cause a cerebral form of beriberi, called Wernicke-Korsakoff syndrome. It is the most common disorder of the central nervous system because of the effects of alcohol on nutritional status.[8,9] The effects of this thiamine deficiency syndrome may cause the loss of memory, extreme mental confusion, and ataxia exhibited by persons with chronic excessive alcohol ingestion. Clinically, care must be taken when a malnourished person is given parenteral fluids containing dextrose. Parenteral fluids should contain a mix of B vitamins; otherwise, the marginal thiamine levels of nutritionally depleted individuals, combined with a sudden increase of glucose to the brain, can initiate Wernicke-Korsakoff syndrome, regardless of the level of alcohol intake.

Others at risk for thiamine deficiency include renal patients undergoing dialysis, patients receiving parenteral nutrition, and individuals with a genetic disorder affecting thiamine use.[7]

ataxia
muscle weakness and loss of coordination

tachycardia
rapid beating of the heart

wet beriberi
thiamine deficiency with edema affecting cardiac function by weakening of heart muscle and vascular system

dry beriberi
thiamine deficiency affecting the nervous system producing paralysis and extreme muscle wasting

Wernicke-Korsakoff syndrome
cerebral form of beriberi that affects the central nervous system

CULTURAL CONSIDERATIONS
Cuban Crisis

In the spring of 1993 a harsh economy and natural disasters played havoc with Cuba's food supply. The breakup of the Soviet Union dissipated a valuable trade network for Cuba. This, combined with the devastating effects of a tropical storm, severely limited the variety of foods available. The consequence? A disease resulting in vision loss and a numbness caused by nerve damage spread primarily among men. The *New York Times* headlines were startling, "26,000 Cubans partly blinded."

There is speculation that the epidemic was caused by nutritional deficiencies of thiamine and/or folate. These deficits were exacerbated by consumption of home-brewed rum. The rum required thiamine to detoxify the alcohol, further decreasing the available thiamine for body functions. Folate levels declined as supplies of folate-containing foods diminished. Increased reliance on naturally available foods, such as cassava root, and the popularity of cigarettes among 95% of Cuban men further affected folate availability. Both are high in cyanide, which uses up folate stores in the body. The epidemic was eventually brought under control when the Cuban government distributed vitamin supplements to provide the missing nutrients.

Application to nursing: Unusual circumstances may precipitate unexpected conditions. We often expect disorders to be the result of new variations of bacteria or viruses, but sometimes simple deficiencies may be the cause. Note that this chapter also discusses instances of rickets (vitamin D deficiency disorder) and pellagra (niacin deficiency disorder) unexpectedly occurring. All factors affecting health should be considered to determine the true cause of symptoms.

Reference: Altman LK: 26,000 Cubans partly blinded; cause is unclear, New York Times, May 21, 1993:A7; and Community Nutrition Institute: Epidemic, Nutrition Week Newspaper 22:8, June 11, 1993.

Toxicity

Excess thiamine is excreted in urine. Although thiamine is nontoxic, there is no rationale for supplementation in healthy people. In acute care settings, supplemental thiamine and other B vitamins may be recommended for individuals with chronic excessive alcohol consumption. In general, the best advice is to take a daily multivitamin supplement containing B vitamins.

Riboflavin (B$_2$)

Have you ever wondered why milk is sold in opaque cardboard or nontransparent plastic containers? These containers protect riboflavin from exposure to light. Riboflavin is sensitive to ultraviolet rays in sunlight and artificial light; much of the riboflavin is destroyed if milk, an excellent source of riboflavin, is sold in clear glass or clear plastic receptacles. Why risk loss of a valuable vitamin?

Function

Like thiamine, riboflavin's main function is as a coenzyme in the release of energy from nutrients in every cell of the body.

Recommended Intake and Sources

The RDA for riboflavin is 1.3 mg for men and 1.1 mg for women. The body's need is related to total kcalorie intake, energy needs, body size, metabolic rate, and growth rate. Conditions requiring increased protein also require increased riboflavin, such as during wound healing or the growth periods of childhood, pregnancy, and lactation.

Riboflavin is found in both plant and animal foods. In the United States, however, milk is a major source, with small amounts coming from other foods such as enriched grain. Good plant sources are broccoli, asparagus, dark leafy greens, whole grains, and enriched breads and cereals. Rich sources of animal origin include dairy products, meats, fish, poultry, and eggs.

As previously mentioned, riboflavin is sensitive to light and irradiation. It can also be lost in cooking water but is heat stable.

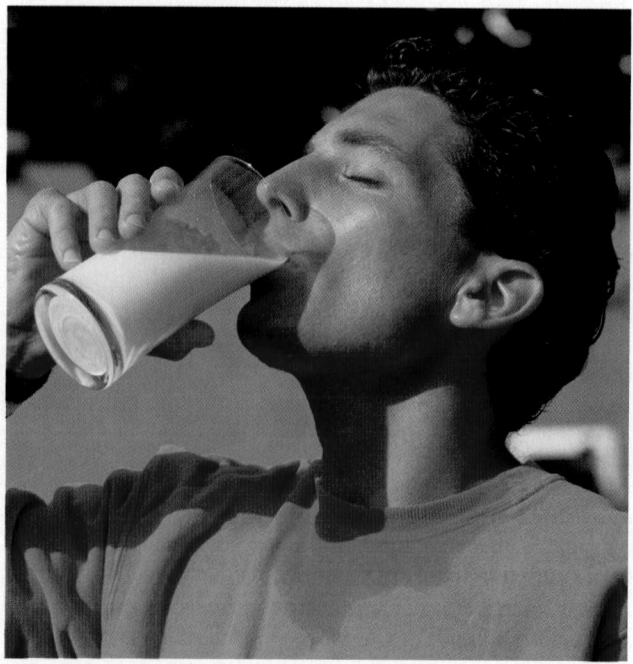

Milk is the major source of riboflavin in the United States. (From PhotoDisc.)

Deficiency

Ariboflavinosis is the name given to a group of symptoms associated with riboflavin deficiency. The lips become swollen; cracks develop in the corners of the mouth (cheilosis). The tongue becomes swollen and purplish-red (glossitis). Seborrheic dermatitis, a skin condition characterized by greasy scales, may occur in the regions of the ears, nose, and mouth. Riboflavin deficiency may also affect the availability and use of pyridoxine and niacin.

Nutritional deficiencies tend to be multiple rather than single, and it is difficult to separate symptoms. If an individual is deficient in a nutrient such as riboflavin, more than likely a deficiency of other nutrients will also be present. For example, esophageal cancer is associated with deficiencies of riboflavin and zinc, particularly in Africa, Iran, and China.[10]

Toxicity

Toxicity to riboflavin has not been reported. Absorption of riboflavin tends to be limited under normal circumstances; excessive absorption is extremely unlikely.[11]

Niacin (B₃)

Niacin occurs naturally in two forms, nicotinic acid and niacinamide. It's hard to imagine, but before niacin was identified, people who were actually suffering from niacin deficiency were so psychologically disoriented that they were sent to mental institutions for treatment. Niacin deficiency can bring on a psychosis that dissipates once sufficient quantities are consumed.

Function

Niacin is involved as a coenzyme for many enzymes, especially those involved in energy metabolism; it is critical for glycolysis and the tricarboxylic acid cycle (TCA).

Recommended Intake and Sources

Niacin is available in foods as the active vitamin or as its precursor, the amino acid tryptophan. That is, tryptophan can be converted to niacin and some niacin can be provided this way. Diets adequate in protein tend to be adequate in niacin.

Niacin requirements are measured in niacin equivalents (NE), reflecting the body's ability to convert tryptophan to niacin. To form 1 mg of niacin, 60 mg of typtophan are needed, both of which equal 1 mg NE. The RDA recommends that men and women consume 16 mg NE and 14 mg NE per day, respectively. The DRI for niacin includes a UL of 35 mg NE per day because of the adverse reactions experienced when excess amounts are taken in supplement form (see "Toxicity").

Protein-containing foods are good sources of both niacin and tryptophan. Meats, poultry, fish, legumes, enriched cereals, milk, and even coffee and tea are sources of niacin.[12]

Deficiency

Pellagra, the niacin deficiency disorder, is characterized by the 3 "Ds":[12]
1. *Diarrhea:* Damage to the GI tract affects digestion, absorption, and excretion of food, leading to glossitis, vomiting, and diarrhea.
2. *Dermatitis:* A symmetrical scaly rash occurs only on skin exposed to the sun (Figure 7-1).
3. *Dementia:* As the central nervous system becomes affected in severe deficiencies, confusion, anxiety, insomnia, and paranoia develop.

In the early 1900s, pellagra was common in the southern United States among the poor who subsisted on corn-based diets. The niacin in corn is in a bound form unavailable for absorption, and many persons subsisting on low incomes had such a limited intake of protein food that neither tryptophan nor preformed niacin was

ariboflavinosis
a group of symptoms associated with riboflavin deficiency

cheilosis
inflammation of the mucous membrane of the mouth and lips (angular stomatitis) caused by riboflavin and other B vitamin deficiencies

glossitis
inflammation of the tongue

pellagra
the deficiency disorder of niacin characterized by diarrhea, dermatitis, and dementia

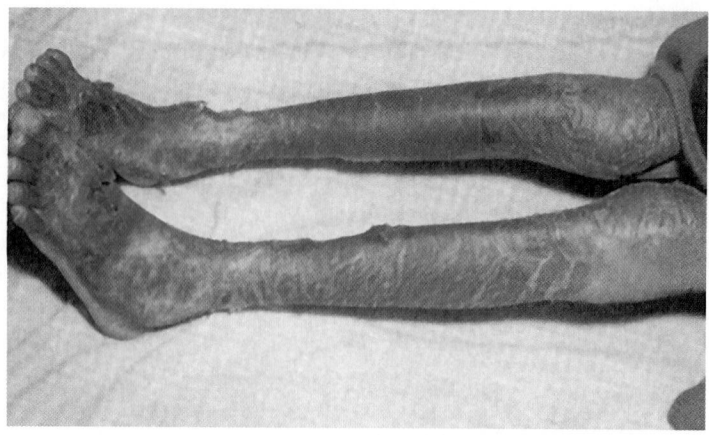

Figure 7-1 Dermatitis in a patient suffering from pellagra. (From McLaren DS: *A colour atlas and text of diet-related disorders*, ed 2, London, 1992, Mosby-Year Book Europe Limited. By permission of Mosby International Ltd.)

available. Since the discovery of the cause of pellagra, flours have been enriched with niacin and the incidence of pellagra has decreased dramatically.

In the United States health professionals need to be vigilant to recognize the symptoms of vitamin deficiencies among patients undergoing specialized treatments or experiencing disorders that may negatively impact their nutritional status. For example, pellagra may develop among persons with chronic excessive alcohol ingestion. Recently, several cases have been reported in which the symptom of dermatitis was not recognized as pellagra. In one situation, the simultaneous use of several alternative remedies initiated pellagra although the individual consumed sufficient dietary niacin.[4] Another report discusses pellagra dermatitis possibly caused by cancer treatment (5-fluorouracil) exacerbating the low niacin levels of the patient.[5] In contrast, in Africa and Asia, pellagra still occurs among the general population.

Toxicity

The UL for niacin is 35 mg NE per day. When preformed niacin and nicotinic acid (but not niacinamide) are consumed in levels above the UL, the vascular system is affected, producing a flushing effect throughout the body. A pharmacologic dose is 3 to 9 grams of niacin, compared with the RDA of 16 mg NE. Niacin has been used therapeutically because megadoses may lower total cholesterol and low-density lipoprotein (LDL) and increase high-density lipoprotein (HDL).[12] These therapeutic doses, however, must be medically administered to guard against liver damage and related gout and arthritic reactions.

Pyridoxine (B$_6$)

Vitamin B$_6$ and pyridoxine are generic terms representing a group of related chemicals. The three main members are pyridoxine, pyridoxal, and pyridoxamine. All three forms can be converted to the coenzyme pyridoxal phosphate (PLP) for use in the body.

Function

The major function of vitamin B$_6$, in the form of PLP, is to act as a coenzyme in the metabolism of amino acids and proteins. These reactions are involved in the formation of neurotransmitters and are essential for proper functioning of the nervous system. PLP is essential for hemoglobin synthesis. It is required for the conversion of tryptophan to niacin. It also serves as a coenzyme for fatty acid and carbohydrate metabolism.

Supplements of B_6, folate, and B_{12} may reduce risk of coronary artery disease (CAD) by lowering homocysteine levels. (This is discussed in the "Overcoming Barriers" section of this chapter.)

Recommended Intake and Sources

The RDA for vitamin B_6 is 1.3 mg for men and women. These amounts are based on protein intake. Vitamin B_6 is found in a wide variety of foods. Particularly good sources include whole grains and cereals, legumes, and chicken, fish, pork, and eggs.

Deficiency

A deficiency of vitamin B_6 rarely occurs alone; it normally accompanies low intakes of other B vitamins. Symptoms include dermatitis, altered nerve function, weakness, poor growth, convulsions, and microcytic anemia (small red blood cells deficient in hemoglobin).

Of the numerous drugs affecting the bioavailability and metabolism of vitamin B_6, oral contraceptive agents (OCAs) may be among the most widely used. Prolonged use of such drugs as isoniazid (for tuberculosis), penicillamine (for lead poisoning, cystinuria, Wilson's disease, sclerosis, and rheumatoid arthritis), cycloserine (for tuberculosis), and hydralazine (for hypertension) may require vitamin B_6 supplements to reduce neurologic side effects and prevent deficiency during treatment.[13,14]

Toxicity

Vitamin B_6 has sometimes been prescribed to relieve the symptoms associated with premenstrual syndrome (PMS); however, there are not adequate data to support this treatment. Although doses of 10 mg, an amount often prescribed, are most likely not harmful (even considering the RDA of 1.3 mg), long-term supplementation in megadose gram quantities has been reported to cause ataxia and sensory neuropathy. The UL of B_6 is 100 mg per day.

Folate

Folate, like other B vitamins, actually consists of several similar compounds. One of these compounds was originally extracted from spinach and was given the name folic acid, from the Latin word *folium*, meaning *leaf*. Folic acid was discovered in 1945 during the search for the nutritional factor responsible for control of pernicious anemia. We now know that vitamin B_{12}, rather than folate, is the nutrient that cures pernicious anemia. Folate and its related compounds, however, play a role in other essential biologic processes. The terms *folate, folic acid, folacin,* and *pteroylglutamic acid (PGA)* are often used interchangeably. Folate is the form of this vitamin found naturally in foods. Folic acid is a synthetic form used in vitamin supplements and for food fortification. Folic acid is actually more available for absorption by the body.

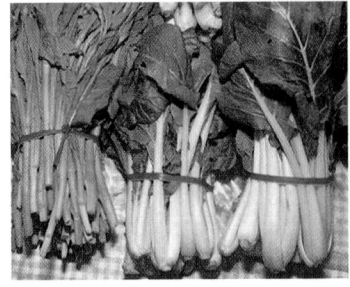

Leafy green vegetables are rich in folate. (From PhotoDisc.)

Function

Folate acts as a coenzyme in reactions involving the transfer of one-carbon units during metabolism. As such, it is required for the synthesis of amino acids, which are the building blocks of protein, and for the synthesis of deoxyribonucleic acid (DNA) and ribonucleic acid (RNA). Blood health also depends on folate to form the heme portion of hemoglobin. For the active form of folate to be maintained for use in the body, vitamin B_{12} must be available.

Attention recently focused on the role of folate in the proper formation of fetal neural tubes.[15] Neural tube birth defects affect brain and spinal cord development, resulting in the disorders of spina bifida and anencephaly. Spina bifida is a congenital defect of the spinal column that causes the spinal cord to be un-

spina bifida
a congenital defect of the spinal column causing the spinal cord to be unprotected, resulting in a range of disabilities including paralysis and incontinence

anencephaly
a congenital defect in which the brain does not develop; death occurs shortly after birth

protected. This results in a range of disabilities including paralysis and incontinence. In cases of anencephaly, a congenital defect in which the brain does not develop, death occurs shortly after birth. Although these disorders result from a combination of genetics and environment, adequate folate levels during the first month after conception appear to greatly reduce the incidence of these serious birth defects. Unfortunately, women of childbearing age are sometimes marginally deficient in folate. They may not know they are pregnant during the first few crucial weeks when the neural tube of the fetus forms.

Recommended Intake and Sources

The RDA reflects that some folate is stored in the liver, but generally daily supplies are needed. The RDA is 400 mcg for men and women. Physiologic state greatly affects folate need. During pregnancy, a woman's blood supply increases. This increase of blood and the growth of other tissues necessitate a greater need for folate. Consequently, the RDA jumps to 600 mcg during pregnancy. While lactating, nutrient needs are elevated because of the nutrient content of the human milk being produced. Therefore, the RDA for folate is 500 mcg for lactation needs.

It is recommended that women of childbearing age increase their folate intake to include 400 mcg of synthetic folic acid to reduce the risks of birth defects, including spina bifida. The increased levels could be provided by natural sources, fortified foods, or supplements[15] (Table 7-1). To ensure adequate access to folic acid, the Food and Drug Administration (FDA) mandates that cereal-grain products be

Table 7-1
Food Sources of Folate

Food	Serving Size	Amount (Micrograms)	% Daily Value*
Chicken liver	3.5 oz	770	193
Breakfast cereals	½ to 1½ cup	100 to 400	25 to 100
Braised beef liver	3.5 oz	217	54
Lentils, cooked	½ cup	180	45
Chickpeas	½ cup	141	35
Asparagus	½ cup	132	33
Spinach, cooked	½ cup	131	33
Black beans	½ cup	128	32
Burrito with beans	2	118	30
Kidney beans	½ cup	115	29
Baked beans with pork	1 cup	92	23
Lima beans	½ cup	78	20
Tomato juice	1 cup	48	12
Brussels sprouts	½ cup	47	12
Orange	1 medium	47	12
Broccoli, cooked	½ cup	39	10
Fast-food French fries	large order	38	10
Wheat germ	2 tbsp	38	10
Fortified white bread	1 slice	38	10

Data from Pennington JAT: Bowes & Church's food values of portions commonly used, ed 17, Philadelphia, 1998, Lippincott-Raven.
*Based on Daily Value for folate of 400 micrograms.

fortified with 140 mcg/100 g folic acid. This means that manufacturers of enriched breads, flours, corn meals, rice, pastas, and other grain products are required to add folate to their products.[16] Fortified product labels may include the claim that adequate intake of folic acid may reduce the risk of neural tube defects.[17]

Although this folic acid fortification assists in meeting the recommended levels for women of childbearing age, healthcare professionals must be prepared to individualize nutrition guidance to ensure daily optimal consumption of folate and folic acid.[18] Clients and patients need to understand that simply consuming fortified cereals and grains does not necessarily provide sufficient amounts of folate. Dietitians should be consulted to ensure the appropriateness of dietary recommendations.

Concern has been expressed regarding the risk and benefits of this fortification to other age groups. In particular, the effects on older adults may be an issue because an excess of folate can mask a B_{12} deficiency for which older adults are at risk.[19] Requiring vitamin supplements that contain folic acid to also contain vitamin B_{12} can reduce this risk. This decreases the risk of the larger folate intakes overshadowing possible deficiencies of B_{12}.[20] Overall, though, the benefits appear to outweigh the risk because the increase in folic acid intake from fortification should also cause decreases in homocysteine blood levels, thereby decreasing the risk of heart disease (Box 7-2). The actual risk, though, will need to be studied as the fortification program progresses.[19]

Folate is widely available in foods, particularly in leafy green vegetables, legumes, ready-to-eat cereals, and some fruits and juices. Folate is affected by heat, oxidation, and ultraviolet light; processing and cooking of fresh foods reduce the amount of folate available. Folate is found in many foods that contain ascorbic acid (vitamin C), such as oranges and orange juice. Ascorbic acid protects folate from oxidation. Diets deficient in folate are often deficient in vitamin C, and vice versa.[15]

Deficiency

Cells whose normal activities require rapid cell growth and division are particularly sensitive to folate deficiency. Examples include red blood cells and the cells that line the GI tract. Folate deficiency results in megaloblastic anemia. This is a form of anemia characterized by large red blood cells that cannot carry oxygen

---

Box 7-2 Homocysteine, Vitamins, and Heart Health

*H*omocysteine is a compound found in blood formed during the metabolism of the essential amino acid methionine. Elevated levels of homocysteine (hyperhomocysteinemia) are associated with an increased risk of coronary artery disease (CAD). There may also be a relationship between elevated homocysteine and increased risk of Alzheimer's disease and/or dementia. The risk of CAD may be caused by increased clotting and damage to the vascular system because of the excess homocysteine. The mechanism of Alzheimer's disease and homocysteine levels has not been determined.

Individuals at high risk for CAD should be screened for hyperhomocysteinemia. High levels of homocysteine have been associated with low consumption of foods containing folate, vitamin B_6, and vitamin B_{12} that results in low serum levels of these vitamins. Treatment recommendations are based on this association between homocysteine levels and intake of the three B vitamins. One treatment approach consists of pharmacologic doses of folic acid (400-1000 mcg/day) and a vitamin supplement containing the DRI for pyridoxine (B_6) and vitamin B_{12}. Another treatment strategy focuses only on levels of folic acid (100% of the DRI) and vitamin B_6 (150% of the DRI). In addition to supplements, consumption of foods high in these vitamins is strongly recommended. Refer to Table 7-1 for specific food sources containing these nutrients.

Studies have found that either approach significantly reduces blood homocysteine levels and reduces risk of CAD. A registered dietitian or healthcare provider should determine levels of supplementation.

Compiled from Molloy AM, Scott JM: Folate and prevention of disease, Public Health Nutr 4(2B):601, Apr 2001; Seshadri S et al.: Plasma homocysteine as a risk factor for dementia and Alzheimer's disease, N Engl J Med 346(7):476, Feb 14, 2002; Tice JA et al.: Cost-effectiveness of vitamin therapy to lower plasma homocysteine levels for the prevention of coronary heart disease: effect of grain fortification and beyond, J Am Med Assoc 286(8):936, Aug 22-29, 2001.

properly. Other deficiency symptoms include glossitis, diarrhea, irritability, absentmindedness, depression, and anxiety.[15,21]

Deficiency may result from any condition that requires cell division to speed up, including infection, cancer, burns, blood loss, GI damage, growth, and pregnancy. Currently about one third of pregnant women worldwide are affected by folate deficiency. Other groups at risk include those with a limited intake and variety of food, including older persons with low incomes and persons with chronic excessive alcohol ingestion. Alcoholic cirrhosis often results in both liver damage (which interferes with storage and metabolism of folate) and excessive losses of the vitamin in feces and urine.[21]

Numerous medications may affect folate absorption or be antagonistic to folate. These drugs include anticonvulsants, oral contraceptives, aspirin, cancer chemotherapy agents, sulfasalazine, nonsteroidal antiinflammatory drugs, and antacids. Long-term use of any medication may affect the body's use of nutrients; folate is one that is particularly vulnerable.

Before folic acid supplementation is administered, the absence of vitamin B_{12} deficiency must be established. Therapy with folic acid in the presence of vitamin B_{12} deficiency will favorably improve blood profiles, decreasing megaloblastic anemia, while damage to the central nervous system from lack of B_{12} continues.

Toxicity

Excess folate or folic acid intake is not recommended or warranted. Consuming amounts beyond the UL of 1000 mcg folic acid (for men and women) has not been studied. Such high levels may mask the presence of pernicious anemia, discussed under the following section on cobalamin.

Cobalamin (B_{12})

Cobalamin and vitamin B_{12} are used as generic terms to refer to a group of cobalt-containing compounds. The common pharmaceutical name, used widely in supplements, is *cyanocobalamin*.

Function

Two cobalamins function as vitamin B_{12} coenzymes in humans. B_{12} has a role in folate metabolism by modifying folate coenzymes to active forms to support metabolic functions, including the synthesis of DNA and RNA. The metabolism of fatty acids and amino acids also requires vitamin B_{12}. In addition, B_{12} develops and maintains the myelin sheaths that surround and protect nerve fibers.

Vitamin B_{12}, in conjunction with consumption of vitamin B_6 and folate, appears to reduce the levels of homocysteine, thereby decreasing the risk of CAD (see Box 7-2).

Recommended Intake and Sources

intrinsic factor
a substance produced by stomach mucosa that is required for vitamin B_{12} absorption

Absorption of vitamin B_{12} relies on an intrinsic factor. The intrinsic factor is produced by stomach mucosa. Both vitamin B_{12} and the intrinsic factor must be present for absorption. Recommended B_{12} levels take into account that some vitamin B_{12} is stored in the liver. The RDA for young adults is 2.4 mcg daily. Foods of animal origin are the only reliable sources of vitamin B_{12}; meat, fish, poultry, eggs, and dairy products are all good sources. For example, one glass of skim milk provides 0.93 mcg of vitamin B_{12}. The vitamin has been reported to be found in legumes (nodules on roots) because of bacteria formation in soil, but they are not a reliable source. Vegans must supplement their intake with vitamin B_{12} supplements or use fortified products.

Deficiency

pernicious anemia
inadequate red blood cell formation caused by a lack of intrinsic factor in the stomach with which to absorb vitamin B_{12}

Deficiencies of B_{12} are usually secondary deficiencies. Pernicious anemia (from B_{12} deficiency) or megaloblastic anemia (from related folate dysfunction) occurs. Additional neurologic effects develop because of damage to the spinal cord as the breakdown of myelin sheath synthesis affects brain, optic, and peripheral nerves.[22]

Older persons are more at risk for deficiency because of a naturally occurring reduction in production of the intrinsic factor by the stomach mucosa. Most older persons, however, remain within normal range. For those who do become deficient, injections to bypass intestinal absorption are warranted. Particularly noted among this population are neuropsychiatric symptoms, including delusions and hallucinations, that may occur in the absence of anemia.[23] These symptoms can be misdiagnosed as senility or other illnesses. To alleviate this risk, the recommendations include that adults older than age 50 consume foods fortified with vitamin B_{12} or take a B_{12} supplement to ensure adequacy of the RDA for B_{12}. Vitamin B_{12} is more absorbable in this form because it is already separated from food.

As was previously discussed concerning relation to folate supplementation, folate levels may disguise a B_{12} deficiency. Blood hematologic damage is masked by folate, but neurologic damage continues.[22]

Toxicity

Toxicity to vitamin B_{12} has not been noted, but there are no benefits to large doses unless deficiency exists.

Biotin

Humans need biotin, a member of the B vitamin complex, in tiny amounts.

Function

Biotin assists in the transfer of carbon dioxide from one compound to another, playing an important role in carbohydrate, fat, and protein metabolism.

Recommended Intake and Sources

Biotin is synthesized in the lower GI tract by bacterial microorganisms. However, the amount produced and its bioavailability are unknown. Although biotin is produced in the body, it is still an essential nutrient. (The human body does not produce biotin, but bacteria hosted in the gut do.) It must also be consumed in foods.

The AI for biotin is 30 mcg. Biotin is widespread in foods. The richest sources are liver, kidney, peanut butter, egg yolks, and yeast.

Deficiency

Deficiency of biotin is unknown among people eating a typical North American diet. When experimentally produced, symptoms of biotin deficiency include a scaly red skin rash, hair loss, loss of appetite, depression, and glossitis.[24]

Biotin deficiency has been produced by consumption of large amounts of avidin, a protein in raw egg whites that binds biotin. You would need to consume many raw egg whites for this to occur; salmonella poisoning would probably strike first. Avidin is denatured by heat, so cooked egg whites pose no problem to biotin status.

Antibiotics are known to reduce the number of biotin-producing bacteria. In addition, clients receiving long-term intravenous feeding are prone to biotin deficiency, therefore their feeding mixtures should contain biotin.

Toxicity

There is no known toxicity.

Pantothenic Acid

Pantothenic acid gets its name from its presence in all living things (from the Greek *pantothen*, meaning *from all sides*).

Function

The principal active form of pantothenic acid functions as part of coenzyme A (CoA for short); therefore it is required for the metabolism of carbohydrates, fats, and protein.

Recommended Intake and Sources

The AI for pantothenic acid is 5 mg per day. Pantothenic acid is widespread in foods and easily consumed in whole grain cereals, legumes, meat, fish, and poultry.

Deficiency

Deficiencies do not naturally occur in humans.

Toxicity

Doses of up to 10 grams daily have been administered with no ill effects. Researchers have reported that daily doses of 10 to 20 grams may produce diarrhea or water retention.

Choline

Function

Choline is needed for the synthesis of acetylcholine, a neurotransmitter, and lecithin, the phospholipid.

Recommended Intake and Sources

The body can actually make choline from the amino acid methionine, but this process does not produce enough choline to meet the needs of the body. Consequently, food sources are still required. This requirement qualifies choline as an essential nutrient. The AI is 550 mg/day for men and 425 mg/day for women with a UL of 3500 mg/day for adults.[1]

Food sources include many commonly consumed foods with rich sources including milk, eggs, and peanuts.

Deficiency

Deficiency of choline is rare.

Toxicity

Toxicity symptoms include sweating, fishy body odor, vomiting, liver damage, reduced growth, and low blood pressure (hypotension).

Vitamin C

Vitamin C is almost a household word. It's hard to believe that it was isolated as a nutrient only around 1930. The discovery of vitamin C is associated with the search for the cause of scurvy, a potentially fatal disease that weakens the body's connective tissues and also causes inflammation to them. As early as the eighteenth century, it was known that eating certain foods, particularly citrus fruits, could control scurvy, but the actual substance responsible for gluing the cells together was not determined until Albert Szent-Gyorgy and Glen King isolated it in 1928 and 1930, respectively.[25] One of the two active forms of vitamin C is ascorbic acid (*ascorbic* meaning *without scurvy*).

scurvy
extreme vitamin C deficiency disorder characterized by inflammation of connective tissues, gingivitis, muscle degeneration, bruising, and hemorrhaging as the vascular system weakens

Function

Vitamin C functions as an antioxidant and as a coenzyme. It can perform different functions in various situations. Collagen formation for bone matrix, teeth, cartilage, and connective tissue depends on ascorbic acid. Vitamin C provides the cement that holds structures together. Wound healing, which necessitates the formation of new tissue, also requires vitamin C.

As an antioxidant, vitamin C protects folate, vitamin E, and polyunsaturated substances from destruction by oxygen as they move throughout the body. An **antioxidant** is a compound that guards others from damaging oxidation by being oxidized itself. Vitamins C and E also work together as antioxidants to destroy substances released as cells age, are oxidized, or become damaged. Their work may prevent damage by free radicals to vascular walls, thereby limiting the development of atherosclerotic plaques.

Among its other functions, vitamin C enhances the absorption of nonheme iron, found in plant foods. Thyroid and adrenal hormone synthesis requires vitamin C. Several conversion processes depend on vitamin C; these include tryptophan to serotonin, cholesterol to bile, and folate to its active form.

Vitamin C may have a role in reducing the risk of cancer development. Epidemiologic studies have uncovered an association between levels of dietary intake of vitamin C and incidence of cancer in the stomach, esophagus, and colon.[10] Because these studies are of dietary intakes of populations, it is not yet known whether the effects are caused by vitamin C or by other, as yet unidentified components of foods containing vitamin C.

Recommended Intake and Sources

The RDA for vitamin C has varied from 45 mg to 60 mg for adults. Currently, the RDA is 90 mg for men and 75 mg for women. Recommendations vary worldwide; the minimum daily requirement to prevent symptoms of scurvy is 10 mg. However, the amount recommended daily to provide enough circulating vitamin C for tissue saturation for good health is open to interpretation.

As more is learned about vitamin C functions, recommendations customized to specific disease and lifestyle behaviors will be determined. For example, cigarette smokers have lower circulating levels of vitamin C compared with nonsmokers, regardless of their dietary intake of vitamin C. The metabolic use of vitamin C by smokers is twice that of nonsmokers. Recognizing this deficit, smokers are advised to increase their vitamin C intake from the 90 mg RDA to 125 mg daily.[1]

Fruits and vegetables provide 95% of the vitamin C we consume. Many foods are excellent sources; some of them include citrus fruits, red and green peppers, strawberries, tomatoes, potatoes, broccoli, and other green leafy vegetables. Servings sizes to meet the RDA are listed in Table 7-2.

Some foods and drinks are fortified with vitamin C. Ready-to-eat cereals have added vitamin C (about 25% of the daily values) and other vitamins not naturally found in grains. Additional vitamin C, often 100% of the daily values, is added to the small amounts naturally found in apple and grape juice.

Vitamin C is destroyed by air, light, and heat. Fruit juices should be stored in an airtight container that holds only the amount that can be consumed in a short time. The vitamin C content of cooked foods can be maximized by cooking in the minimal amount of water or, even better, by microwaving (see the Teaching Tool box, "Vegetable Victories").

Deficiency

Although vitamin C deficiency is rare in developed countries in the West, it may still occur among persons who are chronic alcohol and drug users and those whose dietary intakes are extremely poor. Older persons may have marginal intake because of difficulty in obtaining and preparing fresh foods. These at-risk groups may experience other vitamin and mineral deficiencies as well.

Scurvy represents the extreme result of vitamin C deficiency. The symptoms are tied to the functions of vitamin C in the body. When the gluelike substance of collagen is not replaced, tissues throughout the body degenerate. Gingivitis causes

antioxidant
a compound that guards other compounds from damaging oxidation

The bulk of evidence does not support the theory that vitamin C reduces the incidence of the common cold. Taking supplemental vitamin C, however, can decrease the duration and reduce the severity of the symptoms.[26]

Recommend that clients who smoke consume 125 mg rather than 90 mg of vitamin C daily.

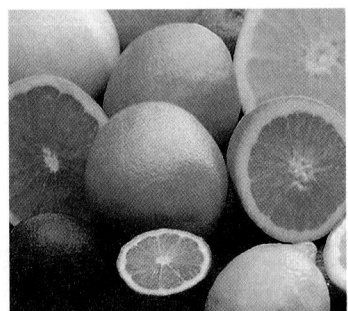

Although citrus fruits are well known for being rich in vitamin C, vegetables such as green peppers, cauliflower, and broccoli are also nutrient-dense sources. (From PhotoDisc.)

Table 7-2
RDA Serving Sizes of Vitamin C (RDA = 75-90 mg)

Food	Serving	Vitamin C
Broccoli	¾ cup	58 mg
Brussels sprouts	¾ cup	48 mg
Cantaloupe	1¼ cup	68 mg
Grapefruit	½ fruit	47 mg
Kiwifruit	1 piece	75 mg
Orange	1 piece	80 mg
Orange juice	¾ cup	93 mg
Peppers, green or red	¾ cup	64 mg
Strawberries	1 cup	64 mg

Data from Pennington JAT: Bowes & Church's food values of portions commonly used, ed 17, Philadelphia, 1998, Lippincott-Raven.

gums to bleed, and teeth come loose; joints and limbs ache from muscle degeneration and lack of new connective tissue formation; bruising and hemorrhages occur as the vascular system weakens, and plaques form as a result of the vascular damage. Death ultimately occurs as functioning of all body systems disintegrates.

TEACHING TOOL
Vegetable Victories

We may focus on teaching clients what vitamins do in their bodies, but this education is pointless unless they relate the information to the foods they actually eat. Some of our clients, who may be willing to experiment with preparing foods (particularly vegetables) in a more nutrient-retaining manner, may be at a loss as to how to proceed. We cannot assume that everyone has grown up naturally knowing how to steam broccoli.

Clients need assistance in achieving vegetable victories. What is a vegetable victory? This is a situation in which individuals learn to prepare the vegetable they most enjoy in a way that still retains the most nutrients possible. With vegetables, most of those nutrients are vitamins, mainly water-soluble vitamins. Because water-soluble vitamins are in the liquid parts of vegetables, if vegetables are cooked or boiled (please don't) the vitamins are either leached into the cooking water or may even be destroyed by the heat. What to do? Nutritional value is reduced by air, heat, water, and light. The following are some preparation pointers:

- To prevent loss from air exposure, use plastic containers to store vegetables and cook with lids.
- To limit vitamin forfeiture from water-related preparation, cook vegetables with as little water as possible or use vegetable cooking water in soups or sauces.
- To reduce destruction from light, keep vegetables in dark places; most should be stored in the refrigerator.
- To reduce heat damage to vitamins, keep vegetables cool and cook only until they are crisp by microwaving, stir-frying, or lightly steaming.

Data from Clark N: Nancy Clark's sports nutrition guidebook, Champaign, IL, 1997, Human Kinetics.

Marginal deficiency symptoms may manifest as gingivitis, poor wound healing, inadequate tooth and bone growth or maintenance, and increased risk of infection as the integrity of tissues throughout the body becomes compromised.

Toxicity

Toxicity from foods high in vitamin C does not occur even if we consume cups of fresh strawberries washed down with a quart of orange juice. Chronic supplement intakes of megadoses from 1 g to 15 g may result in cramps, diarrhea, nausea, kidney stone formation, and gout. The effects of anticlotting medication may also be affected.[1]

Taking supplements of vitamin C seems benign, but the body adapts to protect itself from harm. If continually inundated with excessive vitamin C, the body develops a mechanism that destroys much of the extra vitamin C circulating in the body. A rebound effect may occur if, after taking megadoses for several months or more, an individual abruptly stops supplementation and consumes a quantity closer to the RDA. The protective mechanism of the body is still in gear and continues to destroy vitamin C. An individual may develop symptoms of scurvy although the RDA is consumed. A newborn exposed to vitamin C megadoses in utero may experience this rebound effect. Although the rebound effect may not occur in every case, withdrawal from vitamin C megadoses should be gradual, over a period of 2 to 4 weeks. Consequently, there is an UL of 2000 mg for adults and 400 mg to 1800 mg for children and adolescents.

Table 7-3 provides a quick reference to water-soluble vitamins.

DRI = Dietary Reference Intakes
RDA = Recommended Dietary Allowance
AI = Adequate Intake
UL = Tolerable Upper Intake Level

FAT-SOLUBLE VITAMINS

Vitamin A

Each year about 250,000 children enter a world of permanent darkness.[10] The cause? Vitamin A deficiency. Extreme vitamin A deficiency is so damaging to corneas that blindness occurs. Although this could be prevented with just a few cents worth of vitamin A per year, there is little money for preventive health measures in areas of the world where food is scarce.

Function

Vitamin A is a group of compounds that function to maintain skin and mucous membranes throughout the body. Specific activities depending on vitamin A are vision, bone growth, functioning of the immune system, and normal reproduction. Our eyes depend on visual purple, technically called *rhodopsin,* to be able to adjust to light variations. Rhodopsin is formed from retinal, a vitamin A substance, and opsin, a protein. Without enough vitamin A, rhodopsin cannot be formed and the retina cannot easily respond to light changes. As a result, night blindness develops (Figure 7-2). Bone growth involves a process of remodeling that reshapes and enlarges the skeleton. Reshaping requires vitamin A to undo existing bone. Vitamin A maintains integrity of epithelial tissues throughout the body, providing protection against infections and assuring optimum function. Hormonelike effects of vitamin A appear to be tied to cell synthesis for reproductive purposes.

night blindness
the inability of the eyes to readjust vision from bright to dim light caused by vitamin A deficiency

Recommended Intake and Sources

Vitamin A is measured as retinol activity equivalents (RAE). The RDA, based on providing optimum storage of vitamin A in the liver, is 900 mcg RAE for men and 700 mcg RAE for women.[1] RAE incorporates both the preformed, active forms of vitamin A called *retinoids* (found in animal foods) and the precursor forms of vitamin A called *carotenoids* (found in plant foods). The carotenoid beta carotene is the primary source of vitamin A from plant foods.

Table 7-3
Water-Soluble Vitamins

Vitamin	Function	Clinical Issues (Deficiency/Toxicity)	Recommended Intakes	Food Sources
Thiamine (B₁)	Coenzyme energy metabolism; muscle nerve action	Deficiency: beriberi (ataxia, disorientation, tachycardia); marginal (headaches, tiredness); wet beriberi (edema); dry beriberi (nervous system); Wernicke-Korsakoff syndrome (alcoholism)	Men: 1.2 mg Women: 1.1 mg	Lean pork, whole or enriched grains and flours, legumes, seeds, and nuts
Riboflavin (B₂)	Coenzyme energy metabolism	Deficiency: ariboflavinosis with cheilosis, glossitis, seborrheic dermatitis	Men: 1.3 mg Women: 1.1 mg	Milk/dairy products; meat, fish, poultry, and eggs; dark leafy greens (broccoli); whole and enriched breads and cereals
Niacin (B₃) (nicotinic acid and niacinamide) precursor: tryptophan	Cofactor to enzymes involved in energy metabolism; glycolysis and TCA cycle	Deficiency: pellegra Toxicity: vasodilation, liver damage, gout, and arthritic reactions	Men: 16 mg NE Women: 14 mg NE (UL 35 mg NE)	Meats, poultry, and fish; legumes; whole and enriched cereals; milk
Pyridoxine (B₆)	Forms coenzyme pyridoxal phosphate (PLP) for energy metabolism; CNS; hemoglobin synthesis	Deficiency: dermatitis, altered nerve function, weakness, anemia; OCAs decrease B₆ levels Toxicity: ataxia, sensory neuropathy	Men: 1.3 mg Women: 1.3 mg (UL 100 mg)	Whole grains/cereals, legumes, poultry, fish, pork, eggs
Folate (folic acid, folacin, PGA)	Coenzyme metabolism (synthesis of amino acid, heme, DNA, RNA); fetal neural tube formation	Deficiency: megaloblastic anemia; many drugs affect folate use Toxicity: megadoses may mask pernicious anemia	Men: 400 mcg Women: 400 mcg Pregnancy: 600 mcg Lactation: 500 mcg (UL 1000 mcg)	Widely available leafy green vegetables, legumes, ascorbic acid–containing foods
Cobalamin (B₁₂)	Transport/storage of folate; metabolism of fatty acids/amino acids	Deficiency: pernicious anemia, CNS damage	Adults: 2.4 mcg	Animal sources
Biotin	Metabolism of carbohydrate, fat, and protein	Deficiency: produced by avidin and long-term antibiotics	Adults: 30 mcg AI	Liver, kidney, peanut butter, egg yolks, intestinal synthesis
Pantothenic acid Choline	Part of Coenzyme A Synthesis of acetylcholine and lecithin	Deficiency: not possible Deficiency: rare Toxicity: body odor, liver damage, hypotension	Adults: 5 mg AI Men: 550 mg Women: 425 mg (UL 3500 mg)	Widespread in foods Widespread—milk, eggs, peanuts
Vitamin C	Antioxidant, coenzyme, collagen formation, wound healing, iron absorption, hormone synthesis	Deficiency: scurvy Toxicity: cramps, nausea, kidney stone formation, gout (1 to 15 g), rebound scurvy	Men: 90 mg Women: 75 mg (UL 2000)	Fruits/vegetables (citrus fruits, tomatoes, peppers, strawberries, broccoli)

AI, *Adequate Intake;* UL, *Tolerable Upper Intake Level.*

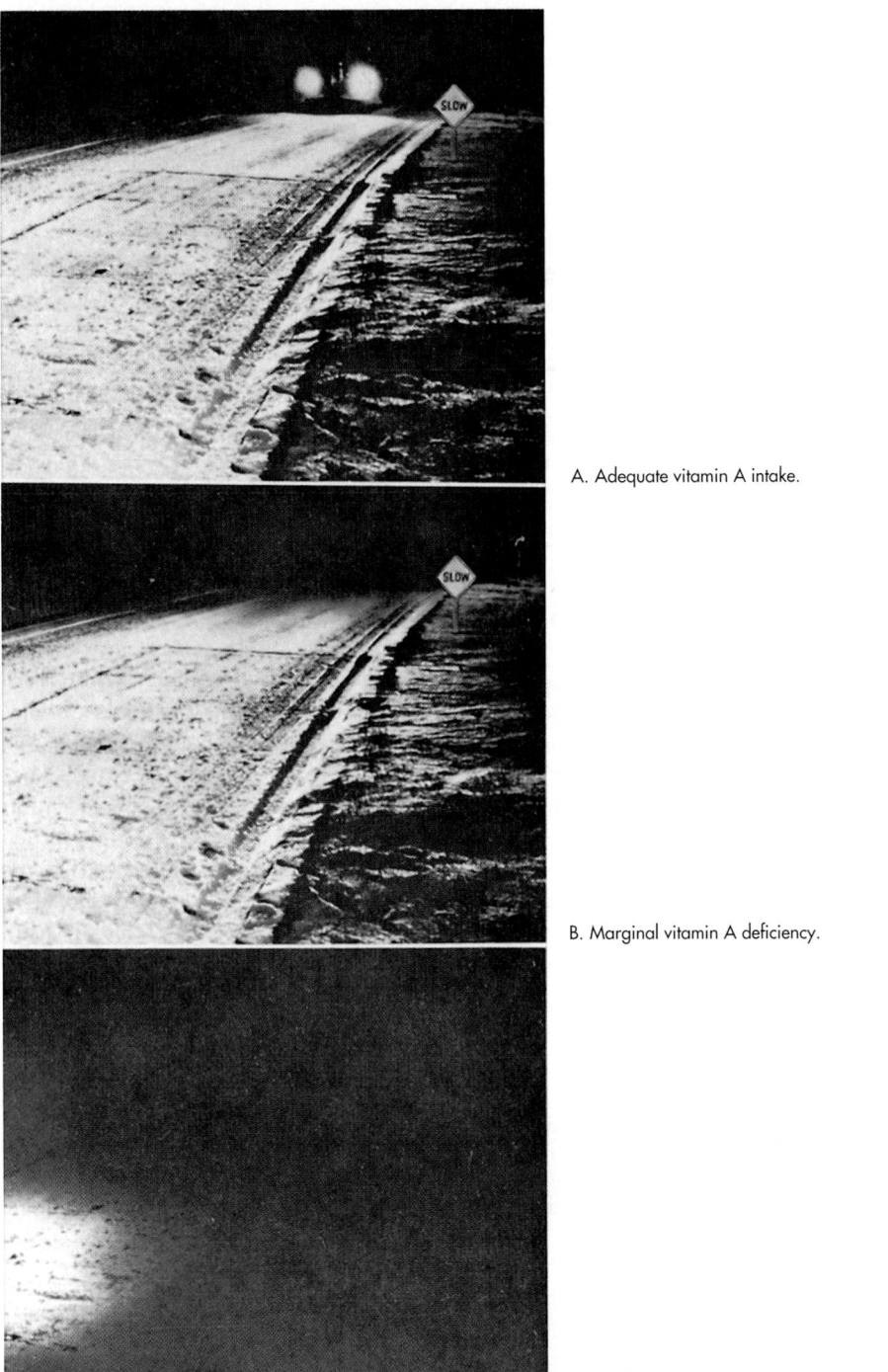

A. Adequate vitamin A intake.

B. Marginal vitamin A deficiency.

C. Vitamin A deficiency resulting in night blindness.

Figure 7-2 Night blindness. These photographs simulate the eyes' slow response to a flash of light at night. (From Pharmacia and Upjohn.)

Because vitamin A (a fat-soluble vitamin) is stored in the body, daily doses are not necessary, but they are desirable. Deficiency of other nutrients affects the absorption and use of vitamin A.[27] Nutrients are interdependent, and imbalances of specific nutrients affect the functioning of others.

Natural preformed vitamin A is found only in the fat of animal-related foods; these include whole milk, butter, liver, egg yolks, and fatty fish. Carotenoids are found in deep green, yellow, and orange fruits and vegetables. The best sources include broccoli, cantaloupe, sweet potatoes, carrots, tomatoes, and spinach (Table 7-4). High consumption of carotenoids recently has been associated with decreased risk of certain cancers and other chronic diseases (see the Health Debate box, "Antioxidants: From Foods or Pills?").

When fats are removed from animal-related foods, preformed vitamin A is also lost. To maintain traditional sources of the vitamin, low-fat, skim, and nonfat milks are fortified with vitamin A. Other fortified products include margarine (which often replaces butter, a natural source of vitamin A), and ready-to-eat cereal, a staple food product commonly fortified with many nutrients.

Deficiency

xerophthalmia
a condition caused by vitamin A deficiency ranging from night blindness to keratomalacia; may result in complete blindness

keratomalacia
a condition caused by vitamin A deficiency in which the cornea becomes dry and thickens from the formation of hard protein tissue

Vitamin A supplements taken internally will not cure or improve acne and are toxic in excess.

Vitamin A deficiency is either primary, caused by lack of dietary intake, or secondary, the result of chronic fat malabsorption. As liver storage becomes depleted, symptoms develop. The effects are closely tied to vitamin A functions. Ocularly, xerophthalmia incorporates a range of symptoms manifested by night blindness progressing to a hard, dry cornea (keratinization) or keratomalacia, resulting in complete blindness. The degeneration of the epithelial tissues protecting the eye itself leads to the effects of xerophthalmia. Compromised epithelial tissues also result in hair follicles developing white hard lumps of keratin (hyperderatosis), respiratory infections, diarrhea, and other GI disturbances. Overall, the immune system is endangered; for children especially, a minor illness or a bout of measles may be deadly. Growth is inhibited because of lack of vitamin A–dependent proteins for bone growth.

In the United States individuals experiencing chronic fat malabsorption are at risk for vitamin A deficiency and deficiencies of other fat-soluble vitamins. These nutrients are incorporated into their overall medical nutrition therapy plans. Although marginal vitamin A deficiency is possible, overt deficiencies are rare. Deficiency is a health threat in parts of the world where food availability is limited.

Table 7-4
Vitamin A/Beta Carotene Sources*

Food	Serving	Vitamin A/Beta Carotene
Apricots	3 medium	277 RAE
Butternut squash	½ cup cooked	714 RAE
Carrots	1 whole	2025 RAE
	½ cup cooked	1915 RAE
Cantaloupe	1 cup	516 RAE
Liver (beef)	3½ oz	10,000 RAE
Spinach	½ cup cooked	737 RAE
Sweet potato	1 whole baked	2488 RAE
Red pepper	1 whole	422 RAE

Data from Pennington JAT: Bowes & Church's food values of portions commonly used, ed 17, 1998, Lippincott-Raven
*RDA = 900 RAE for men; 700 RAE for women.
RAE, Retinol activity equivalents.

Toxicity

Hypervitaminosis A occurs only from preformed vitamin A from either an acute or chronic intake of supplements. Most food sources of preformed A do not contain high enough levels to ever result in toxicity. The only exception noted is polar bear liver and the livers of other large animals. Explorers who feasted on polar

---

HEALTH DEBATE
Antioxidants: From Foods or Pills?

To live is to use oxygen. As our bodies use oxygen to provide energy for all our needs, the process may result in unstable forms of oxygen, such as singlet oxygen or free radicals. In this form, the single oxygen atom is unstable and ready to hook up with other substances. Any substance hooked up with the singlet oxygen is destroyed. Free radicals are byproducts of oxidation at the cellular level, such as the singlet oxygen. They may also develop as part of metabolic process in cells or from the effects of environmental or external factors on the body.

Depending on the effect of external factors, the body's response to free radicals may be overwhelmed and health may be compromised. External factors may include exposure to smoke, ozone, car exhaust, ultraviolet light, radiation such as radiographs, and especially tobacco smoke. Intense physical activity, burns, and other injuries also produce free radicals. But some of these free radicals, such as those produced in physical activity, are "good" free radicals. Other good free radicals are those produced by the white blood cells to protect the body against bacteria and viruses. Aging also causes an increase in the production of free radicals as the maturing body responds differently to cell renewal.

Effects of excess free radicals may include damage to arterial walls, which can lead to atherosclerosis and coronary artery disease. Low-density lipoprotein cholesterol may get oxidized, further damaging the vascular system. If the deoxyribonucleic acid (DNA) of a cell is damaged, cell replication is flawed, and this can lead to cancer development. If free radicals damage cell DNA, the aging process may occur more rapidly.

The body doesn't just stand idly by and let free radicals take over. Antioxidants act as cellular guards. Like any guard, antioxidants can be viewed as protecting membranes and other cell components, including DNA. This protection may prevent damage by the free radicals. Instead of the cellular components being oxidized by free radicals, the antioxidant is oxidized.

Several vitamins function as antioxidants. They are vitamins C and E and carotenoids (vitamin A precursors), including beta carotene, lycopene, alpha carotene, and other forms of carotenoids. Selenium, a mineral, also has antioxidant function. Other forms of antioxidants are produced by the body and perform a variety of antioxidant functions. Because the antioxidant vitamins and selenium are contained in foods, we can increase our intake of these nutrients and possibly increase available levels of antioxidants in the body.

The controversy over antioxidants from nutrients is whether we can consume sufficient amounts through our dietary intake of foods, particularly from fruits and vegetables. Medical experts disagree as to whether supplementation with antioxidants should be recommended. Those in favor of supplementation maintain that the amount of antioxidants needed for disease prevention is more than Americans could reasonably consume from foods. Those opposed believe supplementation is premature and has associated risks such as iron overload from large doses of vitamin C. More research is needed before general recommendations to the public are advocated. Table 7-5 lists sources of the major antioxidants.

What is your opinion? Should we turn to supplements or just increase consumption of foods that contain these nutrients?

Compiled from Should you take vitamin C and E supplements? Wellness Letter *17(9), 2001; Beta carotene pills: might help, might hurt,* Wellness Letter *16(6), 2000; Does this mineral prevent cancer?* Wellness Letter *16(9), 2000; Kanter M: Free radicals, exercise and antioxidant supplementation,* Proceedings of the Nutrition Society *57(1):9,1998.*

Table 7-5
Antioxidants

Antioxidant	Antioxidant Functions	Major Food Sources	Adult RDA	Daily Recommended Supplementation
Beta carotene (pre-Vitamin A)	May decrease risk of some cancers and CAD	Sweet potatoes, winter squash, carrots, red bell peppers, dark green vegetables, apricots, mangos, cantaloupe	No RDA (1 sweet potato = 15 mg, 1 carrot = 10 mg)	6-15 mg, nontoxic, higher doses may give skin a harmless orange cast (not recommended for smokers)
Vitamin C	May decrease risk of certain cancers and CAD	Kiwi, citrus fruits, berries, cantaloupe, honeydew, bell peppers, tomatoes, cabbage family vegetables	75-90 mg (1 kiwi = 150 mg, 1 cup broccoli = 115 mg, 1 orange = 70 mg)	250-500 mg, more may cause diarrhea (UL 2000 mg)
Vitamin E	May decrease risk of cancer and CAD; may also prevent or delay cataracts	Vegetable oil, nuts, seeds, margarine, wheat germ, olives, leafy greens, avocado, asparagus	15 mg α-TE (1 tbsp oil = 9 mg, 1 tbsp margarine or 1 oz nuts = 2 mg)	300-600 mg (200-400 IU) daily* for all adults, higher doses may cause headaches and diarrhea (UL 1000 mg)
Selenium	Prevents cell and lipid membrane damage	Meat, fish, eggs, whole grains	55 mcg	Same as RDA; not more than 200 mcg; higher very toxic with severe liver damage, vomiting, diarrhea, metallic aftertaste (UL 400 mcg)

Data from Wellness Letter, Sept 2001, June 2000, Mar 2000.
*Contraindicated for those with hypertension or who take warfarin (Coumadin) and other drugs to inhibit blood clots.

The acne medications isotretinoin (Accutane) and tretinoin (oral forms) are non-nutritive sources of vitamin A that cause birth defects when used by pregnant women. Advise women who take either of these drugs to use a highly reliable birth control method.

bear liver developed hypervitaminosis A; in fact, the way we learned about the toxic effects of vitamin A was through their misfortune.[10] Apparently, the livers of hibernating animals store an extraordinary quantity of vitamin A to provide sufficient amounts for a long winter without nourishment. When humans consume the preformed vitamin A of these livers, the quantity is toxic.

Toxicity does not occur from the carotenoid precursor in foods. If carotenoids are consumed in excess, either from foods or supplements, the skin takes on an orange hue, which dissipates when carotenoid consumption is reduced.

Immediate symptoms of vitamin A toxicity include blistered skin, weakness, anorexia, vomiting, headache, joint pain, irritability, and enlargement of the spleen and liver; long-term effects include bone abnormalities and liver damage.[27]

Vitamin D

With sufficient exposure to ultraviolet light or sunshine, the body can manufacture its own supply of vitamin D. The exposure of skin to ultraviolet light begins the conversion process of the vitamin D precursor 7-dehydrocholesterol (found in our skin) to cholecalciferol, the active form of vitamin D. Because the body can produce vitamin D, it is technically a hormone. However, when vitamin D is supplied by the diet, it is technically a vitamin. Regardless of how it is classified, vitamin D is a substance necessary for a variety of the body's regulating processes as well as normal development of bones and teeth.

Function

Intestinal absorption of calcium and phosphorus depends on the action of vitamin D. This vitamin also affects bone mineralization and mineral homeostasis by helping to regulate blood calcium levels.

Recommended Intake and Sources

The AI for vitamin D is 5 mcg. The DRI includes new AI recommendations for vitamin D for people ages 51 through 70; the suggested new level jumps from 5 mcg (200 International Units [IU]) a day to 10 mcg (400 IU). After age 70, the recommended levels jump again to 15 mcg (600 IU). These levels reflect that older adults are less efficient at synthesizing vitamin D from sun exposure. If these amounts are not consumed from foods or obtained from sunlight, supplement use may be appropriate. Before beginning supplementation, a dietitian should be consulted; these amounts may already be contained in multivitamin mineral supplements formulated for individuals older than 51 years of age. The UL for vitamin D is 50 mcg (2000 IU). The effects of intakes higher than the UL are discussed in the section on toxicity.

Vitamin D is available through body synthesis or from dietary sources. Cholecalciferol, the active form of vitamin D, can be synthesized. Ultraviolet irradiation from sunlight affects the vitamin D precursor 7-dehydrocholesterol in our skin, and this cholesterol derivative is transformed by the liver and kidneys into cholecalciferol. The amount of vitamin D produced depends on length of exposure to ultraviolet irradiation, atmospheric conditions, and skin pigmentation. Geographic regions and seasons that are particularly cloudy and rainy diminish the quantity of vitamin D synthesized. Darker skin pigmentation also reduces the effect of radiation on the skin, as does sunscreen and concealing clothing. Aging may lessen the amount of vitamin D to be formed from sunlight exposure.[10]

The few sources of natural preformed vitamin D are the fat of the animal-related foods of butter, egg yolks, fatty fish, and liver. Milk, although containing fat, is not a good source; it is, however, a good vehicle for vitamin D fortification because it contains calcium and phosphorus, which need vitamin D for absorption. Because vegans consume no animal foods, they may require supplements or regular sunlight exposure to ensure formation of cholecalciferol. Appropriate guidance should be sought from a primary healthcare provider or dietitian.

Deficiency

A deficiency of vitamin D can lead to the disorders of rickets (Figure 7-3) and osteomalacia. Because of insufficient mineralization of bone and tooth matrix, rickets in children leads to malformed skeletons, characterized by bowed legs unable to bear body weight, oddly angled rib bones and chests, and abnormal tooth formation. In adults, osteomalacia, or bad bones, is characterized by soft bones that are at risk for fractures.

It has been thought that rickets occur rarely among well-nourished populations. However, recent reports reveal the risk of rickets has increased among well-fed African American children of families following the dietary and dress customs of the Muslim faith.[28] Other instances are documented in Alaska among breastfed African American and Alaska native children between the ages of 11 to 20 months. The increased risk for these children is caused by several factors, including darker pigmentation, use of heavier clothing by children that limits exposure of the skin to vitamin D synthesis, and limited consumption of dietary sources of fortified vitamin D dairy products by children or women who are breastfeeding infants. Healthcare providers initially misdiagnosed cases of rickets among these children because the disease is more common in instances of famine, neglect, malabsorption, or restricted dietary intakes.[5,28]

Among older adults who may have a diminished ability to produce vitamin D, osteomalacia may develop when marginal intakes of vitamin D or calcium exist for a number of years. Calcium absorption may also be affected by the aging

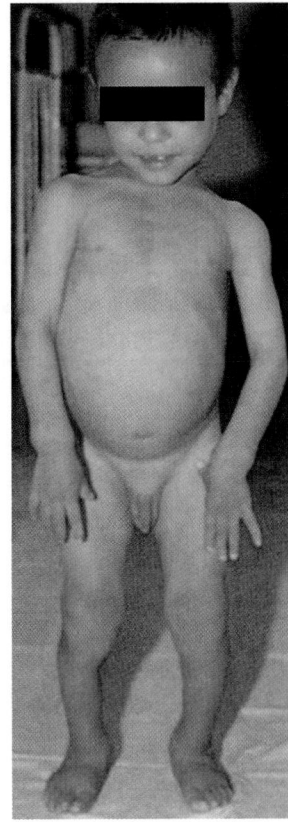

Figure 7-3 Rickets. This child has characteristic bowed legs. (From McLaren DS: *A colour atlas and text of diet-related disorders,* ed 2, London, 1992, Mosby-Year Book Europe Limited. By permission of Mosby International Ltd.)

rickets

a childhood disorder caused by vitamin D or calcium deficiency that leads to insufficient mineralization of bone and tooth matrix

osteomalacia

an adult disorder caused by vitamin D or calcium deficiency characterized by soft, demineralized bones process and contribute to osteomalacia risk. Older women are more at risk than men because of the effects of repeated pregnancies and lactation on bone density. Symptoms of osteomalacia include weakness, rheumatic-like pain, and an awkward gait. Because bones are weakened, fractures of the spine, hips, and limbs may occur.

The use of sedatives and tranquilizers as well as anticonvulsant therapy in persons with epilepsy has also been associated with increases in the incidence of rickets and osteomalacia.[22]

osteoporosis

a multifactorial disorder in which bone density is reduced and remaining bone is brittle, breaking easily

Another disorder of the skeleton is osteoporosis. Osteoporosis is a condition in which bone density is reduced and the remaining bone is brittle and breaks easily. Because vitamin D is crucial for absorption of calcium and the mineralization of bone, chronic vitamin D deficiency may be one of the risk factors of this disorder. Osteoporosis is discussed in detail in Chapter 8.

Outright deficiency of vitamin D is rare in the United States because milk and related food products are fortified. Deficiency is a concern when a lack of exposure to sunlight occurs as a result of (1) environmental limitations, (2) cultural clothing customs that conceal the body, or (3) the inability of older adults or persons with disabilities to get outdoors or to the store, resulting in malnourishment. These conditions may require vigilance in the consumption of fortified dietary sources, or supplements may be appropriate.[10]

Toxicity

High intakes of vitamin D can result in hypercalcemia (high blood levels of calcium) and hypercalciuria (high calcium level in urine), which affect kidneys and may cause cardiovascular damage. Toxicity symptoms occur when dietary intake of vitamin D is just above the UL of 50 mcg or 2000 IU, making vitamin D the most toxic of vitamins.

Vitamin E

During the 1970s vitamin E supplements were a popular aphrodisiac. Male virility, in particular, was thought to be enhanced by taking extra vitamin E. There was only one problem. Vitamin E increased the libido of male rats, not of humans. Research conducted on rats about the effects of vitamin E noted that male rats were able to reproduce better with additional intake of vitamin E. Although research conducted on rats is often applicable to humans, in this instance the results could not be generalized to humans. However, vitamin E is an essential nutrient performing vital functions; we are still learning more about its role in relation to disease prevention.

Function

Vitamin E acts as an antioxidant, protecting polyunsaturated fatty acids and vitamin A in cell membranes from oxidative damage by being oxidized itself. This function is particularly important in protecting the integrity of lung and red blood cell membranes, which are exposed to large amounts of oxygen. Other antioxidative functions of vitamin E are performed as part of a system in conjunction with selenium and ascorbic acid (vitamin C).

Recommended Intake and Sources

Vitamin E is the name given to a family of compounds called *tocopherols*, which are found in plants. Alpha-tocopherol is the most widely occurring form of tocopherol and is also the most active. Vitamin E is measured in terms of alpha-tocopherol equivalents (a-TE). The RDA for vitamin E is 15 mg a-TE for men and women. (The older unit of measurement, International Units [IU], may still be in use on dietary supplements: one mg a-TE equals 1.49 IU). A positive relationship exists between dietary intake of polyunsaturated fats and vitamin E requirements.

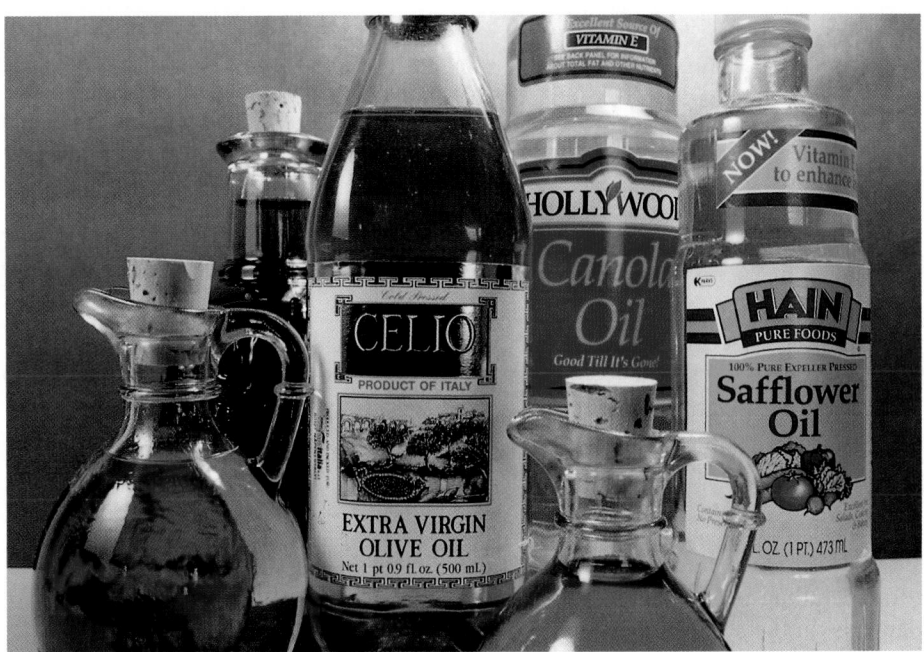

Vegetable oils provide vitamin E. (From Joanne Scott/Tracy McCalla.)

As our dietary intake of polyunsaturated fats increases, we need more vitamin E to protect the integrity of these fats from oxidation.

For vitamin E to function as an antioxidant protecting against heart disease and possible reduced risk of prostate cancer, higher levels—30 to 70 mg a-TE (50 to 100 IU)—are recommended These amounts cannot be consumed through dietary means and suggests the use of supplements. These amounts are most often measured as IU. Although a number of studies support the use of vitamin E in this manner, use of vitamin E at these levels for antioxidant function is not part of the RDA recommendations.[29] Some of the studies used levels of 400 to 800 IU. The optimum level is still being studied. Because no UL has been set yet, it is important to check with a primary healthcare provider before supplementing with vitamin E, especially if an individual has hypertension. Vitamin E may increase the risk of stroke for those with hypertension. It is also contraindicated for individuals taking warfarin (Coumadin) or other medicines that inhibit blood clots because vitamin E may affect the efficacy of the medications.[26,30]

The best sources of vitamin E are vegetable oils (e.g., corn, soy, safflower, and cottonseed) and margarine. Whole grains, seeds, nuts, wheat germ, and green leafy vegetables also provide adequate amounts of vitamin E. Processing of these foods may decrease the final vitamin E content.

Deficiency

A primary deficiency of vitamin E is rare. Secondary deficiencies occur in premature infants and others who are unable to absorb fat normally. Some chronic fat absorption disorders in which deficiencies may occur are cystic fibrosis, biliary atresia, other disorders of the hepatobiliary system, or liver transport problems. Symptoms of vitamin E deficiency include neurologic disorders resulting from cell damage and anemia caused by hemolysis of red blood cells (hemolytic anemia).

cystic fibrosis
a genetic disorder in which excessive mucus is produced, primarily affecting respiratory airways; also limits fat absorption in the digestive system; most common among Caucasian populations

biliary atresia
a congenital condition in which the major bile duct is blocked, limiting the availability of bile for fat digestion

Toxicity

There is no evidence of toxicity associated with excessive intake of vitamin E.[31] Intakes of about 70 to 530 mg a-TE (100 to 800 IU) per day appear to be tolerated, but the value of such doses has not been determined.[32] Megadoses of vitamin E can exacerbate the anticoagulant effect of drugs taken to reduce blood clotting; vitamin E supplementation is not recommended in persons who receive anticoagulant therapy, have a coagulation disorder, or have a vitamin K deficiency. A UL of 1000 mg a-TE has been set.

Vitamin K

Discovered by a Danish scientist, vitamin K was called *koagulationsvitamin* for its blood clotting properties. Later research revealed that vitamin K is several related compounds with similar functions in the body.

Function

Vitamin K's main function is as a cofactor in the synthesis of blood clotting factors, including prothrombin. Protein formation in bone, kidney, and plasma also depends on the actions of vitamin K.

Recommended Intake and Sources

The AI for vitamin K is 120 mcg for men and 90 mcg for women. This amount provides for sufficient storage of vitamin K in the liver. Vitamin K actually consists of compounds in different forms in plant and animal tissues. All are converted by the liver to the biologically active form of menaquinone called vitamin K.

Vitamin K is available through dietary sources and can be synthesized by microflora in the jejunum and ileum of the digestive tract. From plants, vitamin K is consumed as phylloquinone; bacterial synthesis produces vitamin K homologues as forms of menaquinones. As noted, phylloquinone and vitamin K homologues are converted to the active form of menaquinone—vitamin K—by the liver.

Vitamin K is still an essential nutrient although bacteria residing in the intestinal tract can synthesize it. The key distinction is that bacteria hosted by the human body produce the vitamin. Additionally, not enough vitamin K is produced by the microflora to ensure adequate levels for total blood clotting needs; dietary intake is still required.[33]

Primary food sources for vitamin K are dark green leafy vegetables. Lesser amounts are found in dairy products, cereals, meats, and fruits.

Deficiency

Deficiency of vitamin K inhibits blood coagulation. Deficiencies may be observed in clinical settings related to malabsorption disorders or medication interactions. Long-term intensive antibiotic therapy destroys the intestinal microflora that produce vitamin K. As with the other fat-soluble vitamins, any barrier to absorption affects the quantity of fat-soluble vitamin absorbed.

Premature infants and newborns are unable to immediately produce vitamin K; their guts are too sterile, free from the microflora necessary to produce vitamin K. Hospitals in the United States routinely give newborns an intramuscular dose of vitamin K to prevent hemorrhagic disease.

Because vitamin K also has a role in bone metabolism, recent research is considering whether vitamin K has a function in the treatment of osteoporosis.[31] Although insufficient data exist to support vitamin K as a formal treatment component for osteoporosis,[34] it does highlight the need to regularly consume at least the AI for vitamin K.

Toxicity

Consumption of foods containing vitamin K produces no problems of toxicity. Certain medications may be affected by vitamin K. The effectiveness of anticoagulant medications such as warfarin (Coumadin) and other blood thinning drugs can be reduced by high intakes of vitamin K whether from foods or supplements. Clients should be advised to moderate their consumption of foods containing vitamin K. Therapeutic administration of vitamin K in the menadione form has caused reactions in neonates, including hemolytic anemia and hyperbilirubinemia. Phylloquinone administration has been acceptable.[11]

Vitamin K supplements should only be used if advised by a registered dietitian or primary healthcare provider. Because vitamin K has a role in blood clotting, excess amounts may decrease clotting time, thereby increasing the potential risk for stroke.

Table 7-6 provides a summary of fat-soluble vitamins.

hyperbilirubinemia
a neonatal condition of excessively high levels of bilirubin (red bile pigment) leading to jaundice, in which bile is deposited in tissues throughout the body

OVERCOMING BARRIERS

Just Swallowing a Pill

Why do vitamins capture the attention of Americans? We generally do not suffer from vitamin deficiencies, and any problems of vitamin toxicity tend to be self-imposed. Considered through a wellness perspective, vitamin consumption is just one of many factors for achieving optimum health. Yet sales of dietary supplements have significantly increased from $500 million in 1972 to $6.5 billion in 1996.[10,35,36] More than half the adult American population uses these products.[36]

Perhaps vitamins are an easier target on which to focus when emphasizing good health. If a person is concerned about vitamin intake, a vitamin pill can always be taken. That's a lot easier than the dietary and behavior modifications required to meet other health factors such as decreasing fat intake or increasing physical activities. There are, though, circumstances that may warrant supplementation.

Rethinking Vitamin Supplementation

Recommendations for vitamin supplementation intend to improve the nutritional status of at-risk groups of the population. These have included adolescent girls, pregnant and lactating women, individuals with limited economic resources, and older persons. Folate, vitamins A and C, and the minerals iron, calcium, and zinc tend to be consumed in inadequate amounts by these at-risk groups.[35]

The purpose of recommendations for the previously mentioned at-risk groups is to address basic deficiency issues. If the adequate levels are not consumed as a result of social, cultural, or economic reasons,[35] then it is the role of health professionals to provide guidance as to how to meet these levels.

Recommendations are now beginning to move beyond the level of nutrient adequacy to issues of health promotion and prevention of disease. For example, folate requirements are vitally important for the development of a healthy fetus. Should the whole population receive folic acid through fortification when only potentially pregnant women have the additional requirement? Is this supplementation of folic acid acceptable although increased folic acid intake is associated with lowering homocysteine levels (see Box 7-2)?

A recommendation from the DRI addresses the issue of availability of vitamin B_{12} and older persons. It recommends that adults older than age 50 use a vitamin B_{12} supplement or foods fortified with the vitamin to ensure adequate bioavailability of the vitamin to prevent potential deficiencies. But what foods

Table 7-6
Fat-Soluble Vitamins

Vitamin	Function	Clinical Issues Deficiency/Toxicity	Requirements	Food Sources
Vitamin A Precursor: carotenoids Preformed vitamin: retinoids	Maintains epithelial tissues (skin and mucous membranes); rhodopsin formation for vision; bone growth; reproduction	Deficiency: xerophthalmia; night blindness; keratomalcia; degeneration of epithelial tissue; inhibited growth (respiratory and GI disturbances) Toxicity: hypervitaminosis A (from supplements) with blistered skin, weakness, anorexia, vomiting, enlarged spleen and liver	Men: 900 mcg RAE Women: 700 mcg RAE UL 3000 mcg RAE	Deep green, yellow, and orange fruits and vegetables; animal fat sources: whole milk, fortified skim, and low-fat milk; butter; liver; egg yolks, fatty fish
Vitamin D Precursor: 7-dehydrocholesterol Active form: cholecalciferol	Calcium and phosphorus absorption; bone mineralization	Deficiency: bone malformation, rickets (children), osteomalacia (adults) Toxicity: hypercalcemia, hypercalciuria	Adults: 5 mcg AI (<51 years 10 mcg) (<70 years 15 mcg) UL 50 mcg	Animal (fat) sources: butter, egg yolks, fatty fish, liver, fortified milk; body synthesis
Vitamin E alpha-tocopherol	Antioxidant for PUFA and vitamin A; antioxidant with selenium and ascorbic acid	Deficiency: primary deficiency rare; secondary deficiency (caused by fat absorption) neurologic disorders Toxicity: none, but supplements contraindicated with anticoagulation drugs	Adults: 15 mg α-TE UL 1000 mg α-TE	Vegetable oil, whole grains, seeds, nuts, green leafy vegetables
Vitamin K Active form: menaquinones	Cofactor in synthesis of blood clotting factors; protein formation	Deficiency: blood coagulation inhibited; hemorrhagic disease (infants) Toxicity: therapeutic vitamin K (menadione form) reactions in neonates, causing hemolytic anemia and hyperbilirubinemia	Men: 120 mcg AI Women: 90 mcg AI	Green leafy vegetables, intestinal synthesis

α-TE, *Alpha-tocopheral equivalent;* AI, *Adequate Intake;* RAE, *Retinol Activity Equivalents;* UL, *Tolerable Upper Intake Level;* PUFA, *polyunsaturated fatty acid.*

should be fortified that older adults are sure to eat? The DRI has also recommended that the level of vitamin D be increased above levels usually consumed, suggesting the use of vitamin D supplements. This marks a significant change in philosophy, because supplements of vitamin D have been discouraged in the past because of toxicity issues. An important question for health professionals to consider is, "How will older adults know of these vitamin B_{12} and vitamin D recommendations and how should they be implemented?"

To use vitamins and minerals as antioxidants often means using doses beyond the suggested levels of the DRI. At the DRI levels, basic antioxidant functions are achieved. At the higher levels, additional health promotion and disease prevention may occur. But we do not yet have definitive answers. So what advice do we give? The Position of the American Dietetic Association on enrichment and fortification of foods and dietary supplements suggests that: "Nutrition education, fortification of staple food products, and nutrient supplements are three complementary approaches to enhance the nutritional adequacy of at-risk segments of the population."[35]

Nutrition education regarding the use of fortified foods and appropriate use of supplements is one means of teaching the target population about nutrient needs. When implemented on a broad scale to the public-at-large, other segments of the population also learn of the nutrient value. For example, women should be taught the value of folic acid during pregnancy, but men can also be aware of this value so that they can support the implementation of the folic acid goal by the women in their lives. In addition, younger women can become aware of the special nutrient needs of the pregnancy years before they enter them so that the importance of nutrition during pregnancy is not something new or an afterthought when they are older.

Food fortification increases the amount of the nutrient in the food supply. By careful selection of the foods to which specific nutrients are added, increased consumption of the nutrient can be achieved with little effort by the target group. This is a public health approach that affects the community-at-large. The newly approved folic acid fortification begins to provide a safety net for women of childbearing age but only if foods containing the additional folic acid are consumed. Supplements may still be warranted.

The third approach of nutrient supplements is an individualized approach.[35] Individuals take the supplements on their own. Ideally, a qualified health professional such as a registered dietitian, licensed nutritionist, or primary healthcare provider guides the individual as to the need and quantity of the nutrient supplements to be regularly taken. This approach requires the individual to take the responsibility for continued consumption, if appropriate, of the supplement.

The optimal approach is the use of all three approaches to achieve nutrient adequacy that takes into account the special needs of subgroups and considers newer issues such as antioxidants.

Role of the Health Practitioner

Recommendations for use of nutrient supplements should be determined by dietetic professionals such as registered dietitians or by primary healthcare providers. Their counseling evaluates the client's current nutrient intake and assesses his or her dietary supplementation practices and possible interactions with prescribed medical treatments and medications. Foremost in importance is that dietary adequacy should first be met by eating a varied diet of foods and by following the basic dietary guidelines of the Food Guide Pyramid.[35]

The role of other health professionals, such as nurses, is to guide clients to the appropriate nutritional counseling to determine the client's actual nutrient status.

After counseling has been completed, nurses can support the recommendations of the dietitian through teaching strategies such as how to incorporate more fruits and vegetables into one's diet and how to reinforce the understanding of potential drug-nutrient interactions.

TOWARD A POSITIVE NUTRITION LIFESTYLE: SOCIAL SUPPORT

Social support extends throughout the life span; it goes beyond having friends and family with whom to socialize. For families with young children, social support may be cooperative meals when illness strikes (e.g., during a flu epidemic) and cooking time becomes compromised. The term *cooperative* may mean cooking double portions to feed a friend's family during bouts of chicken pox or childhood ear infections. The kindness would then be reciprocated in the future. Both families gain nutritious meals at times when merely thinking about cooking seems overwhelming.

Support for older persons, as mentioned earlier in this chapter, may mean assistance with food shopping or foods delivery. Neighbors or relatives may provide this social support. In some communities, local Red Cross chapters and other charitable organizations have developed car or bus services specifically to provide transportation for older residents. This enables individuals to safely shop in food stores and have the convenience of being driven to their homes and assisted with carrying groceries into their kitchens. Healthcare professionals working with older clients should be aware of these services or perhaps help community organizations initiate similar programs.

SUMMARY

Vitamins are organic molecules that perform specific metabolic functions and are required in very small amounts. As essential nutrients, they must be provided through dietary intake. Vitamins are divided into the two categories of water-soluble and fat-soluble vitamins. Solubility of vitamins affects the processes of absorption, transportation, and storage of vitamins in our bodies.

Water-soluble vitamins are vitamin C, choline, and the B complex vitamins (thiamine, riboflavin, niacin, folate, pyridoxine [B_6], vitamin B_{12}, pantothenic acid, and biotin). The B vitamins function as coenzymes. Choline is part of a neurotransmitter and lecithin. Vitamin C serves as an antioxidant in addition to its coenzyme ability. Water-soluble vitamins are easily absorbed into blood circulation. Because excesses are excreted, toxicity is less likely, however they may occur with pyridoxine and vitamin C.

Fat-soluble vitamins are vitamins A, D, E, and K. These vitamins serve structural and regulatory functions throughout the body. Fat-soluble vitamins are absorbed the same as lipids; bile is required, and the nutrients enter the lymphatic system. Because they are retained in fatty substances in the body, toxicity from supplemental intakes is possible.

THE NURSING APPROACH
Vitamin and Chronic Alcohol Use Case Study

Alcoholism is probably the primary cause of vitamin and other nutrient deficiencies in the United States. Nutritional problems arise because the person substitutes alcohol for food and alcohol is toxic to all cells. Anorexia (loss of appetite) may occur because of complications of alcoholism such as gastritis, hepatitis, or pancreatitis. In addition, alcohol can also impair the storage of nutrients, thereby increasing nutrient catabolism and excretion. Chronic alcohol abuse is associated with liver disease.

Any patients suspected of chronic excess alcohol use should undergo a thorough nutritional assessment.

CASE STUDY:

Joseph, age 53, was brought to the emergency room because he fell down in the street and was found by the police. He was unable to recite his name or address. He had alcohol on the breath (AOB), appeared disheveled, and thought he was in jail. The nurse practitioner recorded the following information.

ASSESSMENT

Subjective

- Experiences muscular and joint pain
- Experiences loss of appetite; has not been eating regularly or taking vitamins
- Feels anxious and irritable
- Unable to remember his address
- Recognizes that he drinks too much; denies he is an alcoholic

Objective

- Decreased muscle strength
- Skin dryness and bruises on knees
- Gingivitis, bleeding gums, and dental caries

NURSING DIAGNOSIS

1. Alteration in nutrition, less than body requirements of thiamine related to alcoholic malnutrition, as evidenced by ataxia and joint pain
2. Alteration in coping as evidenced by alcohol abuse

IMPLEMENTATION

The treatment regimen should include the following:
1. Vitamin supplements
2. High-caloric and high-protein diet
3. Treatment of vitamin deficiency symptoms
4. Weekly weight measurements
5. Recording of daily food diaries
6. Teaching the importance of food variety and Food Pyramid principles

EVALUATION

The goals will be achieved as evidenced by the following:
- Decrease in joint pain within 3 months
- Increase in caloric intake to 2000 kcalories daily by 1 month
- A daily food diary that reveals food selections adequate in vitamin, proteins, and minerals
- Attendance in an alcohol recovery program

APPLYING CONTENT KNOWLEDGE

Mark, age 3, is having his yearly health examination. His mom, rather proudly, tells you that Mark eats one apple and carrot sticks every day. She says that means that he gets all the vitamins he needs. How do you respond?

Web Sites of Interest

InteliHealth Nutrition
www.intelihealth.com/
This is the Harvard Medical School Consumer Information site that provides a variety of information and links to other health-related sites. To reach the nutrition section, scroll to the nutrition topic in the upper right corner and visit topics on vitamin supplements, nutrition for specific health problems, what's in your food, and many others.

National Center for Complementary and Alternative Medicine
www.nccam.nih.gov/
This center is a branch of the National Institutes of Health, which conducts and supports research and training and distributes information on complementary and alternative medicine to health professionals and the public.

U.S. FDA Center for Food Safety and Applied Nutrition
www.cfsan.fda.gov/
This site provides FDA policies, rules, and FDA Talk Papers pertaining to supplements and health claims on foods.

References

1. Institute of Medicine, Food and Nutrition Board: *Dietary reference intakes series,* Washington, DC, 1997, 1998, 1999, 2000, 2001, National Academy Press.
2. Pagana KD, Pagana JT: *Mosby's diagnostic and laboratory test reference,* ed 4, St Louis, 1999, Mosby.
3. Fain O, Mathieu E, Thomas M: Scurvy in patients with cancer, *Br Med J* 316:1661, 1998.
4. Wood B et al.: Pellagra in a woman using alternative remedies, *Australas J Dermatol* 39(1):42, Feb 1998.
5. Gessner BD et al.: Nutritional rickets among breast-fed black and Alaska Native children, *Alaska Med* 39(3):72, 1997.
6. Talalay P et al.: *The proceedings of the National Academy of Sciences,* Apr 12, 1994.
7. Tanphaichitr V: Thiamin. In Shils ME eds.: *Modern nutrition in health and disease,* ed 9, Baltimore, 1999, Williams & Wilkins.
8. Jeffery DR: Nutrition and diseases of the nervous system. In Shils ME eds.: *Modern nutrition in health and disease,* ed 9, Baltimore, 1999, Williams & Wilkins.
9. Baker KG et al.: Chronic alcoholism in the absence of Wernicke-Korsakoff syndrome and cirrhosis does not result in the loss of serotonergic neurons from the median raphe nucleus, *Metab Brain Dis* 11(3):217, 1996.
10. National Academy of Science: *Diet and health: implications for reducing chronic disease risk,* Washington, DC, 1989, National Academy Press.
11. McCormick DB: Riboflavin. In Shils ME eds.: *Modern nutrition in health and disease,* ed 9, Baltimore, 1999, Williams & Wilkins.
12. Cervantes-Laurean D, McElvaneyn G, Ross J: Niacin. In Shils ME eds.: *Modern nutrition in health and disease,* ed 9, Baltimore, 1999, Williams & Wilkins.
13. Morgan SL, Weinsier RL: *Fundamentals of clinical nutrition,* ed 2, St Louis, 1998, Mosby.

14. Chongtham DS, Ram T, Jain S: Acute isoniazid poisoning: presenting as seizure, *Indian J Ches Dis Allied Sci* 39(4):255, 1997.

15. Locksmith GJ, Duff P: Preventing neural tube defects: the importance of periconceptional folic acid supplements, *Obstet Gynecol* 91(6):1027, 1998.

16. US Department of Health and Human Services: FDA announces name changes for lower-fat milks and folic acid fortification for bakery products, *HHS News*, Dec 31, 1997.

17. US Food and Drug Administration: Folic acid fortification, US Food and Drug Administration, Office of Public Affairs, *Fact Sheet*, Feb 29, 1996.

18. Tinkle M: Folic acid and food fortification: implications for the primary care practitioner, *Nurse Pract* 22(3):105, 1997.

19. Tucker KL et al.: Folic acid fortification of the food supply. Potential benefits and risks for the elderly population, *J Am Med Assoc* 276(23):1879, 1996.

20. Oakley GP Jr, Adams MJ, Dickinson CM: More folic acid for everyone, now, *J Nutr* 126(3):751S, 1996.

21. Herbert V: Folic acid. In Shils ME eds.: *Modern nutrition in health and disease,* ed 9, Baltimore, 1999, Williams & Wilkins.

22. Weir DG, Scott JM: Vitamin B$_{12}$ "Cobalamin." In Shils ME eds.: *Modern nutrition in health and disease,* ed 9, Baltimore, 1999, Williams & Wilkins.

23. Liddenbaum et al.: Neuropsychiatric disorders caused by cobalamin deficiency in the absence of anemia or macrocytosis, *N Engl J Med* 318:1720, 1988.

24. Marshall MW et al.: Effect of low and high fat diets varying in ratios of polyunsaturated to saturated fatty acids on biotin intakes and biotin in serum, red cells and urine of adult men, *Nutr Res* 5:801, 1985.

25. Jacob RA: Vitamin C. In Shils ME eds.: *Modern nutrition in health and disease,* ed 9, Baltimore, 1999, Williams & Wilkins.

26. Liebman B: 3 vitamins and a mineral: what to take, *Nutrition Action Health Letter,* May 1998.

27. Ross AC: Vitamin A and retinoids. In Shils ME eds.: *Modern nutrition in health and disease,* ed 9, Baltimore, 1999, Williams & Wilkins.

28. Tortorella K: Rickets, a relic shows up again, *New York Times,* sec 13:1, Mar 12, 1995.

29. Weber P, Bendich A, Machin LJ: Vitamin E and human health: rationale for determining recommended intake levels, *Nutrition* 13(5):450, 1997.

30. Smigel K: Vitamin E reduces prostate cancer rates in Finnish trial: U.S. considers follow-up, *J NAH Cancer Inst* 90(6):416-417, 1998.

31. Weber P: Management of osteoporosis: is there a role for vitamin K?, *Int J Vitam Nutr Res* 67(5):350, 1997.

32. Bendich A, Machlin LJ: Safety of oral intake of vitamin E, *Am J Clin Nutr* 48:612, 1988.

33. Olsen RE: Vitamin K. In Shils ME eds.: *Modern nutrition in health and disease,* ed 9, Baltimore, 1999, Williams & Wilkins.

34. Vermeer C et al.: Effects of vitamin K on bone mass and bone metabolism, *J Nutr* 126(4 Suppl):1187S, 1996.

35. American Dietetic Association, Position of the American Dietetic Association: Food fortification and dietary supplementation, *J Am Diet Assoc* 101:115, 2001.

36. Kurtzweil P: An FDA guide to dietary supplements, *FDA Consumer* Oct 1998, revised Jan 1999.

CHAPTER 8

Water and Minerals

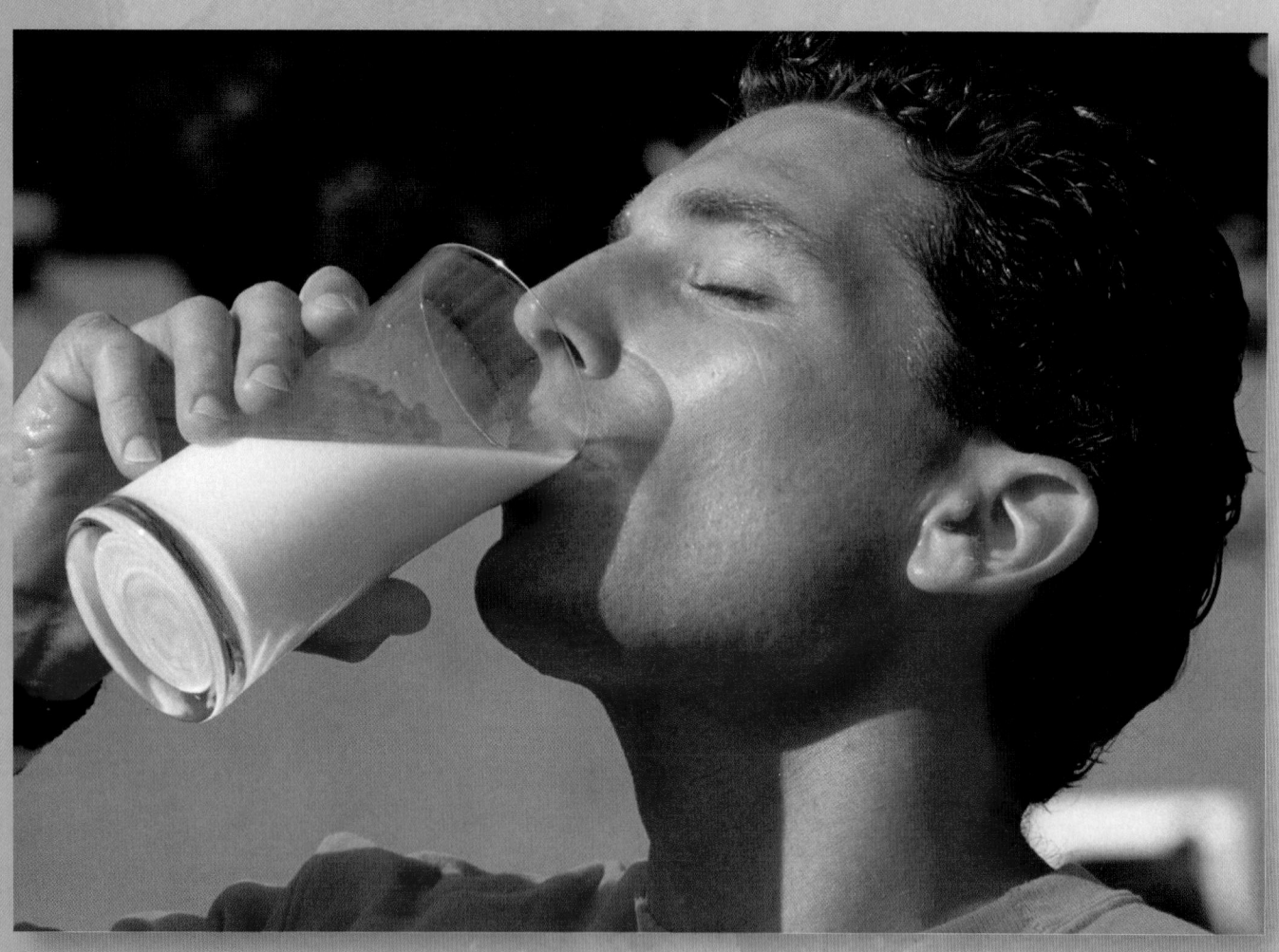

An ever-circulating ocean of fluid bathes all the cells of our bodies; this fluid allows for chemical reactions, transmission of nerve impulses, and transportation of nutrients and waste products throughout the body.

ROLE IN WELLNESS

An ever-circulating ocean of fluid bathes all the cells of our bodies; this fluid allows for chemical reactions, transmission of nerve impulses, and transportation of nutrients and waste products throughout the body. The fluid is not simply water, although water is its primary constituent. Some fluid in the body is used to form blood, lymph, and structure for cells. Minerals circulating in our body fluids create the setting for biochemical reactions to occur.

Water and minerals affect every system of our bodies as well as our five dimensions of health. Physical health depends on adequate levels of these nutrients. Intellectual health is compromised when iron levels are low; iron deficiency affects cognitive abilities and thus diminishes the ability to learn. Emotional health may rely on our being sufficiently hydrated with fluids; cases of fluid volume deficit or dehydration have been mistaken as senility when the thirst acuity of older adults diminishes. Social health may be affected if older adults become debilitated by bone fractures or osteoporosis caused by chronic calcium deficiencies; social mobility may be limited as their physical movement is inhibited. Vegans who consume no animal-derived foods because of spiritual beliefs need carefully designed eating plans to provide adequate levels of zinc, iron, and calcium to avoid deficiencies.

Although water and minerals are primary components of body fluids, each performs other functions as well. This chapter explores water and minerals in the context of their nutritional requirements and physiologic roles for achieving nutritional wellness.

WATER

We can live several weeks without food but can survive only a few days without water or fluids. Although our bodies use stored nutrients to fuel energy needs, a minimum intake of water is required for cell function and as a solution through which waste products of the body are excreted in urine.

Food Sources

If we drank only water and no other liquids, we could meet our body's need for fluid. Most of us, however, consume fluids in addition to water throughout the day. Some fluids also contain other nutrients. Consider the wealth of nutrients found in milk (skim or whole), fruit juices, and soups. Some fruits and vegetables contain as much as 85% to 95% water. Watermelon, grapes, oranges, lettuce, tomatoes, and zucchini have high water content. Most foods contain water, but some are better sources of fluids than others. Generally, we depend on beverages as our main source of fluids.

Water intake recommendations developed to accompany the Dietary Reference Intakes (DRI) suggest that adults consume 1 to 1.5 ml of water for each kcalorie expended under normal conditions (about 2 liters [2 qts] per 2000 kcalories), which equals about 8 glasses of water a day.[1] Although the minimum amount needed by healthy adults is about 4 glasses, higher amounts may be optimum considering an individual's physiologic status and energy output.

Our primary source of water should be the liquids we drink (Box 8-1). Notice that coffee, tea, alcohol, and soft drinks are not listed as primary sources. Although they do contain water, coffee, tea, and alcohol act as diuretics, which cause an increase in water loss via the kidneys as urine. Soft drinks add fluid to the body, but they contain solutes (sugar, salt, various chemicals) that must be diluted as they enter the bloodstream. Drinking a soda increases the concentration of these solutes in the blood. The body responds by pulling fluid from the cells into the bloodstream to dilute the sugar and salt. The body loses the increased fluid in the blood-

DRI =	Dietary Reference Intakes
RDA =	Recommended Dietary Allowance
AI =	Adequate Intake
UL =	Tolerable Upper Intake Level

Box 8-1 Foods as Sources of Water (By Percentage)

FOOD	PERCENT WATER	FOOD	PERCENT WATER
DAIRY PRODUCTS		**VEGETABLES**	
Milk	88-91	Asparagus	91
Cheddar cheese	37	Carrots	88
Cottage cheese	79	Cucumber	96
Ice cream, ice milk	61-66	Lettuce	96
		Potato	75
FRUITS		Spinach	90
Apples	84	Sweet potato	73
Grapefruit	90	Tomatoes	94
(whole or juice)		**MISCELLANEOUS**	
Grapes	81	Beans (cooked)	60-70
Melons	90	Bread	30-40
Oranges	88	Fruit punch	88
(whole or juice)		Gelatin	84
		Meats	50-60
		Oatmeal (cooked)	85
		Poultry	65
		Soups	85-98

From Nutrient Data Laboratory; *www.nal.usda.gov/fnic/foodcomp/.*

stream when it is excreted as urine. In addition, the body responds to the increased solutes and decreased fluid content by once again triggering the thirst mechanism.

Bottled water has become a mainstay in U.S. beverage selections and an economic force. Sales of bottled water reached almost $5.7 billion in 2000.[2] Products range from imported sparkling mineral waters to spring waters to waters treated from nearby reservoirs. Although the price range is equally broad, the common denominator is that Americans enjoy the convenience of water as a beverage when available in portable containers and single portions.

Water Quality

The minerals found naturally in water vary. Hard water refers to water that contains high amounts of minerals such as calcium and magnesium. Drinking this water can provide a significant amount of these nutrients. Nonnutrition-related problems from hard water can develop; mineral deposits may damage appliances and other machinery that interacts with water, and soap suds are reduced. To reduce these problems, a filtration process can be installed to soften water by replacing some minerals with sodium chloride (salt). Soft water containing sodium, however, can be a problem for sodium-sensitive individuals, such as those at risk for hypertension. To prevent health problems, water softeners may be used on only the hot tap in kitchens, leaving the cold tap unsoftened for consumption.

Another aspect of water quality is contamination. For example, many older buildings have pipes with lead solder joints that can release lead into the water that sits in or runs through them. If the level of lead in water is more than 15 parts per billion (PPB), pregnant women, infants, and children are advised to drink bottled water because even low levels of lead can seriously impair normal development. The local health department can recommend a competent laboratory that tests household water quality.

Water treatment processes can remedy some contamination concerns. Others, such as industrial pollution, can be difficult to identify. Complications of bacterial contamination or inadvertent exposure of water to carcinogenic industrial sub-

hard water
water that contains high amounts of minerals such as calcium and magnesium

soft water
water that has been filtered to replace some of the minerals with sodium

To reduce the chance of lead leaking into drinking and cooking water, do the following:
- Run the water for 2 minutes after it has been standing in the pipes.
- Use only cold water for drinking, cooking, and preparing baby formula (cold water absorbs less lead than hot).

stances can lead to health problems that range from simple gastroenteritis to cancer. Municipal and regional water processing plants take great care to ensure the safest water supply possible. Some water sources (private wells, surface water, springs, and cisterns), however, may exceed the maximum contaminant levels set by the Environmental Protection Agency.[3]

The most severe water-related threats such as cholera and typhoid are no longer public health hazards in North America. Other potential industrial and environmental pollutants, however, can enter our water supply and endanger our health. Small suppliers may not have the financial means to improve technologic surveillance. The Environmental Health Objective 5 of *Healthy People 2010* is to address this need and increase the percentage of Americans who receive the safest water possible by meeting the Safe Water Act Regulations.[3]

Poorer countries throughout the world continue to struggle with unsafe water supplies. Without the financial and technologic knowledge and resources, many people become ill by consuming bacteria-contaminated water. Increased incidence of stomach cancer is associated with exposure to *Helicobacter pylori*, which is sometimes found in contaminated waters.[4]

Water as a Nutrient within the Body

Structure

The structure of water—two hydrogen atoms bonded to one oxygen atom—allows it to provide a base for biochemical reactions in the body and to easily move through the various compartments of cells and body systems. As the basis of body fluids, water can host other substances of different electrical charges and characteristics. **Intracellular fluids** (within the cell) are composed of water plus concentrations of potassium and phosphates. **Interstitial fluids** (between the cells) contain concentrations of sodium and chloride. **Extracellular fluids** include interstitial fluid and encompass all fluids outside cells including plasma and the watery components of body organs and substances (Box 8-2).

intracellular fluid
fluid within the cells composed of water plus concentrations of potassium and phosphates

interstitial fluid
fluid between the cells containing concentrations of sodium and chloride

extracellular fluid
all fluids outside cells including interstitial fluid, plasma, and watery components of body organs and substances

Digestion and Absorption

Because water is inorganic, it is not digested. It passes quickly to the small intestine. Once there, most water is absorbed; the rest is regulated by the colon and is either absorbed or excreted with feces.

Metabolism

Although not metabolized or broken down by the gastrointestinal (GI) tract processes, water is an integral component of metabolic processes. In some reactions, the water of metabolism is water released as a byproduct of oxidative reactions; in others, water may be a part of the process to release energy from adeno-

---

Box 8-2 Body Fluid Compartments

INTRACELLULAR FLUID		EXTRACELLULAR FLUID	
PROTEINS	MINERALS	MINERALS	PROTEINS
Enzymes	Potassium	Sodium	Blood proteins
Hemoglobin	Magnesium	Chloride	Antibodies
	Phosphorus	Bicarbonate ions	
		CARBOHYDRATES	LIPIDS
		Glucose	Lipoproteins
65% of body water		35% of body water	

FUNCTIONS OF WATER

- Provides shape and rigidity to cells
- Helps to regulate body temperature
- Acts as a lubricant
- Cushions body tissues
- Transports nutrients and waste products
- Acts as a solvent
- Provides a source of trace minerals
- Participates in chemical reactions

insensible perspiration
water lost invisibly through evaporation from the lungs and skin

solvent
the liquid in which another substance (the solute) is dissolved to form a solution

reactant
a substance that enters into and is altered during a chemical reaction

homeostasis
a state of physiologic equilibrium produced by a balance of functions and of chemical composition within an organism

solute
a substance dissolved in another substance

sine triphosphate (ATP), which is discussed in greater detail in Chapter 9. The released water may be excreted as waste or used elsewhere in the body. Glycogen in muscle and the liver contains water in the structure of glycogen molecules. When glycogen is used for energy, the water becomes available for body functions.

Functions

Water performs a variety of vital functions in the body. It is an important structural component of the body, giving shape and rigidity to cells. It assists in regulating body temperature. Water conducts heat, absorbing and distributing it throughout the body, keeping body temperature stable from day to day. Water also helps cool the body by evaporating invisibly from the lungs and the surface of the skin, carrying off excess heat. This type of water loss is called insensible perspiration.

Water acts as a lubricant in the form of joint fluid and mucous secretions. It forms a shock-absorbing fluid cushion for body tissues such as the amniotic sac, spinal cord, and eyes.

Water is a major component of blood, lymph, saliva, and urine. As such, it delivers nutrients and removes waste products. Acting as a solvent, it enables minerals, vitamins, glucose, and other small molecules to be moved throughout the body.

Water may also supply trace minerals such as fluoride, zinc, and copper. Sometimes it is a source of too many minerals, including potentially toxic metals such as lead, cadmium, and incidental substances from pesticides and industrial waste products.

In addition to serving as a medium for biochemical reactions, water also participates as a reactant. For example, large molecules such as polysaccharides, fats, and protein are split into smaller molecules in which water participates and is changed by the process.

Ultimately, no growth or cell renewal occurs without water; it is part of every cell and is necessary as a medium for reactions and transporter of supplies.

Regulation of Fluid and Water in the Body

Our bodies have delicate but efficient mechanisms for maintaining appropriate fluid levels. The intake of fluids is balanced with the output through urine, sweat, feces, and insensible perspiration (Figure 8-1). Regulation of fluid in the body is of physiologic importance because most of our body weight is composed of water. Water composes 50% to 60% of the weight of an average adult; the percentages are even higher for infants—their body weight is 75% to 80% water (Figure 8-2). Fortunately, all we need to do is take in enough fluids and our bodies' natural systems take care of the rest.

Homeostasis is maintained by electrolytes that include minerals and blood proteins. Two of the most important minerals are sodium and potassium. The extracellular distribution of fluid depends on sodium, and potassium influences intracellular water. Water moves within and between the cells in interstitial fluids in response to the levels of these minerals. An imbalance is corrected by mechanisms that cause thirst and regulate the ability of the kidneys to release or retain fluids.

Thirst, a dryness in the mouth, stimulates the desire to drink liquids. We often ignore our thirst until mealtimes. The thirst mechanism is controlled by the hypothalamus and involves several steps. As the water level in the body gets low, the sodium and solute level in blood increases. This causes water to be drawn from the salivary glands to provide more fluid for the blood. The mouth then feels dry because less saliva, which keeps the mouth moist, is produced. This sensation, thirst, stimulates the drinking process. If the thirst mechanism is faulty, as it may be during illness, physical exertion, or aging, hormonal mechanisms also help conserve water by reducing urine output.

The mechanisms of the kidneys regulate the amounts of water excreted. Obligatory water excretion of at least 500 ml (1 pint) must be excreted daily, regardless of the amount ingested, to clear the body of waste products. The mechanism relies

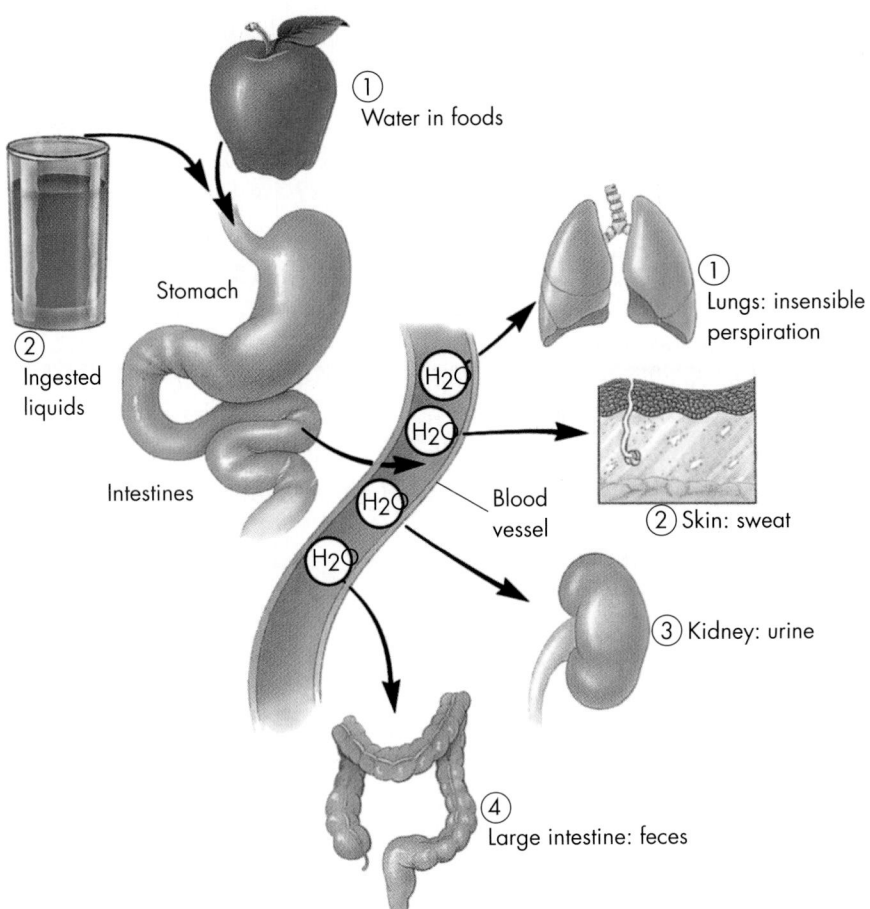

Figure 8-1 Intake of fluids is balanced with output. (Joan Beck; modified from Thibodeau GA, Patton KT: *The human body in health and disease,* ed 2, St Louis, 1997, Mosby.)

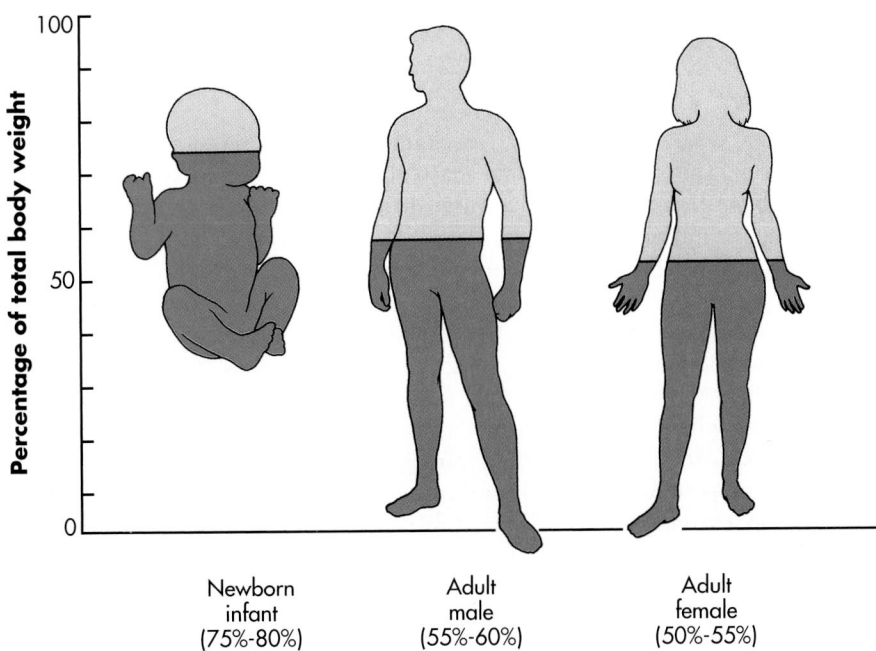

Figure 8-2 Percentage of body weight represented by water in infants compared with adults. (Rolin Graphics; From Thibodeau GA, Patton KT: *Structure and function of the body,* ed 10, St Louis, 1997, Mosby.)

antidiuretic hormone (ADH)
a hormone secreted by the pituitary gland in response to low fluid levels; affects kidneys to decrease excretion of water; also called *vasopressin*

aldosterone
a hormone secreted by the adrenal gland in response to sodium levels in kidneys; affects kidneys to balance fluid levels as needed

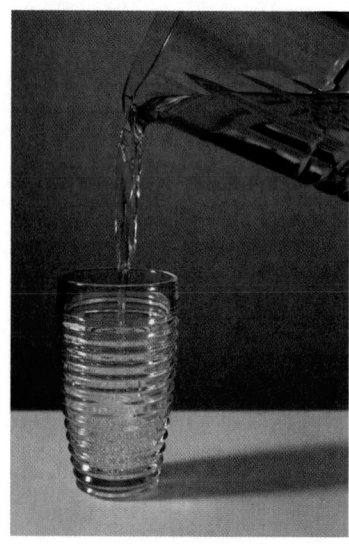

We need water in our diets every day. (From Photodisc.)

fluid volume deficit (FVD)
the state in which a person experiences vascular, cellular, or intracellular dehydration

polyuria
excessive urination

on the combined actions of the brain, kidneys, pituitary gland, and adrenal gland. When fluid in the body becomes low, the hypothalamus stimulates the pituitary gland to release **antidiuretic hormone (ADH)**. ADH is secreted in response to high sodium levels in the body or too low blood pressure or blood volume. The target organ of the hormone is the kidney. The kidneys then conserve water by decreasing excretion of water, and the retained fluid is recycled for use throughout the body.

When the sodium concentration in the kidneys gets high (too much fluid excreted), another process kicks in to counteract the lowered blood volume and pressure. The kidneys release renin, an enzyme that activates the blood protein angiotensin. Angiotensin raises blood pressure by narrowing blood vessels; it is a vasoconstrictor. Angiotensin also prompts the adrenal gland to release the hormone **aldosterone**. The target organ of aldosterone is the kidney. The effect is to decrease excretion of sodium, causing the kidneys to respond by retaining fluid in the body.

Fluid and Electrolytes

Dissolved in body fluids are minerals and other organic molecules required for the regulation of both intracellular and extracellular fluid distribution. Fluids follow salt concentrations; this means that cells can control fluid balance by directing the movement of mineral salts.

Electrolytes are minerals that carry electrical charges or ions (particles) when dissolved in water. These minerals separate into positively charged ions (cations) or negatively charged ions (anions). The primary extracellular electrolytes in body fluids are sodium (NA^+/cation) and chloride (Cl^-/anion), and the primary intracellular electrolyte is potassium (K^+/cation). To maintain fluid balance, cells control the movement of electrolytes. Water will follow sodium concentration. To move electrolytes in and out of the cell membrane requires transport proteins. The sodium/potassium pump is a transport protein that works to exchange sodium from within the cells for potassium. Other ions are also exchanged.

In addition to water regulation, the kidneys also regulate electrolyte levels. If body levels of sodium are low, aldosterone directs the kidneys to reabsorb or retain more sodium. This in turn results in potassium being excreted so the balance of electrolytes is maintained.

Imbalances

What happens when our regulatory mechanisms are unable to maintain the balance? Abnormal shifts in fluid balance may cause a deficit or excess in fluid volume.

Fluid Volume Deficit. In fluid volume deficit (FVD), a person experiences vascular, cellular, or intracellular dehydration. Severe FVD, when body fluid levels fall by 10% of body weight, is a medical emergency.[5]

FVD can occur from diarrhea, vomiting, or high fever—symptoms often experienced with stomach and intestinal viral infections or influenza. Other causes of excessive fluid loss may be sweating, diuretics, or polyuria. Whenever we lose fluid and have difficulty taking in additional fluids, we are at risk for FVD.

Determining whether symptoms are caused by dehydration or illness can be difficult. Characteristics of FVD include infrequent urination, decreased skin elasticity, dry mucous membranes, dry mouth, unusual drowsiness, light-headedness or disorientation, extreme thirst, nausea, slow or rapid breathing, and sudden weight loss. The person will be less able to maintain blood pressure immediately after rising from a sitting or lying position (called *orthostatic hypotension*). For any illness lasting more than a few days that causes loss of body fluids, a primary healthcare provider should be consulted. In moderate or severe FVD, intravenous (IV) therapy is indicated to replace fluids.

FVD can also happen when we are not ill. Strenuous physical activity, either athletic or work-related, that causes excessive sweating can lead to FVD. Hot, dry weather also can overwork the body's cooling mechanisms. Drinking fluids throughout the day despite a low level of thirst sensation can alleviate these risks.

Older adults and infants are the groups most at risk for FVD. Older adults have decreased fluid reserves and diminished thirst mechanism acuity. FVD symptoms may be misdiagnosed as senility. Reminding older clients to drink even when thirst is not experienced is appropriate to ensure adequate intake of fluids. In infants, water makes up a larger percentage of body weight than in adults and a greater percentage is extracellular fluid; dehydration from fluid loss can occur rapidly. In addition to other signs of FVD, infants may have a depressed fontanelle (soft spot) in the skull.

Fluid Volume Excess.   Fluid volume excess is a condition in which a person experiences increased fluid retention and edema. It is associated with a compromised regulatory mechanism, excess fluid intake, or excess sodium intake.

Edema is excess accumulation of fluid in interstitial spaces caused by seepage from the circulatory system, which results in the retention of about 10% more water than normal. Some of us may notice that if we eat meals that are particularly high in sodium, we may feel bloated and our weight may even rise a few pounds the next day. This weight gain is not true weight gain but simply water retention that occurs in response to the excess intake of sodium. Within a few days, weight and water levels in the body return to their usual levels.

Edema can be a symptom of a health risk in certain situations. Sodium-sensitive individuals not only retain fluid when consuming high levels of sodium but also experience an increase in blood pressure, leading to hypertension. Reducing excess water retention through a reduction in sodium consumption is a first step to treat this type of hypertension. A more serious form of edema occurs in victims of kwashiorkor when the protein levels in the body are so low that cellular fluid levels are imbalanced. Inappropriate levels of interstitial fluid accumulate in the stomach, face, and extremities.

Water intoxication refers to the consumption of large volumes of water within a short time. It causes muscle cramps, decreased blood pressure, and weakness. Water intoxication is possible if there is extensive loss of electrolytes because of dehydration, and rehydration is accomplished using only water, without the addition of replacement electrolytes. Generally, this condition tends to occur only among psychiatric patients who have lost the ability to respond to physiologic cues to stop drinking.

MINERALS

Minerals serve a variety of functions in our bodies. Structurally, minerals provide rigidity and strength to the teeth and skeleton; the skeletal mineral components also serve as a storage depot for other needs of the body. Minerals, allowing for proper muscle contraction and release, influence nerve and muscle functions. Other functions of minerals include acting as cofactors for enzymes and maintaining proper acid-base balance of body fluids. Minerals are also required for blood clotting and for tissue repair and growth. (The Cultural Considerations box, "A Chinese Study: Applicable to Americans?," discusses potential links between vitamin and mineral supplementation and decreased cancer incidence and mortality.)

Mineral Categories

Based on the amount of each mineral in the composition of our bodies, the 16 essential minerals are divided into two categories: major and trace minerals. To maintain body levels of major minerals, these minerals are needed daily from dietary sources in amounts of 100 mg or higher. In contrast, trace minerals are required daily in amounts less than or equal to 20 mg (Box 8-3). Although the required amounts differ greatly between the major and trace minerals, each is

fluid volume excess
the state in which a person experiences increased fluid retention and edema

edema
excess accumulation of fluid in interstitial spaces caused by seepage from the circulatory system

major minerals
essential nutrient minerals required daily in amounts of 100 mg or higher

trace minerals
essential nutrient minerals required daily in amounts less than or equal to 20 mg

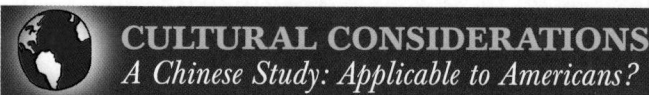

CULTURAL CONSIDERATIONS
A Chinese Study: Applicable to Americans?

*I*n Linxian, China, the death rate from esophageal cancer is 100 times higher than in the United States; other cancers are high as well. As a joint effort, the National Cancer Institute, Chinese Academy of Medicine Sciences, and Rutgers University conducted a study to assess the effects of vitamin/mineral combinations on decreasing cancer incidence and mortality. Thirty thousand subjects, ages 40 to 69, received supplements daily for 5 years. Doses ranged from one to two times the RDA for various nutrients. Results revealed that the risk of death was lower in groups receiving beta carotene, vitamin E, and selenium. The effects appeared 1 to 2 years after the start of supplementation and were significant for esophageal and gastric cancers.

Application to nursing: Are these results applicable to Americans? Yes and no. This prospective clinical trial supports primary disease prevention in a general population through the use of chemo-prevention (use of drugs to prevent disease).

However, the diets of the Chinese peasants studied were significantly different from the typical American's intake. The Chinese intake is low in fruits, meat, and other animal products. Even their average blood levels of vitamins and minerals are lower than those of Americans. Possible underlying deficiencies, not found in Westerners, may be responsible for the etiology of cancer and mortality rather than the effects of additional quantities of specific nutrients. Nonetheless, these results highlight the potential role of antioxidants in the reduction of disease and mortality.

References: Blot WJ et al.: Nutrition intervention trials in Linxian, China: supplementation with specific vitamin/mineral combinations, cancer incidence, and disease-specific mortality in the general population, J Nat Cancer Inst 85:1483, 1993; and Blumberg JB: Comment: nutrition intervention trials in Linxian, China: supplementation with specific vitamin/mineral combinations, cancer incidence, and disease-specific mortality in the general population. In Chernoff R, ed.: Persp Appl Nutr 1(3):31, Winter 1993.

absolutely necessary for good health. The dietary reference intakes (DRIs) listed in this chapter for minerals are those for young adults ages 19 to 24.[6] Levels for other groups are noted when special mention is needed. Keep in mind that because nutrition is a relatively young science, new functions of minerals as nutrients in the human body are still being discovered.

Food Sources

The prime sources of minerals include both plant and animal foods. Valuable sources of plant foods include most fruits, vegetables, legumes, and whole grains. Animal sources consist of beef, chicken, eggs, fish, and milk products. The discussions of individual minerals highlight the best food choices.

In contrast to vitamins, minerals are stable when foods containing them are cooked. As inorganic substances, they are indestructible. Minerals may leach into cooking fluids but are still able to be absorbed if the fluid is consumed.

Box 8-3 Essential Minerals in the Human Body

MAJOR	TRACE
Calcium	Chromium
Chloride	Copper
Magnesium	Fluoride
Phosphorus	Iodine
Potassium	Iron
Sodium	Manganese
Sulfur	Molybdenum
	Selenium
	Zinc

Although plants may contain an abundance of various minerals, some minerals in plants are not easily available to the human body. *Bioavailability* refers to the level of absorption of a consumed nutrient and is of nutritional concern. Binders such as phytic and oxalic acids may bind some minerals to the plant fiber structures. Binders are substances in plant foods that combine with minerals to form indigestible compounds, making them unavailable for our use. The amount of plant minerals available for absorption may depend on minerals in soils in which the plants are grown.

Minerals from animal foods do not have the same bioavailability issues. In fact, minerals from animal foods can be absorbed more easily than those from plants. However, fat content may be an issue for some animal foods. Lower fat sources of dairy and meat products are usually available and provide the same levels of minerals at a higher nutrient density. Liver is often cited as a good source of minerals such as iron and zinc. Liver is also high in cholesterol and saturated fats and may contain toxins to which the animal may have been exposed. These factors, combined with liver's somewhat unusual taste, often leaves the impression that good nutrient intake depends on eating healthy food that tastes bad. Other sources of each nutrient may be more appealing and equally as nutritious.

Food processing may reduce the amount of minerals available for absorption. Processing oranges into orange juice does not affect potassium levels naturally contained in oranges. However, processing whole wheat flour into white flour does cause significant losses of minerals because the whole grain is not used. Iron is the only mineral returned to white flour through enrichment; zinc, selenium, copper, and other minerals are permanently lost.

Because we have difficulty obtaining high enough levels of some minerals naturally, fortification of manufactured foods has become commonplace. It is in this manner that food processing can serve the nutrient needs of consumers while still addressing the issues of convenience and taste appeal. Salt fortified with iodine is available; dry cereals have added minerals such as iron and an assortment of vitamins and other minerals.

Minerals as Nutrients within the Body

Structure

Minerals are inorganic substances. As elements, they are found in the rocks of the earth. Their tendency to gain or lose electrons makes them electrically charged. Thus they have special affinities for water, which itself carries positive and negative charges. As we consume plant and animal foods containing minerals, we can incorporate them into our body structures (bones), organs, and fluids.

Digestion and Absorption

During the process of digestion, minerals (as inorganic substances) are separated from the foodstuff in which they entered our bodies. Digestion does change the valence states of some minerals, which changes their ability to be absorbed. However, their structure is not changed, to prepare them for absorption.

As noted earlier, bioavailability affects the level of minerals we actually absorb. Generally, consuming a variety of whole foods ensures an adequate intake of minerals. Mineral deficiencies for which Americans tend to be at risk are iron, calcium, and zinc. Concerns and strategies for consuming appropriate amounts of these nutrients are discussed later in this chapter.

Metabolism

Because minerals are inorganic and do not provide energy, they are not metabolized by the human body. Instead some minerals assist as cofactors of metabolic processes.

DRI = Dietary Reference Intakes

RDA = Recommended Dietary Allowance

AI = Adequate Intake

UL = Tolerable Upper Intake Level

parathormone
a hormone that raises blood calcium levels; secreted by the parathyroid gland in response to low blood calcium levels

calcitriol
active vitamin D hormone that raises blood calcium levels

calcitonin
a hormone that reacts in response to high blood levels of calcium; released by the Special C cells of the thyroid gland

calcium rigor
a condition of hardness or stiffness of muscles when blood calcium levels get too high

calcium tetany
a condition of spasms and nerve excitability when blood calcium levels get too low

MAJOR MINERALS

Calcium

Function

Calcium is the most abundant mineral in the body. Almost all of the calcium in the body, about 99%, is found in our bones, serving structural and storage functions. The other 1% of body calcium is released into body fluids when blood passes through bones; this constant interaction of blood with bone allows calcium to be distributed throughout the body. Other functions that depend on calcium include (1) function of the central nervous system, particularly nerve impulses; (2) muscle contraction and relaxation, when needed; (3) formation of blood clots; and (4) blood pressure regulation.

Regulation.   Our dietary intake of calcium influences the deposition of calcium in our bones. Blood calcium levels, however, do not depend on a daily dietary calcium intake. Instead the skeletal supply of calcium provides the source of calcium to be distributed throughout the body through the circulatory system. If calcium blood levels get too low, three actions can occur to reestablish calcium homeostasis: (1) bones release calcium, (2) intestines absorb more calcium, and (3) kidneys retain more calcium.

Hormones that regulate the level of calcium in body fluids control the release of calcium from bones. Hormones affecting blood levels include parathormone (parathyroid hormone), calcitriol (active vitamin D hormone), and calcitonin. Parathormone is secreted by the parathyroid gland in response to low blood calcium levels. It raises blood calcium levels by stimulating all three ways of providing calcium to body fluids. Vitamin D has a hormonelike effect as calcitriol and also increases blood calcium levels by acting on all three systems. The third hormone involved, calcitonin, is released by the Special C cells of the thyroid gland. Calcitonin reacts in response to high blood levels of calcium by lowering both calcium and phosphate in the blood.

Reactions of very low or extremely high blood levels could occur if regulatory mechanisms are hindered by a lack of vitamin D or hormone malfunction. If calcium blood levels get too high, calcium rigor (with symptoms of hardness or stiffness of muscles) may occur. Conversely, if levels are too low, a person may experience calcium tetany, with spasms caused by muscle and nerve excitability.

Recommended Intake and Sources

Calcium Adequate Intakes (AIs) for men and women range from 1300 mg (ages 9 through 13) to 1000 mg (ages 19 through 50). Levels increase to 1200 mg for men and women older than 50 years. The AI during pregnancy and lactation is 1000 mg.

Concerns have been raised regarding the calcium intake of those most at risk for deficiency—youths age 11 through 24 and pregnant and lactating women. During these times, calcium needs are still high, although actual consumption of calcium may decrease. To this end, *Healthy People 2010* proposes that 90% of the population of individuals age 2 and older meet these dietary recommendations.[3] For many Americans, this means increasing their number of servings of calcium-rich foods to at least three or more a day. Other issues surrounding calcium intake and children will be discussed in Chapter 12.

Primary sources of calcium are dairy products, mainly milk (whole, low fat, and skim) and milk-based products such as ice cream, ice milk, yogurt, frozen yogurt, cheeses, and puddings (Figure 8-3). Although butter, cream cheese, and cottage cheese are dairy products, they are not good sources of calcium; butter and cream cheese are predominately fat, and cottage cheese loses calcium through processing. Nondairy sources include green leafy vegetables (broccoli, kale, and mustard greens), small fish with bones (sardines and salmon canned with processed edible bones), legumes, and

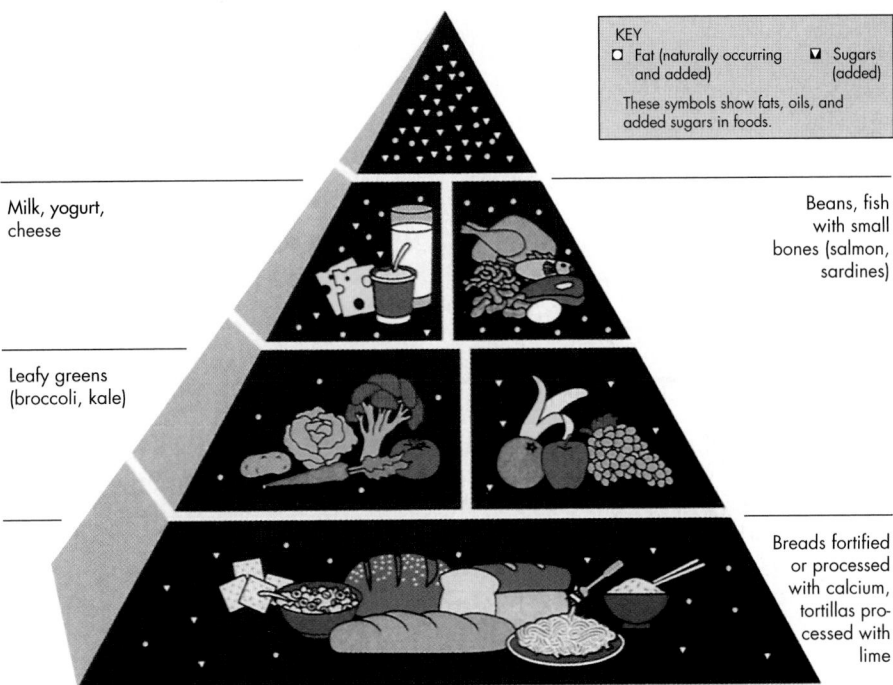

Figure 8-3 The Food Guide Pyramid, highlighting calcium-rich foods. (From US Department of Agriculture: *Human Nutrition Information Pub No 249*, Washington, DC, 1992, revised 1996, US Government Printing Office; www.usda.gov/fcs/cnpp.htm.)

tofu processed with calcium. In addition, a variety of calcium-fortified foods are available, ranging from fortified orange juice to bread products. Box 8-4 gives examples of foods that boost calcium intake, and the Teaching Tool box, "Visualizing the Calcium Values of Foods," provides education strategies for working with clients with low literacy skills.

Some leafy green vegetables, in particular spinach, collards, Swiss chard, and escarole, contain oxalic acid, a binder that reduces the calcium absorbed. Plant foods containing oxalic acid cannot be considered a trustworthy source of calcium. Tea contains oxalic acid as well as tannins (also found in coffee), both of which may affect the absorption of calcium in foods consumed with tea. With the increased consumption of iced tea beverages, this effect should be considered, particularly for female adolescents and young adults.

Box 8-4 Suggestions for Boosting Calcium Intake

DAIRY

Powdered milk added to baking mixes, soups, puddings, gravies, hamburgers, and meat loaves
Sliced apples and pears with cheese wedges
Broccoli with melted cheese
Soups made with low-fat or skim milk
Calcium-fortified milk
Smoothies (fruit drinks made with milk, yogurt, and fruits)

NONDAIRY

Bean soups (split pea or lentil soup)
Tofu (made with calcium carbonate), fresh or in frozen meals and desserts
Chicken cacciatore (chicken with bones cooked in tomato sauce; acid of tomatoes pulls calcium from bones)
Juices fortified with calcium
Bean burritos
Breads fortified with calcium

Food charts that show the calcium values of different foods may be helpful to most people. But these charts may be meaningless to clients who may not read English or who have minimal literacy skills. Consider this innovative teaching strategy for visualizing the calcium content of commonly consumed foods (e.g., skim milk, yogurt, hard cheese).

1. SELECT four calcium-rich foods and four low-calcium foods (e.g., cottage cheese, broccoli, pinto beans).
2. FILL plastic resealable bags with small marshmallows to represent the calcium content of each of the selected foods. Each marshmallow can represent 10 mg of calcium. In addition, fill a large plastic resealable bag with 100 marshmallows (1000 mg or 100% Daily Value) as a reference.
3. MATCH the bag of "calcium" with the appropriate food model (or picture). Have the participants do the matching.
4. DISTRIBUTE a pictorial representation of this activity with additional foods along with their bag of "calcium."

Used with permission of Gayle Coleman, MS, RD, Michigan State University Extension.

Some calcium supplements are poorly absorbed because they don't dissolve in the stomach. If a calcium tablet doesn't readily dissolve when stirred into cider vinegar, it probably will not dissolve in the body.

Many adults are lactose intolerant. Lactose intolerance occurs when the body does not produce enough lactase, an enzyme necessary for the digestion of lactose, the carbohydrate found in milk. (Lactose intolerance is detailed in Chapter 4.) Persons experiencing lactose intolerance need to regularly incorporate sources of calcium other than dairy products into their dietary patterns. For some people, calcium supplements may be indicated; a registered dietitian or qualified nutritionist may be consulted.

Absorption Factors. Our bodies absorb calcium based on physiologic need. During childhood growth phases, we may absorb up to 75% of calcium consumed, compared with absorption rates of 30% to 60% once we complete our prime growth years. Similarly, during pregnancy and lactation, percentages of absorption are higher based on physiologic need.[7] In addition to physiologic needs, other factors also seem to enhance the levels of calcium absorbed. They include the following:

- *Lactose.* Found naturally in milk (an excellent source of calcium), lactose appears to increase calcium absorption.
- *Sufficient vitamin D.* Vitamin D is involved in the synthesis of a protein that allows calcium to pass through the intestinal wall into the bloodstream.
- *Acidity of digestive mass.* Calcium is more soluble in acidic substances, so it is better absorbed when ingested as part of a meal. Generally, enough hydrochloric acid passes from the stomach to the intestine for calcium absorption. As we age, the amount of hydrochloric acid in digestive juices may decrease, causing less calcium to be absorbed.

Other factors may decrease calcium absorption. They include the following:

- *Binders.* Naturally occurring substances in plant foods may bind with calcium in plant foods; two common calcium binders previously mentioned are phytic and oxalic acids (also called *phytates* and *oxalates*). Human digestive processes may be unable to separate calcium from the binder; both are then excreted, reducing the calcium available for absorption.
- *Dietary fat.* Dietary fat can form insoluble soaps with calcium; the insoluble soaps are harder to digest, making calcium less accessible for absorption. Moderate and low dietary fat intakes discourage the formation of this insoluble mass.
- *High-fiber intake and laxatives.* Excessive fiber consumption or laxative abuse results in foodstuff moving through the GI tract too quickly for minerals, particularly calcium, to be absorbed.

FACTORS FAVORING CALCIUM ABSORPTION

Body's need for higher amounts (as in pregnancy), lactose, sufficient vitamin D, acidity of digestive mass

FACTORS HINDERING CALCIUM ABSORPTION

Binders such as phytic acid and oxalic acid, dietary fat, dietary fiber, excessive phosphorus intake, aging, laxatives, sedentary lifestyle, drugs

- *Excessively high intakes of phosphorus or magnesium.* Excessively high intakes of these minerals disturb the balance of calcium in the body. Calcium is best absorbed when moderate or recommended levels of phosphorus and magnesium are ingested in proportion to calcium intake.
- *Sedentary lifestyle.* Being a couch potato has its consequences. A physically inactive lifestyle leads to less bone density. In contrast, weight-bearing exercise that pulls the muscle against the bone enhances calcium deposits in the bone matrix. This action occurs during running, brisk walking, biking, and strength training.
- *Drugs.* Some medications, including anticonvulsants, tetracycline, cortisone, thyroxine, and aluminum-containing antacids, are associated with reduced calcium absorption.

Deficiency

Deficiency of calcium primarily affects bone health. During the growing years, inadequate intake of calcium reduces the density of bone mass and, if severe, can stunt growth.

For adults, long-term calcium deficiency may be one of the risk factors of *osteoporosis,* a multifactorial disorder. This condition takes many years to develop, and overt symptoms appear late in life. Osteoporosis is a condition in which bone density is reduced and the remaining bone is brittle and breaks easily.

One of the most recognizable characteristics of osteoporosis is the dowager's hump; as vertebrae in the spine collapse from weakness, the spine is no longer able to support the weight of the head. The back bows and the head becomes angled down. Most significantly, the internal organs affected by the curvature are unable to function efficiently and other health difficulties develop.

In contrast to *osteomalacia,* osteoporosis is multifactorial and all the factors are tied to bone mineral density. These factors include genetics, diet, and lifestyle determinants.[8] Bone density builds through early adulthood. Peak bone density is reached by about age 20, although some additional bone mineralization continues into the 30s.[1] The more density built early in life, the less potential risk encountered. Factors that affect bone density but cannot be modified include genetic determinants of race, gender, and family history.[8]

- *Race.* Osteoporosis is more common in Caucasian and Asian women than among African and African American women. This is because of racial differences in the skeletal density, possibly caused by hormonal differences.
- *Gender.* Men have greater bone density than women. They enter the later years when bone demineralization begins with a larger storage of calcium. The fact that men have more lean body mass or muscularity may cause more calcium to be deposited and retained in comparison with women. Women lose greater amounts of bone calcium during the first few years after menopause. The drop in estrogen levels appears to initiate the calcium loss. To slow the loss and to provide additional protection against heart disease, many primary healthcare providers prescribe hormone (estrogen) replacement therapy for postmenopausal women.

Osteoporosis, however, does occur in men and women. For men, osteoporosis tends to be a result of secondary causes that affect peak bone mass development or speed the loss of bone density. These causes may include steroid therapy, hypogonadism, skeletal metastasis, multiple myeloma, gastric surgery, and anticonvulsant treatment.[9] Men and women who undergo organ transplants are more at risk for osteoporosis, particularly during the first year after surgery. The loss of bone density is probably caused by the medications used to prevent organ rejection, such as glucocorticoids, that disturb bone and mineral homeostasis.

Osteoporosis prevention can begin before transplantation if bone density is marginal, or therapy can be implemented immediately following transplantation. Rates are lowest among patients receiving kidney transplants and highest among those receiving liver transplants.[10]

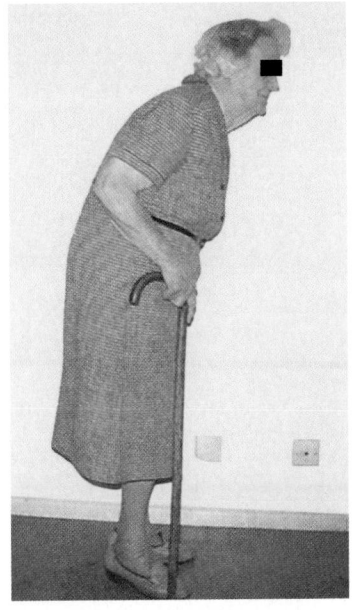

Typical posture in osteoporosis. (From Shipley M: *A colour atlas of rheumatology,* ed 3, London, 1993, Mosby-Year Book Europe Limited. By permission of Mosby International Ltd.)

- *Family history.* A predisposition to lower bone density may be genetically passed between generations, particularly from mother to daughter. If a close family member develops osteoporosis, care should be taken to reduce the effects of other risk factors.

Factors related to development of osteoporosis that can be adjusted include nutrition, particularly calcium intake, and lifestyle determinants.

- *Nutrition/calcium intake.* Dietary calcium intake is of concern throughout the life span. In particular, the growth years (when calcium is deposited in the bone matrix) and the postmenopause years of bone mineralization loss are the periods when calcium intake appears crucial. Although the AI for calcium provides sufficient amounts, many individuals consume less than these levels. Female adolescents often consume levels of kcalories and nutrients well below the AI while attempting to control body weight. These eating patterns often continue through adulthood. This long-term marginal deficiency of calcium may set the stage for future bone disorders. The issue is even more complicated for older adults. When they consume calcium-containing foods, less calcium may be absorbed because of decreased gastric acidity and reduced levels of available vitamin D.

  For others, the risk may be related to genes. A specific gene appears to predispose individuals to absorb less calcium. Changes occur in receptor sites for vitamin D, reducing the availability and functioning of vitamin D in relation to maintaining bone density.[11] It is not yet known what sets off the changes in the receptor sites.

- *Alcohol.* Long-term excessive intake of alcohol appears to reduce bone density. Alcohol may directly depress bone formation or may take the place of more nutritious foods, producing marginal deficiencies.

- *Smoking.* Cigarette smoking has been associated with a higher risk of osteoporosis. Smokers tend to be of lower weight (less bone density) than nonsmokers and appear to lose more bone mineralization after menopause.

- *Caffeine.* Caffeine consumption has been tied to urinary excretion of calcium. Reasonable use of caffeinated beverages, however, may be acceptable.[12] More than likely, the relationship of caffeine to lower levels of body calcium concerns caffeinated beverages that replace those containing calcium such as skim milk. One study found that although caffeinated coffee consumption affected bone density of postmenopausal women, one glass of skim milk per day overcame the effects of the coffee.[13] A recent study showed that consuming dietary caffeine regularly did not affect bone mineral density of the hip or of the total body.[14]

- *Sedentary lifestyle.* As noted earlier, a physically active lifestyle not only enhances calcium absorption but also helps to maintain bone matrix mineralization. However, excessive exercise that results in extremely low body fat levels for women may be detrimental to bone density. If amenorrhea (abnormal cessation of menses) occurs because of excessive exercise, the resulting premature drop in estrogen may limit or decrease bone mineralization during the prime growth periods. Similarly, women with a smaller body size, including those experiencing anorexia nervosa, may have a greater risk of hip fracture later in life compared with those of larger body size.[15] Although no standards have been determined, it is likely that a body mass index (BMI) greater than 26-28 may provide reduced risk, whereas a lower BMI of less than 22-24 increases the risk of osteoporosis.[16]

Although the risk factors for osteoporosis may seem overwhelming, several can be reduced by following basic recommendations for achieving wellness. By consuming the serving amounts recommended on the Food Guide Pyramid and engaging in regular physical exercise, most of the risk can be minimized. See the Teaching Tool box, "Calcium: By Any Means Possible," for tips on educating clients on appropriate calcium intake.

Low levels of calcium intake have also been associated with an increased risk of colon cancer and hypertension.

TEACHING TOOL
Calcium: By Any Means Possible

*T*he Adequate Intake (AI) for calcium ranges from 1000 mg to 1300 mg, depending on a person's age. The best sources are calcium-rich foods. But what if a client is lactose-intolerant or just doesn't like many calcium-containing foods?

Because the potential ramifications of chronic calcium deficiency are serious—fractures and other complications of osteoporosis—calcium supplementation may be appropriate. Here are some suggestions and cautions for client education:

- Calcium supplementation may increase the dietary intake of calcium, but it does not alleviate other risk factors associated with osteoporosis. Other nutrients and lifestyle behaviors also affect the level of risk. Popping a calcium pill does not mean a person is osteoporosis-free.
- Many people have problems with compliance; the regularity of calcium intake, not an occasional dose, builds dense bones. It is better to rely on food sources.
- The source of calcium affects the amount of actual calcium available. Tablets composed of calcium carbonate contain more elemental calcium (often 500 to 600 mg) than those made of calcium citrate or lactate (usually 200 mg per tablet), and it takes fewer pills to achieve the AI. Calcium citrate, however, is more easily absorbed by the digestive tract, even if more pills are needed.
- Be aware that calcium is always combined with another substance to form the tablet. A tablet may contain 1200 mg of calcium carbonate but only 500 mg of elemental calcium. The supplements to avoid are those made from dolomite, bone meal, and oyster shell; they may be contaminated with lead and other toxic metals.
- Although the tablets are supplementing dietary intake, it's best to take them with meals. The acid of the digestive process also helps in the breakdown and absorption of the calcium tablet(s), and tying the supplement to meals works as a reminder system. This also helps to spread supplementation throughout the day. One large dose will not be absorbed as well as two or three smaller doses.
- Calcium supplements often contain added vitamin D. The new vitamin D recommendation doubles after age 50 and triples after age 70, so that the added vitamin D may be age appropriate. If other sources provide sufficient amounts of vitamin D, such as from multivitamin/mineral supplements or from foods or cereals fortified with 100% of the Daily Value for vitamin D, then the added D is not necessary.
- Before supplementing, keep track of sources and amounts of dietary calcium for several days. Intake may be adequate. If not, first contemplate ways to increase intake with foods, then consider supplementation.

Toxicity

Calcium toxicity from consuming foods that contain calcium is not a concern. Problems may occur when supplements of calcium and other nutrients are used instead of foods. Over-supplementation may cause constipation, urinary stone formation that affects kidney function, and reduced absorption of iron, zinc, and other minerals.[7] The general guideline for calcium supplements is that levels should not exceed the AI for calcium. In addition, a UL of 2500 mg has been established.

Phosphorus

Function

Most of the phosphorus in the body (85%) is in our bones and teeth as a component of hydroxyapatite. The other 15% of body phosphorus has functions (1) in energy transfer; (2) as part of the genetic material of deoxyribonucleic acid (DNA) and ribonucleic acid (RNA); (3) as a buffer in the form of phosphoric acid, which balances body acid-base levels; and (4) as a component of phospholipids used for transportation and structural functions.

hydroxyapatite
a natural mineral structure of bones and teeth

Recommended Intake and Sources

The RDA for phosphorus is 700 mg for men and women age 19 years and older. Phosphorus is widely available in foods. Particularly good sources are protein-rich foods such as dairy foods, eggs, meat, fish, poultry, and cereal grains. Because of the processing of convenience foods and soft drinks, both are also sources of phosphorus.

Deficiency

Deficiency of phosphorus is unknown. It is part of the genetic material of every cell of the body.

Toxicity

Excessive amounts of phosphorus, usually only possible from phosphorus supplements, cause calcium excretion from the body. Very high phosphorus intakes could affect the calcium/phosphorus ratio, possibly reducing the amount of calcium absorbed. This is a problem only if calcium intake is inadequate. Because phosphorus-containing soft drinks and convenience foods have replaced milk beverages and less processed foods for many American teens and adult women, this may be a dietary concern. A UL of 4000 mg has been determined for phosphorus.

Magnesium

Function

As with calcium and phosphorus, most of the magnesium in the body is found in our bones, providing structural and storage functions. Magnesium assists hundreds of enzymes throughout the body. It also regulates nerve and muscle function, including the actions of the heart, and has a role in the blood clotting process and in the immune system.

Recommended Intake and Sources

The RDAs for magnesium are 420 mg for men and 320 mg for women. Many commonly eaten foods contain magnesium. Particularly good sources are most unprocessed foods including whole grains, legumes, broccoli, leafy green vegetables, and other vegetables. Hard water can be a significant source of magnesium.

Deficiency

Magnesium deficiency tends to be related to secondary causes, rather than to a primary lack of magnesium consumption. These secondary causes may include excessive vomiting and diarrhea caused by pathologic conditions. A GI tract disorder may affect magnesium absorption, or kidney disease may inhibit retention of the mineral. Malnutrition and alcoholism may also have a negative impact on magnesium levels in the body. Similarly, drug interference or artificial feeding solutions deficient in magnesium may influence total body levels of magnesium. Whenever body fluids are lost, so is magnesium. Individuals on long-term regimens of diuretics are also potentially at risk for deficiency. In addition, if magnesium intake levels are borderline and intake of calcium is high, such as from calcium supplements, magnesium absorption may be limited.

Symptoms of magnesium deficiency include twitching of muscles, muscle weakness, and convulsions. In children, magnesium deficiency may also be associated with growth failure.

Toxicity

Toxic effects of magnesium have not been studied or observed, but a UL of 350 mg, from supplemental sources, has been set.

Sulfur

Function

Sulfur is a component of protein structures. It is present in every cell of the body and is part of several amino acids, thiamin, and biotin. Sulfur is also involved with maintaining the acid-base balance of the body.

Recommended Intake and Sources

No DRI has been established for sulfur. Diets adequate in protein provide sufficient amounts of sulfur. Sulfur is found in all protein-containing foods.

Deficiency

Deficiencies of sulfur do not occur; sulfur is so basic to the structure of the human cell that deficiencies cannot develop.

Toxicity

Toxicity to sulfur is not a health issue.

ELECTROLYTES: SODIUM, POTASSIUM, AND CHLORIDE

Sodium, potassium, and chloride are major electrolytes of the body. As electrolytes, these minerals serve specific functions. The acid-base balance of body fluids depends on regulated distribution of these minerals, proteins, and other electrolytes. Electrolytes also have a role in the normal functioning of nerves and muscles. In addition, each mineral serves other specific functions in the body.

Sodium

Function

Sodium performs a variety of important functions in the body. Blood pressure and volume are maintained by the characteristics of sodium as the major cation in extracellular fluid. Transmission of nerve impulses relies on body sodium levels. As the major extracellular electrolyte, sodium has a role in the regulation of body fluid levels in and out of cells. This movement affects blood volume as well, which is tied to the thirst mechanism and total body fluid levels. The blood proteins, such as albumin, that prevent the development of some types of edema, also regulate blood volume.

Recommended Intake and Sources

There is no DRI for sodium. Instead, estimated minimum requirements (EMR) have been set for sodium and for the other electrolytes. This dietary recommendation is based on the known minimum intake required for good health. It also acknowledges that it is not possible to determine disadvantages to consumption of large amounts of these nutrients except in particular circumstances discussed under toxicities. The EMR for sodium is 500 mg for adults, or about 1/4 teaspoon.

Health-related associations have set guidelines for appropriate and safe levels of sodium. The National Research Council Recommendations and *Healthy People 2010* Nutrition Objective 10 suggest limiting daily salt intake to less than 6 g; this equals 2400 mg of sodium (Figure 8-4).[3] As a guideline, a teaspoon of salt (approximately 2 g) contains 800 mg of sodium.

Most sodium enters our diet as sodium chloride (table salt). Sodium occurs naturally in many foods. It is also added to foods as salt during the cooking process

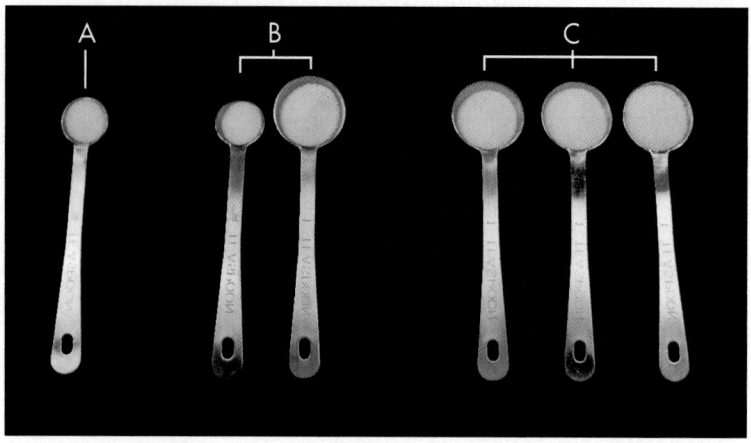

Figure 8-4 Daily salt intakes: **A**, minimum (1/4 tsp salt: 500 mg sodium); **B**, maximum (1 1/4 tsp salt: 2400 mg sodium); and, **C**, typical (3 tsp salt: 6000 mg sodium). (From Joanne Scott/Tracy McCalla.)

and right before consumption (see the Cultural Considerations box, "A (Cooking) History of Salt"). Processing of foods, particularly quick-serve foods, often adds substantial amounts of sodium (Box 8-5 and the Myth box, "Sodium Comes Only from the Salt Shaker"). Processed foods are carriers for other additives that often contain sodium. The sodium adds flavor that may be lost in processing.

Deficiency

Depletion of sodium can develop through dehydration or excessive diarrhea. Because of concern over the relationship between sodium and hypertension, some people may overly restrict sodium and thus be at risk. Typical athletic activity or physical labor that produces excessive sweating may cause dehydration and loss of sodium, but drinking fluids and consuming foods soon restore body levels of sodium. Salt tablets, once a common remedy, are not recommended and may be dangerous.

Symptoms of sodium deficiency include headache, muscle cramps, weakness, reduced ability to concentrate, and loss of memory and appetite. It is rare for sodium

 CULTURAL CONSIDERATIONS
A (Cooking) History of Salt

The course of history has been influenced by salt. Nations explored the world in search of salt because of its value in preserving foods. Bacterial and mold cells are inhibited from growing when placed in a concentrated salt solution. This decreases food spoilage. Though salt is no longer needed to preserve foods, we continue to value its ability to transform the taste of a dish from bland to sublime. Salt's importance to the human body cannot be denied because we have specialized taste buds to identify its consumption. Salt as a compound of sodium chloride contains two essential minerals without which the human body cannot survive.

Recognition of the importance of salt to human life began early. In the Old Testament of the Bible, salt was identified as an offering to God. Later on, Roman soldiers were given a stipend, called *salarium,* to buy salt. Today we can buy salt with our "salaries," a term that is derived from *salarium.* "Salt of the earth" was a phrase used by Jesus to describe his followers who were pure and of the earth.

Application to nursing: Although salt has its virtues, it also has drawbacks. Health professionals continue to recommend moderate intakes of sodium to reduce the risk of hypertension. The amounts recommended for cooking vary because an amount that is pleasing to one person may differ for another. Amounts of salt listed in a recipe can usually be modified to suit the health and taste requirements of the cook and the eaters.

References: McGee H: On food and cooking: the science and lore of the kitchen, *New York, 1997, Firestone;* and O'Neill M: *Let it pour,* New York Times Magazine, *p. 77, Oct 22, 1995.*

Box 8-5 Processing Effects on Food Sodium Content

POTATOES

Baked potato (1)	16 mg
French-fried potatoes (10 strips)	108 mg
Scalloped potatoes from dry mix (1 cup)	835 mg

CHICKEN

Baked chicken (3 oz)	64 mg
Batter-fried chicken (3 oz)	231 mg
Chicken nuggets (6 pieces)	542 mg

OATS

Oatmeal prepared with water (1 cup)	2 mg
Oatmeal bread (1 slice)	124 mg
Ready-to-eat oat cereal (1 cup)	307 mg

APPLES

Apple (1)	Trace
Applesauce (1 cup)	8 mg
Apple pie (1 slice)	476 mg

Data from Pennington JAT: Bowes & Church's food values of portions commonly used, *ed 17, Philadelphia, 1998, Lippincott-Raven; and* Nutrient Data Laboratory, *www.nal.usda.gov/fnic/foodcomp/.*

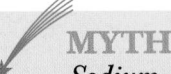

MYTH
Sodium Comes Only from the Salt Shaker

𝒟o you salt your food first, and then taste it? Some habits are hard to break but are worth the effort. However, breaking the salt shaker habit will reduce sodium intake only 15% for most Americans; most of the sodium we eat comes from processed foods.

The more a foodstuff is processed, the higher the sodium content becomes. More nutrients are also lost along the way. Which is saltier, or to be more exact, which contains more sodium—a bowl of corn flakes or a large order of fast-food fries? The corn flakes win, containing 290 mg of sodium compared with 200 mg for the fries. Of course, the fries contain a lot more fat and calories.

Consider the potato. A plain baked potato contains only 16 mg of sodium. Fixed up at a local fast-food restaurant, a baked potato with cheese sauce and broccoli skyrockets to more than 400 mg of sodium and a lot of fat. A cheese or sour cream mix prepared at home is even higher in sodium—close to 600 mg. The sodium in plain mashed potatoes from a mix (dehydrated and then reconstituted) jumps from 8 mg in its original whole form to over 300 mg, and that's without butter or gravy. The point is that processing foods adds invisible sodium as sodium chloride; in fact it's so invisible that we can no longer taste the saltiness.

Sodium enjoys widespread use in the American diet as a flavoring agent (sodium chloride, monosodium glutamate [MSG], sodium saccharin), dough conditioner (baking powder, baking soda), and preservative (sodium sulfite). Because of consumer demand, lower sodium versions of many products are available. Nutrition labeling information must include sodium content. This is powerful information that allows us to compare the sodium content of similar products.

References: Pennington JAT: Bowes & Church's food values of portions commonly used, *ed 17, Philadelphia, 1998, Lippincott; and Liebman B:* The salt shake out, *Nutrition Action Health Letter 21(2):1, 5, 1994.*

deficiency to occur because we get enough sodium naturally from foods. These symptoms are similar to those of fluid volume deficit, which is more common.

Toxicity

An excess sodium intake is difficult for the body to handle. The kidneys have the primary responsibility to flush out the excess sodium. Some individuals are sodium sensitive and may develop hypertension and edema in response to high intake of sodium. Levels consumed in diets based on highly processed foods and high-sodium foods may be enough to initiate hypertension in sodium-sensitive individuals. Although others may not experience negative ramifications from high-sodium intakes, there are no benefits either. This is one of the few nutrients that we can overdose on from foods consumed.

An occasional very salty meal may produce edema but not hypertension. The best remedy for occasional edema is simply to drink more water to equalize the sodium concentration of body fluids. The kidneys take care of the rest by filtering out the excess sodium.

Potassium

Function

Although sodium as a cation maintains the fluid levels extracellularly, potassium, as the primary intercellular cation, maintains fluid levels inside the cells. Potassium is also crucial for normal functioning of nerves and muscles, including the heart.

Recommended Intake and Sources

The EMR for potassium is 2000 mg. Whole unprocessed foods, particularly bananas, oranges, and other fruits, vegetables, dairy products, meats, and legumes are good sources of potassium.

Deficiency

Similar to magnesium deficiency, potassium deficiency may be caused by dehydration from vomiting or diarrhea, diuretics, and misuse of laxatives. If long-term use of diuretics is warranted to reduce edema associated with hypertension, particular attention should be paid to consuming adequate levels of potassium from foods. Some diuretics are potassium wasting; some are potassium sparing. Supplementation when using a potassium-sparing diuretic could be dangerous. Potassium supplements should be taken only when prescribed by a primary healthcare provider.

Symptoms associated with potassium deficiency include muscle weakness, confusion, loss of appetite and, in severe cases, cardiac arrhythmias.

Toxicity

In general, potassium toxicity occurs only from supplements, not from consuming excess from foods. Toxicity doesn't usually occur with foods as long as a person has properly functioning kidneys. For individuals with renal disease, high-potassium foods are toxic. Even patients on dialysis may still be at risk for potassium toxicity. Symptoms of toxicity are similar to those of a deficiency. They include muscle weakness, vomiting and, at excessively high levels, cardiac arrest.

Chloride

Function

As the key anion of extracellular fluids, chloride assists in maintaining fluid balance inside and outside cells. In addition, chloride is a component of hydrochloric acid, an indispensable gastric juice produced by the stomach.

Recommended Intake and Sources

The EMR for chloride is 750 mg for adults. This requirement is easily met by consumption of sodium chloride; foods that provide sodium usually provide chloride as well.

Deficiency

Deficiency of chloride is rare; adequate amounts are easily consumed. Although deficiency is possible, it would occur from the same circumstances as sodium deficiency or from excessive vomiting.

Toxicity

Chloride toxicity may occur because of dehydration, causing an imbalance of chloride to the other electrolytes. However, the other effects of dehydration are more severe than those of chloride toxicity.

Table 8-1 provides a summary of the major minerals.

Table 8-1
Major Minerals

Mineral	Function	Clinical Issues Deficiency/Toxicity	Recommended Intakes*	Food Sources	Absorption Issues
Calcium (Ca)	Bone and tooth formation; blood clotting; muscle contraction/relaxation; CNS; blood pressure	Deficiency: reduced bone density; osteoporosis Toxicity: constipation; urinary stones; reduced iron and zinc absorption	AI Adults: 1000-1200 mg Pregnancy/lactation: 1000 mg UL 2500 mg	Milk (whole, low-fat, skim), milk-based products, green leafy vegetables, legumes	Absorption based on need: increased by vitamin D; decreased by binders, inactivity coffee/tea
Phosphorus (P)	Bone and tooth formation (component of hydroxyapatite); energy metabolism (enzymes); acid-base balance	Deficiency: rare Toxicity: increased calcium excretion	RDA Adults: 700 mg Pregnancy/lactation: 700 mg UL 4000 mg	Dairy foods, egg, meat, fish, poultry	Absorbed with calcium
Magnesium (Mg)	Structure/storage; cofactor; nerve and muscle function; blood clotting	Deficiency: secondary with muscle twitching, weakness, convulsions from FVD	RDA Men: 420 mg Women: 320 mg Pregnancy/lactation: 320-360 mg UL 350 mg	Whole grains, legumes, green leafy vegetables (broccoli), hard water	
Sulfur (S)	Component of protein structures	Deficiency: only if protein malnourished	Protein-adequate diets contain adequate levels	Protein-containing foods	

*Ages 19-30.

AI, Adequate Intake; CNS, central nervous system; EMR, Estimated Minimum Requirement; FVD, fluid volume deficit; RDA, Recommended Dietary Allowance.

Continued

Table 8-1
Major Minerals—cont'd

Mineral	Function	Clinical Issues Deficiency/Toxicity	Recommended Intakes	Food Sources	Absorption Issues
Sodium (Na)	Major extracellular electrolyte for fluid regulation; body fluid levels; acid-base balance; nerve impulse and contraction; blood pressure/volume	Deficiency: FVD with headache; muscle cramps, weakness, decreased concentration, memory and appetite loss Toxicity: sodium-sensitive hypertension	EMR Adults: 500 mg	Table salt; naturally in many foods; processed foods	
Potassium (K)	Major intracellular electrolyte for fluid regulation; muscle function	Deficiency: muscle weakness, confusion, decreased appetite, cardiac arrhythmias caused by FVD from vomiting/diarrhea or diuretics Toxicity: from diet or supplements if renal disease present	EMR Adults: 2000 mg	Unprocessed foods, fruits, vegetables, dairy products, meats, legumes	
Chloride (Cl)	Acid-base balance; gastric hydrochloric acid for digestion	Deficiency: FVD caused by vomiting/diarrhea	EMR Adults: 750 mg	Table salt	

AI, Adequate Intake; CNS, central nervous system; EMR, Estimated Minimum Requirement; FVD, fluid volume deficit; RDA, Recommended Dietary Allowance.

DRI = Dietary Reference Intakes

RDA = Recommended Dietary Allowance

AI = Adequate Intake

UL = Tolerable Upper Intake Level

hemoglobin
oxygen-transporting protein in red blood cells

myoglobin
oxygen-transporting protein in muscle

TRACE MINERALS

Trace minerals as a group of nutrients function primarily as cofactors by performing metabolic and transport functions.

Iron

Function

Iron is responsible for distributing oxygen throughout our bodies. Oxygen depends on the iron in hemoglobin of red blood cells (erythrocytes) to bring oxygen to all cells. Myoglobin holds oxygen in the muscle cells for quick use when needed. Because of its ability to change ionic charges, iron also assists enzymes in the use of oxygen by all cells of the body.

Iron is conserved and recycled by the body. When red blood cells are old or damaged, the spleen removes their iron component. Some iron is kept in the spleen for later use, and the rest is sent to the liver for processing. From the liver, iron is transported as transferrin to bone marrow and recycled for use in new red blood cells. Some iron is lost through the shedding of tissue cells in urine and sweat and when bleeding occurs; this lost iron must be replaced by dietary sources.

Recommended Intake and Sources

The RDA for iron is one of the few that is higher for females than for males. When red blood cells break down, the iron in the hemoglobin is recycled to the liver and used to form new red blood cells. Whenever blood is lost from the body, iron is lost as well and cannot be recycled. Internal bleeding, such as from acute ulcers, can be a deceptive cause of iron loss. More obvious is the loss of blood by women from menstruation. Based on this monthly loss and the increased iron demands of pregnancy, women's overall need for iron is higher than men's. The RDA for men is 8 mg and 18 mg for women. During pregnancy the requirement is 27 mg; the blood supply of a pregnant woman is 1.5 times greater than her normal level.

The RDA allows for the unusual absorption rate of dietary iron. Only about 10% to 15% of dietary iron consumed is absorbed; this amount increases up to 20% if body levels are deficient. Higher percentages are absorbed during pregnancy and during periods of growth.

Intestinal mucosal cells contain two proteins that assist in absorption of dietary iron. One protein, *mucosal transferrin*, moves iron to a protein carrier in blood transferrin. This allows for the movement of iron through blood to bone marrow and tissues as needed. The second, *mucosal ferritin*, stores iron in the mucosal cells as a reserve if iron is needed. If not used, mucosal cells are replaced every few days so a continuous short-term supply of iron is available.

The RDA is also set to provide adequate storage levels of iron in the liver; iron is also stored in the spleen and bone marrow. In these organs, iron is contained in the proteins ferritin and hemosiderin. Ferritin is always being made and is easily available as an iron source. Hemosiderin is made when iron levels are high. Although it is a source of iron, its availability from storage to be used by the body takes longer than ferritin.

Iron is found in both plant and animal sources (Figure 8-5). Heme iron, found in animal sources of meat, fish, and poultry, is more easily absorbed than nonheme iron found in plant foods. Animal sources of iron also contain nonheme iron in ad-

heme iron
dietary iron found in animal foods of meat, fish, and poultry

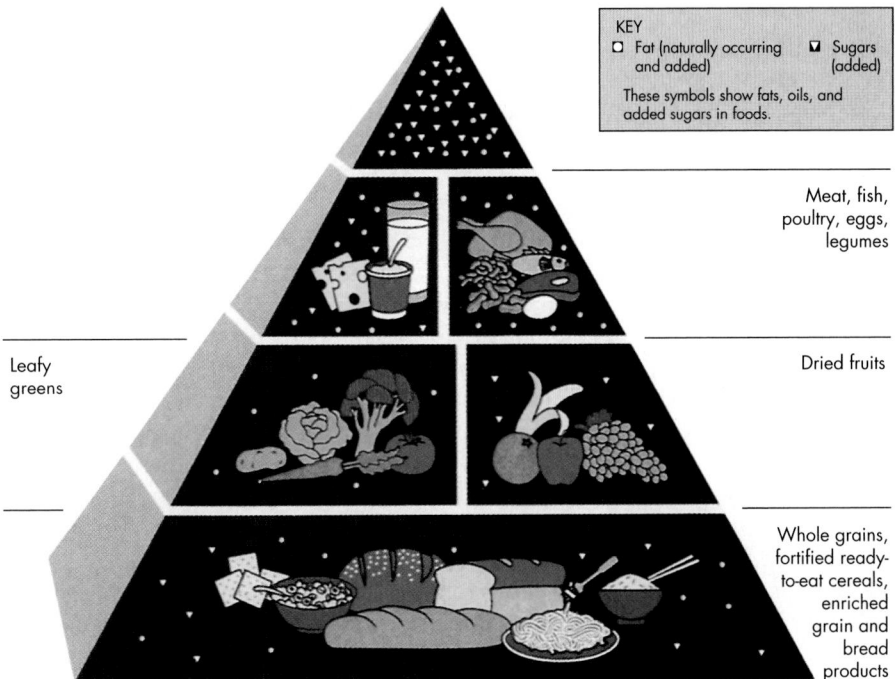

Figure 8-5   The Food Guide Pyramid, highlighting iron-rich foods. (From US Department of Agriculture: *Human Nutrition Information Pub No 249*, Washington, DC, 1992, revised 1996, US Government Printing Office; www.usda.gov/fcs/cnpp.htm.)

nonheme iron
dietary iron found in plant foods

Another way to increase dietary iron intake is to cook foods in cast iron skillets. Iron in the skillet leaches into the foods, providing an easy means for boosting iron intake.

dition to heme iron. Although egg yolks contain iron, the iron is not absorbed as well as other heme sources. **Nonheme iron** sources include vegetables, legumes, dried fruits, whole grain cereals, and enriched grain products, especially iron-fortified dry cereals.

Increased absorption of iron occurs when dietary sources are consumed with foods containing ascorbic acid (vitamin C). For example, drinking orange juice or eating slices of cantaloupe with meals increases the amount of nonheme iron absorbed.[17] Absorption of nonheme iron increases in the presence of heme iron. This means that consuming iron from several sources improves absorption of the total iron amounts of heme and nonheme iron.

Factors that inhibit iron absorption include consumption of foods that contain binders (e.g., phytates) and oxalates that keep the dietary iron from separating from plant sources. Tannins in plants, most notably in teas and coffee, can also interfere with iron absorption. Continuous use of antacids and excessive intake of other minerals competes with the absorption sites for iron. Pica, the consumption of nonnutritive substances, creates health problems. When the nonnutritive substances are excreted from the body, minerals are also excreted, which decreases mineral absorption. Pica is discussed in the next section.

Deficiency

Iron deficiency has been a public health problem for many years. Although the incidence has decreased in the United States, most likely because of increased fortification, it is still common for iron deficiency and iron deficiency anemia to occur among young children, teenage girls, and women of childbearing ages. These disorders are more common among minority women of low income who have had many children.[18] In other parts of the world, it is still the most widespread nutrient deficiency, primarily in the developing world.[19] Children and women of childbearing age are most at risk. The effects of iron deficiency can be subtle and may be assigned to other causes. A range of symptoms accompanies different degrees of deficiency. All levels of iron deficiency affect the availability of oxygen throughout the body.

Iron deficiency occurs when there is reduced supply of iron stores available in the liver. If neither the diet nor body stores can supply the iron needed for hemoglobin synthesis, the number of red blood cells decreases in the bloodstream. The blood hemoglobin concentration also falls. When both the percentage of red blood cells (called *hematocrit*) and the hemoglobin level fall, a healthcare provider should suspect iron deficiency.

In severe deficiency, the hemoglobin and hematocrit levels fall so low that the amount of oxygen carried in the blood is decreased and the person is pale, tired, and anemic. Iron deficiency anemia is characterized by microcytes or small, pale red blood cells. Physical activity or work may be difficult to perform because not enough oxygen is available for use by the muscles. Cognitive functioning is compromised. For children, developmental delays and learning problems may develop; an iron-deficient child is easily distracted and unable to focus on learning tasks. A person may have a sensation of always feeling cold, as if body temperature cannot be regulated appropriately. The immune system is compromised as well, reflected in decreased wound-healing ability. During pregnancy, iron deficiency anemia caused by inadequate dietary intake is associated with greater risk of premature delivery and low birth weight.[20]

Because infants have received more iron during the past 3 years, a decline in iron deficiency anemia among American children has occurred. However, prevalence has remained constant among women of childbearing ages. Recent Centers for Disease Control and Prevention (CDC) recommendations were established for use by primary healthcare providers to prevent, detect, and treat iron deficiency. The guidelines focus on adequate iron nutrition for infants and young children, screening for anemia among women of childbearing age, and the value of low-dose iron supplements for pregnant women.[21] Nutrition Objectives 11 and 12 of *Healthy People 2010* also support the recommendations of the CDC to reduce the iron deficiency among these at-risk-groups.[3]

A form of anemia called *sports anemia* occurs among endurance athletes. As the body adapts to aerobic development from intense exercise, the individual's volume of blood expands. This expansion lowers hemoglobin concentration, producing an appearance of anemia. This condition, however, is not an illness but a positive adaptation of the body.

To alleviate iron deficiency, the cause of the deficiency (either internal loss of blood or lack of dietary intake) needs to be addressed. Children may lack sufficient intake of iron foods. Toddlers may develop iron-deficiency anemia from drinking too much milk, a poor source of iron, which fills them up and keeps them from eating other iron-containing foods. Women tend to be doubly at risk because of dieting habits and female physiology. Chronic dieting may affect the intake of iron-rich foods; loss of blood through menses and the high iron demands of pregnancy combine to greatly increase female iron requirements. The recent increased consumption of iced tea as a popular soft drink may also affect women's iron levels. The tannin in tea reduces iron absorption. For adults in the United States, iron deficiency is rarely caused by dietary deficiency; instead, it usually results from the blood loss of menstrual bleeding or internal bleeding in the GI tract, perhaps from bleeding ulcers or hemorrhoids.

An unusual behavior associated with iron deficiency is pica. Pica is characterized by a hunger and appetite for nonfood substances including ice, cornstarch, clay, and even dirt. These substances contain no iron and may even lead to loss of additional minerals, particularly when clay and dirt are consumed. Although *geophagia* (pica of clay or dirt) and *amylophagia* (pica of corn and laundry starch) are primarily recognized among women of rural lower socioeconomic groups, *pagophagia* (excessive ice consumption) has been noted among all socioeconomic levels. Of particular concern is the practice of pica during pregnancy when the risk and implications of iron deficiency anemia are most severe. A challenge to obstetric nurses is to elicit information about this type of dietary behavior when assessing clients.

If increases in dietary sources of iron-rich foods do not raise hematocrit levels, supplements may be prescribed. Determination of dose is made based on physiologic requirements as assessed by primary healthcare providers. Long-term compliance is necessary to adequately restore iron storage levels in the body. Client education and support by nurses are advantageous.

Toxicity

Hemosiderosis, storing too much iron in the body, is a health concern. This condition may be caused either by **hemochromatosis,** a genetic disorder that allows more dietary iron to be absorbed than usual, or by consumption of very high levels of iron-containing foods, perhaps through iron fortification. The resulting iron overload can damage tissues cells when storing excess iron. Bacterial microorganisms may thrive on the excessive amounts of iron circulating in the blood. These effects are manifested in vague symptoms of weakness and fatigue. More specific symptoms include liver and heart damage, diabetes, arthritis, and discoloration of skin.[22]

Those at risk include men, persons with chronic excessive alcohol consumption, and individuals who are genetically at risk for hemochromatosis. Because men lose no iron through menstruation or childbirth and may consume more foods fortified with iron, their bodies can potentially store more iron than needed. Excessive consumption of alcohol puts people at risk because their livers are affected by alcohol and may malfunction, absorbing too much iron. Individuals with diabetes may also be at higher risk.[22]

IRON SUPPLEMENT TIPS

- Drink a glass of orange juice when taking an iron supplement to maximize iron absorption.
- Avoid taking iron supplements with milk because the calcium in milk interferes with iron absorption.
- Use of iron supplements may cause stools to turn black and constipation to result.

pica
a condition characterized by a hunger and appetite for nonfood substances

hemosiderosis
a condition in which too much iron is stored in the body

hemochromatosis
a genetic disorder causing excessive dietary iron absorption

Hemochromatosis alters iron metabolism allowing excess iron to be absorbed from food and supplements. CDC estimates are that as many as 1 in 200 Americans may have this disorder.[22] Treatment for hemochromatosis is blood removal by giving blood regularly and by decreasing dietary intake of iron-containing foods. This disorder is sometimes misdiagnosed as diabetes or as liver disorders. Although they are caused by hemochromatosis, these disorders are treated as individual ailments, rather than addressing the underlying iron overload. However, awareness of hemochromatosis is increasing among primary healthcare providers and other health professionals. Screening during regular checkups is recommended for those older than age 30, particularly if they have diabetes. Screening is conducted by a blood test to assess transferrin saturation.[22]

A final concern about iron toxicity is less a nutritional issue and more of a public health and safety issue. Accidental iron poisoning of children who consume iron supplements or vitamin/mineral supplements containing iron is a medical emergency. As few as 6 to 12 pills can be lethal, depending on the dose and age of the child. All supplements, even the fruit-flavored shapes formulated for children, should be treated as medicinal drugs and be kept out of the reach of children.

Zinc

Function

More than 200 enzymes throughout the body depend on zinc. Zinc affects our growth process, taste and smell ability, healing process, immune system, and carbohydrate metabolism by assisting insulin function.

Recommended Intake and Sources

The zinc RDA for men and women is 11 mg and 8 mg, respectively. During pregnancy and lactation, suggested levels for women increase to a range from 11 mg to 12 mg.

Zinc-containing foods include meat, fish, poultry, whole grains, legumes, and eggs. In the United States, a variety of zinc sources are easily available. In parts of the world where animal foods are not regularly consumed and grains are a primary zinc source, deficiencies may develop because of the low bioavailability of zinc from fibrous whole grain plant foods. Grains contain phytic acid that remains bound to zinc in the intestinal tract; human digestive juices cannot break this bond. Use of leavening agents such as yeast to prepare whole grain food products breaks this bond, making zinc available. Zinc deficiency still occurs in parts of the world where food sources may be limited and whole grains are consistently consumed as unleavened breads.

Deficiency

Deficiency symptoms are related to zinc's functions in the body. Symptoms include impaired growth, reduced appetite, and immunologic disorders. Severe zinc deficiency during the growth years may result in dwarfism and hypogonadism (reduced function of gonads) leading to delayed sexual development. Reduced appetite is most likely related to reduced ability to taste (hypogeusia) and smell foods (hyposmia). The difficulty is that once appetite is reduced, fewer potential sources of zinc may be consumed, which causes the zinc deficiency to worsen. Marginal deficiencies among children categorized as picky eaters have been noted to negatively affect height status.[23] Among older persons, inadequate dietary intake resulting in reduced zinc intake appears to affect wound healing, taste and scent ability, and immune functions.[24]

Toxicity

Zinc toxicity from inappropriate supplementation produces GI distress leading to vomiting and diarrhea, fever, and exhaustion. The symptoms appear similar to those of the flu. Continual use of supplements decreases iron and copper levels in the body and reduces levels of high-density lipoprotein (HDL), thereby increasing risk of coronary artery disease. Intake should be no higher than the RDA unless directed by a primary healthcare provider; individuals should not self-medicate. Consequently, the UL of 40 mg should be observed.

Iodine

Function

Iodine is part of the hormone thyroxine produced by the thyroid gland. Thyroxine is involved with regulating growth and development, basal metabolic rate, and body temperature.

Recommended Intake and Sources

The RDA for iodine is 150 mcg for both men and women. Many sources of iodine provide inconsistent amounts. Water may contain some iodine, but the amounts vary. Seafood is a good source, and dairy products and eggs may contain some iodine depending on the feed the animals consumed. Surprisingly, sea salt does not contain iodine; the iodine is lost in processing. The amount of iodine in plant foods depends on the amount in the soil in which the food is grown. Incidental sources of iodine are cleaning products whose residues adhere to cooking and baking equipment and dough conditioners. To ensure the population receives adequate amounts of this nutrient, salt in the United States may be purchased fortified with iodine.

Deficiency

Iodine deficiency reduces the amount of thyroxine produced. Symptoms of iodine deficiency then reflect the effects of reduced thyroxine, including sluggishness and weight gain. Severe iodine deficiency during pregnancy causes cretinism of the fetus that results in permanent mental and physical retardation.

Goiter, enlargement of the thyroid gland, occurs during extended iodine deficiency (Figure 8-6). The thyroid gland works to compensate for the low iodine levels and expands; the goiter frequently remains even after iodine intake is again sufficient.

The incidence of goiter in certain populations has been endemic or regionally defined. In the past, a goiter belt existed in the Midwestern states. Iodine was unavailable in the soil and water of the area because this region is untouched by oceans; oceans provide a natural source of iodine. Since then, fortification of salt with iodine and the wider availability of seafood because of improved refrigeration and transportation systems have reduced this deficiency. Goiter, although extremely rare in North America, may still occur in parts of Europe, Africa, and South and Central America. To eliminate iodine deficiency globally, the United Nations Joint Commission on Health Policy recommended universal salt iodization, which is now being implemented in countries in which iodine deficiency is a public health concern.[25]

Goiter may also be caused by the action of goitrogens. When consumed as a staple component of dietary intake, goitrogens (substances in the root vegetable cassava and in cabbage) suppress the actions of the thyroid gland. Although the thyroid gland swells as in iodine deficiency goiter, the iodine level is not the initiating agent; instead, substances in these vegetables suppress the actions of the thyroid gland. To control these iodine deficiency disorders (IDD) in areas such as South

goiter
enlargement of the thyroid gland caused by iodine deficiency

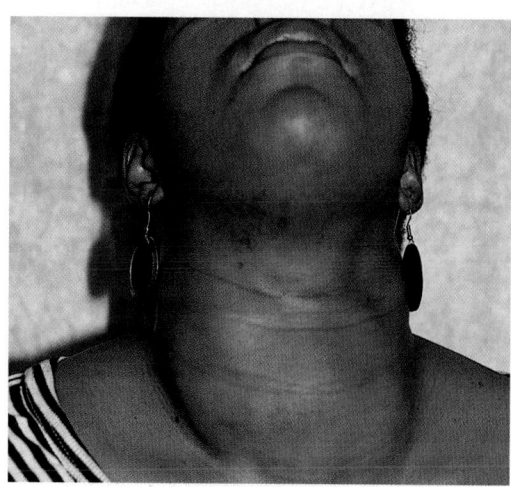

Figure 8-6 Goiter caused by iron deficiency. (From Swartz MH: *Textbook of physical diagnosis history and examination*, ed 3, Philadelphia, 1998, WB Saunders.)

Ethiopia, programs are conducted to teach villagers how to reduce cassava toxicity by using safer preparation techniques.[26]

Toxicity

thyrotoxicosis
iodine-induced goiter

Too much iodine can cause iodine-induced goiter called thyrotoxicosis, therefore the UL is set at 1100 mcg.

Fluoride

Function

Fluoride increases resistance to tooth decay and is part of tooth formation. Skeletal health also depends on fluoride for bone mineralization.

Recommended Intake and Sources

The AI for fluoride is 4 mg for men and 3 mg for women.

Sources of fluoride vary. The most consistent is fortified water to which fluoride has been added. Tea, seafood, and seaweed are other reliable sources. Unfortunately, these are not regularly consumed, particularly by children during tooth formation years.

An inadvertent source of fluoride is toothpaste. Most toothpaste has fluoride added as a topical agent to strengthen tooth enamel. However, some fluoride is ingested during the rinsing process, providing a kind of dietary source of fluoride. Children can ingest a lethal dose of fluoride if a tube of toothpaste is consumed.

Deficiency

Low levels of fluoride increase the risk of dental caries. Other factors of hygiene, food choices, and possibly genetics also affect plaque and subsequent dental caries.

Toxicity

fluorosis
a condition of mottling or brown spotting of the tooth enamel caused by excessive intake of fluoride

Too much fluoride causes fluorosis. Fluorosis consists of mottling or brown spotting of the tooth enamel; severe fluorosis may also cause pitting of the teeth. A UL of 10 mg reduces the risk of toxicity.

Selenium

Function

Selenium is part of an enzyme that acts as an antioxidant. Vitamin E and selenium work together to prevent cell and lipid membrane damage from oxidizing substances. Selenium is also associated with thyroid function. It is found extensively throughout the body.

Recommended Intake and Sources

The RDA for selenium ranges from 55 mcg to 70 mcg per day. Meats, fish, eggs, and whole grains are good sources of selenium. It is a nutrient for which the RDA is easily met.

Deficiency

Deficiency of selenium may predispose individuals to heart disease, particularly Keshan disease. Keshan disease was first noted in China, primarily in children and women of childbearing age. The symptoms of the disease include cardiomyopathy and other features common to selenium deficiency, including muscle pain and tenderness. It is difficult, however, to separate other environmental factors specific to China that may also affect long-term nutritional status. Deficiencies of nutrients other than selenium may have a role in the etiology of Keshan disease. Keshan disease differs from the form of heart disease common in the United States because the myocardium of the heart is affected. In the United States most heart disease is coronary artery disease.[27] Therefore selenium deficiency is probably not a factor affecting the American incidence of heart disease.

However, low dietary levels of selenium or reduced blood levels of selenium may be associated with an increased risk of cancer among Americans. The relationship of cancer to selenium consumption is probably caused by selenium's antioxidant functions combined with other antioxidants in the body. This relationship continues to be explored.

Toxicity

Selenium can be toxic at levels as low as five times the RDA of 55 mcg. Effects of toxicity include severe liver damage, vomiting, and diarrhea. Additional symptoms include metallic aftertaste, respiratory distress with lung edema and bronchopneumonia, and garlic-scented breath and sweat.[28] The toxicity of selenium highlights the delicate nature of the body's use of trace minerals. Although selenium is proposed as an antioxidant supplement, the amounts suggested are those of the RDA for selenium. To avoid toxicity, a UL of 400 mcg has been established.

Copper

Function

Although the body requires minute amounts, copper performs many functions. Some roles of copper include action as (1) a coenzyme involving antioxidant reactions and energy metabolism, (2) a component of wound healing, (3) a constituent of nerve fiber protection, and (4) a required element for iron use.

Recommended Intake and Sources

The RDA for copper is 900 mcg for adults. Good sources include organ meats (liver), seafood, green leafy vegetables, legumes, whole grains, dried fruits, and water, if it flows through copper pipes.

Deficiency

Copper deficiency causes bone demineralization and anemia; this form of anemia can also be caused by zinc toxicity reducing body levels of copper. Copper deficiency does not occur in the United States.

Toxicity

Toxicity occurs from supplementation. Common toxic response consists of vomiting and diarrhea. Wilson's disease, an inherited disorder, results in the excessive accumulation of copper in the liver, brain, and cornea of the eye. Eventually the disorder can lead to cirrhosis, chronic hepatitis, liver failure, and neurologic disorders. Worldwide, the incidence of copper toxicity appears tied to use of brass and copper pots to prepare and store foods. Nutritional treatment for copper toxicity, whether caused by Wilson's disease or dietary sources, is through dietary restrictions and chelation therapy that initiates excretion of excess copper from the body.[29,30] In addition, 10,000 mcg is the UL for copper.

Chromium

Function

Chromium has a role in carbohydrate metabolism as a constituent of the glucose tolerance factor (GTF) that facilitates the reaction of insulin.

Recommended Intake and Sources

The AI of chromium is 35 mcg for men and 25 mcg for women. Found in animal-related foods, eggs, and whole grains, chromium is lost in food processing, particularly when wheat is refined to white flour.

Studies are exploring the effects of chromium supplementation on increasing HDL and decreasing glucose and insulin levels. The findings may have implications for populations who consume refined foods and for those who are exposed to stressors that increase the need for chromium; these may include infections, trauma, and diets high in simple sugars.

Deficiency

Although chromium is lost through food processing, outright deficiencies of chromium are unusual. Inadequate chromium status may be responsible in part for some cases of impaired glucose tolerance, hyperglycemia, hypoglycemia, and unresponsiveness to insulin.[31]

Toxicity

Toxicity has been noted from environmental contaminants in industrial settings rather than from excessive dietary intakes.

OTHER TRACE MINERALS

The amount needed of the following trace minerals is so low that it is easy to meet these amounts through ordinary consumption of foods. All are problematic in large doses; supplements are contraindicated.

Manganese is a component of enzymes involved in metabolic reactions. The AI for manganese is 2.3 mg for men and 1.8 mg for women. Found in whole grains, green vegetables, legumes, and other foods, manganese deficiency in humans is unknown. A UL of 11 mg for manganese exists.

Molybdenum functions as a coenzyme. The RDA of 45 mcg is easily consumed through typical dietary selections. Deficiencies have not been recorded except under medical circumstances in which dietary intake has been greatly altered. The UL for molybdenum is 2000 mcg.

Other trace minerals found in our bodies that may have a role in human health include *silicon, boron, nickel, vanadium, lithium, tin,* and *cadmium.* The amounts required are so small we naturally consume enough and are never deficient in these nutrients.

Table 8-2 provides a quick reference to the trace minerals.

Table 8-2
Trace Minerals

Mineral	Function	Clinical Issues Deficiency/Toxicity	Recommended Intakes	Food Sources	Absorption Issues
Iron (Fe)	Distributes oxygen in hemoglobin and myoglobin; growth	Deficiency: microcytic anemia (children and women at risk) Toxicity: hemosiderosis; hemochromatosis	RDA Men: 8 mg Women: 18 mg Pregnancy: 27 mg Lactation: 9 mg UL 45 mg	Heme sources: meat, fish, poultry, egg yolks Non-heme sources: vegetables, legumes, whole grains, enriched grains	Conserved and recycled; absorption 10%-15% of dietary iron consumed
Zinc (Zn)	Cofactor for more than 200 enzymes; carbohydrate metabolism (insulin function)	Deficiency: decreases wound healing; decreases taste and smell; impaired sexual and physical development; immune disorders Toxicity: similar to flu with vomiting/diarrhea/fever/exhaustion	RDA Men: 11 mg Women: 8 mg UL 40 mg	Meat, fish, poultry, whole grains, legumes, eggs	Binders may decrease absorption in whole grains
Iodine (I)	Thyroxine synthesis (thyroid hormone) regulates growth and development; BMR regulation	Deficiency: decreases thyroxine, causing sluggishness and weight gain, goiter, cretinism (if during pregnancy) Toxicity: thyrotoxicosis	RDA Adults: 150 mcg UL 1100 mcg	Iodized salt, seafood	
Fluoride (Fl)	Bone and tooth formation; increases resistance to decay; decreases mineralization	Deficiency: increases dental caries Toxicity: fluorosis	AI Men: 4 mg Women: 3 mg UL 10 mg	Fluoridated water, tea, seafood, seaweed	

AI, Adequate Intake; CNS, central nervous system; EMR, Estimated Minimum Requirement; FVD, fluid volume deficit; RDA, Recommended Daily Allowance.

Continued

Table 8-2
Trace Minerals—cont'd

Mineral	Function	Clinical Issues Deficiency/Toxicity	Recommended Intakes	Food Sources	Absorption Issues
Selenium (Se)	Antioxidant cofactor with vitamin E; prevents cell and lipid membrane damage	Deficiency: possible Keshan disease/cancer Toxicity: liver damage, vomiting, diarrhea	RDA Adults: 55 mcg UL 400 mcg	Meat, fish, eggs, whole grains	
Copper (C)	Coenzyme in antioxidant reactions and energy metabolism; wound healing; nerve fiber protection; iron use	Deficiency: bone-demineralization and anemia (not in U.S.) Toxicity: Wilson's disease or with supplements producing vomiting/diarrhea	RDA Adults: 900 mcg UL 10,000 mcg	Organ meats (liver), seafood, green leafy vegetables	
Chromium (Cr)	Carbohydrate metabolism, part of glucose tolerance factor	Deficiency: possible link with cardiovascular disorders; hypoglycemia, hyperglycemia, and unresponsive insulin	AI Men: 35 mcg Women: 25 mcg	Animal food, whole grains	
Manganese (Mn)	Part of metabolic reaction enzymes	Deficiency: unknown	AI Men: 2.3 mg Women: 1.8 mg UL 11 mg	Whole grains, green leafy vegetables, legumes	
Molybdenum (Mo)	Coenzyme	Deficiency: unknown	RDA Adults: 45 mcg UL 2000 mcg	Many foods	

AI, *Adequate Intake;* CNS, *central nervous system;* EMR, *Estimated Minimum Requirement;* FVD, *fluid volume deficit;* RDA, *Recommended Daily Allowance.*

OVERCOMING BARRIERS

Overcoming barriers to wellness pertaining to individual mineral status has already been addressed in this chapter. Hypertension appears to be affected by the actions of several minerals and therefore is explored here.

Hypertension

Continuing research appears to suggest that adequate levels of calcium and magnesium have roles in the maintenance of appropriate blood pressure levels. Population studies point to lower intakes of these nutrients among individuals who are hypertensive. Marginal intake of these nutrients, combined with other lifestyle factors such as lack of exercise, excessive weight, cigarette smoking, and sodium sensitivity, sets the stage for hypertension to occur. Sodium sensitivity reflects the need to avoid excesses even if marginally higher intakes than recommended are consumed safely by most of the population.

Consumption levels of calcium, magnesium, and sodium are based on recommendations to consume foods as whole as possible. It is through processing that minerals are lost and sodium levels in foods escalate.

Two recent studies have further supported the value of long-term lifestyle changes to reduce blood pressure among individuals with hypertension. The 1998 findings of a multicenter clinical trial, the Trial of Nonpharmacologic Interventions in the Elderly (TONE), revealed that lifestyle changes including reduction of dietary salt, weight loss, or the two combined resulted in reduced blood pressure in older patients. For those with hypertension, medications were reduced. [32] A previous study conducted in 1997, the trial of Dietary Approaches to Stop Hypertension (DASH), studied complete eating plans. A diet lower in fat and higher in fruits, vegetables, and low-fat dairy foods in which salt was not controlled reduced blood pressure levels ranging from normal to slightly elevated. Additional analysis has continued to affirm the value of the DASH program as an effective foundation for the reduction and prevention of hypertension.[32]

The dietary recommendations of these two clinical trials continue to validate the need to consume fewer processed foods, with the focus on increasing fruits and vegetables while consuming low levels of dietary fat as a means to either lower or maintain normal blood pressure levels.

TOWARD A POSITIVE NUTRITION LIFESTYLE: PROJECTING

Projection is placing responsibility for our own unacceptable feelings or behaviors on others. In relation to health, we may attribute our poor eating patterns to hectic schedules and possibly to roommates or family members who don't want to shop for food or prepare meals. We project our unacceptable behaviors on others, rather than take responsibility for our own health.

One mineral for which projection sometimes occurs is iron. Because iron deficiency is often manifested with tiredness, paleness, and frequent infections, it is frequently self-diagnosed as the pathologic cause of poor health. Accurate diagnosis of iron deficiency is based on blood analysis, not on self-reporting. As an aspect of client education, we can help clients clarify the actual cause of their symptoms if they are not clinically iron deficient. Often these symptoms are caused by poor health habits—not enough sleep, irregular meals, and too little exercise. Rather than projecting ill health on the mineral iron, clients can take responsibility and modify their own health behaviors.

SUMMARY

In this chapter, water and minerals are explored through their nutritional requirements and physiologic roles for achieving nutritional wellness. Although water and minerals are primary components of body fluids, each performs other functions as well.

Water supports a variety of functions, including acting as a structural component of the body, a temperature regulator, a lubricant, a fluid cushion, a transportation vehicle, a trace mineral source, and a medium for and participant in biochemical reactions. About four to eight 8-oz servings of water per day (1 to 1.5 ml per kcal of energy expended) are required to meet basic physiologic needs. Sources may include beverages and foods with high water content, although the best source is water in its pure form.

Minerals also fill diverse roles. Structurally, minerals provide rigidity and strength to the teeth and skeleton; the skeletal mineral components also serve as a storage depot for other needs of the body. Minerals allowing for proper muscle contraction and release influence nerve function. Minerals also assist enzymes, maintain proper acid-base balance of body fluids, and are required for blood clotting and wound healing.

The 16 essential minerals are divided into two categories: major and trace minerals. Major minerals, needed daily in amounts of 100 mg or higher, include calcium, phosphorus, magnesium, sulfur, and the electrolytes of sodium, potassium, and chloride. Trace minerals, required daily in amounts less than or equal to 20 mg, include iron, zinc, iodine, fluoride, selenium, copper, chromium, manganese, and molybdenum.

Prime food sources of minerals include both plants and animals. Valuable plant sources include most fruits, vegetables, legumes, and whole grains. Animal sources consist of beef, chicken, eggs, fish, and milk products. Although minerals are stable when cooked, the bioavailability of some minerals may be limited depending on the source. Some plant minerals are not easily available to the human body because of binders inhibiting absorption. Generally, minerals from animal foods are able to be absorbed more easily than those from plants. Whatever the specific food source, dietary patterns consisting primarily of whole foods provide an adequate supply of minerals.

THE NURSING APPROACH
Fluid Volume Deficit Case Study: The Nursing Process

Sal, age 82, resides in a long-term care facility. One night he develops nausea, vomiting, diarrhea, and fever from a gastrointestinal virus that has affected several other residents. After 8 hours of repeated vomiting and diarrhea, the nurse is concerned that Sal may develop fluid volume deficit. The nurse uses nursing process skills to investigate and handle the problem as follows.

ASSESSMENT

Objective

- Dry mucous membranes
- Normal filling of hand veins
- Pulse rate increase from 80 to 86
- Respiration rate increase from 20 to 24
- Blood pressure in normal range for patient
- Temperature 101.6° F (38.6° C)
- Warm extremities
- Drowsiness

Subjective

- Thirst
- Dry mouth
- Generalized weakness

NURSING DIAGNOSIS

Mild fluid volume deficit related to vomiting and diarrhea as evidenced by dry mucous membranes, thirst, and elevated pulse and respiratory rates

THE NURSING APPROACH–cont'd
Fluid Volume Deficit Case Study: The Nursing Process

PLANNING

The nurse sets goals in consultation with Sal to achieve the following outcomes:
1. No further fluid loss
2. Fluid balance restored to normal within 36 hours

IMPLEMENTATION

1. Obtain orders for antiemetic and antidiarrheal drugs.
2. Obtain order for acetaminophen for temperature above 101° F (38.3 ° C)
3. Monitor vital signs every 2 hours.
4. Try sips of ginger ale and broth beginning 1 hour after antiemetic.
5. Promote oral fluids hourly.
6. If needed, initiate oral rehydration therapy by providing formulated solutions containing glucose and electrolytes (2-3 liters/day) such as Resol and Ricelyte.

EVALUATION

Goals must be evaluated to see if the outcomes have been met as evidenced by:
- Moist mucous membranes in 36 hours
- Balanced intake and output in 36 hours

APPLYING CONTENT KNOWLEDGE

The camp nurse gives a talk to the camp staff about the signs of fluid volume deficit. She encourages the counselors to be sure the campers drink fluids throughout the day. One counselor responds, "Oh, that's no problem. The kids guzzle flavored ice tea all day long." How should she respond?

Web Sites of Interest

American Hemochromatosis Society (AHS)

www.americanhs.org

The American Hemochromatosis Society provides support for individuals with hereditary hemochromatosis and information on diagnosis, genetic testing for hereditary hemochromatosis, pediatric hereditary hemochromatosis, and research relating to hereditary hemochromatosis/iron overload.

Dietary Approaches to Stop Hypertension (DASH)

www.nhlbi.nih.gov/health/public/heart/hbp/dash

This site presents a comprehensive guide to implementing DASH dietary plans including research and results, the DASH Diet, DASH publications, and DASH Centers.

National Osteoporosis Foundation (NOF)

www.nof.org/

This site of the NOF provides resources on causes, prevention, detection, and treatment of osteoporosis. It includes links for professionals, the press, and support groups, along with cutting-edge reports and advocacy information.

References

1. National Research Council, Food and Nutrition Board: *Recommended dietary allowances,* ed 10, Washington, DC, 1989, National Academy Press.
2. *Bottled water industry overview,* Bottled Water Web, 2002; www.bottledwaterweb.com/indus.html.
3. Department of Health and Human Services, Public Health Service: *Healthy People 2010,* ed 2, Washington, DC, 2000, US Government Printing Office; www.health.gov/healthypeople.
4. Correa P: Is gastric carcinoma an infectious disease? *N Engl J Med* 325(16):1170, 1991.
5. Mans OH, Uribarri J: Electrolyte, water, and acid-base balance. In Shils ME et al., eds.: *Modern nutrition in health and disease,* ed 9, Baltimore, 1999, Williams & Wilkins.
6. Institute of Medicine, Food and Nutrition Board: *Dietary reference intakes for calcium, phosphorus, magnesium, vitamin D, and fluoride,* Washington, DC, 1997, National Academy Press.
7. Weaver CM, Heaney RP: Calcium. In Shils ME et al., eds.: *Modern nutrition in health and disease,* ed 9, Baltimore, 1999, Williams & Wilkins.
8. Wardlaw GM: Putting osteoporosis in perspective *J Am Dietetic Assoc* 93(9):1000, 1993.
9. Scane AC, Sutcliffe AM, Francis RM: Osteoporosis in men, *Baillieres Clin Rheumatol* 7(3):589, Oct 1993.
10. Rodino MA, Shane E: Osteoporosis after organ transplantation, *Am J Med* 104(5):459, 1998.
11. Mundy GR: Boning up on genes, *Nature* 367(6460):216, Jan 20, 1994.
12. Massey LK: Caffeine, urinary calcium, calcium metabolism and bone, *J Nutr* 123(9):1611, 1993.
13. Barrett-Connor E, Chang JC, Edelstein SL: Coffee-associated osteoporosis onset by daily milk consumption: The Rancho Bernardo Study, *J Am Med Assoc* 271(4):280, Jan 26, 1994.
14. Lloyd T et al.: Dietary caffeine intake and bone status of postmenopausal women, *Am J Clin Nutr* 65(6):1826, 1997.
15. Ensrud KE et al.: Body size and hip fracture risk in older women: a prospective study. Study of Osteoporotic Fractures Research Group, *Am J Med* 103(4):274, 1997.
16. Wardlaw GM: Putting body weight and osteoporosis into perspective, *Am J Clin Nutr* 63(3 Suppl):433S, 1996.
17. Jacob RA: Vitamin C. In Shils ME et al., eds: *Modern nutrition in health and disease,* ed 9, Baltimore, 1999, Williams & Wilkins.
18. Looker AC et al.: Prevalence of iron deficiency in the United States, *J Am Med Assoc* 277(12):973, 1997.
19. Viteri FE: A new concept in the control of iron deficiency: community-based preventive supplementation of at-risk groups by the weekly intake of iron supplements, *Biomed Environ Sci* 11(1):46, 1998.
20. Scholl IO, Hediger MI: Anemia and iron-deficiency anemia: compilation of data on pregnancy outcome, *Am J Clin Nutr* 59(2 suppl):429s, Feb 1994.
21. Centers for Disease Control and Prevention: Recommendations to prevent and control iron deficiency in the United States, *MMWR Morb Mortal Wkly Rep* 47(Rr-3):1, 1998.
22. Don't let iron overload hide behind other diseases, *Envir Nutr* Apr 1998.
23. Sanstead HH: Zinc deficiency: a public health problem? *J Disease in Children* 145:853, 1991.
24. Greger JL: Potential for trace mineral deficiencies and toxicities in the elderly. In Bales CW, ed.: *Mineral homeostasis in the elderly: current topics in nutrition and disease,* vol 21, New York, 1989, Alan Liss.
25. van der Haar F: The challenge of the global elimination of iodine deficiency disorders, *Eur J Clin Nutr* 51 Suppl 4:S3, 1997.
26. Abuye C, Kelbessa U, Wolde-Gebriel S: Health effects of cassava consumption in south Ethiopia, *East Afr Med J* 75(3):166, 1998.
27. McLaren D: Clinical manifestations of human vitamin and mineral disorders: a resume. In Shils ME et al., eds.: *Modern nutrition in health and disease,* ed 9, Baltimore, 1999, Williams & Wilkins.
28. Bedwal RS et al.: Selenium—its biological perspectives, *Med Hypotheses* 41(2):150, Aug 1993.

29. Turnland JR: Copper. In Shils ME et al., eds.: *Modern nutrition in health and disease,* ed 9, Baltimore, 1999, Williams & Wilkins.

30. Giacchino R et al.: Syndromic variability of Wilson's disease in children: clinical study of 44 cases, *Ital J Gastroenterol Hepatol* 29(2):155, 1997.

31. Stoecker BJ: Chromium. In Shils ME et al., eds.: *Modern nutrition in health and disease,* ed 9, Baltimore, 1999, Williams & Wilkins.

32. National Institutes of Health, National Heart, Lung, and Blood Institute: *Statement on sodium intake and high blood pressure,* Press Release, Aug 17, 1998.

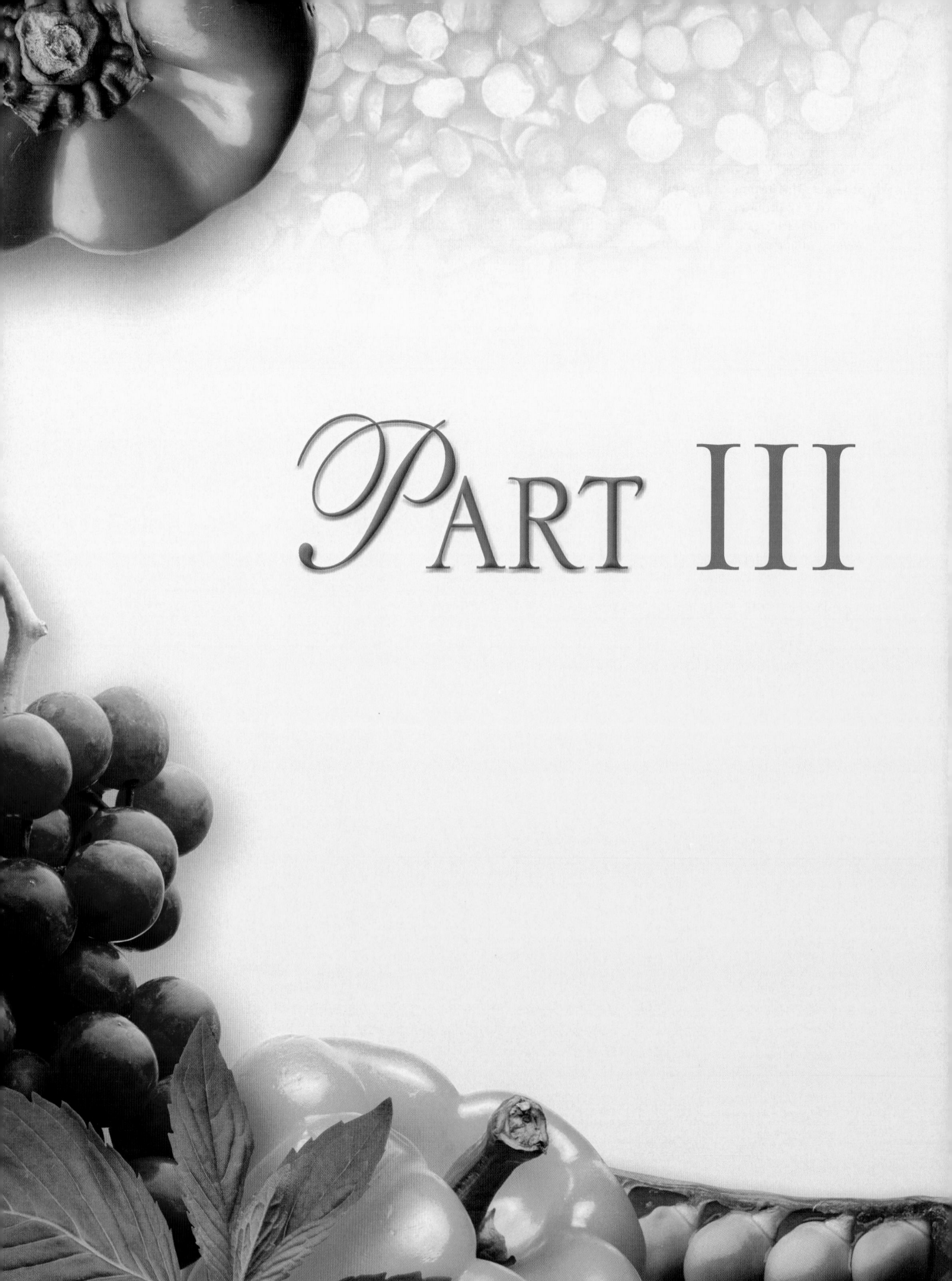

PART III

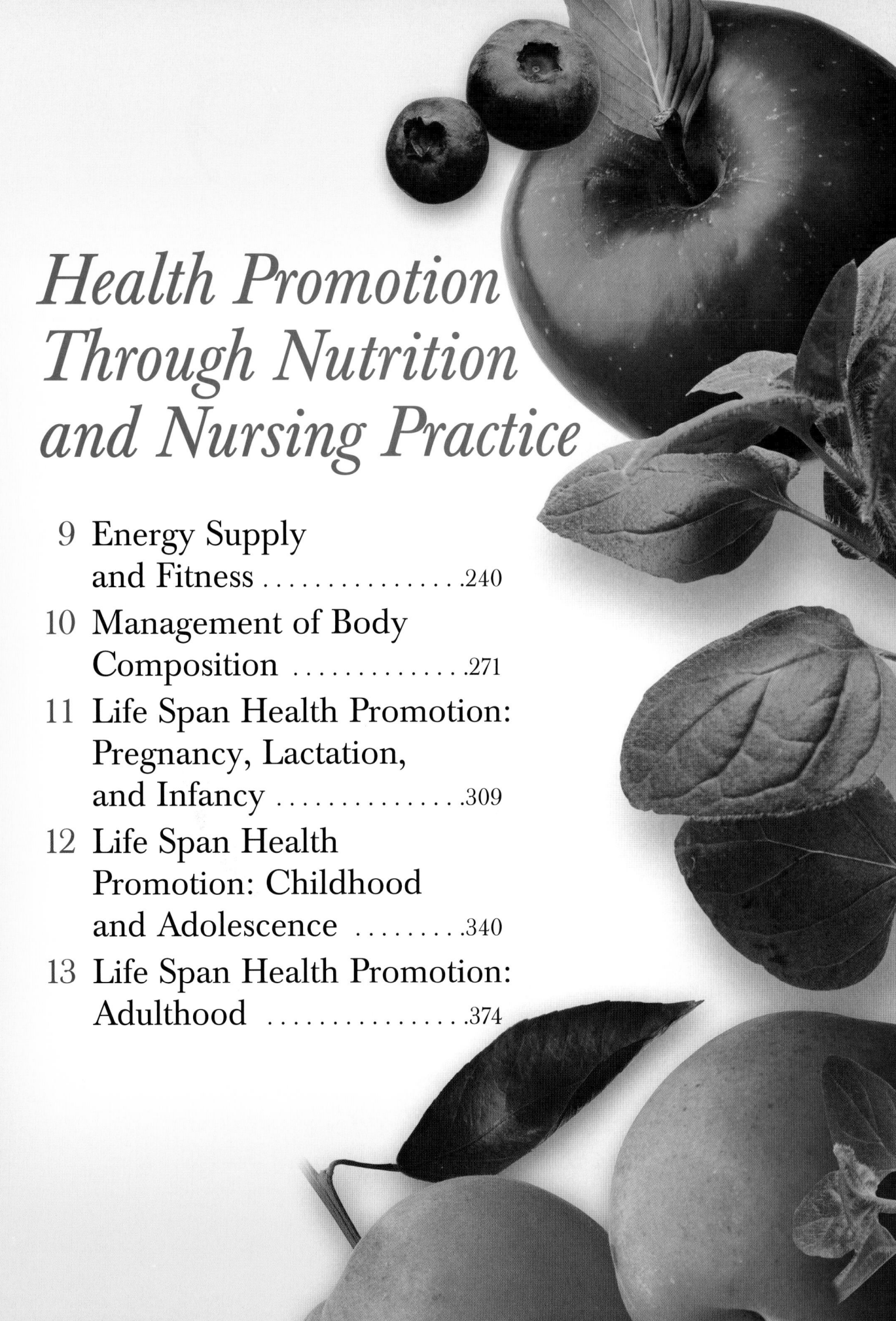

Health Promotion Through Nutrition and Nursing Practice

CHAPTER 9

Energy Supply and Fitness

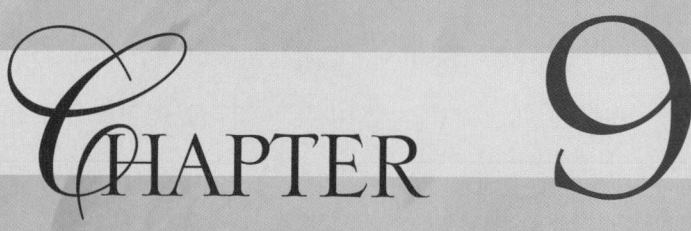

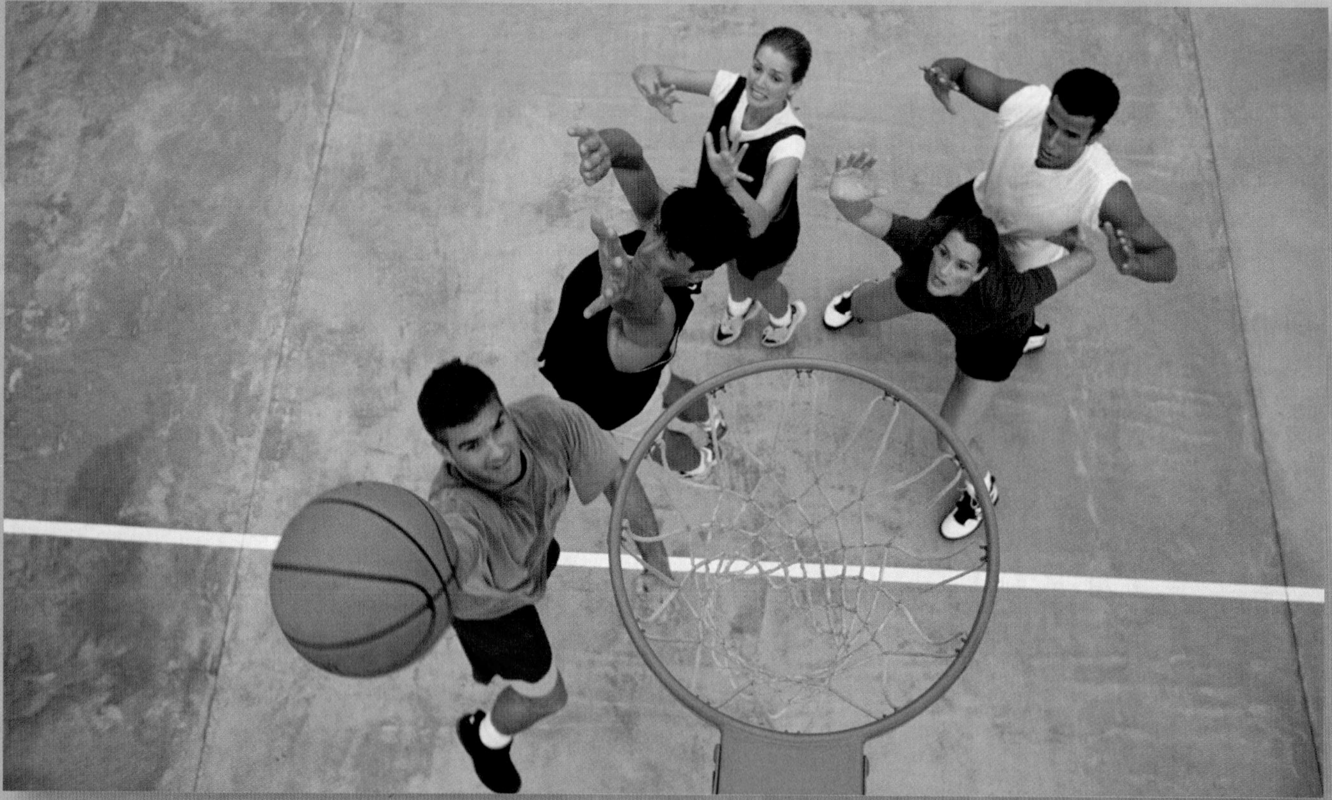

The abilities to perform work, produce change, and maintain life all require energy.

ROLE IN WELLNESS

Consideration of the five dimensions of health guides our understanding of the value of energy supply and fitness. To achieve optimal physical health and fitness, dietary intake and regular physical activity are essential. Exercise affects all muscles; even the muscles of our gastrointestinal tract function better when we regularly exercise. To strengthen our intellectual dimension of health, the old saying, "A sound body makes for a sound mind," still holds true. By being physically fit, we may be able to devote our full intellectual capacity to our work. The emotional health dimension may be supported by fitness because for some persons, depression seems to lift if they regularly engage in sustained aerobic activities. Even if we are not depressed, our general state of mind improves with daily physical exercise. Group sports provide an excellent opportunity for social activity while pursuing healthful goals that enhance social health. A sense of belonging and sharing occurs whether the group is a formal organization, such as a running club, or consists of friends who bike together. Respecting and caring for our bodies by engaging in regular physical activity reflects the understanding of the unique nature of the human body, which reflects spiritual health.

Physical activity has always been recognized as a component of health. Within the past decade, this importance has increased because an inverse relationship between level of fitness and risk of development of chronic degenerative disorders is becoming better understood. This means that the less physical activity a person experiences, the greater the risk of developing disorders such as diabetes, coronary artery disease (CAD), cancer, and hypertension. This chapter addresses the health benefits of exercise as complementing optimum nutrition to decrease risk factors and as improving quality of life. In the nursing profession, we may also work with athletes of all ages who will benefit from our knowledge of their physical requirements. Consequently, this chapter discusses specific nutrient issues that affect the athlete—"a person who is trained or skilled in exercises, sports, or games requiring physical strength, agility, or stamina."[1] Finally, as nurses we have a responsibility to maintain our own fitness levels as role models for our clients and for our own benefits to function comfortably in our sometimes physically demanding profession.

ENERGY

The abilities to perform work, produce change, and maintain life all require energy. Energy exists in many forms, such as mechanical, chemical, heat, electrical, light, and nuclear energies. The laws of thermodynamics tell us that each type of energy can be converted from one form to another. As our bodies function, chemical energy from food is converted to mechanical energy and heat.

The ultimate source of energy is the sun. Sunlight is used by plants to produce chemical energy in the form of carbohydrates, proteins, or fats. These foods possess stored energy. People are not capable of doing this. We must convert the chemical energy from the foods we eat into forms useable by the human body.

The energy released from food is measured in kilocalories (thousands of calories), or Calories. Technically, a calorie is the amount of heat necessary to raise the temperature of a gram of water by 1° C (0.8° F). As first noted in Chapter 1, to ensure accuracy, the term *kilocalories* is used throughout this text, abbreviated as *kcalories* or *kcal*.

Two methods are used to determine the energy a food contains. One is through the use of a bomb calorimeter (Figure 9-1). This instrument is designed to burn a food while measuring the amount of heat or energy released. This provides an estimate of the energy available to humans. Because the bomb calorimeter method is

---

Jaime S. Ruud, MS, RD, contributed this chapter in the first and second editions of this text.

more efficient than the human body, the kcalorie value assigned to a food item is adjusted to reflect the limitations of the human system. Amounts listed in food tables reflect this adjustment.

The other method of assessing food energy is proximate composition, which determines the grams of carbohydrates, proteins, and fats of a food item. The grams are then multiplied by the energy value of each (carbohydrates × 4 kcal/g; proteins × 4 kcal/g; fats × 9 kcal/g). The sum of these calculations equals the total energy content of a specific food.

Energy Pathways

The processes of digestion, absorption, and metabolism for each of the three energy-supplying nutrients—carbohydrates, fats, and proteins—have been presented in previous chapters. (Alcohol also provides energy but is not considered a nutrient category.) Carbohydrate digests to glucose, triglycerides (fats) to fatty acids and glycerol, and protein to amino acids. Here we continue to follow their journey as they are used for energy in individual cells.

adenosine triphosphate (ATP)
an energy-rich compound used for all energy-requiring processes in the body

The nutrients release energy when they are catabolized (broken down), forming carbon dioxide and water. The released energy becomes caught within adenosine triphosphate (ATP), the *fuel* for all energy-requiring processes in the body (Figure 9-2).

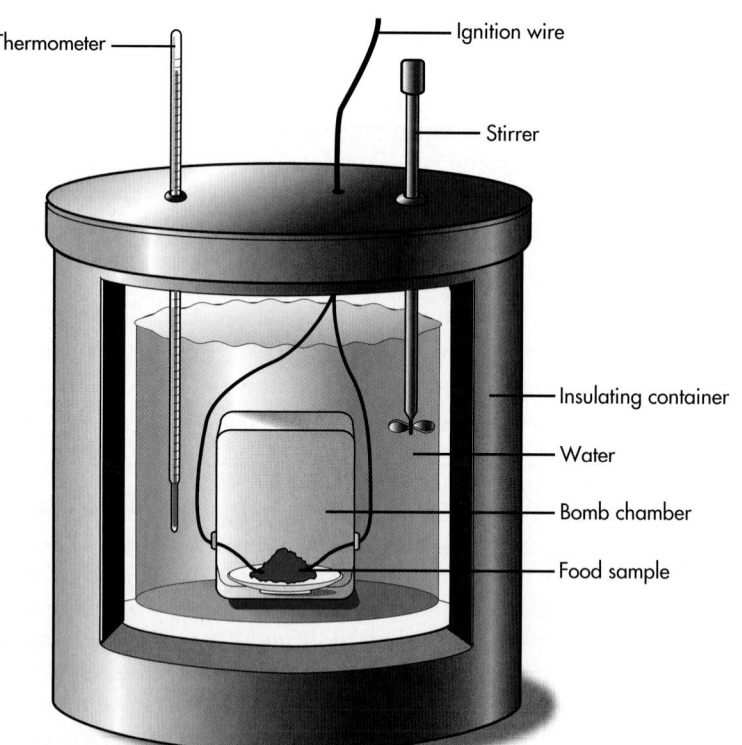

Figure 9-1 Cross-section of a bomb calorimeter. To determine energy, a dried portion of food is burned inside a chamber charged with oxygen that is surrounded by water. As the food is burned, it gives off heat. This raises the temperature of the water surrounding the chamber. The increase in water temperature indicates the number of kcalories contained in the food. One kcalorie equals the amount of heat needed to raise the temperature of 1 kilogram of water by 1° C (0.8° F).

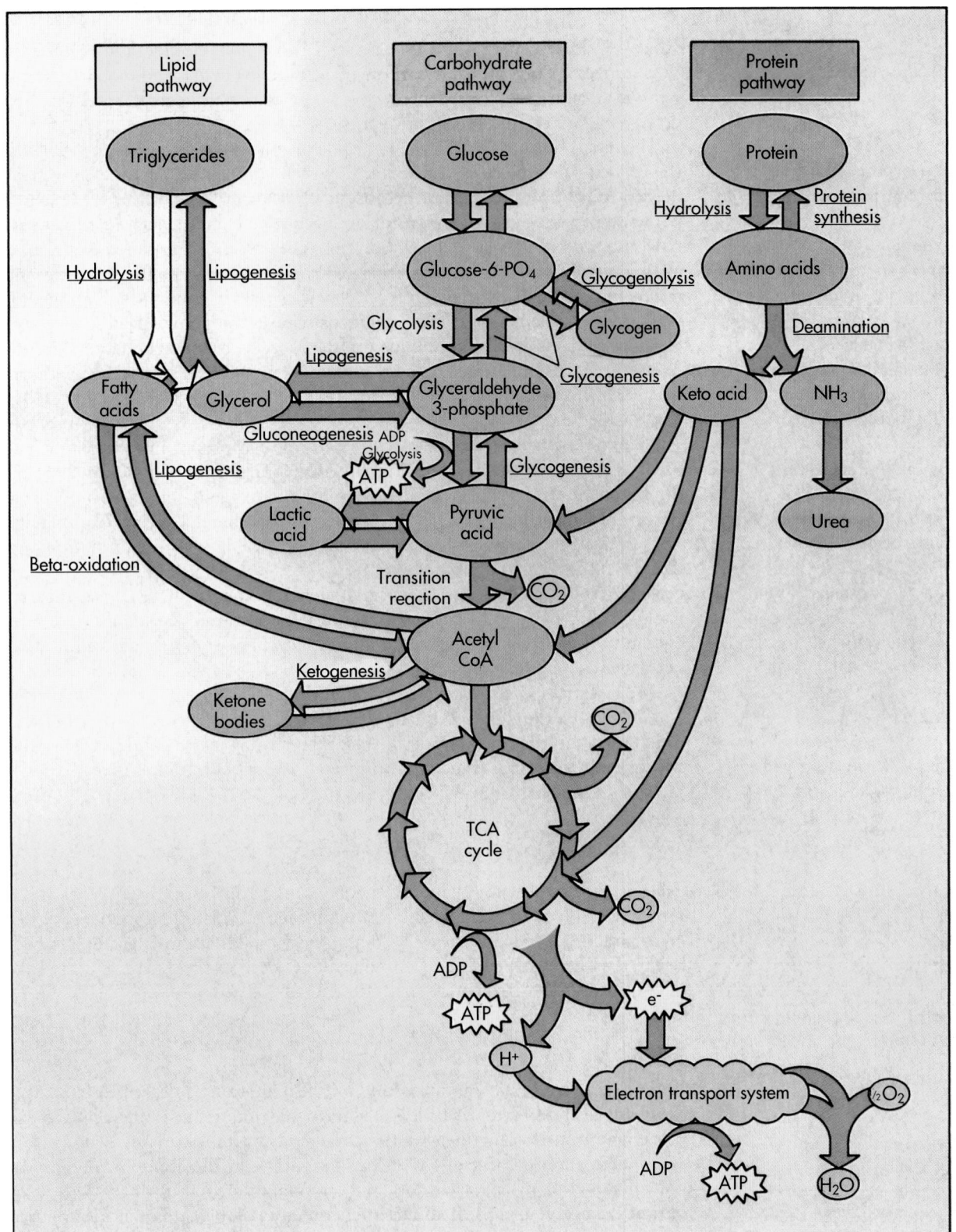

Figure 9-2 Summary of key steps in the metabolism of glucose, fatty acids, glycerol, and amino acids. *ADP,* Adenosine diphosphate; *ATP,* adenosine triphosphate; *TCA,* tricarboxylic acid cycle. (Rolin Graphics; from Thibodeau GA, Patton KT: *Anatomy and physiology,* ed 4, St Louis, 1999, Mosby.)

Carbohydrate as a Source of Energy

Glucose releases energy and is converted to carbon dioxide and water through three processes: glycolysis, tricarboxylic acid cycle (TCA), and oxidative phosphorylation. These complicated processes are reviewed in general here; the intricate details are beyond the scope of this text.

Through glycolysis, a glucose molecule produces pyruvic acid and ATP. Part of this process depends on niacin and other B-complex vitamins. Oxygen is not needed for glycolysis to occur because it is an anaerobic pathway. The anaerobic pathway provides energy for sprint or speed-type exercise such as soccer, basketball, and football. We also depend on this energy source to run for the train, chase after toddlers, or bound across the room to answer the phone. This type of exertion is limited because oxygen is not available quickly enough to continue its support. Instead, the incomplete use of glucose causes the pyruvic acid to be converted to lactic acid. As lactic acid builds up, the muscles become sore and stiff. Consequently, the exertion ceases because of pain. Within a few minutes, enough oxygen is available to break down the lactic aid, relieving the physical discomfort. The effect is called oxygen debt.

Anaerobic glycolysis takes place in the cell cytoplasm, but oxygen-dependent aerobic glycolysis (the aerobic pathway) occurs in the mitochondria of the cell. In the mitochondria, pyruvic acid (made without oxygen) reacts with coenzyme A (CoA) creating acetyl CoA. The energy process continues as acetyl CoA reaches the TCA cycle. The reactions that are part of that cycle lead to the formation of additional ATP and carbon dioxide.

The aerobic pathway is the primary energy source for exercise that is low enough in intensity to be carried on for at least 5 minutes or longer. This includes endurance-type exercise (e.g., swimming, bicycling, running) as well as walking and most of our daily activities.

The last process of glucose conversion to energy is oxidative phosphorylation. A number of actions lead to the release of hydrogens in the forms of water and additional energy that is captured in ATP. The term *oxidative* reflects the combination of hydrogen with oxygen to form water; *phosphorylation* is the creation of the phosphate bond to form ATP.

Fat as a Source of Energy

The first step in the use of fat for energy is the hydrolysis into glycerol and three fatty acids. Glycerol is changed into pyruvic acid and is used for energy. The fatty acids undergo a process known as *beta-oxidation,* which involves the breakdown of the fatty acids into acetyl CoA molecules that enter the TCA cycle and proceed like the acetyl CoA from carbohydrate (glucose).

Protein as a Source of Energy

Amino acids are first catabolized through deamination as described in Chapter 6. While the liver and kidneys process the nitrogen-containing amino acid groups, the other amino acid components enter the energy metabolism pathway, with each component entering at a different location. Some of the amino acid components are converted to pyruvic acid; others become intermediaries of the TCA cycle or part of the acetyl groups. If sufficient energy is available, amino acids are used for protein synthesis rather than for energy.

It is important to note that just as all three nutrients (carbohydrate, protein, and fat) can be used for energy when consumed in excess, they can also be stored as fat in the body. Likewise, when too little energy is consumed, these processes reverse. Energy that is consumed is used immediately, regardless of its source. The first stored energy used is glycogen, followed by the energy reserve of body fat in adi-

glycolysis
the conversion of glucose to carbon compounds

anaerobic pathway
a form of energy production that does not require oxygen

oxygen debt
the amount of oxygen required to clear lactic acid buildup from the body

anaerobic glycolysis
the conversion of glucose to pyruvate to provide energy in the absence of oxygen

aerobic glycolysis
the conversion of glucose to ATP for energy when oxygen is available

aerobic pathway
a form of energy production that depends on oxygen and increases the use of fat

pose cells. Glucose must be available to the brain. Only a small portion of triglycerides (glycerol) can yield glucose, and continuous use of this source results in a buildup of ketones and the potential imbalance of the body pH (see Chapter 6). The body prefers to spare protein for its more important function, that of building and repairing cells and tissues.

Anaerobic and Aerobic Pathways

How do anaerobic and aerobic energy pathways work together to supply energy? For the first minute or two of exertion, oxygen has not arrived at the muscles and therefore energy must come from anaerobic sources. After several minutes the aerobic pathway takes over. However, as the exertion or exercise continues, there is a constant interchange or use of energy sources.

The energy source that muscles use during exercise depends on the intensity and length of exercise, the person's fitness level, and the foods eaten. Short-term, high-intensity activities such as sprinting rely mostly on the anaerobic pathway for energy, and only carbohydrates (primarily from muscle glycogen) can be used. On the other hand, exercise of low to moderate intensity is supported primarily by the aerobic system, and both carbohydrate and fats are used. Fats are an important energy source during exercise because, unlike carbohydrates, fatty acids are abundant in the body and their use spares muscle glycogen.

The length of activity also determines what type of fuel the muscles will use during exercise. As the duration of exercise increases, glycogen stores become depleted and fat becomes the primary source of energy (Figure 9-3). A sedentary person breaks down glycogen faster and as a result accumulates more lactic acid in the tissues. The lactic acid causes muscle fatigue. A physically fit person has a higher aerobic capacity (the ability of the heart to supply oxygen) so that oxygen is available sooner and in greater quantity; this allows use of the aerobic pathway of energy,

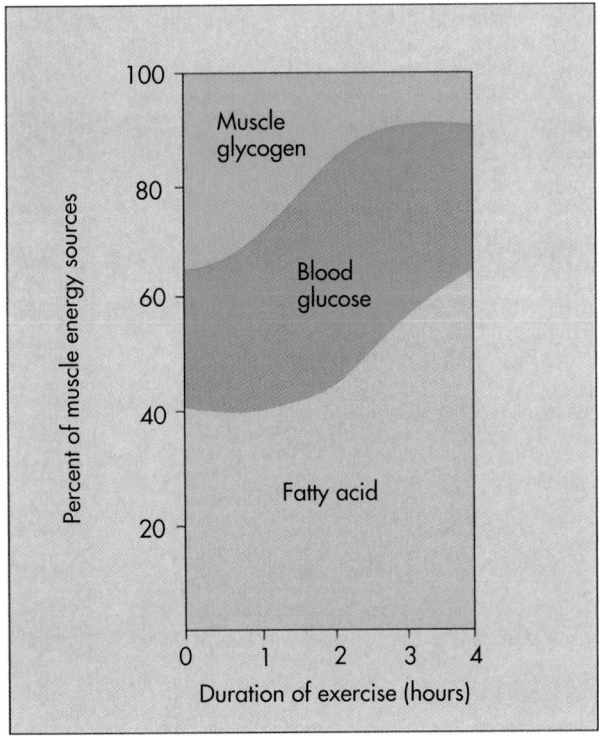

Figure 9-3 Relative use made of energy sources in the body as exercise continues. (Pagecrafters; from Guthrie HA, Picciano MF: *Human nutrition,* New York, 1995, McGraw-Hill.)

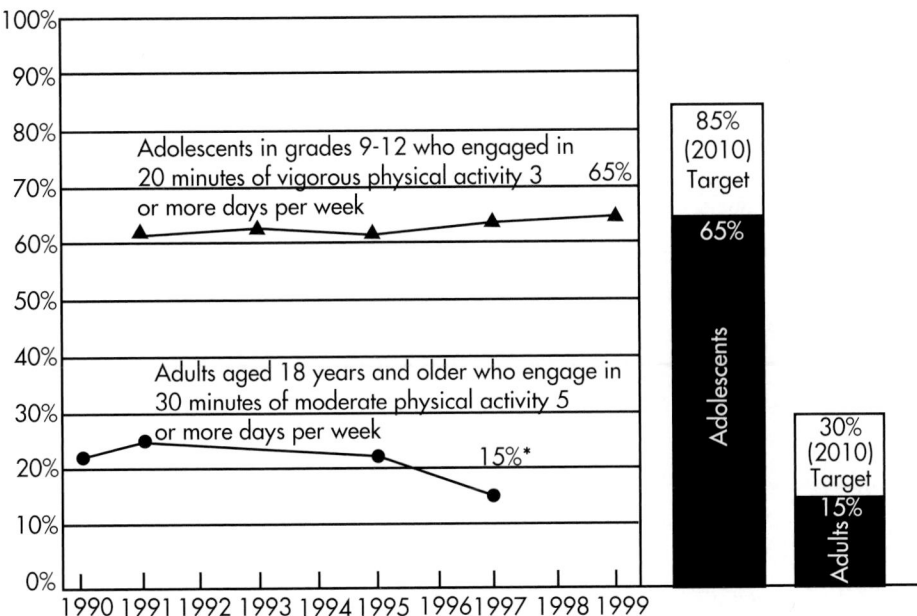

*The definition of moderate physical activity was changed in 1997.

Figure 9-5 Participation in regular physical activity, United States, 1990-1999. (From *Healthy People 2010*. Sources: Centers for Disease Control and Prevention, Youth Risk Behavior Surveillance System, 1991-97; Centers for Disease Control and Prevention, National Center for Health Statistics, National Health Interview Survey, 1990-99.)

Physical activity need not be strenuous to achieve healthful benefits. Even people who are usually inactive can improve their health by becoming moderately active on a regular basis. As we counsel clients and patients in community and acute care settings, we can incorporate suggestions for simple fitness activities into care plans (see the Health Debate box, "What Kind of Exercise Is Best?").

HEALTH DEBATE
What Kind of Exercise Is Best?

Guidelines for physical fitness recommended by the American College of Sports Medicine are 20 to 60 minutes of aerobic activity, three to five times a week. The lower numbers of 20 minutes, three times a week, apply to more intense forms of exercise such as running. The higher numbers of 60 minutes, five times a week are applicable for less intense activities such as continuous brisk walking.

Some health experts maintain that formal programs may not be necessary. It is possible to be physically fit by doing a variety of tasks throughout the day that produce an adequate level of fitness. For example, if within 1 day a person takes a 15-minute walk to the store, gardens actively for 30 minutes, and vacuums the house for another 15 minutes, the person has completed the recommended 60 minutes without disrupting or changing his or her lifestyle.

Other health experts believe a formal fitness program produces more consistent measurable results of improved cardiovascular endurance and overall physical conditioning. The amount of time required is not great and can be individualized to fit a person's lifestyle.

To address all concerns, the Physical Activity Pyramid has been developed. Six types of activity divided into four levels are based on the associated health benefits of activity. The six types of activity are (1) lifestyle physical activity, (2) active aerobics, (3) active

Continued

HEALTH DEBATE–cont'd
What Kind of Exercise Is Best?

sports and recreation, (4) flexibility exercises, (5) muscle fitness exercises, and (6) inactivity. Activities from Level 1 or Level 2 can provide general health and wellness advantages, although performing activities from all three levels is most recommended (see the Pyramid).

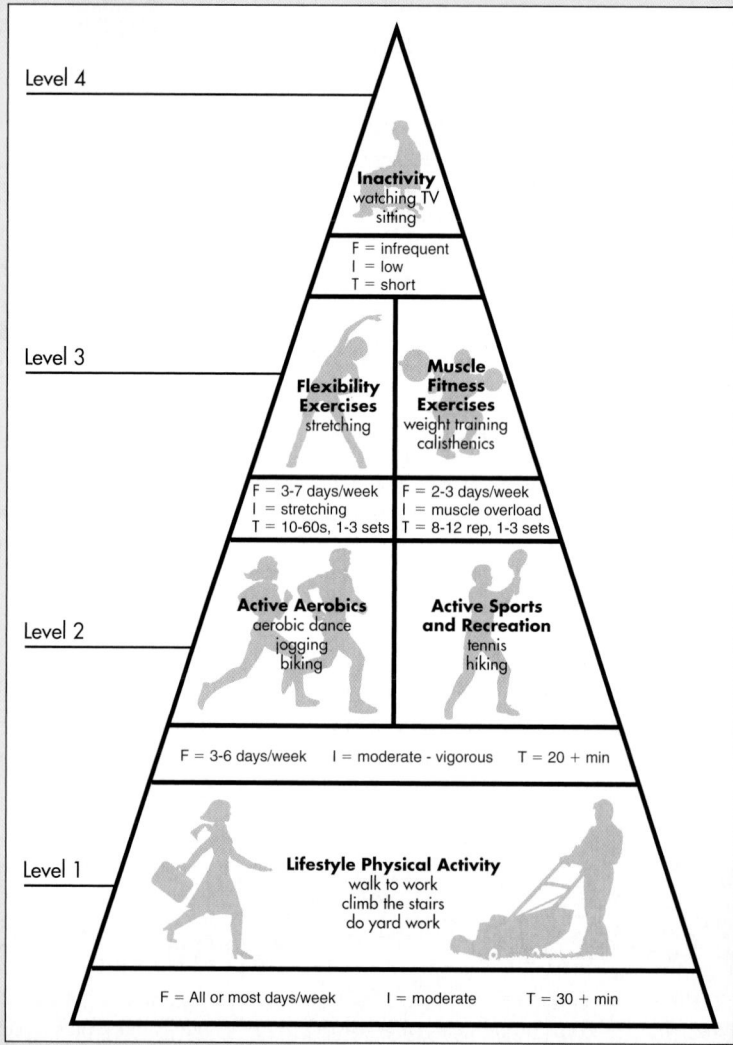

Physical Activity Pyramid. *F,* Frequency; *I,* intensity; *T,* type. (From Scott Foresman: Fitness for life, ed 4, by Charles B. Corbin and Ruth Lindsey. Copyright © 1997 by Scott, Foresman, and Company. Reprinted by permission of Addison-Wesley Educational Publishers, Inc.)

What do you think? Which approach works best? How do you achieve physical fitness through a variety of tasks or by formal fitness activities?

Data from Corbin CB, Pangrazi RP: Physical Activity Pyramid rebuffs peak experience, ACSM's Health & Fitness Journal 2(2):12, Jan/Feb 1998.

The National Institutes of Health (NIH) makes the following recommendations regarding the quantity, intensity, and type of exercise for cardiovascular fitness and muscular strength and endurance[2]:
1. *Frequency and duration of exercise.* Thirty minutes or more of moderate-intensity exercise on most, or preferably all, days of the week (Box 9-1).

Box 9-1 Examples of Moderate Amounts of Activity*

Washing and waxing a car for 45-60 minutes
Washing windows or floors for 45-60 minutes
Playing volleyball for 45 minutes
Playing touch football for 30-45 minutes
Gardening for 30-45 minutes
Wheeling self in wheelchair for 30-40 minutes
Walking 1 3/4 miles in 35 minutes (20 min/mile)
Shooting basketballs for 30 minutes
Bicycling 5 miles in 30 minutes
Dancing fast (social) for 30 minutes
Pushing a stroller 1 1/2 miles in 30 minutes
Raking leaves for 30 minutes
Walking 2 miles in 30 minutes (15 min/mile)
Water aerobicizing for 30 minutes
Swimming laps for 20 minutes
Playing wheelchair basketball for 20 minutes
Playing basketball for 15-20 minutes
Bicycling 4 miles in 15 minutes
Jumping rope for 15 minutes
Running 1 1/2 miles in 15 minutes (10 min/mile)
Shoveling snow for 15 minutes
Walking stairs for 15 minutes

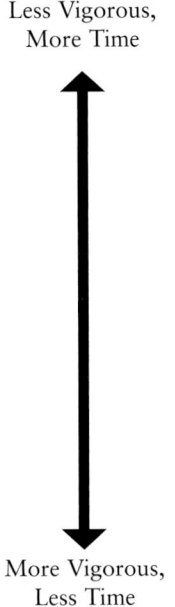

Less Vigorous,
More Time

More Vigorous,
Less Time

From US Department of Health and Human Services, Public Health Service, Centers for Disease Control and Prevention: Report of the Surgeon General: physical activity and health, Washington, DC, 1996, U.S. Government Printing Office.
*A moderate amount of physical activity is roughly equivalent to physical activity that uses approximately 150 Calories (kcal) of energy per day, or 1000 Calories per week. Some activities can be performed at various intensities; the suggested durations correspond to expected intensity of effort.

Shorter sessions of activity (at least 10 minutes), including occupational, nonoccupational, or everyday activities like shopping, running errands, or cleaning the house, also have health benefits if performed at a level of moderate intensity.

2. *Intensity of exercise.* This is influenced by several factors, including needs, goals, health status, availability of exercise, and personal preference. Higher intensity exercise could be performed three times a week, whereas low intensity activities should be performed more frequently to achieve cardiovascular benefits.

3. *Type of activity.* This is best determined by the individual's preferences and what will be sustained. Developing muscular strength and joint flexibility is also important to improve an individual's ability to perform tasks and to reduce the risk of injury.

Sedentary Persons

Generally, sedentary individuals can do little activity without the early onset of fatigue or discomfort. For these individuals, it is best that physical activity be included as part of their lifestyle. For example, taking a 10-minute walk three times a day plus stretching and strengthening activities provides adequate physical activity without the strain of fatigue or discomfort.

Moderately Active Persons

Moderately active individuals are those who can participate in 30 minutes of physical activity with minimum fatigue. They are generally interested in improving cardiovascular health; however, many of these individuals may wish to decrease body fat or increase muscle mass. If the goal is to lose fat, the total kilocalories expended are more important than the intensity level of the activity.[9] Moderately active individuals should also engage in resistance exercises that involve major muscle groups (Box 9-1). The American College of Sports Medicine (ACSM) recommends a minimum of 8 to 10 exercises for the upper and lower body 2 days per week.[10]

Vigorously Active Persons

This category generally includes recreational athletes, competitive athletes, and elite and Olympic-level athletes. These individuals not only want to develop cardiovascular fitness but also look to enhance their performance and move to the next level in their sport. In most cases, the training intensity should match the intensity of the sport. For example, a cyclist works primarily on aerobic training. The basketball player would perform some aerobic and anaerobic training.

Special Populations

Pregnant women and those individuals with physical disabilities or health problems such as diabetes, hypertension, or cardiovascular disease can follow the same principles of prescribing intensity with a few exceptions[9]:
- The more severe the condition, the lower the intensity of exercise.
- Pregnant women should not participate in high-intensity exercise after their first trimester because of the increase in body core temperature (see Chapter 11 for exercise guidelines during pregnancy).
- Individuals who have diabetes or hypertension need to be more aware of their conditions and carefully monitor their exercise intensity. Depending on the frequency and intensity of exercise, levels of medications may need adjustment.

Strength Training

Strength training has become a popular way to stay in shape. It is an integral part of an overall exercise program. Strength training involves lifting various types of weights to build muscle strength and endurance. It may differ from weightlifting. With strength training, improvement is gauged by increased muscle mass. In contrast, weightlifting may be a competitive sport in which individuals lift weights in specific body weight divisions.

Proper strength training exercise programs can reliably increase muscle size and strength in men and women of all ages. The stimulus for muscle growth is overload—resistance greater than that to which the muscle has been accustomed must be imposed. Beginners may start with 3-lb weights and progress to higher weights as strength increases. Research shows that moderately active persons can achieve significant gains in strength by performing one set of 8 to 12 repetitions.[11]

Most of us know that aerobic exercise, such as running and cycling, is good for the heart, making it stronger and more efficient. However, strength training has benefits for cardiovascular health, too. It can help improve blood cholesterol levels, burn fat, and contribute to our well-being. Strength training may also protect against back problems, osteoporosis, and minor injuries. Recent studies show that strength training builds muscle mass of adults in their 80s. Increased muscle mass improves strength and flexibility, both of which reduce the risk of injuries caused by poor muscle coordination and resulting falls.[12]

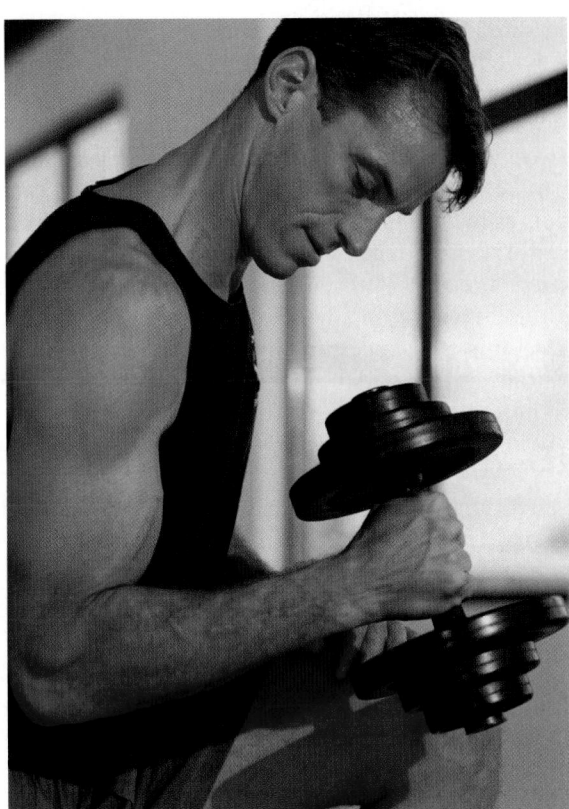

Weight-bearing exercises, including strength training, are beneficial for bone health. (From PhotoDisc.)

Bone responds to the force of gravity and to muscular contraction. Physical exercise forces bone to adapt to the stresses imposed upon it. When stressed, bones become larger and stronger. Weight-bearing exercises (e.g., walking, jogging, weight [strength] training) are beneficial for bone health. The density and health of bone tissue are of particular concern for women. Being physically fit through aerobic and weight-bearing exercise is a good defense against osteoporosis, for which women are at greater risk. Fortunately, this can be accomplished through daily brisk walking or jogging. Other strategies for reducing the risk of osteoporosis are listed in Chapter 8.

For some clients, the development of a simple strength-training program with a certified exercise physiologist may be appropriate as a valuable addition to individual healthcare plans. Such a program may also be beneficial for nursing professionals as well.

Bodybuilding

In recent years there has been increased interest and participation in bodybuilding. Bodybuilders work to develop muscle mass, strength, and muscle definition through a combination of diet, weight training, and aerobic exercise. Unlike weightlifting and other traditional sports that involve strength, bodybuilders exercise to improve their physique as a form of athletic performance.

To prepare for competition, bodybuilders diet and exercise to reduce their body fat. Unfortunately, many bodybuilders follow a number of dietary practices that may place them at risk for health problems.[13] Bodybuilders are susceptible to misinformation about muscle growth and development because they want quick results and may not understand the dietary requirements of muscle gain. Instead, they may consume protein or amino acid powders and supplements in the belief they will provide extra energy and increase muscle mass and strength. These beliefs are reflected in endorsements for a variety of protein and amino acid supplements found in popular fitness and strength magazines. Claims for fast muscle development are made for everything from bee pollen to specific types of exercise equipment.

The composition of muscle is approximately 70% to 75% water, 15% to 22% protein, and 5% to 7% other materials, including inorganic salt, lipids, glycogen, enzymes, and minerals. There is no evidence that extra dietary protein increases muscle mass (see the discussion in Chapter 6 regarding the potential harm of excess protein). Exercise is the single most important factor in increasing the size, strength, and endurance of muscles.

FOOD AND ATHLETIC PERFORMANCE

Physical activity and nutrition have been associated with health since the time of ancient Greece. Hippocrates said, "All parts of the body which have a function, if used in moderation and exercised in labors in which each is accustomed, become thereby healthy, well-developed, and age more slowly, but if unused and left idle they become liable to disease, defective in growth and age quickly."[14] Today, more than 2000 years later, this advice is still consistent with our knowledge about nutrition, physical fitness, and health.[14]

Physically active people of all ages and levels of competition are seeking information to enhance their training and achieve a competitive edge. They want to know what kinds of foods to eat and specific dietary regimens to follow. The nutritional needs of athletes are basically no different from nonathletes, with the exception of kcalories and fluids. A diet that provides a variety of foods supplying 55% to 65% of the kcalories from carbohydrates, 10% to 15% from protein, and no more than 30% from fat is recommended for health and performance.[15] However, some forms of heavy training increase the requirement for certain nutrients. For example, carbohydrates are an important source of energy during endurance exercise, and therefore runners, cyclists, and swimmers may need more carbohydrates (60% to 70% of their total kcalorie intake) than other individuals.

Nutrition can affect an athlete in many ways. At the most basic level, nutrition is essential for normal growth and development and for maintaining good health. By staying healthy, an athlete will feel better, train harder, and be in better condition. Among comparable athletes, good eating habits can be the factor that determines the winner. However, these good habits do not come from the pregame meal or even from what the athlete eats the week before competition. They are built daily over a long period.

A number of dietary patterns will provide good nutrition. The Food Guide Pyramid can be a useful outline for athletes of what to eat every day. Each food group provides some—but not all—of the nutrients an athlete needs. Foods in each of the six food categories in the Food Guide Pyramid provide kcalories from different combinations of carbohydrate, protein, and fat (see Figure 1-2). For example, fruits provide kcalories from carbohydrates, and milk products contain carbohydrate, protein, and varying amounts of fat.

Athletes should eat at least the minimum number of servings for each group daily to meet energy needs. Depending on their body size and level of training, some athletes may need more than the larger number of servings (Box 9-2).

Nurses and other health professionals should have a basic understanding of the nutritional needs of athletes to provide fundamental information and to conduct a simple assessment or screening of nutritional status as influenced by athletic activities. Referrals to a registered dietitian with expertise in sports nutrition is appropriate for athletes and coaches with more specific concerns, such as the creation of individualized eating plans to support training and competitive needs.[16]

Box 9-2 Benefits of Snacking

*S*nacking provides the following benefits:

- Helps the athlete get enough kcalories without having to eat large amounts of food at any one meal; this is especially important for staying awake in class and helping curb hunger pains during practice. Snacking supports academic and physical performance.
- Helps to replace muscle glycogen stores and fluids lost during practice or competition.

- Supplies vitamins and minerals the athlete may not get in regular meals.

Whatever kind of snacker you are, ask yourself these questions:

- What nutrients do snacks provide?
- Do I need the extra calories?
- How can these snacks fit into the total day's diet?

Kcalorie Requirements

As noted earlier, kcalorie requirements vary greatly from person to person and are affected by activity level, body size, age, and climate. Body size affects kcalorie requirements more than any other single factor. The smaller the athlete, the lower the kcalorie requirement.

Some sports demand high-energy expenditure; others do not. A frequently asked question is, "How many kcalories should I consume?" Athletes are consuming enough kcalories if they are maintaining their best competitive yet healthy weight. Ideally, kcalorie intake should balance energy expended. If intake is consistently above or below an athlete's requirement, weight gain or weight loss will occur, both of which can affect performance.

Many athletes are concerned about their appearance and thus eat less to keep their body weight and percentage of body fat low. However, restricting kcalories can have a negative impact on health and performance. As kcalorie intake decreases, so does nutrient intake. A minimum kcalorie requirement for college athletes is 1800 to 2000 kcalories a day. Eating less than this amount can leave the athlete feeling weak and listless and may lead to iron deficiency, stress fractures, and, for women, *amenorrhea* (lack of menstruation) and osteoporosis.

On the other hand, increasing kcalorie intake to gain weight may also be difficult for athletes. Too much food can cause discomfort, especially if a workout takes place soon after eating. Furthermore, when balancing school, work, and practice, little time is available to eat. Small meals and snacks become an important source of nutrients. How often you snack depends on body size and kcalorie needs.

Water: The Essential Ingredient

Water is the nutrient most critical to athletic performance. Without adequate water, performance can suffer in less than an hour. Water is necessary for the body's cooling system. It also transports nutrients throughout the tissues and maintains adequate blood volume.

During exercise there is always the risk of becoming dehydrated *(fluid volume deficit)*, especially when the temperature is hot. When athletes sweat, they lose water. Although sweat rates vary among people, losing as little as 2% to 3% of weight via sweat can impair performance.[17] When the water lost via sweat is not replaced, blood volume falls and body temperature rises, causing confusion and loss of coordination. To replace the lost water, athletes must consume extra fluids.

The athlete's sense of thirst is not the best indicator that the body needs water; fluid needs may be greater than thirst can gauge. Adequate water intake before, during, and after an event or practice session is of utmost importance. The following guidelines by the American College of Sports Medicine ensure adequate fluid replacement, leading to optimal performance.[17]

- Eat a nutritionally balanced diet and drink adequate fluids during the 24-hour period before an event.
- Consume 2 cups (16 oz) of fluid 2 hours before exercise followed by another 2 cups 15 to 20 minutes before exercise and 4 to 6 oz of fluid every 10 to 15 minutes during exercise.
- Drink cool beverages to reduce body core temperature. Cool beverages are best for activities lasting less than 1 hour.
- Consume sport drinks to enhance fluid intake and absorption and help delay fatigue in endurance events lasting longer than 1 hour.
- After exercise, consume sport drinks to enhance palatability and further promote fluid replacement.

How can athletes be sure they are well hydrated? One criterion of hydration is that urine should be basically clear in color throughout most of the day. Athletes should also weigh themselves before and after workouts. For every pound lost, an athlete needs to drink 2 cups of fluid (see Chapter 8 for effects of fluid volume deficit).

Stress the importance of adequate fluid intake. Clients should weigh themselves nude before and after exercise to determine fluid replacement needs. Sweat loss of 1 lb (2.2 kg) of body weight is equal to 2 cups (480 ml) of water.

Sport Drinks

Athletes often wonder which is better for replacing fluids during exercise—water or sport drinks. The number one goal is to remain well hydrated. Whether the athlete drinks water or a sport drink is his or her choice. Cool water is what the body really needs during activities lasting less than 1 hour. However, athletes participating in endurance events requiring more than 90 minutes of continuous moderate to heavy exercise, such as distance running or cycling, may benefit from sport drinks that contain carbohydrate and electrolytes (sodium and potassium). Sports drinks provide fluids to keep the athlete well hydrated and provide extra carbohydrate for energy.

A major consideration in fluid replacement is how quickly the fluid empties from the stomach. To hydrate the total body, the fluid needs to leave the stomach quickly to be distributed throughout the body. Although larger volumes of fluid empty more rapidly from the stomach, many athletes cannot exercise with a full stomach. Cool fluids empty faster from the stomach than warm fluids. Kcalorie content is also important. The greater the kcalorie content of a beverage, the slower the emptying rate.

Carbohydrate: The Energy Food

Carbohydrate stores in the body (glycogen) are limited, and research has shown that low levels of muscle glycogen can impair performance.[18] Consuming carbohydrates before and during exercise will delay the onset of fatigue and allow the athlete to compete for a longer period.

How much carbohydrate should an athlete eat each day to replace muscle glycogen? It depends mostly on body size. An athlete with more muscle mass will require more carbohydrate. Carbohydrate requirements also depend on intensity and level of training. Athletes participating in high-energy sports that require short bursts of energy (e.g., basketball, tennis, football, soccer) need about 5 grams of carbohydrate per kilogram of body weight daily to maintain muscle glycogen stores. Endurance athletes who train aerobically for more than 90 minutes daily may need up to 10 grams of carbohydrate per kilogram of body weight to replace glycogen.[17] Individuals who exercise regularly to maintain conditioning do well with general guidelines of high complex carbohydrate diets as represented by the Food Guide Pyramid. The Teaching Tool box, "How Much Carbohydrate Do You Need?," shows how to calculate carbohydrate requirements.

> ## ✦ TEACHING TOOL
> ### *How Much Carbohydrate Do You Need?*
>
> 1. Divide body weight in pounds by 2.2 lb/kg to determine body weight in kilograms. For example:
>
>   154 lb ÷ 2.2 lb/kg = 70 kilograms body weight
>
> 2. Multiply each kilogram of body weight by 5 grams to determine the number of grams of carbohydrate needed daily. For example:
>
>   70 kg × 5 g = 350 g of carbohydrate daily

Carbohydrate is found in foods in two forms: complex carbohydrates and simple sugars (see Chapter 4). Both types are effective in replenishing glycogen in the muscles. However, complex carbohydrates provide vitamins, minerals, and fiber as well. Examples of complex carbohydrates include bread, potatoes, pasta, cereal, fruits, and fruit juices. Simple sugars include maple syrup, molasses, honey, and table sugar.

Carbohydrate Loading

Carbohydrate loading is the process of changing the type of foods eaten and adjusting the amount of training to increase glycogen stores in the muscle. This concept first became of interest around 1939 when scientists studied the effects of dietary manipulation on the ability to perform prolonged hard work. They found that men consuming a high-carbohydrate diet for 3 days could perform heavy work twice as long as men fed a high-fat diet for the same 3 days.[19] Since then, researchers have investigated several techniques for increasing glycogen levels in the muscles.

To achieve maximum muscle glycogen stores through carbohydrate loading, athletes should consume a high-carbohydrate diet as part of their regular training program. At least 60% (preferably 60% to 70%) of their total kcalories should come from carbohydrate. For the athlete eating 3000 kcalories a day, this represents a minimum of 450 grams of carbohydrate daily. Three days before competition, exercise should taper off to allow muscles to rest. Dietary carbohydrates should be increased to 60% to 70% of total kcalories. This technique of combining rest and increased carbohydrate intake encourages greater glycogen storage. Kcalorie intake may need to be reduced to compensate for less training.

Carbohydrate loading is usually recommended only for athletes engaged in continuous exercise lasting more than 90 minutes, although benefits may be gained for shorter events as well.[20] It is not recommended for athletes participating in short-term events such as sprints or in sports such as football, baseball, and wrestling; nor should individuals with diabetes or hypoglycemia consider this dietary pattern that affects carbohydrate metabolism. Furthermore, the degree of benefit from carbohydrate loading varies among individuals. Therefore athletes should determine before competition the value of this regimen for them and should refer to specific resources for detailed recommendations. The potential negative side effects of carbohydrate loading include increased water retention and weight gain, stiffness, cramping, and digestive problems.[21]

A more practical concern is whether athletes are eating enough carbohydrate on a daily basis to maintain adequate levels of muscle glycogen for training and workouts. See the Web Sites of Interest at the end of this chapter for sites that determine adequate carbohydrate intake to maximize muscle glycogen stores.

Protein

The importance of protein for athletes has been a subject of controversy for many years. Many athletes and coaches believe that a high-protein diet supplies extra energy, enhances athletic performance, and increases muscle mass. There is no evidence, however, that eating more protein than needed improves athletic ability.

Although carbohydrate and fat are the major fuels used for energy, studies indicate that protein use increases during exercise, and under certain conditions protein may contribute significantly to energy metabolism.[21] Two factors that influence the use of protein as an energy source are the length of exercise and the carbohydrate content of the diet. The body may depend on protein for an increased percentage of energy in prolonged exercise (greater than 90 minutes), particularly when carbohydrate intake is low.

The Dietary Reference Intake (DRI) for protein for sedentary adults is 0.8 grams per kilogram of body weight per day.[22] Research suggests that athletes need between 1.5 and 2.0 grams of protein per kilogram of body weight per day.[17] For a 150-lb (68 kg) athlete (runner), this amounts to 102 to 136 grams of protein per day. Factors such as kcalorie intake, protein quality, and type and intensity of the sport are important considerations. The lower the kcalorie intake, the higher the protein requirements. This is one reason why protein intake is often a concern among female athletes because many do not consume enough calories.

The type of protein eaten also affects the amount of protein needed. The 1.5 to 2.0 grams of protein per kilogram of body weight recommendation is based on a diet containing animal foods. Athletes who eat meat, fish, poultry, eggs, milk, or cheese will have little problem meeting their protein needs. Strict vegetarian athletes, however, will need to plan their diets more carefully to ensure that their protein needs are met. Protein bars may be used to supplement protein and energy intakes for athletes. Products should be carefully chosen to avoid excess intake of protein and simple sugars masked as dietary supplement bars (Box 9-3).

Protein and Amino Acid Supplements

The use of protein and amino acid supplements is a common practice among athletes. Various combinations of individual amino acids are sold to athletes with the promise that the acids will stimulate the release of growth hormone and thus increase muscle mass. Promoters claim that amino acids can build muscle, aid fat loss, provide energy, speed up muscle repair, and improve endurance. Others claim that they are more readily digested and absorbed than the protein consumed in foods.

Box 9-3 Is a Snack Bar *Just* a Snack Bar?

Do you grab a snack bar before heading to the gym? Why? Is it high in protein? Or high in energy?

Snack or energy bars tend to be either high in protein or high in energy. They are often expensive and may not be necessary. If the "snack" is to provide some quick energy before exercise, then the bar should be high in carbohydrate energy. Having a high-protein bar that may also be high in fat before exercise won't provide you with quick energy; it takes a longer time for the protein and fat to be digested and absorbed.

Protein bars are appropriate if one's protein intake is low or if the bar is a meal replacement. Popular among body-builders, protein bars are considered a way to maintain protein intake throughout the day. For some, the bar functions as a mini-meal in addition to regularly planned meals. Most likely, most bodybuilders consume an adequate protein intake even for muscle-building purposes.

Perhaps the bottom line is to determine which type of snack bar fulfills a particular need at an appropriate cost and whether it is edible (tastes good). And remember that a well-planned snack, such as a piece of fruit plus some raisins and nuts, may provide the same nutrients for a lot less cost.

Data from Energy bars or protein bars? Penn State Sports Medicine Newsletter *6(9):6, May 1998.*

The question is: Do athletes need to take these supplements or can they get the protein they need from food alone? Many athletes eat more than the recommended amount of protein (and thus amino acids) from food alone. Amino acids as building blocks of all proteins are found in a wide variety of foods, from pork chops to bread and from beans and peas to milk and tacos. Because the body cannot store extra protein, excess protein and amino acids are broken down and used for energy or stored as fat. If protein or amino acid supplements provide more nutrients than needed for protein functions, the body treats supplements the same as any excess source of protein.

It is safer and cheaper to take amino acids in a glass of milk, a turkey sandwich, or other protein-rich foods. Muscle size and strength increase only after weeks of work. If athletes want to gain muscle mass, they need to become involved in a resistive strength training program and consume a diet rich in carbohydrates.

Fat

In athletic performance, carbohydrate and fat are the major sources of energy. The amount of fat used during exercise depends on the duration and intensity of exercise, degree of prior training, and the composition of the diet. Exercise performed under aerobic conditions will promote fat use as a source of energy. There is a good reason to increase your body's ability to burn fat as fuel—using fat as a source of energy will spare muscle glycogen.

Athletes need a certain amount of fat in their diets and on their bodies for optimal health and performance. The challenge is eating a diet that provides the right amount. The position of the American Dietetic Association, Dietitians of Canada, and The American College of Sports Medicine recommends moderate energy intake of 20% to 25% energy from fat.[16] Because each athlete is different, some may eat less and some slightly more than the recommended range of kcalories from fat. Many athletes cannot get the kcalories they need without eating a little extra fat. However, fat intakes greater than 35% of total kcalories have been associated with increased risk of certain diet-related diseases (e.g., heart disease, obesity, cancer).

To lower fat intake, athletes should choose lean meats, fish, poultry, and low-fat dairy products. Fat and oils should be used sparingly in cooking, and fried foods and high-fat snacks should be eaten in moderation (see Chapter 5 for strategies to lower dietary fat intake).

Vitamins and Minerals

A balanced diet generally supplies enough vitamins and minerals to meet the needs of most athletes, and consuming more has not been shown to improve performance. Nevertheless, surveys of athletes show that 41% of high school and 51% of college athletes take supplements.[23] Use is even higher among elite athletes. Female athletes reportedly use vitamin/mineral supplements more than men, and patterns also tend to exist among sport groups.[24] For example, bodybuilders, cyclists, and runners are bigger supplement users than gymnasts, wrestlers, and basketball players.

There are reportedly many reasons why athletes take vitamin/mineral supplements, such as for extra energy, to make up for a poor diet, to recover quicker after exercise, and for general well-being. The problem is that athletes may view supplements as "good" and therefore harmless. Such beliefs can lead to excessive intakes. For many athletes, the level of nutrients consumed from food alone is greater than 200% of the DRI. With the addition of a supplement, combined food and nutrient intakes can exceed 1000% of the DRI. Toxicity and adverse health effects can occur from consuming high doses of vitamins and minerals over a long period.

On the other hand, athletes in "thin-build" sports (e.g., gymnastics, figure skating, wrestling, distance running) often consume low-calorie intakes and thus are at risk for vitamin and mineral deficiencies. For these athletes, supplementation with a multivitamin/mineral providing 100% of the DRI can be beneficial.

Ergogenic Aids

ergogenic aids

drugs and dietary regimens believed by some (but not proven) to increase strength, power, and endurance

In athletics, the term ergogenic aids is used to describe drugs and dietary regimens believed by some to increase strength, power, and endurance (Table 9-5). Because winning is often a matter of a split second, it is easy to see why athletes are continuously looking for the competitive edge. The fact that more and more nutritional supplements are marketed to athletes presents a challenge to coaches, trainers, nutritionists, and healthcare providers to provide sound nutrition information.

The nutritional supplements used by athletes constantly change. Often, as athletes find that one doesn't work, they search for another. Today commonly used nutritional aids include creatine monohydrate (a protein), chromium picolinate, beta-hydroxy-beta-methylbutyrate (HMB) and dehydroepiandrosterone (DHEA).

Table 9-5
Ergogenic Aids Marketed to Athletes

Substance	Description	Claims	Actual Effect
Arginine, lysine, ornithine	Amino acids	Stimulate release of human growth hormone	No proven effect
Antioxidant vitamins C, E, beta-carotene	Compounds that may prevent free-radical damage	Prevent muscle damage from oxidation following high-intensity exercise	Some evidence of proven benefit
Caffeine*	Stimulant	Improves performance; increases fatty acid; oxidation; spares glycogen	Some evidence of proven benefit
Carnitine	Facilitates the transfer of long-chain fatty acids into the mitochondria	Enhances energy levels; decreases body fat	No proven effect
Creatine	Protein/amino acids	Increases intramuscular creatine; increase power output; promote increase in lean body mass	Some evidence of proven benefit
DHEA	Hormone	Increases energy, increase muscle mass, decreases body fat	More research is needed to confirm these observations
Ephedra	Ephedrine alkaloids	Increases energy, decrease body weight, increase athletic ability	Adverse effects on central nervous system and heart
Ginseng	Extract of ginseng root	Reduces fatigue and improves endurance, strength, and recovery from exercise	No proven effect
HMB	Metabolite of the amino acid leucine	Increases in lean body mass, decreased body fat, increased strength	More research is needed to confirm these observations

*The use of caffeine is considered a form of doping by the International Olympic Committee (IOC). The IOC has set an upper limit of 12 micrograms per milliliter of caffeine in the urine.

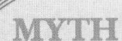

MYTH
Ephedra: A Stimulant By Any Other Name Is Still . . . a Stimulant

*W*ant the best workout ever? Lose weight without any effort? Be energized? These are the types of claims made by the manufacturers of products that contain ephedrine alkaloids, commonly called *ephedra*. Ephedrine alkaloids are amphetamine-like chemicals having a powerful stimulant effect on the central nervous system and the heart. The substance occurs naturally in plants, such as in ephedra herbal species. It is also known as *ma huang,* a traditional Chinese medicine. The ephedrine alkaloids can be synthesized in a laboratory.

In the United States products that contain ephedra are used in dietary supplements to presumably increase energy, achieve weight loss, and increase athletic ability. Although ephedra is naturally derived from plants, safety is not guaranteed. A number of serious adverse reactions—even deaths—have been reported to the Food and Drug Administration (FDA). Ephedrine alkaloids can cause blood pressure to spike, leading to strokes in young, healthy individuals. Other adverse reactions may include rapid or irregular heartbeat, chest pain, severe headache, shortness of breath, dizziness, loss of consciousness, sleeplessness, and nausea. Banning ephedra is being considered by the FDA.

These adverse side effects are too serious to ignore. The best way to experience increased energy, improved athletic ability, and weight loss is to get sufficient rest, train regularly to achieve athletic goals, and consume fewer calories than energy expended.

The U.S. Department of Health and Human Services (USDHHS) reviewed the safety of ephedrine alkaloids in herbal products and tracked the illegal distribution of synthetic ephedrine alkaloid products. The review was completed in fall 2002. For the most up-to-date information, visit www.hhs.gov or nccam.nih.gov. To report adverse effects of products that contain ephedrine-related products, visit www.fda/medwatch.

From Consumer Advisory: Ephedra to be researched more closely, *National Center for Complementary and Alternative Medicine (NCCAM), National Institutes of Health (NIH), June 20, 2002, nccam.nih.gov/health/alerts/ephedra; Press release, HHS announces plans to study ephedra; steps up enforcement of illegal ephedrine marketing,* HHS News, *June 14, 2002; www.hhs.gov/news/press/2002pres/20020614.html.*

Although the use of DHEA is banned in some states, athletes still use it. With the exception of creatine, research has not shown these supplements to have a significant effect on performance. Ephedra use has potentially serious side effects, but the energy boost it provides appears to cause users to disregard these effects (see the Myth box above, discussing ephedra). Despite a lack of scientific basis for the claims associated with these products, their widespread use continues.

Nutritional supplements are a multimillion-dollar business. Athletes are a prime target for the marketers of these products. Athletes make good consumers because, like many Americans, they believe that if a little is good, a lot is better. It is not uncommon for an athlete to consume five or six different supplements a day and not know what substances are in them. Many of the supplements athletes purchase from specialty nutrition stores and mail-order catalogs are not subject to the regulations established by the Food and Drug Administration (FDA), and this presents another concern. Athletes have no way of knowing whether these nutritional supplements are safe.

Taking several different supplements at one time, or one that contains a large amount of one nutrient such as vitamin A, can be toxic. There is also the risk of nutrient-nutrient interactions, in which an excess of one nutrient can interfere with the body's ability to use another nutrient. This may occur when excessive amounts of one amino acid are consumed; the body's use of other amino acids may be affected.

OVERCOMING BARRIERS

American "Couch Potatoes"

The term "couch potatoes" became part of our slang terminology several years ago. The term refers to people who just sit on the couch and vegetate (do nothing) while watching television, viewing movies, or playing video games. Those of us who do more sitting rather than doing, often end up soft and fluffy like mashed potatoes. How did we fall into such habits?

 More than likely, couch potatoes have always existed. Habits that develop during childhood and adolescence may predispose us to lead sedentary lifestyles (see the Cultural Considerations box, "Does Ethnicity Affect Physical Activity Levels in Children?"). If as children our favorite activities involved watching television and sports events rather than playing sports or being physically active, we may end up as couch potato adults. If our parents were also sedentary, we did not have fitness role models.

What has changed is that more focus is being placed on the health benefits of physical fitness. We now know a sedentary lifestyle puts us more at risk for heart disease, some cancers, diabetes, hypertension, and obesity. Even if our body weight is low, we are still at risk for health problems if we are sedentary. These chronic diseases drain the productive and economic resources of our society. Now is a good time for couch potatoes to transform their ways and turn into roadrunners.

Exercise Makes You Hungrier: Myth or Fact?

Does exercise make us hungrier? Do we have a greater physiologic need for food when using our bodies more? Or is the hunger psychologic?

During and immediately after exercise our digestive system basically slows down. Blood flow through the main digestive organs slows; the blood concentrates on reaching the large muscles that need all the nutrients and oxygen possible to do their work. This means that any foodstuff in the digestive tract takes longer to be processed. When we complete and recover from exercising, the digestive process resumes.

However, we may experience low blood glucose levels depending on how long ago we ate and the amount of exercise we completed. Until the body recovers from the exercise, a glass of juice or other light snack best serves the needs of the body to raise blood glucose to a comfortable level.

CULTURAL CONSIDERATIONS
Does Ethnicity Affect Physical Activity Levels in Children?

Does ethnicity affect the amount of physical activity children experience? Researchers addressed this question in a recent study. Predictors of physical activity and fitness of 107 children ranging in age from 6 to 13 years in a longitudinal study of childhood obesity in Birmingham, Alabama, were analyzed. Various methods of physical activity were examined, such as TV viewing, exercising vigorously, exercising in school, participating on sports teams, and performing aerobic activities.

The results showed there were few ethnic differences in childhood physical activity. What the study did find was higher TV viewing and vigorous exercise among children from single-parent families.

Application to nursing: The implications from this study stress that ethnicity alone is not a predictor of physical activity in children. Other social factors must be taken into consideration. Nurses can incorporate suggestions regarding physical activity as part of health and nutrition education. The social and physical benefits of exercise can be explained to parents and children in the context of their everyday lives.

Reference: Lindquist D, Reynolds D, Goran M: Sociocultural determinants of physical activity among children, Preventive Med 29(4):305, 1999.

Sustained regular exercise does cause a physiologic need for more food. The work of exercise uses additional kcalories. Although we may be hungrier and take in more kcalories, we also use more kcalories. The equation of kcalorie input and output can still balance. The bonus is that we will have stronger bodies with more stamina.

TOWARD A POSITIVE NUTRITION LIFESTYLE: MODELING

Want to begin a fitness routine but don't know how to get started? Although motivation is essential, sometimes the basic steps of getting started are the hardest. Should exercise be done in the morning, at lunch, or at night? Every day? Three times per week? How is this done?

A technique to assist in changing behavior is called *modeling;* modeling can be used as an education strategy with patients or may be personally applied to our own lifestyles. Modeling is replicating or imitating the behavior of someone else.

For simplicity, let's apply this technique to you. You are modeling your behavior to be similar to that person's behavior. Approaches to modeling include visualization by imagining you doing what the other person does or discussion with the person to discover how the desired behavior is performed.

Application to a fitness routine could use both approaches. Perhaps a friend has an established fitness routine, and you would like to begin to work out also. To use visualization, first imagine the friend preparing for the workout, exercising, and resting afterwards. Then substitute yourself for the friend. Imagine getting your exercise clothes ready, setting the alarm clock, getting dressed to exercise, exercising, and then resting afterwards. Do this for several days and then actually exercise.

The other approach is to talk with friends or family members who exercise regularly. Find out how they prepare for workouts. What motivation techniques to maintain a fitness program do they use? How many times per week do they exercise? How do they deal with everyday interruptions to their exercise program such as examinations, sick children, or work crises? After adjusting their techniques to your circumstances, actually exercise.

SUMMARY

The ability to perform work, produce change, and maintain life all require energy. ATP is the fuel for all energy-requiring processes in the body. We convert the energy from the food we eat into ATP energy.

There are two related energy pathways. The aerobic pathway depends on oxygen; the anaerobic pathway functions without oxygen. The physical demands of different sports require specific sources of energy. Carbohydrate in the form of glucose is the only fuel to be used anaerobically without oxygen to produce ATP. During low- to moderate-intensity exercise, muscles cells mainly use fat for fuel.

Our daily energy requirement depends on three major components: basal metabolism, physical activity, and the energy to metabolize food. Each of these components is affected directly or indirectly by many factors including our age, gender, and body size. Physical exercise is important to our long-term health and well-being because increased physical activity leads to improved fitness and other physiologic changes that may reduce the risk of chronic diseases such as heart disease, cancer, diabetes, and obesity. A combination of aerobic exercise and strength training is recommended for overall fitness.

The nutritional needs of athletes are generally no different from those of nonathletes, with the exception of kcalories and fluids. Many different dietary patterns can meet the athlete's nutrition needs. Carbohydrate is an important nutrient for both health and athletic performance. Athletes should eat enough carbohydrate on a daily basis to maintain adequate levels of muscle glycogen for training and workouts.

Protein requirements of athletes may be slightly greater than that of sedentary individuals. Most athletes, however, get enough protein in their diets. There is no need for them to take protein powders or amino acid supplements. For the most part, research has shown that nutritional supplements including vitamins and minerals have little effect on performance in athletes who consume a balanced diet.

THE NURSING APPROACH
Nutrition and Fitness Case Study

Phoebe, a college freshman, has a meal plan at the college cafeteria during the week and generally eats what she likes. At the encouragement of her brothers, she recently tried out for the soccer team. She wasn't active in high school, but she thought soccer would be good exercise and some of her friends are on the team. Phoebe sustained an injury during practice and was recently discharged from the hospital on crutches with a closed transverse fracture of the right leg. Phoebe seeks your advice as the school nurse. She is interested in exercising and asks, "What should I do?"

ASSESSMENT

Objective

- Height: 5'5"
- Weight: 123 lbs.
- Right leg in a soft cast

Subjective

- Expresses no pain and "getting used to crutches"
- Says "I know I don't eat like I should"

NURSING DIAGNOSIS

Knowledge deficit between the relationship between nutrition and fitness

PLANNING

Short-term Goal

Provide information concerning nutrition and fitness for the next 6 to 8 weeks.

Long-term Goal

Plan for a regular nutritional and fitness program.

IMPLEMENTATION

Short-term Implementation (6 to 8 Weeks While on Crutches)

1. Assessment
   - 24- to 48-hour food diary
   - Overall knowledge of nutrition
   - Exercise program before accident
   - Overall schedule of activity including classes
2. Provide information on the relationship of nutrition and fitness.
3. Explain the benefits of physical exercise.
4. Discuss the options for physical activity with the cast on such as active and passive exercises with demonstration.
5. Discuss a plan for nutrition during the next 6 to 8 weeks to increase healing by increasing her intake of proteins.
6. Explain the Food Guide Pyramid and kcalories requirements.

Long-term Implementation (After 8 Weeks)

1. Discuss her preferences for physical exercise (e.g., individual or team).
2. Explain the relationship of moderate level of exercise and benefits at a regular schedule.

THE NURSING APPROACH–cont'd
Nutrition and Fitness Case Study

3. Discuss the need for warm-ups before exercising and cool down after exercise.
4. Discuss a plan for food choices for meals and healthy snacks with vitamin supplements.
5. Encourage her to drink fluids daily and plan when exercising.

EVALUATION

Short-term Ealuation

- Phoebe explains the relationship between nutrition and fitness.
- Phoebe explains the benefits of exercise.
- Phoebe implements a plan for physical activity while on crutches.
- Phoebe explains her intake of a balanced meal with increased protein foods for healing.

Long-term Evaluation

- Phoebe states her plan for a type of regular physical exercise.
- Phoebe explains her plan for food choices for meals and snacks.

APPLYING CONTENT KNOWLEDGE

Darren, a college student, just started an aerobic exercise plan to lose some "fat." Because he feels tired, he stops by the college health center and chats with a nurse practitioner about his exercise program. He asks, "If my muscles use simple carbohydrates for energy, why isn't it okay for me to have a soda and a candy bar rather than a regular meal? It's all kilocalories, isn't it?" How might the nurse practitioner respond?

Web Sites of Interest

The Physician and Sportsmedicine Online
www.physsportsmed.com
This sports medicine site provides clinical and personal health resources including articles on nutrition, prevention, personal fitness, exercise, and rehabilitation. It also includes information on sports medicine clinics and fellowship lists. This online site of *The Physician and Sportsmedicine* journal includes links to many related sites.

Gatorade Sports Science Institute
www.gssiweb.com
This institute supports and educates people about sports nutrition, exercise science, and physically active lifestyles. The institute helps health professionals (e.g., athletic trainers, dietitians, coaches, physical scientists, educators) in the exercise sciences by providing service and supporting research for educational purposes.

Healthwise Columbia University
www.goaskalice.columbia.edu/
Go Ask Alice!, a service of Columbia University, lets participants ask questions about nutrition and diet, drugs, stress, sex, alcohol, and other health-related issues. Selected questions are answered on the site.

References

1. *Webster's Dictionary,* www.webster.com/cgi-bin/dictionary.
2. National Institutes of Health Consensus Conference: Physical activity and cardiovascular health, *J Am Med Assoc* 276:241, 1996.
3. Powell KE et al.: Physical activity and chronic disease, *Am J Clin Nutr* 49:999, 1989.
4. Rosato FD: *Fitness and wellness: the physical connection,* ed 3, St Paul, Minn, 1995, West Publishing.
5. US Department of Health and Human Services, Public Health Service: Leading Health Indicators, *Healthy People 2010,* ed 2, Washington, DC, 2000, US Government Printing Office; www.health.gov/healthypeople.
6. Berlin JA, Colditz GA: A meta-analysis of physical activity in the prevention of coronary heart disease, *Am J Epidemiol* 132:612, 1990.
7. US Department of Health and Human Services, Public Health Service, Centers for Disease Control and Prevention: *Report of the Surgeon General: physical activity and health—persons with disabilities,* Washington, DC, 1996, U.S. Government Printing Office.
8. US Department of Health and Human Services, Public Health Service: *Healthy People 2010,* ed 2, Washington, DC, 2000, US Government Printing Office; Chapter 22; www.health.gov/healthypeople.
9. Franks BD, Welsch MA, Wood RH: Physical activity intensity: how much is enough? *ACSM's Health & Fitness,* 1:14, Nov/Dec 1997.
10. American College of Sports Medicine: *ACSM's guidelines for exercise testing and prescription,* ed 6, Baltimore, 2000, Williams & Wilkins.
11. Starkey DB et al.: Effect of resistance training volume on strength and muscle thickness, *Med Sci Sports Exerc* 28:1311, 1996.
12. Takeshima N, et al.: Water-based exercise improves health-related aspects of fitness in older women, *Med Sci Sports Exerc* 34(3):544, March 2002.
13. Walberg-Rankin J: A review of nutritional practices and needs of bodybuilders, *J Strength Cond Res* 9:116, 1995.
14. Simopoulos AP: Opening address: nutrition and fitness from the first Olympiad in 776 BC to 393 AD and the concept of positive health, *Am J Clin Nutr* 49:921, 1989.
15. Reimers KJ, Ruud JS, Grandjean AG: Sports nutrition. In Mellion MB, ed.: *Office sports medicine,* Philadelphia 1996, Hanley & Belfus.
16. Nutrition and Athletic Performance—Position of the American Dietetic Association, Dietitians of Canada, and the American College of Sports Medicine, *J Am Diet Assoc* 100:1543, 2000.
17. American College of Sports Medicine: Position stand: exercise and fluid replacement, *Med Sci Sports Exerc* 28:i, 1996.
18. Sherman WM, Wimer GS: Insufficient dietary carbohydrate during training: does it impair performance? *Int J Sports Med* 1:28, 1991.
19. Christensen E, Hansen O: Arbeitsfahigkeit and Ernahrung, *Skand Arch Physiol* 81:160, 1939.
20. Applegate L: *Eat smart, play hard: customized food plans for all your sports and fitness pursuits,* Emmaus, Penn, 2001, Rodale Inc.
21. Williams MH: *Nutrition for fitness and sport,* ed 6, New York, 2001, McGraw-Hill.
22. Institute of Medicine, Food, and Nutrition Board: *Dietary Reference Intakes for energy, carbohydrate, fiber, fat, fatty acids, cholesterol, protein, and amino acids,* Washington, DC, 2002, National Academy Press.
23. Sobal J, Marquart LF: Vitamin/mineral supplement use among athletes: a review of the literature, *Int J Sport Nutr* 4:320, 1994.
24. Marquart LF: Vitamin/mineral supplement use among high school athletes, *Adolescence* 29:835, 1994.

CHAPTER 10

Management of Body Composition

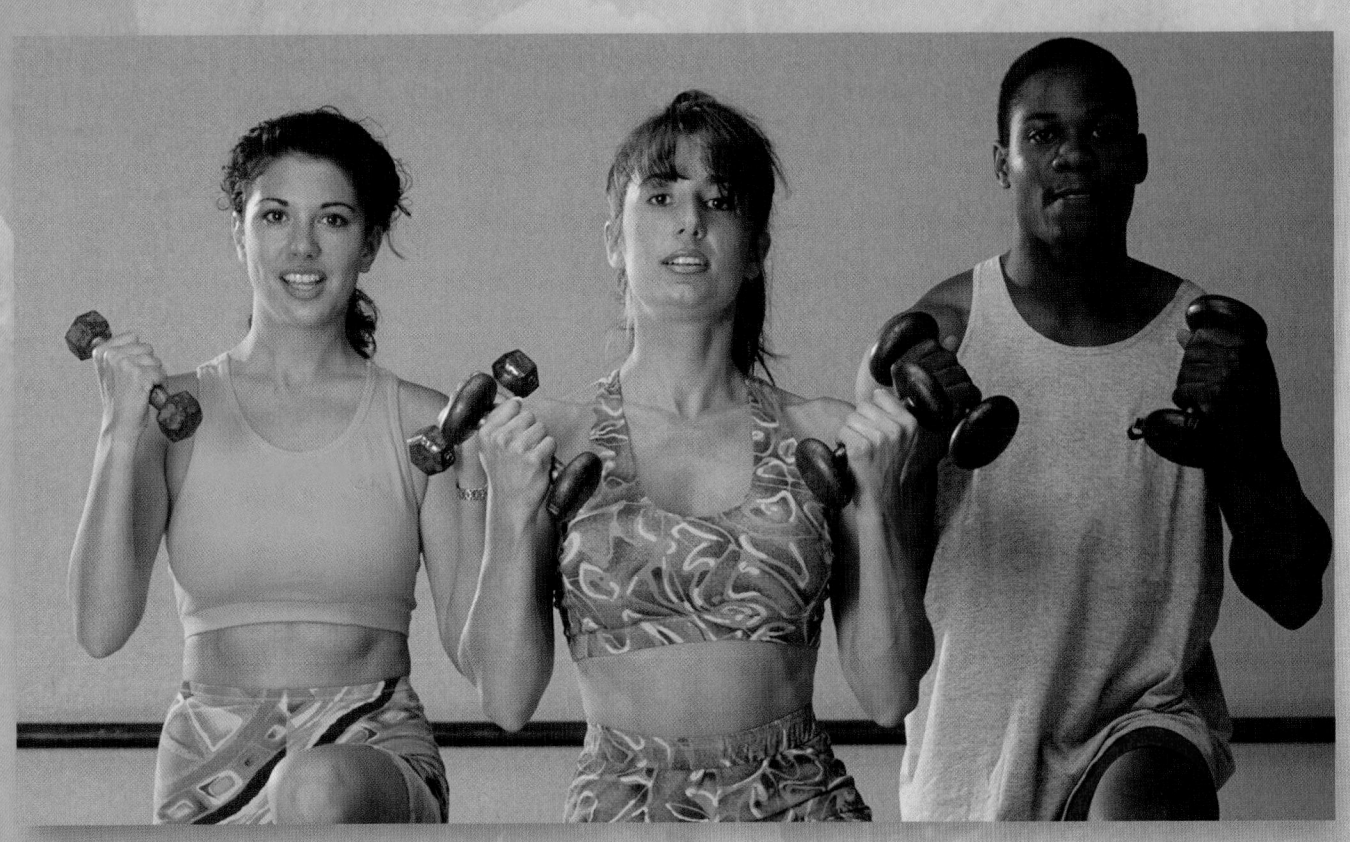

Lifelong management of body fat levels provides a more holistic health approach to body size than does body weight.

ROLE IN WELLNESS

What does weight or fatness mean to us as members of our contemporary culture? We step on the scale frequently, we read the numbers, and we often seem to get a message that extends beyond the simple mass of heaviness of our bodies. What message does the scale deliver? For some members of our culture, the figures on the scale convey something about their physical health. For others, the scale measures attractiveness. Sometimes it measures a sense of empowerment, of being in control of our lives. How can one simple assessment convey so many powerful interpretations? This chapter explores the meanings of weight or fatness in our contemporary culture and challenges these meanings and how they relate to wellness.

Because it is body fat that is really the issue, our focus is on fat rather than on weight. In addition, we use the approach of *management of body composition, specifically body fat levels,* rather than achievement of ideal body fatness. In this context, *management* is defined as the use of available resources to achieve a predetermined goal. This definition recognizes that individuals differ in the resources available to them and in the goals they set.

Consideration of the five dimensions of health helps emphasize that managing body composition is more than just counting calories. Managing body composition levels by decreasing or increasing body fat or lean body mass is, if appropriate, an aspect of the physical dimension of health. Adequate levels of body fat allow the body to function most efficiently. The intellectual dimension of health provides the skills to understand and critique the role of society in molding our attitudes toward the shapes of our bodies. Regardless of our body size, our emotional health depends on our developing positive self-esteem. The social dimension of health may not be affected by body fat levels, although those at either extreme of body size may need to develop a circle of friends and family who accept their size differences. The spiritual dimension of health is sometimes tested as a belief in a higher being who provides support for some individuals struggling with behavior changes relative to the quantity and emotional meanings of food consumed.

BODY COMPOSITION, BODY IMAGE, AND CULTURE

Body Image

The phrase *body image* refers to the perceptions we have of our bodies. Although body image can refer to the functioning of the body, most often it deals with our ideas, feelings, and experiences about the physical appearance or attractiveness of our bodies. Individuals have a distorted body image when their perceptions are inconsistent with reality. For example, most people with anorexia nervosa view their bodies as disgustingly fat when in fact they are emaciated. Body image is important because it may affect how we feel about ourselves and how we behave.

Body Perception

All of us have notions as to what makes a body attractive. Thank goodness we all don't agree on some of the fine distinctions. In general, however, from where did our notions of attractiveness come? Why do we think men should look strong and women soft? Many of our notions of attractiveness are so ingrained that we are unaware of them. Apparently, biology and culture interact to set the standards. Certainly biology plays a role by arranging our genetic inputs so that men and women develop body characteristics that attract the opposite sex and thereby per-

---

Ellen S. Parham, MSEd, PhD, RD, LPC, contributed this chapter in the first and second editions of this text.

petuate the species.[1] It is probably this biologic influence that causes us to admire an appearance of strength in men and soft curves in women. Genetics also determine the potential for other characteristics of appearance, such as height, color of skin, shape of nose, and texture of hair.

However, within these biologically determined characteristics we make great distinctions as to what is attractive and desirable. At different times and places, humans have had widely differing notions of what constitutes an attractive man or woman. As far as fatness is concerned, a rotund figure has often in the past been considered evidence of fertility and well-being. Prehistoric figures of women with massive breasts and hips have been unearthed all over Europe and are believed to have been symbols of good fortune and fertility. Over time, styles in attractiveness would come and go, sometimes favoring a full figure, other times favoring slenderness. Both fatness and thinness were viewed as unhealthy when carried to an extreme, but generally there was not a great deal of interest in weight.

As America entered the twentieth century, things changed. There developed a preference for slenderness that has not abated. Why this change in perception of attractiveness occurred and endured is not completely clear. Probably it was the coming together of several factors. These include concerns about the effects of an increasingly sedentary lifestyle, a heightened interest in fashion, the development of the medical profession, and increased knowledge of nutrition, as well as the self-interests of various promoters who saw profit to be gained by creating an anxiety about fatness.[2]

After World War II, we entered an era of especially strong cultural influences. Mass media created a web of communication of a magnitude and efficiency that was never before possible. Now notions of attractiveness are shared quickly around the globe. Furthermore, sales promotion is a motive that underlies much of the communication. The outcome has been a view of beauty that homogenizes individual differences into a general sameness, decreeing the same size and shape for all.

Body Image: Illusions vs. Reality

The effect of these conflicting cultural pressures are bewildering and, for some individuals, overwhelming. Physical attractiveness is narrowly defined as thinness and firmness and becomes, for some, the expression of personal worth. There follows an urgency to be sure one is thin enough. This concern is compelling for those fat and thin alike.

Most of us weigh ourselves regularly and have a good idea of our current weight. The figure on the scale, however, does not always agree with how fat we feel. Figure 10-1 shows an example of the type of instrument that investigators use to assess differences between actual, perceived, and preferred body size. The investigator instructs the subjects to mark the figure that is most like the way they feel at that time, as well as the figure that they consider ideal for themselves. When these figures are compared with an objective assessment, regardless of their actual size, the subjects usually have greatly overestimated their size.

Body Preferences: Gender Concerns

Investigators also use figure rating scales to determine how men and women differ in size preferences; they ask you which figure is most like how you would like to be, which is most like how you currently are, and which you think is most attractive to the opposite sex. Ideally, the answers to these three questions would be closely clustered, indicating that you are fairly satisfied with your size. For men, that is usually the case. Women, however, on average feel much fatter than they think is ideal. Originally it was assumed that the women's dissatisfaction represented a desire to appear more slender and, therefore, more attractive to men. Usually, however, women's personal ideal is thinner than the figure they think men

Which one is most like you?

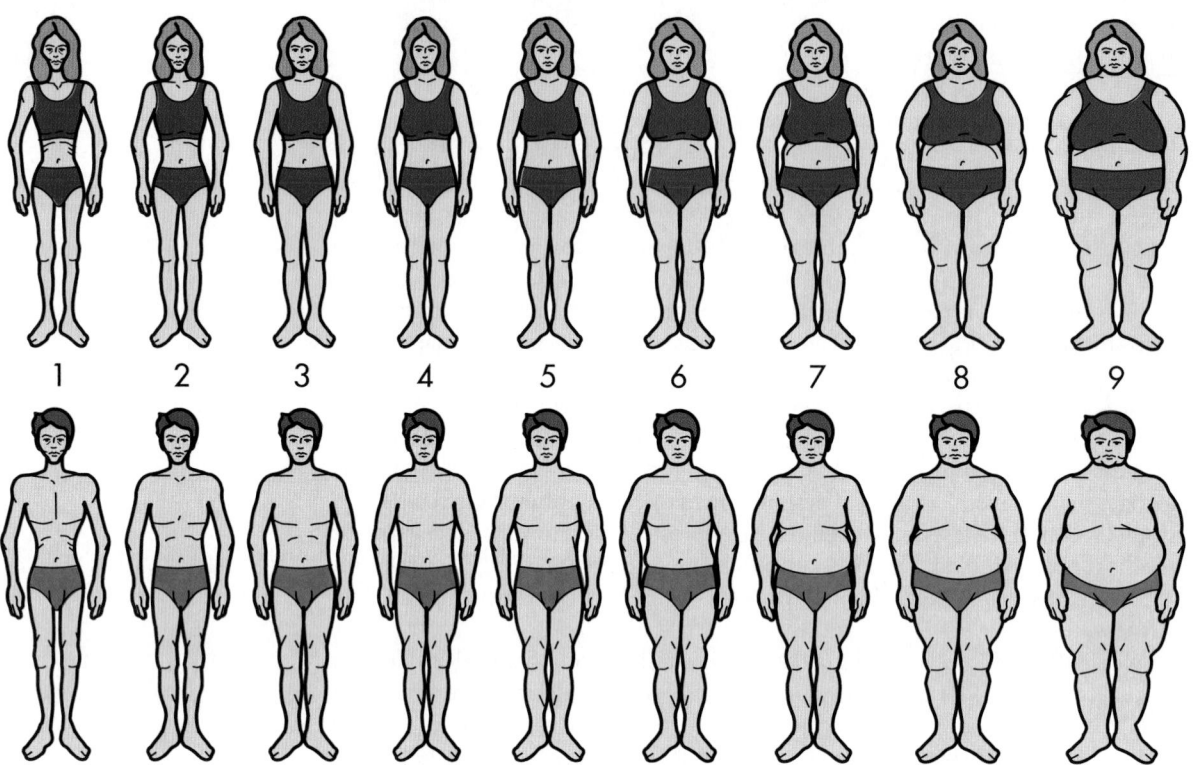

Figure 10-1 An example of a figure rating scale. (Modified from Stunkard AJ, Sorensen T, Schulsinger F: Use of the Danish adoption register for the study of obesity and thinness. In *Genetics of neurological and psychiatric disorders*, New York, 1983, Raven Press. From ARNMD Series, Vol. 60.)

would choose, challenging the assumption that women want to be thin to attract men. An alternative interpretation is that both men and women interpret a slender body as evidence of being in control of one's life.[3]

Body Acceptance: A Key to Wellness

Why is body image important? A negative body image may affect how we feel about ourselves generally: *body image* tends to become *self-image*. Furthermore, a negative body image may influence our health behaviors. We may feel defeated that because our bodies are so bad, it is not worth working hard to improve our health. At other times, we may feel drawn to various kinds of risky behaviors in a frantic attempt to make our bodies more acceptable. We may strive mightily to meet the societal standards of attractiveness and thinness, but given our individual genetic makeup, we cannot all succeed. Although humans have an awesome potential for growth and development, there are limits to the changes we can make and sustain in our body size and shape.[3]

If we have a healthy and positive body image, we evaluate various aspects of our bodies fairly realistically, finding some characteristics positive and others less so. Those we consider weak or unattractive, we accept in a dispassionate way, much the same that we accept that we don't all have beautiful singing voices or the ability to throw a great curve ball. We understand that our bodies have multiple aspects, that there is more to our bodies than their size and shape. Our healthy

*W*e live in a world where fat intolerance or fat phobia (fear of fat) is the last socially acceptable prejudice. "Fatism" even seems to have similarities with racism. As a society, we are committed to self-improvement. Consequently, it may feel wrong to question the directive that all those who deviate from the ideal size and shape should dedicate themselves to rectifying the situation. Our fat intolerance may be motivated by the best intentions to be helpful to ourselves and to others, but like all prejudices, it diminishes the people to whom it is applied.

This prejudice is especially problematic when it exists among health professionals. Obese people often report they feel degraded by their healthcare encounters and therefore avoid seeking medical help. The traditional medical model holds the patient responsible for the existence of a health problem; this moralistic philosophy tends to justify blaming the patient for choosing to be fat or thin. Although this prejudice could be expected to interfere with their effectiveness, health professionals seem to possess high levels of fat intolerance; one study found that among medical students, 57% characterize obese individuals as lazy, 52% as sloppy, and 62% as lacking self-control. Encouragingly, the same author found when medical students participate in a program to increase understanding, their negative stereotypes diminish.

What about you? Have you been successful in questioning and replacing your own prejudices? Are you able to accept yourself and your body? As a future health professional, are you prepared to empower your patients to work toward total wellness, including healthy nondieting habits?

Compiled from Achterberg C, Trenkner LL: Developing a working philosophy of nutrition education, J Nurs Educ 22:189, 1990; *Crandall CS: Prejudice against fat people: ideology and self-interest,* J Personality Assess 66(5):882, 1994; *Parham ES: Fear of fat: attitudes toward obesity,* Nutrition Today, *Jan/Feb 26, 1990; Parham ES: Is there a new weight paradigm?* Nutrition Today *31:155, 1996; and Wiese HJC et al.: Obesity stigma reduction in medical students,* International J Obes 16:859, 1992.

---

body image is influenced by our awareness of how our bodies function and how they look. This image affects and is affected by sociodemographic factors. Body image satisfaction may be related to the degree of overweight and to psychologic distress represented by depression and low self-esteem.[4] We are more able to undertake and sustain healthy behaviors. Understanding and accepting what we can and cannot expect to achieve in pursuit of the ideal body is a key to wellness. Only with this understanding can we establish goals that will guide our behaviors toward health (see the Social Issues box).

MANAGEMENT OF BODY FAT COMPOSITION

If we say that individuals must choose their own values and goals, it is impossible to state one goal for everyone. Nevertheless, we can identify some probable commonalities. Surely most of us would define a goal of maximizing the quality and length of our lives. We probably can go further and say that our goal is to achieve the best possible health, including emotional, social, intellectual, physical, and spiritual aspects. This chapter proceeds on the premise that we can agree on some version of this goal. Most of us would also agree that too little and too much fat are likely to compromise physical health. In addition, we assume that the relationship between fatness and well-being is limited. That is, being slender does not guarantee happiness and health in all its aspects nor is being heavy a sentence of unhappiness and illness.

Association of Body Fatness with Health

Physical Health

Most of our evidence of the association between fatness and physical health comes from epidemiologic studies. Epidemiologic research investigates the distribution of disease in a population and seeks to explain associations between causative-factors and the disease. This type of research usually involves thousands of subjects and may be longitudinal (i.e., involving observations over a number of years). Because it is not practical to measure fatness in these large studies, weight is usually measured instead. Weight is most meaningful when considered in relationship to height. A convenient way to possibly determine fatness is to calculate body mass index (BMI), a value derived by dividing one's weight in kilograms by the square of one's height in meters (Table 10-1). This formula for BMI results in a value that may correlate well with body fatness.

If we were to plot the findings of epidemiologic studies of the association of BMI and the risk of certain diseases or mortality from all causes, we would usually produce a U-shaped curve such as that shown in Figure 10-2.[5] This curve means that individuals at both extremes of fatness—those very thin and those very

Table 10-1
Body Mass Index Chart*

Height (inches)	19	20	21	22	23	24	25	26	27	28	29	30	31	32	33	34	35
	\	\	\	\	\	\	\	Body Weight (pounds)									
58	91	96	100	105	110	115	119	124	129	134	138	143	148	153	158	162	167
59	94	99	104	109	114	119	124	128	133	138	143	148	153	158	163	168	173
60	97	102	107	112	118	123	128	133	138	143	148	153	158	163	168	174	179
61	100	106	111	116	122	127	132	137	143	148	153	158	164	169	174	180	185
62	104	109	115	120	126	131	136	142	147	153	158	164	169	175	180	186	191
63	107	113	118	124	130	135	141	146	152	158	163	169	175	180	186	191	197
64	110	116	122	128	134	140	145	151	157	163	169	174	180	186	192	197	204
65	114	120	126	132	138	144	150	156	162	168	174	180	186	192	198	204	210
66	118	124	130	136	142	148	155	161	167	173	179	186	192	198	204	210	216
67	121	127	134	140	146	153	159	166	172	178	185	191	198	204	211	217	223
68	125	131	138	144	151	158	164	171	177	184	190	197	203	210	216	223	230
69	128	135	142	149	155	162	169	176	182	189	196	203	209	216	223	230	236
70	132	139	146	153	160	167	174	181	188	195	202	209	216	222	229	236	243
71	136	143	150	157	165	172	179	186	193	200	208	215	222	229	236	243	250
72	140	147	154	162	169	177	184	191	199	206	213	221	228	235	242	250	258
73	144	151	159	166	174	182	189	197	204	212	219	227	235	242	250	257	265
74	148	155	163	171	179	186	194	202	210	218	225	233	241	249	256	264	272
75	152	160	168	176	184	192	200	208	216	224	232	240	248	256	264	272	279
76	156	164	172	180	189	197	205	213	221	230	238	246	254	263	271	279	287

From National Institutes of Health/National Heart, Lung, and Blood Institute: Clinical guidelines on the identification, evaluation, and treatment of overweight and obesity in adults: the evidence report, June 1998.

*To use the table, find the appropriate height in the left-hand column. Move across to a given weight. The number at the top of the column is the BMI at that height and weight. Pounds have been rounded off. Additional BMI listed in Appendix E.

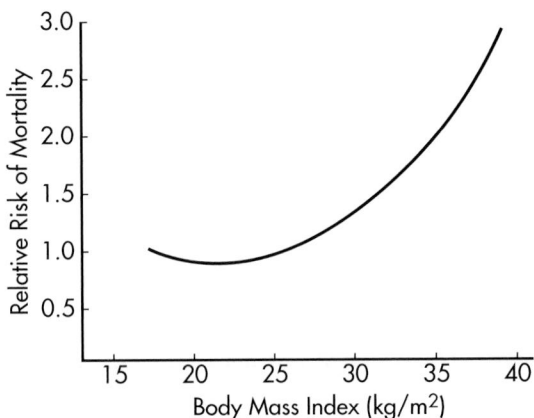

Figure 10-2 U-shaped relationship between BMI to excess mortality in adults. Relative risk was defined as 1.0 for adults with BMIs between 20 and 25. (From Stipanuk MH: *Biochemical and physiological aspects of human nutrition*, Philadelphia, 2000, WB Saunders.)

fat—are at increased risk. Those at a more moderate fatness level have the lowest risk for the four leading causes of death in the United States: heart disease, some types of cancer, stroke, and diabetes. It is a surprise to many people that the low end of the fatness range, or underweight, shows an increased risk, which provides strong evidence that one can be too thin.

It is possible that the lowest BMI in these types of curves reflects low levels not of fat but of the lean body components.[5] The higher risks at the low BMI levels probably reflect some degree of body wasting, including lean body mass, possibly caused by smoking or the effects of disease. To understand the effect of fat on mortality, we need to measure body composition (fat and lean) and not rely on weight alone. Although the factors contributing to this increased risk of extremely low weight are not completely clear, they are thought to differ from the factors associated with increased risk of heavy individuals.

Obesity and Physical Health

Because we have far more overfat people in this country than underfat ones, let's consider first the impact of excess fat or obesity on physical health. Obesity can be defined as excessive fatness. More quantitative definitions traditionally used in medicine and the popular press are that weights greater than 110% of desirable weight equal overweight and weights greater than 120% of desirable weight equal obesity. These definitions assume a precision in interpreting risks of fatness that is simply not available. Use of BMI provides another tool for providing a quick assessment of weight in relationship to height. But, as will be discussed, BMI does not account for distribution of body fat, nor is it accurate for muscular individuals.

As research has extended beyond merely relating BMI to mortality risk, we have become aware that, between extreme emaciation and great obesity, just knowing how fat a person is doesn't tell us much about their health. If we consider how the body fat is distributed, we can improve our understanding. Without knowing the individual's total fatness or BMI, we can still make fat-mediated predictions about health risk. For example, Figure 10-3 shows how health risk is related to one's age and to the ratio of the size of one's waist to one's hips (waist/hip ratio). Higher levels of body fat around the waist seem to be more dangerous than fat in the buttocks and thighs. Fat located within the abdominal area is called visceral fat and seems to be especially related to risk. Persons with high levels of visceral fat are prone to a cluster of metabolic risk factors including high blood pressure (hypertension), distorted levels of certain blood lipids (elevated very low-density lipoproteins and low high-density lipoproteins), and

visceral fat
fat that is within the abdominal cavity

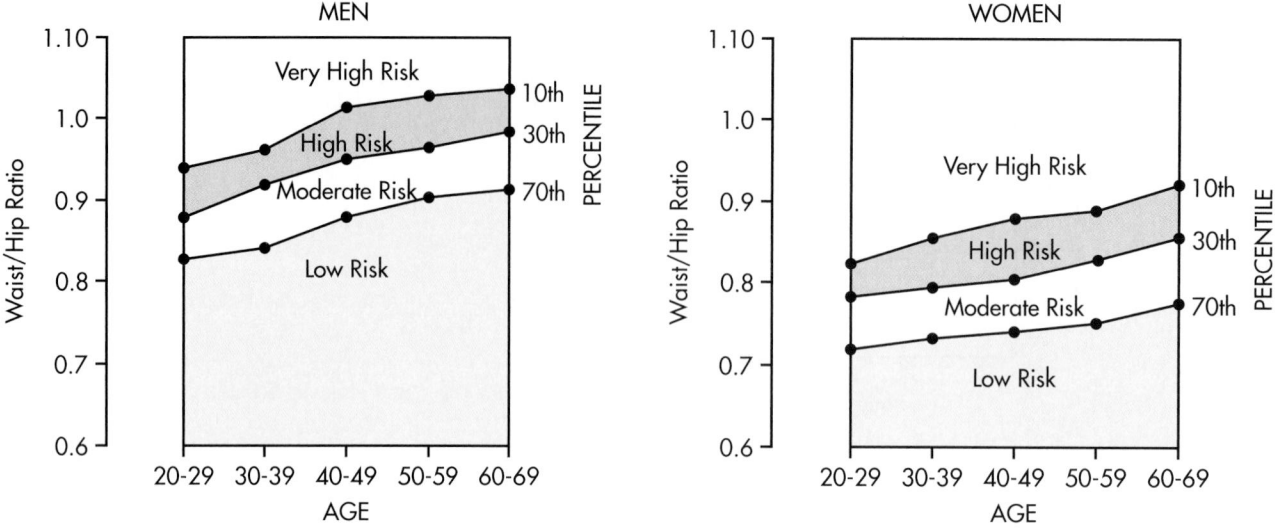

Figure 10-3 Waist/hip ratio and age related to health risk. (From Bray GA, Bouchard C, James WPT: *Handbook of obesity,* New York, 1998, Marcel Dekker.)

more resistance to insulin.[6] Investigators refer to this group of conditions as *syndrome X,* or the *metabolic syndrome.*[6]

The metabolic syndrome, apparently the result of complex endocrine interactions, increases the risk of atherosclerosis, heart disease, stroke, and diabetes mellitus. Diabetes mellitus (DM) is characterized by inadequate insulin activity. In the metabolic syndrome, levels of insulin are usually normal or even elevated, but obese persons have developed a resistance to their own insulin. Although they have high levels of this hormone in their blood, the insulin fails to control blood glucose levels. As a result, type 2 diabetes mellitus (DM) develops. Type 2 DM is the most common type and is highly, but not exclusively, associated with obesity.

Figure 10-4 shows three curves relating risk factors associated with the metabolic syndrome to the risk of ill health.[5] The top curve shows the same relationship of BMI to risk that we saw in Figure 10-2, whereas the next two curves reflect the effects of specific components of the metabolic syndrome, serum lipids levels (here represented by cholesterol), and diastolic blood pressure. Notice that the lower two curves show a stronger relationship, the relative risk increasing fourfold with extremely elevated cholesterol levels and fivefold with extremely high blood pressures. If we had a fourth curve that related the amount of visceral fat to risk, we could expect that it would show a stronger relationship than that shown by BMI alone. It is important to remember that not all heavy persons have high levels of visceral fat and that not all persons with hypertension, type 2 DM, and elevated serum lipids are heavy. The deleterious effect of fatness is stronger in young to middle-aged adults than among older individuals.[7]

Obesity also increases the risk of health conditions that affect well-being but aren't usually life threatening. Examples include menstrual irregularities, infertility, gallbladder disease, and some types of arthritis.

Lastly, we should bear in mind that obesity does not increase all types of health risks (see the Health Debate box). In fact, risks of some types of cancer and of osteoporosis are lower, and risks of other conditions (e.g., infectious diseases, chronic lung disease, liver disease, injuries) are no higher among obese people than the general population.

Unanswered Questions. Up to this point, we have shown some convincing evidence that obesity compromises physical health. However, to get a balanced perspective, we must consider some important issues and unanswered questions. First, we must recognize that most studies show considerable variability in the effect of fatness on health. Three factors identified that may be involved in the

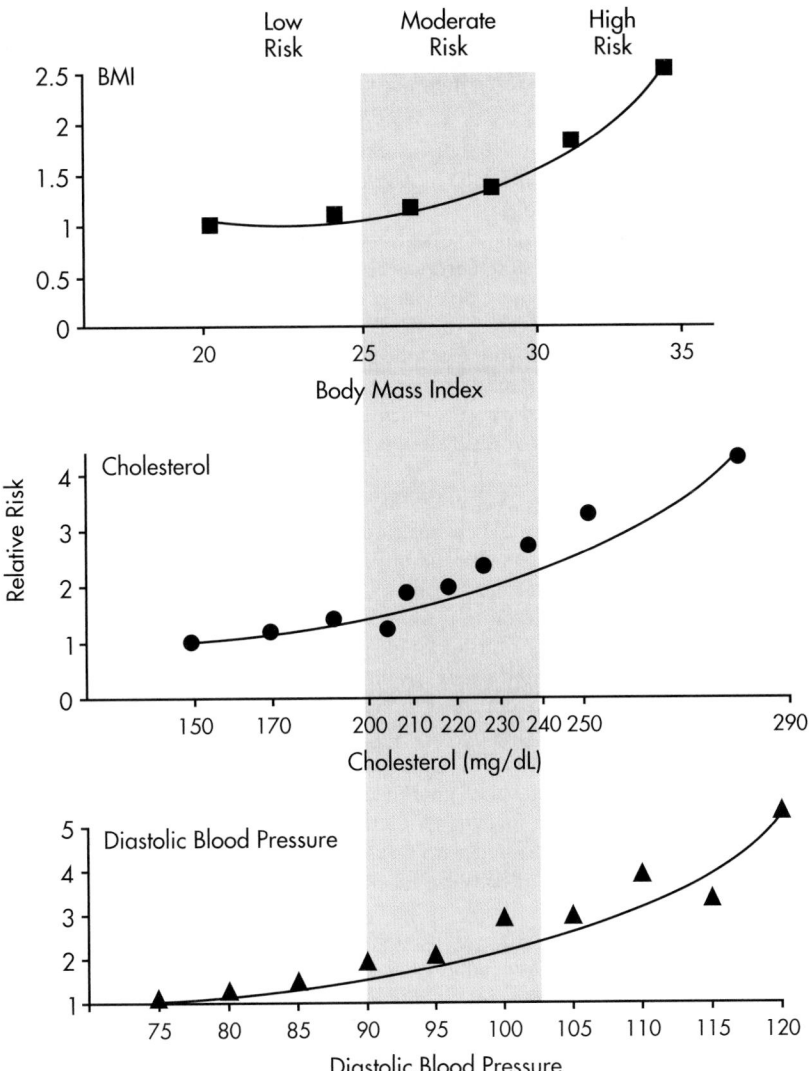

Figure 10-4 Relationship of BMI, cholesterol, and blood pressure to risk of ill health. (Copyright George A. Bray, 1995.)

variability are fat distribution, age, and sex. Even considering these factors, however, we still find a lot of variability in risk. For example, it is widely agreed that obesity increases the risk of developing type 2 DM, but little consideration is given to the fact that more than 90% of obese adults do not develop diabetes.

What accounts for this variability? Why is obesity more of a risk to young adults than to older ones? How do risks differ between men and women? Most large-scale studies of risk have included Caucasians living in the United States or Canada as subjects. What about risks of other ethnic groups? The limited information available indicates that racial and ethnic factors may be important. In addition, why is it that in recent decades, Americans have gotten fatter, yet rates of mortality caused by heart disease have dropped significantly? As scientists sort out the various genetic influences on fatness and on vulnerability to various diseases, many of these questions will be answered.

Does losing weight make health risks go away? And what about weight gain? We don't have strong evidence that weight loss reduces health risk. The literature is mixed about the long-term health effects of weight loss; some epidemiologic studies show increased risks following weight loss,[9] whereas others show no effect or a diminished risk.[7] Important factors seem to be whether the weight was lost in response

HEALTH DEBATE
Is Obesity a Chronic Disease?

*I*s obesity a chronic disease? Or do some people simply weigh more than others? And if the latter is true, is health possible at any size? There are social and medical implications of both positions.

The basis of obesity as a chronic disease is its association with illness and death from other diseases such as hypertension, coronary artery disease, and diabetes. To qualify as a chronic disease, the disorder must be of slow onset, continue over a long period, may reoccur, and have symptoms affecting the whole body. If obesity becomes medicalized—recognized as a chronic disease—there can be reimbursement by health insurance companies for treatment and additional funds for research. At this time, obesity treatment, if prescribed by a primary healthcare provider, may be reimbursed. Treatment generally continues to be of the associative disorders rather than directly of the excessive body weight.

The flip side of the medicalization of obesity is whether it is possible to be "healthy" and "fit" at any size or body weight. If health determinants other than weight are used to assess health, then it is possible. Criteria of physical fitness, normal range blood lipid, blood cholesterol, blood glucose, and blood pressure readings and the absence of weight-associated diseases may provide more health than continual weight-loss regimens. The physical and psychologic stress of attempting weight loss among individuals who are healthy based on the above criteria may be more harmful than remaining at a higher, though stable, weight. Over the course of time, attempts to lose weight often result in the cycle of weight loss/weight gain or yo-yoing, which increases body weight. The goal of weight management is good health achieved through stable weight. For many, it is more realistic to realize the benefits of good health at higher than average weights than to be unhealthy struggling with inadequate dietary intakes in addition to the other negative behaviors and effects associated with weight-loss dieting.

What do you think? Should obesity be considered a chronic disease or can health be achieved at every size?

Reference: Dalton S: The dietitians' philosophy and practice in multidisciplinary weight management, J Am Dietetic Assoc 98(suppl2):S49, 1998.

---

to a voluntary effort, the health condition of the persons initially, and the pattern of weight changes (many gains and losses, one sustained loss, or other patterns).[7]

Most epidemiologic studies include only initial weight, final weight, and mortality. This level of evidence is inadequate to illustrate the effect of sustained weight changes. One of the studies attempting to provide the needed information is the Nurses' Health Study, which has monitored for 20 years the health of more than 100,000 female nurses. This study shows that nurses who gained 22 pounds or more after the age of 18 had increased mortality risk in middle age.[8]

Chronic Dieting and Risk.   One issue of contemporary concern is the effect of repeated or chronic dieting on risk. Given our cultural concern about fatness and the extremely limited success of most weight-loss attempts, there is a high likelihood that an overweight or obese adult will have tried to lose weight many times. Is it possible that some of the observed negative effects of obesity are really the outcomes of a lifetime of unsuccessful dieting? Although animal studies and some limited observations of humans give support to this hypothesis, recent reviews of the evidence have concluded that the risks were not strong enough to justify discouraging people from making repeated attempts to lose weight.[9]

Obesity and Emotional/Social Health.   For many years investigators have searched for a psychopathology that would fit most obese people and would help explain their fatness. Their efforts have failed, for although a minority of overweight people suffer from a variety of mental health problems, no set of psychologic problems typical of obesity has been identified.[10] What these investigators have found is that our culture's extreme stigma against fatness extracts a tremendous toll on people who are obese. Social, economic, and other types of discrimination against obese persons are widely practiced. This may lead to impaired self-image and feelings of inferiority, which in turn may contribute to social isolation. Some people feel so guilty about their fatness that they hide away and put their lives on hold until they can achieve slenderness.

Other people (both obese and slender) concerned about their weights develop a characteristic known as *restrained eating*.[10] Restrained eaters try to use willpower to restrict their eating to a level below their natural appetite. Their restraint is susceptible to disruption by various disinhibitors, especially stress. When disinhibited, restrained eaters usually binge.[11] The binge may be a response to the hunger denied for days or weeks. It may be guided by black and white thinking, such as, "If I can't be perfect, I might as well give up." Thus restrained eating makes management of body composition harder.

As is the case with threats to physical health, the psychosocial risks are not uniform. Many people who are obese feel good about themselves and lead active, productive lives with a variety of positive relationships with other people.

appetite
desire for food

hunger
a physiologic need for food

Underweight and Physical Health

Although the number of individuals struggling with being underweight is a fraction of those concerned with being overweight, we still need to consider issues related to physical health and underweight. Underweight is defined as 15% to 20% below weight standards. BMIs of 18.5 or lower are considered underweight and are associated with illness and greater risk for mortality as BMI decreases further. The causes of underweight may include genetics, malabsorption of nutrients, metabolic disorders caused by wasting diseases such as cancer, extreme psychologic or emotional stress, excessive expenditure of energy in athletics, and/or voluntarily restricting dietary intake as in anorexia nervosa.[12]

Health problems may be associated with underweight if they are caused by undernutrition or disease. A medical and nutritional assessment should be conducted. These health problems may include malfunctioning of the adrenals, pituitary, thyroid, and gonads. Disruption of the menstrual cycle may also occur in addition to decreased immune system functions.[12] Extreme underweight caused by illness is called the *wasting syndrome* and is most often associated with human immunodeficiency virus (HIV) and acquired immunodeficiency syndrome (AIDS). This syndrome is discussed in Chapter 22.

In contrast, healthy underweight individuals may find that their level of underweight is problematic and they wish to gain weight. Medical nutrition therapy can be beneficial for both categories—healthy underweight and underweight caused by illness—by providing an analysis of dietary intake patterns and by assisting with eating strategies to ensure regular meals and planned snacks to increase the overall kcalorie and nutrient intake.[12]

Strategies may include simple changes such as choosing juices and milk beverages over water, exercising to build lean body mass for physical and psychologic benefits, and individualizing eating plans to accommodate the foods most enjoyed.[12]

HEALTHY BODY FAT

Functions of Fat

Although we tend to think of body fat as something to be avoided, it serves a number of vital functions.[1] As discussed in Chapter 5, we could not live without some body fat. For most people, the major portion of body fat is storage fat (Figure 10-5). A layer of this fat under our skin provides protection from extremes of environmental temperatures, and cushions of fat defend many internal organs against physical trauma. Storing fat provides an efficient means of stockpiling energy so that we can endure moderate fasts. In addition to this storage fat, there is

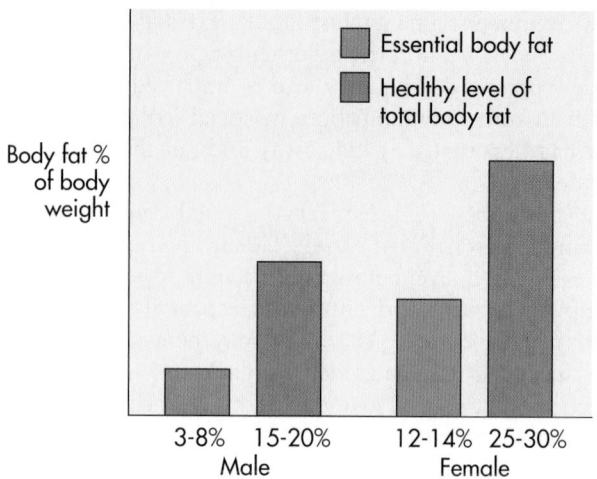

Figure 10-5 Male and female body fat levels. *Essential body fat,* minimum level of body fat for biologic functions; *total body fat,* range of level of body fat that provides for biologic functions but that does not have potential to negatively affect health. (From Rolin Graphics.)

essential fat
certain components of body fat that are essential for life

storage fat
layers and cushions of fat providing stored energy and protection from extremes of environmental temperatures; also protects internal organs against physical trauma

a small amount of fat that serves vital functions such as membrane integrity; this minimal amount of fat is termed *essential.* Although we must always allow for individual differences, **essential fat** in men seems to be 3% to 8% of their body weight. When appropriate amounts of **storage fat** are added to essential fat for men, we derive a recommended range for total fat of 15% to 20% of body weight.[13] In women, the concept of essential fat must be expanded to include gender-specific fat in their breasts, pelvic region, and buttocks that is apparently an evolutionary feature that provides energy during childbearing and lactation. Thus for women the minimum levels of fatness compatible with health are based on the essential fat plus the gender-specific fat and are in the range of 12% to 14% of body weight; healthy levels of total fat range from 25% to 30%.[13]

Sometimes athletes and dancers may strive for body fat levels below these ranges. There is concern that low body fat levels may be responsible for the menstrual irregularities experienced by many athletic women.[13] Amenorrhea is associated with bone loss and increased risk of fractures. Early work indicated that most girls do not begin menstruation unless their bodies are at least 17% body fat and do not continue regular periods without 22% body fat. Modern methods of assessing body composition do not support these exact fatness levels as predictive of menstrual performance for all physically active women, but body fatness is considered an important factor. The fat level associated with the best athletic performance may not be the best level for all-around long-term health. Working to achieve a lower percent body fat can be tempting; the desirability of doing this should be carefully assessed, considering the effect on strength, general health, menstruation, and other individual factors.

Body Fat Distribution

From both a health and an appearance perspective, it is not only the amount of fat but also its location that is important. Spend a few minutes at a popular swimming pool and notice the diverse patterns of fat distribution. Differences related to gender, age, and stage of development become apparent. Fat patterns may also vary among ethnic groups.[14] These distinctions are genetically determined and, although the amount of exercise can affect the tone of the underlying muscle, it cannot change the pattern of distribution.

Imagine the various adult shapes seen at the swimming pool; try to classify them as either apples or pears. Apples (android body type) are biggest around the waist, and pears (gynoid type) are biggest in the hips, buttocks, and upper thighs. Although some evenly proportioned people will fit neither category, probably most of the pears are women and most of the apples are men and older women. Although this swimming pool visualization may seem frivolous, it focuses attention on the location of fat, which largely determines its effect on health. As discussed earlier, fat that is within the abdominal cavity seems to be much more dangerous than is the lower body fat or fat under the skin in the abdominal area.

Although some sophisticated techniques accurately assess fat distribution patterns, a good estimate is possible by comparing waist circumference to that of hips (Figure 10-6).[15] For men it is healthier to have a waist-to-hip ratio of less than 0.95

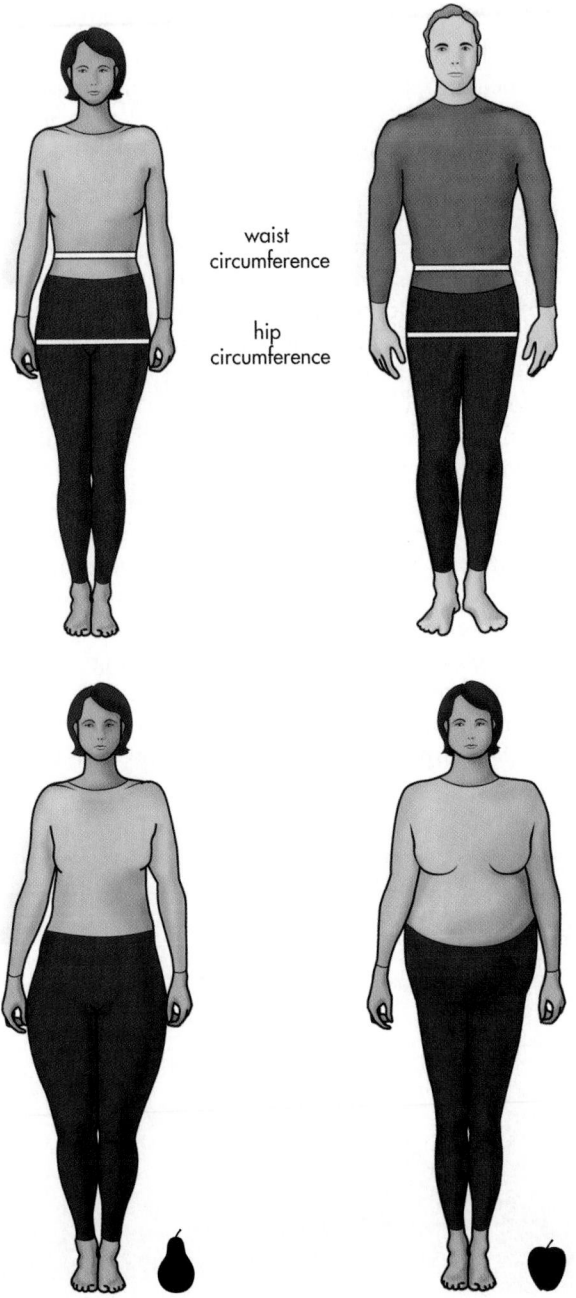

Figure 10-6 Apple (android) and pear (gynoid) body shapes. To estimate your fat distribution, measure the circumference of your waist and your hips. Divide your waist measurement by your hip measurement. You are an apple if you are a man and your waist-to-hip ratio is greater than 0.95 to 1.0 or if you are a woman and your waist-to-hip ratio is greater than 0.8. You are a pear if you are a woman and your waist-to-hip ratio is less than 0.8.

to 1.0, whereas women should have a ratio of 0.8 or less. The diameter of your waist alone provides a good estimate of the fat within your abdominal area; persons who have waist measurements in excess of 39 inches are at greater risk for the various chronic diseases associated with obesity.[16]

The two types of fat distribution also differ in their rate of turnover, with visceral fat being much more easily lost and also more quickly regained than subcutaneous abdominal fat or lower body fat. This is one of the factors contributing to men's apparent greater ease in losing and regaining fat. It is ironic that although the typical female fat pattern of lower body obesity is more benign, women tend to be more concerned with their fatness than do men.

Body Fat Storage

adipocytes
cells specialized for storage of fat

Most of the fat in our bodies is stored in special cells called **adipocytes.** These cells have a nucleus, mitochondria, and other organelles just as other cells do, but as Figure 10-7 illustrates, these features are usually squeezed over to the side to make room for the droplet of stored fat.

The fat in this droplet is in the form of triglycerides, the same type of molecule that makes up most of the fat we eat. These triglycerides are synthesized from glucose, glycerol, fatty acids, and some amino acids that are carried to the adipocyte by the bloodstream. The stored fat is in a constant state of flux, with some triglycerides breaking down while others are built. The net effect of this flux—that is, how much fat is in storage—is the result of our energy balance at that time. If we need energy, the balance shifts to favor breakdown and release of fatty acids and glycerol to be transported to various cells where they are oxidized or converted to other needed molecules. When we have a ready supply of energy, especially shortly after a meal, the balance tilts toward storage.

hyperplasia
an increase in the number of cells occurring during the growth spurts accompanying normal development

hypertrophy
an increase in the size of cells

At birth, most of us have relatively small numbers of adipocytes, but during the next few years, these cells increase in number (a type of growth known as hyperplasia) and in size (hypertrophy). Hypertrophy occurs whenever we continue in positive energy balance for any time. Hyperplasia, however, is more specialized, occurring during the growth spurts that accompany normal development. These growth-related times of hyperplasia occur during infancy, the preschool years, adolescence, and pregnancy. The adolescent increase in the number of fat cells is much more pronounced among girls than in boys, and it results in the higher level of body fat normal for girls in comparison with boys.

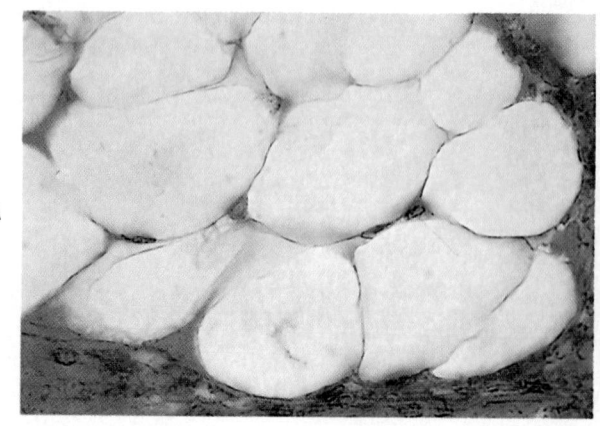

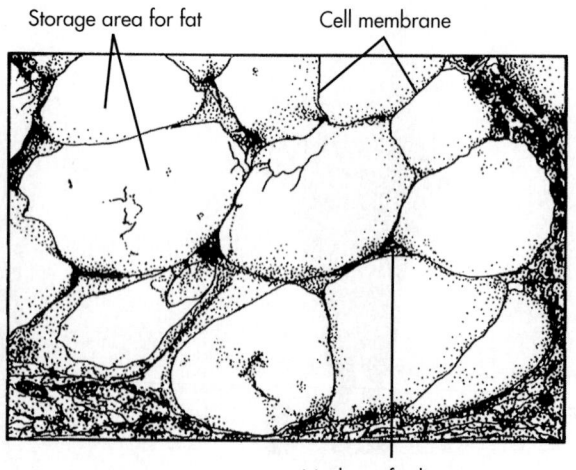

Storage area for fat   Cell membrane

Nucleus of adipocyte

Figure 10-7 Filled adipocytes. **A,** Photomicrograph. **B,** Sketch of photomicrograph. Note the large storage spaces for fat inside the adipocytes. (*A,* from Ed Reschke; *A* and *B,* in Thibodeau GA, Patton KT: *Anatomy and physiology,* ed 4, St Louis, 1999, Mosby.)

Most evidence indicates that once these cells form the process of adipocyte hyperplasia, there is no natural means of reducing the number. Knowing that there are predictable times of adipocyte hyperplasia, scientists once thought that if we carefully controlled our energy balance during those critical periods, we would have lifetime insurance against becoming too fat. Unfortunately, we now know that this is not true. We can form new adipocytes at any stage of life if the conditions are right.[17]

If more energy is consumed than expended, fat storage will go on until the fat droplet reaches its maximum size. If the positive energy balance continues, the body will make new adipocytes, thereby expanding the storage capacity. The stored fat is relatively equally divided so that all cells contain less than their maximum capacity. We are then able to continue to expand our storage capacity as long as the positive energy balance persists.

When fat is lost, whether through reduced intake, increased physical activity, or illness, fat is mobilized from adipocytes to meet energy needs. This reduces the size of the droplet of stored fat, producing a smaller adipocyte. If we have been obese and then lose a lot of fat, our adipocytes may become quite tiny—smaller than the cells of people who were never fat. Our bodies seem to monitor the size of adipocytes, interpreting the shrunken cells as evidence of imminent starvation. We may then feel compelled to eat more. Although the response mechanisms are not fully understood, clearly the effects on metabolism and drive to eat have developed as a means to reverse the threat of further loss. This set of responses is a major part of the theory of set point, discussed later in this chapter.

Measuring Body Fatness

Body weight is the most common way to estimate fatness. Weight is used although our bodies are made up not only of fat but also bone, muscle, and other nonfat tissue known as *lean body mass*. Weighing works fairly well as a means to determine fatness because usually the lean body mass changes only slowly. Therefore we assume that if the scale says we are a pound heavier this week than we were the last, the change is caused by a gain of fat.

There are several situations in which weight is not a good measurement of fatness. One involves fluctuations in body fluid; fluid retention that occurs before menstruation or during hot weather may be interpreted as fat gain, and losses in a sauna may appear to be fat losses. In these circumstances, normalizing the fluid balance makes the apparent fat change promptly disappear. On the other hand, the scale is also misleading for anyone whose amount of lean body mass deviates from what is expected. A bodybuilder will have a higher portion of lean body mass than the average person and thus will weigh more at the same height. Someone who has suffered from a wasting disease will have less lean tissue.

Because weighing is so convenient, it remains a useful assessment. However, if we really need to know how fat we are, we must resort to other means, which generally involve other measurements of the size of the body (anthropometric measurements) or assessments that distinguish between fat and other body components on the basis of their physical differences. Of the latter group, underwater weighing (densitometry) is the most widely accepted and is often used as a standard to assess the validity of other measures. Unfortunately, densitometry apparatus is bulky and expensive, and not everyone is willing or able to be submerged.

A practical alternative is bioelectric impedance analysis (BIA), a method often offered at health fairs and health and fitness centers. This method uses electrodes placed at the wrists and ankles to monitor the ease of passage of a mild electrical current.[18] Fat is a poor conductor of electricity; the conductivity occurs through the nonfat parts of the body. BIA actually estimates the amount of lean body mass, and then the amount of fat is calculated from the difference between the lean body mass and the total weight. BIA is safe, inexpensive, easily performed, and reason-

densitometry
underwater weighing

bioelectric impedance analysis (BIA)
a method using a mild electric charge to estimate lean body mass to determine body fat composition

ably accurate, but it is not considered sensitive enough to detect day-to-day changes experienced by someone trying to gain or lose fat. Other methods of assessing fat level include triceps skinfold and mid-upper arm circumference (see Chapter 14), but likewise these are unable to detect day-to-day changes.

Interpreting Body Fatness Measures

To interpret fatness measures, we have to agree on some criteria. Because our focus is achieving wellness rather than current fashion standards, we direct our attention to health-related criteria. Before we consider various measurement systems, let us emphasize the importance of individual interpretations. All systems are based on averages; however, we're all aware that there is no average person. Consider these factors that affect our clients' and our own body configurations, our values, our personal and family health history, the fatness level at which we feel best, and what we find achievable. The systems we review should not be construed as iron-clad laws but merely guidelines.

Interpreting Weight

A convenient way to interpret weight is to determine BMI. As mentioned earlier, BMI is calculated by dividing the weight in kilograms by the square of the height in meters. This yields a value that can be interpreted without further reference to height. BMI can be determined and related to the associated health risk by consulting Table 10-1. BMI levels apply equally well to men and women without adjustment. BMIs between 19 and 25 to 28 are associated with the least health risks.[19,20] Although some controversy exists as to whether the standards should be increased with age, health risk evidence supports increasing the recommended range by one unit for each decade beyond 24 years.[5] Thus for people aged 25 to 34 years, the recommended range would be 20 to 25 BMI.

Bear in mind that although BMI is widely used and convenient, it is still a measure of weight and has all the shortcomings of using weight to estimate fat. When both weight and fat are measured on the same men and women, there are usually some individuals who have weight-to-height ratios that are considered normal but levels of body fat that are beyond what is recommended—they are normal weight to height but obese. On the other hand, there are other individuals who are overweight but not overfat; this group is most likely to include very physically active persons.

BMI CLASSIFICATIONS[20]

>18.5	underweight
18.5-24.9	normal
25.0-29.9	overweight
30.0-39.9	obese
≥40.0	extreme obesity

REGULATION OF BODY FAT LEVEL

Our bodies form fat as a way of storing energy between eating episodes. When excess energy is available, we synthesize triglycerides and store them in adipose cells. When we have a shortage of energy, those stored triglycerides break down and the energy stored in them is used. Thus the bottom line in adjustment of body fat levels is the status of the body's energy balance: when energy intake exceeds expenditure, we gain fat; when it is less than expenditure, we lose fat. Sounds simple, doesn't it? In fact, it's not simple at all. Our bodies are much more complex than the teeter-totter that is often used to illustrate energy balance. Many factors affect the rate of energy intake and expenditure. We all are familiar with the concept that some cars get good gas mileage and others don't. Humans have many systems that regulate the mileage we get from our food energy. The previous chapter explored some of these factors.

Changes in Body Fatness

Levels of body fatness change when a disequilibrium in energy balance is established and maintained for a period. A pound of body fat is roughly equivalent to 3500 kcalories. Thus a cumulative positive balance of that magnitude should cause an estimated weight gain of one pound, whereas a negative balance of the same size should result in the loss of about a pound of fat. Recall that energy balance is determined by the relationship of the energy intake to the energy expenditure. The intake side of the equation is simple: it represents the kcaloric value of the food and drink consumed. The expenditure side is more complex, including the energy required to just keep the body going when at rest (resting energy expenditure, or REE), the energy cost of exercise, and the energy expenditures incurred by eating (called the *thermic effect of food [TEF]*). The levels of these expenditures are major factors in determining whether we will gain weight, lose weight, or stay the same weight on a given level of intake.

 Chapter 9 considered how changes in one's physical activity change the energy balance, an important factor when one is trying to achieve healthy levels of fatness. In addition to the effect of physical activity, our rate of energy expenditure is affected by a number of factors that cause individuals to vary significantly in the efficiency of their energy use. Difference of REE may occur because of ethnicity. African Americans may have lower REE than Caucasians. This may impact efforts to prevent childhood/adolescent obesity among this group.[21] Although factors that affect BMR and TEF are of interest, there is no safe and practical way to alter them. Nevertheless, understanding these influences helps us interpret what we see in the outcomes of the weight management efforts (see the Cultural Considerations box).

Genetic Influences on Body Size and Shape

In the mid-1990s the media in the United States was all abuzz about a series of new discoveries about fatness.[22] Mutations in a recessive gene named the *ob/ob gene* were found to produce early and massive obesity in mice. One exciting discovery was made after another as scientists announced success in cloning not only the gene but also the hormone product—leptin—that it produced. Then the gene was cloned in humans and leptin was found in in humans. In normal mice, leptin is produced in increasing quantities as the animal stores fat; leptin seems to function as a messenger to tell the rest of the body that the fat cells are full and that regulatory adjustments in eating and exercise should be made to cease fat storage. The *ob/ob* mouse lacks effective leptin, fails to make the adjustments, and continues to

---

CULTURAL CONSIDERATIONS
Dietary Patterns, BMI, and Ethnic Background

A Hawaiian study investigated the relationship between dietary patterns and body mass index (BMI) among 514 women of different ethnic backgrounds. Four significant dietary patterns emerged of meat, vegetable, bean, and cold foods. The "meat" pattern was characterized by high intake of processed and red meats, fish, poultry, eggs, fats and oils, and condiments. The "vegetable" pattern consisted of a variety of different vegetables. The "bean" pattern included consumption of legumes, tofu, and soy proteins. The "cold foods" pattern was fruit, fruit juice, and cold breakfast cereals.

The researchers found there were considerable differences in mean BMI, with Native Hawaiian women reporting the highest BMI, Caucasians reporting intermediate levels, and Chinese and Japanese women reporting the lowest BMI. Analysis shows that the "meat" pattern was predominant among Native Hawaiian women whereas the "bean" pattern was more common among Japanese and Chinese women.

Application to nursing: This study suggests the type of dietary pattern is associated with levels of BMI. In addition, genetic predisposition as well as physical activity may contribute to dietary patterns and obesity. Food choices based on cultural patterns are important in weight control. Consequently, nurses can assess the impact of ethnic influences on dietary patterns and BMI by assessing ethnic food choices of clients rather than the commonly used nutrient-based methods of dietary education or counseling.

Reference: *Maskarinec G, Novotny R, Tasaki K: Dietary patterns are associated with body mass index in multi-ethnic women.* J Nutr *130(12):3068, 2000.*

store fat. Furthermore, several other types of obese mice were found to have a defect in their ability to use leptin (although they were able to make it).

This was exciting information. People declared that now we knew the answers about obesity and predicted that this would be the end to problems of overfatness—we could just administer leptin when a person was concerned about getting too fat and the problem would be solved. Unfortunately, this has not proved to be the case. Despite much searching, scientists have not been able to show that mutations in these genes are causes of human obesity.[22]

Another hormone of interest is *ghrelin,* which increases food intake of humans (and rodents). When weight is lost, changes in appetite and energy use occur. Ghrelin circulating in plasma is part of the adaptive response of the body to weight loss by leading the body to regain lost weight. As such it acts as a long-term regulator of body weight. Consequently, depending on genetic predisposition, ghrelin may make maintaining weight loss harder—especially when the weight loss is through restrictive dieting. Its effect is less so when weight loss is through the severe stomach bypass intervention probably because the stomach, under that circumstance, is unable to produce ghrelin.[23]

Although the studies of leptin and ghrelin are not definitive and are ongoing, they have contributed greatly to the understanding of the chemistry of appetite control and have demonstrated that there are genetic factors in obesity. The work has also served to remind us that human fatness is complex, influenced by the interaction of many factors, both genetic and environmental.

The efforts of these scientists reveal that the role of genetics in fatness is complex. There is no single gene for human fatness or thinness. True, there are a couple of rare syndromes (e.g., Prader-Willi and Bardet-Biedl) where obesity is clearly determined by a genetic factor that also produces mental retardation. In these rare cases, there is a gene that is necessary for the production of the syndrome. These genes are called *necessary genes;* the syndrome cannot occur in their absence. Otherwise, fatness must be considered a **multifactorial phenotype**; that is, the displayed characteristic (phenotype) is the product of numerous genetic and environmental factors. The main genetic influences come from susceptibility genes—genes that do not in themselves produce a certain characteristic but rather affect the susceptibility to other factors (Figure 10-8). Interactions between genes and gene-environmental influences as well as nongenetic influences complete the scheme of factors that contribute to differences in fatness levels.

Regardless of one's genetic makeup, one's fatness is also influenced by nutritional, psychologic, economic, and social factors. In addition, there are many different types of obesity and thinness. When a family is characterized by a marked degree of fatness or thinness, casual observations are unable to distinguish between the effects of a shared environment, shared genetics, or both. By extensive study of

multifactorial phenotype
a characteristic that is the product of numerous genetic and environmental factors

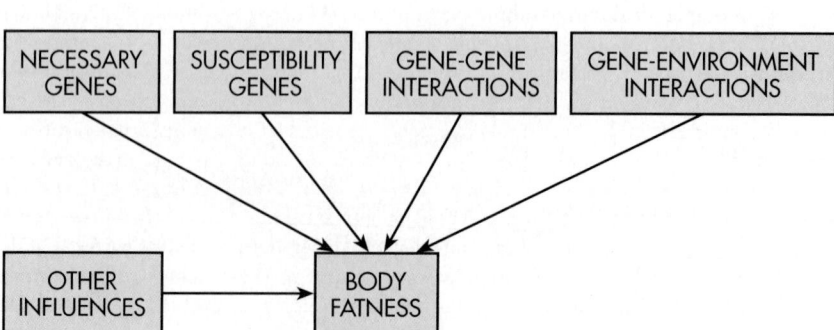

Figure 10-8 Genetic factors and causes affecting body fatness levels. (Modified from Bouchard C: Genetic factors and body weight regulation. In Dalton S, ed.: *Overweight and weight management,* Sudbury, Mass., 1997, Jones and Bartlett Publishers, www.jbpub.com. Reprinted with permission.)

large numbers of people, geneticists have learned that a significant amount of the influence on one's fatness (and characteristics such as metabolic efficiency that contribute to fatness) is genetic. Somewhat more influence comes from cultural or environmental influences shared by a family, and the remaining influence is related to factors beyond the shared genes and shared environment within a family.[24]

How would genes affect the amount and distribution of fat? Research suggests that there is a strong genetic influence on certain components that make up the energy balance equation: basal or resting metabolic rate, TEF, and the energy cost of light exercise (see Chapter 9). Investigators have also found genetic influences on the ability to use ingested fat for energy, on taste preferences, and on the ability to achieve a high level of physical conditioning. These findings help explain why people differ in their ease of gaining or losing weight. Nevertheless, for almost every component studied, there were not only genetic but also environmental factors involved. Although genetics play a part in the level of body fatness, they are not the only factor. The extent of their influence probably varies from person to person.

Set Point and Body Fatness

Many of our body characteristics are regulated so that they are maintained at a constant level or within a narrow range. This is true of body temperature, the level of glucose in our blood, blood pressure, the acidity of body fluids, and many other features. Departure from the usual levels of these variables is usually a clear indication that something is wrong. Usually when the problem is corrected, the characteristic returns to its usual level. This usual or natural level is called the set point. Actually, this term usually indicates not a single point but rather a narrow range that defines the natural level for the characteristic. The adjustments our bodies make to return to the set point are called *defending the set point*. Thus we can define set point as a natural level (of some characteristic) that the body regulates or defends.

Because energy is a high priority for the body, the level of energy stores is not left to chance without regulation. Indeed, as described previously, the weight (and body fatness) of most adults is remarkably stable, returning to the usual level after minor gains and losses. In spite of minor gains over the years, this is true of fat people and thin people alike.

For the most part, our adult weights are pretty constant. Something regulates them; there is evidence that we defend a set point.[25] This regulation is skewed toward prevention of weight loss rather than avoidance of weight gain. Furthermore, it is clear that among adult humans there is quite a range of set points for body fatness.

Any theory describing set point mechanisms must be able to describe three components: (1) some characteristic that the body monitors, (2) some kind of messenger to carry the information to the central nervous system, and (3) some mechanism of response to exert the control. Evidence suggests that fatness, lean body mass, and body mass in general are all monitored.

Our major attention will be on the possible mechanisms of response, the actual regulation. The only options for exerting this control are (1) changing the amount of energy ingested, (2) changing the level of physical activity, or (3) changing the efficiency with which we use ingested and stored energy. These options are exercised through overlapping neural, endocrine, and metabolic mechanisms to exert both short- and long-term adjustments.[25] Defending our bodies' fat stores is a matter of some complexity. Undoubtedly, this complex system with lots of checks and balances and backup schemes reflects the fact that energy is of prime importance to our survival.

The concept of a set point for body weight or composition is still controversial. Some of the controversy involves the question of set point vs. set range. Other experts debate what characteristic (weight, fat, or lean body mass) is under regulation. Still others resist the concept because they feel it discourages individual re-

set point
a natural level (of some characteristic) that the body regulates or defends

sponsibility for one's own health behaviors. The importance of these controversies is that they do not refute the basic concept.

Food Intake Adjustments

In discussing the regulation of food intake, one aspect of set point control was identified. When an individual's weight or fatness is below what the body perceives as appropriate, the drive to eat is activated.[25] Although the person will experience short-term satiety, this long-term hunger drive apparently is maintained as long as the lower weight exists. Although an individual may learn to ignore this drive, there is no evidence that it goes away. The individual is vulnerable to disinhibition, leading to potential excessive food intake or binge eating. It seems to take effort and attention to resist this hunger drive. People don't always have the psychologic energy to devote to this resistance.

Some people come back from a holiday or other situation during which they overate and gained weight, saying, "I ate so much then that I'm just not hungry now." Unfortunately, this type of hunger adjustment is rare. It is much more common for people to experience their usual degree of hunger and usual intake even after a period of overeating. The regulation system works poorly, if at all, in limiting food intake in this situation. Fortunately, the energy use efficiency part of regulation works somewhat better.

Adjustments in Energy Use

The body can adjust the efficiency of energy use in numerous ways; we will examine only a few here. A fundamental mechanism of control is the rate of energy metabolism. This is implemented primarily in adjustments in the resting energy expenditure (REE). The level of the TEF and the energy cost of a given amount of physical activity are probably affected as well. REE is a major component of total energy expenditure and usually accounts for at least half of total energy expenditure. Researchers in numerous laboratories have demonstrated that reduced food intake produces a prompt and significant depression in REE. REE drops promptly and stays depressed throughout the period of lowered intake.[26,27] If the reduction in intake is not too great, the drop in REE may be sufficient to prevent weight loss—this a successful defense of set point. With greater dietary restriction, weight is lost, producing a departure from set point (at least temporarily). When weight is lost, there is less body to use energy; this also depresses REE. Thus these adjustments greatly slow the rate of weight loss. Most often the weight is then regained.

Figure 10-9 shows the total energy expenditure responses of obese and nonobese individuals who overate or dieted under carefully monitored conditions. When the

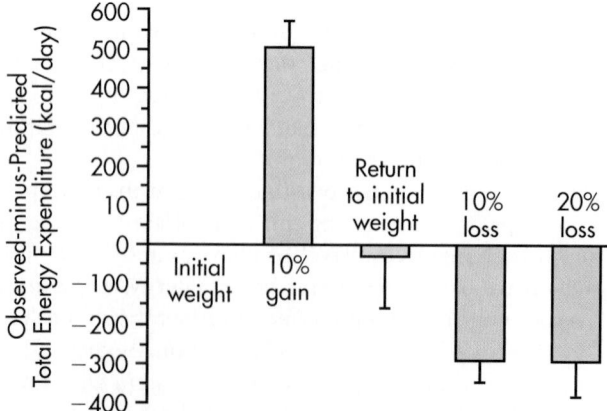

Figure 10-9 Mean (±SD) observed-minus-predicted total energy expenditure *(shaded bars)* based on the regression of total energy expenditure in a model with a variable combining fat-free mass and fat mass in the same subjects at their initial weight. (From Leibel et al.: Changes in energy expenditure resulting from altered body weight, *N Engl J Med* 332:621, 1995. Copyright © 2002, Massachusetts Medical Society.)

individuals overate so that they increased their body weight by 10%, their total energy expenditure was significantly increased. When they dieted so that they lost the extra weight, their energy expenditure returned to the initial level. When the obese members of the group continued dieting until losses of 10% to 20% were achieved, their energy expenditure dropped well below the baseline level.

The energy effect shown in Figure 10-10 occurs whenever food intake is reduced significantly—in dieters, in victims of disasters, in those suffering from illness, in anyone whose food intake is reduced. There is some concern that yo-yo dieters, persons who repeatedly diet and lose weight only to regain, may lose the ability to raise their REEs during the regain phase, making it harder to lose weight again and to maintain the loss. At this time there is not good evidence from research to demonstrate that this failure of REE recovery occurs.

Longer studies have shown that the REE and total energy expenditure stay depressed as long as the weight loss is maintained. This means that one's usual amount of food will go further than it did before. One will now gain weight on intakes that previously supported a steady weight. The body is fighting to preserve itself, defending its set point. Although the amount of the decrease in REE seems relatively small to have such an effect, the REE represents energy expenditure in every second of every day; it adds up fast.

As shown by the first bar in Figure 10-9, excursions into overeating trigger an increase in energy expenditure. In many people this increase is sufficient that they can overeat periodically without gaining weight. In that case the set point had been successfully defended. On the other hand, there are limits to the ability to expand energy expenditure, and if over consumption is sustained, weight gain usually occurs and the set point is reestablished at a higher level.

Before leaving Figure 10-9, note one more point: the vertical lines that extend beyond each bar represent the variability in the response of the subjects. The magnitude of the range from the greatest to least value is a reminder of the high level of individual variability in energy efficiency.

Total energy expenditure is also reduced when we reduce our level of physical activity. Restriction of food intake usually produces a reduction in the level of voluntary activity. This phenomenon was first observed in naturally occurring famines

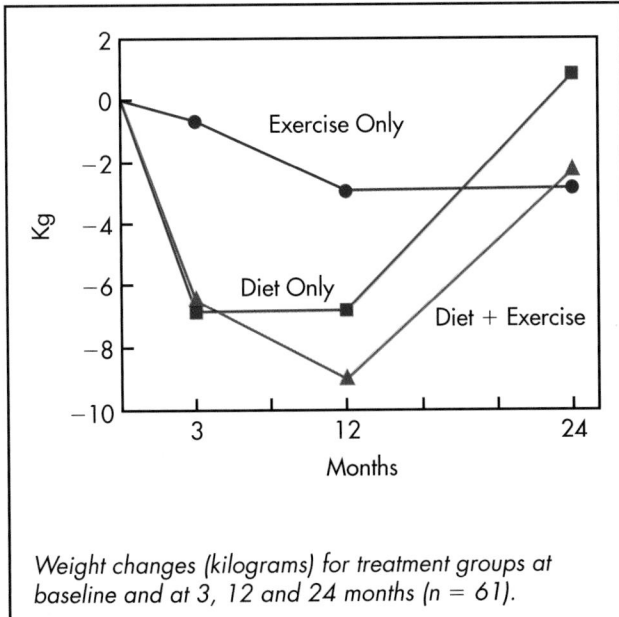

Weight changes (kilograms) for treatment groups at baseline and at 3, 12 and 24 months (n = 61).

Figure 10-10 Typical outcome of serious attempts to lose weight. (From Skender et al.: Comparison of 2-year weight loss trends in behavioral treatments of obesity: diet, exercise, and combination interventions, *J Am Dietetic Assoc* 96:342, 1996.)

where the starved were seen to reduce their activity to the lowest possible level, moving only as absolutely necessary. This seems to be a natural way to conserve the limited energy supply; it occurs whether the restriction is the product of a natural disaster or a self-imposed diet.

✿ Determinants of Set Point Ranges

Are we born with our regulatory systems set for slenderness or fatness? Exactly what is it that determines set point? Definitive answers are not available yet, but here are some probable answers. Observations of weight histories suggest that set point ranges are mainly a matter of the body's adjustment to the maximum size or fatness achieved. The combination of each person's genetic makeup, cultural heritage, environmental experience, and voluntary behavior leads to the development of his or her adult body size and composition. The body seems to assess this size and composition and uses it to establish set point.

This is easiest to understand in the case of adipocytes. Once formed they are maintained for life. If their size becomes smaller than usual (because the person has lost fat), the body sets in motion the mechanisms previously described to refill the cells to their usual size. This means that set point can easily be adjusted upward. One's set point may be at a level of fatness that seems too high or too low. Clearly, set point weight or fatness is not synonymous with what we usually consider ideal or desirable levels.

Changing Set Point

The previous discussion has shown that the set point regulatory mechanisms dampen the effects of conscious changes in eating and exercise. However, we have also seen that the set point effects can be overridden by consistent changes in voluntary behaviors of eating and exercise. If these behaviors lead to a consistent positive energy balance, we will gain fat and adjust our set points upward. Usually this seems to be a true change in set point; the new level of fatness becomes one that we can maintain without a great deal of effort, and we return to it after minor excursions above and below.

✿ Unfortunately, the situation related to a negative energy balance is not parallel. As we have shown, those rare enduring weight losses seem to be maintained only through continuing effort. A recent study illustrated the magnitude of the effort required by assessing the energy expenditures of women who were attempting to maintain weight they had lost.[26] Only those who had a high level of exercise were successful in sustaining their losses for one year; the amount of exercise these women performed was the equivalent of 80 minutes daily of moderate exercise, such as brisk walking, or 35 minutes daily of vigorous aerobic exercise.

✿ Another investigation has studied the food intake of people enrolled in the National Weight Control Registry.[27] To be included in this registry, a person must have maintained a weight loss of at least 30 pounds for a year or more. These successful maintainers reported that they continued to diet, the women consuming an average of about 1300 kcalories a day and the men slightly less than 1700 kcalories. Both men and women ate very low levels of fat, about 24% of their kcalories. Achieving such low levels of fat intake requires constant attention to one's food choices. These studies are encouraging in that they show that some people are successful in altering their environment and in changing their habits so that the effort required is manageable. On the other hand, the level of effort is significant and may explain why many people are unable to withstand the set point pressure.

Various pharmacologic substances that have been proposed to aid weight loss by reducing the appetite or increasing energy expenditure are sometimes described as having the ability to adjust the set point downward. These substances have only temporary effects. As soon as the medication is discontinued, the effect disappears and the set point forces are reestablished.[25] Furthermore, some individuals have found that the medication loses its effectiveness over time.

Nevertheless, in 1996 alone at least 20 million prescriptions for weight loss medications were written.[28] This wild enthusiasm waned, however, when the popular combination of two medications, phentermine and fenfluramine (phen-fen), were shown to be associated with serious health problems, including damage to the valves of the heart. The manufacturers withdrew the products.

Scientists have looked for factors that would change set point by affecting the rate of breakdown or synthesis of storage fat in adipocytes. Many enzymes and other factors influence these processes, but the search for a factor that could be externally controlled without bodily harm has not been successful to date.

Set Point Is Not the Whole Story

This discussion of set point has focused on physiologic factors that regulate fatness. As important as these factors are, we must not lose sight of the fact that one's level of fatness is influenced by environmental and psychosocial influences as well. In fact, because the physiologic influences are basically beyond our control, we usually focus on these other factors. Nevertheless, set point often helps us understand what is going on with our weights.

When Body Fatness Deviates from Usual

In spite of these various regulatory systems, our population includes many people whose fatness deviates from usual, resulting in obesity or emaciation. Obesity and emaciation have both been tied to disordered eating, resulting in the development of clinically diagnosable eating disorders. Binge eating disorder may result in obesity, whereas anorexia nervosa may lead to emaciation. Obesity and emaciation in these instances represent a continuum of disordered eating. The eating disorders of anorexia nervosa, bulimia nervosa, and binge eating disorder are discussed in Chapter 12. This section considers deviation of body fatness not caused by eating disorders but from other determinants of health.

Incidence of Obesity

If someone asks, "What is the incidence of obesity or overweight in the United States?" the answer would depend on the definition of obesity and the age, gender, and ethnicity of those studied. If we use an obesity definition of BMI 27.3 for women or 27.8 for men (definitions that include not only those frankly obese but also those with mild obesity) and apply that definition to adult Americans in general, we find that roughly 33% of those older than 20 years of age meet the criterion.[29] This incidence of fatness represents a significant upturn in levels that had been relatively stable since 1960. Generally, more women than men are overfat, especially African American and Hispanic American women. The incidence usually increases with age up to about age 50, and then levels off until age 60, at which age it declines.[29] The higher incidence among ethnic minorities seems to reflect combined genetic and environmental influences. Generally, the incidence of obesity is inversely related to socioeconomic status.

It is especially alarming that the incidence of obesity among children and adolescents has increased sharply in recent decades. The latest available data show that 14% of children aged 6 to 11 years and 12% of adolescents had BMIs that exceeded the 95th percentile.[29] Compared with the prevalence of fatness among adults, these figures do not seem startling. However, these figures represent an increase of two- to threefold over the last 20 years. There is considerable ethnic influence of obesity among young people, roughly paralleling that found among adults in this country.[29] Significant portions of obese young people grow to be obese adults. Add to early-onset obese persons those who become obese as adults and it appears that the incidence will continue to increase.

When researchers analyzed data from a large longitudinal study to see who was most likely to experience significant weight gains over 7 years, the findings included the following[30]:

• Individuals averaged gains of about 6 lbs (Caucasian men) to 11 lbs (African American women) over the 7 years.
• People who are already somewhat overfat are most likely to gain more weight than those who are not; however, the most common weight change over 7 years was a gain, regardless of the original weight status.
• At the end of the 7 years, all groups reported less physical activity and had lower levels of measured physical fitness. These changes explained most of the change in weight.
• Although food intake increased over the 7 years, it was not associated with weight change.

Success of Attempts to Lose Weight

Ironically, during the time reflected in the statistics presented earlier, Americans were busily engaged in trying to lose weight, primarily through diet and exercise but also through surgery, jaw wiring, pills, hypnosis, acupuncture, sweating devices, and other systems. Actually, the number of people who describe themselves as being "on a diet" has decreased somewhat in the last 10 years or so. Data from 1996 showed 24% of Americans dieting.[31] However, when you consider that 144 million Americans use low-calorie or sugar-free foods and beverages,[31] it becomes clear that restricting one's intake has become an accepted way of life. Furthermore, remember that 20 million prescriptions for weight loss medications were also written in 1996.[28] Unquestionably, there is a high level of weight-loss activity occurring. Yet the incidence of obesity is at an all-time high.

Considering these facts, what is the success of weight-loss attempts? Many of the commercial programs and products don't release data on the long-term effectiveness of their systems. None of those for which data is available produce significant weight losses that are sustained for more than a year in the majority of people who try them. If we ignore the downright fraudulent methods and consider only those systems designed to induce a negative calorie balance through reduced intake or increased activity, we find that although losing weight is not easy, maintenance is the real pitfall.[32]

The typical outcome of serious attempts to lose weight is shown in Figure 10-10. In a group setting, these individuals followed a low-calorie diet, exercised, or did both for 3 months, and then did the same things on their own for another 9 months.[33] Then they tried to maintain their losses over a year, but at the end of this time their weights were not significantly different from when they started.

Repeat Dieting.   Do you know someone who has dieted repeatedly, who never eats without feeling guilty, and yet who remains fat? Dieting changes the act of eating from a simple, enjoyable process into something complicated and laden with guilt and other moral overtones. Hunger is interpreted as temptation, and responding to it becomes evidence of weakness or even sin. After repeatedly denying the call of hunger, most dieters lose touch with the sensations of hunger. Hunger becomes confused with being tired, bored, sad, or other feelings. Dieters rarely eat to satiety; they either force themselves to stop short of satisfaction or they become disinhibited and eat far beyond satiety. Their physiologic regulatory cues are completely tuned out. They usually develop two lists of foods: virtuous ones that they eat when they are being "good" and forbidden foods that are constant pitfalls. Rather than increasing the ability to regulate food intake to meet body needs, dieting makes this regulation more precarious.

Certainly one of the harmful aspects of repeated dieting is the sense of personal failure that accompanies the almost inevitable weight gains. Dieters feel pressured not only by those with a commercial interest but also by healthcare professionals, friends, and family to try every new weight-loss plan that comes along. Most plans do produce initial losses, and dieters are lured into thinking that significant and lasting losses are obtainable. Dieters ignore the powerful and automatic adjustments in metabolism and hunger drive that weight loss triggers. Bodies naturally adjust to restore the lost fat. When the weight comes back, dieters may internalize the failure of their diets and suffer feelings of inadequacy that spread to other areas of their lives.

Gain/loss cycles are not benign. They may lead to nutritional inadequacies, confused food habits, loss of sensitivity to physiologic hunger cues, diminished self-confidence, and loss of self-esteem. Furthermore, as more data about the effect of weight changes become available, we may find that they exacerbate the health risks associated with obesity.

It Is Time for Some New Approaches

This book takes a nontraditional stance regarding attempts to change body composition. We as healthcare professionals, convinced that diets (even the good ones) don't work, have instead chosen to share an approach that emphasizes acceptance of diversity in body size and shape and puts emphasis, not on achieving ideal body composition, but instead upon promotion of wellness, personal satisfaction, and well-being. It is our philosophy that, except for acute medical conditions, it is inappropriate to give weight-loss advice. This is an attitude shared by increasing numbers of healthcare professionals.[34,35] Instead, all people—the fat, the thin, and the in-between—can benefit by adopting attitudes and behaviors that over time should promote the body composition appropriate to each individual's genetic makeup and contribute to true wellness. To emphasize the lifelong nature of this approach, we will refer to maintenance approaches rather than to efforts to change body composition.

DEVELOPING A PERSONAL APPROACH

Gain, Lose, or Maintain: A Wellness Approach

Although it is untrue that we can mold our bodies to any size or shape we desire, we do have the power to change our attitudes and behaviors if needed so that we can achieve satisfaction and wellness at the body composition most natural for each of us. This section describes some guidelines that are equally applicable to nurses and to their patients who are fat, thin, or just right. We draw on ideas advanced by a number of specialists who support what they call a *nondiet approach*.[34,36-40] All of the behaviors recommended focus on long-term changes. Those who adopt these attitudes and implement these behaviors can expect to feel more comfortable with their bodies and probably better about themselves in general. If we eat well and are physically active, we will look and feel good. Body fatness may or may not change. Although this approach may seem discouraging, the harmful and disheartening effects of diets and other programs that promise a lot but deliver only worse problems will be avoided. Appendix F, "Kcalorie-Restricted Dietary Patterns," provides dietary procedures for those few people who have a serious health condition that justifies the risks of traditional weight-loss efforts.

Establishing Realistic Goals

In setting goals, we must consider two almost opposing factors: (1) our unique and individual values, needs, and characteristics and (2) the limits to the extent of control we have over our bodies and our level of fatness. It is fashionable to deny any limits to this control, but objective observation will reveal the fallacy in that thinking. Aspiring to total control is neither realistic nor healthy for most of us. In goal-setting we need to consider what is practically feasible.

Changing Behavior

The most important goals are those related to changes in behavior. By choosing appropriate behaviors for change, we can work toward establishing habits that will become almost self-sustaining. The behavioral goals should be related to each person's unique needs. For example, in examining his lifestyle, one person may discover that he is always out of food and running out to grab whatever he can find, usually pizza and convenience store items. He may try to establish a habit of planning and shopping for the next week every Sunday afternoon. For him, this behavior change automatically leads to better food choices. For a different person, this particular goal might be irrelevant.

The Teaching Tool "Principles of Behavior Change" outlines basic principles of behavioral modification applicable to choosing appropriate changes. In recent decades it has become popular to make superficial use of the principles of behavioral change in weight-loss programs. These techniques have had limited success because they were presented as just a list of handy hints (e.g., eat on a smaller plate, put down the fork between bites) rather than the individualized system described in the box. Don't confuse these principles with those hints having little to do with the original concepts.

Normalizing Eating

The goal here is to reclaim eating as a comfortable and natural process. It involves being in tune with the needs of one's body and its signals about those needs.

Enjoying Eating

Normal eating should be enjoyable. Eating is a very sensual process and has the potential to be highly pleasant. Unfortunately, the ubiquitous dieting mentality dictates a love-hate relationship with food. Those foods we most love, we label sinful

---

TEACHING TOOL
Principles of Behavior Change

Set a positive, specific, and achievable objective. It is helpful to frame a goal in terms of the exact behavior to be practiced. Objectives like "I want to eat better" or "I don't want to be so inactive" fail to give you any guidance about how to achieve them and what constitutes success. On the other hand, an objective such as eating vegetarian meals five times per week can orient you in a helpful direction right from the start. It is easier to replace a behavior with a new one than to just stop doing it. Break major behaviors down into smaller, less daunting parts and try only a few changes at a time.

Establish a system for monitoring the behavior to be changed. This observation helps to assess success in changing the behavior and assists in determining what contributes to and detracts from mastery.

Modify the environment so that it supports the change. If you were trying to eat more vegetarian meals, for instance, it would be helpful if the environment included vegetarian cookbooks and ingredients and opportunities to be with vegetarian friends.

Set up a plan for rewarding successes. Be sure to choose rewards that will be appreciated but are appropriate to the magnitude of the achievement. The reward should be as immediate as possible. Long-range rewards can seem immediate by awarding points toward the reward.

Recruit support from friends and family. These people may want to be helpful but may not be skilled at it. Tell them of your objectives and how they can help, but do not make them responsible for personal behavior.

Allow enough time for a new behavior to become habit. A simple new behavior, like taking smaller bites, practiced faithfully for 3 weeks, should be well on the way to becoming habit. More complex lifestyle behaviors take much longer to change, usually at least 4 months. Under stress, most of us revert to old habits, so have a plan for how to deal with this.

and declare off-limits. Then we long for them and feel dissatisfied with the more ordinary foods we allow ourselves.

In normalizing eating we strive to retain the enjoyment of the process. This involves eating with awareness, relaxation, and without guilt, allowing ourselves to eat, in appropriate quantities, all the foods we enjoy. It may also involve expanding our pleasure by learning to enjoy a wider variety of foods.

Enjoyment can be enhanced by keeping meals and snacks simple enough that the true flavors of each item can be tasted. Not only do toppings, sauces, and the like usually involve the addition of extra sugars and fats, but they also obscure flavors.

In spite of all this emphasis on enjoyment, normal eating does not mean depending on food as a major source of pleasure. Just as drinking a long, cool glass of water is a joy when we are thirsty (but is without appeal when we're not thirsty), eating should be a natural source of pleasure and not a preoccupation. We are not advocating that we all live to eat.

Letting Hunger and Satiety Guide Eating

As discussed earlier, most of us guide our eating not only by physiologic cues to hunger and satiety but also by environmental and cognitive factors. Of these three sets of stimuli, only the physiologic cues are triggered by the body's needs. Therefore normalizing eating involves letting hunger and satiety guide eating. It means eating when hungry even if it is not a traditional meal time, and it means stopping with the first signs of satiety even if there is still food on the plate.

Although it would seem that eating this way would be easy, trying to implement this advice is actually challenging. A person may fear that if the cognitive control that tells us what we should be eating is relinquished, all control will be lost and huge amounts eaten. A few people actually do go through such a period—a pretty scary experience. Nevertheless, when they trust that they can eat again as soon as hunger dictates, most find that they are no longer driven to continue eating such large quantities.

A great many people actually have a different problem: they have ignored their hunger/satiety cues for so long that they no longer sense them. Reversing this lack of awareness involves relearning how to feel and identify the body's signals for satiety. An individual can start this process by carefully noting feelings when several hours pass without eating. Then the person should interrupt a meal midway through it and examine body sensations for satiety cues. A few minutes will be needed to perceive the satiety. If there are no cues to satiety, eating should continue but be stopped again to assess satiety after a few more bites.

Most people are less aware of their satiety signals than of hunger cues. Eating slowly may enhance awareness of satiety. Keeping meals and snacks simple may help, too. Some research indicates that there is a component of satiety tied to specific tastes: the greater the variety, the more food is required to reach satiety because each component is activated by the array of sensations. This may be responsible for eating behaviors at generous buffets.

Sensations of hunger are often confused with those of tiredness, anxiety, relief of anxiety, and other states. Distinguishing the difference may require work. It may be helpful to keep a journal of the various sensations observed.

Minimizing the Use of Food to Meet Emotional Needs

Probably all humans use food and eating to help them deal with emotions. We use food for expressing positive feelings, celebrating good fortune, rewarding hard work, and creating a sense of companionship. Eating as a means of handling negative emotions such as boredom, frustration, anger, or loneliness is especially problematic for many people. Compared with some other ways of responding to strong emotions, eating may be relatively benign, but when we rely on it as our main means of coping, our consumption patterns may have little or no relationship to our physiologic needs. This emotion-driven eating often is followed by feelings of guilt that may feed into the original negative feelings, creating a destructive cycle.

Minimizing emotional eating requires being aware of feelings and any associated eating. For personal understanding or as an adjunct to patient education, a journal or eating record can help achieve this awareness by monitoring feelings, hunger, and eating. Records kept for several weeks catch a range of moods. Examine the records from both the perspective of what triggered eating and of how the feelings were expressed or handled.

When we practice eating in response to hunger, we will probably use food less to meet emotional needs. However, if a pattern of eating in response to feelings rather than to hunger still occurs or if we regularly use food to deal with certain emotions, we need to learn some alternative ways to respond to emotions. We can often be our own best resource for discovering alternative responses by using the records to identify coping behaviors that are already working and that can be used more often. Books are available that deal with making these kinds of changes. Counseling can also help.

Although we are probably never going to completely give up using food to meet emotional needs, it is worth considering how to do so effectively so that we may increase awareness of how food consumption and emotions are connected. The following guidelines may help:

- Be aware of the reasons behind food use. Verbalize the intended function of the food. Eat food slowly and with concentration.
- Eat without guilt. If this type of eating occurs only rarely, there is nothing about which to feel guilty.
- Arrange a safe circumstance for eating. If some rich, creamy chocolate is just the thing needed, that's fine. Have some, but make sure there is no danger of overdoing it. Buy just one piece, eat in public, or do whatever is necessary to ensure that a reasonable amount can be enjoyed without feeling at risk of bingeing.

Eating Regularly and Frequently

Our bodies have evolved so that we function best when we eat several times a day at times spaced throughout our waking hours. Unfortunately, our modern hurried lifestyle often makes eating balanced meals inconvenient. We tend to snack on what is handy early in the day and do most of our eating between 5 PM and bedtime. This pattern has several undesirable effects:

- It puts the greatest food intake at the least active time of day. This means that the energy ingested must be stored as fat to await use the next day. Because many individuals do not efficiently mobilize stored fat for energy, they probably feel sluggish and curtail their activity the next day.
- It may mean long stretches of time with little food. During these times we often find it too inconvenient to eat, and therefore we deny our hunger or stave it off with inadequate snacks. By late afternoon our hunger, now joined by tiredness and frustrations of school and work, overwhelms us, and we eat frantically, often far more than we need. Thus this pattern runs counter to our goal of hunger-directed eating. Furthermore, with little or nothing to break the overnight fast, it's hard to get a good start in the morning.
- The quick meals or snacks we grab during the day usually are high in sodium and fat with little nutritive value.

There is nothing magical about three meals a day. Five may be better. Fewer than three meals results in long fasting times and may induce the problems described earlier. Whatever pattern works best, it should space food throughout active hours and should not produce overwhelming hunger or the drive to consume excessively. For most of us, how often we eat has to reflect the difficulties of providing ourselves with nourishing options throughout the day. Normalizing eating involves planning ahead to ensure that we don't get caught without any alternatives to chips and candy bars. Consider the suggestions provided in the Teaching Tool box, "Making Healthy Food Choices."

Adopting an Active Lifestyle

Does physical exercise help maintain a desirable body composition? The conclusions from research are contradictory and confusing. A lot of the confusion disappears when distinguishing between what is possible in a controlled laboratory experiment and what is probable in the reality of most people's lives. Although exercise is not a panacea, it is one of the few factors consistently associated with success in maintaining a healthy body composition.

Increase Energy Expenditure

Exercise is mechanical work that requires energy—it takes more energy to stand than to sit, to walk than to stand, and so on. Furthermore, vigorous exercise has the potential to increase the rate at which energy is used, even beyond the period of activity. However, for the level of exercise most people are able to accommodate in their lives, the daily effect on energy expenditure is in the range of a few hundred kcalories. The American College of Sports Medicine[41] recommends an exercise goal of three sessions a week, each expending 200 to 300 kcal per session (300 to 500 kcal for the more fit). Most authorities believe that the beneficial health effects of exercise are far greater than can be accounted for by the direct effect on energy balance of these few hundred kcalories.

Maintain Lean Body Mass

Many factors conspire to reduce our levels of lean body mass. These include aging, sedentary lifestyles, wasting caused by illness, and dieting. Exercise reduces the effect of these factors by increasing or maintaining the muscles of the body that directly affect lean body mass levels.

TEACHING TOOL
Making Healthy Food Choices

A major characteristic of normal, nondiet eating is the attention given to making healthy food choices. The Food Guide Pyramid is a helpful guide in making such choices, conveying the idea that some types of food (at the base of the Pyramid) should be eaten in much greater quantities than those at the top of the Pyramid (see Figure 2-2). When helping clients toward more healthful management of body composition, consider using the Food Guide Pyramid.

The Pyramid emphasizes low-fat foods as the mainstay of dietary intake. Because high-fat foods have such high energy content, it is difficult to gauge the amount needed to satisfy hunger; minor errors in estimation mount up quickly. Therefore an effective food plan should be relatively low in fat, with about 30% of kcalories coming from fat. If a person has energy needs of 1600 kcalories, that person would limit fat intake to about 50 grams, whereas another person needing 2200 kcalories would aim for no more than 73 grams of fat. Leaf through the food composition table in Appendix A to get an idea of how various foods contribute to the fat content. The nutrition label also describes fat content in easy-to-understand terms.

Low-fat, low-sugar foods should be chosen from each Pyramid section. Ideally, hunger should guide decisions as to the number of servings to eat each day.

Many people are surprised that the pyramid contains so many servings of starchy foods and so little meat. This makes sense when considering that carbohydrate and protein are equal in kcaloric value and that, unlike most meats, starchy foods are usually low in fat (unless fat is added). Eating according to the Pyramid guidelines means choosing more meatless meals and making sure that vegetables and fruits are available. This takes planning, but it can become a way of life.

No food is excluded from the Pyramid, but there are definite distinctions between everyday foods and occasional foods that tend to be lower in nutrient density and higher in sugar and fat. Most of us have our own personal list of occasional foods, ones that we want to continue to enjoy only at infrequent times because of their cost, difficulty to find or prepare, or low nutritive value.

Improve Many Health Conditions

Exercise reduces a variety of risk factors for hypertension, coronary artery disease, and diabetes mellitus. These conditions are associated with increased obesity. Yet even without changes in body fat levels, exercise can decrease heart rate, reduce blood pressure, and improve the blood lipid profile.

Change Our Outlook

Practically every investigation studying people who are successful in long-term maintenance of a healthy body fatness level finds that exercise is an important factor. Its influence cannot be accounted for on the basis of a direct effect on energy balance because the amount of kcalories used may not be high. Instead, exercise seems to help because it changes how people feel about themselves and about their ability to be in charge of their own lives. Regular, enjoyable exercise increases our awareness and level of comfort with our own body. It provides a good time for thinking and problem solving. It reinforces our commitment to wellness and increases the likelihood that other wellness behaviors will be maintained.

Differences in Responses to Exercise

Two friends exercise together regularly. Only one of them seems to be changing size. They probably differ in their individual response to exercise. In a study of such differences, 31 obese women faithfully exercised for 90 minutes a day four or five times a week.[42] They didn't change their way of eating. After 6 months, two thirds of the women had decreased levels of body fat, whereas the other women had increased levels. Both groups had improved cardiorespiratory fitness, carbohydrate metabolism, and blood lipid profiles. In addition, women in both groups deserved to feel proud of their accomplishments.

Differences in the response to exercise may be related to gender, fat distribution patterns, ability to exercise vigorously, and appetite response to exercise. Our bodies respond differently, and our level of fatness is a poor indicator of the beneficial effects of exercise.

Individualized Exercise

Most of the health benefits of exercise are maintained only as long as the exercise is continued regularly. Therefore it is alarming that most people who start an exercise program drop out. Although many factors undoubtedly contribute to this picture, a major one involves attempting exercise that is too difficult for one's physical condition. This is especially true for older or heavier individuals. Driven by sayings such as "It doesn't count if it isn't aerobic" or "No pain, no gain" regimens may be attempted that are initially too demanding. The goal is to do 30 minutes or so of aerobic exercise three or more times a week. Time can be taken to work up to that level. An exercise diary is a good way to monitor one's progress. We are more likely to exercise if we have access to a variety of activities we enjoy, such as walking, swimming, biking, gardening, sports, or even housecleaning; there are many options.

OVERCOMING BARRIERS

Prospects for the Future

During our lifetime, will the day arrive when no one will have to worry about being too fat, too thin, or too displeasingly shaped? There are several avenues leading to such a future: we could learn how to prevent deviations from healthy amounts and distributions of fat, we could learn how to effectively treat them, or we could become so accepting of individual differences that deviations were no longer defined as problems. All avenues will probably be important, but even when considered together, they will probably be insufficient to lead to such a future.

Some Trends Are Alarming

Recently we have learned of some alarming trends among the children of this country. Children in even the lowest grades of school are already obsessed with their weight and frequently place themselves on diets, yet there is a significantly increased incidence of obesity among our children. Parents, teachers, and healthcare professionals usually feel at a loss as to how to deal with this combination. The instinctive response is to restrict the child's intake, but the evidence overwhelmingly indicates that this response only creates a terror of not getting enough to eat and contributes to a sense of being ugly and generally unacceptable.

It is not clear what has led to these trends among children, but many suspect that physical inactivity accompanied by a rather generalized passivity may be involved. Furthermore, children are not free of the cultural messages that equate slenderness with happiness; thus the practice of dieting early in life.

Americans want to be physically active, but we are working longer hours and spending more time getting to work or school. When our work days are over, concerns about the safety of our neighborhoods may keep us inside and inactive. It will be interesting to see the impact on physical activity of new communication technologies that allow more people to work at home.

As our country's demographics change, we will have more ethnic diversity. We know that there are major ethnic differences in the incidence of obesity and of eating disorders. However, what causes these differences is unclear, and we certainly are not prepared to deal with them at this time.

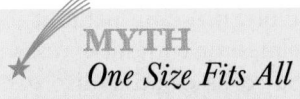

MYTH
One Size Fits All

*H*ealth professionals may not be aware of ways that their practices fail to meet the needs of their large patients. To assist these professionals, the National Association to Advance Fat Acceptance (NAAFA) has developed the following suggestions:

OFFICE ENVIRONMENT

- Provide chairs that are sturdy and armless, with sufficient space between the chairs to accommodate large patients.
- Use wide examining tables bolted to the floor or wall; this prevents tipping when a larger patient sits or gets off the table.
- Offer a solid, secure stool to assist patients getting onto the examining table.
- Have super-large examining gowns available. (One size does not fit all.)

MEDICAL AND WEIGHT PROCEDURES

- Have blood pressure cuffs available in several sizes to prevent false readings.
- Have access to longer needles and tourniquets to draw blood appropriately.
- Provide lavatories with split seats in front to allow large patients to more easily gather urine for specimen collection.
- Weigh patients only if necessary. Do so in a private setting and record weight without commentary. Do not assume that weight is the cause of the patient's condition or the focus of the health visit.

Reference: National Association to Advance Fat Acceptance: Guidelines for health care providers in dealing with fat patients, *Sacramento, Calif., 1994, NAAFA.*

Multiple Etiologies Complicate Treatment and Prevention

"Coming soon: a drug to cure fatness." This title may appear in the tabloids, but the likelihood of a medication that could reverse all types of obesity (or emaciation) is unlikely because there are too many different causes. More than 40 different models of obesity have been demonstrated in laboratory animals.[43] Humans living in the real world are much more complex. Even within a single individual there are numerous factors contributing to fatness level. At one time, doctors thought giving thyroid hormone would reverse all obesity, but experience proved that only a small proportion of individuals were good candidates. Some people lost weight with thyroid treatments, only to regain in response to other factors. The administration of medications may be helpful in some situations, but a pharmaceutical cure-all is unlikely. Likewise, prevention efforts will have to be multifaceted to address all the factors involved.

Acceptance through Prevention Efforts

At this time, it seems prevention is our best hope for a better future concerning fatness. Effective prevention has to encourage behaviors that promote total wellness on a long-term basis. Experience is demonstrating that this requires people to view themselves as valuable and worthy of effort. The Vitality campaign mounted by the Canadian Ministry of National Health and Welfare is a good example of this approach.[44] Designed to promote healthy weights, the Vitality program urges Canadians to feel good about themselves, eat well, and be active (see Appendix D).

Although programs in the United States are generally more traditional in their pressure to lose weight, we have begun to see some changes. The American Health Foundation has begun not only to speak of healthy (slender) weights but also to recognize that for the many persons who are unable to achieve slenderness, a goal of a *healthier weight* is more realistic.[45] A healthy weight may be viewed as a weight at which a person can physically move comfortably, maintain without restricting food intake (but following healthy eating guidelines) or without excessive exercise, and live without experiencing any weight-related associative disorders such as diabetes, hypertension, coronary artery disease, or high blood lipid levels. If associative disorders do develop, lifestyle changes can be initiated to achieve a *healthier weight*. The definition of healthier weight involves a weight loss of 10 to 16 lbs accompanied by healthy lifestyle behaviors.

Nutritionists in California have incorporated similar concepts in a statewide cooperative effort to change perspectives about children and weight. The Cooperative Extension Service in California designed a statewide specialist position in obesity. The job description for this position focuses not on encouragement of dieting and weight loss but rather on prevention of obesity and promotion of healthy eating and exercise habits.[46] Thus as more such programs are launched, we may see that good prevention campaigns also lead toward greater acceptance of individual differences in body size, shape, and fatness.

Role of Nurses

Approaches to weight and body composition management are being reformulated. Recognition that traditional weight-loss approaches to eat less and exercise more are not successful and are often counter-productive is growing and is forcing health professionals to consider alternative and adjunct approaches. Some of these approaches were presented in this chapter. Acceptance of genetic limitations and redefining weight management goals provide health professionals and their clients with potentially achievable objectives to achieve and maintain health.

Within these changes, the role of the dietitian is evolving from a counselor/educator who gives only dietary advice to a therapist who practices advanced counseling skills that use psychodynamic models of therapy to assist and coach clients. This new view that expands medical nutrition therapy involves a shift from a short-term to a long-term approach. Weight management is a lifelong process and so incorporates broader lifestyle skills to achieve healthy weight goals. Dietitians can coach clients about the process of food choice shifting the responsibility of decision-making about food and portion control to the client who is then armed with skills and support from dietetic counseling. The goal is to assure enjoyment of eating while still maintaining a healthy lifestyle. Everyone should be able to enjoy their favorite foods but make conscious choices about where, when, and how much of the food is eaten.[47]

Dietitians are often part of multidisciplinary teams that incorporate primary healthcare providers, physicians, nurses, behavior therapists, exercise therapists, and psychologists. Nurses can provide support during the formal and informal interactions within the healthcare system. An important aspect of this support involves nurses considering their attitudes toward their own bodies and toward clients who struggle with their weight, body image, and possible associated health concerns. In addition, nurses need to be knowledgeable about the lifestyle changes and choices to achieve long-term body composition management to further support client success. This may necessitate further specialization as a member of a multidisciplinary health team.

TOWARD A POSITIVE NUTRITION LIFESTYLE: EXPLANATORY STYLE

In his book *Learned Optimism*, Dr. Martin Seligman, a psychologist and professor, explores applications of explanatory styles to everyday life situations.[48] As a component of personal control, explanatory style is the way in which a person regularly explains why events happen. An individual with a pessimistic explanatory style spreads learned helplessness by having a pervasive negative view that, no matter what he or she does, nothing will change. In contrast, a person with an optimistic explanatory style feels able to stop the reaction of learned helplessness and understands events in a more positive way. An optimistic person feels competent that he or she can change the course of events.

Explanatory style has been studied in relation to health and wellness. A person's approach to dealing with issues of physical health can be helped or hindered by cognitions about personal control over health conditions and maintenance. As Seligman notes:
- The way we think, especially about health, changes our health.
- Optimists catch fewer infectious diseases than pessimists do.
- Optimists have better health habits than pessimists do.
- Our immune system may work better when we are optimistic.
- Evidence suggests that optimists live longer than pessimists.

How does this information apply to body fat management? Having an optimistic explanatory style may mean accepting one's body as it is and acting in ways to improve health by attempting to eat well and exercise regularly. A pessimistic explanatory style would judge one's body negatively and would not attempt behaviors to improve body composition because physical attributes would be understood to be permanent and thus unchangeable. Consider other ways that explanatory styles affect the approach of our patients toward their illnesses and the effect of our explanatory styles on strategies of nursing care.

SUMMARY

Lifelong management of body fat levels provides a more holistic health approach to body size than does body weight. Management is defined as the use of available resources to achieve a predetermined goal. This definition recognizes that individuals differ in the resources available to them and in the goals they set. Goals for body fat levels must take into account an individual's genetic and family factors as well as those of society and health.

Ways of measuring body fat composition include densitometry and bioelectric impedance analysis. In addition to simple body weight, BMI provides another way to interpret weight levels. Weight may be maintained by set point, through which the body regulates its most natural weight.

Body size, as an issue of health status, is still a concern among many health professionals. Individuals at both extremes of fatness, those very thin and those very fat, are at increased risk for certain health-related disorders. Obesity, however, does not increase all types of health risks nor are all obese individuals ill. Risks of some types of cancer and of osteoporosis are lower for the obese than for others.

Body acceptance is a key to wellness. Biology and culture interact to set standards of body image, perceptions, and social models of attractiveness. Because of individual genetic makeup, different body types and sizes may not fit the cultural ideals. The goal is to reclaim eating as a comfortable and natural process. This means being in tune with one's body's needs and its signals about those needs. A part of body composition management is the incorporation of regular exercise. Exercise increases energy expenditure, promotes maintenance of lean body mass, improves many health conditions, and changes one's outlook. Differences in bodies' responses to exercise may be related to gender, fat distribution patterns, ability to exercise vigorously, and appetite response to exercise. Future considerations of body composition management include prevention of deviations from healthy levels and distributions of fat, development of effective treatments, and the cultivation of acceptance of individual differences.

THE NURSING APPROACH
Teaching Others

As a requirement for a nursing course, Jeff is conducting a service-learning project and chooses nutrition as its focus. He speaks with the nurse practitioner, the director of the college Wellness Center, who suggests designing an informational brochure on weight management for students. Jeff decides to create a brochure to teach healthy eating with the emphasis on reducing dietary fat to achieve or maintain appropriate body composition (healthy weight).

He wants to highlight information that is applicable to traditional students (ages 18 to 24) and to nontraditional students (ages 25 and older). Jeff begins with what he knows of the college population who are overweight, obese, or struggling with weight issues. He identifies strengths and areas for improvement.

ASSESSMENT

Strengths

- Student population has an active lifestyle.
- Students are active learners.
- The college environment offers opportunity for application of learning.
- Most students have a need for peer group.

Areas for Improvement

- College students have irregular eating patterns, including habits such as snacking frequently and eating high-calorie foods.
- Overweight and obesity are common problems among college students.
- College students may lack the knowledge or skills to reduce dietary fat intake.

THE NURSING APPROACH–cont'd
Teaching Others

Objectives of the Brochure
- Teach the need for nutrients and appropriate calorie intake.
- Provide simple instructions for reducing dietary fat and caloric intake.
- Teach lifelong health benefits of weight maintenance based on wellness nutrition and physical activity.

PLANNING

1. Design a colorful and attractive brochure.
2. Avoid use of terms such as "obesity," "obese," or other words associated with excessive weight.
3. Provide simple instructions how to choose healthier foods to reduce dietary fat and caloric intake.
   Sample instructions to reduce dietary fat and caloric intake include the following:
   - Choose meats grilled, baked, broiled, or microwaved instead of fried.
   - Substitute fruit, popcorn, or pretzels instead of potato chips, cheese puffs, corn chips, and nuts.
   - Limit desserts high in fat, such as candy, ice cream, cake, and cookies.
   - Substitute hard candies for chocolate bars.
   - Use skim milk or reduced fat milk instead of whole milk.
   - Use less butter or margarine on breads; substitute jam.
   - Eat less red meat and more fish and poultry.
   - Use less salad dressing or use low-fat dressing or lemon juice on salads.
   - Read labels on all processed cans and packages for fat, sugar, and caloric content.
   - Limit portion sizes according to energy and physiologic need.
4. Provide referral to the college Wellness Center for additional dietary information.

IMPLEMENTATION

1. Write brochure and incorporate art.
2. Review brochure with several students; revise based on their comments.
3. Publish brochure.
4. Distribute brochures in the cafeteria, nutrition classes, nursing classes, and college Wellness Center over a 2-week period.

EVALUATION

The success of the brochure will be measured by the following:
- The number of brochures distributed
- The number of students contacting the college Wellness Center regarding their dietary intakes during the 2 weeks before and after brochure distribution
- Survey results gathered in nutrition and nursing classes regarding the brochure

APPLYING CONTENT KNOWLEDGE

Carol eats a moderately low-fat diet, doesn't overeat, and exercises three to four times a week. Her body fat level is about 32%. Her friend, Barbara, also eats a moderately low-fat diet, doesn't overeat, and exercises three to four times a week. However, compared with Carol, Barbara's body fat level is in the low range of 22%. Explain how their body fat levels could differ.

Web Sites of Interest

Healthy Weight Network
www.healthyweightnetwork.com
The mission of the Healthy Weight Network is to provide a critical link between research and practical application of weight and eating issues. This site provides Web sites on eating disorders, size acceptance, and weight management through nondieting approaches to promote good health at any size. The site also features articles from *Healthy Weight Journal.*

Hugs International
www.hugs.com
This site aims to shift our consciousness from dieting and weight loss to attitudes that support size acceptance and healthier lifestyles. Messages are communicated through books, workshops, and other products.

Mayo Health Oasis
www.mayohealth.org
Updated every weekday, this site, prepared and reviewed by a team of Mayo Clinic physicians and scientists, gives access to a variety of medical topics including healthy weight topics. This extensive database provides information on treatment of illnesses and disease prevention.

National Association to Advance Fat Acceptance (NAAFA)
www.naafa.org
NAAFA, a nonprofit human rights organization, works toward improving the quality of life for fat people and eliminating size discrimination through public education, advocacy, and member support.

References

1. Norgan NG: The beneficial effects of body fat and adipose tissue in humans, *Int J Obes* 21:738, 1997.
2. Stearns PN: *Fat history: bodies and beauty in the modern West,* New York, 1997, New York University Press.
3. Brownell KD: Personal responsibility and control over our bodies: when expectation exceeds reality, *Health Psychol* 10:303, 1991.
4. Friedman KE et al.: Body image partially mediates the relationship between obesity and psychological distress, *Obes Res* 10(1):33, 2002.
5. Bray GA: Classification and evaluation of obesity. In Bray GA, Bouchard C, James WPT, eds.: *Handbook of obesity,* New York, 1998, Marcel Dekker.
6. Lopez-Canales A: Metabolic syndrome X: a comprehensive review of the pathophysiology and recommended therapy, *J Med* 32(5-6):283, 2001; Church TS et al.: Relative association of fitness and fatness to fibrinogen, white blood cell count, uric acid, and metabolic syndrome, *Int J Obes Relat Metab Disor* 26(6):805, 2002.
7. Williamson DF, Pamuk ER: The association between weight loss and increased longevity. A review of the evidence, *Ann Intern Med* 119:731, 1993; Ditschuneit HH et al.: Lipoprotein responses to weight loss and weight maintenance in high-risk obese subjects, *Euro J Clin Nutr* 56(3):264, 2002.
8. Manson JE et al.: Body weight and mortality among women, *N Engl J Med* 333:677, 1995.
9. Atkinson RL, Stern JS: Weight cycling: definitions, mechanisms, and problems with interpretation. In Bray GA, Bouchard C, James WPT, eds.: *Handbook of obesity,* New York, 1998, Marcel Dekker.
10. Stunkard AJ, Sobal J: Psychological consequences of obesity. In Brownell KD, Fairburn CG, eds.: *Eating disorders and obesity,* New York, 1995, Guilford Press.
11. Polivy J, Herman CP: Dieting and its relation to eating disorders. In Brownell KD, Fairburn CG, eds.: *Eating disorders and obesity,* New York, 1995, Guilford Press.
12. Mahan LK, Escott-Stump S: *Krause's food, nutrition, & diet therapy,* ed 9, Philadelphia, 1996, WB Saunders.

13. McArdle WD, Katch FD, Katch VL: *Essentials of exercise physiology,* Philadelphia, 1994, Lea and Febiger.

14. Kumanyika SK: Obesity in minority populations. In Bray GA, Bouchard C, James WPT, eds.: *Handbook of obesity,* New York, 1998, Marcel Dekker.

15. *Guidance for treatment of adult obesity,* Bethesda, Md., 1996, Shape Up America! and American Obesity Association.

16. Rippe JM: The case for medical management of obesity: a call for increased physician involvement, *Obesity Res* 6:23S, 1998.

17. Ailhaud G, Hauner H: Development of white adipose tissue. In Bray GA, Bouchard C, James WPT, eds.: *Handbook of obesity,* New York, 1998, Marcel Dekker.

18. Pierson RN, Wang N, Boozer CN: Body composition and resting metabolic rate: new and traditional measurement methods. In Dalton S, ed.: *Overweight and weight management: the health professional's guide to understanding and practice,* Gaithersburg, Md., 1997, Aspen.

19. Meisler JG, St Jeor S: Summary and recommendations from the American Health Foundation's Expert Panel on Healthy Weight, *Am J Clin Nutr* 63:474S, 1996.

20. National Institutes of Health/National Heart, Lung, and Blood Institute: *Clinical guidelines on the identification, evaluation, and treatment of overweight and obesity in adults: the evidence report,* Washington, DC, June 1998, U.S. Government Printing Office.

21. Tershakovec AM et al.: Age, sex, ethnicity, body composition, and resting energy expenditure of obese African American and white children and adolescents, *Am J Clin Nutr* 75(5):869, 2002.

22. Gura T: Obesity sheds its secrets, *Science* 275:751, 1997.

23. Cummings DE et al.: Plasma ghrelin levels after diet-induced weight loss or gastric bypass surgery, *N Engl J Med* 346(21):1623, 2002.

24. Bouchard C: Genetic factors and body weight regulation. In Dalton S, ed.: *Overweight and weight management: the health professional's guide to understanding and practice,* Gaithersburg, Md., 1997, Aspen.

25. Vasselli JR, Maggio CA: Mechanisms of appetite and body weight regulation. In Dalton S, ed.: *Overweight and weight management: the health professional's guide to understanding and practice,* Gaithersburg, Md., 1997, Aspen.

26. Schoeller DA, Shay K, Kushner RF: How much physical activity is needed to minimize weight gain in previously obese women? *Am J Clin Nutr* 66:551, 1997.

27. Shick SM et al.: Persons successful at long-term weight loss and maintenance continue to consume a low-energy, low-fat diet, *J Am Diet Assoc* 98:408, 1998.

28. Hirsch J: The treatment of obesity with drugs, *Am J Clin Nutr* 67:2, 1998.

29. US Department of Health and Human Services, Public Health Service: Leading Health Indicators, *Healthy People 2010,* ed 2, Washington, DC, 2000, US Government Printing Office; www.health.gov/healthypeople.

30. Lewis CE et al.: Seven-year trends in body weight and associations with lifestyle and behavioral characteristics in Black and White young adults: the CARDIA study, *Am J Public Health* 87:635, 1997.

31. Calorie Control Council: Trends and statistics, www.caloriecontrol.org/dietfigs.html, April 4, 1998.

32. American Dietetic Association: Position paper: weight management, *J Am Diet Assoc* 97:71, 1997.

33. Skender ML et al.: Comparison of 2-year weight loss trends in behavioral treatments of obesity: diet, exercise, and combination interventions, *J Am Diet Assoc* 96:342, 1996.

34. Parham ES: Is there a new weight paradigm? *Nutrition Today* 31:155, 1996.

35. Kassirer JP, Angell M: Losing weight—an ill-fated New Year's resolution, *N Engl J Med* 338:52, 1998.

36. Foreyt JP, Goodrick GK: *Living without dieting,* Houston, 1992, Harrison Publishing.

37. Omichinski L: *You count, calories don't,* Winnipeg, Manitoba, 1993, Tamos Books.

38. Hirschmann JR, Munter CH: *When women stop hating their bodies,* New York, 1995, Fawcett Columbine.

39. Tribole E, Resch E: *Intuitive eating,* New York, 1995, St Martin's Press.

40. Kratina K, King N, Hayes, D: *Moving away from diets,* Lake Dallas, Texas, 1996, Helm Seminars.

41. American College of Sports Medicine: *ACSM's guidelines for exercise testing and prescription,* ed 6, Baltimore, 2000, Williams & Wilkins.

42. Lamarche B et al.: Is body fat loss a determinant factor in the improvement of carbo-hydrate and lipid metabolism following aerobic exercise training in obese women? *Metabolism* 41:1249, 1992.
43. Björntorp P, Brodoff BN, eds.: *Obesity,* Philadelphia, 1992, Lippincott.
44. Vitality: *What and why,* Vitality webpage, www.hcsc.gc.ca/main/hppb/nutrition/pube/vtkl/vitlk0.3.htm, April 23, 1998.
45. Meisler JG, St Jeor S: Summary and recommendations from the American Health Foundation's Expert Panel on Healthy Weight, *Am J Clin Nutr* 63:474S, 1996.
46. Department of Nutritional Sciences: *Cooperative Extension nutrition specialist position in obesity,* University of California, Berkeley, e-mail announcement, Feb 3, 1998.
47. Dalton S: The dietitians' philosophy and practice in multidisciplinary weight management, *J Am Dietetic Assoc* 98(suppl2):S49, 1998.
48. Seligman MEP: *Learned optimism,* New York, 1991, Alfred A. Knopf.

CHAPTER 11

Life Span Health Promotion: Pregnancy, Lactation, and Infancy

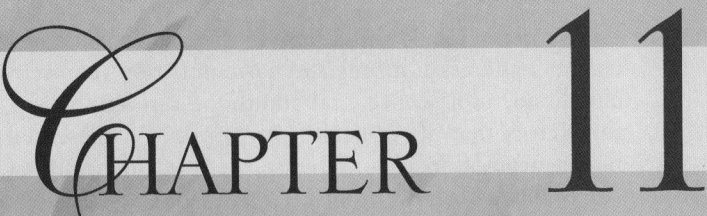

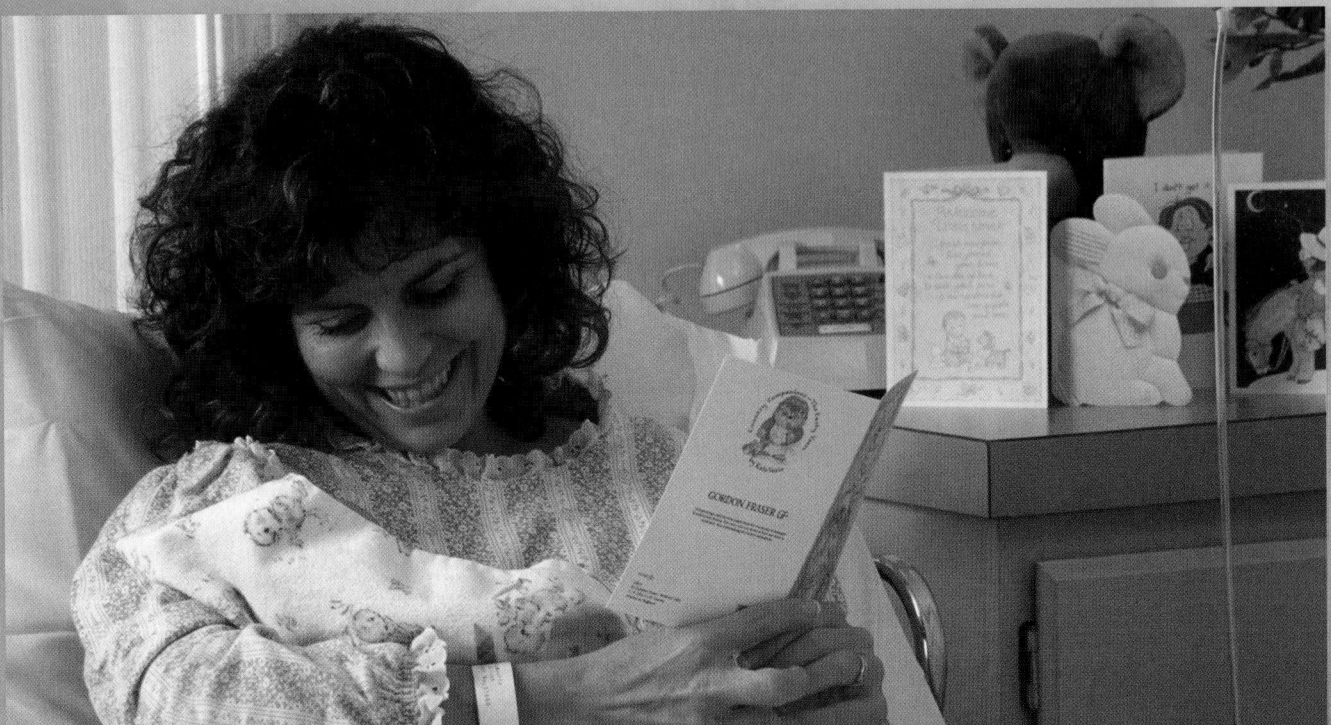

Following conception and continuing until parturition (childbirth), many metabolic, anatomic, hormonal, psychologic, and physiologic changes take place in the mother.

Chapters 11, 12, and 13 cover the topics of life span health promotion. These chapters address not only the basic nutrition requirements of pregnancy, infancy, childhood, adolescence, and adulthood through older adulthood but also consider the factors that affect health promotion. As presented in Chapter 1, the goal of health promotion is to increase the level of health of individuals, families, and communities. Health promotion strategies often focus on lifestyle changes leading to new, positive health behaviors.

Development of these behaviors may depend on knowledge, techniques, and community supports. Knowledge is learning new information about the benefits or risks of health-related behaviors. Techniques are strategies used to apply new knowledge to everyday activities. By applying our knowledge, we modify lifestyle behaviors. Community supports are available (environmental or regulatory measures) that support new health-promoting behaviors within a social context.

ROLE IN WELLNESS

The prenatal period is characterized by numerous physiologic, psychologic, and social changes in the mother in preparation for birth and care of the young. It is a time when a woman often expresses interest and motivation in improving her eating habits, realizing she is the sole source of nourishment for her developing infant. Following birth, lactation leads to changes for the mother. Although providing human milk for one's infant is exhilarating, the 24-hour demands of a newborn lead to a reorganization of everyday life and can sometimes be overwhelming. Societal and cultural influences may also affect the acceptability of breastfeeding.

The goal of health promotion is to prepare a woman for these changes by helping her become knowledgeable and responsible for her own health and the well-being of her infant. Few experience this alone. A spouse, significant other, and family members can be sources of support to further the goals of health promotion. A father-to-be often needs guidance as he grapples with his own expectations of his future responsibilities. Health professionals can use this opportunity to assist individuals to establish healthful habits, such as eating well, being physically active, and avoiding alcohol and drug use.

This chapter explores pregnancy, lactation, and infancy through the framework of nutritional requirements and health promotion. The five dimensions of health provide insight into the issues associated with these topics. The physical health of the newborn depends on the nutrients consumed by the expectant mother and on the teratogens avoided. Preparation before conception to take on the responsibilities of pregnancy and future parenting requires application of knowledge that exercises the intellectual health dimension. Emotional health may be strained as some women develop postpartum depression after delivery; recognition and treatment of this disorder is crucial to the well-being of mother and child. The social health relationships of mothers and fathers may be altered as lifestyle changes occur because of their new social status as parents. Spiritual dimension of health is affected because the creation of new life is one of life's miracles regardless of one's religious or humanistic beliefs.

NUTRITION DURING PREGNANCY

Although the influence of nutrition on the course of pregnancy had been presumed for some time, it was not until the twentieth century when research provided a scientific basis to substantiate such assumptions. During the last 20 years, research on the role of nutrition during pregnancy has increased substantially, including the publication *Nutrition during Pregnancy,* published by the Institute of Medicine of

Marian L. Stone Neuhouser, PhD, RD, contributed this chapter in the first and second editions of this text.

the National Academy of Sciences.[1] Successful pregnancy outcomes include a viable infant of acceptable birth weight, an infant free of congenital defects, and a favorable long-term health outlook for both mother and infant.

Body Composition Changes during Pregnancy

Following conception and continuing until parturition (childbirth), many metabolic, anatomic, hormonal, psychologic, and physiologic changes take place in the mother. This chapter focuses on those most affected by or affecting nutrient intake.

Hormones of Pregnancy

There are numerous steroid hormones, peptide hormones, and prostaglandins that influence the course of pregnancy. Some of them, such as the placental hormones *human placental lactogen* and *human growth hormone,* are produced only during pregnancy. Others, including insulin, glucagon, and thyroxine, are present in altered amounts compared with the nonpregnant state and have profound influences on metabolism throughout gestation.

Progesterone and estrogen have a particularly strong influence on pregnancy. The action of progesterone promotes development of the endometrium and relaxes the smooth muscle cells of the uterus. This relaxation serves both to help the uterus expand as the fetus grows and to prevent any premature contractions of the uterus. The same effect also influences other smooth muscle cells, such as the gastrointestinal (GI) tract. The resulting slowing of the GI tract during pregnancy may increase the absorption of several nutrients, most notably iron and calcium. One perhaps annoying consequence of this decreased gut motility is the promotion of constipation. Progesterone causes increased renal sodium excretion during pregnancy. The body compensates for this sodium-losing mechanism by increasing aldosterone secretion from the adrenal gland and renin from the kidney. Sodium restriction during pregnancy, once thought to prevent hypertensive disorders of pregnancy, is actually harmful because it reduces plasma volume and cardiac output.[2]

Estrogen promotes the growth of the uterus and breasts during pregnancy and renders the connective tissues in the pelvic region more flexible in preparation for birth.

endometrium
mucous membrane of the uterus

Metabolic Changes

There are profound changes in maternal metabolism during pregnancy, and successful adaptation to these changes is necessary for a favorable pregnancy outcome. The basal metabolic rate (BMR) rises during pregnancy by as much as 15% to 20% by term. This increase is caused by the increased oxygen needs of the fetus and the maternal support tissues. There are alterations in maternal metabolism of protein, carbohydrate, and fat. The fetus prefers to use glucose as its primary energy source. Changes occur in maternal metabolism to accommodate this need of the fetus. The adaptation allows the mother to use fat as the primary fuel source, thus permitting glucose to be available to the fetus.[3] Increased macronutrient and micronutrient intake by the mother during pregnancy ensures that these increased metabolic needs are met.

Anatomic and Physiologic Changes

Plasma volume doubles during pregnancy, beginning in the second trimester. Failure to achieve this plasma expansion may result in a spontaneous abortion, a stillbirth, or a low birth weight infant. One of the results of this increase in plasma volume is a hemodilution effect. In other words, measured components in the plasma such as hemoglobin, serum proteins, and vitamins will appear to be at lower levels during pregnancy because there is a greater volume of solvent (the plasma) relative to concentrations of solute (the components). Cardiac hypertrophy occurs to accommodate this increased blood volume, accompanied by an increased ventilatory rate.

hemodilution
dilution of the blood

In the kidneys, the glomerular filtration rate (GFR) increases to accommodate the expanded maternal blood volume being filtered and to carry away fetal waste products. As a result of this increase in GFR, small quantities of glucose, amino acids, and water-soluble vitamins may appear in the urine. Although minor losses may be acceptable, a woman who excretes large amounts of protein may experience a more serious problem called *pregnancy-induced hypertension*, which needs strict medical monitoring. Pregnancy-induced hypertension is described in more detail later in the chapter.

As previously mentioned, progesterone may slow GI motility during pregnancy, leading to constipation, heartburn, and delayed gastric emptying. In late pregnancy, these problems may be exacerbated by the weight of the uterus and fetus as they compress the abdominal cavity.

Weight Gain in Pregnancy

There are three components to maternal weight gain: (1) maternal body composition changes including increased blood and extracellular fluid volume; (2) the maternal support tissues such as the increased size of the uterus and breasts; and (3) the products of conception, including the fetus and the placenta. Inadequate weight gain by the mother during pregnancy suggests she may not have received the proper nutrients during pregnancy. Poor weight gain may then lead to intrauterine growth retardation in the infant. Infants born small for gestational age (SGA) or low birth weight are more likely to require prolonged hospitalization after birth or be ill or die during the first year of life. Additionally, infant mortality rate, which in part reflects maternal weight gain, is regarded as one measure of a country's health and well-being. Although the 1998 infant mortality rate for the United States continued an all-time low first reached in 1996 (7.2 per 1000 live births),[4] it still remains far greater than other developed countries. Infant mortality rates are higher among African Americans (14.3/1000 in 1998) than among Caucasians.[4]

There is strong evidence that the pattern of weight gain is just as important as the absolute recommended weight gains shown in Table 11-1. Failure to gain adequately during the second trimester of pregnancy is associated with poor infant birth weight, even if the net gain falls with the recommendations.[5]

small for gestational age (SGA)
having a lower birth weight than expected for the length of gestation

low birth weight
weighing less than 5.5 pounds (2500 g) at birth

Table 11-1
Recommended Total Weight Gain Ranges for Pregnant Women, by Prepregnancy Body Mass Index (BMI)

Weight-for-Height Category	Recommended Total Gain	
	kg	lb
Low (BMI of <19.8)	12.5-18	28-40
Normal (BMI of 19.8-26.0)	11.5-16	25-35
High* (BMI of >26-29)	7-11.5	15-25

Young adolescent and African-American women should strive for gains at the upper end of the recommended range. Short women (<157 cm or 62 in) should strive for gains at the lower end of the range.

From *National Academy of Sciences*: Nutrition during pregnancy: weight gain and nutrient supplements, *Washington, DC, 1990, National Academy Press.*
*The recommended target weight gain for obese women (BMI of >29.0) is at least 6 kg (13 lb).

A balance must be struck regarding weight gain during pregnancy. Although women who are underweight or normal weight (as defined by body mass index [BMI]) are counseled to eat sufficiently to promote adequate gain, caution must be observed in counseling women who enter pregnancy overweight or obese. Overweight and obese women should gain enough weight to support the fetus and maternal support tissues but without increasing total body fat. There are increased risks for operative delivery, increased maternal postpartum weight, gestational diabetes, and other long-term health consequences when maternal weight goes beyond the guidelines, particularly among women who are obese before pregnancy.[6,7] In addition, there may be subpopulations such as minorities and low-income women who need special guidance regarding weight gain during pregnancy.

Energy and Nutrient Needs during Pregnancy

The dietary reference intakes (DRIs) recommend increases during pregnancy of all nutrients *except* vitamin D, vitamin E, vitamin K, phosphorus, fluoride, calcium, and biotin. There are separate dietary recommendations for adolescents who are pregnant (Table 11-2).

Table 11-2
DRIs to Meet Needs of Pregnancy and Lactation

	Adult Women (25-49 Years of Age)	Pregnant Women (Third Trimester)	Lactating Mothers*
Energy (kcal)	2200	2500	2700
Protein (g)	50	60	65
Vitamin A (RE)	800	800	1300
Vitamin D (mcg)†	5	5	5
Vitamin E (mg α-TE)	8	10	12
Vitamin C (mg)	60	70	95
Thiamin (mg)	1.1	1.4	1.5
Riboflavin (mg)	1.1	1.4	1.6
Niacin (NE mg)	14	18	17
Vitamin B$_6$ (mg)	1.3	1.9	2.0
Folate (mcg)	400	600	500
Vitamin B$_{12}$ (mcg)	2.4	2.6	2.8
Calcium (mg)†	1000	1000	1000
Phosphorus (mg)	700	700	700
Iron (mg)‡	15	30	15
Zinc (mg)	12	15	19
Iodine (mcg)	150	175	200
Selenium (mcg)	55	65	75

Data from National Academy of Sciences: Dietary Reference Intakes (five reports), Washington, DC, 2002, National Academy Press.
NE, Niacin equivalent; RE, retinol equivalent; TE, tocopherol equivalent.
*During the first 6 months of lactation.
†Adequate Intake
‡The increased iron requirement for pregnancy cannot be met by the usual American diet or from body stores; thus a supplement of 30 to 60 mg of elemental iron is recommended.

Energy

It is difficult to estimate the true energy cost of pregnancy, but the best estimates place the total energy cost somewhere between 68,000 kcalories and 80,000 kcalories. The increase accommodates the rise in maternal BMR during pregnancy as well as the synthesis and support of the maternal and fetal tissues.[8] The current recommendation is for a woman to consume an extra 300 kcalories per day during the second and third trimesters of pregnancy. Although she is eating for two, the expectant mother need not and should not double her food intake. An extra sandwich and a glass of milk can easily provide the additional 300 kcalories per day, providing she was eating well before pregnancy. Personal preference may guide particular food choices to provide the extra kcalories, as long as the foods are nutritious.

What happens if a pregnant woman fails to increase her energy intake during pregnancy? The best known example in the twentieth century occurred in Holland during World War II. Infants born during the famine of 1944 and 1945 had smaller birth weights and birth lengths when compared with infants born either before or after the famine.[9] Recent research shows that when women who begin pregnancy in energy deficit (e.g., those who are chronically undernourished in developing countries) are provided with energy supplementation throughout the course of pregnancy, there is a positive effect on maternal weight gain and infant birth weight.[10] On the other hand, some research suggests that women in the United States who are well nourished do not increase their total energy intake by a full 300 calories per day and still have a positive pregnancy outcome.[11] Most likely, in the third trimester, many women decrease their energy expenditure in pregnancy by decreasing activity, thereby giving a net increase in energy intake.

Pregnancy is not a time to restrict kcalories or to lose weight, even if the mother begins the pregnancy as overweight. This may be particularly important to emphasize to the adolescent population. The mother should be encouraged to eat at least the minimum number of servings from the Food Guide Pyramid (Table 11-3). Sample menus can be helpful in showing the pregnant woman how the Pyramid should be used (Box 11-1).

Protein

The Recommended Dietary Allowance (RDA) for protein during pregnancy is 60 grams per day for adolescent and adult women. Women can easily obtain this in the American diet; the use of special protein powder supplements is not recom-

Table 11-3
Changes in the Daily Food Guide Pyramid during Pregnancy and Lactation

Food Group	Nonpregnant	Pregnant or Lactating
Milk, yogurt, and cheese	2-3 servings	3-4 servings*
Meat, poultry, fish, dry beans, eggs, and nuts	2-3 servings	3 servings
Fruit	2-4 servings	2-4 servings (1-2 citrus)
Vegetables	3-5 servings	3-5 servings (1-2 green leafy)
Bread, cereal, rice, and pasta	6-11 servings	7-11 servings

Data from U.S. Department of Agriculture: Food Guide Pyramid, Human Nutrition Information Pub No 249, Washington, DC, Revised 1996, U.S. Government Printing Office.
*4-5 servings for pregnant adolescents.

Box 11-1 Sample Menu for Pregnant Women

BREAKFAST

Whole grain toast
Banana
Oatmeal
Skim milk or orange juice

LUNCH

Roast beef (lean) sandwich on whole
  grain bread with lettuce and tomato
Green salad
Orange wedges
Skim milk†

DINNER

Sesame chicken (or fish) with broccoli
  and pasta
Mixed salad (carrots, tomatoes, spinach,
  romaine lettuce)
Italian bread and butter
Fresh fruit salad
Skim milk

SNACK*

Cereal (ready to eat)
Skim milk

SNACK

Apple with cheese, or fruit and yogurt
  shake

SNACK

Fig or oatmeal raisin cookies or open-
  face peanut butter sandwich

Snacks are all interchangeable.
†*Assumes water consumed throughout the day as a beverage in addition to skim milk.*

---

mended. Pregnant patients may be counseled to include appropriate sources of protein that provide vitamins, minerals, and moderate amounts of fat. Patients from low-income populations may need counseling or other assistance to ensure protein intake is sufficient; these clients may qualify for food vouchers through the USDA's Special Supplemental Food Program for Women, Infants, and Children (WIC) (see the Social Issue box, "Providing the Essentials").

SOCIAL ISSUE
Providing the Essentials

Nutrient-dense foods are the foundations for healthy expectant mothers and their offspring. Women at low socioeconomic levels may have difficulty affording these essentials. One way to ensure adequate nutrition is through a federal government program, such as the USDA's Special Supplemental Food Program for Women, Infants, and Children (WIC).

The WIC program began in 1972 and currently operates through approved clinics in all 50 states. Eligible participants must live in an area served by WIC, meet federal income guidelines (income no greater than 185% of U.S. poverty level), and have a nutritional risk factor such as anemia, poor weight gain during pregnancy, previous low birth weight infant, or inadequate diet. Pregnant and postpartum women (up to 12 months postpartum if breastfeeding, 6 months if not) are eligible to participate, as well as infants and children up to 5 years of age.

WIC provides vouchers for foods high in protein, vitamin C, vitamin A, iron, and calcium—nutrients having shown to be lacking in this population. Participants are offered nutrition education or nutrition counseling, receive testing for anemia, receive routine anthropometric monitoring, and obtain referrals to other healthcare resources.

Community healthcare nurses can refer clients to local WIC programs for assistance. Contacting the city, county, or state health departments can identify the closest WIC clinic.

The increase in protein intake over the nonpregnant state is necessary to build and maintain the variety of new tissues of pregnancy. A woman experiencing nausea and vomiting in the first trimester of pregnancy may find it difficult to increase sources of protein in her diet, particularly if meats (which have a strong cooking odor) aggravate the nausea. If this is the case, she should consume small amounts of high-quality protein as tolerated.

Vitamin and Mineral Supplementation

The DRIs are increased during pregnancy for most vitamins and minerals. Vitamins of concern are vitamins A and D. As little as 10,000 IU preformed vitamin A per day[12] and excessive vitamin D during pregnancy can each cause birth defects. Micronutrient needs may be met with a balanced diet, with a few notable exceptions including folate and iron. All supplementation during pregnancy should be in the form of prenatal type multivitamin-mineral supplements as recommended by primary healthcare providers or dietitians.

Folate.   Substantial research has demonstrated that folate is important for the prevention of neural tube defects (NTDs) such as spina bifida and anencephaly, one of the most common congenital malformations in the United States.[13] Approximately 2500 to 3000 infants are born with NTDs each year in the United States, with an equal number likely lost to pregnancy termination and additional unknown numbers of spontaneous abortions. The U.S. Public Health Service and the American Academy of Pediatrics now recommend all women of childbearing age who are capable of becoming pregnant receive a daily intake of 400 mcg of synthetic folic acid (from vitamin supplements, fortified grains, and other foods). Although fortification has been implemented, education continues to be needed to encourage awareness of folic acid intake by women of childbearing age. During pregnancy the Dietary Reference Intakes (DRI) increase to 600 mcg dietary folate equivalents (DFE) per day.[14]

Iron.   The RDA for iron during pregnancy is 30 mg/day. This level may be difficult to achieve with a normal diet, which maintains recommended fat and kcaloric guidelines. Therefore all women should take a supplement with 30 mg ferrous iron daily beginning in the second trimester to prevent iron deficiency anemia in pregnancy[1] (see the Cultural Considerations box).

CULTURAL CONSIDERATIONS
Ethnicity and Prepregnancy Eating Habits

Energy intake, selected nutrients, health status, and nutrition practices of women were examined 3 months before pregnancy. The sample consisted of 462 California women who delivered normal infants. About 35% of the subjects were Latina. Of these Latina women, 58% were foreign born.

The findings show that energy intakes in all ethnic groups exceeded 2000 kcal/day, but fewer than half the women consumed the recommended five servings of fruit and vegetables a day. Half of the women failed to consume the Recommended Dietary Allowance (RDA) for iron, and one quarter were below the AI/RDA for calcium, magnesium, and zinc.

The diets of the foreign-born Latina women were lowest in total fat as a percentage of total energy intakes but highest in carbohydrate, cholesterol, fiber, grain products, protein, folate, vitamin C, iron, and zinc. Approximately 25% of all the subjects used some type of vitamin/mineral supplement in the 3 months before pregnancy. Vitamin/mineral supplements were common among Caucasian non-Latina women (34%) but rare among foreign-born Latina women (5%). This study suggests ethnicity is one possible predictor of prepregnancy eating habits.

Application to nursing: This study shows that women, regardless of ethnicity, tend not to take vitamin/mineral supplements before pregnancy. Nurses working with women during the first trimester of pregnancy can guide them to consider regularly taking vitamin/mineral supplements as prescribed by their healthcare providers. Because the foreign-born Latina women were least likely to use vitamin/mineral supplements before their pregnancy, special attention can be made to use cultural messages and nutritional counseling for this subgroup to achieve compliance.

Reference: Schaffer D et al.: Ethnicity and prepregnancy eating habits J Am Dietetic Assoc 98(8):876, 1998.

Iron deficiency anemia is one of the most common complications of pregnancy. The iron requirement increases secondary to the expansion of the maternal red cell volume. Iron deficiency anemia can mean impaired oxygen delivery to the fetus, which may have severe consequences. In addition, during the last trimester, the fetus stores iron in its liver to use during the first 4 months of life.

As discussed in Chapter 8, an unusual behavior associated with iron deficiency is pica. *Pica* is characterized by a hunger and appetite for nonfood substances including ice, corn starch, clay, and even dirt. These substances contain no iron and may lead to loss of additional minerals, particularly when clay and dirt are consumed. Intestinal blockages caused by consumption of these substances may be life-threatening. Of particular concern is the practice of pica during pregnancy when the risk and implications of iron-deficiency anemia are most severe. Although more common among African American women, pica has been diagnosed among all ethnic groups within all socioeconomic levels. A challenge to obstetric nurses is to elicit information about this type of dietary behavior when assessing clients.

Calcium.   The Adequate Intake (AI) for calcium is 1000 mg/day for women and 1300 mg/day for adolescents, neither of which is an increase over the non-pregnant state.[15] Although calcium needs are great during pregnancy, particularly for mineralization of the fetal skeleton, changes occur in maternal calcium homeostasis, which results in an increase in intestinal calcium absorption.[16] Many women, particularly adolescents, may not consume the AI for calcium *before* pregnancy. Women who are unable to consume rich sources of calcium may need to seek advice from a dietitian/nutrition specialist to determine whether supplements are necessary.

Nutrition-Related Concerns

A number of nonnutritive substances that women may be exposed to during pregnancy may have the capability to act as teratogens. A teratogen is an agent that is capable of producing a malformation or a defect in the unborn fetus. Some anomalies are apparent at birth or shortly after, such as NTDs or a cleft lip or palate. Other defects such as delayed growth or learning deficits may not be noticeable for several months or even years. Potential teratogens include caffeine, drugs, alcohol, and tobacco. Other concerns affecting the course and outcome of pregnancy include strenuous exercise, maternal age, and medical conditions requiring nutrition intervention such as hypertension, diabetes, phenylketonuria, and human immunodeficiency virus (HIV) infection. Although not nutritional in nature, the effect of teratogens on the course of pregnancy may be so serious as to warrant at least a brief review.

teratogen

an agent capable of producing a malformation or a defect in the unborn fetus

Caffeine

Whether a woman should refrain from caffeine consumption during pregnancy has been a matter of debate. Caffeine (1-, 3-, 7-trimethyxanthine) may alter deoxyribonucleic acid (DNA) and, in some individuals, may alter circulating levels of neurotransmitters and increase blood pressure.[17] It has been argued that any or all of these effects may have direct adverse consequences on the developing fetus. However there is now enough evidence stating that caffeine is not a human teratogen, and even at modest doses (<300 mg/day or about 2 cups or less of coffee), there is no increased risk of spontaneous abortion or preterm labor. It doesn't affect birth weight, gestational age, or fetal growth.[17,18] There may be small reductions in birth weight at very high levels of consumption. The important issue may be that heavy use of nonnutritive substances such as coffee, tea, and cola may displace needed nutrients in the diet and thus interfere with prenatal development. Moderation of caffeine use during pregnancy as opposed to complete elimination is reasonable advice.

Drugs

A pregnant woman should not consume any over-the-counter or prescription medications unless prescribed by her primary healthcare provider. The growing fetus, particularly during the period of organogenesis in the first trimester, is highly susceptible to insult.

Although not a direct nutrient concern, the acne medication isotretinoin (Accutane) contains high levels of retinoic acid in the form of a vitamin A analogue. This medication causes fetal malformations such as craniofacial abnormalities and microcephaly when ingested in the periconceptional period. The current recommendation is that women of childbearing age not use isotretinoin for the treatment of acne.

This recommendation is consistent with a large body of animal data that shows that consumption of large quantities of preformed vitamin A during pregnancy results in an excess of malformations such as anencephaly (defective brain development), cleft palate, spina bifida, webbed fingers or toes, and facial malformations. Vitamin A crosses the placenta by simple diffusion. Because it is fat-soluble, the excess vitamin A can accumulate in the fetal tissues and may cause damage by interfering with cellular growth and differentiation during critical periods of development.[12]

Alcohol

fetal alcohol syndrome (FAS)/fetal alcohol spectrum disorders (FASD)
a disorder caused by alcohol consumption during pregnancy that produces a range of specific anatomic and central nervous system defects

The use of alcohol during pregnancy may produce fetal alcohol syndrome (FAS) or fetal alcohol spectrum disorder (FASD) in the infant. Symptoms include specific anatomic defects such as a low nasal bridge, short nose, flat midface, and short palpebral fissures (Figure 11-1).

There is no safe level of alcohol intake during pregnancy. FAS is not confined to heavy drinkers; anyone who uses alcohol during pregnancy places the infant at risk of this preventable syndrome. Therefore *all* pregnant women should be urged to

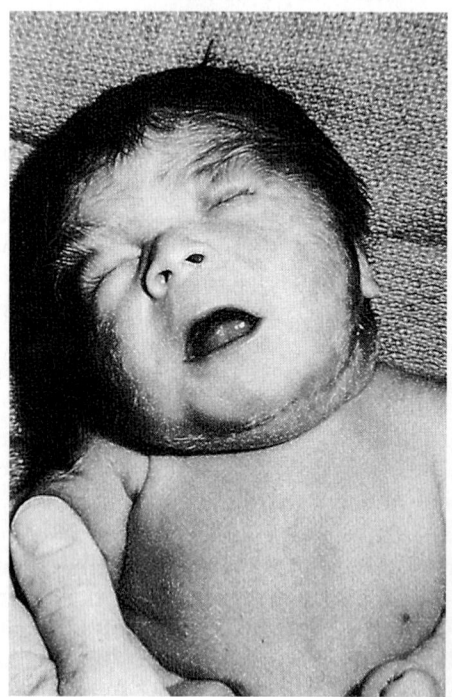
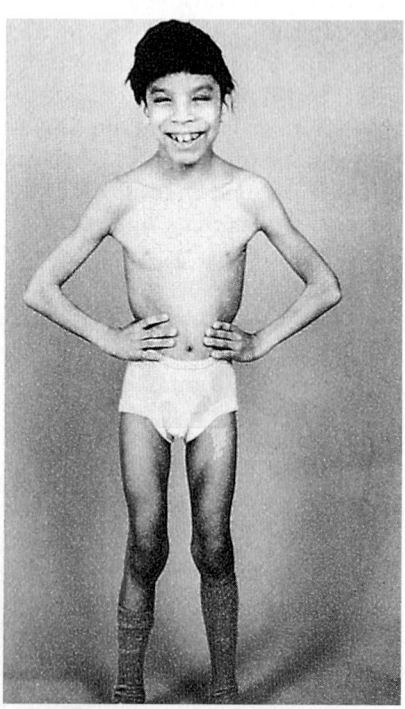

Figure 11-1 Child with FAS at day 1 and 8 years. This child was diagnosed at birth and has spent all his life in a foster home where his care has been excellent. His IQ has remained stable at 40 to 45. (From Dr. Ann P. Streissguth, University of Washington, Seattle; In Streissguth AP, Clarren SK, Jones KL: Natural history of the fetal alcohol syndrome: a 10-year follow-up of eleven patients, *The Lancet* 2:85, July 1985. Reprinted with permission from Elsevier Science.)

cease consumption of *all* alcoholic beverages. A *Healthy People 2010* health objective is to increase the number of pregnant women not consuming alcohol during pregnancy to 94%. Because alcohol use by pregnant women increased between 1991 and 1995, healthcare providers should screen women for alcohol use and counsel clients appropriately.[19]

Tobacco

Considerable research has been conducted on the effects of cigarette smoking during pregnancy. Women who smoke during pregnancy are at greater risk for several adverse outcomes including the following: prematurity, low birth weight, SGA, stillbirth, placenta previa (location in lower uterine area), placentae abruptio (separation from uterine wall), and postnatally, sudden infant death syndrome (SIDS). Smoking during pregnancy may cause prolonged effects of impaired intellectual performance and decreased attention span in the offspring. Poor nutrition during pregnancy will compound the risks associated with smoking.[20]

Women should avoid saunas, hot tubs, and very hot baths during pregnancy to decrease the risk of raising maternal (and fetal) temperatures above normal.

Exercise

Women with normal pregnancies should stay active during pregnancy, but the intensity of exercise is a matter of debate. Strenuous exercise was thought to divert blood to the exercising muscles and thus reduce the blood supply to the fetus.[21] There was also speculation that intense exercise would place the mother at risk for premature labor. More recent research shows that the short-term metabolic changes associated with exercise pose no problem for the fetus. In a longitudinal study, Clapp and colleagues found that infants born to women who exercised throughout pregnancy weighed slightly less and had less body fat compared with infants of nonexercising women. At 1 year of age, though, there were no differences in growth or development of the infants between the two groups.[22] On the other hand, strenuous work conditions may pose risks for adverse pregnancy outcome. Heavy lifting and a heavy work pace may increase the risk of low birth weight infants.[23]

Based on these recent studies, there is no reason for women to discontinue established exercise programs during pregnancy. However, it is not the best time to begin a new exercise program. If a woman chooses to exercise during pregnancy she must remember to drink fluids before, after, and, if necessary, during exercise and to choose nutritious snacks before and after exercise. General guidelines for exercise during pregnancy are listed in the margin.

GUIDELINES FOR EXERCISE DURING PREGNANCY:

- Limit workouts to 15 minutes.
- Keep pulse rate below 140 beats per minute.
- Drink plenty of fluids before, after, and during exercise.
- Do not exercise lying on your back after the fourth month.
- Avoid exercising in hot, humid weather.
- Consume enough kcalories to meet the extra needs of pregnancy plus the exercise performed.

Maternal Age

Adolescents and women older than 35 years of age are at higher risk for poor pregnancy outcome.[1] When assessing the nutritional status of the pregnant teen, there are several important factors to consider. These include the growth pattern of the mother, the psychologic maturity of the mother, the lack of economic resources to provide for the infant, and delay in seeking medical care. Dietary factors to assess are the poor dietary habits that are typical of many teens, frequency with which meals are eaten away from home each day, and the possible preoccupation with weight gain during pregnancy. There is growing evidence that the nutrition intervention targeted specifically for this age group is highly effective at reducing the risk of adverse outcomes commonly seen among this group.[24,25]

Women who become pregnant after the age of 35 years have distinct nutritional needs, reflecting their longer medical history, potential long-term use of oral contraceptives (which may affect folate levels) and the possibility of a longer history of poor eating habits.[1] In addition, older women are at risk for nutrition-related complications such as gestational diabetes. Careful nutritional evaluation of these patients can be useful in providing guidance to reduce the risk of nutritional imbalances that cause pregnancy complications.

pregnancy-induced hypertension (PIH)
a sudden rise in arterial blood pressure accompanied by rapid weight gain and marked edema during pregnancy; formerly known as *toxemia of pregnancy*

Preeclampsia

Preeclampsia, known as pregnancy-induced hypertension (PIH), is a complex syndrome of deficient vascularization, platelet dysfunction, hyperlipidemia, and altered cytokine levels.[26,27] Although clinical diagnosis is usually after 28 weeks of gestation, it is now appreciated that the origins of preeclampsia are early in pregnancy.[26] Clinically, the mother experiences a sudden and severe rise in arterial blood pressure, rapid weight gain, and marked edema, often necessitating immediate delivery of the fetus to save the life of both mother and infant.

Preeclampsia may occur in as many as 5% to 15% of all pregnancies and is one of the leading causes of prematurity and maternal and fetal death. Risk factors for preeclampsia are listed in Box 11-2.

Nutrition support during preeclampsia includes provision of a well-balanced diet with generous sources of protein to replace losses in proteinuria and with adequate vitamins and minerals. It should supply a sufficient amount of energy. Energy intake should not be limited in an attempt to restrict maternal weight gain.

Currently there is much research on prevention of preeclampsia. Uses of low-dose aspirin, calcium supplements, and omega-3 fatty acids from fish oil have been suggested as agents to prevent this disorder.[26-28] Because the use of these supplements is still experimental, supplements should only be used when recommended by a physician.

Diabetes Mellitus

Women with preexisting diabetes mellitus (DM) (type 1 and type 2 DM) require specialized care during pregnancy. Approximately 5% to 10% of all infants of diabetic mothers are born with congenital anomalies. Other complications include fetal macrosomia, dystocia, operative delivery, neonatal hypoglycemia, and neonatal respiratory distress syndrome. The major defects reported include cardiac defects, nervous system defects including NTDs, kidney malformations, and skeletal anomalies.[29]

These infants may experience hypoglycemia after birth. The maternal source of glucose is no longer available, and because glucose readily crosses the placenta, levels of glucose in utero tend to be high, especially if the diabetes has been poorly controlled. Without quick treatment, this condition can be fatal in neonates. Infants born to mothers with diabetes require immediate monitoring in the neonatal intensive care unit. Additionally, the mother with diabetes is at greater risk for preeclampsia, retinopathy, and neuropathy during pregnancy.[30,31]

Box 11-2 Risk Factors and Symptoms of Preeclampsia

PREPREGNANCY FACTORS THAT MAY LEAD TO THE DEVELOPMENT OF PREECLAMPSIA INCLUDE THE FOLLOWING:

- No previous pregnancies
- Inadequate dietary intake
- Diabetes mellitus (type 1; type 2)
- Age at conception: 20 years or younger
                       35 years or older
- Family history: hypertension, vascular disease
- Medical history of hypertension or renal or vascular disease
- Preeclampsia in earlier pregnancies
- Poverty that affects access to prenatal care

SYMPTOMS DURING PREGNANCY INCLUDE THE FOLLOWING:

- Hypertension (change compared with usual level)
- Headaches (continuous and severe)
- Dizziness and blurred vision
- Edema of hands and face
- Sudden weight gain
- Upper abdominal pain
- Slowed fetal growth
- Protein in urine (proteinuria)

Modified from Worthington-Roberts BS, Williams SR, eds.: Nutrition throughout the life cycle, ed 3, New York, 1996, McGraw-Hill.

Fortunately, there may be a decreased prevalence of many of the maternal and fetal complications associated with DM when normal blood glucose level (normo-glycemia) is achieved before conception and maintained throughout pregnancy. The current recommendation is for women to achieve tight glucose control *before* conception to maximize the likelihood of a healthy mother and infant, while avoiding perinatal risks. Control includes prudent blood glucose monitoring, adherence to diet, moderate exercise, and strict adherence to the prescribed insulin regimen.[32] Total energy intake and energy distribution will likely need modification during pregnancy because of the increased energy needs of pregnancy. Insulin dosages will require adjustment because many of the hormones of pregnancy, such as estrogen, progesterone, human chorionic, somatotropin, and maternal cortisol, act in an antagonistic fashion with insulin.

Oral hypoglycemic agents may have teratogenic effects on the fetus and should be discontinued in women with type 2 DM who previously had used them for glucose control.[33] All women with diabetes should discuss drug treatment options with their physician before conception.

Gestational diabetes mellitus (GDM) is a form of diabetes that occurs during pregnancy—most commonly after the twentieth week of gestation. Patients experience abnormal carbohydrate metabolism in a manner similar to other persons with diabetes. Of all forms of diabetes during pregnancy, GDM is the most common, affecting 2% to 3% of all pregnancies.[34] All women should undergo screening for GDM during the second trimester, with repeat testing for women who may be borderline.

Treatment of GDM consists primarily of dietary control combined with moderate exercise leading to an appropriate weight gain. Insulin may be required if glycemic control is not achieved through dietary control and exercise. Risk factors for GDM include delivery of a previous large infant, a prior perinatal death, glycosuria, and maternal age greater than 30 years. The majority of women with GDM have normal glucose tolerance following delivery, but they may remain at risk for type 2 DM later in life.

gestational diabetes mellitus (GDM)
a form of diabetes occurring during pregnancy, most commonly after the twentieth week of gestation

Maternal Phenylketonuria

Phenylketonuria (PKU) is an inborn error of metabolism characterized by extremely low levels of the enzyme phenylalanine hydroxylase, which catalyzes the conversion of phenylalanine to tyrosine. Absence of this crucial enzyme causes a failure in the metabolism of the amino acid phenylalanine and low levels of tyrosine. Successful treatment of this disorder occurs by adhering to a strict diet low in phenylalanine and supplemented with tyrosine beginning in the first week of life. Failure to detect the disease or a lack of compliance with the dietary therapy results in irreversible mental retardation.

Thirty years ago, most patients with PKU did not conceive and bear children. However, with the advent of neonatal PKU testing in all 50 states, diagnosis and treatment of the disorder have allowed many young women to lead normal, productive lives, including the desire to have children. Women with PKU require specialized nutrition care during pregnancy. Maternal PKU, particularly if not well controlled at the time of conception, poses a great risk to the unborn offspring. Mothers with untreated PKU have a high likelihood of experiencing spontaneous abortion or having an infant born with microcephaly, mental retardation, congenital heart defects, or intrauterine growth retardation, even if the infant does not have the genetic defect. Conscientious adherence to a low-phenylalanine diet may lessen, but not completely eliminate, the risk of an adverse pregnancy outcome. Total nutrient intake and maternal weight gain should be monitored throughout pregnancy.[35]

All young women with PKU should continue their low-phenylalanine diets throughout the childbearing years. Family planning is strongly encouraged to establish safe phenylalanine levels before conception and to educate women regarding the high risk of poor pregnancy outcome, even with good dietary control.

HIV Infection

In the United States approximately 85% of female cases of HIV infection are among women of childbearing age.[36] Of women who give birth, about 1.6/1000 are HIV infected.[37] Pregnancy may put an additional strain on the already fragile immune system because the hormones and proteins of pregnancy (including estrogen, progesterone, human chorionic gonadotropin, alfafetoprotein, corticosteroids, prolactin, and alphaglobulin) have immunosuppressive effects.

The HIV-infected woman who experiences an opportunistic infection during pregnancy will have increased needs for kcalories, protein, vitamins, and minerals. Weight gain must be strictly monitored, although there are no specialized weight gain recommendations for this population.

Overcoming Barriers: Relief from Common Discomforts during Pregnancy

The following information discusses the common discomforts during pregnancy and methods of relief.

Nausea and Vomiting

Nausea and vomiting during the first trimester of pregnancy can be annoying, but it generally begins to subside by the beginning of the second trimester. Symptoms of morning sickness may actually occur at any time throughout the day, though vomiting tends to be more common between 6 A.M. and noon. Although the etiology of nausea and vomiting during pregnancy is unknown, it may be caused by hormonal factors such as a rise in estrogen or the placental hormone human chorionic gonadotropin (HCG). Stress or fatigue may exacerbate the condition. There is no cause for alarm unless the mother begins to lose weight or becomes severely dehydrated. If she cannot retain either foods or fluid for 6 hours or longer, a physician should be contacted.

If nausea or vomiting persists into the second trimester or severely interferes with the mother's life, it may be a more serious condition. Hyperemesis gravidarum is severe and unrelenting vomiting and usually requires intravenous replacement of nutrients and fluids. If the mother receives total parenteral nutrition or nasogastric tube feedings for the treatment of hyperemesis gravidarum, appropriate levels of vitamins and minerals should be included, with careful monitoring and follow-up.

There are no specific foods to avoid, but many women find it is helpful to eat small, frequent, meals; drink liquids between rather than with meals; and avoid fried and greasy foods. Some women find it helpful to reduce coffee intake and to prepare meals near an open window to avoid cooking odors. If nausea upon getting out of bed in the morning is a problem, dry toast or crackers eaten before getting out of bed may provide relief. Snacks to keep handy while working or traveling might include dried fruit, crackers, and small cans of juice.

hyperemesis gravidarum
severe and unrelenting vomiting in the second trimester or vomiting that severely interfers with the mother's life; a serious condition usually requiring intravenous replacement of nutrients and fluids

Heartburn

In late pregnancy, when the fetus rapidly grows in size, the uterus pushes up against the stomach, which may cause a feeling of fullness in the mother. Additionally, because of the action of progesterone (which can cause relaxation of smooth muscles), a relaxation of the gastroesophageal sphincter may occur, resulting in some reflux of gastric contents into the lower esophagus. This is the cause of the heartburn so common during the final weeks of pregnancy. The best dietary remedies include eating small frequent meals, avoiding foods high in fat, drinking fluids between rather than with meals, limiting spicy foods, and avoiding lying down for 1 to 2 hours after eating. Many women find relief by wearing loose-fitting clothing around the abdomen. Expectant mothers should not take antacids without approval of a primary care provider. Heartburn generally disappears after delivery of the infant.

Constipation

As mentioned earlier, constipation is common during the first and third trimesters of pregnancy. During the first trimester, progesterone (which slows GI motility) may be responsible. In the third trimester, the growing fetus crowds the other internal organs, again possibly slowing GI motility. Although bothersome, constipation responds well to dietary treatment. A generous intake of fiber, such as whole grain cereals, fresh fruit, and raw vegetables, as well as inclusion of plenty of fluids should alleviate constipation. Moderate exercise such as a daily walk may also help. The recommendations for alleviating constipation also help prevent hemorrhoids. Over-the-counter laxatives or enemas should not be used unless prescribed by a physician.

NUTRITION DURING LACTATION

All sexually mature female mammals possess milk-producing mammary glands and are able to produce milk specifically formulated to provide optimum growth and development for their offspring. Although there are historical accounts of wet nurses and even artificial feeding implements dating back to Greek and Roman times, breastfeeding (lactation) was the primary mode of infant feeding until this century in the United States and around the world.[24]

Since World War II, however, there has been a dramatic decline in the incidence and duration of breastfeeding worldwide. Currently close to 60% of mothers in the United States initiate breastfeeding at hospital discharge, but by 5 to 6 months after birth, only about 20% of American infants are breastfed.[38,39] In many developed countries, such as Sweden, all women initiate breastfeeding and continue for most of the infant's first year of life. Although there is not one isolated cause for poor breastfeeding rates in the United States, it can be attributed to a multitude of causes. These include the advertising of breast-milk substitutes, lack of support for the breastfeeding mother, lack of knowledge of lactation by healthcare professionals, short postpartum hospital stays, and the rise in maternal employment without appropriate facilities to nurse infants or pump and store breast milk.[40]

The American Dietetic Association and the American Academy of Pediatrics have policy statements advocating exclusive use of human milk as the preferred feeding choice for infants for at least the first 4 to 6 months of life.[38,40] Ideally, breastfeeding should occur for the entire first 12 months accompanied by appropriate weaning foods. Breastfeeding offers advantages for both infant and mother (Box 11-3).

Box 11-3 Benefits of Breastfeeding

- Provides immunologic protection to the infant against many infections and diseases (especially respiratory and gastrointestinal)
- Offers uniquely suited nutrient composition with high bioavailability
- Reduces risk of food allergy in the infant
- Promotes infant oral motor development
- Offers convenience: always fresh, available, and at the right temperature
- Is generally less expensive than formula feeding
- May protect infant against some chronic diseases such as type 1 diabetes and childhood leukemia
- Promotes mother-infant bonding
- Facilitates uterine contractions and controls postpartum bleeding
- Promotes return to prepregnancy weight

Anatomy and Physiology of Lactation

SIGNS INFANT IS GETTING ENOUGH TO EAT:

- Six or eight wet diapers a day; breastfed infants often have one or two stools a day for the first few weeks and sometimes as many as one every feeding
- Feeding every 1 1/2 to 3 hours, after which infant seems content
- Adequate weight gain
- Good skin color and tone

oxytocin

a hormone that initiates uterine contractions of labor and has a role in the ejection of milk in lactation

prolactin

a hormone responsible for milk synthesis

The human breast begins its development in utero and goes through two further stages of change after birth: at puberty and during pregnancy. The mature human breast consists of a system of alveoli and ducts. Myoepithelial cells surround the milk-producing glands, located in the alveoli. The ductules emerge from the alveoli to carry the milk to the lactiferous ducts, which eventually empty into the lactiferous sinuses. The lactiferous sinuses are located behind the areola, or the darkened area of the nipple where the infant latches on during nursing (Figure 11-2).

Throughout the course of pregnancy, the breast tissue undergoes considerable development. Under the influence of progesterone, the lobules or alveoli increase in size and number, while estrogen stimulates proliferation of the ductal system. Together, these changes render the breast completely capable of milk production after delivery. An uncommon occurrence is a failure of the breasts to undergo development during pregnancy. A women who does not notice any changes in her breasts during pregnancy, particularly if she is pregnant for the first time, should receive postnatal assistance to determine her ability to fully lactate. Most women are able to fully lactate with no problems. Actual size of breast has no bearing on ability to breastfeed.

Lactation is a normal process beginning when various hormones interact following delivery of the infant. Before the onset of labor, there is a rise in serum levels of oxytocin. This hormone is instrumental in initiating the uterine contractions of labor that bring about birth. Oxytocin and another hormone, prolactin, set off the lactation process. Prolactin is primarily responsible for milk synthesis; oxytocin is involved with milk ejection from the breast.

As an infant is allowed to suckle after birth, a nerve impulse is sent to the mother's hypothalamus. This stimulates the anterior pituitary to secrete prolactin, which then stimulates milk production in the alveolar cells (Figure 11-3). The infant sucking stimulus initiates the release of oxytocin from the posterior pituitary. The flood of oxytocin into the breast tissue causes the myoepithelial cells around the glands to contract, thereby ejecting the milk into the infant's mouth. This is called the *let-down reflex*, or the *milk-ejection reflex*. Many women report feeling a tingling sensation in their breasts when the let-down occurs. Additionally, if a mother hears her infant's cry or sees another infant, she may experience a let-down accompanied by a rush of milk ejecting from her breasts. Deterrents to the let-

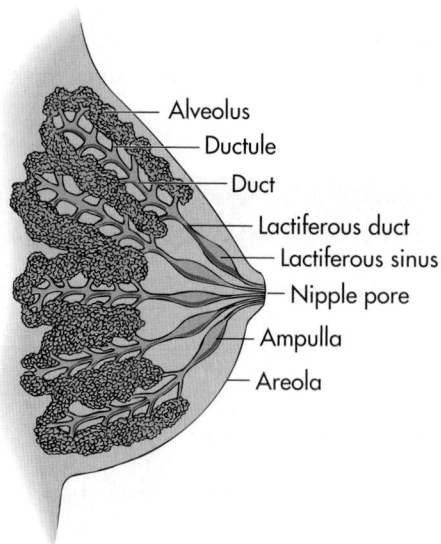

- Alveolus
- Ductule
- Duct
- Lactiferous duct
- Lactiferous sinus
- Nipple pore
- Ampulla
- Areola

Figure 11-2 Detailed structural features of human mammary gland. (From Rolin Graphics.)

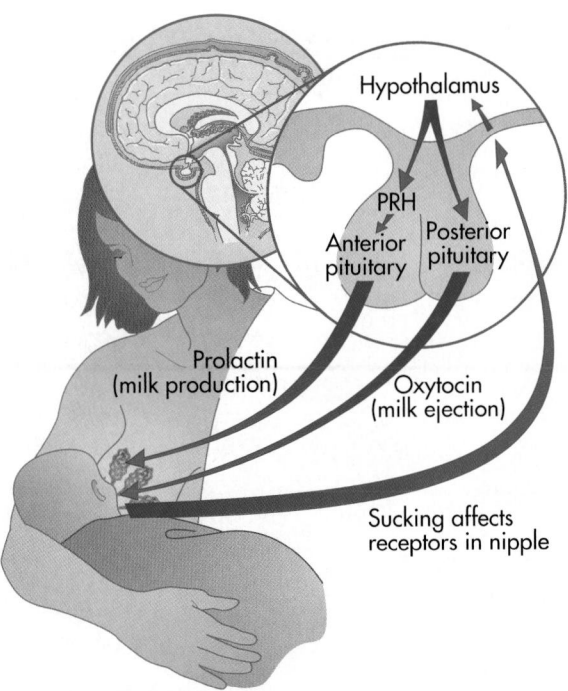

Figure 11-3 Maternal breastfeeding reflexes. (From Mahan KL, Escott-Stump S: *Krause's food, nutrition, and diet therapy,* Philadelphia, 2000, WB Saunders.)

down reflex may include fatigue, stress, alcohol, smoking, and some prescription medications.

An important point to note is that milk production is a supply-and-demand mechanism. The more an infant is allowed to nurse, the more nerve stimulation there will be, resulting in a rise in prolactin levels followed by increased milk production. There should be no restrictions placed on the number of times an infant, particularly a newborn, nurses per day.[40]

Promoting Breastfeeding

To increase the incidence and duration of breastfeeding in the United States and around the world, healthcare professionals must take measures ensuring that appropriate breastfeeding policies are adopted and practiced in hospitals providing maternity care. In 1991 the World Health Organization and UNICEF launched the Baby Friendly Hospital Initiative. The initiative includes "Ten Steps to Successful Breastfeeding" that the hospital must be willing to take to become infant friendly. Among the steps is breastfeeding education for all mothers, no separation of mother and infant following birth except for medical reasons, and no supplemental feedings unless medically indicated.[41] Nurses play a key role in prenatal counseling and in postpartum support to help mothers successfully establish and maintain lactation. Obstetric nurses should consult a lactation specialist if an infant or mother has difficulties initiating breastfeeding.

Another influence on successful lactation is acceptability of lactation within the cultural and ethnic communities of which the mother is a part. Cultures in which breastfeeding is common include Chinese, Finnish, Indian, Saudi Arabian, Muslim, South African, and Swedish. In the following cultures, breastfeeding is common, but infants are not given colostrum because it is considered bad or unclean: Cambodian, Filipino, Haitian, Japanese, Korean, Laotian, Mexican, and Vietnamese.[42] Socioeconomic and education levels are influences that help or hinder a mother's attempt at successful lactation. Organizations such as La Leche League or

colostrum
the fluid secreted from the breast during late pregnancy and the first few days postpartum; contains immunologic active substances (maternal antibodies) and essential nutrients

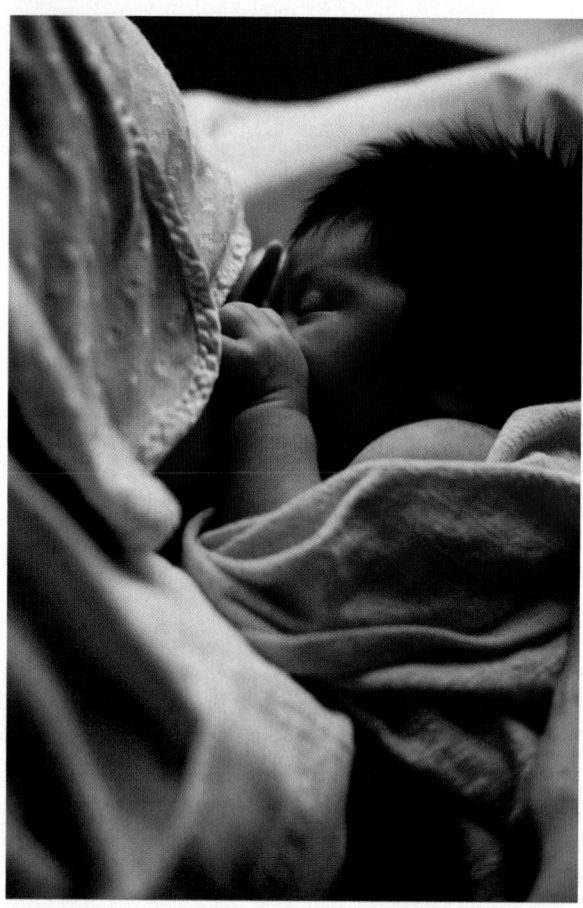

Successful breastfeeding depends on the health and nutritional status of the mother, her attitude toward breastfeeding, and support from healthcare providers and family. (From PhotoDisc.)

community-based mothers' groups may provide invaluable support to nursing mothers, particularly those nursing for the first time.

Energy and Nutrient Needs during Lactation

A large proportion of the energy stores laid down as adipose tissue during pregnancy are mobilized in lactation. Both BMR and maternal activity return to their prepregnant levels. The energy cost of milk production is approximately 500 to 800 kcalories per day depending on the volume of milk production. The RDA recommends increases for protein (65 g/day for the first 6 months of lactation and 62 g/day for the second 6 months of lactation) and for most of the vitamins and minerals over the normal adult levels. The mother can meet most of these increases by consuming a well-balanced diet (see Table 11-3).

A woman need not avoid certain foods while breastfeeding unless a problem occurs. For example, some infants are fussy following the mother's consumption of gas-producing vegetables such as cabbage, onions, and broccoli.

Adequate fluid intake is important during lactation. The average woman produces 750 to 1000 ml of milk per day. She can replace this fluid through consumption of water or juice. Coffee or cola drinks should be avoided or used on a minimal basis. They act as diuretics in the mother's body and caffeine, a stimulant, passes into breast milk in small amounts. The old myth stating that alcohol helps a mother relax and enhances milk production should not be followed. Alcohol not only passes into milk, becoming available to the infant, but also may inhibit oxytocin, consequently reducing the let-down reflex.

Despite the desire of most women to return to their prepregnancy weight quickly, rapid weight loss should not be encouraged while breastfeeding. Recent research shows that women achieve weight loss, without compromising their nutritional intake or the infants, when breastfeeding without the use of supplementary formula continues for at least 6 months. The amount of fat loss is highly variable between women (see the Health Debate box, "Lactation: A Natural Way to Lose Weight?").[43]

Contraindications to Breastfeeding

Common colds, the flu, and even most illnesses requiring short-term antibiotic therapy do not require cessation of breastfeeding. A number of maternal illnesses or conditions are contraindications to breastfeeding (see note in margin).

Most medications for mild illnesses are safe for the mother to take while breastfeeding. Mothers should always remind their healthcare providers they are nursing an infant should the need for a medication arise. The American Academy of Pediatrics has classified medications into five categories based on safety considerations. For mild illnesses as well as for chronic diseases, a medication compatible with breastfeeding can usually be found and substituted for one that is contraindicated. The amount of the maternal dose of drug actually secreted into the milk depends

CONTRAINDICATIONS TO BREASTFEEDING:
- Active tuberculosis
- HIV/AIDS
- Herpes simplex lesions on the maternal breast
- Maternal alcoholism
- Maternal drug addiction
- Malaria
- Maternal chicken pox (first 3 weeks postpartum only)
- Maternal breast cancer requiring treatment

HEALTH DEBATE
Lactation: A Natural Way to Lose Weight?

Considerable controversy surrounds the role of lactation in postpartum weight loss. It is generally believed that women who breastfeed their infants return to their prepregnancy weight more easily than those who do not because of the additional energy required for milk production.

Several studies, however, show little or no increase in postpartum weight loss for lactating women when compared with nonlactating women. Some of these studies may suffer from poor methodologic design. Difficulties in quantifying kcaloric intake and levels of physical activity affect the overall validity of results. One review of many studies found gestational weight gain is the most significant factor that affects weight and body fat change. This finding supports the idea, regardless of the feeding process; biologic mechanisms naturally lead the body to restore prepregnancy body weight and fat composition.

Other studies show that when infants are breastfed for at least 6 months, mothers lose significantly more body fat as measured by triceps skinfold thickness and body weight than controls who were matched on age, education, prepregnancy weight, parity, and pregnancy weight gain. Weight loss of lactating women may be slower or equal to nonlactating women who may diet to lose weight. The difference is the quality of weight lost by lactating women—body fat rather than lean body mass is better to lose in terms of overall health goals.

What do you think? Should lactation be promoted as a way to lose postpregnancy weight?

Compiled from Butte NF, Hopkinson JM: Body composition changes during lactation are highly variable among women, J Nutr 128(2 Suppl):381S, 1998; Dewey KG: Effects of maternal caloric restriction and exercise during lactation, J Nutr 128(2 Suppl):386S, 1998; Janney CA, Zhang D, Sowers M: Lactation and weight retention, Am J Clin Nutr 66(5):1116, 1997; Dewey KG, Heinig MJ, Mommsen LA: Maternal weight-loss patterns during prolonged lactation, Am J Clin Nutr 58:162, 1993; Potter P et al.: Does infant feeding method influence maternal postpartum weight loss? J Am Dietetic Assoc 91:441,1991.

on the route of administration, the size of the molecule, ionization, the pH of the medication, solubility, and protein binding.[44] Healthcare providers might keep this information in mind as they consider prescription medications for nursing mothers.

The Centers for Disease Control and Prevention recommend that all women in the United States infected with HIV not breastfeed their infants.[45] In developing countries where the risk of death from diarrhea caused by inappropriate bottle feeding is far greater than the risk of transmission of HIV via human milk, the World Health Organization recommends that breastfeeding continue in these situations. The woman with active acquired immunodeficiency syndrome (AIDS) and opportunistic infections is unlikely to have the physical strength to successfully lactate.[46]

Because of the advent of hepatitis B vaccinations given at birth, hepatitis B is no longer a contraindication to breastfeeding. However, there is mother-to-infant transmission of hepatitis C[45] and therefore, mothers with hepatitis C should not breastfeed.[47]

Nutrition during Infancy

Energy and Nutrient Needs during Infancy

Dramatic changes in growth and development occur during the first 12 months of life. In the first year, a human infant is expected to triple its birth weight and increase its length by 50%. In addition, after birth, organs such as the kidney and brain continue to develop and mature. In no other period of life do growth and development occur so rapidly. To support this rapid growth and development, the appropriate balance of all nutrients is essential. At the same time, parents, caregivers, and healthcare professionals must realize that infants have specialized nutrient needs. Advice appropriate for adults, and even older children, is inappropriate for infants, particularly with regard to fat and fiber intake and weight gain patterns.[48]

Energy

The World Health Organization suggests that infants receive 108 kcal/kg/day for the first 6 months of life and 98 kcal/kg/day from 6 months until the first birthday.[49] Adequate energy intake will be reflected in satisfactory gains in length and weight as plotted on a National Center for Health Statistics (NCHS) growth chart (see Appendix G). Infants should not have a restricted fat intake. Well-meaning parents should not place their infants on low-fat diets. Human milk, in fact, is high in cholesterol and fat content. Omega-3 fatty acids are plentiful in human milk, particularly if the mother includes fish in her diet on a regular basis. These fatty acids have been found to be essential for proper brain and nervous system development.[50,51]

Protein

Protein needs of infants have been hard to determine because of the difficulty of performing nitrogen balance studies on this population. Requirements are estimated based on the intake and growth rates of normal, healthy breastfed infants. Protein requirement is highest during the first 4 months of life when growth is the most rapid. It is suggested that infants receive 2.2 g/kg/day from birth to 6 months of age and 1.6 g/kg/day for the second half of the first year.[51] An excess of protein in an infant's diet can be problematic. Protein has a significant influence on renal solute load. The infant kidney is immature and unable to handle the large renal solute loads of an adult. Therefore increasing a normal infant's protein intake above the recommended amount should be avoided.

Vitamins and Mineral Supplementation

The DRIs may be consulted for appropriate levels of vitamins and minerals for infants. Breast milk or commercial formula should provide infants with all the vitamins and minerals needed for proper growth and development (Table 11-4).

Table 11-4
Recommended Supplementation of Infant Diets

Type of Feeding	Iron	Vitamin D	Fluoride	Vitamin K
Human milk	1 mg/kg/day*	10 μg/day	0.25 mg/day	Single intramuscular dose of 0.5 to 1 mg or oral dose of 1 to 2 mg
Formula	Iron-fortified formula	—	0.25 mg/day†	Single intramuscular dose of 0.5 to 1 mg or oral dose of 1 to 2 mg

From Committee on Nutrition, American Academy of Pediatrics, Handbook of Pediatric Nutrition, ed 4, Elk Grove Village, Ill, 1998, American Academy of Pediatrics.
*If an iron-fortified cereal is not used after 6 months of age.
†If fluoride content of water is less than 0.3 parts per million.

During the third trimester of pregnancy, the fetus stores iron in its liver to be used during the postnatal period. By 4 months of age, this supply of iron is usually depleted. The iron in breast milk, although lower in absolute amounts, is more bioavailable than iron from commercial formula. Many breastfed infants do not need to be supplemented with iron. However, their iron levels should be assessed periodically. Infants who consume commercial formula should use the iron-fortified variety to prevent iron deficiency anemia.

Humans are able to manufacture vitamin D through exposure to the sun; many young infants may not receive enough sun exposure for adequate synthesis. Breast milk contains vitamin D, but it may not be present in levels sufficient to prevent vitamin D–related rickets. There are several documented cases of vitamin D–related rickets, particularly among fully breastfed infants who receive little or no sunlight exposure.[52,53] Therefore it is recommended that all breastfed infants receive a daily oral supplement of vitamin D, unless they receive substantial sunlight exposure. Vitamin D can be toxic, so the recommended dosage should not be exceeded. Because vitamin D is present in commercial infant formula, formula-fed infants need not receive a supplement. Use of milk alternatives such as rice beverage ("rice milk") and soy health food beverage have also resulted in rickets. These alternatives, which are low in protein, calcium, and vitamin D, are not nutrient dense in comparison with breast milk, formula, or cow's milk.[54] Healthcare providers need to emphasize to caregivers that although the term "milk" is used in reference to these beverages, they are not nutritionally equal to milk produced by humans or by animals.

The water supply of most major cities in the United States contains fluoride as a preventive measure against tooth decay. The availability of fluoride may be particularly important for infants and young children whose teeth are developing. Routine fluoride supplementation is not recommended for infants less than 6 months of age. Older infants may need to receive fluoride if their local water supply is not fluoridated, but an assessment of total exposure to fluoride (via water, or juice prepared from local water source) should be made before systemic fluoride is prescribed.[55] For example, many rural families who rely on well water should have water supplies assessed for fluoride content. Excess fluoride can result in fluorosis, or mottling of tooth enamel; consequently the dosage should be followed precisely.[56]

Newborns are vulnerable to vitamin K deficiency (and thus hemorrhaging) in part because they lack intestinal bacteria to synthesize the vitamin. As a preventive measure, U.S. hospitals routinely give infants 0.5 to 1.0 mg of vitamin K by injection or 1 to 2 mg orally, once shortly after birth.

Food for Infants

The ideal food for the first 4 to 6 months of life is exclusive use of breast milk. As mentioned previously, breast milk has the correct balance of all the essential nutrients as well as immunologic factors that protect the infant from acute and chronic disease. The breast should be offered at least 10 to 12 times per 24 hours in the first several weeks. As the infant develops a stronger suck, more milk will be extracted with each nursing session and the frequency of feeding may decline. Although there is no specified time the infant should stay on the breast, between 10 to 15 minutes per breast (offering both breasts per session) is a good recommendation. It is important to realize this is a *general* guideline because all infants have different nursing styles. It may in fact be more appropriate to watch the *infant*—not the *clock*—in an effort to allow the infant to dictate when satiety is reached. The Teaching Tool box offers some suggestions to facilitate successful breastfeeding.

If a mother chooses not to breastfeed or if she has a medical condition contraindicating breastfeeding, a variety of formulas made from either cow's milk or soy are available. In addition, a number of specialty formulas, such as protein hydrolysate formulas, are available for infants with medical problems. The parents should consult their primary healthcare provider or nutrition care specialist to identify the most appropriate formula for their infant.

Formulas are either ready-to-feed, where no mixing is required, or are a powder or liquid concentrate to be mixed with water. To reduce the chance of lead leaching into water, tap water should be run for 2 minutes after it has been standing in the pipes and only cold water should be used for formula preparation. The formula should be mixed exactly as stated on the package, unless otherwise directed by a primary healthcare provider. Adding insufficient water can result in a high renal solute load, placing strain on the immature infant kidneys; overdiluting will precipitate undernutrition.

For parents or caregivers who may be non-English speaking or have low literacy skills, pictorial mixing instructions may be useful. Alternatively, asking the caregiver to demonstrate appropriate formula mixing may be suitable. Formula should never be heated in a microwave oven because microwaves heat food unevenly. Contents of a bottle appearing to be cool on testing may actually have portions that could scald an infant. All unused formula at the end of a feeding should be discarded if not used within 2 hours because of contamination by saliva enzymes and bacteria. Home-prepared formulas made from evaporated milk, popular in some cultures, are likely to be low in iron, vitamin C, and other essential nutrients and should be avoided.[57]

FORMULA PREPARATION

1. Clean all necessary equipment and wash hands before preparing formula.
2. Read formula label and dilute formula exactly as recommended by the manufacturer.
3. Use cold tap water for preparation of concentrated or powdered formula, unless directed otherwise by physician or nurse.
4. Never heat formula in a microwave oven.
5. Discard unused formula after 2 hours.

TEACHING TOOL
Guidelines for Successful Breastfeeding

Although breastfeeding is the most natural and easiest way to feed infants, mothers who decide to breastfeed will welcome the following suggestions:

- Offer both breasts at each nursing session.
- Open infant's mouth wide to latch on correctly.
- Place at least 1/2 inch to 3/4 inch of the areola in the infant's mouth, not just the nipple.
- Check that the infant's lips make a tight seal around the breast.
- Sore nipples are usually caused by incorrect positioning; position the infant correctly in a tummy-to-tummy fashion or in a "football hold." Support a newborn's head and back with extra pillows on the mother's lap or with the mother's arm cradling infant.
- Do not limit nursing time in the first several days. This does not prevent sore nipples and may hinder milk production.
- Remember: milk is produced by supply and demand—the more often the infant nurses, the more milk produced.
- Expect growth spurts at approximately 10 days, 2 weeks, 6 weeks, and 3 months. At these times, expect a fussy infant who wants to nurse frequently.
- Offer no bottles of formula or water while the milk supply is being established. The artificial nipple may confuse the infant, and substitute feedings that replace breast stimulation may diminish milk production.
- Learn your infant's cues for satiety.

Before 1 year of age, cow's milk, regardless of fat content or form (evaporated, liquid, or dried), should not be fed to infants. The fat in cow's milk is less digestible than the fat in breast milk or formula and contains less iron and more sodium and protein. These higher levels of solutes may lead to dehydration caused by increased urine volume to reduce solute levels in the body. Deficiencies of other nutrients, such as vitamin C, essential fatty acids, zinc, and possibly other trace minerals, develop because cow's milk is a poor source of these nutrients.

Cow's milk may be introduced after 1 year of age when at least two thirds of energy needs are fulfilled by foods other than milk. The delay in cow's milk consumption reduces the risk of developing a milk allergy. Reduced fat and nonfat milk is not recommended until age 2.

Introduction of Solid Foods.   Solid foods may be added to the infant's diet between the ages of 4 and 6 months. Infants who are introduced to solid foods before this time may be prone to excessive kcaloric intake, food allergies, and GI upset. Many parents and even some healthcare professionals believe offering an infant cereal in the evening will promote sleeping through the night. This belief, however, is not supported by research.

There are two basic issues when considering the introduction of solid foods to the infant's diet: (1) how to introduce them and (2) what to introduce.

How to Introduce Solid Foods.   Parents and other caregivers may be anxious to introduce foods other than breast milk or formula to their infant's diet. Health professionals can assure them that it's best for the infant to be developmentally ready for solid foods. The infant should be able to sit with some support; move the jaw, lips, and tongue independently; be able to roll the tongue to the back of the mouth to facilitate a food bolus entering the esophagus; and show interest in what the rest of the family is eating. For example, the infant may try to reach and grab an item off of a family member's plate at mealtime. Likewise, parents should become familiar with satiety cues so as not to overfeed the infant. To indicate fullness the infant may turn her head to the side, refuse to open her mouth, or grimace when the spoon comes close to her mouth. The caregiver should respect these cues. The infant should never be force-fed. If the infant is overtired or is not interested in food, she ought to be removed from the high chair and the foods offered again later.

When an infant reaches the age of 9 to 12 months, he may enjoy self-feeding. Although this may be a messy process, caregivers should encourage the development of these skills through food exploration.

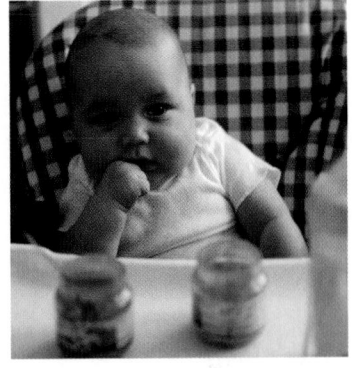

Solid foods should be introduced one at a time. (From PhotoDisc.)

Appropriate Solid Foods during the First Year of Life.   The second half of the first year of life should be thought of as a transitional period; breast milk or formula is still the primary food, and the solid foods are complementary.[48] Solid foods should be introduced gradually and one at a time with a 4- to 5-day interval between new foods. This timing is crucial because if the infant has any type of allergic reaction such as GI upset, upper respiratory distress, or skin reactions (e.g., eczema, hives), the offending food may be easily identified. Families with a documented history of allergies should delay introduction of solid foods until the infant is about 6 months old. If solid foods are introduced too early, the large protein molecules of the offending food may cross the intestinal barrier and elicit an immunologic response in the infant. As the gut matures, it is less likely to allow large unhydrolysed proteins to cross the mucosa.

Solid foods offered to the infant need not be commercial. Home-prepared foods are a good, practical alternative. There should be strict attention to sanitary food preparation procedures. Although infants should not be offered excessive sweets, naturally sweet fruits such as peaches offer them a taste satisfaction. Although salt should not be added to an infant's food, complete elimination of sodium from foods in the diet is neither practical nor recommended.[48]

A variety of textures, colors, and tastes is important for infants, whether they receive home prepared or commercial infant foods. General guidelines for infant feeding are listed in Table 11-5.

Table 11-5
Solid Foods during the First Year of Life

Age	Food	Foods to Avoid in the First Year of Life
4-5 months	Iron-fortified infant cereal	Honey (may cause infantile *Clostridium botulinum* poisoning); hot dogs, grapes, hard candies, raw carrots, popcorn, nuts, peanut butter (choking hazards); skim milk (insufficient calories); cow's milk (potential allergen, may replace breast milk or formula); egg whites (potential allergen)
5-6 months	Strained fruits and vegetables	
6-8 months	Mashed or chopped fruits and vegetables	
	Juice from a cup	
9-12 months	Crackers, toast, cottage cheese, plain meats, egg yolk, finger foods	

Beverages during the First Year of Life.   Fruit juice, particularly apple juice, is offered to many infants. Fruit juice can make an important contribution to the diet as a source of vitamin C, water, and possibly calcium. Its use, though, may need to be monitored. Excess fruit juice (greater than 12 fluid ounces per day) may lead to diarrhea from carbohydrate malabsorption, growth failure, or, in some children, obesity caused by excess calories.[58] All fruit juice given to infants (and children) should be pasteurized.

Baby Bottle Tooth Decay

Baby bottle tooth decay (BBTD), also known as *nursing bottle caries, nursing bottle mouth,* and *nursing bottle syndrome,* is a distinctive pattern of tooth decay in infants and young children. It most commonly affects the maxillary incisors, although other teeth may be affected as well. From 5% to 15% of all children may be affected, but precise prevalence figures are difficult to obtain.[59,60] For BBTD to develop, the mouth requires the presence of fermentable carbohydrate and a pathogenic organism.

BBTD commonly occurs in infants who are allowed to sleep with a bottle of milk, juice, or other sweetened liquid. As the infant falls asleep, the vigorous suck-swallow pattern that normally occurs during feeding diminishes. Moreover, saliva production decreases, resulting in a loss of saliva's buffering action in the mouth. Liquid pools in the infant's mouth, particularly behind the central incisors, becoming a ready source of fermentable carbohydrate for the bacteria colonizing the oral cavity. The acid produced by bacterial metabolism then destroys tooth enamel and initiates caries.

Prevention of BBTD is important for long-term dental health. Infants should never be put to bed with a bottle of milk, formula, juice, or other sweetened liquid. If a bottle is needed at bedtime, it should be plain water only. Oral hygiene may begin as soon as teeth erupt by a daily gentle cleaning of the tooth surfaces with gauze or a washcloth. Finally, sharing of food and utensils between adults and infants should be discouraged, and weaning from the bottle should occur as soon as the child can drink from a cup.

Special Nutritional Needs

The nutrition requirements of children with congenital or acquired health problems deserve special attention. These infants often have increased nutrient requirements, increased losses, or malabsorption. Significant drug-nutrient interaction often takes place as well. Although it is beyond the scope of this chapter to describe all of the children's special needs one might encounter in practice, a few of the major disorders are outlined. In all of these cases, a registered dietitian should be a part of the medical team.

The Premature and Low Birth Weight Infant

An infant is considered premature if he or she is born before 37 weeks' gestation. Low birth weight infants may be full term or premature but weigh 2500 grams or less at birth. As medical technology becomes increasingly sophisticated, infants are surviving at younger ages and lower weights. However, their developmental outlook may still be tenuous. Nutrition support of these infants plays a crucial role in successful long-term outcome. The major issues of concern in the premature infant are low birth weight, immature lung development, poor immune function, immature GI and neurologic function, insufficient production of digestive enzymes, inadequate bone mineralization, and minimal energy and mineral reserves.

Because the coordinated suck-swallow reflex is not fully developed until an infant reaches 34 weeks' gestation, initial feeding of the premature infant may need to be via total parenteral nutrition, tube feeding, or gavage feeding. Many criteria influence the route of nutrient delivery, and thus each infant should receive an individualized nutrition assessment by a registered dietitian who specializes in high-risk pediatrics.

Premature infants have increased needs for protein, kcalories, calcium, phosphorus, sodium, iron, zinc, vitamin E, and fluids. The best feeding choice for a premature infant is mother's milk with the addition of "human milk fortifier," which adds additional minerals and protein needed by the premature infant. Although the infant may not suckle well or may tire easily at the breast, the nurse can play a key role in helping the mother pump and store her milk in the neonatal nursery. The milk may then be given by gavage even when the mother is not present.[61] If the mother chooses not to breastfeed, a variety of specialized infant formulas are available to meet the special nutritional requirements of the infant.

Recent research suggests these formulas should be fortified with long chain fatty acids to mimic what would be delivered via the placenta. Long chain fatty acids are essential for proper retinal and neurologic development. Premature and low birth weight infants require continual nutrition follow-up after discharge for at least the first year of life because they are at risk for feeding problems, developmental delays, and growth retardation.

Cystic Fibrosis

Cystic fibrosis (CF) is an autosomal recessive disorder and is the most common genetic disorder among Caucasian populations, affecting roughly 1 in 2000 live births. Clinical features of the disease include chronic pulmonary disease, pancreatic exocrine insufficiency, and increased sweat chloride. The nutrition considerations facing children with CF include growth failure and energy and protein malnutrition. The chronic pulmonary dysfunction leads to malnutrition caused by an increased metabolic rate, increased energy requirement, and frequent use of antibiotics, which can cause anorexia. Steatorrhea, maldigestion, and malabsorption are common because of the lack of lipase secretion in the pancreas. Because of these increased needs as well as greater losses, patients are not always able to meet nutrition needs.

To prevent frank protein and energy malnutrition and resulting growth failure, the Consensus Committee of the Cystic Fibrosis Foundation recommends all CF patients receive a comprehensive nutrition assessment every 3 to 4 months. Care of the CF patient should be multidisciplinary, and each nutrition assessment plan should be individualized to promote optimal growth and development.[62] Further nutrition interventions are discussed in Chapter 18.

Failure to Thrive

Failure to thrive (FTT) is defined as a fall of two standard deviations in weight gain over an interval of 2 months or longer for infants less than 6 months of age or over an interval of 3 months or longer for infants greater than 6 months of age.[63] An alternative definition is a weight-for-length measurement less than the fifth percentile or weight for age below the third percentile.[64]

FTT may have organic causes such as an underlying metabolic disorder. Congenital heart disease or HIV infection may cause such an increased energy requirement that oral intake is not able to keep up with metabolic need.

Nonorganic FTT may be diagnosed when no medical reason for poor growth can be recognized. There may be psychosocial causes of the FTT such as inadequate maternal-infant bonding, poverty, child abuse, or neglect. Treatment for nonorganic FTT must include nutrition intervention to promote weight gain and therapy to correct developmental delays and any psychosocial problems in the home environment.[65]

Inborn Errors of Metabolism

Phenylketonuria.   All 50 states have newborn screening programs to detect PKU. When discovered early, dietary therapy can begin immediately and long-term prognosis is good. Without treatment, phenylalanine and its metabolites reach toxic levels in the blood, resulting in damage to the central nervous system including mental retardation. Likewise, because phenylalanine cannot be converted to tyrosine, low or absent tyrosine may contribute to the mental retardation.

Treatment consists of a low-phenylalanine diet to be followed throughout the individual's life. In infancy the use of a special formula such as Lofenalac is recommended. Partial breastfeeding is permitted, but phenylalanine levels in the infant's blood must be monitored carefully.[66] As PKU children are introduced to solid foods and make the transition to table foods, meals require careful planning. The use of low-protein breads and pastas is advised. This condition requires close monitoring of dietary intake by specialized dietitians.

galactosemia
an autosomal recessive disorder resulting in an inability to metabolize galactose and lactose milk products

Galactosemia.   Galactosemia is another rare, autosomal recessive disorder caused by an enzyme deficiency and is part of the newborn screening panel. Absence of the enzyme galactose 1-phosphate uridylyltransferase results in an inability to metabolize galactose. Because the milk sugar lactose is a disaccharide of glucose and galactose, these infants are unable to tolerate any milk products containing lactose. Manifestations include diarrhea, growth retardation, and mental retardation. Treatment is dietary therapy excluding all milk products, including human milk. Soy formulas and casein hydrolysate formulas are acceptable. Even with lifelong diet therapy, there may be long-term health consequences such as nervous system or ovarian dysfunction.[67] Specialized pediatric dietitians closely monitor the diet of infants and children who have this disorder.

Other inborn errors of metabolism requiring nutrition therapy include urea cycle disorders, maple syrup urine disease, and homocystinuria.

TOWARD A POSITIVE NUTRITION LIFESTYLE: REFRAMING

Reframing means to change the way a situation or concept is understood to a different frame that equally suits and explains the situation. Pregnancy and all of the recommendations in this chapter could be viewed as a worrisome burden to the expectant mother. Her body will swell in size, and others may tease her for the weight she gains. Based on what she hears about pregnancy, it sounds as if every action and every morsel of food consumed will affect the health of her unborn child. Anxiety replaces excitement over the beginning of a new life.

Reframing pregnancy can improve the well-being of the expectant mother physically and emotionally. Nurses can encourage mothers to view the weight gain of pregnancy as a natural feminine process enhancing fetal growth and development. Dietary and lifestyle suggestions can be presented as proactive behaviors to support the nutrient needs of the expectant mother and those of the fetus. A more positive frame of pregnancy provides a reassuring gestational period full of anticipatory excitement.

SUMMARY

From before conception and through infancy, health promotion concepts are intricate components of wellness. Good nutrition habits form a foundation for proper growth and development. The importance of nutrition during pregnancy, the benefits of breastfeeding, and the establishment and maintenance of positive eating styles during infancy are crucial to overall health goals. Nutrition services should play a role in all healthcare delivery systems, not only as a vehicle to prevent chronic disease but also as an important part of comprehensive healthcare for chronic disease such as DM, inborn errors of metabolism, and CF.

Women need to be knowledgeable of dietary patterns providing for nutritional requirements of pregnancy. They should understand the impact of smoking, drugs, and alcohol on the course of fetal development. Health professionals need to review risk factors and never assume the public is knowledgeable of these dangers. Women whose pregnancies are at high risk, such as those complicated by DM, should have early and regular nutrition services provided during routine prenatal care; specific education may be needed to sensitize them to their special medical and nutritional needs.

Lactation is a natural, physiologic process beginning shortly after delivery. It completes the cycle of the female body from pregnancy through motherhood. Human milk is the best health promoter for the neonate. The majority of women can successfully breastfeed when given proper instruction, support, and follow-up. The nursing professional is in a good position to provide such care. Breastfeeding should begin immediately after birth and continue every 2 to 3 hours during the initial weeks postpartum.

Lactating women should continue to consume a diet with adequate sources of protein, energy, vitamins, and minerals. Despite the desire of most women to return to their prepregnancy weight quickly, rapid weight loss should not be encouraged while breastfeeding.

Health promotion, attending to the needs of the total person, begins as soon as an infant is born. Sound nutrition practices during the first year of life lay the foundation for good health. The ideal food for the first 4 to 6 months of life is breast milk. Supplemental foods may be introduced one at a time at 4 to 6 months of age. Breast milk (or formula) should continue until the infant reaches 1 year of age. Children with medical problems may require specialized nutrition support.

THE NURSING APPROACH
Pregnancy Case Study

Helen, who is in her first trimester of pregnancy, and her husband are excited about having their first child. At her first prenatal visit with her obstetrician, as an obstetric nurse, you interview Helen to determine her health history. She begins to ask you many questions regarding what would be healthy for her to eat.

Continued

SPECIAL NEEDS POPULATIONS

Special considerations are needed for the following cases:

- Adolescents
- Vegetarians
- Women older than 35 years of age
- Women who are underweight
- Women who are overweight
- Women with phenylketonuria
- Women with multiple pregnancies
- Women who smoke or use drugs or alcohol
- Women with concurrent medical problems

THE NURSING APPROACH—cont'd
Pregnancy Case Study

ASSESSMENT

Subjective
- Nausea in the morning
- Fatigue
- Frequency of urination
- Patient states, "I feel hungry all the time now; I hope I eat enough to be healthy for my infant and me."

Objective
- Height: 5'6"
- Weight: 134 lbs.
- Vital signs: B/P: 100/76
                 Respirations: 16
                 Resting pulse: 68

NURSING DIAGNOSIS

Knowledge deficit regarding increased nutrition intake and concern about choosing appropriate foods

PLANNING

Goals
- Client will verbalize body requirements needed during pregnancy.
- Client will chose appropriate foods during her pregnancy.

IMPLEMENTATION

1. Assess a total nutrition history.
2. Teach and review the Food Guide Pyramid.
3. Assist and encourage her to make a daily food plan based on her family, financial, and cultural considerations.
4. Discuss special concerns for pregnant women, including the need for vitamin B_{12}, increased intake of calcium and vitamin D, and possible food sources for these nutrients.
5. Reinforce the importance of taking a daily prenatal vitamin/mineral supplement to ensure adequate iron and folic acid intake.

EVALUATION

The goals will be achieved as evidenced by the following:
- At the next prenatal visit, Helen will verbalize knowledge of protein and calcium sources and keep a weekly menu including three main meals and two snacks per day.

APPLYING CONTENT KNOWLEDGE

Elena, age 18, is a client at the city Special Supplemental Food Program for Women, Infants, and Children (WIC) program; she is beginning her third trimester of pregnancy. She attended nutrition education classes taught by the WIC nutritionist. The nutritionist, though, is concerned because Elena has not been gaining sufficient weight to support her pregnancy but is otherwise healthy. The nutritionist suspects that Elena does not understand the relationship between her dietary intake and the health of her fetus. The nutritionist asks you as a WIC nurse to reinforce these concepts when Elena comes in for her monthly checkups. What will you discuss with Elena?

Web Sites of Interest

BabyCenter

www.BabyCenter.com

This colorful Web site provides a full range of topics ranging from preconception through infancy and gives sound nutrition advice.

La Leche League

www.lalecheleague.org

The La Leche League is an international, nonprofit, nonsectarian organization that advocates breastfeeding through education, information, and support through publications, conferences, and local chapter meetings.

March of Dimes

www.modimes.org

This is the national site of March of Dimes, an organization devoted to safeguard the health of American children through the prevention of birth defects. It provides information and resources on all aspects of pregnancy, genetic disorders, and birth defects.

References

1. National Academy of Sciences: *Nutrition during pregnancy: weight gain and nutrient supplements*, Washington, DC, 1990, National Academy Press.
2. Van der Post JA et al.: Vasopressin and oxytocin levels during normal pregnancy: effects of chronic dietary sodium restriction, *J Endocrin* 152:345, 1997.
3. Lockitch G: Clinical biochemistry of pregnancy, *Crit Rev Clin Lab Sci* 34:67, 1997.
4. Guyer B et al.: Annual summary of vital statistics: trends in the health of Americans during 20th century, *Pediatr* 106(6):307, 2000.
5. Muscati SK, Gray-Donald K, Koski KG: Timing of weight gain during pregnancy: promoting fetal growth and minimizing maternal weight retention, *Int J Obstet Related Metab Disord* 20:526, 1996.
6. Lederman SA et al., Pregnancy-associated obesity in black women in New York City, *Matern Child Health J* 6(1):37, 2002.
7. Thorsdottir I et al.: Weight gain in women of normal weight before pregnancy: complications in pregnancy or delivery and birth outcomes, *Obstet Gynecol* 99(5):799, 2002.
8. Brown JE, Kahn ESB: Maternal nutrition and the outcome of pregnancy, *Clin Perinatol* 24:433, 1997.
9. Smith C: The effect of wartime starvation in Holland upon pregnancy and its product, *Am J Obstet Gynecol* 53:599, 1947.
10. Brown HL, Watkins K, Hiett AK: The impact of the Women, Infants, and Children Food Supplement Program on birth outcome, *Am J Obstet Gynecol* 174:1279, 1996.
11. Murphy SP, Abrams BF: Changes in energy intakes during pregnancy and lactation in a national sample of US women, *Am J Pub Health* 838:1161, 1993.
12. Rothman KJ et al.: Teratogenicity of high vitamin A intake, *N Engl J Med* 333:1369, 1995.
13. Williamson R: Prevention of birth defects: folic acid. *Biol Res Nurs* 3(1):33, 2001.
14. Food and Nutrition Board: *Dietary reference intakes for thiamin, riboflavin, niacin, vitamin B_6, folate, vitamin B_{12}, pantothenic acid, biotin, and choline*, Washington, DC, 1998, National Academy of Sciences.
15. Food and Nutrition Board: *Dietary reference intakes for calcium, phosphorus, magnesium, vitamin D, and fluoride*, Washington, DC, 1997, National Academy of Sciences.
16. Ritchie LD et al.: A longitudinal study of calcium homeostasis during human pregnancy and lactation and after resumption of menses, *Am J Clin Nutr* 67:693, 1998.
17. Hinds TS et al.: The effect of caffeine on pregnancy outcome variables, *Nutr Rev* 54:230, 1996.
18. Clausson B et al.: Effect of caffeine exposure during pregnancy on birth weight and gestational age, *Am J Epidemiol* 155(5):429, 2002.
19. MMWR: Alcohol use among women of childbearing age—US 1991-1999, *MMWR Morb Mortal Wkly Rep* 51(14):308, Apr 12, 2002.

20. Muscati SK, Koski KG, Gray-Donald: Increased energy intake in pregnant smokers does not prevent human fetal growth retardation, *J Nutr* 126:2984, 1996.

21. Sternfeld B: Physical activity and pregnancy outcomes: review and recommendations, *Sports Med* 23:33, 1997.

22. Clapp III JF et al.: The one-year morphometric and neurodevelopmental outcome of the offspring of women who continued to exercise regularly throughout pregnancy, *Am J Obstet Gynecol* 178:594, 1998.

23. Wergeland E, Strand K, Bordahl PE: Strenuous working conditions and birthweight, *Acta Obstetricia et Gynecologia Scand* 77:263, 1998.

24. Dubois S et al.: Ability of the Higgins Nutrition Intervention Program to improve adolescent pregnancy outcome, *J Am Dietetic Assoc* 97:871, 1997.

25. Pope JF, Skinner JD, Carruth BR: Adolescents' self-reported motivations for dietary changes during pregnancy, *J Nutr Ed* 29:137, 1997.

26. Ghidini A, Salafia CM, Pezzullo JC: Placental vascular lesions and likelihood of diagnosis of preeclampsia, *Obstet Gynecol* 90:542, 1997.

27. Williams MA et al.: Omega-3 fatty acid in maternal erythrocytes and risk of preeclampsia, *Epidem* 6:232, 1995.

28. Parazzini F et al.: Risk factors for pregnancy induced hypertension in women at high risk for the condition, Italian study of aspirin in pregnancy group, *Epidem* 7:306, 1996.

29. Oberhoffer R et al.: Cardiac and extracardiac complications in infants of diabetic mothers and their relation to parameters of carbohydrate metabolism, *Eur J Pediatr* 156:262, 1997.

30. Mironik M et al.: A class of diabetes in mother, glycemic control in early pregnancy and occurrence of congenital malformations in newborn infants, *Clin EXP Obstet Gynecol* 24:193, 1997.

31. Rudge MV et al.: Hypertensive disorders in pregnant women with diabetes, *Gynecol Obstet Invest* 44:11, 1997.

32. El-Sayed YY, Lyell DJ: New therapies for the pregnant patient with diabetes, *Diabetes Technol Ther* 3(4):635, 2001.

33. Reece EA, Homko CJ: Diabetes mellitus in pregnancy: what are the best treatment options? *Drug Safety* 18:209, 1998.

34. Bowes SB et al.: Measurement of glucose metabolism and insulin secretion during normal pregnancy and pregnancy complicated by gestational diabetes, *Diabetologia* 39:976, 1996.

35. Michals K et al.: Nutrition and reproductive outcome in maternal phenylketonuria, *Eur J Pediatr* 155(suppl):S165, 1996.

36. Anonymous: ACOG educational bulletin: human immunodeficiency virus infections in pregnancy, American College of Obstetricians and Gynecologists, *Intern J Gynecol Obstet* 57:73, 1997.

37. Davis SF et al.: Prevalence and incidence of vertically acquired HIV infection in the United States, *J Am Med Assoc* 274:952, 1995.

38. Work group on breastfeeding, American Academy of Pediatrics: Breastfeeding and the use of human milk, *Breastfeed Rev* 6(1):31, 1998.

39. Visness CM, Kennedy KI: Maternal employment and breastfeeding, *Am J Pub Health* 87:945, 1997.

40. Position of the American Dietetic Association: breaking the barriers to breastfeeding, *J Am Diet Assoc* 101(10):1213, 2001.

41. Ebrahim GJ: The baby friendly hospital initiative, *J Trop Pediatr* 39:2, 1993

42. Blaumslag N: Breastfeeding: cultural practices and variations. In Hamosh M, Goldman AS, eds.: *Human lactation 2: maternal and environmental factors*, ed 9, New York, 1986, Plenum Press.

43. Dewey KG: Effects of maternal caloric restriction and exercise during lactation, *J Nutr* 128(2 Suppl):386S, 1998.

44. Bailey B, Ito S: Breastfeeding and maternal drug use, *Pediatr Clin N Am* 44:41, 1997.

45. Public Health Service Task Force: Recommendations for the use of antiretroviral drugs in pregnant women infected with HIV-1 for maternal health and for reducing perinatal HIV-1 transmission in the United States, *MMWR* 1998; 47(No. RR-2); www.cdc.gov/mmwr/preview/mmwrhtml/00053202.htm

46. World Health Organization: *WHO Statement: Effect of breastfeeding on mortality among HIV-infected women*, June 7, 2001; www.who.int/child-adolescent-health/New_Publications.

47. Ni Yh et al.: Evolution of hepatitis C virus quasispecies in mothers and infants infected through mother-to-infant transmission, *J Hepatol* 26:967, 1997.

48. Glinsman WH, Bartholmey SJ, Coletta F: Dietary guidelines for infants: a timely reminder, *Nutr Rev* 54:50, 1996.

49. National Academy of Sciences: *From death to birth,* Washington DC, 1998, National Academy Press.

50. Gibson RA, Makrides M: Long-chain polyunsaturated fatty acids in breastmilk: are they essential? *Adv Exp Med Biol* 501:375, 2001.

51. Avestad N et al.: Growth and development in term infants fed long-chain polyunsaturated fatty acids, *Pediatrics* 108(2):372, 2001.

52. Binet A, Kooh SW: Persistence of vitamin D-deficiency rickets in Toronto in the 1990s, *Can J Pub Health* 88:10, 1996.

53. Eugster EA, Sane KS, Brown DM: Minnesota rickets: need for a policy change to support vitamin D supplementation, *Minn Med* 79:29, 1996.

54. Carvalho NF et al.: Severe nutritional deficiencies in toddlers resulting from health food milk alternatives, *Pediatrics* 107(4):E46, 2001.

55. Kuman JV, Green EL: Recommendations for fluoride use in children: a review, *NY St Dental J* 64:40, 1998.

56. Riordan PJ: The place of fluoride supplements in caries prevention today, *Austral Dental J* 41:335, 1996.

57. Lo CW, Kleinman RE: Infant formula, past, present and future: opportunities for improvement, *Am J Clin Nutr* 63:646S, 1996.

58. American Academy of Pediatrics: The use and misue of fruit juice in pediatrics, *Pediatrics* 107(5):1210, 2001.

59. Mohan A et al.: The relationship between bottle usage/content, age and number of teeth with mutans streptococci colonization in 6-24 month old children, *Commun Dent Oral Epidemiol* 26:12, 1998.

60. Hicks TW et al.: Infant feeding caries, part II: the simcoe and muskoka-parry sound health unit project, *Ontario Dentist* 72:24, 33, 1995.

61. Tudehope DI, Steer PA: Which milk for the preterm infant? *J Paediatrics Child Health* 32:275, 1996.

62. Creveling S et al.: Cystic fibrosis and the health care team, *J Am Dietetic Assoc* 97:S186, 1997.

63. Wright C et al.: New chart to evaluate weight faltering, *Arch Dis Childhood* 78:40, 1998.

64. Batchelor JA: Has recognition of failure to thrive changed? *Child: Care, Health and Development* 22:235, 1996.

65. Moores J: Non-organic failure to thrive—dietetic practice in a community setting, *Child: Care, Health and Development* 22:251, 1996.

66. Duncan LL, Elder SB: Breastfeeding the infant with PKU, *J Hum Lactat* 13:231, 1997.

67. Widhalm K, Miranda da Cruz BD, Koch M: Diet does not ensure normal development in galactosemia, *J Am Coll Nutr* 16:204, 1997.

CHAPTER 12

Life Span Health Promotion: Childhood and Adolescence

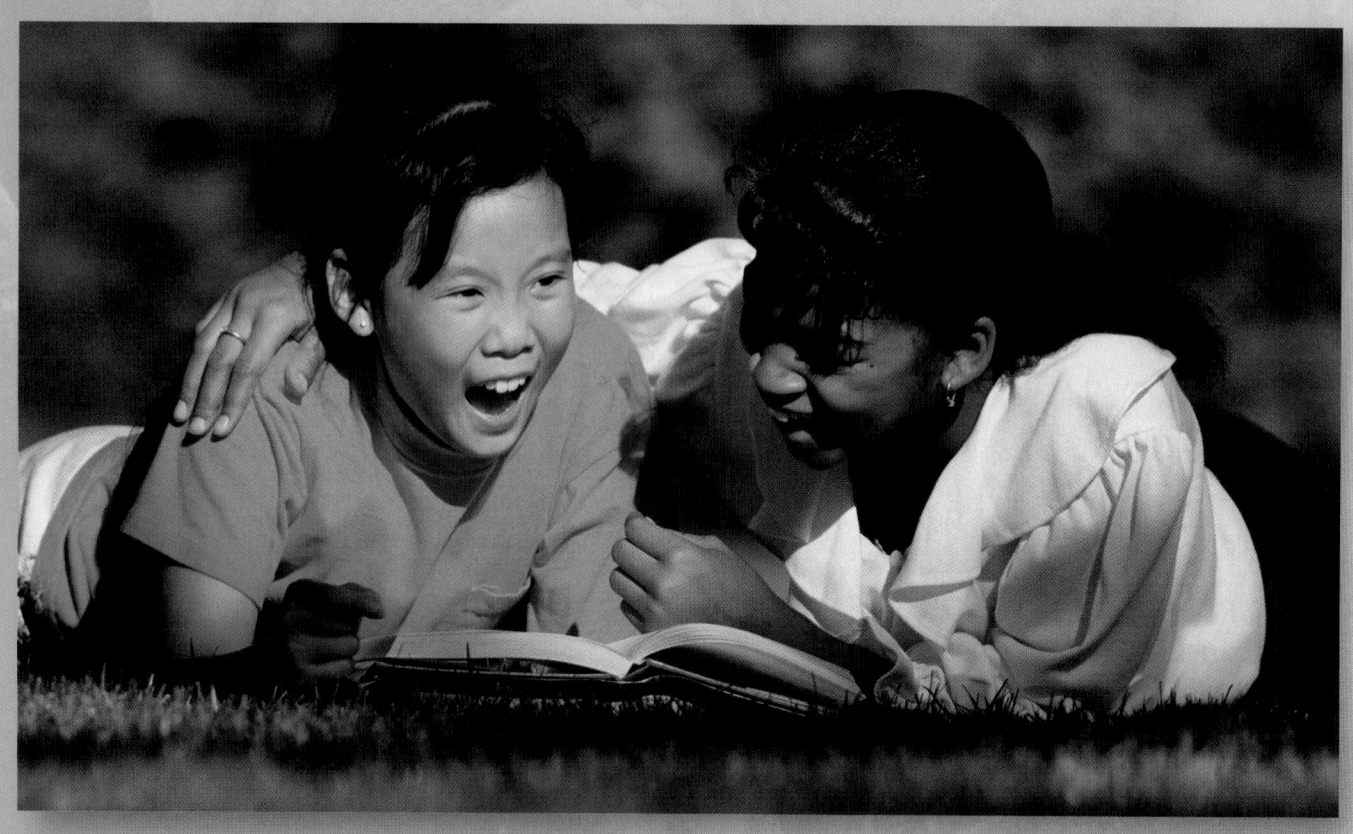

Once we pass the specific nutrition and health necessities of pregnancy and infancy, the rest of the life span categories share more similarities than differences regarding nutrient intake and dietary patterns.

This chapter continues the exploration of the life span categories of childhood and adolescence. Once we pass the specific nutrition and health necessities of pregnancy and infancy, the rest of the life span categories share more similarities than differences regarding nutrient intake and dietary patterns. In striving to increase the level of health of individuals, families, and communities, the degree of knowledge appropriate at each stage varies and the techniques reflect these limitations. Community supports reveal the commitment of the society regarding health issues.

ROLE IN WELLNESS

The nutrient requirements of humans are basically the same throughout the life span. What differs, depending on age, are the amount of nutrients required and frequency of food consumption (dietary patterns) recommended; these differences are caused by physiologic and psychosocial needs. For example, consider the amount of food individuals are able to consume at one time. Toddlers can eat only small amounts at one time. They depend on planned snacks to provide their full assortment of nutrients. Adolescents, however, can eat large quantities but also need time throughout the day to eat. In contrast, older adults still have high nutrient needs but require less energy and therefore need more nutrient-dense foods.

The five dimensions of health also apply to the nutrition needs of children and adolescents. Knowledge of the relationship between adequate nutrient intake and good health empowers children to practice health-promoting behaviors that enhance physical health. Children can use their intellectual skills to make decisions about their food choices. Caregivers should provide guidance for children to use food for nourishment and enjoyment, not as a means of emotional comfort. The social dimension of health is strengthened by including children in the preparation of food, which teaches children the social skills of cooperation. The spiritual dimension is developed by sharing meals with others as a form of communication and bonding.

LIFE SPAN HEALTH PROMOTION

Stages of Development

The life span stages reflect psychologic and physiologic maturation. Approaches to health promotion take into account these stages and their impact on nutrient requirements, eating styles, and food choices.

Childhood (1 to 12 Years)

The accelerated growth of infancy slows down by about age 1, marking the transition to childhood. Growth then occurs unevenly until puberty heralds the onset of adolescence. This growth deceleration during childhood results in varying hunger levels that reflect physiologic need. Awareness of these fluctuations by parents and caregivers allows children to stay in tune with their internal hunger cues.

Nurses sensitive to normal growth patterns as affected by genetics and environmental influences can assist families to understand the growth curves of their children. Height, weight, and head circumferences are used with the standard growth charts from the National Center for Health Statistics to monitor growth (www.cdc.gov/growthcharts). See Chapter 14 for a detailed description of clinical nutrition assessment procedures.

Childhood categories are based on a combination of psychosocial and physiologic developmental stages. Physiologic requirements are the basis of the age and gender divisions of the Dietary Reference Intakes (DRIs). This discussion highlights the nutrients of concern-protein, iron, calcium, and zinc. For other specific age-related nutrient recommendations, refer to the DRI tables inside the front cover.

feeding relationship
the interactions or patterns of behaviors that surround food preparation and consumption within a family

Children depend on adults for the provision of food. A discussion of the nutrient needs of the growing body is not complete without a discussion of the role of adults in nourishing children. Children are influenced by adults and model the behaviors of adults. Adults control all the quantity and quality of foods prepared and the environment within which foods are presented for consumption. The children themselves, however, control the actual amount consumed.

Ellen Satter, a registered dietitian and therapist, describes the feeding relationship as the interactions or patterns of behaviors that surround food preparation and consumption within a family. This description reveals the contextual nature of food preparation and consumption. Her advice to parents and caregivers is about "the division of responsibility. You are responsible for what your child is offered to eat, but he is responsible for how much of it he eats and even whether he eats."[1]

Adults are responsible for not only what meals are offered but also *when* meals are offered. Regularity of mealtimes at home-breakfast and dinner-helps support success at school. Breakfast supplies energy in the morning for school learning (see the Teaching Tool box, "What's the Best Breakfast?"); dinner supports the ability to complete homework, study, and relax before bedtime. Most children eat lunch away from home and either bring a prepared lunch from home or purchase meals through a school lunch program (school lunches are discussed later in "Community Supports page 349").

Snacks boost daily nutrient intake; for children whose energy and general dietary intake are adequate, snacks may sometimes include sweets such as cookies and even an occasional candy bar. A common myth is that sugar makes children hyperactive, yet studies have shown no convincing evidence that consumption of sugar causes attention-deficit hyperactivity disorder.[2] High-sugar-containing foods, however, can displace more nutritious foods and contribute to nutrient deficiencies. No food should be forbidden; frequency and quantity are the guides.

Children too young for school may attend day care programs if their parents work. The impact on their nutrition may be positive or negative depending on the quality and attitude of the programs toward nutrition and meal times. Most young children, regardless of parental employment, attend some form of preschool; for

TEACHING TOOL
What's the Best Breakfast?

Foods considered best for breakfast have changed. Although traditional breakfasts consist of eggs, bacon, white toast, and whole milk, this combination is now recognized as being too high in fat and protein. In addition, in the rush of morning preparation, few of us have the time to prepare this type of meal. Nonetheless, breakfast, which breaks our fast, is an important contributor of nutrients and energy.

As we teach clients and their families about nutrition and optimum dietary intake patterns, we can assure them that breakfast can be simple, yet still provide appropriate levels of nutrients. Here are some ideas for parents to use to ignite their children's breakfast appetites:

- For children (and adults) who eat and run, have quick foods available such as fruit, granola bars, muffins, and raisins.
- For older children, offer to prepare a simple breakfast. Although they are able to prepare their own meal, the extra nurturing and time saved will be appreciated.
- For creating appetites, toast bread while family members are dressing. The enticing scent will spark their taste buds.
- For picky eaters, create small smorgasbord plates with several choices such as a small container of yogurt, crackers with cheese, and some pear slices.
- Many of the healthy snacks listed in Box 12-1 can alternate as breakfast foods for everyone.
- Be a role model by also eating breakfast yourself.

many, the food and social experiences broaden acceptance to a variety of foods and eating styles.

Although adults may have predominant influence over the eating behaviors of children, another primary influence for some children is television. The influence of TV commercials has been studied extensively and is most often condemned as negatively influencing children's food choices. In addition, watching television when eating family meals appears to impact the types of foods served, which results in consumption of foods higher in fat and lower in fiber. This possibly reflects the categories of foods most often advertised on television.[3] Parents and caregivers can watch television with their children to assess the type of products advertised and then discuss their nutritional value. As more healthful products are marketed, even if targeted at adults, acceptance by children may increase. Occasional treats of advertised products may lessen their appeal if children are accustomed to high-quality snacks and meals.

The recommendations given by the *Dietary Guidelines for Americans* (see Figure 2-1) are considered appropriate for ages 1 through 10, particularly in regard to fat intake; 30% kcal from fat or less is the general goal for the population at large. A level of about 30% may also assist with obesity prevention and emphasize fruits, vegetables, and complex carbohydrates. It is easier to enjoy whole foods that are naturally low in fat throughout childhood than to convert one's eating style as an adult. The American Heart Association, the American Health Foundation, and the National Institutes of Health Consensus Development Panel recommend application of the 30% goal to the age group from years 1 to 2 and older. The Committee on Nutrition of the American Academy of Pediatrics, however, has expressed concern that 30% or less of kcalories from dietary fat would overly increase the intake of bulky plant foods, possibly precluding consumption of enough nutrients by young children. Consequently, the Committee accepts a 30% to 40% dietary fat intake for age 2 and older.[4] Levels higher than the 30% to 40% recommendation may actually cause fat to crowd out other nutrients.

Despite national dietary recommendations, the U.S. Department of Agriculture's Continuing Surveys of Food Intakes by Individuals (1989-1991) reveals that for children ages 2 to 11, the average number of servings per day was below the minimum recommendations for all food groups except for the dairy group. Roughly 16% did not meet any food group recommendations, whereas only 1% consumed recommended amounts for all food groups. Those who did meet dietary recommendations had intakes that were high in fat.[5] These findings indicate that nutrition education is still needed for parents and their children. (The Cultural Considerations box offers suggestions for educating foreign-born parents about their child's health.)

CULTURAL CONSIDERATIONS
Child Health Education for Foreign-Born Parents

Providing child health education for foreign-born parents presents special concerns related to language and culture. An innovative, culturally relevant approach should be used to present basic child health information in English, with translators present as facilitators. Foreign-born parents who need a partial or complete language interpretation then have readily available access to translation support. Parents can ask questions, provide comments and suggestions, and evaluate the presentation through the translator. Because participants can be grouped with an appropriate translator, each presentation can accommodate more than one language.

The presentation, conducted in English, is paced to allow for discussions. Childcare is provided in a nearby setting. This allows parents to focus on the presentation without the concern of childcare. Vocabulary relative to healthcare is developed from English into the parents' primary language with the support of the translator.

Application to nursing: This is an example of one cultural-specific strategy used to meet minority and ethnic health needs. Nurses are also encouraged to provide translated health education materials for the populations whom they teach.

Reference: Baker R: Child health education for the foreign-born parent, Issues Comp Ped Nurs 24:45, 2001.

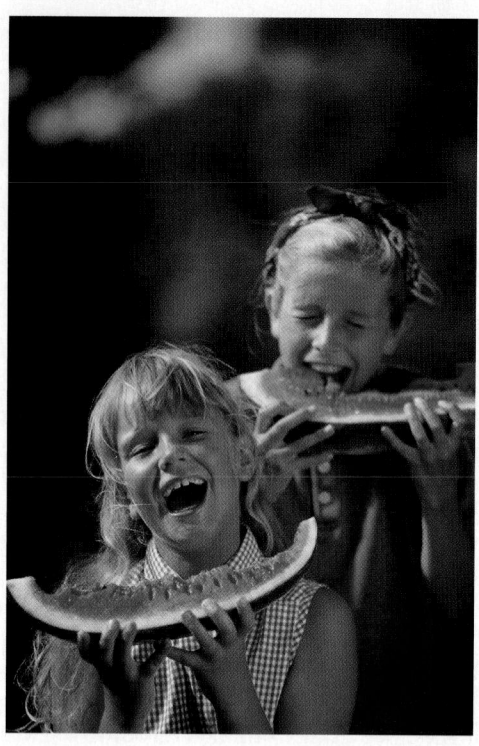

Making low-fat foods a habit throughout childhood is easier than trying to change one's eating style as an adult. (From PhotoDisc.)

Health professionals need to use careful wording when discussing nutrient restriction or reduction for children. Several infants have developed failure to thrive, not because of neglect or lack of food, but because of parental overzealousness about fat, both dietary and body.[6]

Stage I: Children 1 to 3 Years Old

Usually referred to as *"toddlerhood,"* the age span of 1 to 3 years old is a busy time for young children. They are dealing with issues of autonomy. Often food and eating create an arena for asserting newly discovered independence. The eating relationship between parent (or caregiver) and child is forming, and adult reaction to autonomy sets the stage for future encounters.[1] Consistency of mealtimes is important. Meals are best accepted when hunger, tiredness, and emotions are still controllable; an overly tired child just cannot eat. Equally important is fostering self-reliance by allowing young children to feed themselves in a manner most appropriate for their psychomotor abilities. Regardless of the messy results, attempts to self-feed provide the roots of self-empowerment crucial to overall physical and psychologic development (Figure 12-1).

Hunger, rather than adult meal schedules, guides the child's perception of time to eat. Meals for toddlers are based on the same design and food selections as adults, only in smaller portions. (Of course, overly spicy foods may not be acceptable to young taste buds.) Snacks are a necessity in addition to meals. Toddlers are able to eat only small amounts at each meal or food encounter. Planned snacks provide required additional nourishment between meals to ensure an adequate dietary intake.

Nutrition Requirements.   Growth, basal metabolic rate (BMR), and endless activity require an energy supply of 1300 kcal/day for ages 1 to 3. Protein needs increase to 16 grams to meet the demands of growing muscles. For ages 1 through 6, a general guideline is one fruit or vegetable serving equals one level-measuring

Young children should not be pushed to "clean their plate" at mealtime if they seem finished eating so as to not override natural feelings of satiety.

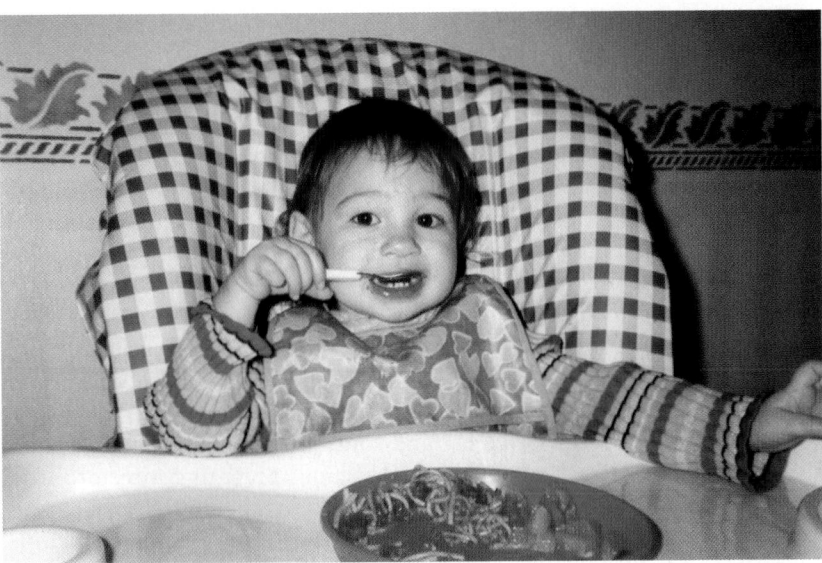

Figure 12-1 Allowing toddlers to feed themselves promotes physical and psychologic development.

tablespoon of fruit or vegetable per year of age. A serving of bread or cereal is equal to about one fourth of an adult's serving. Up to age 3, children should consume two to three 8-oz cups of milk per day or about 16 to 24 oz per day, and meats or meat substitutes can be offered at least twice per day.[4] Caregivers should be advised that alternative milk products such as rice milk and soy milk may not provide the same quality of nutrients as animal-derived foods.

This age span of 1 to 3 years old is the time to begin introducing lower-fat versions of commonly eaten foods. As previously mentioned, fat-containing foods should not be obsessively restricted; however, high-fat foods are often filling and may displace other nutrient-containing foods.

This is also a prime time to introduce toddlers to a variety of foods. Toddlers imitate the adults around them. Therefore adults can model behavior by eating a variety of foods themselves. Clever introductions to foods are always helpful to catch the attention and appetite of toddlers. Broccoli is not just a vegetable; cut up, it looks like little trees. Peas steamed in their pods are not just peas but green pearls waiting to be discovered.

Although breast milk or formula is the milk of choice until age 1, toddlers should drink breast milk, whole milk, or formula until age 2, after which low fat or skim milk is best. Sometimes toddlers consume too much milk or juice, particularly if they are given an unlimited number of servings. Perhaps drinking from feeding bottles throughout the day simply becomes a habit. Unfortunately, the child fills up on milk or juice, both low sources of iron, and then does not have an appetite for iron-containing foods such as meat, fish, poultry, eggs, or legumes. Iron deficiency anemia may develop. Additionally, apple juice is sweet tasting and has few nutrients beyond carbohydrate kcalories. Frequent consumption may habituate young children to sweet drinks. Later, apple juice may be replaced with sugar-laden sodas, which displace more nutrient-dense beverages. One possible solution is to dilute juices with water. Milk can be served with meals and diluted juices drunk between meals. Parents and caregivers can view bottles as cups or glassware. Few of us drink from a cup continuously while watching television, reading, or playing games. Similarly, once past infancy, young children's use of feeding bottles should be viewed as beverages, with the use of cups encouraged.

Stage II: Children 4 to 6 Years Old

The stage of 4 to 6 years old is characterized by independent eating styles, although modeling of adults still occurs. Children of this age clearly understand the time frame of meals and can save their appetite for meals. Snacks are still an integral part of the child's nutrient intake. Far from the messy eating styles of toddlers, these children accept foods more easily if presented separately, not mixed in a casserole style. Variations of hunger and appetite levels may confuse parents and caregivers. The most practical approach is to be respectful of these variations of hunger; this diffuses power plays over food consumption.

New foods can continue to be introduced. For some families, back-up meal plans can encourage trying new foods. For instance, if a child does not accept a new dish after a reasonable attempt, the child may be allowed to prepare a meal of a peanut butter sandwich or cereal and fruit. By establishing back-up meals in advance, parents avoid becoming short-order cooks preparing three or more individualized meals for dinner.

Another approach is to have at least one meal (eaten at home) include new foods along with favorite foods. When the child looks at his or her plate, he or she recognizes some familiar foods in addition to the new foods. A meal can consist of a sampling of food items; several will probably be acceptable.

At this stage children can develop a sense of responsibility for healthful food selections. They can understand that although all foods are okay, some foods such as fruits, vegetables, and low-fat foods can be eaten more often than others. After participating in a 3-month nutrition education demonstration project to decrease cholesterol and cardiovascular risk, some of the children ages 4 to 10 reduced their caloric intake of fat by about 9 percent by replacing higher fat food with lower fat foods within the same food group. These same children also increased their overall intake of fruits, vegetables, and very-low-fat desserts. Their total calorie and nutrient intake remained appropriate.[7]

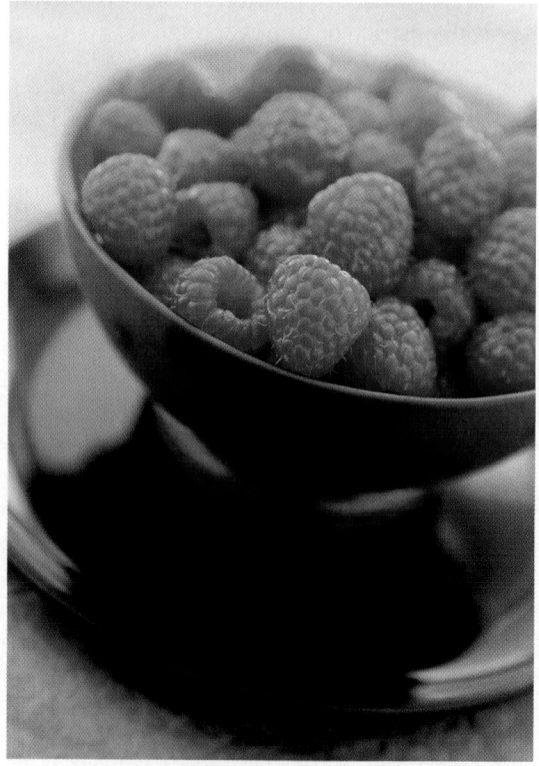

Snacks can play an important role in nutrition. (From PhotoDisc.)

Sometimes children develop food jags, wanting to eat only a narrow range of foods. Parents and teachers can educate the child that each food contains a different assortment of nutrients and offer substitute choices that contain additional nutrients, with the child making the final selections. Eventually food jags diminish and the child consumes a broader selection of foods.

Nutrition Requirements.   Energy requirements jump to 1800 kcal/day at 4 to 6 years of age, reflecting continued growth and activity levels. Protein needs increase to 24 grams.

Stage III: Children 7 to 12 Years Old

The years from 7 to 12 are tumultuous. Although actual growth may slow down, the body is preparing and seemingly storing up for the puberty growth spurt. Puberty may begin for girls from around age 9 and on; boys may reach puberty in the early teen years. This prepuberty time may be reflected by weight buildup; an increase in chubbiness is not alarming if moderate eating and physical activities are maintained. Adults must be careful not to overreact or they may plant the seeds of eating disorders. To rule out overeating, children can be asked if they are really hungry for food or if they are just tired or thirsty. These are different sensations. A child can be reminded to "stop eating when you are full." If hunger returns, a snack can be provided. By taking time to consider these sensations, children can stay in touch with internal cues of true hunger.

Exposure to other dietary patterns takes place as children spend more time away from home at school and socializing with friends. Peer influence at school lunchtime increases; having the right kind of lunch may be as important as wearing the right kind of clothes. Adults need to be sensitive to these issues. As long as a basic lunch of some protein, complex carbohydrates, and a beverage (preferably milk, juice, or water) is consumed, missing nutrients can be adjusted for later in the day, especially through after-school snacks.

It is at this age, when midmorning school snacks disappear and school lunch scheduling has more to do with numbers of students than with actual lunchtime appetites, that after-school hunger may intensify. This is the time to provide healthful snacks or at least stock the kitchen shelves with an assortment of nutrient-dense treats (Box 12-1). If children purchase snacks away from home, adults can develop guidelines with children this age to maintain positive eating styles.

Nutrition Requirements.   Energy needs for 7 to 12 year olds increase to 2000 to 2200 kcal/day. Protein requirements rise to between 28 grams to 46 grams depending on sexual maturity. Sexual maturity leads to an increase of lean body mass, particularly for boys. Lean body mass requires more dietary protein for growth and maintenance.

DRI = Dietary Reference Intakes

RDA = Recommended Dietary Allowance

AI = Adequate Intake

UL = Tolerable Upper Intake Level

Box 12-1   Healthy Snacks

- Ready-to-eat cereals: reserve presweetened cereals as special snack treats or mix a sweet cereal with a less sweet cereal–the best of both worlds
- Snack smorgasbord: cut-up apples and oranges, popcorn, cheese, crackers, and cookies
- Fruit juice packs
- Low-fat chocolate milk packs
- Open-face peanut butter sandwich (child-made) with cut fruit, jelly, coconut, and raisins
- Fresh or canned fruit (in fruit juice) with cottage cheese (in 4-oz sizes)
- English muffins (oat bran, raisin, and whole wheat)
- Healthier Danish: a slice of toasted bread reheated with low-fat ricotta cheese and preserves
- Bagels with a spread of whipped cream, margarine/butter, or peanut butter; freeze a variety of bagels
- Smoothies or fruit shakes made with skim milk or fruit juice, plain or fruit-flavored yogurt, fresh or frozen fruit–just mix in a blender
- Leftovers from lunch or dinner; a bowl of soup with bread for dipping instead of a prepackaged snack

Mineral needs increase as well. Because of increased bone growth and mineralization, calcium Adequate Intake (AI) recommendations jump from 800 mg/day at age 8 to 1300 mg/day throughout adolescence. Iron and zinc allowances increase as well. Well-chosen dietary intakes will provide sufficient amounts of these nutrients. Marginal intakes of zinc have been noted among school children who are finicky eaters; low zinc intakes can affect growth rates.[8]

Childhood Health Promotion (1 to 12 Years)

Knowledge

The growth cycle of this age span is important for parents and children to understand. Attention to issues related to weight, appropriate appetite, and meal patterning are crucial for the development of positive eating relationships and may prevent the development of eating disorders in the future. By understanding the relationship of nutrients and kcalories to their growth needs, children possess sufficient information to take responsibility for certain aspects of their food choices and dietary patterns. Children with special needs who are challenged by physical and/or mental limitations may require additional support to achieve nutritional adequacy (Box 12-2). Ultimately, however, adults must provide nourishment for children and guidance as to positive health behaviors.

Techniques

Use of the Food Guide Pyramid to visualize and comprehend the variety and number of servings of foods that constitute a balanced nutrient intake works for both parents and children. A Food Guide Pyramid for Young Children ages 2 to 6 is now available (Figure 12-2). The "5 A Day" approach to consume at least five

---

Box 12-2   Nutrition Needs of Children with Special Needs

*A*lthough the basic nutrition needs of all children are the same, some children may be challenged by the limitations of physical and mental differences and the physical and pharmacologic consequences of chronic disease treatment. The ability to self-feed may be highly related to life expectancy. Enhancing feeding skills to the greatest extent possible is an involved procedure. Nutrition education has valuable skills and experiences to offer. Keep the following issues in mind:

- All children can enjoy working together to prepare foods. The process of measuring, mixing, arranging, and *eating* food that they helped to prepare enhances self-esteem and provides the acquisition of other skill competencies such as math, science, and interpersonal skills of cooperation.
- Positioning of children with physical handicaps may require adaptive equipment and alternative eating strategies for special conditions. Oral stimulation before eating may be required for children with low muscle tone and certain textures of foods may be better received than others. If chewing and swallowing are problematic, textures of foods may need adjustment.

- Low muscle tone may also affect functioning of the large intestine and require adequate fiber and water to reduce the risk of constipation.
- Medications may increase or decrease appetite. Caregivers and teachers should be aware of these effects and time meals and snacks to be offered when hunger is the strongest.
- Children with sensory integration difficulties may be sensitive to textures, temperature, and even colors of foods. Accommodate preferences when possible to ensure adequate nutrition and to provide the children a sense of control over food choices.
- Children experiencing growth retardation or malnutrition should be reassessed by a registered dietitian to determine if alternative feeding strategies can improve the child's nutritional status. Parents should regularly receive assessments of nutritional status to fully understand their children's conditions.
- Periodic nutritional assessments of children with special needs should be conducted by registered dietitians who have the expertise to evaluate nutritional status and offer practical strategies for everyday eating situations.

From Fung EB et al.: Feeding dysfunction is associated with poor growth and health status in children with cerebral palsy, J Am Dietetic Assoc 102(3):361, 373, 2002; and correspondence on Society for Nutrition Education (SNE) list/serv February 19, 1998, from Susan Piscopo, Associate Professor, University of Malta; Sharon Davis, Education Director, Home Baking Association; Collette Janson-Sand, Associate Professor, University of New Hampshire, and others.

fruits and vegetables a day is also ideal for use by children. For young children, however, the five servings would be of smaller sizes.

Community Supports

Community supports for children are currently divided into two categories based on location and services or education offered: (1) school-food service and (2) classroom nutrition education.

School-Food Service.   The National School Lunch Program (NSLP) was established to protect the health and wellness of American children. Formalized in 1946, the program provides lunches at varying costs, depending on family income, to all school children at public and nonprofit private schools and residential child

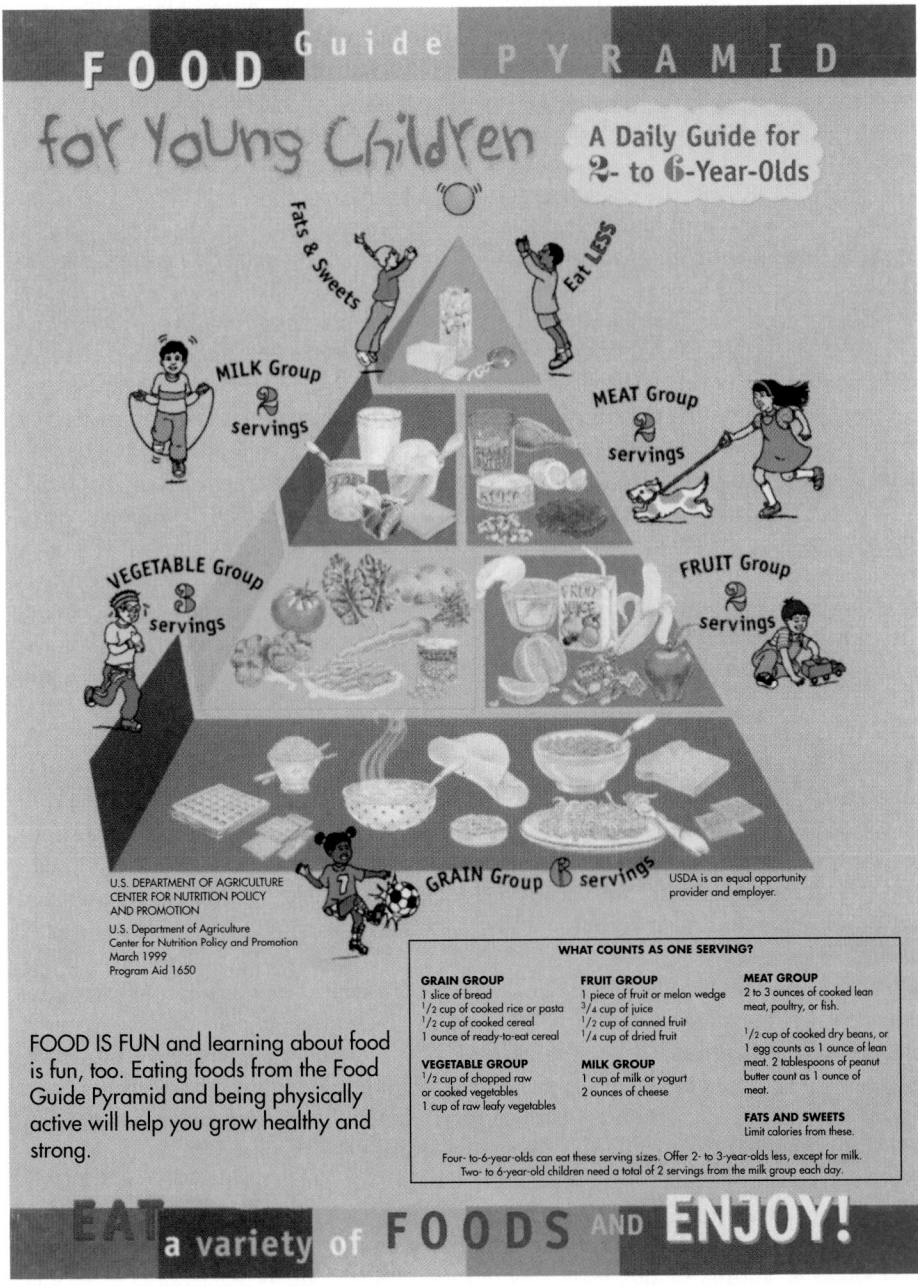

Figure 12-2 Food Guide Pyramid for Young Children: A daily guide for 2- to 6-year-olds. (From US Department of Agriculture, Center for Nutrition Policy and Promotion, March 1999, Program Aid 1650.)

care institutions. At the federal level the program is administered by the Food and Nutrition Service (FNS) of the U.S. Department of Agriculture (USDA), at the state level by various agencies, and locally by school boards. As an entitlement program, the NSLP provides funds to all schools that apply and meet the criteria of eligibility. Currently, more than 95,000 schools participate in this program.[9]

Reduced-price meals are offered to children whose household income is below 185% of the federal poverty level; free meals are available to those falling below 130% of poverty. During the 1999-2000 school year, NSLP served meals daily to 26.8 million children. About 60% of these children received free or reduced-price lunches daily.[9]

Specific nutrient guidelines regulate the meals served through this program. At times the definition of these guidelines has been controversial because of their nutritional impact on children and their economic impact on the farmers and food producers supplying the food. Some foods are available at reduced cost because of federal surplus commodities programs. Although wholesome, these may contain higher fat contents than would otherwise be used in the preparation of school lunches. Fresh fruits and vegetables may be passed over for canned fruits and vegetables that are not as acceptable to children and at times not as nutritious. Whole milk, cheeses, and high-fat meats may be served more often because of economics, despite the health objectives of consuming lower-fat foods. Meals served may not meet the lower fat and higher fruits and vegetable consumption recommendations of the *Dietary Guidelines for Americans*. Consequently, a *Healthy People 2010* objective addresses this concern:

> *Increase the proportion of children and adolescents 6-19 years of age whose intake of meals and snacks at school contributes to good overall dietary quality.*[10]

Basically, lunch must provide approximately one third of the Recommended Dietary Allowance (RDA) and include the four food groups: dairy, protein, vegetables and/or fruits, and grains, bread, or pasta. For low-income children participating in the program, this provides one third to one half of their daily intake.[9]

The School Breakfast Program was created in 1966 to support schools by providing morning meals in areas where children ride buses to school and/or most mothers are in the workforce, particularly in economically disadvantaged areas. The program has reduced tardiness and decreased absenteeism. It is administered through the same governmental offices as the School Lunch Program and is also an entitlement program. During the 1999-2000 school year, 71,180 schools participated in the School Breakfast Program, serving 7.6 million children. More than 80% of the participants qualify for free or reduced-priced meals. More than 42% of the children from low-income families receive both school lunch and school breakfast.[9]

An assortment of foods can comprise breakfast, but the program requires milk (either as a beverage or with cereal), a serving of fruit (either whole or as juice), and two servings of a bread/cereal product or meat/meat alternative or a combination of bread and meat servings. The breakfast is designed to provide one fourth of the DRI.

During summer, the Summer Food Service Program for Children (SFSP) functions through a range of eligible organizations including schools, summer camps, and community agencies as well as various federal, state, and local government departments. The purpose is to serve meals to school-age children when schools are not in session in communities where children depend on school meals as an essential component of their daily nourishment. During the summer of 2000, this program served more than 2 million children at 30,000 sites sponsored by 3600 organizations nationally.[9]

School nurses and community health nurses should be aware of these programs as a valuable source of nutrition. Sometimes children do not participate because school payment policies create a stigma associated with participation. Intervention by a health professional may be required to ensure that children's health needs are met in a socially sensitive manner. As health advocates, nurses may be able to highlight the importance of school lunch and breakfast programs to educational administrators and the community at large.

Classroom Nutrition Education.   Health has been taught for many years in most school systems. What vary are the depth of school health curricula and the qualifications of the instructors. Both may affect the quality of the nutrition education. Although basic nutrition facts can be taught within a short-term health course, lifestyle changes that affect dietary patterns take longer to achieve. Unless they have special preparation, instructors may not feel comfortable teaching the intricate and ever-changing discipline of nutrition. This may lead to either poor quality teaching or the imparting of negative attitudes toward nutrition and food selections.

To further the goal of increasing the level of nutrition education throughout the country, a *Healthy People 2010* objective addresses this concern within the school health curriculum:

> *Increase the proportion of middle, junior high, and senior high schools that provide school health education to prevent health problems in the following areas: unintentional injury; violence; suicide; tobacco use and addiction; alcohol and other drug use; unintended pregnancy, HIV/AIDS, and STD infection; unhealthy dietary patterns; inadequate physical activity; and environmental health.[10]*

Adolescence (13 to 19 Years)

The adolescent years are marked by change. Not only does puberty initiate growth acceleration, but emotional and social developmental struggles also occur as academic and personal responsibilities escalate. Adults often assume the attitude that teenagers can take care of themselves. Although teens need to take responsibility for their behavior and overall health status, they still need the guidance and nurturing of caring adults. There is a fine line between allowing adolescents to be responsible and neglecting their needs. Adult involvement is still necessary to provide physical and emotional support during the stressful years of adolescence.

Part of the physical and emotional support includes creating guidelines for dietary patterns and providing food for consumption. Creating guidelines means maintaining a household in which meals are available, even if family members may not be able to eat together. Knowing that dinner just needs to be reheated means someone was thinking of the welfare of all family members. Of course, shared responsibility for meal preparation may be an appropriate component of family duties. A kitchen stocked with nourishing snack foods and ingredients for simple meals helps to make stressful, chaotic teenage schedules more manageable.

Older teens may be adjusting to the new demands of the college environment, including adapting to dining hall meals. Some campuses provide flexible meal plans with several locations for meal acquisition around campus. Others offer salad bars and food "stations" to provide a variety of selections. Individuals needing special dietary requirements such as kosher meals or lactose-reduced meals should discuss these issues with food service staff or with student service personnel.

As their sense of social awareness develops, some teens may adopt a vegetarian dietary pattern. Creative planning on the part of the teen and the family meal planner can result in meals that meet everyone's nutritional needs without compromising personal convictions.

Discussions of the eating habits of teens tend to be critical of their fast-food consumption. Fortunately, most teens can afford the extra kcalories that typically higher-fat foods of hamburgers, fries, and pizza may contain. If teens have grown up accustomed to well-balanced meals, they will more than likely still prefer those meals to high-fat delights. Eating in fast-food restaurants, where prices tend to be

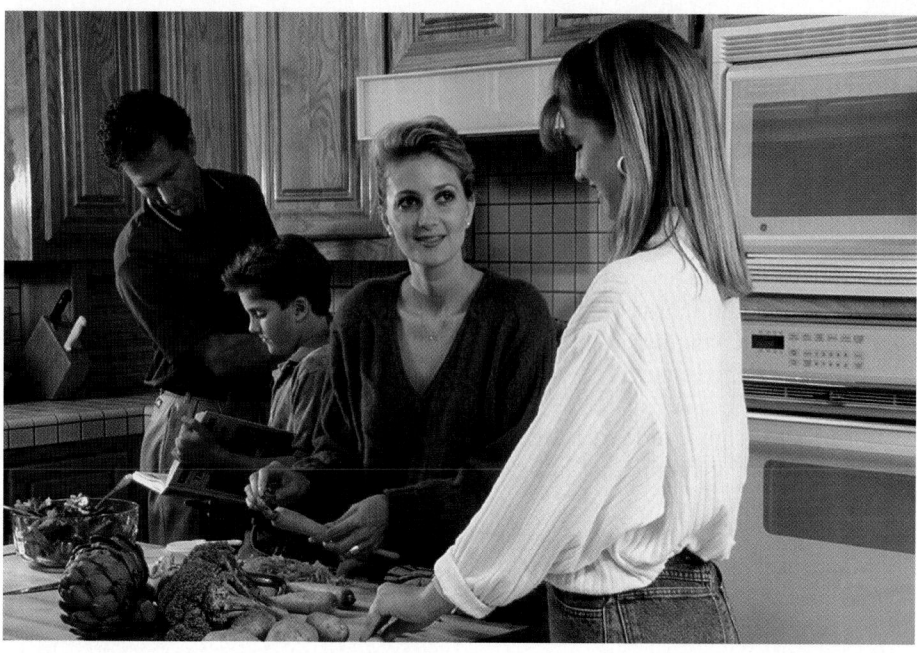

Teens can help plan meals that meet the whole family's nutritional needs while incorporating alternative food styles. (From PhotoDisc.)

inexpensive, may have more to do with socializing with peers than with nutrient values.

When fast foods become the mainstay of an individual's diet, regardless of age, then some nutrients such as vitamin A and C may be lacking and overconsumption of dietary fats and kcalories may occur. Although teens may be seen at such restaurants, most other customers consist of families with young children as well as older adults. Fast foods affect the nutrient intake of all ages (see the Teaching Tool box, "Fast-Food Choices").

Nutrition Requirements

Because of the natural physiologic differences between adolescent males and females, nutrient requirements from age 9 and older are divided by gender. Females need about 2200 kcalories and 45 grams of protein daily. Recommendations for males are 2500 to 2900 kcalories and 45 to 59 grams of protein daily. These values for kcalories and protein reflect the increased lean body mass developing in males. They do, however, only represent suggested amounts; physical activity, either work or athletic endeavors, affects the actual nutrient needs for both males and females.

Calcium AI recommendations are the same for both genders, 1300 mg per day, to allow for skeletal growth (particularly for boys) and for bone mineralization, a prime physiologic function during adolescence. Bone mineralization for girls is a concern because teenage girls often underconsume calcium-rich foods.

Teenage girls and sometimes teenage boys are at risk for dieting-related disorders and eating disorders. By regularly underconsuming nutrients during a time when the human body is completing maturation, girls are at risk for various deficiencies as they progress toward adulthood and the nutrient requirements of potential pregnancies. In addition to calcium, iron allowances are important to fulfill, particularly for girls who begin menstruation; iron is also needed by boys, whose accelerated growth necessitates an increased blood volume and lean body mass.

DRI = Dietary Reference Intakes

RDA = Recommended Dietary Allowance

AI = Adequate Intake

UL = Tolerable Upper Intake Level

TEACHING TOOL
Fast-Food Choices

We might as well accept it: fast-food restaurants are part of our everyday lives. Because they provide quickly prepared foods that are usually reasonably priced and in convenient locations, fast-food chains are here to stay. Although many health professionals complain about the high-fat, high-sodium, and calorie-laden foods provided, consumers continue to flock to these locales. Rather than fight a losing battle, we serve the needs of our clients best by providing guidelines for making healthier selections when time is short and hunger great.

Choose plainer food items such as a plain hamburger instead of a specialty burger that has more fat-laden toppings or select a grilled chicken sandwich rather than a fried chicken sandwich. A request for "no sauce" can lower the fat content significantly.

INSTEAD OF:

Specialty burger*
570-660 kcal; 280-360 kcal fat
(32-40 g fat)

Fried chicken sandwich*
710 kcal; 390 kcal fat (43 g fat)

SOMETIMES CHOOSE:

Quarter-pound burger
430 kcal; 190 kcal fat (21 g fat)

Bacon cheeseburger (regular size)
400 kcal; 200 kcal fat (22 g fat)

Grilled chicken sandwich†
450-530 kcal; 160-230 kcal fat
(18-26 g fat)

Grilled chicken sandwich†
450-530 kcal; 160-230 kcal fat
(18-26 g fat)

Fried chicken sandwich without
mayonnaise
500 kcal; 180 kcal fat (20 g fat)

Reference: Fast Food Facts, www.kenkuhl.com/fastfood/.
*There are also other specialty sandwiches that are much higher in kcalories and fat content than these.
†Order without mayonnaise sauce to save 110 kcal.

Adolescence Health Promotion (13 to 19 Years)

Knowledge

The adolescent body benefits from a dietary intake most similar to an adult's; however, some nutrient needs are greater. Energy requirements are higher than at any other time of life, especially for adolescents involved in competitive athletics. Calcium recommendations increase to ensure adequate mineralization of bones. Tolerance for alternative food styles enhances overall dietary intake and allows for the acceptance of dietary suggestions to maintain appropriate nutrient consumption.

Teenagers can comprehend the body's physiology and nutrient needs. Ideally this information should be taught within family life, health, or science curricula in schools. This knowledge provides a rationale for consumption of nutrient-dense foods, especially as preparation for sport activities. Although adults may supply provisions for meals and snacks, especially those that can be reheated, ultimately most adolescents take responsibility for their own nutrient intake.

Awareness of the risk factors and symptoms of disordered eating and drug/alcohol abuse should be provided through health classes or interactions with health and educational professionals and parents. Even mild substance abuse in the face of the increased nutritional needs of adolescence can compromise nutritional status. For example, alcohol adversely affects absorption of folate and zinc, two nutrients required for normal growth. Nurses need to be aware of the indicators of substance abuse so they can guide adolescents into treatment (Box 12-3). Nutrition assessment, intervention, and support are part of comprehensive physical and psychologic rehabilitation of all substance abusers.

Techniques

Similar to techniques for children, the concepts of the Food Guide Pyramid and 5-A-Day provide a basis for adolescent food choices. Often the forces that override good food choices are lack of time and scheduling demands. One strategy accommodating both is to ensure the availability of simple meals that are easily eaten and reheatable. Scheduling of meals in a home or institutional setting (e.g., school cafeterias, dining halls) can take into account school, sports, work, and recreational agendas. To improve the quality of food choices, adolescents should be included in meal planning and food preparation.

Community Supports

Except for federal government programs serving children and adults, no food programs are specifically targeted at adolescents.[11] At a time when teens are developmentally ready to be empowered to take care of themselves, society provides few supports. In fact, school, sports, and work schedules often hinder adolescents from taking responsibility for their health behaviors. Television, radio, and print messages rarely promote healthy behaviors. Although the increased interest in physical pursuits of basketball, soccer, biking, skateboarding, in-line skating, and other recreational sports enhances fitness, the nutrition component is often overlooked or cloaked in misinformation. This is an area to which all health professionals should be sensitive.

One of the few community supports is a comprehensive school health program. The depth of health issues covered varies and may not include sufficient nutrition guidance, but at the least, these programs highlight basic concerns of nutrition and health. *Healthy People 2010* includes a separate objective for middle/junior and senior high schools to increase the number of schools that offer nutrition education to decrease unhealthy dietary patterns.

Box 12-3 Signs of Substance Abuse: Drugs and Alcohol

Behavior characteristics associated with substance abuse include the following:
- Abrupt changes in work or school attendance, quality of work, work output, grades, and discipline
- Unusual flare-ups or outbreaks of temper
- Withdrawal from responsibility
- General changes in overall attitude
- Deterioration of physical appearance and grooming
- Wearing sunglasses at inappropriate times
- Continual wearing of long-sleeved garments, particularly in hot weather, or reluctance to wear short-sleeved attire when appropriate
- Association with known substance abusers
- Unusual borrowing of money from friends, co-workers, or parents
- Stealing small items from employer, home, or school
- Secretive behavior regarding actions and possessions; poorly concealed attempts to avoid attention and suspicion (e.g., frequent trips to storage rooms, restroom, basement)

From Signs and symptoms: behavior characteristics associated with substance abuse. Copyright © 1996-2003. David A. Brocato, BCSAC, ICADC; www.addictions.org/signs_htm.

OVERCOMING BARRIERS

Food Asphyxiation

Asphyxiation from food is possible at any point along the life span, but toddlers and older adults tend to be more at risk. (Older adults are discussed in Chapter 13.) As toddlers first become accustomed to a variety of food textures and substances, they sometimes misjudge the size of food being chewed or may be too active when eating and accidentally swallow before sufficient chewing has taken place. Some foods that are potential problems are peanut butter (large clumps can stick in the throat), peanuts, popcorn, hot dogs, hard candies, gum, grapes, and foods containing bones (e.g., beef, poultry, fish). Efforts by parents and caregivers to serve appropriate foods to young children can prevent choking incidents. Children can be reminded to chew food well and sit quietly while eating.

Lead Poisoning

Lead poisoning can be an invisible health hazard. Found in old paint dust or chips, enameled porcelain fixtures (bathtubs), and soil or air from industrial and transportation pollution, excessive amounts of lead can be absorbed into the body.[12] Children are most at risk; they naturally absorb greater amounts of minerals than adults. Nutritional deficiencies of iron, calcium, and zinc tend to increase the absorption of lead. Lead poisoning and iron deficiency anemia are sometimes diagnosed concurrently. Excessive exposure to lead can permanently affect cognitive and perceptual abilities. These reduced functions affect learning ability.[13]

Role of Nurses

School and community nurses in high-risk areas should be sensitive to this risk to both physical and intellectual health. High-risk areas for children include lower socioeconomic areas with poor housing conditions. Once lead poisoning is determined through blood testing, local health departments work with families to ascertain the sources of contamination in the home or school environment while physicians implement lead-reduction therapy.

Overall levels of lead in the environment are lower than in the past because of standards established and enforced by the Environmental Protection Agency. Levels of lead in some communities, however, are still high enough by Centers for Disease Control and Prevention standards that primary prevention activities to further reduce lead poisoning should remain a community-wide goal.[14]

Obesity

The prevalence of obesity among American children and adolescents increased substantially over the past 30 years. A comparison of skinfold measurements and body mass index (BMI) from the National Health Examination Surveys (NHES) from 1963 to 1970 with NHES measurements from 1980 and 1990 revealed that one in five children and adolescents is overweight. Severe obesity has increased more quickly than even the increases of moderate over fatness.[15]

The etiology of these changes is not obvious but may be considered multifactorial. Eating more food as snacks and meals away from home may be a subtle factor for children and adults. These food portions tend to be larger and higher in calories and dietary fat than those eaten at home. Another factor may be the increase of sedentary lifestyles. Physical activity has decreased, with a related decline of fitness. Although TV watching has not increased substantially over the years, children may be more sedentary than in the past because they play video and computer games and "surf" the Internet. Physical and behavioral environmental influences also affect the level of physical activity. If facilities are not available or not safe to use, activity is limited. Concerns over increasing numbers of latchkey children (grade-school children arriving home without adult supervision until the evening) focus on the use of food for emotional comfort and security. All of these factors impact the effect of genetics, which may predispose children toward heavier weights and should be considered as interventions are considered.

Clinical assessment of obesity consists of completing a health history including the pattern of weight gain, emotional health status, and physical activity patterns. If BMI is greater than 30, a further discussion of weight issues may be appropriate, but first a consultation with parents or guardians may be appropriate to determine if intervention is warranted.

As with adults, intervention regarding weight should only be initiated when the patient is motivated or is experiencing weight associative disorders. Conducting a 24-hour recall provides an opportunity to engage in a discussion of dietary intake patterns such as excessive or imbalanced intake of nonnutrient-dense foods such as sodas, sweets, and fast foods. (This type of discussion may be appropriate regardless of the child's weight.) Physical examinations need to be sensitive to the child regarding his or her weight and body issues. If weight is excessive, the assessment can determine if weight causes physical symptoms such as sleep apnea. Morbidly obese adolescents may require a more comprehensive physical examination and intervention approaches.

Treatment, if warranted, must include the family. The goal is to maintain the current weight of the child while growth continues. Children should not be "dieting," but guidance can be provided to the child and caregivers as to healthier eating patterns. Education about dietary patterns such as the Food Guide Pyramid and food choices to restructure dietary intake patterns may be sufficient and should be conducted by a dietitian who has the expertise to work with children and their families. The goal of treatment should not be to reach an "ideal weight" but to develop and maintain a healthy lifestyle that includes acceptance of diverse body sizes.

Role of Nurses

Nurses support the goals of health promotion of obese children by being sensitive to the emotional, social, and physical dimensions associated with weight and body composition. As allies, nurses create an affirming medical environment for large children by awareness of their own behavior when conducting physical examinations, such as quietly recording weight rather than announcing weight aloud in a medical office or school setting. Pediatric offices should also have examining gowns large enough to adequately be used by larger pediatric patients.

Iron Deficiency Anemia

For children, poverty is a significant risk factor for iron deficiency anemia. Economically deprived children of inner cities are most at risk because of the dual risk of lead poisoning, which reduces the amount of iron absorbed by the body, and chronic hunger that limits the intake of adequate nutrients. Lead poisoning and iron deficiency each contribute to learning failure. Ability to learn is decreased because cognitive and motor abilities are altered and this limits the ability to explore, focus, and benefit from the education environment. Although poor Americans of any group are at risk, African American, Hispanic American, and Native American children are most likely to have inadequate intakes of iron.

Malnourished children may be developmentally delayed and unable to benefit from educational experiences. The effects of iron deficiency anemia may begin in childhood and carry through adolescence and into adulthood, limiting the productivity and potential accomplishments of individuals.

Although iron deficiency has been recognized as a public health issue for many years, it is still a concern. It is possible that federal government programs to increase nutrition status among poor Americans may actually work against decreasing iron deficiency. For example, the U.S. Federal Commodity Food Program releases cheese and butter to the poor. Not only are these foods high in fat but they also are particularly poor sources of iron and may contribute to the continuing prevalence of iron deficiencies.[16] Another contributing factor may be that in 1997, the USDA began to allow the School Lunch Program to substitute yogurt for meat/protein requirements.[15] For the general population, the effect on iron intake may be minimal, but for economically disadvantaged children, the amount of iron consumed through school lunch servings of meat, poultry, fish, and beans is significant. The effects of chronic poverty and malnutrition are so intertwined that simple nutritional intervention will not overcome the deficits of social deprivation.[17]

Role of Nurses

Nurses, particularly school nurses, can educate teaching staff about the relationship between iron deficiency and learning ability. Children may be labeled as slow learners and "behavior problems" when iron deficiency may be the cause of learning difficulties.

Food Allergies and Food Intolerances

Food allergies and food intolerances pose nutritional and social challenges for children, their families, and caregivers. Although adults may also experience adverse responses to foods, infants and children are most commonly affected. About 6% to 8% of children and 0.5% to 2% of adults have documented food allergies.[18] Commonly affected individuals are those with asthma and hay fever.

Food Allergy

A food allergy is the overreaction of the immune system to a food protein or other large molecule that has been absorbed and interacts with the immune system that produces a response. The body produces antibodies to protect itself from the foreign substance, the protein allergen. The reaction causes a variety of physical symptoms that occur immediately (less than 2 hours), intermediately (2 to 24 hours), or delayed (over 24 hours).[18] The most common food allergies experienced by children are peanuts, milk, eggs, and wheat. Seafood and peanuts are more common among older children and adults. Cross reactivity also occurs. For example, if a person is affected by a ragweed allergy, reaction to melons and bananas may occur.[19]

Symptoms may include skin, respiratory, and gastrointestinal reactions (Box 12-4). Reactions may affect breathing ability if the upper airway becomes obstructed because of swelling. If the symptoms are treated as asthma, instead of a true food allergy, the misdiagnosis may trigger more serious physical responses and a continuation of symptoms because the offending food may continue to be consumed.

Reactions for a small number of individuals may be so severe as to be life threatening. This type of reaction is called anaphylaxis and may occur immediately after eating the food substance. Peanuts, eggs, shellfish, and nuts may cause anaphylaxis in sensitive individuals. Symptoms may include hives, breathing difficulties, and unconsciousness. It requires immediate medical care or a plan of action in case inadvertent consumption of the offending food occurs. Caregivers, whether parents, school officials, family, or friends, must be aware of the potential reaction and the appropriate and immediate treatment for the anaphylaxis response.[20]

Risk Factors. Risk factors include heredity, gastrointestinal permeability, and environmental factors. Heredity is a risk factor because if parents have allergies, their children are most at risk. Gastrointestinal permeability affects the amount of the antigen inappropriately absorbed. Environmental factors can increase food allergic responses. Environmental factors include increased exposure to inhalant seasonal allergies such as pollen and cold weather and other environmental allergens of dust, mold, dust mites, smoke, and stress.

asthma
a chronic respiratory disorder characterized by airway obstruction caused by excessive mucus production and respiratory mucosa edema; may be triggered by infection, cold air, vigorous exercise, stress, or inhalation of environmental allergens or pollutants

food allergy
the overreaction to a food protein or other large molecule that produces an immune response

anaphylaxis
a severe immune system response to an allergen

Box 12-4 Potential Symptoms of Food Allergies

GASTROINTESTINAL SYSTEM

Nausea
Abdominal cramping
Vomiting
Gastroesophageal reflux
Gastrointestinal bleeding
Oral and pharyngeal pruritus (itchiness)

RESPIRATORY SYSTEM

Rhinitis (inflamed nasal membranes and discharge)
Cough
Hoarseness
Asthma
Stridor (high-pitched sound from trachea/larynx obstruction)
Chest tightness
Dyspnea (shortness of breath)

NEUROLOGIC SYSTEM

Headache (migraine)
"Feeling of impending doom"

DERMATOLOGIC SYSTEM

Itching
Contact dermatitis
Flushing
"Goose-bumps"
Eczema (itchy, crusty rash)
Erythema (redness of skin/mucous membranes)
Urticaria (itchy skin eruptions)

CARDIOVASCULAR SYSTEM

Syncope (brief lapse of consciousness)
Hypotension (abnormally low blood pressure)
Dizziness
Loss of consciousness

GENITOURINARY SYSTEM

Uterine bleeding
Uterine cramping

Compiled from Sampson HA: Diagnosis and management of food allergies. In Shils ME eds.: Modern nutrition in health and disease, *ed 9, Philadelphia, 1999, Williams & Wilkins; Schepers A: Nutritional care in food allergy and food intolerance. In Mahan LK, Escott-Stump S, eds.:* Krause's food, nutrition, & diet therapy, *ed 9, Philadelphia, 2000, WB Saunders; and Smith LJ, Munoz-Furlong A: Management of food allergy. In Metcalfe DD, Sampson HA, Simon RA, eds.:* Food allergy: adverse reactions to food and food additives, *ed 2, Cambridge, Mass, 1997, Blackwell Science.*

food intolerance

an adverse reaction to a food that does not involve the immune system

Food Intolerance

In contrast to a food allergy, food intolerance is an adverse reaction to a food that does not involve the immune system. The symptoms are triggered by a reaction of the body to a food. Pharmacologic properties of foods (e.g., tyramine in aged cheese, theobromine in chocolate), metabolic disorders (e.g., lactose intolerance), or idiosyncratic responses may cause the reaction.[21] Lactose intolerance is an example of a food intolerance (see Chapter 3). The lack of the enzyme lactase limits the digestion of lactose, leading to physical symptoms of bloating, flatulence, diarrhea, and nausea. The resulting symptoms can be similar to and mistaken as a food allergy. Treatment, though, is different than if a true allergy. For lactose intolerance, products are available that contain reduced lactose, or there are pills (e.g., Lactaid) that break down lactose, thus easing digestion. In contrast, if the symptoms are caused by a food allergy, the offending substance in milk (the milk proteins) are not affected by the reduction of lactose (a carbohydrate) and the immune system response and symptoms would still occur.

Diagnosis

Determination of whether a reaction is caused by a food allergy or by intolerance requires consultation with a healthcare provider specializing in allergies. Diagnosis involves a health history and physical examination, food and symptom diary, biochemical and immunologic testing, and a food elimination procedure.[18] The health history records symptoms, including the reaction time from ingestion to symptoms, and a family allergy history, in addition to traditional information of health histories. The physical examination assesses weight and height patterns to determine whether potential malnutrition may be present because of the effects of the food allergies. Related allergenic symptoms such as eczema are noted. A food and symptom diary keeps track of amounts of food consumed, time and day of consumption, and any resulting symptoms. This information is valuable to begin to isolate potential food allergens. Biochemical testing such as a complete blood count rules out symptoms caused by conditions unrelated to food allergies. Immunologic testing through skin pricking of individual foods assists in identifying potential food allergens based on reactive immunologic adverse reactions, such as swelling and welts at the site of the skin prick.

A food elimination process consists of not eating foods suspected of being allergenic for 2 weeks to allow the person to become symptom-free. Guidance during this phase is crucial to ensure complete compliance. Adequate nutrition can be sustained by substitution of other foods to provide nutrients lost by the elimination of allergenic foods. A registered dietitian or qualified nutritionist should be consulted for appropriate elimination diets. To ensure the accuracy of the diagnosis, a food challenge is implemented. This consists of consuming the allergenic food and assessing the responsive symptoms. Severe reactions are possible. Consequently, food challenges should be conducted in an appropriate healthcare setting. Another protocol is to conduct a double-blind, placebo-controlled food challenge. Rechallenges may be conducted after several years to assess if the food allergy is still present.[18]

Treatment

The only way to treat a food allergy is to avoid consumption of the food. Referral to a registered dietitian for nutrition counseling is important, and family and caregivers should be included in the nutrition counseling process. Nutrition counseling identifies alternative sources of nutrients to assure appropriate substitutions for the foods eliminated. Nutrition counseling also assists in teaching how to use food labels to recognize the different terms of allergenic items (Box 12-5). Valuable assistance is provided

Box 12-5   Label Terminology for Milk, Wheat, and Soy Ingredients

Milk, wheat, and soy may be contained in the following ingredients:

MILK	WHEAT	SOY
Buttermilk solids	Enriched flour	Corn syrup
Caramel color/flavoring	Flour	Hydrogenated oils
Casein	Gluten	Soy
Caseinate	Graham flour	Soy flour
Cream	Hydrolyzed vegetable protein	Soy protein
Curds	Malted cereal syrup	Soybean oil
Lactalbumin	Seminola	Vegetable broth
Milk	Starch	Vegetable shortening
Milk solids	Gelatinized starch	Vegetable starch
Natural flavoring	Modified starch	Vegetable gum
Sodium caseinate	Modified food starch	
Whey	Vegetable starch	
	Vegetable gum	
	Wheat	
	Wheat bran	
	Wheat germ	
	Wheat starch	

Compiled from Schepers A: Nutritional care in food allergy and food intolerance. In Mahan LK, Escott-Stump S, eds: Krause's food, nutrition, & diet therapy, ed 9, Philadelphia, 2000, WB Saunders; and Smith LJ, Munoz-Furlong A: Management of food allergy. In Metcalfe DD, Sampson HA, Simon RA, eds.: Food allergy: adverse reactions to food and food additives, ed 2, Cambridge, Mass, 1997, Blackwell Science.

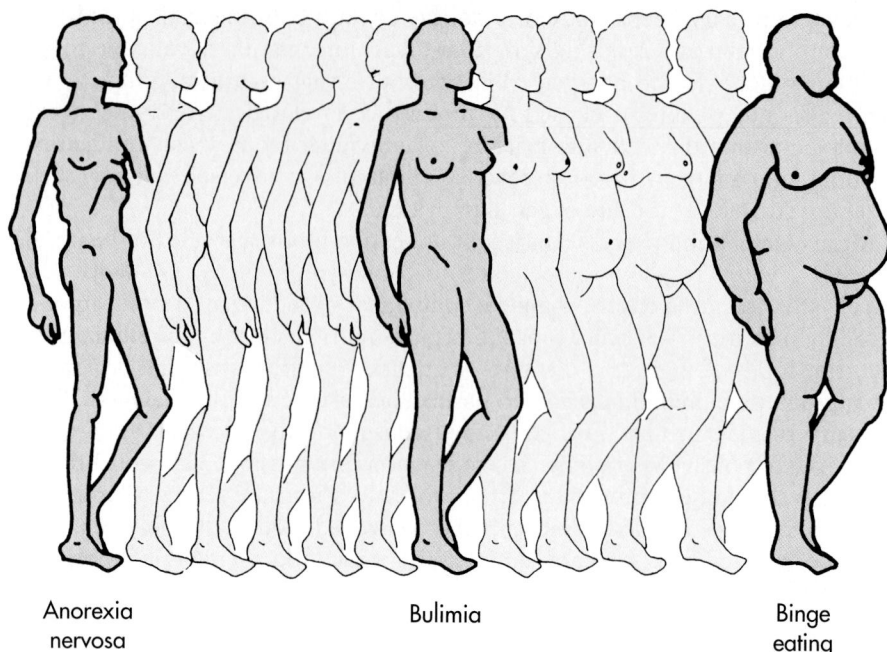

Anorexia
nervosa

Bulimia

Binge
eating

Figure 12-3 Continuum of eating disorders. Although physical conditions vary, underlying psychologic characteristics are held in common across the continuum. (From Worthington-Roberts BS, Williams SR: *Nutrition throughout the life cycle*, ed 4, New York, 2000, McGraw-Hill. Reprinted with permission.)

by organizations such as the Food Allergy Network, which provides a newsletter, informational Web site, and other educational supports. Planned nutrition counseling follow-up sessions should be considered to assess progress in complying with dietary recommendations.

Role of Nurses.   Awareness of food allergies and the nutrition adequacy issues associated with specific food elimination supports the health promotion goal of clients. Appropriate referrals to nutrition counseling can assist in avoiding nutrient deficiencies and frustrations with compliance.

Eating Disorders

eating disorders
a group of behaviors fueled by unresolved emotional conflicts, symptomized by altered food consumption

Eating disorders are a group of behaviors fueled by unresolved emotional conflicts, symptomized by altered food consumption. Disorders include anorexia nervosa, bulimia nervosa, and binge eating. These represent a continuum from the starvation of anorexia nervosa to the uncontrollable excessive food intake of binge eating disorder (Figure 12-3). Most individuals with eating disorders are women; however, men are also susceptible.

Although disordered food consumption is the overt symptom of eating disorders, changed nutrient intake is not the cause. Nourishment becomes a symbolic issue when individuals experiencing eating disorders are not able to deal directly with their emotions and instead nourish their psyches by either excessively restricting food or consuming extremely large quantities of foods that may then be purged. Eating properly cannot cure eating disorders. Underlying psychologic concerns must first be addressed. Nurse-client relationships often provide informal opportunities to discuss dietary patterns; if early signs of dis-

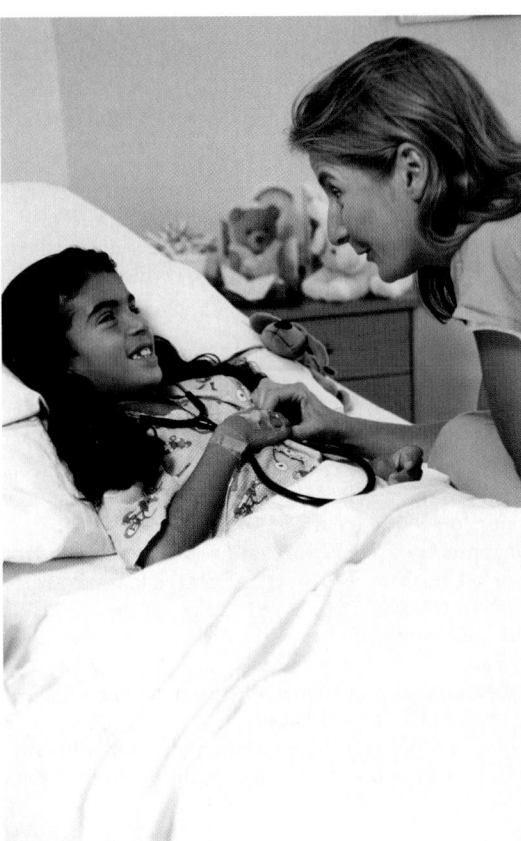

Figure 12-4 Nurse-client relationships often provide informal opportunities to discuss dietary patterns; if early signs of disordered eating are detected, further assessment or treatment can be initiated. (From PhotoDisc.)

ordered eating are detected, further assessment or treatment can be initiated (Figure 12-4).

Etiology

The etiology of eating disorders tends to be assigned to our Western obsession with thinness. For many American women, dieting (restrictive food intake) is a way of life from early adolescence on. Most who are caught in the web of the culture of thinness experience chronic dieting syndrome. Chronic dieting syndrome can be described as a lifestyle inhibited or controlled by a constant concern about food intake, body shape, or weight that affects an individual's physical and mental health status.[22] Only a small percentage of these chronic dieters manifest eating disorders. Additional risk factors must be present for eating disorders to evolve. Common risk factors include low self-esteem, depression, participation in appearance or endurance sports, history of sexual abuse, or self-regulatory difficulties. The influence of risk factors is cumulatively mediated by the context of the individual in relation to societal and familial variables (see the Teaching Tool box, "Are You at Risk for an Eating Disorder?").

Anorexia Nervosa and Related Eating Disorders, Inc. (ANRED) is an organization dedicated to the education, prevention, and dissemination of treatment resources on many disordered eating conditions. They provide the following self-assessment.

chronic dieting syndrome a lifestyle inhibited or controlled by a constant concern about food intake, body shape, or weight that affects an individual's physical and mental health status

TEACHING TOOL
Are You at Risk for an Eating Disorder?

ARE YOU AT RISK? TAKE A SELF-TEST

The following questionnaire can help you decide if you have an eating disorder, or if you are at risk of developing one. The easiest way to take the test is to print it out (www.anred.com) and then check the items that describe you. Then read the explanatory paragraph at the end. The test and your visit to the Web site are anonymous.

- Although people tell me I'm thin, I feel fat.
- I get anxious if I can't exercise.
- [Woman] My menstrual periods are irregular or absent.
  [Man] My sex drive is not as strong as it used to be.
- I worry about what I will eat.
- If I gain weight, I get anxious and depressed.
- I would rather eat by myself than with family or friends.
- Other people talk about the way I eat.
- I get anxious when people urge me to eat.
- I don't talk much about my fear of being fat because no one understands how I feel.
- I enjoy cooking for others, but I usually don't eat what I've cooked.
- I have a secret stash of food.
- When I eat, I'm afraid I won't be able to stop.
- I lie about what I eat.
- I don't like to be bothered or interrupted when I'm eating.
- If I were thinner, I would like myself better.
- I like to read recipes, cookbooks, calorie charts, and books about dieting and exercise.
- I have missed work or school because of my weight or eating habits.
- I tend to be depressed and irritable.
- I feel guilty when I eat.
- I avoid some people because they bug me about the way I eat.
- When I eat, I feel bloated and fat.
- My eating habits and fear of food interfere with friendships or romantic relationships.
- I binge eat.
- I do strange things with my food (e.g., cut it into tiny pieces, eat it in special ways, eat it on special dishes with special utensils, make patterns on my plate with it, secretly throw it away, give it to the dog, hide it, spit it out before I swallow).
- I get anxious when people watch me eat.
- I am hardly ever satisfied with myself.
- I vomit or take laxatives to control my weight.
- I want to be thinner than my friends.
- I have said or thought, "I would rather die than be fat."
- I have stolen food, laxatives, or diet pills from stores or from other people.
- I have fasted to lose weight.
- In romantic moments, I cannot let myself go because I am worried about my fat and flab.
- I have noticed one or more of the following: cold hands and feet, dry skin, thinning hair, fragile nails, swollen glands in my neck, dental cavities, dizziness, weakness, fainting, and rapid or irregular heartbeat.

As strange as it seems in our thin-obsessed society, none of the above behaviors is normal or healthy. The more items you have circled, the more serious your problem may be. Please check with your physician or a qualified mental health counselor to prevent medical and psychologic problems. You could show the person this questionnaire and the items you have circled as a way to begin the conversation.

People do recover from eating disorders, but almost all of those who do need professional help to get back on track. We know this is hard, and we appreciate your courage as you take the first step by calling today to make an appointment with your physician or counselor.

⚠ **Please Note:** ANRED information is not a substitute for medical or psychological evaluation and treatment. For help with the physical and emotional problems associated with eating disorders, talk to your physician and a mental health professional.

Page reprinted with permission of ANRED: Anorexia nervosa and related eating disorders, Inc., http://www.anred.com

Diagnosis

Uniform criteria for these psychiatric disorders are established by the American Psychiatric Association and published in the *Diagnostic and Statistical Manual of Mental Disorders,* fourth edition (DSM-IV).[23] Periodic revisions allow for updating disorder criteria and for adding newly recognized conditions. The DSM-IV criteria for clinical diagnosis of anorexia nervosa, bulimia nervosa, and binge eating disorder are listed in Boxes 12-6 through 12-8 (see also the Myth box, "Eating Disorders Affect Only Teens and Young Women").

Box 12-6 Diagnostic Criteria for Anorexia Nervosa

A. Refusal to maintain body weight at or above a minimally normal weight for age and height (e.g., weight loss leading to maintenance of body weight less than 85% of that expected; or failure to make expected weight gain during period of growth, leading to body weight less than 85% of that expected).

B. Intense fear of gaining weight or becoming fat although underweight.

C. Disturbance in the way in which one's body weight or shape is experienced, undue influence of body weight or shape on self-evaluation, or denial of the seriousness of the current low body weight.

D. In postmenarcheal women, amenorrhea (i.e., the absence of a least three consecutive mentrual cycles). (A woman is considered to have amenorrhea if her periods occur only following hormone [e.g., estrogen] administration.)

SPECIFY TYPE
RESTRICTING TYPE

During the current episode of anorexia nervosa, the person has not regularly engaged in binge-eating or purging behavior (i.e., self-induced vomiting or the misuse of laxatives, diuretics, or enemas).

BINGE-EATING/PURGING TYPE

During the current episode of anorexia nervosa, the person has regularly engaged in binge-eating or purging behavior (i.e., self-induced vomiting or the misuse of laxatives, diuretics, or enemas).

Reprinted with permission from the Diagnostic and Statistical Manual of Mental Disorders, Fourth Edition, Text Revision. Copyright 2000, American Psychiatric Association.

Box 12-7 Diagnostic Criteria for Bulimia Nervosa

A. Recurrent episodes of binge eating. An episode of binge eating is characterized by both of the following:
  1. Eating, in a discrete period (e.g., within any 2-hour period), an amount of food that is definitely larger than most people would eat during a similar period of time and under similar circumstances
  2. A sense of lack of control over eating during the episode (e.g., a feeling that one cannot stop eating or control what or how much one is eating)

B. Recurrent, inappropriate compensatory behavior to prevent weight gain, such as self-induced vomiting; misuse of laxatives, diuretics, enemas, or other medications; fasting; or excessive exercise.

C. The binge eating and inappropriate compensatory behaviors both occur, on average, at least twice a week for 3 months.

D. Self-evaluation is unduly influenced by body shape and weight.

E. The disturbance does not occur exclusively during episodes of anorexia nervosa.

SPECIFY TYPE
PURGING TYPE

During the current episode of bulimia nervosa, the person has regularly engaged in self-induced vomiting or the misuse of laxatives, diuretics, or enemas.

NONPURGING TYPE

During the current episode of bulimia nervosa, the person has used other inappropriate compensatory behaviors, such as fasting or excessive exercise, but has not regularly engaged in self-induced vomiting or the misuse of laxatives, diuretics, or enemas.

Reprinted with permission from the Diagnostic and Statistical Manual of Mental Disorders, Fourth Edition, Text Revision. Copyright 2000, American Psychiatric Association.

Box 12-8 Research Criteria for Binge Eating Disorder

A. Recurrent episodes of binge eating. An episode of binge eating is characterized by both of the following:
   1. Eating, in a discrete period (e.g., within any 2-hour period), an amount of food that is definitely larger than most people would eat in a similar period of time and under similar circumstances.
   2. A sense of lack of control over eating during the episode (e.g., a feeling that one cannot stop eating or control what or how much one is eating).
B. The binge-eating episodes are associated with three (or more) of the following:
   • Eating much more rapidly than normal
   • Eating until feeling uncomfortably full
   • Eating large amounts of food when not feeling physically hungry
   • Eating alone because of being embarrassed by how much one is eating
   • Feeling disgusted with oneself, depressed, or guilty after overeating
C. Marked distress regarding binge eating is present.
D. The binge eating occurs, on average, at least 2 days a week for 6 months. **Note:** The method of determining frequency differs from that used for bulimia nervosa; future research should address whether the preferred method of setting a frequency threshold is counting the number of days on which binges occur or counting the number of episodes of binge eating.
E. The binge eating is not associated with the regular use of inappropriate compensatory behaviors (e.g., purging, fasting, excessive exercise) and does not occur exclusively during the course of anorexia nervosa or bulimia nervosa.

Reprinted with permission from the Diagnostic and Statistical Manual of Mental Disorders, Fourth Edition, Text Revision. Copyright 2000, American Psychiatric Association.

MYTH
Eating Disorders Affect Only Teens and Young Women

Although most individuals with eating disorders are in their teens and early 20s, these disorders can strike at most any age. Particularly difficult is anorexia nervosa, for which the struggle to recover may be lifelong. Family members may be affected psychologically and physically as their loved ones experience this disorder. Consider the following experiences of Mark Stuart Ellison:

GROWING UP WITH AN ANOREXIC MOTHER

"A hamburger on whole wheat toast and don't cut it." Those words are indelibly etched in my mind. That's how my mother would order whenever she ate out. Although the hamburger was never to her liking and she would never eat the toast, the order was always the same. I recall the extraordinary patience and compassion of waiters and waitresses trying to please someone who was unpleasable. My mother had anorexia nervosa.

My mother died of anorexia at age 49; I was 17. As an attractive young woman, my mother, at 5'4", weighed a voluptuous 135 lbs. During the course of her illness, she weighed as little as 60 lbs, while exercising to exhaustion. The circumstances surrounding her illness had caused me to become socially withdrawn years earlier. I am now 34 years old and have only recently begun to emerge from that isolation.

When I was 9, I witnessed a horrifying scene. The bathroom door in our apartment was slightly ajar. My mother was in the bathroom, squirming on the toilet seat, my father struggling to hold her on the bowl. I was terrified. I didn't know what was happening.

A few minutes later, paramedics took her to the hospital on a stretcher. Mom had had one too many enemas and suffered the consequences on that day. From then on, my mother was in and out of hospitals for the rest of her life and never lived with me again.

As an anorexic she was ever-present; as a mother, she was absent. I have only begun to fill in the blanks in my own life.

From Ellison MS: Growing up with an anorexic mother, AABA Newsletter, Summer 1995.

Anorexia Nervosa.   Anorexia nervosa is characterized as refusal to maintain normal body weight through self-imposed starvation. Because of distorted body images, individuals who experience this disorder do not see themselves as underweight and continue to restrict their food intake, often in a ritualistic manner. Some experience binge-eating episodes that are also associated with bulimic behaviors. Psychologic characteristics include obsession with body shape and weight and an intense phobia of obesity. Chronic restrictive dieting is coupled with self-imposed limitation of food selection, hoarding, or hiding of food. Although their personal food intake is restricted, anorexics often prepare food for others; otherwise they avoid food-related events. When questioned about their food intake, they deny the disorder and weight loss. Anorexics tend to be overly perfectionist *model children* who are introverted, reserved, or possibly socially insecure. A profile of low self-esteem or a family history of anorexia or depression often exists, as well as compulsive behaviors in areas other than food intake. Other areas of compulsion may include excessive exercise, ritualized personal hygiene habits, and intensive study and work behaviors. Bingeing behaviors, if present, are similar to those of bulimia nervosa.

Physical dimensions may include amenorrhea; fatigue yet appearance of hyperactivity; dehydration; electrolyte imbalances including abnormally low levels of magnesium, zinc, phosphorus, and calcium in circulating blood; and metabolic alkalosis or metabolic acidosis caused by laxative abuse. Cardiovascular problems may develop such as hypotension (abnormally low blood pressure), arrhythmias, and sinus bradycardia (unusually slow heartbeat). Also present may be hormonal imbalances of reduced levels of estrogen or testosterone, hypothermia, and hypertension. Lanugo (soft white hair covering the body) is a late-stage effect as is edema not caused by premenstrual conditions or other medical conditions. Other physical conditions may include metabolic changes, constipation, and symptoms associated with starvation including loss of muscular strength, endurance, aerobic capacity, speed, and coordination. Vitamin, mineral, and protein deficiencies may also develop, leading to loss of bone mass and permanent damage to body organs. Approximately 0.2 to 1.3% of the general population is affected. Mortality for anorexia nervosa is between 5% and 10%.[24,25]

Bulimia Nervosa.   Bulimia nervosa is called the *binge and purge syndrome;* bulimic behaviors include experiencing repetitive food binges accompanied by purging or compensatory behaviors. Bingeing is defined as feeling out of control when eating, resulting in the consumption of excessive amounts of food. In response to bingeing, the individual with bulimia purges using laxatives, diuretics, or self-induced vomiting or uses inappropriate compensatory behaviors of fasting, diet pills, or excessive exercise. Bingeing is one of the primary characteristics of bulimia. A *binge* consists of the consumption of excessively large quantities of food in a short period of time with a feeling of being unable to control the amount consumed. An average of two binges per week for 3 months accompanied by several other psychologic and physical dimensions constitutes a diagnosis of bulimia nervosa. Binge foods tend to be of high-kcaloric value and require minimal preparation. Sleep, abdominal pain, or self-induced or drug-induced vomiting terminates the binge.

Purging and other compensatory behaviors to counteract binges are other characteristics of bulimia. Compensatory behaviors include self-induced vomiting and the use of emetics, diuretics, and laxatives as purging agents. Fasting or restrictive dieting, appetite suppressants, and excessive exercise may serve as compensatory behaviors. The use of emetics in particular to induce vomiting may have serious medical consequences; fatal incidences associated with bulimia have been reported.[26]

Psychologic dimensions of bulimia encompass obsessions with body shape and weight associated with chronic restrictive dieting. Binge eating and purging are *triggered* by stressful events or initiated as a group activity as part of a social event.

anorexia nervosa
a mental disorder characterized by self-imposed starvation; may include binge-eating episodes associated with bulimic behaviors

bulimia nervosa
a mental disorder characterized as the *binge and purge syndrome;* includes experiencing repetitive food binges accompanied by purging or compensatory behaviors

bingeing
feeling out of control when eating, resulting in the consumption of excessive amounts of food

emetics
substances that cause vomiting

Episodes of bingeing are accompanied by a loss of self-control and low self-esteem. Individuals tend to lack the ability to apply appropriate coping skills. Addictive disorders, depression, and family history of obesity, bulimia nervosa, or sexual abuse may be present.

Physical characteristics may include weight fluctuation, amenorrhea, and fatigue. Dental health is affected because dental caries (from excessive simple-sugar consumption) develops and dental enamel erosion (from acidic vomitus) occurs. Purging may lead to dehydration and electrolyte imbalances, particularly with abnormally low levels of chloride, sodium, and calcium in circulating blood; laxative abuse may result in metabolic acidosis. Recurrent episodes of vomiting may cause metabolic alkalosis, bruising of the dorsal surface of the hands (from inducing vomiting), sore throat, swollen salivary glands (especially parotid glands), hormonal imbalances, blood-shot eyes (particularly after vomiting), and broken blood vessels on the face. Rare complications may include gastric rupture, esophageal tears, and cardiac arrhythmias. Chronic use of emetics may lead to cardiac and skeletal abnormalities.

binge eating disorder (BED)
a mental disorder characterized by frequent binge eating behaviors, not accompanied by purging or compensatory behaviors; commonly called *compulsive overeating*

Binge Eating Disorder.   The third eating disorder, binge eating disorder (BED), is commonly called *compulsive overeating*. Individuals with this disorder frequently engage in binge eating behavior not accompanied by purging or compensatory behaviors.

Psychologic dimensions are reflected by binges *triggered* by stressful events or dysphoric moods including anxiety and depression. The binge eating may occur in secret or private settings and be accompanied by a sense of loss of control. Individuals appear to lack appropriate coping skills. After bingeing episodes, they experience low self-esteem, shame, remorse, or depression. Other addictive disorders may be present in addition to obsessive behaviors in nonfood areas. A family history of obesity, depression, or addictive disorders is likely.

Physical characteristics may include obesity with increased risk of joint pains, breathing difficulties, coronary artery disease, elevated blood cholesterol levels, hypertension, and gastrointestinal tract disturbances. BED, however, is not the only etiologic factor of obesity. Obesity may also be caused by excessive kcaloric consumption not associated with emotional turmoil, poor eating habits, sedentary lifestyle, or genetic factors. Conversely, BED may be present in the absence of obesity if the criteria of recurrent binges associated with emotional upset and a sense of loss of control occur.

Nutritional Therapy

Dietary patterns in eating disorders may be fractured to a point at which meals are nonexistent or so redefined as to lose all meaning. A challenge in treatment is the relearning of meal patterns.

medical nutritional therapy
the use of specific nutrition services to treat an illness, injury, or condition

Medical nutritional therapy is the use of specific nutrition services to treat an illness, injury, or condition. It involves assessment and treatment including diet therapy, counseling, and the use of specialized nutrition supplements. Because medical nutritional therapy is an integral component of eating disorder recovery, knowledge of the process of nutritional care is beneficial for all healthcare professionals who interact with patients who have eating disorders. As the medical, nursing, and psychologic staffs implement their therapeutic approaches, they will be aware of the medical nutritional therapy objectives. Although underlying psychologic issues are worked on through psychologic therapy, the registered dietitian works with the patient to bring about changes in the patient's food-and-weight-related behaviors. This collaborative effort occurs in various phases of outpatient or inpatient therapy and constitutes nutrition intervention.

Nutrition intervention consists of two phases: the educational phase and the experimental phase. According to the position paper on eating disorders of the

American Dietetic Association (ADA), all registered dietitians are trained to implement the educational phase, but specialized training and experience in eating disorder counseling are required for the experimental phase.[26]

The educational phase provides a knowledge foundation to support the behavioral changes of the experimental phase. The dietitian shares nutrition information about dietary patterns and nutritional adequacy. The interaction is brief and relatively impersonal; the emotional dynamic surrounding food intake as an aspect of eating disorders is not explored in this phase.[26]

The experimental phase does incorporate such issues. Through a long-term counseling relationship, the registered dietitian as a member of a multidisciplinary team works directly with the patient to mediate eating behaviors. The intervention may be a psychonutritional approach through which the dietitian discusses emotional issues of eating with the patient. To do so, the registered dietitian should be supervised by and communicate with the multidisciplinary team because formulating appropriate therapeutic boundaries is crucial.

Based on the position of the ADA, there are five objectives of the nutrition education phase: (1) collect relevant information through detailed assessment of the diverse eating disorder population; (2) establish a collaborative relationship between the person with the eating disorder and the registered dietitian; (3) define and discuss relevant principles and concepts of food, nutrition, and weight regulation; (4) present examples of hunger patterns, typical food intake patterns, and the total kcaloric intake of a person who has recovered from an eating disorder; and (5) educate the family.

Primary objectives for the experimental phase have also been established. They include: (1) separate food- and weight-related behaviors from feelings and psychologic issues; (2) change food behaviors in an incremental fashion until food intake patterns are normalized; (3) slowly increase or decrease weight; (4) learn to maintain a weight that is healthful for the individual without using abnormal food- and weight-related behaviors; and (5) learn to be comfortable in social eating situations.

The effectiveness of the multidisciplinary approach to treatment is caused by the recognition that the complex etiology of eating disorders requires the expertise of various health professionals. With the dietitian addressing the food- and weight-related behaviors, the psychologic team members can focus on the psychologic issues while the medical and nursing personnel rectify the physical ramifications of the disorder.

Role of Nurses.   Nurses are members of the therapeutic multidisciplinary team along with physicians, psychiatrists, psychologists, and dietitians. The therapeutic orientation of nursing care depends on the philosophy and clinical modalities of individual treatment programs. Although nurses are central to the staffing of inpatient programs, their participation in outpatient programs may be marginal. If outpatient treatment is within a holistic clinic attending to medical and psychologic concerns, the role of nurses is integral. Most outpatient treatment tends to be direct care between the client and a health specialist such as a psychologist or dietitian.

Nurses have an educational role in the prevention of eating disorders. By providing information about nutrition and normal eating patterns to parents, caregivers, and children, healthier feeding relationships can evolve.[27] This can help diffuse the behavior of using food as an emotional outlet. Additionally, nurses can be accepting of all body types, taking care to be sensitive to issues of weight and size when providing basic healthcare. Nurse-client relationships often provide informal opportunities to discuss dietary patterns; if early signs of disordered eating are detected, further assessment or treatment can be initiated before a clinically diagnosable disorder develops (see the Social Issue box). Referral to a dietitian with special training in eating disorders should be considered.

SOCIAL ISSUE
When an Eating Disorder Is Suspected: Who Is Responsible for Intervention?

*P*erhaps it is a daughter, son, sibling, friend, or roommate. An eating disorder is suspected; too much weight is lost, little is eaten or too much is eaten, and vomiting and other purging is observed. What should you do?

Too often, denial occurs, not only by the person with disordered eating but by her family and friends as well. It's easier to ignore what is happening than to risk becoming involved. On the other hand, sometimes over-involvement happens when family and friends become so embroiled in the battle to eat or not eat that the disorder becomes the center of relationships. Few relationships can survive well based on struggling with eating issues.

When an eating disorder is suspected, the first action is to talk directly to the person about it. She may be waiting for someone to confront her and tell her these behaviors are not okay; such an encounter may be a trigger for her to seek professional help. If that is not sufficient, friends may choose to contact family members who may have more influence and responsibility for the health of the individual. In a college dormitory setting, resident life personnel should be contacted. They are often specially trained to assist students with eating disorders. It is unfair for the eating disorder of a roommate to negatively affect the lives of the others. Roommates can best help the person by intervening, however risky such actions may be to the friendship.

Once intervention begins, new rules often have to be negotiated. Food and related eating behaviors can no longer be the focus of relationships. Each person becomes responsible for her own intake of nourishment. Although meals may be shared, food policing needs to be curtailed. Parents will need to refrain from pushing food to their child who is anorexic; friends may need to ignore second helpings of a friend who is bulimic. Other rules may evolve; if an individual still binges, she must replace the food she consumes. If the binge is followed by purging, she must completely clean the bathroom after vomiting. The goal is that the person must be responsible for her or his own actions without interfering with the rights of others. Though friends and family may analyze how their behaviors might have supported this illness, ultimately the struggle to heal is the individual's alone.

Reference: Siegel M, Brisman J, Weinshel M: Surviving an eating disorder: strategies for family and friends, New York, 1997, Harper Perennial.

TOWARD A POSITIVE NUTRITION LIFESTYLE: PSYCHOSOCIAL DEVELOPMENT

Psychosocial development occurs during childhood through adolescence. This continual process is most often assessed through the work of Erik Erikson. Erikson's Stages of Ego Development considers the emotional, cultural, and social forces that mold an individual's personality. Divided into stages, this process involves the resolution of psychosocial conflicts. The resolution for children from ages 2 to 3 years is self-confidence and self-control; 4 to 5 years is independence; 6 to 11 years is competence; and 12 to 18 years is sense of self and loyalty.[28]

Each resolution skill has applicability to food preparation and consumption. Children 2 to 3 years of age attain self-confidence and self-control by using acceptable social skills when eating with others and only taking appropriate portions to allow enough for everyone. Allowing children to choose and prepare safe and appropriate snacks can encourage independence for 4- to 5-year-olds. Competence is exhibited by 6- to 11-year olds by preparation of simple meals and by assistance in the meal preparation for the family. A sense of self among teens occurs as they successfully negotiate complicated school schedules, extracurricular activities, or work schedules while still allowing time and energy for adequate nutrition because they value the importance of health promotion behaviors.

SUMMARY

The nutrient requirements of humans are basically the same throughout the life span. Overall, the issues of health promotion and disease prevention apply regardless of age. This chapter focuses on those issues most tied to nutrition-related concerns such as prevention of diet-related disorders (e.g., coronary artery disease, some cancers, type 2 diabetes melllitus, and obesity) and emphasizes dietary patterns rather than specific nutrients.

The life span stages reflect psychologic and physiologic maturation. They include childhood (ages 1 through 12), adolescence (ages 13 through 19), and adulthood. Approaches to health promotion take into account these stages and their impact on nutrient requirements, eating styles, and food choices. Health promotion depends on knowledge, techniques, and community supports. Each stage of development requires different approaches and is supported in various ways by the larger community. Barriers to health promotion during childhood and adolescence may include food asphyxiation, lead poisoning, obesity, iron deficiency anemia, food allergies and intolerances, and eating disorders.

THE NURSING APPROACH
Case Study #1: Toddler

Tracy, age 18 months, is visiting the family nurse practitioner (FNP) for her annual checkup. After the physical examination, the FNP asks Tracy's mom how she is eating. Tracy's mother replies, "I'm concerned; Tracy doesn't seem to be eating very well." Upon further interview, the FNP listed the mother's concerns.

"She used to eat a lot before she started walking."
Because growth slows abruptly after the first year of life, the toddler's appetite is smaller than is the infant's.

"How will I know she is getting enough food?"
The actual amount of food eaten daily will vary from one child to another. It is recommended that parents place small amounts of food on a plate and allow the child to eat it and then ask for more rather than serve a large portion that he or she cannot finish. One level tablespoon of each food per year of age served is a good start.

"What should I be primarily concerned with at this age?"
The primary dietary concern is the prevention of iron deficiency anemia. Sources of iron such as meat may be rejected. Cooked eggs, specifically the yolk, offer a valuable source of iron that can be incorporated easily.

"Are the jars of prepared foods healthy?"
The use of prepared toddler foods during the transition from infancy to early childhood presents special concerns. These products may not provide the nutrient or food range needed by the child. It is important to read the information label of all prepared foods.

"Tracy doesn't seem interested in eating."
The eating behavior and habits of the young child present one of the major barriers in providing adequate nutrition. The toddler often begins to use the meal event as an occasion to assert individuality, control of the environment, and simple exploration of food textures and qualities. Definite food preferences and food fads emerge.

Continued

THE NURSING APPROACH–cont'd
Case Study #1: Toddler

"What can I do to get her to eat?"
- Offer simple, single foods. Toddlers often reject mixtures of foods.
- Offer a variety of foods but repeat the same foods often enough so that the toddler recognizes them.
- Do not use food as a reward or punishment for behavior.
- Schedule meals and sleep periods so that the child is awake and alert during meal-time.
- Serve small portions and offer seconds after the first portion is eaten.
- Do not offer raw carrots, celery, peanuts, or other such foods that could be easily aspirated.
- Allow the toddler to self-feed; this is a major way to strengthen independence.
- Offer finger foods and allow a choice between two types of food to help promote independence.
- Serve nutritious finger foods such as pieces of chicken, slices of bananas, and pieces of cheese and crackers.

Case Study #2: Teen

Meg is a senior in high school. Her physical education teacher stopped by one day to talk to the school nurse about Meg. The teacher noticed that Meg lost a lot of weight during the school year, and although she has not missed any time from school, she appears thin, pale, introspective, and generally unhealthy. The nurse says she will call Meg in and talk to her.

When Meg arrives in the office, the nurse makes the following assessments by means of observation, Meg's health record, and some information supplied by Meg, although it is difficult to get her to talk about herself.

ASSESSMENT

Subjective
- Has lost some weight because she has been on a diet
- Believes she needs to lose more weight because she is still fat
- Feels tired but has kept up usual activity
- Claims she eats well
- Has not had her menstrual cycle for a while

Objective
- Height: 5'5"
- Weight: 125 lbs a year ago
- Current weight: 105 lbs
- Hair dull and straight
- Skin pale

NURSING DIAGNOSIS

Altered nutrition, less than body requirements, related to unwarranted desire to lose weight, as evidenced by undesirable weight loss.

The school nurse does not have enough information to confirm anorexia nervosa as the cause of the problem, but she strongly suspects that it is. She feels she has enough information to make the following plans, which she shares with Meg.

PLANNING

The nurse will call Meg's mother to share her concerns about Meg's dieting and will try to negotiate the following goals. Meg and her mother will do the following:
1. Discuss her dieting and weight loss.
2. Attempt to stop the intentional weight loss.
3. Consult with their primary care physician.

THE NURSING APPROACH–cont'd
Case Study #2: Teen

IMPLEMENTATION

1. Call Meg's mother and discuss the findings and possible dangers; find out what the parents' reaction has been to Meg's weight loss.
2. Enlist the help of Meg's mother to monitor Meg's diet until she can get professional help for Meg; encourage her to give Meg a balanced diet, even if the portions are small.
3. Ask Meg's mother to check her weight twice a week (at the same time of day and with the same clothing) until they see a physician.
4. Impress upon Meg's mother the importance of getting professional help immediately, first with the primary care physician, with possible need for a therapist specializing in eating disorders.

EVALUATION

The goals will be evaluated in 2 weeks to see if they have been met, as evidenced by the following:

- Meg's mother states that she has discussed the dieting behavior with Meg.
- No further weight loss (Meg weighing no less than 105 lbs) has occurred as measured by Meg's mother.
- An appointment has been scheduled with the primary care physician.
- The school nurse will continue to follow Meg's case to make sure she receives the help she needs.

APPLYING CONTENT KNOWLEDGE

Daphne is upset about the way her young children eat. "Although I have the nanny prepare meals for them, they just don't sit still to eat. They seem to want to just grab foods from the time they get home from school until they go to sleep." When Daphne was asked about her eating style and that of her husband, she responded, "Oh, we both work crazy hours so we don't have time to eat regular meals. We just grab a bowl of cereal or have leftovers from takeout orders." What strategies would you share with Daphne to change the eating styles of her young children?

Web Sites of Interest

The Food Allergy & Anaphylaxis Network (FAAN)
www.foodallergy.org
FAAN is a nonprofit organization devoted to educating the public about food allergies and anaphylaxis responses by providing support; research; publications such as monthly newsletters, videos, cookbooks, and "How to Read a Label" cards; and special product alert notices to assist individuals, families, and health professionals.

Kids Food CyberClub
www.kidfood.org
This site provides fun activities for kids and teens about healthy foods; lesson plans for teachers to incorporate nutrition and the Internet; and strategies for parents to help children eat well and be healthy. Sponsored by the Connecticut Association for Human Services.

KidsHealth
www.kidshealth.org
This Web site provides information for children, teens, and parents on all aspects of health, food, and fitness including games and colorful animations. It was created by the medical staff of The Nemours Foundation and is a sister site of KidsHealth at the American Medical Association.

References

1. Satter E: *How to get your kid to eat...but not too much,* Palo Alto, Calif, 1987, Bull Publishing.
2. American Dietetic Association: *Sugar myths—a trick or treat,* www.eatright.org/feature/100198.html.
3. Coon K et al.: Relationship between use of television during meals and children's food consumption patterns, *Pediatrics* 107:e7, 2001.
4. Heird WC: Nutritional requirements during infancy and childhood. In Shils ME eds.: *Modern nutrition in health and disease,* ed 9, Philadelphia, 1999, Williams & Wilkins.
5. Munoz KA et al.: Food intakes of US children and adolescents compared with recommendations, *Pediatrics* 100(3 Pt 1):323, 1997.
6. Parental health beliefs may cause failure to thrive, *Nutr Rev* 46(6):217, 1988.
7. Dixon LB et al.: The effect of changes in dietary fat on the food group and nutrient intake of 4- to 10-year-old children, *Pediatrics* 100(5):863, 1997.
8. Sanstead HH: Zinc deficiency: A public health problem? *J Diseas Childr* 145:853, 1991.
9. Food Research & Action Center, National School Lunch Program (Oct 2001); School Breakfast Program (May 2001); Summer Food Service Program for Children (Feb 2002), www.frac.org/html/federal_food_programs/federal_index.html.
10. US Department of Health and Human Services, Public Health Service: *Healthy People 2010,* ed 2, Washington, DC, 2000, US Government Printing Office; www.health.gov/healthypeople.
11. Food Research & Action Center: Federal Food Programs. www.frac.org/html/federal_food_programs/federal_index.html.
12. Revich BA: Lead in hair and urine of children and adults from industrialized areas, *Arch Environ Health* 49(1):59, 1994.
13. Brown MJ et al.: Lead poisoning in children of different ages, *N Engl J Med* 323(2):135, 1990.
14. Gottlieb K, Koehler JR: Blood lead levels in children from lower socioeconomic communities in Denver, Colorado, *Arch Environ Health* 49(4):260, 1994.
15. Dietz WH: Childhood obesity. In Shils ME eds.: *Modern nutrition in health and disease,* ed 9, Philadelphia, 1999, Williams & Wilkins.
16. Fairbanks VF: Iron in medicine and nutrition. In Shils ME eds.: *Modern nutrition in health and disease,* ed 9, Philadelphia, 1999, Williams & Wilkins.
17. Karp R: Malnutrition among children in the United States: the impact of poverty. In Shils ME eds.: *Modern nutrition in health and disease,* ed 9, Philadelphia, 1999, Williams & Wilkins.
18. Anderson JA: Tips when considering the diagnosis of food allergy, *Top Clin Nutr* 9(3):11, 1994.
19. Schepers A: Nutritional care in food allergy and food intolerance. In Mahan LK, Escott-Stump S, eds.: *Krause's food, nutrition, & diet therapy,* ed 9, Philadephia, 1996, WB Saunders.
20. Smith LJ, Munoz-Furlong A: Management of food allergy. In Metcalfe DD, Sampson HA, Simon RA, eds.: *Food allergy: adverse reactions to food and food additives,* ed 2, Cambridge, Mass, 1997, Blackwell Science.
21. Sampson HA: Diagnosis and management of food allergies. In Shils ME eds.: *Modern nutrition in health and disease,* ed 9, Philadelphia, 1999, Williams & Wilkins.
22. Grodner M: Forever dieting: chronic dieting syndrome, *J Nutr Ed* 24(4):207, 1992.
23. American Psychiatric Association: *Diagnostic and statistical manual of mental disorders (DSM-IV TR 2000),* ed 4, Washington, DC, 2000, American Psychiatric Association.
24. Hobbs WL, Johnson CA: Anorexia nervosa: an overview, *Am Fam Physician* 54(4): 1273, 1996.

25. Food and Nutrition Board, National Research Council: *Diet and health: implications for reducing chronic disease risk*, Washington, DC, 1989, National Academy Press.
26. American Dietetic Association, Position of the American Dietetic Association: Nutrition intervention in the treatment of anorexia nervosa, bulimia nervosa, and eating disorders not otherwise specified, *J Am Dietetic Assoc* 101:810, 2001.
27. Chitty KK: The primary prevention role of the nurse in eating disorders, *Nurs Clin North Am* 26:789, 1991.
28. Cowan M: Children's Health. In Stanhope M, Lancaster J, eds.: *Community health nursing: promoting health of aggregates, families, and individuals*, St Louis, 1996, Mosby.

CHAPTER 13

Life Span Health Promotion: Adulthood

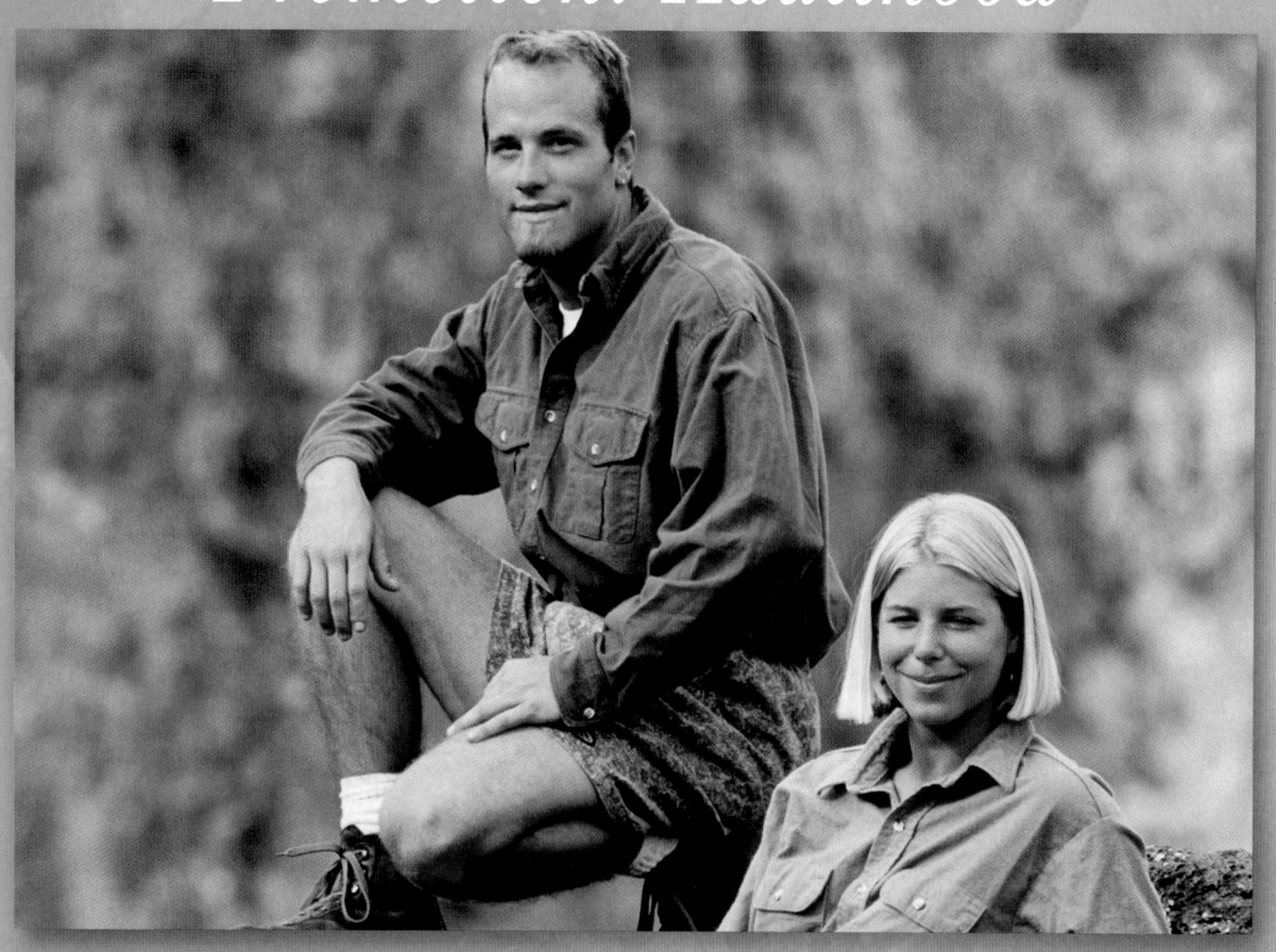

Aging is a gradual process that reflects the influence of genetics, lifestyle, and environment over the course of the life span.

ROLE IN WELLNESS

By the time young adults reach their early 20s, growth levels off and the body achieves a state of homeostasis. Mental capacity is fully developed as young people begin to assume their roles in adult society. How this transition is experienced depends on cultural views of growing older. Does growing older confer social privileges of respect and authority? Or does it mean the loss of youth and good times? How we accept new responsibilities within family and intimate relationships may affect our overall health status and level of wellness.

Layered on cultural perceptions of aging is the complexity of today's world. Through telecommunications we are exposed to and influenced by numerous world and local events in ways unimaginable to previous generations. Similarly, educational and employment opportunities seem endless; yet some adults are caught in cycles of underemployment and unemployment as the marketplace evolves, and others, through economic misfortune, are homeless. Additionally, each stage of adulthood presents particular life stressors. How we cope with these stressors and those of society affects adult nutritional status.

The five dimensions of health affect the health promotion of adulthood. Beginning health-promoting habits early in life and continuing them through older adulthood maintains physical health. Our intellect provides the ability to change and adapt as circumstances vary according to age and related responsibilities for our health. The symbolic representation and occasions defined by certain foods are often tied to our emotional well-being. Food provides a means of communication; customs surrounding eating behaviors vary between cultures and ethnic groups; exposure to these differences is rewarding and enhances social health. The support of our spiritual communities provides an added dimension to health promotion and to recovery from disease and illness.

Although previous chapters have addressed nutrition for adults, this section addresses the different influences on nutritional lifestyles through the adulthood stages of the early years (20s and 30s); the middle years (40s and 50s); the older years (60s, 70s, and 80s); and the oldest years (80s and 90s).

AGING AND NUTRITION

Aging is a gradual process that reflects the influence of genetics, lifestyle, and environment over the course of the life span. Beginning around age 30, the purpose of cell creation changes. No longer supplying new cells for growth and development, cell metabolism slows down and instead creates new cells to replace old cells. At older ages, this process of cell replication slows even more, and the effects of aging on body organs begin to appear. Some body systems are more affected than others, and the changes may begin to affect nutritional status. Other organ functions that may be altered include taste and smell, saliva secretions, swallowing difficulties, liver function, and intestinal function.[1] For example, the gastrointestinal tract functions are diminished by reduced production of gastric juices such as hydrochloric acid, which results in decreased absorption of nutrients.[1] The systems and the effects of aging are listed in Table 13-1.

How an individual body responds to these changes reflects health status across the life span. Consequently, everyone ages differently. The role of nutrition during the life span categories of adolescence through the middle years (40s and 50s) provides a foundation to adequately support body processes to effectively deal with the effects of lifestyle and environmental factors. Nutrient intake and dietary patterns directly influence the risk of developing the chronic disorders of osteoporosis, coronary artery disease, diabetes, hypertension, and obesity. The effect of nutrient intake, though, is mediated by lifestyle behaviors including physical activity, stress, smoking, alcohol consumption, and exposure to environmental factors. For example, how a young woman eats and the amount of exercise she performs affect the density of her bones

Table 13-1
Effects of Aging

Effect on Nutritional Status	Caused by	Organ Involved
↓Ability to taste salt and sweets ↓Palatability of food ↓Food intake ↓Taste and smell	↓Taste buds ↓Taste and olfactory nerve endings	Tongue and nose
Reduced sense of thirst/dry mouth Difficulty chewing	↓Saliva production	Salivary glands
Minor effects on swallowing (but may progress to dysphagia)	Muscle contractions may malfunction	Esophagus (and swallowing process)
↓Bioavailability of vitamins, minerals, proteins ↓Absorption of vitamin B_{12} and folate	↓HCl secretion and intrinsic factor ↓Pepsin	Stomach
↓Drug doses (adjustments possible to avoid overdosing)	↓Production of drug-metabolizing enzymes	Liver

Modified from Rosenberg IH, Russell RM, Bowman BB: Aging and the digestive system. In Munro HN, Danford DE, eds.: Nutrition, aging, and the elderly, New York, 1989, Plenum Press.

and the level of lean body mass of her body. If her nutrient intake is adequate and the exercise is weight bearing, she may reduce her risk of osteoporosis (as well as the risk of the other chronic disorders) decades later when she is in her 60s or 70s.

Productive Aging

The concept of productive aging considers the many psychosocial influences on successful aging. *Productive aging* refers to an overall process of aging that is dependent on attitudes and skills developed over the course of one's life. These attitudes and skills prepare an individual to adapt to the transitions of life and maintain a personal sense of experiencing a productive, meaningful life.[2] Box 13-1 lists factors of healthy aging that apply to everyone regardless of age. This list is based on the perspectives offered by intergenerational focus groups.[2] Successful aging considers that different criteria of success apply during the older years compared

Box 13-1 Factors for Healthy Aging

MEANINGFUL INVOLVEMENT

Keeping active
Functioning as a productive citizen
Remaining involved in community
Volunteering
Continuing to learn
Continuing to travel
Experiencing new things
Having meaningful work

POSITIVE MENTAL OUTLOOK

Developing good mental outlook
Feeling optimistic and hopeful
Maintaining mental and physical health
Being happy
Being joyful
Keeping an active mind
Exercising self-discipline
Being glad for every day

RELATIONSHIPS WITH OTHERS

Giving to others
Having friends
Expressing an interest in others
Displaying kindness toward others
Spending time with family
Showing concern for those with less
Helping make the world a better place

From Kerschner H, Pegues JM: Productive aging: a quality of life agenda, J Am Dietetic Assoc 98(12):1445, 1998.

Box 13-2 Fifteen Ways to Promote Successful Aging: Suggestions from Older Adults

Simplify your life; identify priorities and set limits.

Pay attention to yourself: your body, your mind, and your spirit.

Continue to teach, continue to learn; teach a class, take a class.

Plan some serious leisure activities (painting, woodwork) and do them.

Let yourself laugh and let yourself cry—both are important.

Be flexible; learn to navigate change.

Be charitable; make it a practice to give (wisdom, experience, money, time, yourself).

Be financially astute; invest early for retirement.

Get a life; you'll live better in retirement if you do.

Practice good nutrition and exercise; discover your internal and external motivators.

Think about your past and future; write your autobiography.

Be involved; discover what has meaning for you.

Be positive; have hope and believe there is a tomorrow.

Link with others—relationships are important.

Become mortal and deal with your mortality.

From Kershner H, Pegues JM: Productive aging: a quality of life agenda, J Am Dietetic Assoc 98(12):1445, 1998.

with those of the earlier life span categories. Box 13-2 is a list of 15 ways to promote successful aging that was developed from suggestions by older adults.[2]

STAGES OF ADULTHOOD

The Early Years (20s and 30s)

Students tend to imagine that once they finish high school or college and enter the working world they will then be able to eat better, sleep more, and generally take better care of themselves than they do during their hectic school years. Unfortunately, that is rarely the experience of young adults. Many find that their lifestyles may be even more time-restricted, and positive health behaviors such as regular meal patterns and exercise may fall by the wayside.

These years mark a transition from one stage of the life span to another; young adults separate from their family of origin, focus on personal and career goals, and often face reproductive decisions. As such, it is a prime time to either refine or establish an eating style that promotes health, possibly preventing future development of diet-related diseases. The 1989-1991 Continuing Survey of Food Intakes by Individuals reports that only 1% of American adults have a food pattern that includes all five food-group recommendations.[3] A self-review or assessment by a nutrition professional can assist in creating a personal schedule that allows time for planning and preparation of simple yet high quality meals.

Many women bear children during these years. The nutrition and health requirements of pregnancy are detailed in Chapter 11. Layered on these needs during this life span stage are often employment and other family commitments, all of which affect nutritional and health behaviors. Physically caring for young children, although eminently rewarding, may be exhausting. Throughout the mother's pregnancy and during childbearing, the father's role in terms of health issues is often ignored. Although the woman's body is nourishing fetal development, the father is under stress as he prepares to support additional responsibilities. Fathers also need to be at optimum health, especially during the first few years of childrearing when physical stamina is put to the test.

Nutrition Requirements

Growth tends to be completed by the late teens for women and early 20s for men, as reflected by the Dietary Reference Intake (DRI) (see the inside front cover). For women, the Recommended Dietary Allowance (RDA) for energy is 2200 kcalories daily; for men, it is 2900 kcalories. This reflects the typical differences in body weight and lean body mass of men and women. When this stage includes a departure from high school or college sports training, energy intake should be reduced to meet actual need, otherwise weight gain could occur. A teenage boy's serious athletic training may require as much as 5000 to 6000 kcalories a day to maintain weight. Switching to a desk job and exercising for 1 hour per day does not equal previous energy requirements.

The RDA for protein increases for women from 46 grams to 50 grams and for men from 58 grams to 63 grams daily; these ranges reflect lean body mass growth that may still occur in both men and women through about age 24. Vitamin and mineral needs do not significantly change. Calcium and phosphorus needs for men and women decline after age 18 because skeletal growth is almost complete. Daily Adequate Intake (AI) recommended calcium levels up to age 18 are 1300 mg, dropping to 1000 mg from 19 years on. For phosphorus, RDA levels up to age 18 are 1250 mg a day, dropping to 700 mg from 19 years on. Maintaining calcium and iron intake continues to be a concern for women because of their often-restricted intake of food during dieting.

The Middle Years (40s and 50s)

The years from 40 to 50 are marked by a continuation of family demands and career involvement. Some middle-year adults may be faced with caring for aging parents; this increased stress and responsibility may be offset by the seemingly reduced parenting of their own children. As older children leave for college or move into their own residences, the resultant "empty nest" necessitates rediscovering preparation of dinners for two or, for single parents, dinners for one. With family meals no longer a requirement, many middle-year adults often have the finances and time for restaurant dining. However, making the transition to food preparation styles and dietary patterns that maintain healthful dietary patterns is crucial.

The impact of continued positive dietary patterns coupled with regular exercise provides continued prevention or delay of diet-related diseases such as type 2 diabetes mellitus (type 2 DM) and coronary artery disease. Increased stamina is an additional benefit from such behaviors.

Nutrition Requirements

During the middle years, cell loss rather than replication occurs. Kcaloric needs decline as lean body mass is lost and replaced by body fat that is less metabolically active. Women in particular experience an increase in body fat composition. Body fat increases can be slowed by exercise and strength training to continue maintenance of lean body mass. After age 50, daily energy needs drop from 2200 kcalories to 1920 kcalories for women and from 2900 kcalories to 2300 kcalories for men. It is a challenge to meet the same nutrient needs with reduced kcaloric intake. Protein needs remain constant for both genders. Iron requirements for women drop from 18 mg to 8 mg, which reflects reduced iron loss because of menopause.

Overall, dietary patterns that are nutrient-dense and feature lower-fat protein foods coupled with fiber-containing fruits, vegetables, and grains best meet the nutrient needs of middle-year adults.

The Older Years (60s, 70s, and 80s)

The United States has never had a population with as high a percentage of older adults as it will soon have. As our life span increases in years, senescence (older adulthood) is for many a time of life for continued professional or career advancement and recreational enjoyment. Others are in transition, adjusting to retirement and settling into new patterns of activities. Gerontology, the study of aging, has provided insights into the emotional, physical, and social aspects of the

senescence
older adulthood

gerontology
the study of aging

later years of life. Preparation for the social and physical transitions of aging actually begins many years earlier, as individual approaches to lifestyle health behaviors, career fulfillment, and leisurely pursuits evolve.

The level of wellness experienced during this stage of life often reflects health behaviors through the several life span stages. A lifetime of physical fitness and good nutrition allows an individual to enter these years with more stamina, cardiovascular conditioning, and solid health-promoting habits that enable him or her to overcome the inevitable slowing down or physical limitation of the later years. Even those who were not always active have been shown to benefit from regular exercise. Strength training has improved muscle tone and stamina of men and women in their 80s.[4]

During these later years, individuals may struggle with the deaths of family members and friends and adjustment to retirement. Although some delight in retirement, others view retirement as a loss of social status. This combination of death and loss of status may lead to isolation and depression. The economic realities of retirement without a solid financial base may thrust some older adults into unexpected poverty, because Social Security and Medicare payments may not be sufficient to adequately cover living and medical expenses. Unless social networking and family supports are strong, these conditions may persist. Older adults may abuse alcohol as a way to deal with these perceived difficult events.

Disorientation or senility often associated with aging may be caused by improper use of medications, marginal nutrient deficiencies (e.g., vitamin B_{12}), or simple dehydration. Older clients may intentionally restrict fluids because of incontinence, nocturia, or inability to get to the toilet on their own. Some older adults lose their sense of thirst and forget to consume enough fluids. Fluid requirements in older adults remain the same as in younger adults (about 8 cups a day) unless a medical condition or medication prescribe otherwise. The signs of dehydration are listed in Box 13-3. Medical diagnosis should be sought to determine the specific etiology of these signs.

Nutrition status may be affected by restricted access to food and ability to prepare meals. Shopping may be difficult without transportation, and mobility to walk through stores may be limited. Funds for food may be constrained, and often food quantities available are beyond the amounts that can be used by individuals living alone. Once foods are purchased, preparation may be affected by physical limitations caused by progressive chronic illnesses such as arthritis. Some older adults may no longer have an interest in cooking. Others have become so frightened about foods that contain too much fat or cholesterol that they become malnourished. For individuals in this age bracket, there is not sufficient evidence to warrant restrictive dietary intake; in actuality, malnutrition and underweight are more detrimental than excess dietary fat and cholesterol intake. Box 13-4 lists strategies to increase food intake and promote good nutrition.

Living arrangements also affect nutritional status. A variety of living arrangements exist for older adults. Although many continue to live in their own homes or with family members, some opt for retirement communities and others, because of health conditions, may reside in long-term care facilities or nursing homes. Living in one's own home provides the freedom to prepare and eat foods whenever

nocturia
excessive urination at night

Box 13-3 Signs of Dehydration in Older Adults

Confusion	Decreased skin turgor (may not be valid
Weakness	finding in older adults)
A hot, dry body	Rapid pulse
Furrowed tongue	Elevated urinary sodium

Box 13-4 Strategies for Overcoming Barriers to Good Nutrition

COUNTERACT DECREASED SENSES OF TASTE AND SMELL

Recommend smokers refrain from smoking at least 1 hour before meals.

Suggest sipping water before and during the meal to moisten a dry mouth.

Amplify flavors with the use of seasonings other than salt.

Recommend chewing food thoroughly to fully release flavor and aroma.

Vary food textures and flavors.

ENCOURAGE SOCIAL INTERACTION

Find others who are willing to share food preparation and mealtimes.

Investigate congregate meal programs available through senior citizen centers, religious organizations, and hospital community outreach programs.

Avoid noisy dining areas if hearing aids are used.

PRESENT FOOD ATTRACTIVELY

Use colorful foods and table settings.

Provide enough lighting to see food clearly.

PROVIDE OUTSIDE SUPPORT

Arrange for Meals-on-Wheels for homebound adults.

Refer eligible clients to the Food Stamp Program, Emergency Food Assistance Program, Child and Adult Care Program, or community food banks or soup kitchens.

Locate grocery stores with delivery service.

Refer to the Expanded Food and Nutrition Education Program (EFNEP) of the Cooperative Extension Service for recipes, meal suggestions, and budgeting assistance.

Refer to home health nurse for routine nutrition screening and appropriate interventions.

---

desired; illness, however, may make shopping for food and preparing it difficult. Retirement communities may provide transportation to food stores and more social events involving meals, although residents still are responsible for their own food preparation. Long-term care facilities usually provide prepared meals, but the style of cooking may not be as appealing or comforting as home-prepared meals.

A challenge for meeting the nutritional needs of institutionalized older adults is that the DRIs used to guide nutrient levels are intended to meet the needs of *healthy* older adults. Adjustments are necessary for individual circumstances of acute or chronic illness to achieve rehabilitation, recuperation, or maintenance to reduce the risk of further complications.[5] Consequently, it is now recommended that diets in long-term care facilities be liberalized to improve dietary intake of this age group.[6]

Dietary patterns and preferences of older adults are the result of long-established habits. When they are ill, lonely, or under stress, older adults may strongly prefer foods they associate with pleasant memories. Ethnic favorites may provide security and comfort. The psychologic and social meanings

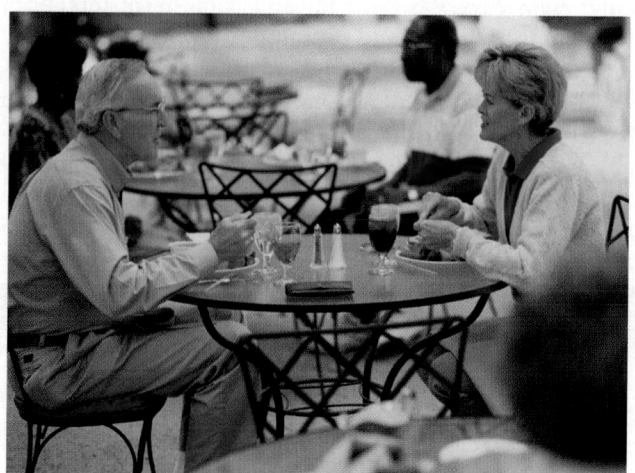

Companionship makes mealtimes more enjoyable for older adults. (From PhotoDisc.)

of foods can play an important part in helping an older client recover from illness or adjust to changed circumstances.

Overall, older adults may be at nutritional risk because of demographic and lifestyle characteristics. Factors may include gender, smoking, alcohol abuse, dietary patterns, educational level, dental health, chronic illnesses, and living situations. Interventions to assist older adults need to account for these influences and should view support services through a continuum of care. Continuum of care provides continuity of care while the older individual moves through different living situations and services as health, medical, and supportive services are provided in suitable care environments. Care settings may range from acute medical settings to community and day care, from assisted-living retirement housing to traditional nursing home facilities and hospices.[6]

Nutrition Requirements

The DRIs remain constant from age 51 and older for men and women, except for vitamin D. What does change is the ability of the body to either process or synthesize certain nutrients. Synthesis of vitamin D is reduced; the AI for vitamin D for individuals older than age 70 increases to 15 mcg a day compared with 10 mcg a day for ages 51 to 70 years. Older adults either need more exposure to sunlight to produce required amounts of vitamin D or require a supplement if so diagnosed by a physician, qualified nutritionist, or dietitian. Because of decreased production of gastric juices and intestinal enzymes, digestion and absorption may be reduced, further highlighting the need for optimum nutrient intake. The production of the intrinsic factor required for vitamin B_{12} absorption may also be reduced, increasing the risk of pernicious anemia. New recommendations suggest the use of vitamin B_{12} supplements or consumption of foods fortified with vitamin B_{12} to meet the RDA of 2.4 mcg per day.

Other factors may affect nutritional status. A marginal deficiency of zinc can alter the sensitivity of taste receptors. This deficiency heightens the ability to taste bitter and sour flavors and reduces sweet and salty sensations; excessive use of sugars and salt to make foods taste appealing may result.

Overconsumption of simple sugars and sodium may exacerbate other diet-related disorders such as diabetes and hypertension. As the muscularity of the digestive system weakens, constipation may be a problem, especially after a lifetime of low-fiber foods. Constipation may be alleviated by slowly increasing consumption of whole-wheat products, fruits, vegetables, and fluids, as well as increasing exercise.

Dental health may also affect the ability of older adults to be well nourished. Loss of teeth caused by periodontal disease limits the ability to chew foods such as meats, a prime source of zinc. Chewing ability for some may still be compromised even after dentures have been fitted to replace missing teeth. Dentures may need to be periodically refitted. When dentures do not fit properly, some people do not use them. Instead, they tend to eat foods that can be gummed rather than chewed.

The Oldest Years (80s and 90s)

As life expectancy increases in years, the number of those in the most golden years rises. Although nutrient needs remain basically stable, the effects of aging may continue to reduce the ability of the body to absorb and synthesize nutrients. Optimum nutrition continues to be critical. The healthiest of the oldest develop individual patterns of dietary intake that most meet their physical and social needs.

Nutrition Requirements

Malnutrition and underweight become concerns during this stage.[4] Risk factors for malnutrition are listed in Box 13-5. As food preparation becomes more physically difficult to accomplish, kcaloric intake may diminish. Illness and accompanying medications may reduce appetite; malnutrition is associated with increased com-

Box 13-5 Risk Factors for Malnutrition of Older Adults

Alcoholism
Anorexia
Chewing and swallowing problems
  (dysphagia)
Consuming only one meal a day
Dental difficulties
Depression or dementia
Diabetes
Diminished physical functioning
Feeding problems

Food purchasing/preparation difficulties
Impaired acuity of taste and smell
Living in long-term care institution
Loss of spouse
Multi-medications
Nerve disorders
Poverty
Pulmonary disease
Surgery

Reference: Chernoff R: Nutrition and health promotion in older adults, J Gerontol Med Sci 56A (Spec Iss 2):M47-M53, 2001. Copyright © The Gerontological Society of America. Reproduced by permission of the publisher.

plications. Relatives, friends, and healthcare professionals can assist in ensuring that adequate meals are available and consumed (see Box 13-4). Those in the oldest years may be most at risk for dehydration. Particularly at risk are African Americans and men. Risk increases because of decreased ability of kidneys to concentrate urine, limited movement, drug interactions, and malfunctioning thirst sensation. Limited ability to move may increase fears of incontinence that leads to decreased fluid intake. Nearly half of older adults hospitalized as Medicare patients experience dehydration.[6]

Although assessment is the responsibility of all healthcare professionals, home health nurses are particularly able to conduct routine nutrition screening and implement appropriate interventions to prevent or halt malnutrition among this population[7] (see the accompanying Teaching Tool box). Government and community meal programs help fill this need and are discussed in "Community Supports" later in this chapter.

ADULT HEALTH PROMOTION

Knowledge

Health promotion integrates nutrition education and focuses on three areas of knowledge: (1) adequate intake of nutrients found in foods (rather than supplements), (2) the relationship between diet and disease, and (3) moderate kcaloric intake coupled with regular exercise for physical fitness and obesity prevention.

Techniques

Several *Healthy People 2010* objectives address the preceding key concepts.[8] Other strategies for adult health promotion include the following.

To promote and maintain positive health status and to reduce risk of diet-related disorders (coronary heart disease, some cancers, type 2 DM, and obesity):[8]

- Schedule routine food shopping so staples such as fruits, vegetables, and grains are available for meal preparation.
- When shopping, occasionally compare fat content of commonly purchased foods to similar products; purchase the lower-fat product.
- Aim to limit visible fat-containing foods.
- Reorganize work and personal priorities if necessary to allow time for meal preparation and consumption; for example, get up earlier for breakfast, pack a lunch or afternoon snack, preplan easy-to-prepare dinner menus.

TEACHING TOOL
Nutrition Screening Initiative

As the risk of malnutrition among older adults become recognized, the American Dietetic Association, the American Academy of Family Physicians, and the National Council on Aging developed the Nutrition Screening Initiative (NSI) project to identify individuals older than 65 who are at nutritional risk. A simple-to-use screening tool is based on key risk factors that may represent determinants of undernutrition or malnutrition. Individuals or caregivers who can consult with a health professional for further guidance can use the tool.

DETERMINE YOUR NUTRITIONAL HEALTH

The warning signs of poor nutritional health are often overlooked. Use this checklist to find out if you or someone you know is at nutritional risk.

Read the statements below. Circle the number in the *yes* column for those that apply to you or someone you know. For each *yes* answer, score the number in the box. Total your nutritional score.

	Yes
• I have an illness or condition that made me change the kind or amount of food I eat.	2
• I eat fewer than two meals per day.	3
• I eat few fruits, vegetables, or milk products.	2
• I have three or more drinks of beer, liquor, or wine almost every day.	2
• I have tooth or mouth problems that make it hard for me to eat.	2
• I don't always have enough money to buy the food I need.	4
• I eat alone most of the time.	1
• I take three or more different prescribed or over-the-counter drugs a day.	1
• Without wanting to, I have lost or gained 10 lbs in the last 6 months.	2
• I am not always physically able to shop, cook, and feed myself.	2
Total	

TOTAL YOUR NUTRITIONAL SCORE

0-2   *Good!* Recheck your nutritional score in 6 months.

3-5   *You are at moderate nutritional risk.* See what can be done to improve your eating habits and lifestyle. Your office on aging, senior nutrition program, senior citizens center, or health department can help. Recheck your nutritional score in 3 months.

6 or more *You are at high nutritional risk.* Bring this checklist the next time you see your doctor, dietitian, or other qualified health or social service professional. Talk with them about any problems you may have. Ask for help to improve your nutritional health.

From the Nutrition Screening Initiative, a project of American Academy of Family Physicians, American Dietetic Association, and National Council on the Aging and funded in part by a grant from Ross Laboratories, a division of Abbott Laboratories.

- Keep track of dietary intake using the Food Guide Pyramid or 5 A Day plan. Review Chapter 5 for other dietary fat-lowering techniques and Chapter 4 for approaches that increase use of complex carbohydrates and fiber-containing foods. For overall bone health and to reduce the risk of osteoporosis:[8]
- Focus on routine dietary habits; for example, drink a glass of milk at lunch each day. A food pattern assessment can assist in creating a practical calcium consumption plan. Review Chapter 8 for other approaches to increasing calcium consumption.

  To reduce risk of coronary artery disease and sodium-sensitive hypertension:[8]
- Check food labels to determine sodium content.

- Learn food categories that are generally salty and either consume them only occasionally or, if available, purchase low-sodium versions of products. See Chapter 8 for other sodium-reducing strategies.
- Reduce overall fat intake, particularly saturated fat.

To attain appropriate body weight and to reduce risk of obesity caused by diet and lifestyle:[8]

- Rather than focusing on food-restricting diets, respond to actual hunger with low-fat, high-fiber foods (with occasional splurges).
- Exercise regularly to increase stamina, strength, and a sense of wellness. Depending on conditioning, incorporate exercise gradually. A 10-minute walk may be comfortable for some; others can begin with more strenuous endeavors.

See Chapters 9 and 10 for related strategies (see also the accompanying Cultural Considerations box).

Community Supports

Government, corporate, and social institutions create the environments and structures that can support lifestyle health promotion behaviors. Although the actions of these institutions affect groups of the public, employees, or communities, it is the individual who can choose to reap the rewards.

CULTURAL CONSIDERATIONS
Diet Quality and Aging

The Healthy Eating Index (HEI), previously introduced in Chapter 2, evaluates the overall quality of an individual's dietary intake based on 10 components. Each component is worth up to 10 points so that the HEI has a range of 0 to 100. The higher the score, the better the dietary intake. The first five components use the *Dietary Guidelines for Americans* and the Food Guide Pyramid as measures of dietary adequacy. The other five components consider the total fat, saturated fat, cholesterol, and sodium intake and the variety of foods consumed.

The most recent HEI (1994-1996) provides assessment of dietary intake based on cultural and racial subgroups. Of these subgroups, the mean score for African Americans is 59 compared with 64 for Caucasians and 65 for other racial groups (i.e., Asian/Pacific Islanders, Native Americans, and native people of Greenland and Alaska). Although most people in all groups consume diets that need improvement, 28% of African Americans have poor diets, while only 16% of Caucasians and 14% of the other racial groups scored in this category. Overall the lower levels of milk products consumed by African Americans, who are more likely to experience lactose intolerance, may affect scores.

All groups have similar scores during the early childhood years. Differences become apparent by the 19- to 50-year-old age groups. These differences become smaller as African Americans enter the 51 and older age group.

Other issues are faced by different subgroups. Older Caucasians are faced with the use of many drugs (polypharmacy) and the inadequate intake of nutrients. Both of these issues relate to the level of functional ability of older adults as influenced by depression, low income, and eating problems. Among African Americans, older urban individuals were at nutritional risk because of dental problems such as tooth pain and chewing difficulties. Intakes of vitamin E, vitamin B_6, calcium, zinc, fiber, and energy were low. Cholesterol and fat intakes were high among a group of older African American women surveyed in a large-scale study. Older Hispanic Americans may be more at risk for inadequate consumption of nutrients because of dental problems, difficulty preparing meals, and limited income. Older Asian/Pacific Islanders from China, Korea, and Japan who reside in senior citizen housing were more likely to be underweight than overweight with particularly low intakes of calcium. Compared with all subgroups, older Native Americans are most at risk for chronic disorders such as types 1 or 2 DM, heart disease, arthritis, cancer, and fractured bones. In particular, the risk of type 2 DM among Native Americans and Inuits is three to five times greater than the general population, with women most at risk.

Application to nursing: Awareness of HEI scores begins to direct our concerns about the nutrient status of our clients. Studies provide details about particular factors that may affect nutritional status of specific subgroups. Although this information has value, we still need to consider the situation of each client as he or she proceeds through the aging process.

Reference: Position of the American Dietetic Association: Nutrition, aging, and the continuum of care, J Am Dietetic Assoc 100:580, 2000; and USDA Center for Nutrition Policy and Promotion: Report card on the diet quality of African Americans, Nutrition Insights, July 1998.

Government agencies such as the Food and Drug Administration create regulations that either provide consumers information for decision making (e.g., nutrition labeling) or that control the quality of foods, which in turn affects the nutrient viability of manufactured products.

Food manufacturers as an institution were challenged by the earlier *Healthy People 2000* to increase to at least 5000 brand items the availability of processed food products that are reduced in fat and saturated fat. This objective was achieved.[8] The intent of this objective was to make it easier for consumers to reduce their intake of fat and saturated fat through manufactured products. Not all health professionals are in favor of this approach. Some suggest that it is better to choose foods that are naturally low in fat than to consume prefabricated foods that may lose other nutritious properties during the manufacturing process.

Another objective of the earlier *Healthy People 2000* objectives concerns eating outside of the home. The purpose of this objective is to increase to at least 90% of the proportion of restaurants and institutional food service operations that offer identifiable low-fat, low-calorie food choices, consistent with the *Dietary Guidelines for Americans*.[8] It has been difficult to assess progress toward this objective because the operational definition of food choices is so broad.

Nonetheless, awareness about lower fat choices has been raised. The American Heart Association has a program called *Heart Healthy*; its purpose is to help the public identify food choices on restaurant menus that are low in fat, sodium, and cholesterol. Health professionals can request that these food choices be available and be highlighted on menus, especially at the food service institutions that serve our patients. Our professional organizations can also request these changes of restaurants, especially of national restaurant corporations. Many retail and food service institutions already meet the guidelines; specific entrees need to be identified as an educative service for consumers and patients.

Corporations can support health promotion activities. This issue is addressed in the *Healthy People 2010* objective to increase the proportion of worksites that offer a comprehensive employee health promotion program to their employees.[8]

This can be accomplished through wellness centers that provide programs about healthy lifestyles. Although most corporations may not be able to provide on-site gyms or similar facilities, some have arranged for corporate discounts at local gym facilities. Perhaps the leader of on-site wellness centers is the Nike corporate headquarters on the Nike World Campus in Beaverton, Oregon. Employees are able to use the Bo Jackson Fitness Center, a state of the art health club facility, for a nominal fee and run on an outdoor jogging trail that encircles the Nike campus. Boats are even available to sail on the lake that is a centerpiece of the corporate headquarters. In addition, employees can take longer lunch breaks, even 2-hour breaks, which allows for complete workouts.[9]

Health departments, through their health officers, often provide community programming that meets the next two objectives.

1. *Increase the proportion of local health service areas/jurisdictions that have established a community health promotion initiative that addresses multiple* Healthy People 2010 *focus areas.*[8]
2. *Increase the proportion of local health departments that have established culturally appropriate and linguistically competent community health promotion and disease prevention programs for racial and ethnic minority populations.*[8]

Government agencies and community groups provide socioeconomic support within the community. Government programs include the Food Stamp Program, Emergency Food Assistance Program, and community food banks and meals.

The Food Stamp Program provides coupons toward the purchase of foods for people with low incomes. By boosting food purchasing power, overall nutrient intake is improved. This program is administered nationally by the U.S. Department

of Agriculture (USDA) and on the state and local levels by welfare or human services agencies. The federal government pays the actual food stamp cost; administration costs are divided among the other agencies.

As an entitlement program, the Food Stamp Program is available to all who are
eligible without restriction of age or family size. Financial and nonfinancial factors
of households are considered to determine eligibility. Financial factors include income and economic resources such as savings or vehicles; nonfinancial considerations consist of a variety of factors such as social security eligibility, citizenship,
and work requirements. Gross incomes must meet certain percentages of the
poverty level based on overall factors; the level of support varies based on family
membership and net income.[10]

The Food and Nutrition Service of the USDA administers the Emergency Food
Assistance Program (TEMFAP). Various local agencies may administer the program. State agencies determine their own criteria for eligibility based on household
income. The program serves two functions: (1) to reduce government-held surplus
dairy commodities and (2) to supplement the dietary intake of low-income households through the distribution of basic commodities. The types of foods distributed vary between actual surplus foods and foods purchased especially for this
program. In addition to dairy products of nonfat dry milk and cheese, TEMFAP
has distributed canned meat, peanut butter, citrus juices, legumes, dried potatoes,
and canned and dried fruit. Some of this program's funds are used by states to fund
emergency feeding programs such as soup kitchens or food banks.[10]

Community food banks and emergency feeding programs may be partially
funded by TEMFAP in addition to support by foundations and other charitable organizations. Some programs also collect food from the surrounding community
and surplus donations from supermarkets and restaurants. Personnel at these facilities are usually volunteers from youth groups, religious organizations, and civic
associations. Food banks often provide a bag of food staples to help bridge the gap
that may occur when food stamps and monthly welfare support are exhausted before the beginning of the next month. Emergency feeding programs such as soup
kitchens may provide hot meals as a safety net to assist individuals among lower
socioeconomic populations to avoid malnutrition.[10]

Supports specifically for older adults include the Child and Adult Care Food
Program and the Senior Nutrition Program. Community groups may sponsor
some of the government programs or may develop their own local programs to
meet the following objective:

*Increase to at least 80% the receipt of home food services by people aged 65
and older who have difficulty in preparing their own meals or are otherwise in
need of home-delivered meals.*[8]

Little progress was made on this objective from *Healthy People 2000*. The number of people served by these programs has not increased significantly since the
early 1990s.[8]

The Child and Adult Care Food Program provides meals and snacks for children up to age 12 and to senior citizens and specific categories of handicapped persons participating in day care programs that are nonprofit, licensed, or receive
agency approval. Reimbursement rates differ for programs that serve children and
adults. Family income of the participants may be considered. Similar to other programs, it is administered on the federal level by the Food and Nutrition Service of
the USDA and on the state level by human services or education departments.
Adult day care programs may be administered locally by a variety of community
sponsors. For children, eligible programs include Head Start, after-school programs, family day care, and other approved sites.[10]

The Senior Nutrition Program serves only older adults and was created to offer
inexpensive meals, education, and socialization. The Congregate Meals Program
and Home-Delivered Meals Program are both part of the Senior Nutrition Pro-

gram. This program provides for those in financial need as well as for those in social need. Eligibility is open to everyone aged 60 years or older; spouses of participants may also be served regardless of their age. To participate in the Home-Delivered Meals Program, individuals must reside in the program service area and be unable to prepare their own meals. Meals are generally provided Monday through Friday. Those receiving meals at home may also be given frozen meals for weekend consumption.[10] Distribution of meals varies among programs.

OVERCOMING BARRIERS

Food Asphyxiation

Older adults may be at risk for asphyxiation of food because of reduced chewing ability from loss of teeth or poorly fitting dentures. Conditions such as Parkinson's Disease and effects of stroke may result in chewing and swallowing difficulties (dysphagia) that may cause asphyxiation. Counseling older adults about problematic foods may avert asphyxiation occurrences. Referrals to a registered dietitian with expertise in these disorders should be considered.

Stress

Stress can affect all aspects of well-being. Although the actual cause of stress may not be related to dietary intake and meal patterns, nutrient intake may be altered. The *normal* stresses of contemporary life may lead individuals to be so busy that they forget to eat or do not make appropriate food selections, particularly for breakfast and lunch. Some may overeat to soothe their nerves, and others may lose their appetite totally. If these actions become habitual, inappropriate eating patterns reduce the ability to cope with stressors.

Other impediments may occur. Stress may lead the gastrointestinal tract to overfunction and thus produce excessive gastric juices. The resulting indigestion may lead to the potential development of peptic ulcers. The anxiety of stress could also cause loss of appetite, which further reduces nutrient intake and can affect the absorption of nutrients, including minerals, protein, and vitamin C. Emotional stress increases the release of some hormones such as adrenaline. Adrenaline has a role in the breakdown of bone tissue during bone remodeling. Excess production of adrenaline in response to repetitive stressors affects bone health and is a potential risk factor for osteoporosis. The stressors of everyday life may occasionally cause an increase of urinary nitrogen output; however, the amount is not significant. Extreme levels of stress caused by environmental or physiologic factors can substantially increase nitrogen loss, requiring therapeutic intervention; these interventions are detailed in Chapter 15.

Women's Health Issues

Adult women must take responsibility for their own nutritional intake, but most often they are also the caregivers and food and nutrition gatekeepers who influence the nutritional status of multiple generations within their families. Consequently, health promotion activities, services, and other medical/educational efforts should support women to adopt appropriate nutritional approaches to achieve health and wellness. The diseases for which women are most at risk include osteoporosis, coronary artery disease, hypertension, certain cancers, diabetes, and potential weight-related disorders.[11] These health problems are most common among minority women who are more at risk for these chronic diseases. Their access to preventive and medical care may be limited by greater incidence of poverty and other socioeconomic factors that further impair their health status.[11] Although these disorders are discussed in detail throughout this textbook, specific concerns for women regarding breast cancer and related issues are presented here.

Breast Cancer

Breast cancer affects one out of nine North American women. Although breast cancer is probably caused by a combination of factors, diet may play a role in preventing or slowing the course of the disorder. The exact relationship of breast cancer to diet has been considered through dietary fat intake, but results are still inconclusive. Theories focus on the consumption of high-fat diets that are associated with more quickly developing breast tumors. A possible connection is that dietary fat increases hormones (estrogen and prostaglandins) that may increase breast cancers. Another view is that the immune system is compromised by the consumption of dietary fat.[11]

Regardless of the mechanism, consumption of fruits, vegetables, and whole grains may decrease the risk of breast cancer while also reducing the risk of colon cancer, another cancer common to women. Although genetics appear to be a factor in the development of colon cancer, studies also show a relationship between colon cancer and dietary fat intake. In particular, dietary intakes high in animal fat and low in dietary fiber increase risk.[11]

Menopause

Recommendations to increase fruits, vegetables, and grains not only possibly reduce cancer risk but also address the increased risk for coronary artery disease for which women are more at risk after menopause. Menopause is characterized by the decreased production of estrogen and progesterone, which results in the termination of menses. For about 3 to 7 years before menopause, a range of symptoms may be experienced, including changes in menstruation, night sweats, hot flashes, insomnia, loss of bone density, and mood swings. This cluster of symptoms is called perimenopause.

Controversy continues regarding whether such symptoms should be treated with hormone replacement therapy (HRT), which often reduces the effects of perimenopause and menopause, or whether to proceed with the natural course of female physiology without the use of HRT. Another alternative approach has been to consume foods containing phytoestrogens, particularly soybean products, which appear to replicate some of the functions of estrogen. This function, though, is not nutritional but is actually pharmacologic. The drawback to this approach is that it does not confer the other protective benefits of HRT. HRT also slows the loss of bone density, decreasing the risk of osteoporosis and possibly decreasing the risk of coronary artery disease to the level of premenopause. Decisions regarding HRT need to take into account a woman's genetic and medical history and personal beliefs about aging because of the possible increase in risk of endometrial and breast cancer from HRT.

Overall, an increased intake of fruits, vegetables, and whole grains—including calcium-containing foods—accompanied by decreased consumption of dietary fat—especially animal-derived fat—is appropriate to provide a solid nutritional basis as women progress through the life span. This dietary pattern provides possible protection for all diet-related chronic disorders.

Men's Health Issues

Although most major health research studies have used men, particularly Caucasian men, as research subjects, the emphasis on male-only health issues is not as great as it is for the female health issues, such as menopause and breast can-

menopause
the end of menstruation because of the cessation of ovarian and follicular function

perimenopause
the time before menopause during which hormonal, biologic, and clinical changes begin to occur

cer. With the exception of testicular cancer and prostate cancer, other health obstacles also affect women as well as men. Consequently, the discussion on alcohol abuse also has significance for women, although it has a higher incidence
among men.

Alcohol

Alcohol is the most commonly used drug in the United States. Although both men
and women use it, the death rate from alcohol abuse is more than twice as high for
men as for women (11.7 per 100,000 for men and only 5.2 for women). African
American men are at even greater risk for alcohol abuse; their alcohol-related
death rate is three times that for women (17.4 and 5.2 per 100,000, respectively).[12]
Native Americans are most at risk for chronic alcohol ingestion problems. Alcohol
abuse is severe among this group and affects the physical, mental, social, and economic well-being of many Native Americans. Excessive alcohol consumption is associated with violent crimes, birth defects, suicide, and sexual and domestic abuse.
The pattern of excessive intake often begins during adolescence and continues
through the adult years.[12]

Chronic consumption of large amounts of alcohol affects nutritional status.
Appetite is diminished and is associated with limited nutrient absorption, metabolism, excretion, and further increases the effects of aging. Other medical and
social problems emerge. Medical conditions include cirrhosis of the liver and
cancer of the liver and gastrointestinal tract, including the mouth, pharynx, larynx, and esophagus.[1] Social problems include impaired driving while intoxi-
cated, which has resulted in significant mortality and morbidity. Family functioning may also be altered when excessive consumption of alcohol begins to
affect an individual's ability to parent and to function in the work setting. Community resources are available to help individuals reduce their consumption of
alcohol.[1]

Prostate Cancer

Although diet-related cancers such as colon cancer are discussed under "Women's
Health Issues," men are also at risk for such cancers. Prostate cancer, of course, affects men only and is most likely a result of multifactorial causes including genetics, hormones, environment, virus, and diet.[12] Prostate cancer is noted for an association with fat intake, particularly saturated fat. It appears that consumption of
animal fat is most closely associated with the aggressive prostate cancer that is
most lethal. As with breast and colon cancer, increased consumption of fruits, vegetables, and whole grains that lowers intake of animal-derived saturated fat may
not only reduce risk of these cancers but is heart healthy and may also help reduce
blood pressure and decrease risk of type 2 DM. Men older than age 40 should be
encouraged to undergo an annual digital rectal examination or other form of
prostate cancer screening because overt symptoms may not occur until the cancer
is advanced. Prostate cancer is the most common cancer among American men,
with an incidence of 89 per 1000 men.[13] African American men have a 45% higher
incidence rate than other Americans.[13]

TOWARD A POSITIVE NUTRITION
LIFESTYLE: RATIONALIZING

Rationalization is one of the psychologic defense mechanisms used to protect our
sense of self when we are under stress. When our behaviors, feelings, or perceptions are irrational or unreasonable, we may use rationalization to assign reasonable explanations to ourselves as to why we behaved as we did.

For example, from adolescence on through the older years, some individuals rationalize their poor eating habits. The list of reasonable explanations may include not enough time to prepare better meals, lack of knowledge of nutrition, or lack of cooking skills. Although these may be reasonable explanations, they do not help improve nutritional status. Often these types of rationalizations make it harder to change unproductive behaviors.

Consider the same explanations in a more positive way.

- Not enough time to prepare better meals but can reorganize schedule to create time.
- Lack of knowledge of nutrition or of cooking skills but can take a nutrition or cooking course or read books on nutrition and use simple cookbooks to learn basic skills.

Instead of continuing negative rationalization, positive rationalization may provide the means to change.

SUMMARY

Aging is a gradual process that is different for each individual depending on the influence of genetics, lifestyle, and environment across the life span. Productive aging takes into account the many psychosocial influences of successful aging. Many of these factors may affect nutrient intake.

The role of nutrition in each of the adult life span categories reflects the value of adequate nutrient intake to reduce the risk of chronic disorders of osteoporosis, coronary artery disease, diabetes, hypertension, and obesity. During the early years (20s and 30s), establishment of positive health behaviors is desirable. These years are the childbearing and childrearing years, with health implications for both women and men. The middle years (40s and 50s) are years of career and family demands. Chronic diet-related diseases, such as type 2 DM and coronary artery disease, may occur during these years. Positive dietary and exercise behaviors may provide protection. Nutrient needs for women change as menopause occurs. In particular, adequate calcium consumption is recommended to offset loss of bone density. The older years (60s, 70s, and 80s) are most reflective of lifestyle behaviors practiced over many years. Psychosocial issues of dealing with the deaths of loved ones, adjustment to retirement, and changes in living arrangements and economic status may affect the adequacy of nutrient intake. During the older years, nutrients remain the same as in earlier years except for vitamin D, for which the AI is increased. During the oldest years (80s and 90s) malnutrition and underweight are of concern.

A variety of techniques and community supports are available to implement the objectives of *Healthy People 2010*. Other barriers to health promotion during the adult years include food asphyxiation, stress, and health issues particular to women and men.

THE NURSING APPROACH
A Geriatric Assessment Program

Healthcare professionals advocate to keep older adults in their homes as long as possible. Avoiding institutionalization is often the best way to maintain quality of life for older adults and to minimize expense associated with nursing homes or other institutional settings. However, older adults who live alone or with their spouses or children may still not have the highest possible quality of life if they suffer from undiagnosed mental or physical problems or if they do not receive the supportive services they need. They may benefit from an assessment of their health, functional abilities, and need for health-related or home maintenance services. Such an assessment is usually done through a local Geriatric Assessment Program sponsored by a hospital or community agency.

A family member or primary care provider on behalf of older adults usually makes the contact with a geriatric assessment team individual. The assessment team is composed, in most instances, of a physician or primary healthcare provider who is a geriatrician, a nurse practitioner, and a social worker. They visit the person in the place of residence and do a complete health assessment, including nutritional assessment, an assessment of activities of daily living, and an evaluation of the physical surroundings and the social support available to the individual.

An example of how this system works is as follows. An older woman lives alone and her family is concerned that she does not adequately care for herself and that there might be safety hazards. Maybe the woman needs to see a medical specialist or needs physical therapy, or she may be depressed and need medication. The team may discover that this client does not eat a balanced diet or does not take in a sufficient quantity of food. She may have significant functional limitations in activities of daily living, making it impossible for her to cook or to shop for groceries often enough to get fresh vegetables, fruit, and milk.

After this thorough assessment is completed, which may take several hours, a written plan is developed for the client and perhaps for the family. In relation to nutrition, the plan may include teaching the client about the need to change her diet or may involve contacting the Home-Delivered Meals Program or providing a community volunteer who can shop for groceries for this older adult. An alternative recommendation might be to hire a home health aide who would cook at least one meal per day for the client.

This type of assessment and planning service is invaluable to many older adults in the community. They and their families know they need help, but they often don't know what they need until they consult health professionals. A geriatric assessment program provides an integrated approach to meeting all of the identified unmet needs in this population and may result in a healthier and happier aging process.

APPLYING CONTENT KNOWLEDGE

Jennifer and Peter are in their late 40s. Recently Peter was diagnosed with high blood cholesterol levels. His doctor told him to cut down on fats and cholesterol, but he is confused about what to order at the daily business lunches he must attend. Jennifer has noticed that she is starting to put on weight and wonders if it has to do with peri-menopause or if she is just eating more than usual. In addition, Jennifer's mother has just moved in with them because she could no longer afford her own home. Jennifer is concerned because her mother seems to eat little during the day. Her mother is alone all day because Jennifer and Peter work. What advice might you give to this family?

Web Sites of Interest

American Optometric Association
www.aoa.org/EyeOnNutrition
The American Optometric Association Web site provides information on age-related macular degeneration (AMD) and cataracts and features an assessment of an individual's dietary intake to ascertain consumption of nutrients and dietary components that may reduce the risk of cataracts and AMD.

Initiative to Eliminate Racial and Ethnic Disparities in Health
www.raceandhealth.hhs.gov
Sponsored by the U.S. Department of Health and Human Services, this site makes available information about a new strategy to eliminate racial and ethnic health disparities in six key areas of health status. This site is intended for use by community and church leaders, healthcare professionals, and provider and minority health experts.

National Women's Health Information Center
www.4woman.org
The U.S. Public Health Service's Office on Women's Health has created this site to be the federal "Woman's Health Central" as a single point-of-entry for federal and private sector sources on women's health issues. The Center can also be reached at (800) 994-WOMAN.

References

1. Ausman LM, Russell RM: Nutrition in the elderly. In Shils ME et al., eds.: *Modern nutrition in health and disease,* ed 9, Philadelphia, 1999, Williams & Wilkins.
2. Kerschner H, Pegues JM: Productive aging: a quality of life agenda, *J Am Dietetic Assoc* 98(12):1445, 1998.
3. Krebs-Smith SM et al.: Characterizing food intake patterns of American adults, *Am J Clin Nutr* 65(4 Suppl):1264S, 1997.
4. Feigenbaum MS, Pollock ML: Strength training: rationale for current guidelines for adult fitness programs, *The Physician and Sportsmedicine* 25(2): Feb 1997.
5. Chernoff R: Nutrition and health promotion in older adults, *J Gerontol A Biol Sci Med Sci* 56 Spec 2(2):47, Oct 2001.
6. Position of the American Dietetic Association: Nutrition, aging, and the continuum of care, *J Am Dietetic Assoc* 100:580, 2000.
7. Millen BE et al.: The elderly nutrition program: an effective national framework for preventive nutrition interventions, *J Am Dietetic Assoc* 102(2):234, Feb 2002.
8. US Department of Health and Human Services, Public Health Service: *Healthy People 2010,* ed 2, Washington, DC, 2000, US Government Printing Office; www.health.gov/healthypeople.
9. Katz D: *Just do it: the Nike spirit in the corporate world,* New York, 1994, Random House.
10. Food Research & Action Center, www.frac.org.
11. Position of the American Dietetic Association and The Canadian Dietetic Association: Women's health and nutrition, *J Am Dietetic Assoc* 99:738, 1999.
12. Kippenbrock T: Men's health. In Stanhope M, Lancaster J, eds.: *Community health nursing: promoting health of aggregates, families, and individuals,* St Louis, 1996, Mosby.
13. US Department of Health and Human Services: *Vital and health statistics: current estimates from the National Health Interview Survey, 1999,* DHHS Pub No (PHS) 94-1517, Hyattsville, Md, 1999, Public Health Services, Centers for Disease Control and Prevention.

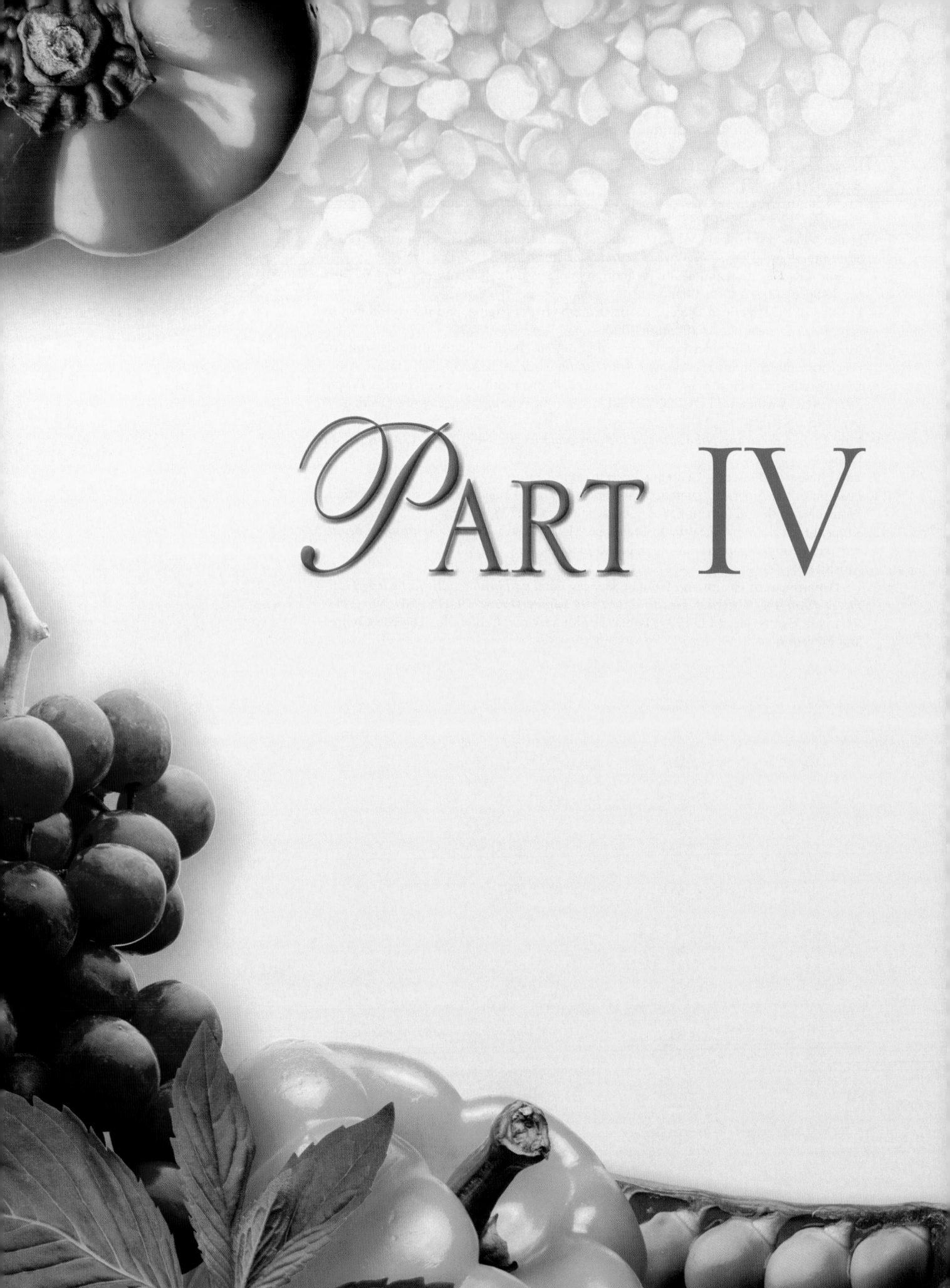

PART IV

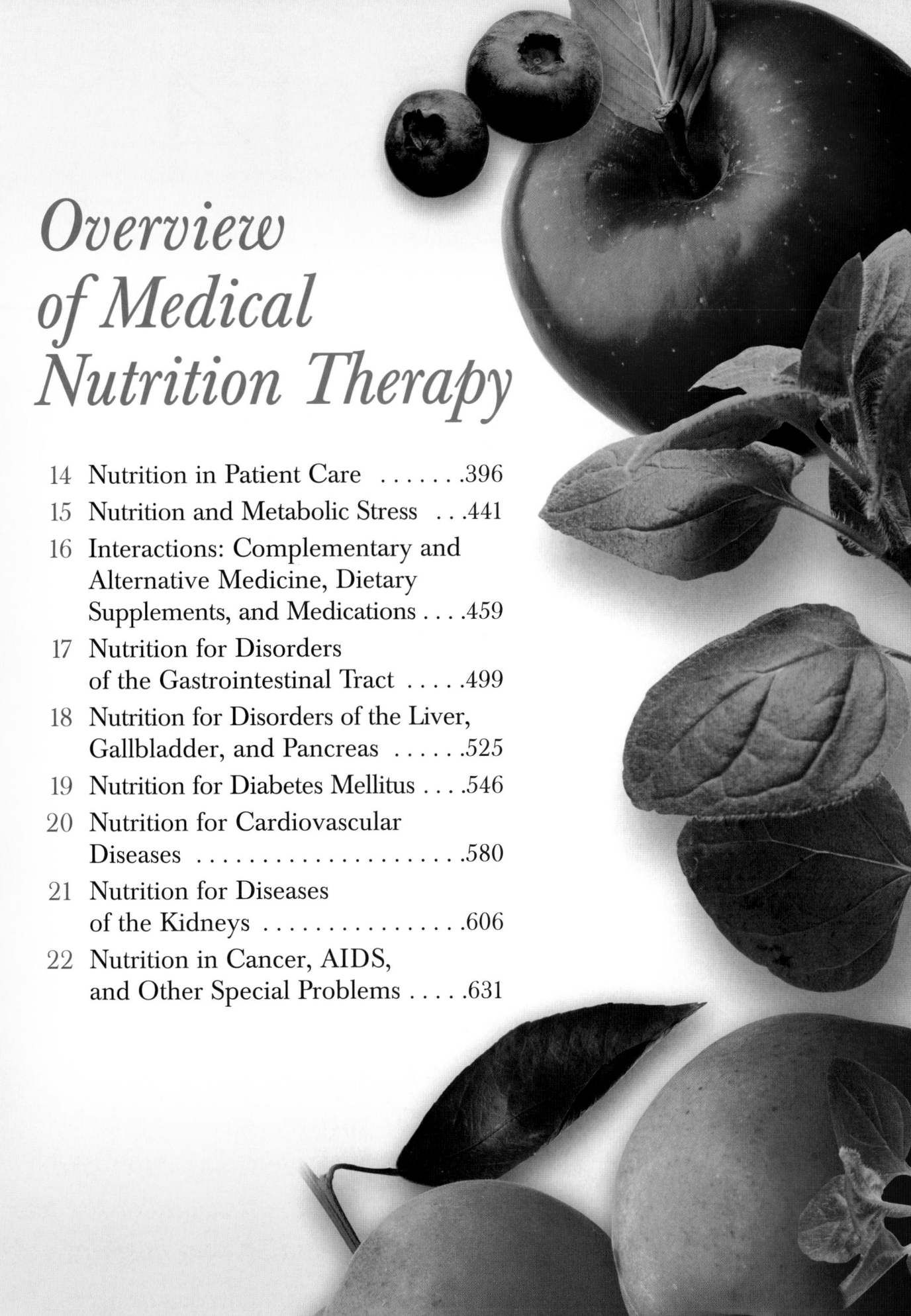

Overview
of Medical
Nutrition Therapy

CHAPTER 14

Nutrition in Patient Care

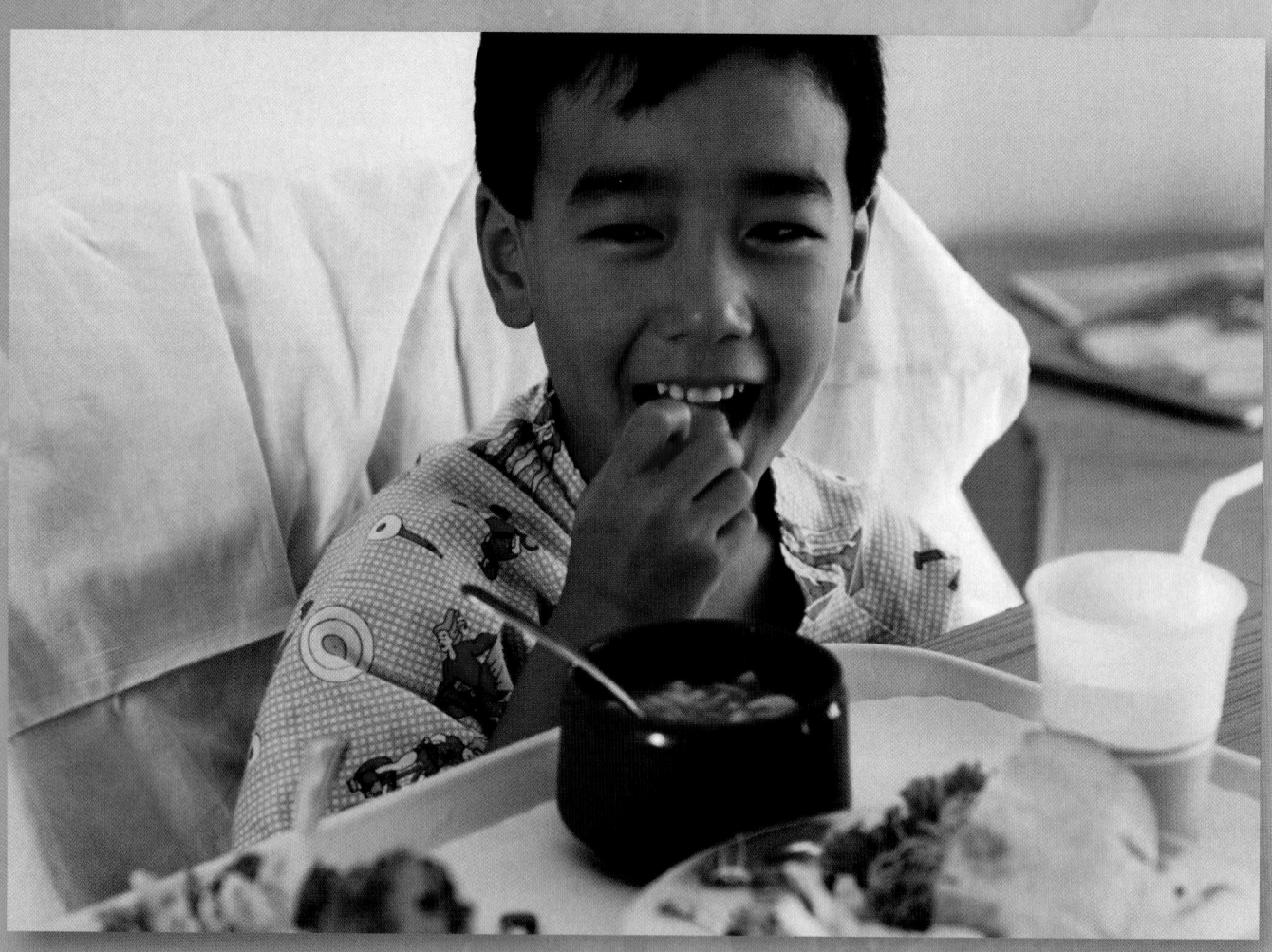

During these trying times for patients and staff alike, food becomes very important, both physiologically and psychologically, to patients because it is often one of the few familiar experiences patients encounter in a hospital.

ROLE IN WELLNESS

The first three parts of this text discuss basic nutrition as it relates to wellness. Part IV, "Overview of Medical Nutrition Therapy," provides information for nursing professionals on how nutrition pertains to the physiologic stresses of disease states.

Although Hippocrates made the link between nutrition and disease almost 3000 years ago, the modern medical community has just recently made the same discovery. The tremendous advances of medical technology are fundamentally important if the recipient is malnourished or is at nutritional risk. Nutritional risk is the potential to become malnourished because of primary (inadequate intake of nutrients) or secondary (caused by disease or iatrogenic affects) factors. The capacity for recovery from illness or disease depends on nutritional status. Poor nutritional status delays or prevents recovery, whereas good nutritional status promotes healing and recovery. It is therefore important to determine the nutritional status of those undergoing medical treatment or cure.

Sometimes dietary modifications are required to allow the body to heal, to adjust to physical disability, to prepare for diagnostic tests, or to prepare for surgical procedures. Medical nutrition therapy may involve changes in dietary intake to liquefied or pureed foods, tube feeding, or intravenous (IV) nourishment. This chapter discusses the promotion of wellness through typical progressive hospital diets, enteral formulas, and parenteral nutrition.

Because wellness is the goal of caring for patients, the five dimensions of health are applicable to the issues of this chapter. The physical health dimension is impacted because dietary alterations may affect overall nutritional status; careful nursing supervision can ensure adequate nutrient intake. The intellectual dimension is tested because nurses and caregivers are in the tricky position of observing patient eating patterns and then assessing whether problems are caused by illness or food availability. Nurses need the intellectual skills to determine when to alert the clinical dietitian. The emotional health dimension can be challenged if the loss of symbolic foods, particularly if modifications are long term or permanent, stresses emotional health. Nurses can be sensitive to this aspect of dietary modification and assist patients to create new symbols to replace the old. The social health dimension may be altered when patients are served meals in their rooms. Feelings of isolation may deprive meal times of their function of social relatedness. The spiritual health dimension is affected because some foods have spiritual or religious significance to individuals, such as bread and wine used for communion or matzoh used during the Jewish holiday of Passover. When such foods are not permitted because of enteral problems, individuals should consult their spiritual or religious advisors.

NUTRITION AND ILLNESS

Nurses are usually the first healthcare workers with whom the hospitalized patient comes into contact. By using information from nursing assessments, they are in a good position to identify patients in need of nutritional services. However, hospital size or staffing may necessitate nursing staff to perform some basic nutrition assessment and nutrition education.

When more in-depth knowledge of aspects of nutritional care beyond basic nutrition interventions is needed, this care is provided by registered dietitians (RDs). They conduct nutritional assessments, provide medical nutrition therapy, and serve as a valuable resource for the nursing staff. Occasionally, RDs may be assisted by dietetic technicians when taking diet histories, collecting information for nutritional screenings and assessments, and working directly with patients who are having problems with foods.

Modern healthcare settings—acute care hospitals—can play havoc with the nutrition status of patients. During their hospitalization, patients admitted in good nutritional status encounter several elements—psychologic and physiologic—that can

nutritional risk
the potential to become malnourished because of primary (inadequate intake of nutrients) or secondary (caused by disease or iatrogenic affects) factors

medical nutrition therapy
definition may be dictated by state laws that license registered dietitians (RDs) but typically this involves provision of nutrient, dietary, and nutrition education needs by RDs based on a comprehensive nutritional assessment

potentially put them at nutritional risk. If patients are admitted in compromised nutrition status, as many are, risks are even greater and of more consequence.

✽ Hospital Setting

Imagine you have been taken to a place where, after answering a multitude of questions about your insurance, financial status, and durable power of attorney, you are whisked off to a sterile-looking room you may share with a stranger. In this room, your clothes are replaced with a thin, flimsy gown with an open back. You answer more questions about your medical history from the nurse who admits you. Once he or she finishes, a resident/intern comes into your room to ask many of the same questions and conduct a physical examination.

During your stay in the hospital, your eating habits are open to scrutiny, possibly provoking guilty feelings. You're away from your own refrigerator, and meals are served on a schedule that may or may not coincide with your personal meal schedule. Although the food is prepared with the utmost care, it will be different from home cooking (just like any food eaten away from home). Depending on your diagnosis, the food is likely to be modified in texture, consistency, nutrients, or energy. When you're waiting for the meals to be served (you still haven't gotten used to eating in bed), different hospital staff routinely enter your room to ask more questions, draw blood, take you elsewhere in the hospital for tests that may or may not be invasive, and ask you about your elimination habits and what you have eliminated, if anything.

Many patients who enter hospitals are miles away from their homes, family, and friends. Although no malfeasance is intended, little privacy is afforded hospital patients while they undergo tests and examinations that may provide them with critical information regarding their prognosis or life expectancy. During these trying times for patients and staff alike, food becomes very important, both physiologically and psychologically, to patients because it is often one of the few familiar experiences encountered in a hospital setting.

Particularly with hospitalized toddlers and adolescents, food can become a battleground because of all its emotional connotations. As you will see in this chapter and those following, food or alternative nourishment can mean the difference between a good or poor prognosis for many patients' morbidity or mortality (see the Cultural Considerations box, "Asking the Right Questions for Cultural Competence").

Bed Rest

Occasionally, complete bed rest is prescribed as part of patients' medical care, or patients may be unable to ambulate because of the severity of their illness or because they are "hooked up" to a multitude of necessary life-saving equipment at bedside. Although it is often necessary or unavoidable, complete bed rest can cause injurious effects on a patient's body.[1] Skin integrity may be compromised after just 24 hours of immobilization, and after 3 days of lying supine in bed, muscle tone, bone calcium, plasma volume, and gastric secretions diminish. In addition, glucose intolerance and shifts in body fluids and electrolytes may also occur. Nursing personnel can provide care that may help prevent or delay the injurious effects of bed rest by frequently turning patients and stimulating the skin and underlying muscles by providing skin care (e.g., applying skin lotion) and passive exercises for the extremities, respectively.

Iatrogenic Malnutrition

Iatrogenic malnutrition has been likened to a closet skeleton.[2] It has been estimated that one third to one half of all patients admitted to hospitals are at nutritional risk. These patients may be experiencing hypermetabolism or have physiologic

durable power of attorney
a legal document in which a competent adult authorizes another competent adult to make decisions for him/her in the event of incapacitation

iatrogenic
inadvertently caused by treatment or diagnostic procedures

hypermetabolic
elevated metabolic rate

*H*ealthcare professionals strive for cultural competence when providing care to patients in a variety of healthcare settings. By doing so, they provide truly comprehensive healthcare. Cultural competence involves understanding the attitudes and knowledge of each cultural group in relation to how foods protect health and maintain wellness.

It is difficult to know all of the specific cultural food practices of diverse groups in North America. The use of the Cultural Nutritional Assessment Guide (below) is essential as part of a patient's health history. The information obtained from the patient or family member by healthcare professionals ensures culturally competent practice.

CULTURAL NUTRITIONAL ASSESSMENT GUIDE

- What nutritional factors are influenced by the client's cultural background? What is the meaning of food and eating to the client?
- With whom does the client usually eat? What types of foods are eaten? What is the timing and sequencing of meals?
- What does the client define as food? What does the client believe comprises a "healthy" vs. an "unhealthy" diet?
- Who shops for food? Where are groceries purchased (e.g., special markets or ethnic grocery stores)? Who prepares the client's meals?

- How are foods prepared at home—type of food preparation, cooking oils used, length of time foods are cooked (especially vegetables), amount and type of seasonings added to various foods during preparation?
- Has the client chosen a particular nutritional practice such as vegetarianism or abstinence from alcohol or fermented beverages?
- Do religious beliefs and practices influence the client's diet (e.g., type, amount, preparation, or delineation of acceptable food combinations [e.g., kosher diets])? Does the client abstain from certain foods at regular intervals, on specific dates determined by the religious calendar, or at other times?
- If the client's religion mandates or encourages fasting, what does the term *fast* mean (e.g., refraining from certain types or quantities of foods, eating only during certain times of the day)? For what period of time is the client expected to fast?
- During fasting, does the client refrain from liquids/beverages? Does the religion allow exemption from fasting during illness? If so, does the client believe that an exemption applies to him or her?

From Boyle J, Andrews M: Transcultural concepts in nursing care, *ed 2, Philadelphia, 1995, Lippincott, Williams & Wilkins.*

stress from injury or illness that increases nutritional needs, further increasing nutritional risk. To add insult to this potential injury, there may be a lack of nutritional screening or monitoring to identify patients at nutritional risk. Additionally, nutritional needs may be further compromised because of, for example, the periodic need for an empty gut for laboratory testing or diagnostic procedures. Nursing personnel can be a fundamental factor in the prevention of iatrogenic malnutrition by paying particular attention to patients' diet orders, recognizing the potential risk when patients have had nothing but clear or full-liquid diets for more than 24 hours, and contacting the RD to evaluate patients' nutritional risk (see the Myth box, "Hospitalized, Yet Malnourished? Impossible!").

NUTRITION INTERVENTION

The tremendous advances of medical technology are fundamentally important if the recipient is malnourished or is at nutritional risk.

Nutritional Care Process

Each patient has special nutritional needs depending on his or her injury or illness. For nutrition intervention to be efficacious and successful, a systematic, logical strategy is necessary. The nutritional care process provides such an approach. Like the nursing process, this process uses a five-step procedure to identify and solve nutrition-related problems (Figure 14-1).

diagnostic related groups (DRGs)

classifications used to determine Medicare payments for inpatient care, based on primary and secondary diagnosis, primary and secondary procedures, age, and length of hospitalization

MYTH
Hospitalized, Yet Malnourished? Impossible!

As noted in Butterworth's classic 1974 article "The Skeleton in the Hospital Closet," more than one third of hospitalized patients are at risk of malnutrition. Sadly, there has not been any data to show this was not just a freak observation. Furthermore, when **diagnostic related groups (DRGs)** became the law of the land and managed care became the norm; hospitalized patients began leaving the hospitals "quicker and sicker." Poorly nourished patients are often discharged from acute care in hospitals. When these patients transfer from hospitals to convalescent facilities, the incidence of malnutrition substantially increases to even epidemic proportions. Obviously, identifying patients who may be at nutritional risk is important. Because nurses are the primary caregivers, they can spot potential problems that they can address themselves or refer to the dietitian. The following indicators should alert a nurse to nutritional problems.

INDICATORS OF POTENTIAL NUTRITIONAL PROBLEMS

- Clear or full liquid diets for more than 3 days without nutrient supplementation or with inappropriate or insufficient nutrient supplementation
- Intravenous feeding (dextrose or saline) or NPO for more than 3 days without supplementation
- Low intakes of prescribed diet or tube feedings
- Weight 20% above or 10% below desirable body weight (accounting for edema)
- Inconsistent growth or weight for height, above or below norms in children
- Pregnancy weight gain deviating from normal patterns
- Diagnoses that increase nutritional needs or decrease nutrient intake (or both): cancer, malabsorption, diarrhea, hyperthyroidism, excessive inflammation, postoperative status, hemorrhage, wounds (large, draining, or infected wounds), burns, infection, sepsis, major trauma (or multisystem injury)
- Chronic use of drugs, especially alcohol, that affects nutritional status
- Alterations in chewing, swallowing, appetite, taste, and smell
- Temperature consistently above 37° C (98.6° F) for more than 2 days
- Hematocrit: <43% in men, <37% in women
- Hemoglobin: <14 g/dl in men, <12 g/dl in women; accompanied by mean cell volume <82 cu or > 100 cu
- Absolute decrease in lymphocyte count (<1500 cells/mm³)
- Elevated (>250 mg/dl) or decreased (<130 mg/dl) total plasma cholesterol
- Serum albumin <3 g/dl in patients without renal disease, liver disease, generalized dermatitis, overhydration

Reference: Butterworth CE: The skeleton in the hospital closet, Nutrition Today 9:4, 1974; Hopkins C: Developing an approach to nutritional assessment. In The American Dietetic Association: handbook of clinical dietetics, ed 2, New Haven, Conn, 1992, Yale University Press; and Thomas DR et al.: Malnutrition in subacute care, Am J Clin Nutr 75:303, 2001.

Step 1: **Assessment** of patient's nutritional status and needs
Step 2: **Analysis** of assessment data to determine nutritional requirements
Step 3: **Planning** intervention to meet nutritional needs
Step 4: **Implementation** of the plan (steps 1 through 3)
Step 5: **Evaluation** of intervention by ongoing assessment (step 1) and making appropriate changes

Nutritional Assessment

The nutritional care process is often performed during a comprehensive nutritional assessment conducted by dietetic professionals. Dietetic professionals work synergistically with nursing personnel to provide this essential component in medical

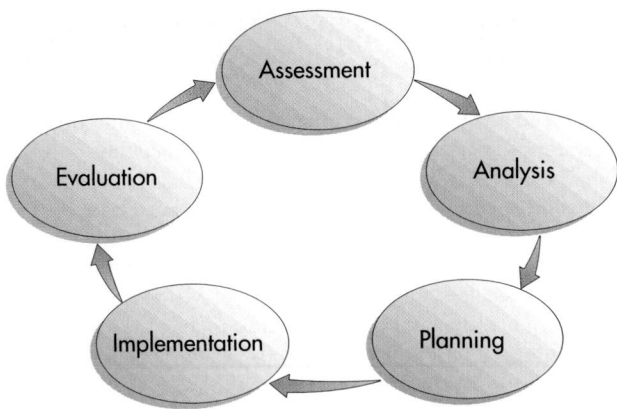

Figure 14-1 Nutritional care process. (From Rolin Graphics.)

care. A **comprehensive nutritional assessment** is a procedure conducted by dietetic professionals to determine appropriate medical nutrition therapy based on the identified needs of the patient. This process uses data collected from several different sources to assess patients' nutritional needs, often using the *ABCD* approach: Anthropometrics, Biochemical tests, Clinical observations, and Diet evaluation. Each part of this process is important because there is no one parameter that directly measures nutritional status or determines nutritional problems or needs. Thus a combination of these parameters must be used to interpret the overall nutrition picture presented by patients within the context of their personal, social, and economic backgrounds.*

Anthropometric Assessment. Anthropometric measurements are determined by simple, noninvasive techniques that measure height; weight; head, arm, and muscle circumferences; and skinfold thicknesses. Effectiveness of single anthropometric measurements is limited, but certain serial measurements can be useful to assess body composition changes or growth over time. Standardized techniques must be used to obtain valid and reliable measurements. Evaluation of anthropometric data involves comparison of data collected with predetermined reference limits or cutoff points that allow classification into one or more risk categories and, in some cases, identification of the type and severity of malnutrition.[3] Discussion of various anthropometric measurements follows.

Height. Stature (height/length) is important in evaluating growth and nutritional status in children. In adults, height is needed for assessment of weight and body size. Height should be measured using a fixed measuring stick or tape on a true vertical, flat surface with no carpeting. If this is not available, the movable measuring arm on platform clinic scales may be used with reasonable accuracy but tends to produce lower measures.[4] The patient should be measured standing as straight as possible, without shoes or head coverings, with the heels together, and looking straight ahead (Box 14-1).

Accurate heights are important in nutritional assessment. Many calculations used to determine energy requirements and needs are based on height and weight. Heights are not always available in the medical records of hospitalized patients. When heights are documented, it is often unclear whether they are reported by the patient or measured. Asking patients about their height does not always produce accurate information. On average when asked, people report being slightly taller than they actually are (approximately 0.6 inches [1.5 cm] taller).[5] Men overstate their height more often than women[5,6] and the extent of overstating height

comprehensive nutritional assessment
a procedure conducted by dietetic professionals to determine appropriate medical nutrition therapy based on the identified needs of the patient

---

*Note that information described in the anthropometric, biochemical, clinical, and dietary assessment data is *not* all encompassing. In an effort to conserve time and space, only parameters of particular interest to nursing are discussed.

Box 14-1   Measuring Height

1. Have patient stand erect with weight equally distributed on both feet.
   a. If the legs are of unequal length, place boards under the short limb to make the pelvis level.
   b. Where possible, make sure the head, shoulder blades, buttocks, and heels all touch the vertical surface.
   c. Instruct patient to let arms hang free at the sides with palms facing the thighs.
2. Have patient look straight ahead (so the line of vision is perpendicular to the body), take a deep breath, and hold that position while the horizontal headboard is brought down firmly on top of the head. (Measurer's eyes should be level with the headboard to read the measurement.)
3. Read the measurement to the nearest 0.1 cm or 1/8 in.

From Lee RD, Nieman DC: Nutritional assessment, *ed 3, New York, 2002, McGraw-Hill.*

---

recumbent measures measurements taken while the subject is lying down or reclining

---

increases as people age.[5] If the height of a patient recorded in the medical record is not a measured height, it should be documented as a stated height.

When measuring infants and children (less than 2 to 3 years) who cannot stand or others unable to stand erect without assistance, recumbent measures can be taken. A recumbent length table can be used. A recumbent length table or board has a fixed headboard, a movable footboard, and a permanent measuring tape along the side (Figure 14-2). To measure a patient, he or she should be placed supine on the board or table with shoulders and legs flat against the measuring board (table) and arms at the sides. The head should firmly touch the headboard while the line of vision is perpendicular to the board or table. Soles of the feet should be vertical, and the footboard should touch the bottom of the feet so that the soft tissue is compressed. Length can be recorded from the measure at the footboard. Two people are often needed to take an accurate measurement (Box 14-2).[4]

When the patient is comatose, critically ill, or unable to be moved for other reasons, taking a recumbent bed height may be possible.[7] Note that when compared with standing height, bed height is significantly greater by at least 2%.[7]

A more accurate measurement for patients who cannot stand is knee height. Knee height is more accurate when measured in a recumbent rather than sitting position.[8] This measurement is minimally affected by aging. In older adults, knee height can be measured to estimate height by using the following formulas[9]:

Male height (cm) = 64.19 − (0.04 × age) + [2.02 × knee height (cm)]

Female height (cm) = 84.88 − (0.24 × age) + [1.83 × knee height (cm)]

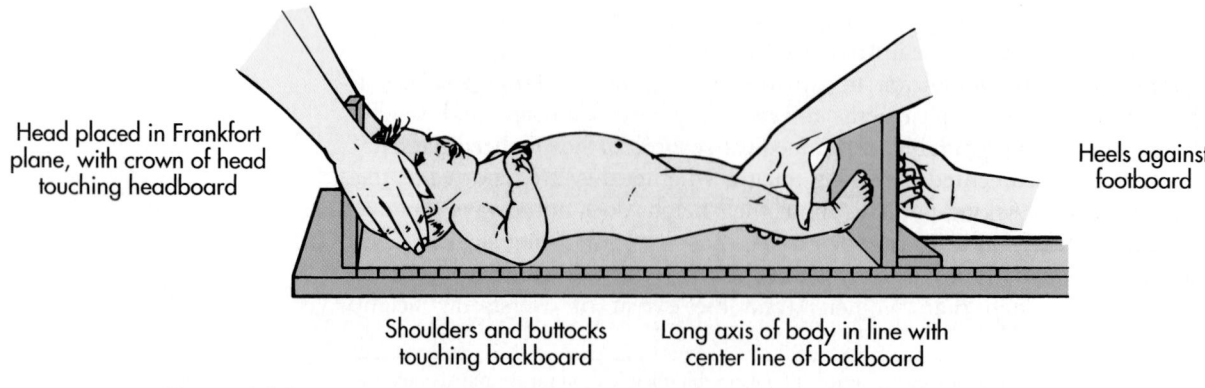

Head placed in Frankfort plane, with crown of head touching headboard

Heels against footboard

Shoulders and buttocks touching backboard

Long axis of body in line with center line of backboard

Figure 14-2 A recumbent length board used to take height measurements vertically. (From Lee R, Neiman D: *Nutritional assessment,* ed 3, New York, 2002, McGraw-Hill.)

Box 14-2 Measuring Recumbent Bed Height

1. Remove pillows and make bed level.
2. Straighten the patient out in bed but with the feet flexed.
3. With a clipboard or ruler, extend perpendicular lines from the top of the head and the bottom of the feet out to the side of the bed.
4. Mark the two positions on the bed sheet and measure the distance between them to the nearest 0.5 cm.

Reference: Gray D: Accuracy of recumbent height measurement, J Parenteral Enteral Nutr 9:712, 1985.

The special calipers necessary for measuring knee height are available from Ross Laboratories in Columbus, Ohio.

Weight.   When accurately measured, body weight is a simple, gross estimate of body composition. In fact, body weight is one of the most important measurements in assessing nutritional status and is used to predict energy expenditure.[10] Beam scales with movable but nondetachable weights or accurate electronic scales are recommended to obtain accurate results.[4] Spring scales are not recommended.[4] If the patient is nonambulatory, wheelchair or bed scales should be used (Figure 14-3).[4] Scales should be checked for accuracy periodically and recalibrated when necessary. Like heights, actual measured weights are more accurate than patients' estimated weights because most people report their weight as slightly less than it actually is (by approximately 2.4 lbs or 5 kg).[5] Women tend to underestimate their weight more than men, and for men and women, the extent of underreporting increases as actual weight increases.[5]

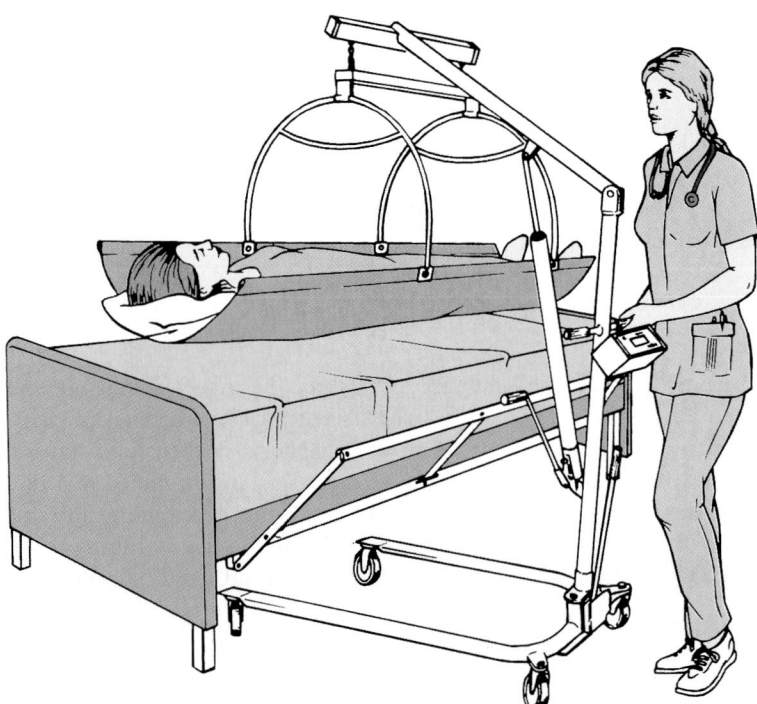

Figure 14-3 If a patient is nonambulatory, a bed scale can be used to measure patient weight. (From Lee R, Neiman D: *Nutritional assessment,* ed 3, New York, 2002, McGraw-Hill.

For accurate weights, patients should be clothed in their underwear or hospital gown. Weights should be measured at the same time of day and after voiding. The patient should stand still with the weight evenly distributed on both feet while weight is recorded to the nearest 0.1 kg or 0.25 lb.[4]

As a nutritional screening tool, weights can be used to recognize changes that may be representative or suggestive of serious health problems. The magnitude and direction of weight change are more meaningful when dealing with sick or debilitated patients than the standardized desirable weight references. Percent weight change is a useful nutrition index and may be computed as follows[11]:

$$\% \text{ weight change} = \frac{(\text{usual weight} - \text{actual weight})}{\text{usual weight}} \times 100$$

For example, Mrs. Welch is admitted to your unit. Her weight on admission is 120 lbs. During the admissions interview, she indicates that 3 months ago she weighed 135 lbs. Her percent weight change from usual weight is:

$$\frac{(135 - 120)}{135} \times 100 = \frac{15}{135} \times 100 = 0.11 \times 100 = 11\% \text{ weight change}$$

Mrs. Welch's (actual) weight is 11% less than her usual weight.

$$\% \text{ weight change from admission weight} = \frac{(\text{usual weight} - \text{actual weight})}{\text{admission weight}} \times 100$$

For example, Mr. Tucker is a patient in the long-term care facility where you work. When he was admitted more than a year ago, he weighed 180 lbs. He has weighed 170 lbs for the past 6 months, but today you weigh Mr. Tucker and he weighs 165 lbs. His percent weight change from admission weight is:

$$\frac{(170 - 165)}{180} \times 100 = \frac{5}{180} \times 100 = 0.0278 \times 100 = 2.78\% \text{ or}$$
$$3\% \text{ weight change}$$

Mr. Tucker's (actual) weight is 3% less than his admission weight.

$$\% \text{ weight change since nutrition intervention} =$$
$$\frac{(\text{usual weight} - \text{actual weight})}{\text{preintervention weight}} \times 100$$

For example, Mrs. Bussard was placed on a feeding tube because her weight has decreased from her usual weight of 130 lbs to 115 lbs. She has been on the feeding tube for 1 week and when you weigh her today, she weighs 122 lbs. Her percent weight change since nutrition intervention is:

$$\frac{(130 - 122)}{115} \times 100 = \frac{8}{115} \times 100 = 0.067 \times 100 = 6.96\% \text{ or}$$
$$7\% \text{ weight change}$$

Mrs. Bussard's weight has increased 7% since the tube feedings were initiated.

Care should be taken to identify patients with ascites, edema, or dehydration because their weight changes may be more a reflection of their fluid status than actual changes in body composition. If more than 1 pound is gained in a day's time, it may be indicative of excess fluid. It is also important to examine any unplanned weight loss the patient might experience as indicated in the margin note. Reported or measured percent weight losses of these magnitudes could be cause for alarm.

Weight Change as an Indicator of Nutritional Status

% Weight Change	Time Period	Nutritional Status
1%-2%	1 week	Moderate weight loss
>2%	1 week	Severe weight loss
5%	1 month	Moderate weight loss
>5%	1 month	Severe weight loss

For older adult patients who cannot be weighed because of the severity of their medical condition, or if bed or chair scales are not available, Chumlea et al.[12] have developed gender-specific equations used to predict body weight in persons 60 to 90 years of age. The estimated weights are based on recumbent measures of arm circumference (AC), calf circumference (CC), subscapular skinfold (SSF), and knee height (KH).

Women: Weight (cm) = [0.98 × AC(in cm)] + [1.27 × CC(in cm)] +
[0.4 × SSF(in mm)] + [0.87 × KH(in cm)] − 62.35

Men: Weight (cm) = [1.73 × AC(in cm)] + [0.98 × CC(in cm)] +
[0.37 × SSF (in mm)] + [1.16 × KH(in cm)] − 81.69

Another challenge in obtaining weights occurs in patients who have missing body parts because of accidents or amputation. Figure 14-4 shows the approximate percent of body weight contributed by individual body segments so desirable weight can be calculated.

Body Mass Index. Body mass index (BMI) has been proposed as an alternative to the traditionally used height-weight tables in assessing obesity.[13] BMI measures weight corrected for height. You can determine BMI by referring to Table 10-1 or by dividing weight in kilograms by height in squared meters using the following steps:
1. Divide weight in pounds by 2.2 to convert it into kilograms.
2. Multiply height in inches by 2.54 and divide the result by 100 to convert height to meters; then multiply height in meters by itself (that is, square it).
3. Divide weight in kilograms (result of step 1) by the square of height in meters (result of step 2). The result is BMI.

$$\text{BMI} = \frac{\text{Weight (kg)}}{\text{Height (m)}^2}$$

body mass index (BMI) a measure that describes relative weight for height and is significantly correlated with total body fat content

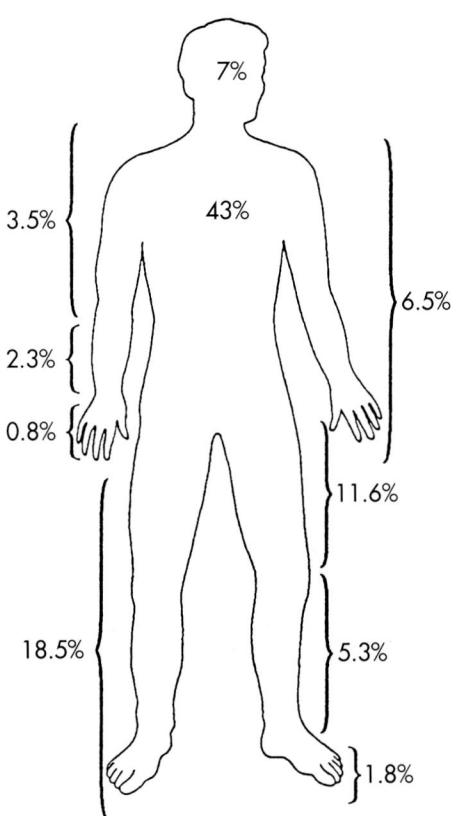

Figure 14-4 Approximate body weight percentages. (Modified from Brunnstrom S: *Clinical kinesiology,* Philadelphia, 1962, FA Davis.)

The desired BMI range for healthy adults is 18.5 to 24.9 kg/m², which reflects a healthy weight for height. Although at low risk for health problems, persons with BMIs of 25 to 29.9 kg/m² are approximately 20% above desirable levels. Persons with BMIs between 30 to 39.9 kg/m² are at high risk, and BMIs greater than 40 indicate very high risk. A BMI of less than 18.5 kg/m² is classified as underweight (Table 14-1) and is associated with risk factors such as respiratory disease, tuberculosis, digestive disease, and some cancers.[14]

Body Measures.   Skinfold thicknesses are often used to estimate subcutaneous fat stores or the pattern of fat distribution. This information can then be used to help determine nutritional status. Skinfold measures are taken by measuring a double layer of skin and subcutaneous fat tissue at specific body sites using a special calibrated instrument. Although eight sites (chest, triceps, subscapular, midaxillary, suprailiac, abdomen, thigh, and medial calf) can be used, the triceps skinfold (TSF)—midpoint at the back of the upper arm—is the most commonly used single site. The only tools necessary are a tape measure and calipers of acceptable quality. Detailed instructions for measuring various body sites have been published elsewhere and should be studied carefully before undertaking the actual measurement.[4] It is important that the person taking the skinfold measures be properly trained and that subsequent measurements be taken by the same person. As with any other measurement of nutritional status, skinfold measurements should be used in conjunction with other parameters and should be followed over time to provide an accurate and thorough assessment.[4] Skinfold measurements should be compared with percentages of standards,[11] be taken from multiple body sites, or be collected as serial measurements to assess changes in fat stores over time.[11]

somatic protein stores
proteins in skeletal muscle

Mid-upper-arm circumference (MAC) provides an indication of skeletal muscle mass (somatic protein), bone, and subcutaneous fat; consequently it is sensitive to any change that can take place in the upper arm. It can be used as a screening tool as well as a method to monitor nutrition intervention over time.[11] It is particularly useful for patients who cannot be weighed.[15] Mid-upper-arm muscle circumference (MAMC) adjusts for subcutaneous fat and reflects somatic protein and bone within the arm. MAMC is estimated using the following equation:

$$MAMC = MAC(mm) - [0.314 \times TSF(mm)]$$

Mid-upper-arm muscle area (MAMA) is a two-dimensional measurement that indicates somatic protein and bone in the arm. It is more responsive to change in somatic protein stores than MAMC. It tends to overestimate muscle area because it does not correct for bone inside the arm.[15]

$$MAMA = \frac{[MAC(mm) - (0.314 \times TSF(mm)]^2}{4 \times 0.314}$$

Table 14-1
Classifications of Overweight and Obesity by Body Mass Index (BMI)

	Obesity Class	BMI (kg/m²)
Underweight		<18.5
Normal		18.5-24.9
Overweight		25.0-29.9
Obesity	I	30.0-34.9
	II	35.0-39.9
Extreme obesity	III	≥40

Corrected mid-upper-arm muscle area (cMAMA) is a two-dimensional measurement that reflects somatic protein within the arm without the bone. It is not valid in older adult or obese patients and may not be sensitive to small changes in somatic protein.[11,16]

$$\text{cMAMA for males} = \frac{[MAC(cm) - (0.314 \times TSF(cm)]^2 - 10}{4 \times 0.314*}$$

$$\text{cMAMA for females} = \frac{[MAC(cm) - (0.314 \times TSF(cm)]^2 - 6.5}{4 \times 0.314*}$$

All mid-upper-arm circumferences and their indexes can be evaluated against reference data such as NHANES I and II tables.[11] Patients' measurements that fall above the 95th percentile or below the 5th percentiles (for age, gender, frame size, or race) indicate the patients are at risk for compromised nutritional status. Measurements between the 5th percentile and 15th percentile may indicate a patient is at risk for depleted nutritional status.[11]

Biochemical Assessment. Many routine blood and urine laboratory tests recorded in patients' charts are useful in providing an objective assessment of nutritional status. However, care should be taken in interpreting test results for a number of reasons. First, there is no single test available for evaluating short-term response to medical nutritional therapy. Laboratory tests should be used in conjunction with anthropometric data, clinical data, and dietary intake assessments. Second, some tests may be inappropriate for certain patients; for example, serum albumin might not be useful in the evaluation of protein status in those patients with liver failure because this test assumes normal liver function. Third, laboratory tests conducted serially will give more accurate information than a single test.[4] Although serial measures can be obtained in long-term care settings, patients in acute care facilities are rarely hospitalized long enough to obtain serial measures. Therefore, it might be more appropriate to compare test results with known standards.

The most important biochemical parameters are visceral protein status and immune function. Visceral protein status is assessed through tests of serum albumin and prealbumin. Immune function is evaluated based on total lymphocyte count (TLC). The test results of these biochemical assessments provide useful information to determine the effects of nutritional factors or of medical conditions on the health status of patients (Table 14-2).

visceral protein
protein contained in the internal organs

Serum Albumin. Serum albumin provides an assessment of visceral protein status. Normal values are within 3.5 to 5.0 g/dl. For nutritional analysis, values between 2.8 and 3.5 g/dl indicate compromised protein status; values less than 2.8 g/dl suggest possible kwashiorkor. This test is most useful when used to monitor long-term nutrition changes because normal values may still be found among patients who are malnourished. In addition, if patients are experiencing dehydration (hemoconcentration) or have received infusions of albumin, fresh frozen plasma, or whole blood serum albumin, levels may appear normal. However, as a tool to assess long-term changes, the effects of dehydration and infusions would dissipate. Alternate causes of abnormally low values may be infection and other stressors (especially with poor protein intake), burns, trauma, congestive heart failure, fluid overload, and severe hepatic insufficiency.[17,18]

Prealbumin. Prealbumin (thyroxine-binding prealbumin) can also provide a measure of visceral protein status assessment. Normal values range from 20 to 50 mg/dl. This test is useful in monitoring short-term changes in visceral protein status because of its short half-life of 2 days. Compromised protein status is indicated when levels are between 10 to 15 g/dl. Possible kwashiorkor is a potential

---

*It should be noted that the equation assumes measurements have been made in cm, and not mm, for conformity with the original reference. (Gibson RS: *Principles of nutritional assessment,* New York, 1990, Oxford Press.)

Table 14-2
Biochemical Parameters and How They Are Tested

Biochemical Parameter	Test Performed
Visceral protein status	Serum albumin
	Prealbumin (thyroxine-binding prealbumin)
	Total iron binding capacity (TIBC)
Somatic protein status	Serum creatinine
	24-hr urinary creatinine
Immune function	Total lymphocyte count (TLC)
Evaluation of protein intake	24-hr urea nitrogen (UUN)
Iron status	Transferrin
	Hemoglobin
	Hematocrit
	Mean corpuscular hemoglobin (MCH)
	Mean corpuscular volume (MCV)

diagnosis when levels are less than 10 mg/dl. A nonnutritional cause of normal values despite patient malnutrition is chronic renal failure. Other factors that result in abnormally low levels of prealbumin include surgical trauma, stress, inflammation, infection, and liver dysfunction.[17,18]

Total Lymphocyte Count.   Total lymphocyte count (TLC) has been used as a measure of immune function. A normal TLC is greater than 1500 cells/mm³. This test should not be used as an absolute indicator of nutritional status but rather considered with other diagnostic assessments. A count of less than 1500/mm³ indicates possible immunocompromise associated with protein-energy malnutrition, especially kwashiorkor. Other causes of abnormal values are not directly related to nutritional status. Abnormally low TLCs may be caused by severe stress (e.g., infections), corticosteroid therapy, renal failure, and cancer. High levels of TLC may indicate infections, leukemia, myeloma, cancer, and adrenal insufficiency.[17,18]

Clinical Assessment.   Clinical assessment incorporates data from several sources: medical history, social history, and physical examination. Many environmental factors can affect nutritional status. This information can be found by reviewing the patient's medical record or through direct interview. Social or family factors may also affect nutrient intake or past or present medical conditions that influence nutrient use. Many physical signs and symptoms associated with malnutrition are also an integral part of assessing nutritional status.

Features associated with nutritional deficiency may be considered through historical and clinical categories.[17,18] Historical findings may include alcohol abuse, poverty, avoidance of specific food groups (e.g., fruits or vegetables), weight loss, drug use (or abuse), family history of inborn errors, and cigarette smoking. Clinical features are extensive, including surgery or wounds; blood loss; dull, dry, pluckable hair; fever; and bleeding gums. Findings may be organized by symptoms of the eyes, face, skin, muscles, tongue, and central nervous system. Table 14-3 provides additional data about historical and clinical features in relation to nutritional status.

Dietary Intake Assessment.   There are several methods for collecting information regarding actual and habitual dietary intake. Most commonly, data are collected using diet/food recall (retrospective) or diet/food records (prospective). Each method has its pros and cons, so it is important to choose a method best suited to the type of information needed. These data provide information regarding intake

Table 14-3
Historical and Clinical Features Associated with Nutritional Deficiency

History or Physical Findings	Nutritional Implication	Possible Deficiency
Alcohol abuse	Inadequate nutrient intake	Kcalories, protein, thiamine, niacin, folate, pyridoxine, riboflavin
	Increased nutrient losses	Magnesium, zinc
Avoidance of fruits, vegetables, grain products	Inadequate nutrient intake	Vitamins A and C, thiamin, niacin, folate
Avoidance of meat, dairy products, eggs	Inadequate nutrient intake	Protein, vitamin B_{12}
Constipation, hemorrhoids, diverticulosis	Inadequate nutrient intake	Dietary fiber
Isolation, poverty, dental disease, food idiosyncrasies	Inadequate nutrient intake	Various nutrients
Weight loss	Inadequate nutrient intake	Kcalories, other nutrients
Drugs (especially antacids, anticonvulsants, cholestyramine, laxatives, neomycin, alcohol)	Inadequate nutrient absorption, decreased nutrient utilization	Various nutrients
Malabsorption (diarrhea, weight loss, steatorrhea)	Inadequate nutrient absorption, increased nutrient losses	Vitamins A, D, K; kcalories; protein; calcium; magnesium; zinc; electrolytes
Parasites	Inadequate nutrient absorption	Iron, vitamin B_{12} (fish tapeworm)
Pernicious anemia	Inadequate nutrient absorption	Vitamin B_{12}
Surgery	Inadequate nutrient absorption	Vitamin B_{12}, iron, folate
gastrectomy		
intestinal resection		Vitamin B_{12} (if distal ileum), iron, others as in malabsorption
Inborn errors of metabolism (by family history)	Decreased nutrient utilization	Various nutrients
Blood loss	Increased nutrient losses	Iron
Centesis (ascitic, pleural taps)	Increased nutrient losses	Protein
Diabetes, uncontrolled	Increased nutrient losses	Kcalories
Draining abscesses, wounds	Increased nutrient losses	Protein, zinc
Nephrotic syndrome	Increased nutrient losses	Protein, zinc
Peritoneal dialysis or hemodialysis	Increased nutrient losses	Protein, water-soluble vitamins, zinc
Fever	Increased nutrient requirements	Kcalories
Hyperthyroidism	Increased nutrient requirements	Kcalories
Physiologic demands (infancy, adolescence, pregnancy, lactation)	Increased nutrient requirements	Various nutrients
Surgery, trauma, burns, infection	Increased nutrient requirements	Kcalories, protein, vitamin C, zinc
Tissue hypoxia	Increased nutrient requirements	Kcalories (inefficient utilization)
Cigarette smoking	Increased nutrient requirements	Vitamin C, folic acid
Dull, dry, sparse, easily plucked hair		Protein, energy, zinc
Spoon-shaped, brittle, ridged nails		Iron
Face		
Rotundness, "moon face" appearance		Obesity, protein
Presence of edema or decubiti		Protein

From Horne M, Swearingen PL: Pocket guide to fluids and electrolytes, St Louis, 1989, Mosby; and Weinsier RL, Heimburger DC, Butterworth CE: Handbook of clinical nutrition, ed 2, St Louis, 1989, Mosby.

Continued

Table 14-3–cont'd
Historical and Clinical Features Associated with Nutritional Deficiency

History or Physical Findings	Nutritional Implication	Possible Deficiency
Face—cont'd		
Nasolabial seborrhea		Riboflavin, zinc
Xerosis (dryness of mucous membranes)		Vitamin A
Pallor, listlessness		Iron
Eyes		
Redness or fissures at corners of eyelids		Riboflavin
Dry cornea, Bitot's spots		Vitamin A
Cloudy, pale conjunctiva		Iron
Periorbital numbness		Phosphorus
Angular lesions at corners of the mouth		Riboflavin
Bleeding, spongy gums		Vitamin C
Tongue		
Magenta in color		Riboflavin
Scarlet, raw, swollen, fissures on tongue		Niacin
Thick tongue, difficulty with speaking		Phosphorus
Goiter		Iodine
Skin		
Scrotal and vulvar dermatosis not accompanied by inflammation		Riboflavin
Swollen skin pigmentation of areas exposed to sun		Niacin
Pinhead size, purplish hemorrhagic spots (petechiae)		Vitamin C
Excessive bruising		Vitamin C or K
Poor wound healing, decubiti		Protein, kcalories
Follicular hyperkeratosis (epidermal hypertrophy causing horny skin formation)		Vitamin A
Muscular system		
Thinness, tissue wasting		Protein, kcalories
Presence of edema		Obesity, protein, sodium
Skeletal system		
Osteoporosis		Calcium, protein
Circumscribed swelling or growth of frontal and parietal areas of skull, bowed legs		Vitamin D
Central nervous system		
Mental irritability		Protein
Hyporeflexia, foot and wrist drop		Thiamine
Psychotic behavior		Niacin
Peripheral neuropathy, forgetfulness		Pyridoxine
Tremor, convulsions, tetany		Magnesium, calcium

of kcalories, protein, carbohydrate, fat, vitamins, minerals, and fluid, which can be calculated manually using food composition tables or analyzed by computer software. More than 100 programs are available to analyze dietary intake. Evaluation of software needs and systems suitable to meet those needs is important when selecting an appropriate software package.[4]

24-Hour Diet Recall.   In this method, the patient is asked by a trained interviewer to report all foods and beverages consumed during the past 24 hours. Detailed description of all foods, beverages, cooking methods, brand names, condiments, and supplements, along with portion sizes in common household measures, is included. Food models, measuring cups, life-size pictures, or abstract shapes (squares, circles, rectangles) are used to assist the patient in estimating correct portion sizes of foods consumed. This method is useful in screening or during follow-up to evaluate adaptation of or compliance with dietary recommendations. The advantages of this method are that it is quick (only 15 to 20 minutes are needed) and it can be used with most age groups. Because it is retrospective, the patient does not modify his or her actual intake. The information can be obtained by face-to-face interview, telephone, or patient self-reporting. Some of the drawbacks for this method are that it relies on the memory, motivation, and awareness of the patient. Because this is only a single day's intake, it may not be representative of the patient's actual diet.

Food Records.   Estimated or measured food records can provide a more realistic picture of a patient's usual intake. All foods, beverages, snacks, and supplements are recorded by the patient, usually over 1 to 7 days using household measures. The patient must be trained with food models, measuring cups, or other measuring devices that will help ensure recording of proper or actual portion sizes. Cooking methods, recipe ingredients, and descriptions need to be recorded as completely and accurately as possible. Often, record keeping like this influences the recorder's standard food choices but only in some cases. In some instances, the recorder is also asked to record locations, times, events, and feelings in addition to foods eaten if information is needed to identify behavioral as well as nutritional patterns. A 7-day food record is considered optimal for gathering this kind of information, but it does tend to be tedious. Shorter periods are less representative of usual intake, but a 3-day record (including 2 weekdays and 1 weekend day) can be acceptable. Obviously for this method of dietary data collection, the patient must be literate, numerate, and well motivated.[4]

Kcalorie Counts.   In an acute or long-term care setting, one of the most common forms of food records is a kcalorie count. This term is a little misleading because in actual practice, all nutrients can be assessed, but kcalorie and protein intakes are parameters usually quantified. Information gathered in this manner is often used to determine the adequacy of patients' daily oral intake or to document need for **nutritional support**. Nursing observations are essential for early identification of malnutrition and prevention of iatrogenic weight loss during the hospital stay. Staff responsible for recording intake must be accurate in their recordings. It is important to record foods and beverages consumed in measurable amounts (e.g., cups, ounces, teaspoons, tablespoons, cc's) or in percentage of amount eaten (50% baked chicken, 75% bread, 25% green beans). Subjective terms such as *two bites, ate well,* or *three swallows* are not useful and cannot provide objective information needed to calculate protein and kcalorie intake.

nutritional support
although commonly used in reference to enteral and parenteral nutrition delivery systems, it can refer to any nutrition intervention used to minimize patient morbidity, mortality, and complications

Nutritional Risk

As mentioned previously, the nutritional care process involves assessing patients' nutritional status, estimating nutritional needs, and planning for nutritional intervention. If done appropriately, it allows for early intervention in both treatment of established malnutrition and prevention of malnutrition among those at high nutritional risk. Areas to consider regarding nutritional risk are age, weight, laboratory test results, (body) systems, and feeding modalities[17] (Table 14-4).

Age: Moderate nutritional risk occurs among adults between ages 65 and 75 and for children older than 5 years of age. Age-related high risk is possible for patients aged 75 years or older; for children, high risk most often occurs for those younger than the age of 5.

Weight: Weight loss is a potential nutritional risk factor depending on its cause. The percentage of body weight lost combined with the evaluation or cause of the loss determines the possible level of risk (see Table 14-4).

Table 14-4
Areas of Nutritional Risk

Data Source	Moderate Risk	High Risk
Age	65-75 years of age Children more than 5 years of age	75 years of age or older Children less than 5 years of age
Weight	Evaluation of loss (i.e., self-induced?)	5% weight loss in 1 month 10% loss in 6 months Length/height for age <5th percentile Weight/height <5th percentile or <80th percentile of standard
Laboratory	Albumin 3.5-3.0 g/dl	Albumin ≤3.0 g/dl TLC ≤1200 cells/mm³ Prealbumin ≤10 mg
Systems*	Heart, antepartum, pain, orthopedics, selected oncology, short stay, chemotherapy	Renal, pancreas, GI, liver, diabetes with pregnancy, eating disorders, oncology, transplants, any condition in children associated with development of protein calorie malnutrition
Feeding modalities	Transitional (stable) Some selected modified diets with education component	Parenteral nutrition, tube feeding, NPO, or clear liquids >3 days

Reference: Grant A, DeHoog S: Nutritional assessment and support, ed 5, Seattle, 1999, Anne Grant/Susan DeHoog.
*Systems for risk depend on the individual patient population at risk.

Laboratory test results: As noted previously, biochemical tests of albumin, TLC, and prealbumin levels provide an assessment of nutritional risk.

Systems: Systems account for conditions of various body systems that present either moderate or high nutritional risk. Moderate nutritional risk may be experienced when a patient undergoes chemotherapy because of its effects on dietary intake. High risk is incurred among individuals with eating disorders or diabetes when pregnant. (Other conditions are listed in Table 14-4.)

Feeding modalities: Moderate nutritional risk is associated with transition from restrictive therapeutic intervention to a regular dietary intake. Risk may also occur when patients are on modified diets that have potential to cause nutrient deficiencies. Patients may be at high risk when they are on parenteral feeding or tube feeding, are NPO (i.e., nothing by mouth), or on clear liquids for more than 3 days.

Nutritional assessment involves examination of (1) anthropometric data, (2) biochemical data, (3) clinical data, and (4) dietary data. It is important to remember that there is no one absolute index for measuring nutritional status. Accurate and meaningful assessment can be made only by incorporating data from several sources.

MEDICAL NUTRITION THERAPY

As will be discussed in the chapters to follow, specific diseases or conditions require modifications of nutritional components of a *normal* diet. Each modified diet has a purpose and rationale, and its use is usually determined by the physician or dietitian. To appreciate modified diets described in the following chapters, it will be helpful to have an understanding of the basis for these diets: the general, regular, or house diet.

The *general diet* is designed to attain or maintain optimal nutritional status in persons who do not require modified or therapeutic diets. Individual requirements for specific nutrients vary and are adjusted depending on gender, age, height, weight, and activity level. This diet is used to promote health and reduce risks for developing chronic diet-related diseases such as cardiovascular diseases or certain cancers.[11] Depending on individual food choices, a regular diet can be adequate in all nutrients.

Dietary modifications of the *regular diet* may be made in two ways: quantitative or qualitative. Qualitative diets include modifications in consistency, texture, or nutrients, such as clear-liquid or full-liquid diets. Quantitative diets include modifications in number or size of meals served or amounts of specific nutrients, such as six small feedings or kcalorie-controlled diets used in the treatment of diabetes mellitus.

Whatever kind of meals or modified diets patients receive, much of patients' acceptance of the food is influenced by nursing personnel. For example, if a patient's primary caregiver expresses criticism about the food service, the patient is likely to do the same (see the Myth box, "All Hospital Food Is Terrible: Not Necessarily"). It is also possible that acceptance of modified diets may also be influenced by whether patients perceive nutrition to be an important part of their medical care and recovery. Patient education can make a difference in patient acceptability of meals. By explaining the rationale of why some foods are allowed and others are to be reduced or avoided, the nurse or dietitian may affect patient compliance with modified dietary intake. It is important to remember that food provides the energy and nutrients that aid in the healing process. Food left on the tray does not help the patient heal.

Food Service Delivery Systems

Because nursing personnel are often on the front line when food is delivered to patients, it is important to understand how meals are prepared and delivered to patients in hospitals and long-term care facilities. Food service in a healthcare setting is the responsibility of the director of the food and nutrition services department. This person may be either a management dietitian or a specially trained food service manager. He or she is responsible for hiring, terminating, and supervising staff; ordering and purchasing food and supplies; delivering food to patients and staff; and overseeing quality assurance issues. Clinical dietitians may work under the supervision of or alongside the food service director to assess patients' nutritional status, plan appropriate diets and nutrition intervention, and provide nutrition education. Other personnel from the food and nutrition service area include cooks, clerks, dishwashers, aids, and dietetic technicians. Clinical dietitians may also be members of a food service department. Their jobs involve direct patient care. Typically, only RDs (management and clinical) and dietetic technicians have the appropriate education and training in clinical nutrition and all of its applications, whether that is the delivery of food or the assessment of nutritional status. Patients are often able to choose (from a menu) foods they will be served at mealtime. Some institutions provide this service for patients who receive regular as well as modified diets. A menu for a modified diet lists only foods that are appropriate for a given type of patient. This practice allows patients to select foods they like and will eat. Although a dietitian can plan the most nutritious meals, if patients do not eat the food, then patients may be at risk in the long term. A selective menu system also affords patients the feeling of some control over their lives while hospitalized (see the Teaching Tool, "Assisting Patients with Menu Selections," for more suggestions).

Some institutions do not offer selective menus. In their place, a standard *house diet* that is adjusted (or modified) according to special nutritional needs is used. Although a selective menu may not be available, efforts can be made to ensure that

MYTH
All Hospital Food Is Terrible: Not Necessarily

Ask anyone about food served in hospitals and you will probably receive a negative response. Our stereotype of hospital food is that it is bland, without much texture and appeal. Is hospital food as terrible as people think? Or is it just unfamiliar? Or do most people lose their appetite when sick, especially when away from home? Why can't patients just have the same foods they eat at home?

Besides the fact that patients' illnesses usually dictate what they can eat, medical technology has also influenced what foods are served from the hospital kitchen. Treatments and procedures like chemotherapy, angioplasty, organ transplants, new drugs, and/or diseases such as AIDS have resulted in modifications of meals and foods served to meet patients' special needs. Some hospitals may serve as many as 15 or 20 different menus to patients.

In addition, each hospital food service must conform to federal, state, and professional standards that dictate nutritional content. There are even regulations that impose timing of meals. Added to this are cultural preferences; all of us have a better comfort level when served foods that are familiar to us. Physical mechanical problems that hinder patients from eating regular food may require that meat be served cubed or ground. Illness, treatments, or medications may alter patients' ability to taste. Chemotherapy drugs often make meats or high-protein foods taste bitter and metallic. Some other drugs may simply dull all sensation or depress appetite altogether. All of these factors affect perceptions of the quality and taste of hospital meals.

Can anything be done to overcome all these obstacles? In fact, it is the hospitals and food service industries themselves who have initiated efforts to overcome these obstacles. In addition to the hospital industry's desire to improve care, the healthcare dollar is shrinking, and many hospitals find themselves in competition for paying patients. Once patients were recognized as customers, any service provided by a hospital became a customer service. Food that is appetizing to the palate and the eyes is good advertisement. Many hospital food services have recruited chefs or hired contract food services to provide gourmet menus. Some hospitals offer meals made from scratch (freshly prepared dishes) and others offer meals on request.

Hospital food prepared from scratch? Yes, all foods served at the Sutter Health Center facilities in Sacramento, California, are cooked from fresh ingredients. Prepackaged frozen meals are not to be found. But to do so, the food service staff requires special training to prepare the quantities of foods necessary. In addition, the staff has studied the quality of life aspects of food presentation and delivery and has returned the responsibility of distributing food trays and menu selections to the nursing staff. This change allows nurses to be more knowledgeable about the nutritional status of the patients.

Meals on request that are made to order at a healthcare facility? If a patient is receiving chemotherapy treatments at the Dana Farber Cancer Institute in Boston, Massachusetts, they can request their meals anytime between 7 AM to 7 PM. A patient can wait for the effects of a treatment to wear off and then request lunch at 3 PM rather than face a cold tray of leftover foods. And that lunch can even be an order of pancakes! All requests are delivered within 30 minutes. Pretty good service by anyone's standards.

Even without chefs, hospital food services can provide good tasting, attractively served food. The dietitian or food service director should be notified when patients are having problems with their meals. Without proper nutrition, recovery can be delayed and relapse may only be a matter of time.

Reference: Bond M: Sticking with scratch for quality: Sutter Health expands cost reduction, staff training efforts, Food Service: Business and Management Practices *15(1):32, 2002; and Wielawski I: Is there a cure for hospital food?* Eating Well *May/June: 50, 1993.*

patient food preferences are met. Simple changes or substitutions are common. Nursing personnel, on behalf of their patients, often interact with staff of the food service system at their facility. It may be beneficial for nurses to familiarize themselves with the organization and food service system staff. Beneficial information includes the following:[19]

TEACHING TOOL
Assisting Patients with Menu Selections

*W*hen we select food items from a restaurant menu while socializing with friends and family, the process is fun. However, choosing foods from the restricted hospital selections, often with little descriptive information, can be a difficult and sometimes intimidating chore when we are ill in a hospital. Some hospitals are going to paperless menus, instead using palmtop computers to read menus to patients for selections. As nurses, we are familiar with hospital forms and computer entries that require us to choose selections quickly; we cannot assume our patients also share that ability. Patients may need our help. Below are potential menu selection problems and possible solutions.

PROBLEM	SOLUTION
Patient has a low literacy level, is illiterate, has reduced visual abilities, or is too ill to read or write.	Read menu items to patient and mark his or her selections.
Patient does not understand the vocabulary used on menu (we cannot assume dietary terms are common knowledge).	Clarify for patient or ask for clarification from dietetic technician, dietitian, or food service personnel.
Patient often must select foods from menu a day in advance, often resulting in choosing too much or too little food (particularly a concern when appetite may be diminished from drug-nutrient interactions or from the effects of the illness).	Remind patients they are selecting food for the next day. If they have not selected enough food, offer them foods kept on the nursing unit for snacks or order additional foods from food service. If they have selected too much food, cover, date, and store appropriate foods for use later in the day.
Patient does not understand why some of his or her favorite foods are not included on the menu or why smaller amounts are served (when ill, familiar foods are most desired and comforting).	Menus are a great teaching tool for modified diets. Discuss dietary concerns of the patient's illness, explaining why specific foods are not included or only limited amounts allowed. Contact the RD to provide education for patient.

- Procedure and telephone numbers to request a physician-ordered diet, make diet changes, or report problems with a patient's tray
- Procedure and telephone number of the clinical dietitian to request nutrition assessment or education
- Time schedule of meal service so requests or changes can be made before meals are delivered to patients
- Location of the diet manual on the nursing unit, which is required in each unit by the Medicare Conditions of Participation for Hospitals and the Joint Commission Accreditation for Health Care Organizations; the diet manual is the reference book (usually in a three-ring binder) that describes the rationale and indications for using a specific diet, lists allowed and restricted foods, and provides sample menus

Most of this information also applies to long-term care facilities, but there are a few additional concerns. Food service provided to residents in long-term care facilities often relies solely upon the food service department for nutritious foods and meals. Repetition and boredom also affect patient acceptance of foods and meals served. Therefore it is of particular importance that these patients receive food they can and will eat because they are often at high nutritional risk.[19]

Basic Hospital Diets

Clear Liquid Diets. Clear liquid diets may be used postoperatively or if a patient is scheduled for diagnostic tests (Box 14-3). A clear liquid diet consists of foods that are clear and liquid at room or body temperature, factors that help

diet manual
the reference (usually in a three-ring binder or on computer) that describes the rationale and indications for using a specific diet, lists the allowed and restricted foods, and provides sample menus

prevent dehydration and keep colon contents to a minimum. Although a good source of fluids and water, this modified diet is desolate when it comes to adequate amounts of protein, fat, and energy. In addition, the clear liquid diet is almost devoid of dietary fiber, which is one of the reasons it is used. Whereas this diet can provide adequate amounts of vitamin C (if an adequate amount of juice is consumed), it is nutritionally inadequate for almost all other required nutrients except water. Because of its limited choices, this diet is boring and does not meet patients' expectations for a meal. Because a clear liquid diet is inadequate in energy and almost all nutrients except water, the diet should not be used for more than 24 hours even when supplemented with low-residue, nutritional products.[11] Use of a clear

colonoscopic examination
examination of the mucosal lining of the colon using a colonoscope (an elongated endoscope)

barium enema
rectal infusion of a radiopaque contrast medium to diagnose obstruction, tumors, or other abnormalities (e.g., ulcerative colitis)

paralytic ileus
decrease in or absence of intestinal peristalsis

Box 14-3 Types of Diets

LIQUID DIETS

INDICATIONS FOR CLEAR LIQUID DIET

Provide oral fluids; before/after surgery; prepare bowel for diagnostic tests (colonoscopic examination, barium enema, and other procedures); minimize stimulation of GI tract; promote recovery from partial paralytic ileus (early refeeding); minimize residue in the GI tract; transition feeding from IV feeding to solid foods; acute GI disturbances; diarrhea

CONTRAINDICATIONS FOR CLEAR LIQUID DIET

Should not be used more than 24 hours; inadequate GI function; nutrient needs requiring parenteral nutrition

INDICATIONS FOR FULL LIQUID DIET

Provide oral fluids; after surgery; transition between clear liquids and solid food; oral or plastic surgery to the face and neck; mandibular fractures; patients who have chewing or swallowing difficulties; esophageal or GI strictures; diarrhea

CONTRAINDICATIONS FOR FULL LIQUID DIET

Dysphagia

PUREED, MECHANICAL, OR SOFT DIETS

INDICATIONS FOR PUREED DIET

Neurologic changes; inflammation or ulcerations of the oral cavity and/or esophagus; edentulous patients; fractured jaw; head and neck abnormalities; cerebrovascular accident

CONTRAINDICATIONS FOR PUREED DIET

Situations where ground or chopped foods are appropriate

INDICATIONS FOR MECHANICAL SOFT DIET

Poorly fitting dentures; edentulous patients; limited chewing or swallowing ability; dysphagia; strictures of intestinal tract; radiation treatment to oral cavity; progression from enteral tube feedings or parenteral nutrition to solid foods

CONTRAINDICATIONS FOR MECHANICAL SOFT DIET

Situations where regular foods are appropriate

INDICATIONS FOR SOFT DIET

Debilitated patients unable to consume a regular diet; mild GI problems

CONTRAINDICATIONS FOR SOFT DIET

Situations where regular foods are appropriate

liquid diet for more than 1 day can lead to compromised nutritional status and possible nutrient deficiencies. If the patient is already nutritionally depleted, insult is added to the injury.

Caution is also necessary in regard to the amount of caffeine patients might receive on clear liquid diets. Because food choices are so limited, patients might easily receive and consume excessive amounts of caffeine in the form of coffee, strong tea, or soft drinks containing caffeine. Excess caffeine consumption could lead to increased hydrochloric acid production in the stomach, leading to an upset stomach, and contribute to sleeplessness.

Although few conditions contraindicate a clear liquid diet, it is important to reiterate that this diet should not be used as the sole means of nutrition for more than 24 hours *in any condition*. This diet should also not be used if the patient does not possess adequate gastrointestinal (GI) function or has nutrient needs such that parenteral nutrition is indicated.[20] Clear liquid diets can be adjusted to accommodate other dietary modifications, such as sodium restriction, if necessary.

There is some thought that unsupplemented clear liquid diets are one of the causative factors in the incidence of hospital malnutrition.[21] One way to prevent this is quality assurance monitoring by the RD. This helps identify patients who have been on clear liquid diets too long, as well as those patients with any nutritional problems that result from use of the diet. Another way to monitor use of clear liquid diets would be to establish a policy that diet orders for clear liquid diets are valid for only 24 hours (similar to the time-restricted orders for antibiotics), thus allowing physicians to reevaluate the patient and the need for this nutritionally deficient diet. Each day the physician can reorder the diet with documented justification, or choose a more appropriate source of nutrition. Along with this method, a mechanism to identify patients who have had clear liquid diets ordered more than three times would be necessary.

Full Liquid Diets.   A full liquid diet is one that consists of foods that are liquid at room temperature. It is used to provide oral nourishment for patients who have difficulty chewing or swallowing solid foods. Unlike the clear liquid diet, the full liquid diet offers more variety, and commercial nutritional supplements can be used to supply adequate amounts of energy and nutrients to make it nutritionally complete.

There are a few potential hazards associated with full liquid diets that have caused this diet to be excluded in widely used diet manuals,[11] but it may still be found in most hospitals. Because all liquids are allowed, lactose-containing (milk-based) foods are included. This is usually not a problem, except for patients who are lactose intolerant. Most patients do not tolerate fat or lactose well after surgery, albeit temporarily. They may experience symptoms of GI distress such as nausea, vomiting, distention, or diarrhea when given lactose-rich liquids. This, plus the growing evidence that supports rapid postoperative progression of the diet, has led to the elimination of the full liquid diet from many hospital settings.[22,23]

If a patient is to receive a nutritionally complete full liquid diet for an extended period, care should be given to reduce the high saturated fat and cholesterol content of the diet. One approach is to avoid excessive use of whole milk products, ice cream, milk shakes, and eggs as protein sources (e.g., in custards). Another special concern is for patients with **dysphagia** who cannot swallow thin liquids. Chapter 17 discusses special adaptations that can be used.

Full liquid diets can be nutritionally complete if they are well planned and include between-meal snacks or nourishment from commercially prepared supplements. Amounts of the diet consumed by patients should be monitored daily to ensure adequate energy and nutrient consumption. One word of caution about possible problems with foodborne illness: raw eggs should *never* be used in the preparation of any food served to patients, and patients and their families should be educated about possible dangers of foodborne illness.

Mechanically Altered Diets.   When a patient has problems chewing or swallowing, foods can be chopped, ground, mashed, and pureed. Consistency of food

dysphagia
the inability to swallow normally or freely or to transfer liquid or solid foods from the oral cavity to the stomach; may be caused by an underlying central neurologic or isolated mechanical dysfunction

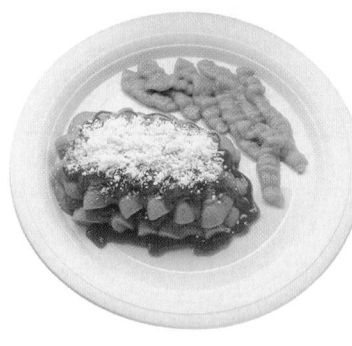

An example of component pureeing: lasagna and green peas, reformed to resemble their original shapes. (Courtesy Bryon Foods.)

component pureeing
each food item is pureed separately (food thickeners may be added to help maintain consistency), then presented in a manner that resembles the original product (e.g., a pork chop can be pureed, then molded into a pork-chop shape and served)

edentulous
toothless

Don't puree the food if ground will do.

Don't grind the food if chopped will do.

Do all you can to make them chew.

enteral nutrition
administration of nourishment via the GI tract

can be varied according to the patient's ability to chew and swallow. The nurse, dietitian, and patient should work together to evaluate the patient's needs for modifying consistency according to the food preferences.

Some foods such as mashed potatoes and ice cream are already of a smooth consistency. For other foods, small amounts of liquids (e.g., broth, milk, gravies) can be added to reach the appropriate consistency needed. Any liquid added to pureed foods should complement the food and not conceal the food's original flavor. Care should be taken to add only enough liquid to achieve desired consistency yet allow nutritional quality of the food to be retained. Butter, margarine, gravies, sugar, or honey may be added to foods to increase kcaloric density. To make pureed foods more attractive, component pureeing may be used. For example, a cake decorating tool (icing bag and tips) can be used to make pureed peas look like regular peas. Molds are also used to shape foods. For example, a pork chop can be pureed and then put into a pork chop–shaped mold and reheated in a microwave oven.

As mentioned previously, exact composition and consistency of a mechanically altered diet will vary depending on the patient's needs. These diets can be modified for additional needs such as low sodium, kcalorie control, or low fat. Care should be taken in evaluating the patient's needs for consistency. Food consistency should be altered only to the degree it is needed. If a patient needs only meats pureed, then only the meats should be pureed. If a patient needs only the foods or meats ground, then they shouldn't be pureed. Sometimes, foods just need to be chopped coarsely or finely. Edentulous patients can often chew solid or soft foods.

Soft Diets.   Soft diets are often used during transition from liquid diets to regular or general diets. Whole foods low in fiber and only lightly seasoned are used. This diet has traditionally been used for patients with mild GI problems. Food supplements or between-meals snacks may be used if needed to add kcalories.

Regular or General Diets.   A regular diet is used for patients who do not need dietary restrictions or modifications. Most hospitals offer self-select menus for regular diets and often for many modified diets. The regular diet serves as the basis for almost all modified diets.

Appendix H lists information about each of the basic hospital diets, which progress from a clear liquid to an unrestricted regular diet. Each step or diet of the progression provides appropriate texture and consistency as GI function increases. As healing proceeds, dietary restrictions decrease toward a regular diet.

Diet as Tolerated.   Occasionally when patients are admitted, the physician writes an order for "diet as tolerated." It is also common for this diet to be ordered postoperatively. This permits patients' preferences and situations to be taken into consideration and also allows for postoperative diet progression at the patient's tolerance. "Diet as tolerated" helps to alleviate prolonged use of clear and full liquid diets. Furthermore, this diet order provides an excellent opportunity for collaboration by the nurse, dietitian, and patient to plan and provide food that is eaten, tolerated, and nourishing.

Enteral Nutrition

Anytime the GI tract is used to provide nourishment, the feeding can be referred to as enteral nutrition. This includes liquid diets, soft and solid food diets, and special nutritionally complete formulas administered orally or via tubes. The consistency of the diet may be modified in progressive steps as in the following discussion and summarized in Appendix H, Foods Recommended for Hospital Diet Progressions. However, when medical personnel talk about enteral nutrition, most often they are referring to specialized formula feedings.

Enteral Feeding by Tube

Frequently, patients are unable or unwilling to orally consume adequate nutrients and kcalories. When this is the case and the GI tract is functioning, nutrients can be provided via feeding tubes placed into the alimentary tract (see the Teaching

Tool, "Tube Feeding the Infant or Child"). In fact, when the GI tract is functional, accessible, and safe to use, enteral feedings are preferred over parenteral nutrition because they are physiologically beneficial in maintaining the integrity and function of the gut.[11] Additionally, enteral tube feedings are much less costly than parenteral nutrition for both patient and the healthcare institution.

Enteral tube feeding can be part of routine care when a patient experiences protein-calorie malnutrition with 5 days of inadequate oral intake or with a reduced oral intake over the previous 7 to 10 days. Other conditions warranting tube feeding are severe dysphagia, major burns, a short gut from small bowel resection, or when intestinal fistulas (abnormal passages between the intestines) are present. Conditions under which enteral tube feedings are helpful, but not routine, include major trauma, radiation therapy, chemotherapeutic regimens, acute or chronic liver failure, or severe renal dysfunction. Enteral feeding is of limited or undetermined value if intensive chemotherapy results in GI tract dysfunction or if adequate postoperative oral intake is expected to resume within 5 to 7 days. Other conditions for which benefit is unclear are acute enteritis secondary to radiation, acute infection, active inflammatory bowel disease, and if less than 10% of the small intestine is intact after surgery.[11,24]

Types of Formulas.   Enteral nutrition by tube has been used since the late 1800s.[25] For years enteral formulas were prepared using foodstuffs, vitamin/mineral preparations, and a blender. Today an extensive variety of commercially prepared formulas are used. Some formulas are nutritionally complete, some are formulated for specific diseases or conditions, and others (modular) provide specific nutrients to supplement a diet or other formula. Commercial products are usually preferred over hospital or home-blended concoctions because they provide a known nutrient composition, controlled osmolality and consistency, and bacteriologic safety. They are also much easier to prepare and store. Many are nutritionally complete if consumed in the volumes recommended by the manufacturers.

osmolality

concentration of electrically charged particles per kilogram of solution

TEACHING TOOL
Tube Feeding the Infant or Child

Parents and caregivers need special support when their infants and children are tube fed. Assure them that the children can still be cuddled and can play without interfering with the tube nourishment. Teach the adults how the process works; they can be allies in helping young children accept and understand these procedures. Be sure to explain the procedures to the children as well. Dolls or stuffed animals can be used to explain how tube feeding helps to speed the healing process.

Every infant and child has individual nutritional requirements based on growth needs and medical conditions. Check with the nurse or dietitian for appropriate rate, concentration, and volume of feedings. The following are some specific techniques to ensure adequate nutrient intake.
- Use additional free water flushes if fluid needs are not met by tube patency flushes.
- Begin feedings with an isotonic formula. Either the strength or the volume of the feeding may be increased every 8 to 12 hours but not both at the same time.
- Check gastric residual before each feeding if you are feeding the infant every few hours. Hold the feeding if the amount is half the volume of the previous feeding.
- Check gastric residual at least every 4 hours if you are feeding with a pump. If residual is equal to the previous hourly rate, hold feedings for 1 hour and recheck. Residual checks are usually not indicated when the tube is placed past the stomach.
- Give medications only in liquid form.
- Elevate the head of the bed 30 to 45 degrees.

Reference: Nelson JK et al.: Mayo Clinic diet manual: a handbook of nutrition practices, ed 7, St Louis, 1994, Mosby.

polymeric formulas
solutions that provide intact nutrients (e.g., whole proteins and long-chain triglycerides) that require a normally functioning GI tract

isotonic
having the same concentration of solute as another solution; therefore, exerting the same amount of osmotic pressure as that solution

hypertonic
having greater concentration of solute than another solution

hypercaloric
more than one kcalorie per ml

elemental formulas
solutions that provide ready-to-absorb basic nutrients, requiring minimal digestion

Standard–Intact Formulas.   Standard–intact formulas (or polymeric formulas) are composed of intact nutrients that require a functioning GI tract for digestion and absorption of nutrients. There are several categories of polymeric formulas that provide 1 to 2 kcalories/ml. Standard–intact formulas can be categorized into blenderized food products, milk-based products, high-kcalorie lactose-free products, and normocaloric lactose-free products.

Normocaloric lactose-free products can be categorized into those that are isotonic, hypertonic, high-nitrogen, and fiber containing. Blenderized formulas (1 kcal/ml) are a blenderized mixture of ordinary foods that usually contain milk products (lactose). They have a high viscosity and moderate osmolality. Blenderized formulas can be made by the dietary staff or in the patient's own home; they are also available commercially. Noncommercial formulas are low in cost but run the risk of bacterial contamination and variation in nutrient composition.[26] Commercial formulas provide a sterile product with a fixed nutrient composition.[26] Extreme caution should be exercised when using noncommercial (home-made) formulas because of the risk of foodborne illness. For patient safety, commercial formulas should be used.

Normocaloric (1 kcal/ml) lactose-free formulas have low osmolality, which generally makes them well tolerated. Hypercaloric (1.5 to 2.0 kcal/ml) formulas are designed to meet kcalorie and protein demands in a reduced volume and have moderate to high osmolality. High-nitrogen lactose-free formulas (1 to 2 kcal/ml) are designed to meet increased protein demands at usual or increased energy needs. They have low to moderate osmolality. Fiber-containing products are low osmolality and are used for patients with abnormal bowel regulation. These formulas contain fiber from natural food sources or soy polysaccharide.

Special Formulas

ELEMENTAL FORMULAS.   Elemental formulas (predigested or hydrolyzed formulas) (1.0 to 1.3 kcal/ml) are composed of partially or fully hydrolyzed nutrients that can be used for patients with a partially functioning GI tract or those who have impaired capacity to digest foods or absorb nutrients, pancreatic insufficiency, or bile salt deficiency. These products are lactose-free and are usually hyperosmolar. They are not palatable and are best suited for administration by tube.

MODULAR FORMULAS.   Modular formulas (3.8 to 4.0 kcal/ml) are not nutritionally complete by themselves because they are single macronutrients such as glucose polymers, protein, or lipids. They are added to foods or other enteral products to change composition when nutritional needs cannot otherwise be met.

SPECIALTY FORMULAS.   These products (1.0 to 2.0 kcal/ml) are designed to meet specialized nutrient demands for specific disease states such as diabetes, renal failure, liver failure, pulmonary disease, or HIV/AIDS. Some formulas may require supplementation with vitamins, minerals, or trace elements. Some are unpalatable, and most formulas are expensive.

Formula Selection.   The numerous types and brands of enteral feeding products on the market can make product selection a complex process. Choosing an enteral feeding formula includes the following considerations[27]:
• What are the patient's digestive and absorptive capabilities?
• Do the patient's fluids need to be restricted?
• Does the patient have high metabolic requirements?

Whether a patient can digest and absorb nutrients indicates whether an elemental or polymeric formula should be used. Individual nutrient requirements determine the type and amount of tube-feeding formula. As with previous components of medical nutritional therapy, ongoing assessment of nutritional status and patients' tolerance of the formula is necessary.[11]

Successful use of enteral feeding depends on the patient's condition, availability of access for feeding, and the patient's tolerance of the chosen enteral formula.[28] Enteral feeding is the feeding route of choice because of benefits provided. Some of these benefits include improved use of nutrients, maintenance of gut mucosa and immunocompetence, decreased catabolic response to injury, administration safety, and lower cost.[28] In fact, McClave insists that the only time enteral feedings should not be used is in the absence of a gut.[29]

Feeding Routes.   In addition to choosing an appropriate tube feeding formula, selecting the appropriate feeding tube and feeding route involves consideration of various factors. Patients' medical status and nutritional status often govern the length of the feeding tube (i.e., the portion of the GI tract into which the formula is delivered). Anticipated length of time that tube feeding will be required dictates whether the feeding tube should be surgically placed. If the tube feeding will be used for short duration, a nonsurgical placement can be made. If the feeding tube will be long-term or permanent, surgical placement is necessary. Routes for tube feeding include the following (Figure 14-5):

- *Nasogastric:* Tube is passed through nose to stomach.
- *Nasoduodenal:* Tube is passed from nose to duodenum (small intestine).
- *Nasojejunal:* Tube is passed through nose to jejunum (small intestine).
- *Esophagostomy:* Tube is surgically inserted into the neck and extends to stomach.
- *Gastrostomy:* Tube is surgically inserted into stomach.
- *Jejunostomy:* Tube is surgically inserted into small intestine.

Placing the feeding tube into the stomach, duodenum, or jejunum through the nose is the simplest and most commonly used tube-feeding technique. This technique is preferred for patients who will resume oral feedings in the near future. Placement into the stomach simulates normal GI function but should be reserved for patients who are alert with intact gag and cough reflexes.[26] Tube placement into the small intestine has less risk of aspiration, but elemental formulas are often

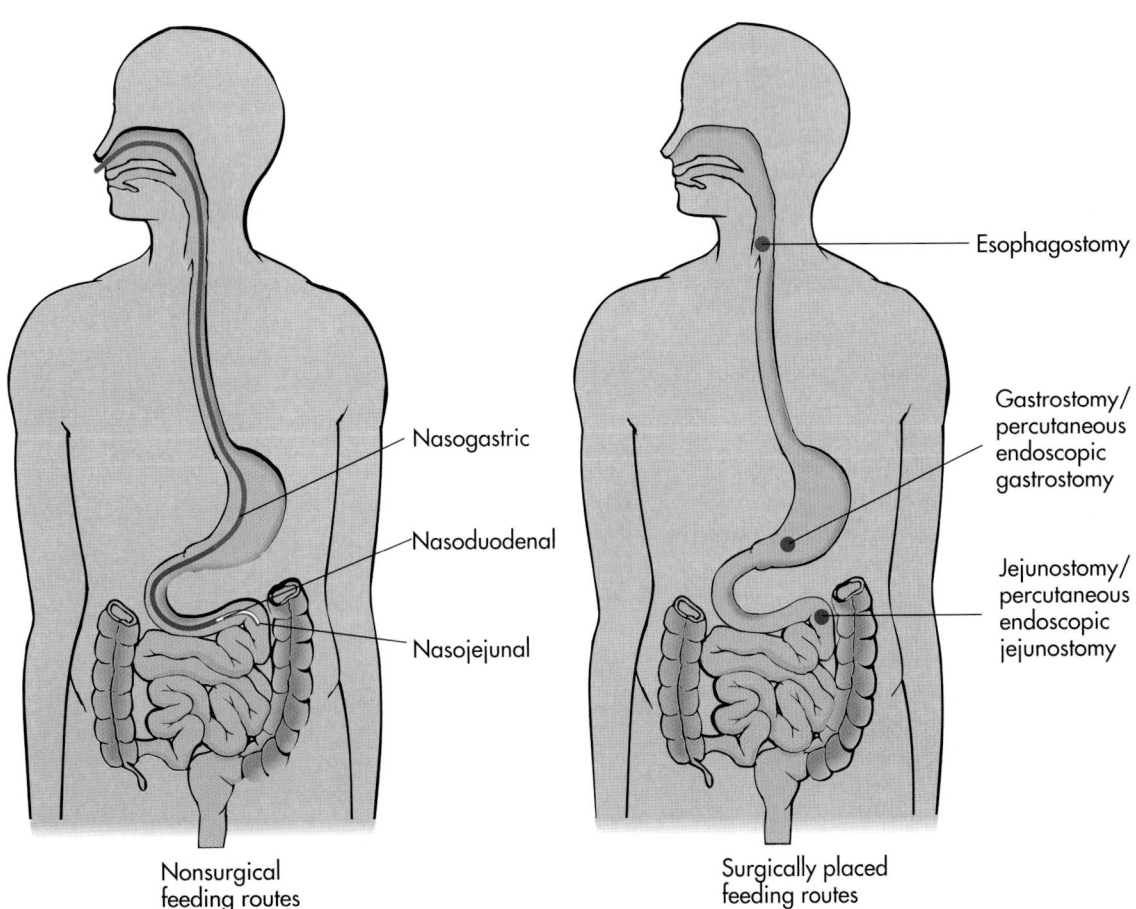

Figure 14-5 Types of enteral feeding routes. (From Rolin Graphics.)

percutaneous endoscopic placement (PEG)
placing feeding tube into stomach via the esophagus and then drawing it through the abdominal skin using a stab incision

required for easier absorption and continuous feedings are better tolerated.[26] Surgical placement of the feeding tube is preferred when long-term use is anticipated or when obstruction makes insertion through the nose impossible. These procedures require surgery with general anesthesia. Percutaneous endoscopic placement of a gastrostomy (PEG) can be performed with minimal sedation and has fewer complications than surgical placement. Table 14-5 describes the classifications, advantages, and disadvantages of feeding routes.

Table 14-5
Advantages and Disadvantages of Enteral Feeding Routes

Feeding Route	Characteristics	Advantages	Disadvantages
Nasogastric	Tube extends from nose into stomach	Easy placement/easy to remove No surgery necessary Less expensive Medications can be administered	Greater risk of aspiration (compared with nasointestinal feeding) Gastric emptying must be monitored
Nasoduodenal or nasojejunal	*Nasoduodenal:* Tube extends from nose through pylorus into duodenum; tube must be advanced by peristalsis or videofluoroscopy *Nasojejunal:* Tube extends from nose through pylorus into jejunum and is usually placed by videofluoroscopy or endoscopy	Lessened risk of aspiration (compared with nasogastric feedings) Helpful in patients with gastroparesis	Requires placement via endoscopy Unable to monitor gastric motility
Gastrostomy or percutaneous endoscopic gastrostomy (PEG)	*Gastrostomy:* Tube placed through incision in abdominal wall into stomach *PEG:* Tube percutaneously placed in stomach under endoscopic guidance, secured by rubber "bumpers" or inflated balloon catheter	Intermediate/bolus feedings possible Patient comfort Size of tube allows medication administration and/or gastric decompression	Increased risk of aspiration in some individuals Stoma care required Potential for dislodgment of tube
Jejunostomy or percutaneous endoscopic jejunostomy (PEJ)	*Jejunostomy:* Types include needle catheter placement, direct tube placement, and creation of jejunal stoma that is catheterized intermittently *PEJ:* Weighted feeding tube (from PEG insertion) into duodenum; peristaltic action advances tube into jejunum	Early postoperative feeding possible Decreased aspiration risk	Smaller tube used, tube may clog easily Stoma care required Intraperitoneal leakage possible Volvulus possible

Modified from American Dietetic Association: Handbook of clinical dietetics, ed 2, New Haven, Conn, 1992, Yale University Press; and American Dietetic Association: Manual of clinical dietetics, ed 6, Chicago, 2000, American Dietetic Association.

Method of Administration. How enteral tube feedings are administered or given to patients is just as important as formula selection and feeding site. Proper administration safeguards delivery of the desired nutrients, enhances tolerance by the patient, and provides optimal nutrition support. Factors affecting decisions about appropriate methods of formula infusion include the patient's medical status, GI function, and feeding route. Tube feedings can be administered by three methods: continuous, intermittent, or bolus infusion.

Continuous infusion is generally the preferred method of feeding.[18] This method provides controlled delivery of a prescribed volume of formula at a constant rate over a continuous period using an infusion pump. Although this method requires use of special equipment, it is preferred, especially when feeding into the small intestine, because it is similar to typical gastric emptying.

Intermittent infusion involves delivering the total quantity of formulas needed for a 24-hour period in 3 to 6 equal feedings. Each feeding is usually delivered by gravity during a 30- to 90-minute period. This method represents a more normal feeding pattern, but patients often do not tolerate this method of feeding if the rate is too rapid. Although equipment needs are minimal, this method is time consuming because feedings must be closely monitored to ensure proper delivery rate.

Bolus feedings involve infusing volumes of formula by gravity or syringe over a short period of time.[5,18] This method requires minimal equipment and time but is associated with increased potential for aspiration, regurgitation, and GI side effects.[26] This method should not be used for intestinal feedings. Table 14-6 summarizes indications for and pros and cons of each feeding method.

Starting the Tube Feeding. Before initiating enteral tube feedings, placement of the feeding tube must be confirmed and documented. This can be done several ways. Aspiration of gastric contents with a large syringe (60-ml) or radiologic confirmation of placement are the most common. The feeding should then be infused at a rate tolerated by the patient. Isotonic formulas can be administered at a rate of 10 to 40 ml/hr[11,26] and can be advanced every 8 to 12 hours until the desired rate is achieved.[11] Most patients can tolerate an advancement of 10 to 20 ml every 12 hours.[11] Hypertonic formulas can be given full strength at 10 to 40 ml/hr and increased gradually as tolerated.[11] The high osmolality of a hypertonic formula can lead to GI distress such as intestinal distention and osmotic diarrhea. Diluting tube feedings will lengthen the amount of time necessary before nutritional requirements can be met by the formula and feeding regimen. Rate of the feedings can be advanced to desired volume, and then concentration can be gradually increased until kcalorie and protein needs are met. Rate and concentration should never be advanced at the same time. If the feeding is not tolerated, rate or concentration can be reduced to the last level of tolerance, then gradually increased again. Other criteria to be considered to ensure optimal tolerance of the formula and safety of the feedings include solution temperature, prevention of bacterial contamination, prevention of aspiration, patency of tubing, administration of medications, and patient monitoring (Table 14-7).

Possible Tube Feeding Complications. Although tube feedings use the GI tract to nourish the patient, they are not without problems. Most are preventable; all are correctable. Tube feeding complications can be categorized three ways according to the type of problem: GI, mechanical, or metabolic. GI problems include diarrhea, nausea and vomiting, cramping, distention, and constipation. Mechanical complications consist of tube displacement or obstruction, pulmonary aspiration, and mucosal damage. Metabolic difficulties involve hyperosmolar dehydration or overhydration; abnormal blood concentration levels of sodium, potassium, phosphorus, and magnesium (too high or too low); hyperglycemia; respiratory insufficiency; and rapid weight gain. Table 14-8 summarizes possible complications, probable causes, and suggested corrective actions.

Diarrhea, a common complication of enteral feedings, was once thought to be caused by hyperosmolar feeding solutions.[18] More recently it has been determined that other factors may contribute to this problem.[30] Patients receiving tube feedings

osmotic diarrhea: diarrhea associated water retention in the large intestine resulting from an accumulation of nonabsorbable water-soluble solutes

Table 14-6
Administration of Enteral Tube Feedings

Method	Indications	Advantages	Disadvantages
Continuous	Patients who have not eaten for a significant period, debilitated patients, those with impaired GI function, patients with uncontrolled type 1 diabetes mellitus, intestinal feedings	Feedings can be administered at constant rate over 24-hr period, feedings can be cycled (allows formula to be delivered over shorter period, allowing patients freedom of movement and to promote oral intake if appropriate), gastric pooling minimized and fewer GI side effects experienced, continuous feeding into jejunum is similar to normal gastric emptying	Requires feeding pump if accuracy of volume delivered is required; continuous drip by gravity is possible, but less accurate
Intermittent	Feedings that are infused at specific intervals throughout the day (total volume of feeding divided and given 4-6 times/day)	Requires only simple equipment, can be used in home settings, may be more physiologic than continuous infusion, feedings can be administered by gravity over 30-90 minutes	In absence of pumps, feedings must be monitored vigilantly, may become time consuming depending on number of scheduled feedings per day, rate of intermittent infusion (rather than volume) seems to be a major reason for intolerance of tube feedings
Bolus	Appropriate *only* for feeding into the stomach, involves feeding large volumes of formula intermittently over short periods, usually by syringe	More manageable for the patient, rate of 30 ml/minute or volume of 500-700 ml per feeding seems to be cutoff of physical tolerance limits	Associated with increased risk of aspiration, regurgitation, and GI side effects; not appropriate for postpyloric feedings

Modified from Nelson JK et al: Mayo Clinic diet manual: a handbook of nutrition practices, ed 7, St Louis, 1994, Mosby; Woolfson AMJ et al.: Prolonged nasogastric tube feeding in critically ill and surgical patients, Postgrad Med J 52:678, 1976; and Heitkemper ME et al.: Rate and volume of intermittent enteral feedings, J Parenteral Enteral Nutr 51:125, 1981.

are frequently placed on liquid forms of medications, and many of these medications contain sorbitol, which can cause diarrhea. Bacterial dysentery caused by *Clostridium difficile* is also a common cause of diarrhea. Diarrhea should not be attributed to tube-feeding formulas until other causes have been ruled out.[18]

Home Enteral Nutrition. Because of changing healthcare reimbursement patterns, demand for home tube feeding has been growing steadily.[31] Although it provides opportunity and convenience for patients, home enteral nutrition (HEN) imparts responsibility that nurses and dietitians must assume and risks that must be anticipated.[31] In addition to criteria already discussed regarding selection of appropriate candidates for tube feedings, other criteria that should be considered when sending a patient home on enteral nutritional therapy include the following[31]:

- Patient's nutritional needs cannot be met orally
- Appropriate enteral access is in place and functioning, and patient is tolerating tube feeding regimen

Text continued on p. 429.

Table 14-7
Criteria for Safe Administration of Enteral Tube Feedings

Criteria	Considerations
Temperature	Administer solutions infused by continuous drip chilled Administer intermittent and bolus feedings at room temperature to decrease incidence of GI side effects
Prevention of bacterial contamination	Use closed feeding containers Prefilled, ready-to-feed, closed systems are available for some products (less chance of contamination) Change extension tubing administration set and bag *daily* Never add new formula to old formula Do *not* hang feedings for longer than 4-8 hours Maintain ice in pouch of bag at all times while formula is running
Prevention of aspiration	Check tube placement before administration Tubes placed into small bowel are associated with decreased risk for aspiration HOB should be elevated 30-45 degrees Consider adding vegetable food coloring to formula to allow for detection of aspirated tube feeding from pulmonary secretions (remember, this does not protect against aspiration)
Patency of tubing	Irrigate tubes every 6-8 hours with 40-50 ml of warm water (continuous feeds) For intermittent or bolus feedings, irrigate tubes after each feeding with 40-50 ml of warm water Flush tube with 40-50 ml of water each time feeding is stopped If tubing clogs, flush with 30-50 ml of warm water Systems are available that allow for self-flushing of the feeding tube (e.g., Ross Laboratories)
Medications	Medications administered through the feeding tube should be in *liquid form* Flush tubing before and after giving the medication with 20 cc of water to prevent clogging If medication is not available in liquid form, consult the pharmacist *before* crushing or diluting the medication (some medications are pharmacologically altered by mechanical manipulation) *Never* crush time-released, liquid-filled capsules or enteric coated medications Do *not* give sublingual medications through the tubing Because hyperosmolar liquid medications (KCl) may cause gastric irritation or diarrhea, dilute with water before administration Supplemental electrolyte preparations (KCl, NaCl, NaPO$_4$) increase the osmolality of the formula and may cause diarrhea Bulk-forming agents cause feeding tubes to clog Do *not* mix together multiple medications and deliver simultaneously unless the compatibility of the medications is known If feeding into the duodenum or jejunum instead of the stomach, check the effect of medication absorption Monitor patient response to medications given through the feeding tube and make changes needed

Monitoring	Confirm tube placement before initiation of feeding and before each intermittent feeding
	Record urine glucose every shift until final feeding rate and concentration are established
	Record gastric residuals every 4 hours (gastric feedings only)
	Record bowel movements and consistency
	Record tolerance to feedings
	Record daily:
	  Weight
	  Intake and output
	Record weekly:
	  Serum electrolytes and blood counts
	  Chemistry profile (including liver function tests, phosphorus, calcium, magnesium, total protein, and albumin)
	  Nitrogen balance, if appropriate
	Reassess nutrition indexes weekly, adjusting energy and protein as needed

Modified from American Dietetic Association: Manual of clinical dietetics, ed 6, Chicago, 2000, American Dietetic Association; and White WT et al.: Contamination of enteral nutrient solution: a preliminary report, J Parenteral Enteral Nutr 3:459, 1979.

Table 14-8
Tube Feeding Complications, Causes, and Corrective Actions

Category	Problem	Possible Cause	Corrective Action
Gastrointestinal	Diarrhea (defined as more than four bowel movements per day or liquid stools greater than 200 g)	Protein energy malnutrition (PEM)	Switch to isotonic formula and feed at slow rate (will allow intestine to adapt to refeeding)
		Infection, microbial contamination of formula	Confirm with stool, blood, or formula cultures; limit hang time of formula to 8-12 hrs, maintain ice in bag's pouch, change bag and tubing every 24 hrs, and rinse after each bolus feeding or before filling bag for continuous feedings; use good handwashing technique
		Malabsorption	Check for pancreatic insufficiency; pancreatic enzymes replacement may be necessary; change to low-fat, lactose-free, or elemental formula; change to continuous feeding
		Bolus feeding, volume overload, rapid administration, dumping syndrome	If infusion rate or concentration was advanced recently, return to previously tolerated rate/concentration; change to continuous feeding; decrease bolus volume and increase frequency of feedings
		Hyperosmolar formula	If started, reduce rate and increase gradually; dilute formula or change to isotonic product; if starting, rate should begin at 25 ml/hr, increasing every 12-24 hours
		Medications	Evaluate types of medications as primary cause (diarrhea has been related to administration of antibiotics and antacids, potassium supplements, cimetidine, and sorbitol-containing drops) and the possibility for change; stool samples should be taken for *Clostridium difficile* culture and toxin; change to fiber-containing formula
		Hypoalbuminemia	Albumin levels <2.5 g/dl result in decreased colloidal osmotic pressure* with accompanying peripheral edema (which may involve GI tract); try peptide-based, low-fat formula with MCT†

Modified from American Dietetic Association: Manual of clinical dietetics, ed 6, Chicago, 2000, American Dietetic Association; Gottschlich MM et al.: Diarrhea in tube-fed patients: incidence, etiology, nutritional impact, and prevention, J Parenteral Enteral Nutr 12:338, 1988; and Edes TE, Walk BE, Austin JL: Diarrhea in tube-fed patients: feeding formula not necessarily the cause, Am J Med 88:91, 1990.

*Pressure difference between the osmotic pressure of blood and that of tissue fluid or lymph; it is an important force in maintaining balance between blood and surrounding tissue and is usually caused by large particles such as protein molecules that will not pass through a membrane. Also called oncotic pressure.

†Medium chain triglycerides (MCTs), distinguished from other triglycerides by having 8 to 10 carbon atoms. MCTs are easily digested.

Table 14-8—cont'd
Tube Feeding Complications, Causes, and Corrective Actions

Category	Problem	Possible Cause	Corrective Action
Gastrointestinal—cont'd		Decreased bulk	Fiber-containing formulas may help control diarrhea by normalizing GI transit time and providing bulk
	Nausea and vomiting, cramping, distention	High osmolality	Dilute formula to isotonic concentration if gastric residuals are consistently high; consider changing to isotonic formula
		Patient position	Reposition patient on right side to facilitate passage of gastric contents through pylorus
		Rapid increase in rate, volume, or concentration	Return to slower rate, and advance by smaller increments; advance only when tolerating current rate
		Delayed gastric emptying	Stop feedings for 2 hrs and check residuals; check residuals every 2-4 hrs (continuous feedings) and before administration (bolus feedings); reduce fat content in tube feeding; consider transpyloric feeding; monitor for drugs or disease that may influence gastric or intestinal motility; ambulation may help
		Lactose intolerance	Change to lactose-free formula
		Cold formula	Warm formula to room temperature
		GI tract obstruction	Stop feeding immediately
		Excessive fat in formula	Change to low-fat formula
	Constipation	Dehydration	Monitor intake and output; add free water if intake not greater than output by 500-1000 ml/day
		Decreased fiber	Use formula with fiber; make sure patient gets adequate water
		Medications	Evaluate medication side-effects; suggest stool softener or bulk-forming laxative
		Inactivity	Increase patient activity if possible
		GI tract obstruction	Stop feedings
Mechanical	Tube displacement	Coughing, vomiting	Replace tube, confirm placement before restarting feeding
		Dislodgment by patient	Replace tube; restrain patient if necessary; consider alternate feeding route
		Inadequate taping of tube	Position tube; tape securely
	Tube obstruction	Improperly crushed medication	Use liquid form of medication, medications should not be crushed without first checking with pharmacy; rinse tube with 20 ml warm water before and after giving medications
		Medications mixed with incompatible formula	Review drug/nutrient interaction guidelines; flush tubing before and after adding medications
		Insufficient tube irrigation; failure to irrigate	Flush tubing with 20-50 ml warm water before and after bolus feeding, every 4-8 hours during continuous feedings, and whenever tube is disconnected or feeding is stopped

Continued

Table 14-8—cont'd
Tube Feeding Complications, Causes, and Corrective Actions

Category	Problem	Possible Cause	Corrective Action
Mechanical—cont'd	Pulmonary aspiration	Patient lying flat	Elevate head of bed 30-45 degrees during continuous feedings and for at least 30-60 minutes after bolus feedings
		Absent or weak gag reflexes	Feed into duodenum or jejunum
		Gastric reflux	May be caused by feeding tube, change to smaller bore tube; feed into duodenum or jejunum
		Delayed gastric emptying	Monitor gastric residual; residual >200 ml in patients with nasogastric tubes and 100 ml in patients with gastrostomy tubes may indicate intolerance; hold feedings, recheck residual in 1-2 hrs
		Improper tube placement	Confirm tube placement with radiology; reconfirm placement before each feeding and periodically during continuous feeding by injecting air into stomach and listening with a stethoscope
	Mucosal damage	Extended use of large-bore tubes	Conscientious mouth and nose care; consider changing to small-bore tubing, or permanent gastrostomy or jejunostomy feeding tubes
		Decreased salivary secretions caused by lack of chewing; mouth breathing	Moisten lips and mouth; let patient chew sugarless gum, gargle, or suck on anesthetic lozenges if appropriate
Metabolic	Hyperosmolar dehydration	Hypertonic formula used without adequate water	Begin hypertonic feedings at slower rate; dilute with free water; or consider isotonic formula
	Overhydration (fluid overload)	Refeeding patients with PEM; fluid overload	Restrict fluids; use concentrated formula
		Prolonged use of overdiluted formula	Advance concentration as tolerated by patient
	Hyponatremia	CHF, cirrhosis, hypoalbuminemia, edema, ascites	Restrict fluids, administer diuretics, use concentrated formulas
		Excess GI losses	Monitor serum Na levels and hydration status, replace Na as needed
	Hypernatremia	Dehydration	Calculate patient's fluid needs: 35 ml/kg can be used unless patient's condition alters fluid needs, <30 ml/kg for the elderly
	Hypokalemia	Refeeding syndrome, insulin administration, diuretics, diarrhea	Monitor electrolytes daily, replete with parenteral potassium

Table 14-8—cont'd
Tube Feeding Complications, Causes, and Corrective Actions

Category	Problem	Possible Cause	Corrective Action
Metabolic—cont'd	Hyperkalemia	Renal insufficiency, metabolic acidosis, anabolic metabolism	Reduce potassium intake, consider changing to a lower potassium tube-feeding formula, assess renal function
	Hyperphosphatemia	Renal insufficiency	Use phosphate binder, consider changing formula
	Hypophosphatemia	Refeeding syndrome, insulin administration	Replace phosphorus with parenteral supplement; monitor serum levels daily; once patient is repleted, monitor weekly
	Hypomagnesemia	Refeeding syndrome, alcoholism	Replete with parenteral magnesium sulfate; monitor serum levels daily; once patient is repleted, monitor weekly
	Hyperglycemia	Diabetes mellitus; temporary insulin resistance or insulin deficiency	Monitor blood sugars frequently, adjust insulin dose; reduce rate of tube feeding until blood sugar controlled; avoid formulas high in simple carbohydrates
	Increased respiratory quotient; excess CO_2 production; respiratory insufficiency	Overfeeding (kcalories), especially in form of carbohydrates	Balance kcalories provided from fat, protein, and carbohydrates; consider using a higher-fat formula or adding modular fat
	Rapid, excessive weight gain	Excess kcalories, excess fluids, electrolyte imbalance	Decrease concentration or amount of formula; evaluate electrolyte status

- Patient and/or significant other is (are) able and willing to perform HEN techniques safely and effectively
- Underlying disease state is stable, and patient is ready for discharge and can be monitored in the home setting
- Affordable HEN supplies are available

Once a patient is considered an appropriate candidate for HEN, the nutrition care plan must be modified to an appropriate home plan that includes tailoring the enteral formula, route and method of administration, and feeding schedule. Amount or type of formula may need to be adjusted to meet the patient's long-term nutritional requirements. Blenderized formulas are strongly discouraged because of reasons previously discussed. Route of HEN administration should also be examined for its ability to meet the patient's long-term needs and adequacy. If at all possible, the patient should be included in this decision. Keeping the functional level of the GI tract and risk of aspiration in mind, method of administration (continuous, intermittent, or bolus) should be altered if necessary according to patient preference, convenience, and cost.[31] Feeding schedules may need to be arranged around family members' schedules or other daily routines. They should be planned to augment patient comfort and convenience and to maximize nutritional benefit.[31]

The patient should be stabilized on the home feeding regimen while still hospitalized before patient education is initiated. Education should include oral instructions, written guidelines, staff demonstration, return demonstration by the patient and significant other, and their assumption of full responsibility for tube feeding before discharge from the hospital.[31] Figure 14-6 is an example of an HEN training checklist.

Patients should also be referred to a source for obtaining supplies such as formula and administration equipment before discharge. Some patients may need help in obtaining financial assistance. Most often, referral to home health agencies provides the necessary supplies, equipment, and staff for home follow-up visits, as well as assistance with third-party payers.[32]

PURPOSE AND INSTRUCTIONS: This checklist will assist in identifying instructional responsibilities and aid in training patients in the skills needed for performing home enteral nutrition (HEN).

The nurse and dietitian will jointly instruct the patient on tube feeding administration and cares.

Date and initial section when instruction/demonstration is completed
RNs: Document training in Nursing Notes.
RDs: Document training in Progress Notes.

STAGE I: INITIATION OF HEN PROGRAM

_____ Patient assessment   (Dietitian-Nurse)
            Medical-social-nutritional history
_____ Plan of care outlined   (Dietitian-Nurse)
_____ Identification of dismissal date _____ (Nurse)
_____ Home enteral coordinator notified   (Dietitian)

STAGE II: IMPLEMENTATION OF HEN TRAINING   (Dietitian)

INTRODUCTION TO HEN PROGRAM   (Dietitian)

_____ Discuss purpose
_____ Introduce manual *Instructions for Tube Feeding at Home*

EQUIPMENT   (Dietitian-Nurse)
Discuss purpose, assembly, use, care, and cleaning of equipment.

	Discuss	Demonstrate	Patient Demonstrate
Feeding tube	_____	_____	_____
Feeding bag	_____	_____	_____
Gavage syringe	_____	_____	_____
Enteral pump (if needed)	_____	_____	_____

FORMULA—FLUIDS   (Dietitian)
_____ Show formula.
_____ Discuss purpose, type, amount, formula concentrations, fluid needs.
_____ Discuss preparation.
_____ Discuss administration schedule.
_____ Discuss weight expectations.

Figure 14-6 Home enteral training checklist. (From Nelson JK, Weckwerth JA: Home enteral nutrition. In Skipper A, ed.: *Dietitian's handbook of enteral and parenteral nutrition*, Rockville, Md, 1989, Aspen.)

Parenteral Nutrition

Fortunately, there are alternatives for providing nutrients to patients when they can't or won't eat and tube feedings are contraindicated. Parenteral nutrition (PN) affords the provision of energy and nutrients intravenously. When infused into a large-diameter vein, such as the superior vena cava or subclavian (Figure 14-7), parenteral nutrition is often called *central parenteral nutrition (CPN)* or *total parenteral nutrition (TPN)*. When a smaller, peripheral vein is used (usually in the forearm), parenteral nutrition is called *peripheral parenteral nutrition (PPN)*. Other terms are also used to characterize parenteral nutrition. These terms include *central venous nutrition (CVN), peripheral venous nutrition (PVN)*, and *hyperalimentation (hyperal)*.

TPN may mean the difference between life and death for patients who cannot be adequately nourished via the GI tract. But because of serious complications that may occur from use of TPN, it should be preserved for severely malnourished patients undergoing chemotherapy and major surgery.[33] Factors that should be considered before initiation of TPN are the nature of the patient's GI dysfunction, severity of malnutrition, degree of hypercatabolism, medical prognosis, and the patient's wishes.[33]

Components of Parenteral Nutrition Solutions

Parenteral nutrition (PN) solutions contain the same nutrients and components you would expect to find in any enteral nutrition source. PN solutions typically contain water, amino acids, dextrose, electrolytes, vitamins, and trace elements. Fat is also included, often by means of piggyback administration or by adding it directly to the PN solution (usually called a *three-in-one solution*, which is discussed later).

Carbohydrates.   The most common carbohydrate used in PN is dextrose monohydrate.[11] Used as an energy source, it yields 3.4 kcal/g because of its hydrated form. Dextrose solutions are available in initial concentrations of 5% through 70%. Higher glucose concentrations are useful when a patient's fluids need to be restricted; lower concentrations are often used to help control hyperglycemia. Concentrations greater than 10% (final concentration) are hypertonic

parenteral nutrition
administration of nutrients by a route other than the GI tract, usually intravenously

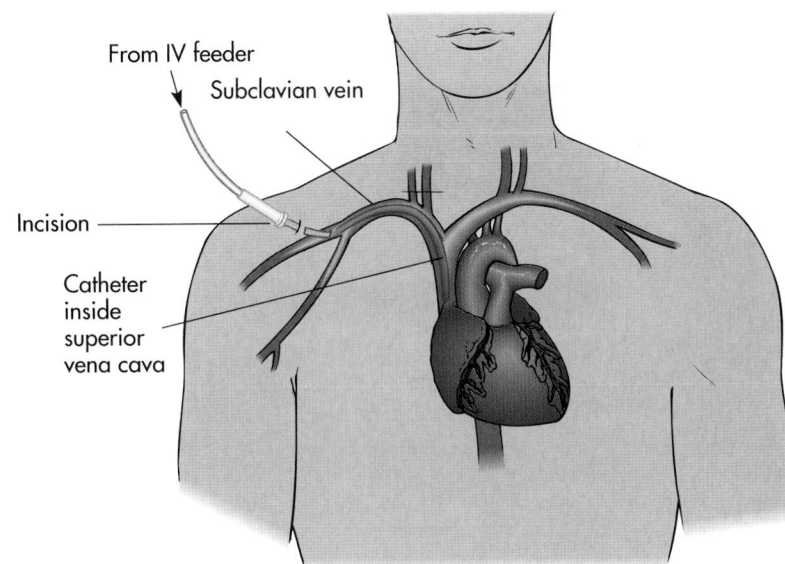

Figure 14-7 Placement of catheter for central parenteral nutrition, via the subclavian vein to the superior vena cava. (From Rolin Graphics.)

and must be delivered via CPN because the larger central vein can dilute the solution rapidly without damaging the blood vessel. Dextrose solutions are mixed with amino acids and other nutrients to form the final solution. Glucose needs and tolerances are important guidelines.

Amino Acids.   Protein is provided in PN solutions as a mixture of essential and nonessential crystalline amino acids that are available with or without added electrolytes.[11] It is important that the amino acids be used for protein synthesis and not be considered part of the solution's kcalorie source. Some facilities will not include protein kcalories when calculating kcalorie content of PN solutions; others will. Amino acid solutions are available in different concentrations as well as in different compositions of amino acids. Amino acid solutions are available for specialized protein needs such as renal failure, liver failure, stress, and trauma, but their efficacy is controversial.[11]

Fats.   IV lipid emulsions are used as a concentrated energy source and to prevent the development of essential fatty acid deficiency.[11,27] Commercial lipid emulsions are formulations of safflower oil, soybean oil, or a combination of the two, with glycerol added for isotonicity and egg phospholipid added as an emulsifying agent.[11] The kcaloric density of lipid solutions is useful when volume restriction is necessary. A 10% fat emulsion yields 1.1 kcal/ml or 550 kcal per 500 ml bottle, and a 20% solution yields 2 kcal/ml or 1000 kcal per 500 ml bottle. Another plus for lipid emulsions is that kcalories can be increased without increasing osmolality of PN solutions.[11]

Traditionally, lipid emulsions have been delivered peripherally using a piggyback system. Although IV lipids are useful in supplying most of the nonprotein kcalories, care should be taken to not exceed 2.5 grams of lipid/kg (adults) or 60% of nonprotein kcalories.[11,34] Baseline serum triglyceride level should be confirmed before administration of IV lipid emulsions and should be monitored according to institutional policy. If a lipid profile is ordered on a patient receiving lipids, the patient should not have received lipid emulsion for the 12 hours before blood is drawn.

Total Nutrient Admixtures.   When lipid emulsions are added to dextrose and amino acid mixtures, the resulting solution is called a *three-in-one mixture* (Figure 14-8) or a *(TNA).*[11] The advantage to this system is that it allows lipid infusion over 24 hours, decreasing carbon dioxide production and reducing hepatic accumulation of fat induced by long-term glucose use.[11,35]

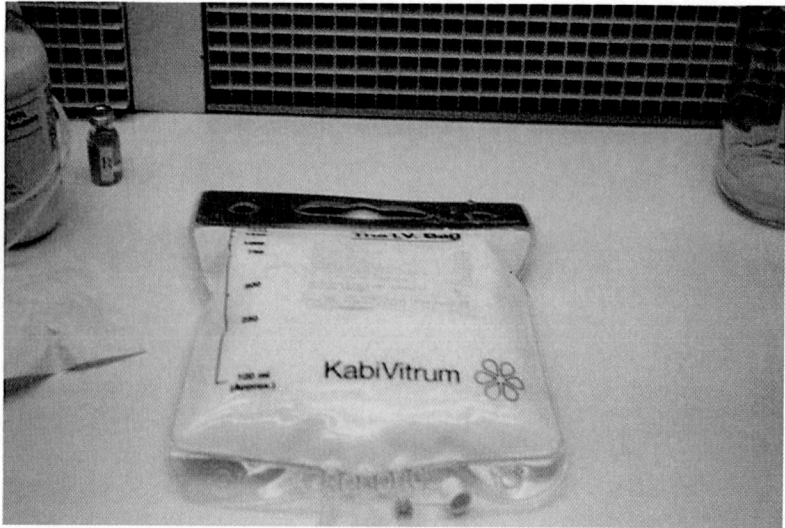

Figure 14-8 A three-in-one solution includes dextrose, amino acids, and lipids. (From Morgan SL, Weinsier RL: *Fundamentals of clinical nutrition,* ed 2, St Louis, 1998, Mosby.)

Electrolytes. Electrolytes and minerals can be provided by the general amino acid solution, as a combined electrolyte concentrate, or added separately as individual salts.[11] Electrolytes and minerals are essential for normal body function and to accommodate excesses and deficiencies of minerals resulting from underlying disease processes. Commercial electrolyte solutions are available. Magnesium, phosphate, and potassium requirements increase in severely malnourished patients during refeeding or when higher levels of dextrose concentrations are used.[11]

Vitamins. Adult and pediatric multivitamin formulations for IV use are available commercially. These products have been formulated according to recommendations of the American Medical Association Nutrition Advisory Group.[36] In the event of frank vitamin deficiency, multiples of daily doses can be given in accordance with clinical status.[11] Vitamin K is not included in adult preparations and must be given either intramuscularly or as an IV injectable added to the PN solution.[11]

Trace Elements. Trace elements are another essential component of PN solutions. Their omission from early formulas led to clinical deficiencies and subsequent recommendations by the American Medical Association.[37] Formulations that include zinc, copper, manganese, chromium, and selenium are available from commercial sources already combined, or institutional pharmacies may develop their own IV injectable formula.

Peripheral Parenteral Nutrition

PN solutions composed of less than 10% (final concentration) dextrose and/or less than 5% (final concentration) amino acids are hypertonic and can be administered only into central veins. PN solutions administered via peripheral veins must be isotonic to prevent damage to the vein. Isotonic PN solutions usually contain 5% to 10% dextrose (final concentration) and 3% to 5% amino acids, plus electrolytes, vitamins, minerals, and fat as needed. These nutrient components can only provide a limited amount of kcalories and protein.[11] PPN is most often used in situations where only short-term nutrition support is needed in nonhypermetabolic conditions.

Monitoring Guidelines

Monitoring needs and protocols will vary among institutions and patient populations. Frequency of baseline parameter readings range from every 6 hours to a one-time baseline reading. Routine frequencies range from every 6 hours to biweekly or as needed. Specific parameters and recommendations for monitoring patients receiving TPN are listed in Box 14-4.

Complications

As with enteral tube feedings, complications can occur with PN. Most can be averted by following the recommendations for monitoring in Box 14-4. Others can be circumvented by adhering to stringent technique. Box 14-5 summarizes possible complications.

Technical complications are related to catheter placement and are not unique to parenteral nutrition. The most common technical complication results in pneumothorax, which can be prevented by careful insertion of the central line using proper technique.[18] Septic complications, like technical complications, are not unique to parenteral nutrition. Infections can be local or systemic, and they usually occur because of poor technique in aseptic catheter care. Metabolic complications are the most common because metabolic requirements (electrolytes and energy) differ from patient to patient. The most common metabolic complication is hyperglycemia, which can be treated by adding insulin to the solution, reducing the dextrose load, or ensuring that the total kcaloric load is not excessive.[18]

Home Parenteral Nutrition

Home parenteral nutrition (HPN) enables selected patients who depend on PN to return to a reasonably normal lifestyle. A specialized catheter is used to reduce possibility of infection (Figure 14-9). The catheter is placed through a tunnel under the

Box 14-4 Recommendations for Monitoring Patients Receiving TPN

EVERY 8 HOURS

Vital signs
Temperature
Urine fractionals

DAILY

Weight
Fluid intake and output
Serum electrolytes, glucose, creatinine, blood urea
  nitrogen until stable; then twice weekly

WEEKLY

Serum magnesium, calcium, phosphorus, albumin
Liver function tests
Complete blood count
Review of actual oral, enteral, and TPN intake

FLUID DISORDERS

Urine sodium or fractional sodium excretion
Serum osmolality
Urine specific gravity

PROTEIN STATUS

Nitrogen balance, serum prealbumin

LIPID DISORDERS

Serum triglycerides or lipid clearance test
Respiratory quotient
Essential fatty acids (if fat-free TPN is necessary)

HEPATIC ENCEPHALOPATHY

Plasma amino acids

GASTROINTESTINAL LOSSES

Serum trace elements
Stool electrolytes

RESPIRATORY COMPROMISE

$Paco_2$
Indirect calorimetry, respiratory quotient

ACID-BASE DISORDERS

Blood pH
Anion gap

LONG-TERM TPN

Body composition measures
Serum trace elements, vitamins

From Lenssen P: Management of total parenteral nutrition. In Skipper A, ed.: Dietitian's handbook of enteral and parenteral nutrition, ed 2, 1998, Jones and Bartlett Publishers, Sudbury, MA, www.jbpub.com. Reprinted with permission.

skin and exits the chest at a place where the patient or caretaker can care for it conveniently.[18] As with HEN, HPN requires the patient and significant other to be willing and able to perform daily procedures involved in administering the PN, which include monitoring laboratory values, temperature, weights, glucose measurements, and fluids.[38] Home healthcare agencies may be used to provide equipment, supplies, and services.

Patients may be scheduled to receive HPN at night during sleep (cyclic TPN) to allow freedom to leave home or even work during the day. If the GI tract is func-

Box 14-5 Complications of Parenteral Nutrition

TECHNICAL COMPLICATIONS

Pneumothorax
Malposition of catheter
Subclavian artery puncture
Carotid artery puncture
Catheter embolism
Air embolism
Catheter obstruction
Thrombosis

SEPTIC COMPLICATIONS

Catheter-related sepsis
Septic thrombosis

METABOLIC COMPLICATIONS

Hyperglycemia
Hyperglycemic hyperosmolar nonketotic
  dehydration
Hypoglycemia
Hyperkalemia
Hypophosphatemia
Hypocalcemia

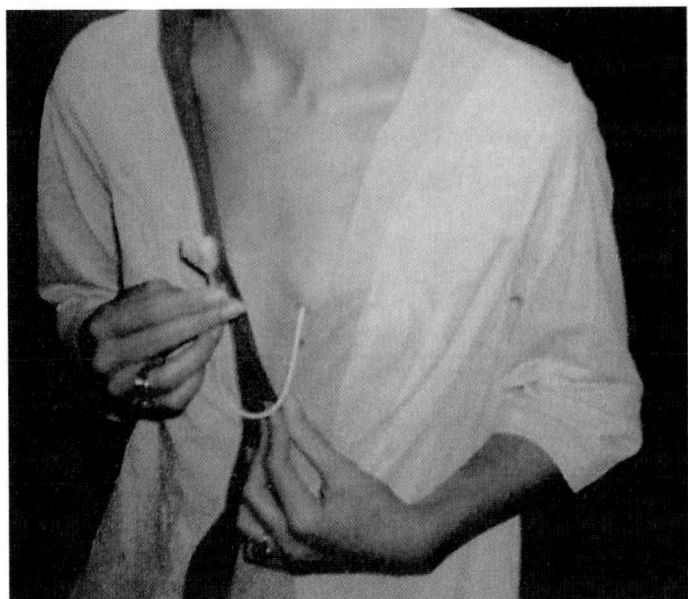

Figure 14-9 Catheter used for home central venous alimentation. (From Morgan SL, Weinsier RL: *Fundamentals of clinical nutrition*, ed 2, St Louis, 1998, Mosby.)

tional, sometimes HPN is administered only selected nights per week to supplement oral intake. Although expensive, HPN costs less than hospitalization, allows the patient to leave the hospital sooner, and in many cases allows the patient to resume a productive lifestyle.[25,38]

Transitional Feedings

A period of adjustment, or weaning, is necessary before discontinuing nutritional support or when converting from one form of nutritional support to another. Transition to an adequate oral intake to maintain nutritional status will differ from patient to patient.[39] Although the GI tract responds quickly to enteral feeding, patients who have been receiving TPN usually have decreased appetites and may take 1 to 2 weeks after complete cessation of TPN before they feel hungry and may experience early satiety.[39] This necessitates gradual weaning from PN as enteral feeding (oral or tube) progresses to ensure continued adequate intake. Moreover, stopping TPN too quickly can result in hypoglycemia.

Parenteral to Oral or Tube Feeding

As mentioned previously, long periods of PN without enteral feedings result in atrophy of the GI tract. If not contraindicated, minimal enteral intake (sips of dilute fruit juice) is encouraged to help maintain normal GI tract physiology and gut mucosal immunity.[39] Before weaning from PN, judicious assessment of GI function is recommended to prevent problems with delayed gastric emptying, nausea, vomiting, or diarrhea.[39] As PN is tapered and oral or tube feeding intake increases, it is important to document actual enteral intake, including fluids. This will facilitate maintenance of nutrient requirements.[39] If oral feedings or isotonic formulas are not well tolerated, an elemental formula may be needed.

Tube to Oral Feeding

In addition to documentation of intake per tube and orally, it will be important to assess the patient's swallowing ability before offering oral feedings. Full liquids are usually offered first, followed by pureed or soft foods. Tube feedings should be stopped at least 1 hour before and after mealtime to promote appetite. As oral intake increases, tube-feeding volume should be decreased. When oral intake consistently exceeds two thirds of energy requirements, the tube feedings can be discontinued.

SUMMARY

Although hospital nurses may perform some basic nutrition assessment and nutrition counseling, RDs can provide more in-depth knowledge of nutritional care, consult individually with patients, and participate in team meetings. Nurses, however, need to recognize that nutritional status of patients may be compromised by their stay in acute care hospitals. Psychologic and physiologic aspects of illness, combined with effects of bed rest and the potential of iatrogenic malnutrition, emphasize the need for nutritional screening or monitoring to identify patients at nutritional risk.

Capacity for recovery from illness or disease depends in part on nutritional status. A comprehensive nutritional assessment is a procedure conducted by dietitians to determine appropriate medical nutrition therapy based on identified needs of the patient. Data are collected from several sources to assess patients' nutritional needs, often using the *ABCD* approach: anthropometrics, biochemical tests, clinical observations, and diet evaluation. The nutritional care process provides for the unique nutritional needs of each patient. This can be accomplished through nutrition intervention to reduce nutritional risk. The nutritional care process uses a five-step procedure to identify and solve nutrition-related problems. The five steps are assessment, analysis, planning, implementation, and evaluation.

All patient nutrition is provided through food service delivery systems of acute care hospitals and long-term care facilities. Staff includes a director of the food and nutrition services department, clinical dietitians, and also cooks, clerks, dishwashers, aides, and dietetic technicians.

To provide medical nutritional therapy, modified diets are developed to meet specific needs of patients as determined by the physician or dietitian. Dietary modifications of the regular diet may be made in two ways: qualitative or quantitative. Qualitative diet changes include modifications in consistency, texture, or nutrients. Quantitative diet changes include modifications in size and number of meals served or amounts of specific nutrients. By working together, nurses and dietetic professionals can most efficiently meet the nutritional and medical needs of patients.

Every patient deserves one of the most basic of all needs—nourishment. For obvious reasons, enteral nutrition (oral or tube feedings) is the preferred method of nutrition support. Feeding patients via the GI tract is safer, easier to administer, aids in maintaining GI tract integrity, and is as much as five times less expensive. An array of commercial tube feeding products that supply intact nutrients is available. When administered in the appropriate volume, 100% of the recommended dietary allowance (RDA) for vitamins and minerals can be provided, as well as adequate amounts of energy and protein.

In those instances when patients are unable to obtain nutrition enterally, use of PN can literally be a life-saving therapy. Peripheral or central infusions of amino acids, dextrose, fat emulsions, vitamins, and minerals can provide the ordinary or extraordinary nutrient needs of patients. Although not without risk, when managed through a team approach and routine monitoring, PN can provide a safe vehicle for meeting patients' nutritional goals.

THE NURSING APPROACH
A Stroke Patient and the Nursing Process

Margaret, age 75, is a widow who suffered a stroke 3 months ago that rendered her semicomatose and left her throat muscles partially paralyzed. She is unable to swallow any solid food and aspirates whenever she is given oral fluids. She was sent home from the hospital with enteral feedings via percutaneous endoscopic gastrostomy tube (PEG), which was inserted 1 week ago. Her family is strongly religious and prefers to have their mother at home where they plan to be active in caring for her instead of her staying at an extended care facility.

She receives intermittent commercially prepared tube feedings four times per day. The formula was changed 2 days ago because she was losing weight. She has begun to have diarrhea. The primary caregivers are concerned about providing these feedings. They expressed their concerns to the home health nurse who makes visits 5 days a week.

ASSESSMENT

Subjective

Family expresses concerns about managing enteral feedings

Objective
- Height: 5'3"
- Weight: 108 lbs
- Temperature: 98.6° F
- Blood pressure, 130/86; pulse, 84; respiration, 24
- Bowel sounds slightly hyperactive
- Skin turgor normal
- Mucous membranes moist
- Loose stools three to four times/day

NURSING DIAGNOSIS #1

Knowledge deficit related to lack of information of enteral feedings as evidenced by caregiver's concerns

PLANNING

Goal

Caregivers will be able to demonstrate the management of enteral feedings at home.

IMPLEMENTATION

1. Allow the family members to discuss concerns and fears regarding feeding.
2. Teach family how to prepare or mix formula feedings for administration.
3. Instruct family on the proper storage of the formula by refrigerating unused formulas.
4. Demonstrate administration of the feeding including proper hand washing, changing the bag and tubing, filling and hanging the bag, operating the infusion pump and adjusting the rate, and making sure the client is properly positioned.
5. Review the management of the enteral access device by site inspection and flushing of the feeding tubes.
6. Reinforce daily monitoring needs, which include temperature, weight, and intake and output (I&O).
7. Advise family to report signs and symptoms of complications such as fever, decreased urinary output, changes in breathing patterns, and level of consciousness.

Continued

THE NURSING APPROACH–cont'd
A Stroke Patient and the Nursing Process

EVALUATION

The goal will be achieved by the following:
- The family expresses a positive attitude toward management of feeding.
- The successful demonstration of preparing, administration, and management of the feeding evidence the achievement of the goal.

NURSING DIAGNOSIS #2

Diarrhea related to hyperosmolar tube feeding as evidenced by three to four loose stools per day.

PLANNING

Goal

Patient will have normal formed stool within 72 hours.

IMPLEMENTATION

1. Clean and dry the skin area and check for skin integrity.
2. Obtain physician's order to reduce rate of tube feeding or to change type of formula.
3. Assess and record consistency and number of stools.
4. After diarrhea subsides, gradually increase rate as tolerated until desired formula is reached.

EVALUATION

The goal will be achieved by evidence of the following:
- Formation of a normal stool after 72 hours.
- Evaluation of vital signs shows no evidence of infection (e.g., increased temperature.

CRITICAL THINKING
Clinical Applications

Advances in medical technology have provided mechanisms to feed or nourish patients who once could not be fed or nourished. However, like most medical advances, it also provides dilemmas and difficult decisions about patient care. Nutrition care dilemmas occur when this technology will keep the patient alive although the patient has no hope of living a normal life. Often, the dilemma involves legal action for resolution. The Karen Ann Quinlan case (1976) was the first case to go to court to withdraw life-sustaining medical care from a permanently incompetent patient. Most recently, a 1988 U.S. Supreme Court decision allowed a feeding tube to be discontinued from Nancy Cruzan, who suffered irreversible brain damage as the result of a car accident in 1983. What are your thoughts about the following circumstances?
- An 85-year-old man who suffers from many physical problems, but is not terminally ill, refuses to be tube fed.
- A 57-year-old woman is hospitalized as a result of a severe psychiatric disorder that prohibits her from speaking or eating. She is bedridden in a fetal position and has a gastrostomy tube. She repeatedly dislodges the feeding tube and is combative when it is replaced.
- A 75-year-old woman's husband has requested termination of her nasogastric feedings. She is brain dead and has no living will.

Modified from Edelstein S: Ethical dilemmas and decisions, *San Marcos, Calif, 1993, Nutrition Dimension.*

Web Sites of Interest

All Health Net
www.allhealthnet.com/Nursing/Telenursing/
This medical search engine site provides medical and health information including telenursing resources, medical help lines, healthcare safety issue Web sites, medical subject listings from NLM MEDLINE *plus* global Web sites, online textbooks, and other Web site lists.

The American Society of Parenteral and Enteral Nutrition (ASPEN)
www.nutritioncare.org
This association is dedicated to patients receiving the most appropriate nutritional therapy. Interactive features on the site allow users to post questions, register for conferences, and view links to other related organizations.

Arbor Nutrition Guide
www.arborcom.com
This site for trained health professionals provides a selection of nutrition links categorized into applied, clinical, food science, search, and home pages.

References

1. Rubin M: The physiology of bed rest, *Am J Nurs* 88(1):50, 1988.
2. Butterworth CE: The skeleton in the hospital closet, *Nutrition Today* Mar/Apr 1974.
3. World Health Organization (WHO): *Physical status: the use and interpretation of anthropometry*, Technical Report Series 854, Geneva, 1995, WHO.
4. Lee RD, Nieman DC: *Nutritional assessment*, ed 3, Boston, 2003, McGraw-Hill.
5. Stewart A: The reliability and validity of self-reported weight and heights, *J Chronic Diseases* 35:295, 1982.
6. Robinson L, Wright B: Comparison of stated and measured patient heights and weights, *Am J Hosp Pharm* 39:822, 1982.
7. Gray D: Accuracy of recumbent height measurement, *J Parenteral Enteral Nutr* 9:712, 1985.
8. Chumlea WC, Roche AF, Steinbaugh ML: Estimating stature from knee height for persons 60 to 90 years of age, *J Am Geriatr Soc* 33:116, 1985.
9. Chumlea WC, Roche AF, Mukherjee D: *Nutritional assessment of the elderly through anthropometry*, Columbus, Ohio, 1984, Ross Laboratories.
10. Blackburn GL, Thornton PA: Nutritional and metabolic assessment of the hospitalized patient, *J Parenteral Enteral Nutr* 1:11, 1977.
11. American Dietetic Association: *Manual of clinical dietetics*, ed 6, Chicago, 2000, American Dietetic Association.
12. Chumlea WC, Shumei G, Roche AF: Prediction of body weight for the nonambulatory elderly from anthropometry, *J Am Dietetic Assoc* 88:564, 1988.
13. National Institutes of Health; National Heart, Lung, and Blood Institute: *The practical guide: identification, evaluation, and treatment of overweight and obesity in adults*, Pub No 00-4084, October 2000, Bethesda, Md, National Institutes of Health.
14. National Institutes of Health; National Heart, Lung, and Blood Institute: *Clinical guidelines of the identification, evaluation, and treatment of overweight and obesity in adults: the evidence report*, Pub No 98-4083, September 1998, Bethesda, Md, National Institutes of Health.
15. Chumlea WHC, Guo SS, Steinbough MI: Prediction of stature from knee height for black and white adults and children with application to mobility impaired or handicapped persons, *J Am Dietetic Assoc* 94:1385, 1994.
16. Heymsfield SB et al.: Anthropometric measurement of muscle mass: revised equations for calculating bone-free arm muscle areas, *Am J Clin Nutri* 36:680, 1982.
17. Heimburger DC, Weinsier RL: *Handbook of clinical nutrition*, ed 3, St Louis, 1997, Mosby.
18. Morgan SL, Weinsier RL: *Fundamentals of clinical nutrition*, ed 2, St Louis, 1998, Mosby.

19. Whitney EN, Cataldo CB, Rolfes SR: *Understanding normal and clinical nutrition,* ed 6, St Paul, 2002, Wadsworth.
20. Philips S: Water and electrolytes in gastrointestinal disease. In Maxwell MH, Klienman CR, eds.: *Clinical disorders of fluid and electrolyte metabolism,* New York, 1979, McGraw-Hill.
21. Murray DP et al.: Survey: use of clear and full liquid diets with or without commercially produced formulas, *J Parenteral Enteral Nutr* 9:732, 1985.
22. Schilder JM et al.: A prospective controlled trial of early postoperative oral intake following major abdominal gynecologic surgery, *Gynecol Oncol* 67(3):325, 1997.
23. Hartsell PA et al.: Early postoperative feeding after selective colorectal surgery, *Arch Surg* 132(5):518, 1997.
24. ASPEN Board of Directors: Guidelines for the use of enteral nutrition in the adult patient, *J Parenteral Enteral Nutr* 17:15A, 1993.
25. Rombeau JL, Barot LR: Enteral nutrition therapy, *Surg Clin North Am* 61:605, 1981.
26. Swearingen PL, Ross DG: *Manual of medical-surgical nursing care,* ed 4, St Louis, 1999, Mosby.
27. DeChicco R, Matarese L: Selection of nutrition support regimens, *Nutr Clin Pract* 7:239, 1992.
28. Chawla KK, Jeske DJ, Renfro AD: *Assessing and managing nutrition status: a complete guide to meeting complex nutritional needs of acutely ill patients,* St Louis, 1994, Barnes and Jewish Hospitals.
29. McClave S, Lowen CC, Snider HL: Immunonutrition and enteral hyperalimentation of critically ill patients, *Dig Dis Sci* 37:1153, 1992.
30. Edes TE, Walk BE, Austin JL: Diarrhea in tube-fed patients: feeding formula not necessarily the cause, *Am J Med* 88:91, 1990.
31. Nelson JK, Weckwerth JA: Home enteral nutrition. In Skipper A, ed.: *Dietitian's handbook of enteral and parenteral nutrition,* Rockville, Md, 1989, Aspen.
32. Westbrook NH: Nutrition support in home care. In Skipper A, ed.: *Dietitian's handbook of enteral and parenteral nutrition,* ed 2, Rockville, Md, 1998, Aspen.
33. Lenssen P: Management of total parenteral nutrition. In Skipper A, ed.: *Dietitian's handbook of enteral and parenteral nutrition,* ed 2, Rockville, Md, 1998, Aspen.
34. Roesner M, Grant JP: Intravenous lipid emulsions, *Nutr Clin Pract* 2:96, 1987.
35. Driscoll DF et al.: Practical considerations regarding the use of total nutrient admixtures, *Am J Hosp Pharm* 43:416, 1986.
36. American Medical Association, Department of Foods and Nutrition: Multivitamin preparations for parenteral use: a statement by the nutrition advisory group, *J Parenteral Enteral Nutr* 3:258, 1979.
37. American Medical Association, Department of Foods and Nutrition: Guidelines for essential trace element preparations for parenteral use: a statement by an expert panel, *J Am Med Assoc* 241:2051, 1979.
38. McCrae JD: Home parenteral nutrition. In Skipper A, ed.: *Dietitian's handbook of enteral and parenteral nutrition,* Rockville, Md, 1989, Aspen.
39. Lenssen P: Monitoring and complications of parenteral nutrition. In Skipper A, ed.: *Dietitian's handbook of enteral and parenteral nutrition,* Rockville, Md, 1989, Aspen.

CHAPTER 15

Nutrition and Metabolic Stress

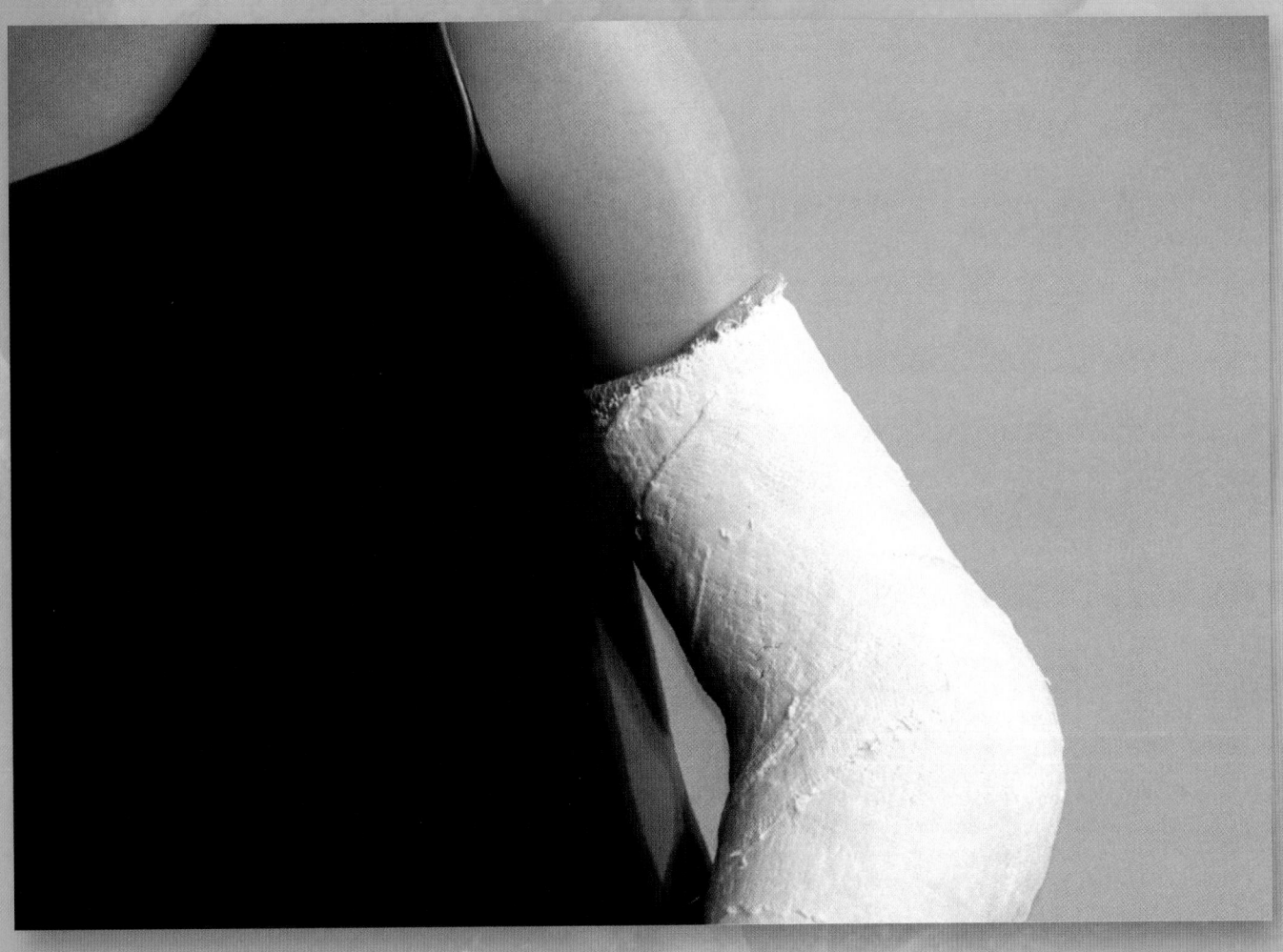

One of the first body functions affected by impaired nutritional status is the immune system.

ROLE IN WELLNESS

In its never-ending quest to maintain homeostasis, the human body responds to stress, physiologic or psychologic, with a chain reaction that involves the central nervous system and hormones that affect the entire body. Magnitude and duration of the stress determine just how the body will react. It is important for nurses to understand metabolic changes that take place in reaction to stress, both in uncomplicated stress that is present when patients are at nutritional risk, and in more multifarious variations that result from severe stress brought about by trauma or disease.

IMMUNE SYSTEM

One of the first body functions affected by impaired nutritional status is the immune system. When metabolic stress develops, hormonal and metabolic changes subdue the immune system's ability to protect the body. This activity is further depressed if impaired nutritional status accompanies the metabolic stress. A deadly cycle often develops: impaired immunity leads to increased risk of disease, disease impairs nutritional status, and compromised nutritional status further impairs immunity. Recovery requires that this cycle be broken.

Role of Nutrition

For the immune system to function optimally, adequate nutrients must be available. A well-nourished body will not be ravaged by infections the way a poorly nourished body will (the Cultural Considerations box presents a multicultural

---

CULTURAL CONSIDERATIONS
The Process of Balance

What is a balanced way of eating for good health? To most Americans, the response is to eat foods from each of the food groups, with particular emphasis on fruits and vegetables. Among other cultures, foods consumed to achieve balance and good health do not follow the American food categories. The Chinese system of *yin-yang* sorts foods into *yin* (bean curd or tofu, bean sprouts, bland and boiled foods, broccoli, carrots, duck, milk, potatoes, spinach, and water) and *yang* (bamboo, beef, broiled meat, chicken, eggs, fried foods, garlic, ginger root, green peppers, and tomatoes). Foods should be selected from each group to achieve balance. Which foods belong in each group may vary by region, but some foods such as rice and noodles are considered neutral. The overall goal is to maintain the harmony of the body with adjustments for climate variations and physiologic factors.

Balance is also the focus of the *hot-cold classification* of foods practiced in the Middle East, Latin American, India, and the Philippines. This concept is derived from the Greek humoral medicine based on the four natural world characteristics of air-cold, fire-hot, water-moist, and earth-dry related to the body humors of hot and moist (blood), cold and moist (phlegm), hot and dry (yellow/green bile), and cold and dry

(black bile). Although this concept is related to the development of disease and their remedies, it also applies to foods. The hot and cold aspects of specific foods are emphasized. This does not relate to the actual temperature of the foods but to their innate characteristics. To achieve balance, eating cold foods offsets hot foods. The list of foods in each category varies among subgroups within each culture. Often, younger generations follow this concept but without knowing that it is based on the hot-cold theory of balance.

Application to nursing: Each of the cultures, subscribing to the yin-yang concept and the hot-cold theory, has sizable populations in the United States. When treating Americans of Chinese, Indian, Latino, Middle Eastern, and Filipino descent, these concepts of food selection to achieve health and harmony may affect client food choices. Although healthy selections are often selected, subtle effects may occur. For example, within the hot-cold theory, pregnancy may be considered "hot" as are vitamins. Consequently, vitamins are not taken during pregnancy because to do so would not restore balance. If a client seems unwilling to follow dietary and supplement recommendations, discussion of these classifications and ways to remedy the situation can be created.

Reference: Kittler PG, Sucher KP: Food and culture in America: a nutrition handbook, *ed 3 Belmont, Calif, 2001, Wadsworth.*

perspective on "balanced" eating for good health). To prove this point, think of the leading causes of death in industrialized countries such as the United States. The majority are chronic diseases associated with lifestyle. In developing countries, however, infections lead to high morbidity and mortality rates, especially in children, largely because of the high rate of protein-energy malnutrition (PEM). The majority of persons in the United States who have serious problems with malnutrition and infections are (1) those with severe medical problems, (2) those who suffer from major metabolic stress, (3) those who suffer from a diseased state that causes metabolic stress and/or decreased nutrient intake and/or nutrient malabsorption, and (4) those who have poor nutritional intakes as a result of socioeconomic conditions (e.g., poverty, homelessness).

Compromised nutritional status creates a vulnerable immune system by making it difficult to mount both a stress response and an immune response when confronted with a metabolic stress. A number of nutrients are known to affect immune system functioning. It is difficult to determine which specific nutrient factor results in symptoms when the patient is malnourished because of overlapping nutrient deficiencies combined with illness and accompanied by weakness, anorexia, and infection.[1]

Immune system components affected by malnutrition include mucous membranes, skin, gastrointestinal tract, T-lymphocytes, macrophages, granulocytes, and antibodies. The effects on the mucous membrane are that the microvilli become flat, which reduces nutrient absorption and decreases antibody secretions. Integrity of the skin may be compromised as it loses density and wound healing is slowed. Injury to the gastrointestinal tract because of malnutrition may increase risk of infection-causing bacteria spreading from inside the tract to outside the intestinal system. T-lymphocytes are affected as the distribution of T-cells is depressed. The effect on macrophages and granulocytes requires that more time be needed for phagocytosis kill time and lymphocyte activation to occur. Antibodies may be less available because of damage to the antibody response. Table 15-1 outlines how specific nutrient deficiencies affect immune system functions; note that fat and water-soluble vitamins, fatty acids, minerals, and protein are important for adequate functioning of most immune system components.[1]

Table 15-1
Role of Nutrients and Nutritional Status on Immune System Components

Immune System Component	Effects of Malnutrition	Vital Nutrients
Mucus	Decreased antibody secretions	Vitamin B_{12}, biotin, vitamins B_6 and C
Gastrointestinal tract	Flat microvilli, increased risk of bacterial spread to outside GI tract	Arginine, omega-3 fatty acids
Skin	Integrity compromised, density reduced, wound healing slowed	Protein, vitamins A and C, niacin, zinc, copper, linoleic acid, vitamin B_{12}
T-lymphocytes	Depressed T-cell distribution	Protein, arginine, omega-3 fatty acids, vitamins A, B_{12}, B_6, folic acid, thiamin, riboflavin, niacin, pantothenic acid, zinc, iron
Macrophages and granulocytes	Longer time for phagocytosis kill time and lymphocyte activation	Protein, vitamins A, C, B_{12}, B_6, folic acid, thiamin, riboflavin, niacin, zinc, iron
Antibodies	Reduced antibody response	Protein, vitamins A, C, B_{12}, B_6, folic acid, thiamin, biotin, riboflavin, niacin

THE STRESS RESPONSE

The body's response to metabolic stress depends on the magnitude and duration of the stress. Stress sets up a chain reaction that involves hormones and the central nervous system that affects the entire body. Whether stress is uncomplicated (altered food intake or activity level) or multifarious (trauma or disease), metabolic changes take place throughout the body.

According to Gould,[2] the body's constant response to minor changes brought about by needs or environment was first noted in 1946 by Hans Selye when he described the "fight or flight" response, or general adaptation syndrome (GAS). The body constantly responds to minor changes to maintain homeostasis. Research following Selye's work has identified that the stress response involves an integrated series of actions that include the hypothalamus and hypophysis, sympathetic nervous system, adrenal medulla, and adrenal cortex.[2] Significant effects of this response to stress are outlined in Table 15-2. These responses to stress produce

Table 15-2
Effects of the Stress Response*

Target Organ	Hormonal Response	Physiologic Response	Signs/Symptoms
Sympathetic nervous system and adrenal medulla	Norepinephrine	Vasoconstriction	Pallor, decreased glomerular filtration rate, nausea, elevated blood pressure
Adrenal medulla	Epinephrine	Vasoconstriction Increased heart rate Vasodilation CNS stimulation Bronchodilation Glycogenolysis, lipolysis, gluconeogenesis	See above Elevated blood pressure Increased skeletal muscle function More alert, increased muscle tone Increased O_2 Increased blood glucose
Adrenal pituitary and cortex	Cortisol (glucocorticoids)	CNS stimulation Protein catabolism, gluconeogenesis Stabilize cardiovascular system Gastric secretion Inflammatory response decreased Allergic response decreased Immune response decreased	 Increased blood glucose, increased serum amino acids, delayed wound healing Enhance catecholamine action Ulcers Decreased WBCs Atrophy of lymphoid tissue, decreased lymphocytes, decreased antibody production
	Aldosterone (mineralocorticoid)		Retain sodium and water, increased blood volume, increased blood pressure
Posterior pituitary	Antidiuretic hormone	Water reabsorbed, increased blood volume, increased blood pressure	
Other feedback mechanisms	Aldosterone and antidiuretic hormone	See above	See above

Data from Gould BE: *Pathophysiology for the health-related professions, Philadelphia, 1997, WB Saunders.*
Possible complications: hypertension, tension headaches, insomnia, diabetes mellitus, infection, heart failure, peptic ulcer, fatigue.

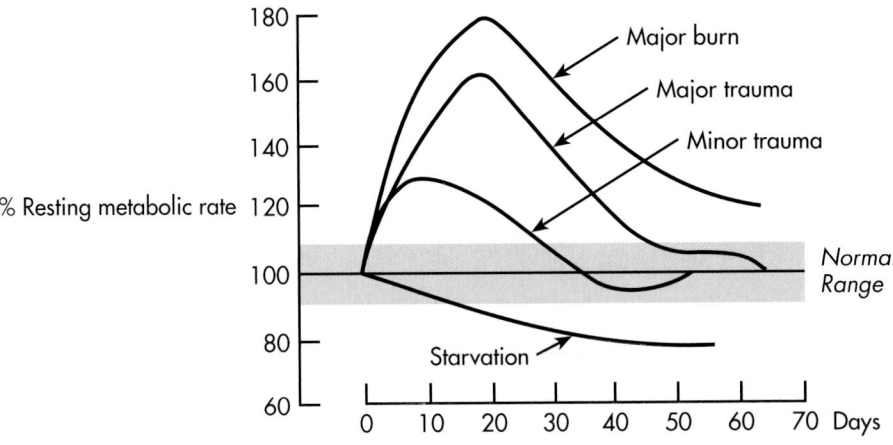

Figure 15-1 Percent resting metabolic rate. (From Kinney JM et al.: *Nutrition and metabolism in patient care*, Philadelphia, 1988, WB Saunders.)

multiple changes in metabolic processes throughout the body. The effect of different levels of stress on metabolic rate is illustrated in Figure 15-1.

Starvation

If someone must involuntarily go without food, that can be defined as *starvation*. If we withhold food from ourselves, such as when we try to lose weight, that can be defined as *dieting* or *fasting*. Whatever the cause of inadequate food intake and nourishment, results are the same. After a brief period of going without food (fasting) or an interval of nutrient intake below metabolic needs, the body is able to extract stored carbohydrate, fat, and protein (from muscles and organs) to meet energy demands.

Liver glycogen is used to maintain normal blood glucose levels to provide energy for cells. Although readily available, this source of energy is limited, and glycogen stores are usually depleted after 8 to 12 hours of fasting. Unlike glycogen stores, lipid (triglyceride) stores may be substantial, and the body also begins to mobilize this energy source. As the amount of liver glycogen decreases, mobilization of free fatty acids from adipose tissue increases to provide needed energy by the nervous system. After about 24 hours without energy intake (especially carbohydrates), the prime source of glucose is from gluconeogenesis.[3]

Some body cells, brain cells in particular, use mainly glucose for energy. During early starvation (about 2 to 3 days of starvation), the brain uses glucose produced from muscle protein. As muscle protein is broken down for energy, the level of **branched-chain amino acids (BCAA)** in circulation increases although they are primarily metabolized directly inside muscle.[3] The body does not store any amino acids as it does glucose and triglycerides, therefore the only sources of amino acids are lean body mass (muscle tissue), vital organs including heart muscle, or other protein-based body constituents such as enzymes, hormones, immune system components, or blood proteins. By the second or third day of starvation, approximately 75 grams of muscle protein can be catabolized daily, a level inadequate to supply full energy needs of the brain.[3] At this point, other sources of energy become more available. Fatty acids are hydrolyzed from the glycerol backbone and both free fatty acids and glycerol are released into the bloodstream. Free fatty acids are used as indicated earlier and glycerol can be used by the liver to generate glucose via the process of gluconeogenesis.

As starvation is prolonged, the body preserves proteins by mobilizing more and more fat for energy. Ketone body production from fatty acids is accelerated, and the body's requirement for glucose decreases. Although some glucose is still vital for brain cells and red blood corpuscles, these and other body tissues obtain the major proportion of their energy from ketone bodies. Muscle protein is still being

branched-chain amino
acids (BCAA)
leucine, isoleucine, and valine

catabolized but at a much lower rate, which prolongs survival. During this period of starvation, approximately 60% of the body's energy is provided by metabolism of fat to carbon dioxide, 10% from metabolism of free fatty acids to ketone bodies, and 25% from metabolism of ketone bodies.[4]

An additional defense mechanism of the body to conserve energy is to slow its metabolic rate, thereby decreasing energy needs. As a result of declining metabolic rate, body temperature drops, activity level decreases, and sleep periods increase—all to allow the body to preserve energy sources. If starvation continues, intercostal muscles necessary for respiration are lost, which may lead to pneumonia and respiratory failure.[4] Starvation will continue until adipose stores are exhausted.

Severe Stress

Whether stress is accidental (e.g., from broken bones or burns) or necessary (e.g., from surgery), the body reacts to these stresses much as it does to the stress of starvation—with a *major* difference. During starvation, the body's metabolic rate slows, becoming hypometabolic. During severe stress, the body's metabolic rate rises profoundly, thus becoming hypermetabolic.

The body's response to stress can be summarized by two phases: ebb phase and flow phase (Table 15-3). The *ebb phase*, or *early phase*, begins immediately after the injury and is identified by decreased oxygen consumption, hypothermia (lowered body temperature), and lethargy. The major medical concern during this time is to maintain cardiovascular effectiveness and tissue perfusion. As the body responds to injury, the ebb phase evolves into the flow phase, usually about 36 to 48 hours after injury.[5] The *flow phase* is characterized by increased oxygen consumption, hyperthermia (increased body temperature), and increased nitrogen excretion, as well as expedited catabolism of carbohydrate, protein, and triglycerides to meet the increased metabolic demands.[5] The flow stage will last for days, weeks, or months until the injury is healed.

Multiple stresses result in increased catabolism and even greater loss of body proteins. Unfortunately, some stresses that patients are obliged to endure are iatrogenic. Think, for example, of the series of stresses a patient admitted for elective surgery might experience. Preoperatively, most surgical patients receive only clear liquids or nothing by mouth (NPO). After surgery, they may remain NPO until the return of bowel sounds, then progress through clear- and full-liquid diets until they can tolerate food.

Table 15-3
Metabolic Responses to Severe Stress

Ebb Phase	Flow Phase
↓Oxygen consumption	↑Oxygen consumption
↓Cardiac output	↑Cardiac output
↓Plasma volume	↑Plasma volume
Hypothermia	Hyperthermia
	↑Nitrogen excretion
↓Insulin levels	Normal or elevated insulin levels
Hyperglycemia	Hyperglycemia
Hypovolemia	
Hypotension	
↑Lactate	Normal lactate
↑Free fatty acids	↑Free fatty acids
↑Catecholamines, glucagon, cortisol	↑Catecholamines, glucagon, cortisol
Insulin resistance	↑Insulin resistance

If the patient is in poor nutritional status before the stress of surgery, he or she is at greater risk to develop pneumonia or a wound infection accompanied by fever as a result of decreased protein synthesis. As in starvation, energy requirements will be met from endogenous sources if exogenous sources are not available or adequate.[4] Thus intercostal muscles may be depleted, leading to pneumonia, or inadequate amino acids may be available to synthesize antibodies, leading to impaired immune response to infection. Either complication has a negative impact on metabolic demands.

Nutrients affected by hypermetabolic stress include protein, vitamins, and minerals, as well as related nutritional concerns for total energy and fluid intake. During moderate metabolic stress, protein requirements have been reported to increase from 0.8 gm/kg body weight (amount recommended for an average healthy adult) to 1.0 to 1.5 gm/kg body weight[6,7] and for severe stress (e.g., thermal injuries exceeding 20% total body surface area) can rise to 1.5 to 2.0 gm/kg body weight.[7] These levels are based on sufficient energy consumption to allow for protein synthesis. Requirements of vitamins and minerals all increase during stress. Tissue repair especially depends on adequate intakes of vitamin C, zinc, calcium, magnesium, manganese, and copper. At the least, Dietary Reference Intake (DRI) levels of nutrients should be consumed, preferably from foods rather than from vitamin or mineral supplements. Achieving requirements through food intake also supports provision of sufficient kcalories to meet increased energy demands during critical illness.

Several formulae have been used to determine energy needs of patients experiencing hypermetabolic stress. One formula (Harris-Benedict) takes into account basal energy expenditure (BEE), activity level, and severity of injury.[8] Activity level considers energy required if the patient is confined to bed or is ambulatory. Severity of injury is a factor based on whether the injury is caused by major or minor surgery, mild to severe infection, skeletal or blunt trauma, or burns (based on percentage of body surface area affected) (Box 15-1).[9]

Registered dietitians, in collaboration with the medical team, use these formulas to determine energy requirements. As factor assessments change, nurses can alert either the registered dietitian or other members of the medical team to ensure adequate energy provision.

Fluid need during hypermetabolic stress is based on age, reflecting age-related modifications of body composition. For adults younger than 55 years old, fluid needs are calculated at 35 to 40 ml/kg body weight. Adults between the ages of 55 to 75 years require a lower amount, 30 ml/kg body weight; and for adults older than age 75, 25 ml/kg body weight is recommended.[7]

endogenous
originating from within the body or produced internally

exogenous
originating outside the body or produced from external sources

Effects of Stress on Nutrient Metabolism

Protein Metabolism

Even if adequate carbohydrate and fat are available, protein (skeletal muscle) is mobilized for energy (amino acids are converted to glucose in the liver). There is decreased uptake of amino acids by muscle tissue, and increased urinary excretion of nitrogen[9,10] (Figure 15-2). Some nonessential amino acids may become conditionally essential during episodes of metabolic stress. During stress, glutamine is mobilized in large quantities from skeletal muscle and lung to be used directly as a fuel source by intestinal cells.[11] Glutamine also plays a significant role in maintaining intestinal immune function and enhancing wound repair by supporting lymphocyte and macrophage proliferation, hepatic gluconeogenesis, and fibroblast function.[11]

Carbohydrate Metabolism

Hepatic glucose production is increased and disseminated to peripheral tissues although proteins and fats are being used for energy. Insulin levels and glucose use are in fact increased, but hyperglycemia that is not necessarily resolved by the use of exogenous insulin[9,10] is present. This appears, to some extent, to be driven by an elevated glucagon:insulin ratio.[10]

Box 15-1 Medical Nutrition Therapy for Metabolically Stressed Patients

$\mathcal{E}$nergy requirements are highly individual and may vary widely from person to person. Total kcaloric requirements are dependent on the basal energy expenditure (BEE) plus the presence of trauma, surgery, infection, sepsis, and other factors. Additionally, age, height, and weight are often taken into consideration.[2]

HARRIS-BENEDICT FORMULA

The Harris-Benedict formula is one of the most useful and accurate for calculating basal energy requirements,[2] although it generally overestimates BEE by 5 to 15%. It is important to remember that this formula uses *current (actual)* weight in the calculation.

$$Wt\ in\ lbs \div 2.2\ kg = wt\ in\ kg$$

$$Ht\ in\ in \times 2.54\ cm = ht\ in\ cm$$

$$Men = 66.5 + (13.8 \times wt\ in\ kg) + (5 \times ht\ in\ cm) - (6.8 \times age)$$

$$Women = 65.1 + (9.6 \times wt\ in\ kg) + (1.8 \times ht\ in\ cm) - (4.7 \times age)$$

Once BEE has been calculated, additional kcalories for activity and injury are added:

$$BEE \times activity\ factor\ (AF) \times injury\ factor\ (IF)$$

PROTEIN REQUIREMENTS

Additional protein is required to synthesize the proteins necessary for defense and recovery, to spare lean body mass, and to reduce the amount of endogenous protein catabolism for gluconeogenesis.

VITAMIN/MINERAL NEEDS

Needs for most vitamins and minerals increase in metabolic stress, however no specific guidelines exist for provision of vitamins, minerals, and trace elements. It is usually believed that if the increased kcaloric requirements are met, adequate amounts of most vitamins and minerals are usually provided. In spite of this, vitamin C, vitamin A or beta carotene, and zinc may need special attention.

FLUID NEEDS

Fluid status can affect interpretation of biochemical measurements as well as anthropometry and physical examination. Fluid requirements can be estimated using several different methods.

MICRONUTRIENT SUPPLEMENTATION

Vitamin C: 500-1000 mg/daily in divided dose
Vitamin A: one multivitamin tablet containing vitamin A, 1-4 times daily
Zinc sulfate: 220 mg, 1-3 times daily

Activity	Activity Factor	Clinical Status	Energy Stress Factor	g Protein/kg Body Wt/Day
Bedrest	1.2	Elective surgery	1.0-1.2	1.0-1.5
Ambulatory	1.3	Multiple trauma	1.2-1.6	1.3-1.7
		Severe infection	1.2-1.6	
		Peritonitis	1.05-1.25	
		Multiple/long bone fractures	1.1-1.3	
		Infection with trauma	1.3-1.5	
		Sepsis	1.2-1.4	1.2-1.5
		Closed head injury	1.3	
		Cancer	1.1-1.45	
		Burns (% BSA*)		1.8-2.5
		0%-20%	1.0-1.5	
		20%-40%	1.5-1.85	
		40%-100%	1.85-2.05	
		Fever	1.2 per 1° C >37°C	

Fluid Requirements Based On		Water (ml)
Weight		100 ml/kg for first 10 kg
		50 ml/kg for next 10 kg
		20 ml/kg for each kg above 20 kg
Age and weight	16-30 yrs (active)	40 ml/kg/day
	20-55 yrs	35 ml/kg/day
	55-75 yrs	30 ml/kg/day
	>75 yrs	25 ml/kg/day
Energy		1 ml/kcal
Fluid balance		Urine output + 500 ml/day

Reference: American Dietetic Association: Manual of clinical dietetics, ed 6, Chicago, 2000, American Dietetic Association; Grant A, DeHoog S: Nutrition assessment and support, ed 5, Seattle, 1999, Anne Grant/Susan DeHoog (publishers); Heimburger DC, Weinsier RL: Handbook of clinical nutrition, ed 3, St Louis, 1997, Mosby; Moore MC: Mosby's pocket guide to nutritional care, ed 4, St Louis, 2000, Mosby; Winkler MF, Manchester S: Nutritional care in metabolic stress: sepsis, trauma, burns and surgery. In Mahan LK, Escott-Stump S, eds.: Krause's food, nutrition, and diet therapy, ed 10, Philadelphia, 2000, WB Saunders.
*Percent of body surface area burned.

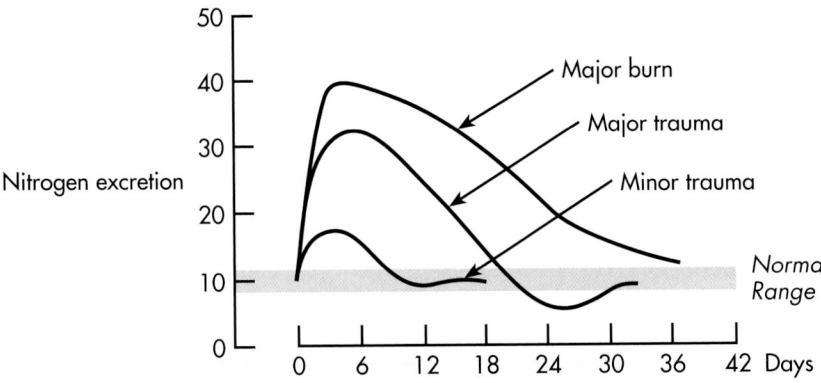

Figure 15-2 Nitrogen excretion. (From Kinney JM et al.: *Nutrition and metabolism in patient care*, Philadelphia, 1988, WB Saunders.)

Fat Metabolism

To support hypermetabolism and increased gluconeogenesis, fat is mobilized from adipose stores to provide energy (lipolysis)[9] as the result of elevated levels of catecholamines along with concurrent decrease in insulin production.[10] If hypermetabolic patients are not fed during this period, fat stores and proteins are rapidly depleted. This malnutrition increases susceptibility to infection and may contribute to multiple organ dysfunction syndrome (MODS), sepsis, and death.[9]

Hydration/Fluid Status

Increased fluid losses can result from fever (increased perspiration), increased urine output, diarrhea, draining wounds, or diuretic therapy.[10]

Vitamins and Minerals

Just as kcaloric needs increase during hypermetabolic conditions, so too do needs for most vitamins and minerals. And if kcalorie needs are met, the patient will most likely receive adequate amounts of most vitamins and minerals. Special attention, however, should be given to vitamin C (ascorbic acid), vitamin A or beta carotene, and zinc.[12] Vitamin C is crucial for the collagen formation necessary for optimal wound healing. Supplements of 500 to 1000 mg/day are recommended.[12] Vitamin A and beta carotene (vitamin A's precursor) also play an important role in the healing process in addition to their role as antioxidants. Zinc increases the tensile strength (force required to separate the edges) of a healing wound. Supplements of 50 to 75 mg/day (orally) when stable are commonly used.[12] Additional zinc may be necessary if there are unusually large intestinal losses (small bowel drainage or ileostomy drainage).[12]

Protein-Energy Malnutrition

Inadequate intake of energy, particularly from protein, can result in acute or chronic protein deficiency, or *protein-energy malnutrition (PEM)*. PEM can be primary or secondary. Primary PEM is the result of inadequate intake of nutrients. Secondary PEM results from inadequate nutrient consumption caused by some disease state that impairs food consumption, interferes with nutrient absorption, or increases nutritional requirements. PEM, kwashiorkor, and marasmus are presented in detail in Chapter 6 and only briefly reviewed here.

Kwashiorkor

The clinical syndrome *kwashiorkor* is diagnosed largely on the basis of results of laboratory tests on patients in the acute state of poor protein intake and stress. Although etiologic mechanisms are not understood, it appears that normal adaptive response of protein sparing seen in fasting fails. Kwashiorkor may develop in as little as 2 weeks.[6]

Patients with kwashiorkor appear to be adequately nourished, tending to have normal fat reserves and muscle mass (or even above normal). However, findings such as easily pluckable hair, edema, skin breakdown, and delayed wound healing are telltale signs of kwashiorkor (Figure 15-3). Characteristic laboratory changes include severely depressed visceral proteins: serum albumin (<2.8 g/dl), transferrin (<150 mg/dl), or reduced iron-binding capacity (<200 ug/dl) and depressed immune function (<1500 lymphocytes/mm³).[6]

Marasmus

Another form of PEM—*marasmus*—is manifested by severe loss of fat and muscle tissue as a result of chronic energy deficiency. Unlike kwashiorkor, an individual with marasmus will appear thin and is weak and listless. Visceral protein stores are preserved at the expense of somatic proteins: skeletal muscle is severely reduced, but laboratory values are relatively unremarkable (serum albumin is usually within normal range).[6] Immunocompetence and wound healing are fairly well preserved in patients with marasmus. Marasmus is a chronic rather than acute condition. Treatment is directed toward gradual reversal of the downward trend. And although medical nutrition therapy or support is necessary, overly aggressive repletion of nutrients can lead to a life-threatening condition called refeeding syndrome (Box 15-2).[6]

Marasmus-Kwashiorkor Mix

This combined form of PEM develops when acute stress (surgery or trauma) is experienced by someone who has been chronically malnourished.[13] The condition becomes life threatening because of the high risk of infection and other complications.

---

visceral proteins
proteins other than muscle tissue; for example, internal organs and blood

somatic proteins
skeletal muscle proteins

refeeding syndrome
physiologic and metabolic complications associated with reintroducing nutrition (refeeding) too rapidly to a person with PEM; these complications can include malabsorption, cardiac insufficiency, congestive heart failure, respiratory distress, convulsions, coma, and perhaps death

---

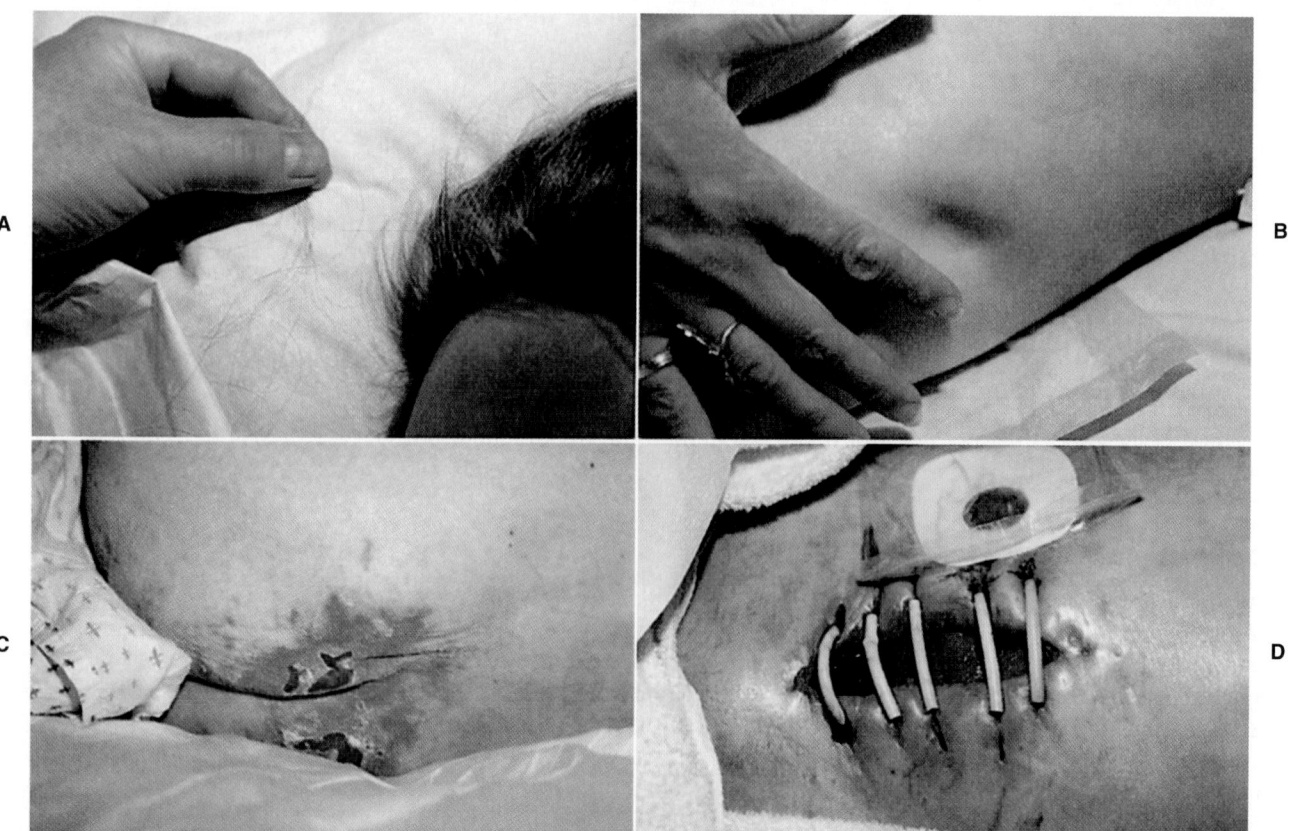

Figure 15-3 Clinical findings in kwashiorkor include (**A**), easy, painless hair pluckability; (**B**), pitting edema; (**C**), skin breakdown; and (**D**), delayed wound healing. (From Morgan S, Weinsier R: *Fundamentals of clinical nutrition,* ed 2, St Louis, 1998, Mosby.)

Box 15-2 Refeeding Syndrome

Refeeding a patient with protein-energy malnutrition can result in many complications if not initiated correctly. In fact, refeeding can be fatal if done too rapidly. The introduction of excess protein and kcalories can overload various enzymatic and physiologic functions that may have adapted during malnutrition. As refeeding is initiated, rapid changes occur in thyroid and endocrine function, causing increased oxygen consumption, cardiac output, insulin secretion, and energy expenditure. Refeeding syndromes are associated more with parenteral nutrition than enteral, but discretion and common sense are of key importance in refeeding semistarved and chronically ill patients. The pathogenesis of refeeding syndrome is as follows.

PHOSPHORUS

During starvation, total body phosphorus is greatly reduced. During refeeding there is an increase in cellular influx of phosphorus, leading to severe extracellular hypophosphatemia. This will occur in enteral and parenteral feeding but can be prevented by a slower rate of nutrient infusion. Hypophosphatemia can also cause cardiac decompensation. (Sodium shifts are thought to play a separate, additional role in cardiac overload.) Additionally, hypophosphatemia can lead to tissue hypoxia and subsequent altered tissue function.

POTASSIUM

Because potassium is greatly reduced from tissue, it is often not reflected in serum levels because extracellular fluid concentrations are maintained. However, during nutritional repletion, potassium is deposited in newly synthesized cells, and serum levels may fall without continued potassium supplementation.

MAGNESIUM

Magnesium is also greatly reduced from tissue, and under anabolic conditions, extracellular fluid levels fall (hypomagnesemia), which in turn can lead to cardiac depression, arrhythmias, neuromuscular weakness, irritability, and hyporeflexia.

GLUCOSE METABOLISM

When glucose is reintroduced via high-glucose or high-volume enteral or parenteral feedings, the starved patient loses the stimulus for gluconeogenesis (an important adaptive mechanism during nutritional depletion). Suppression of gluconeogenic glucose production leads to a corresponding decrease in amino acid use and negative nitrogen balance. Additionally, hyperglycemia can precipitate osmotic diuresis, dehydration, hypotension, hyperosmolar nonketotic coma, ketoacidosis and metabolic acidosis. Hyperosmolar nonketotic coma and ketoacidosis are discussed in Chapter 20.

FLUID INTOLERANCE

Refeeding with carbohydrate results in sodium and water excretion. With concurrent sodium ingestion, this can lead to a rapid expansion of extracellular fluid volume, which will result in fluid retention and subsequent weight gain. This enhanced fluid retention seen with carbohydrate refeeding may in turn be exacerbated because of the loss of tissue mass resulting from starvation.

PREVENTING REFEEDING SYNDROME

Nutrients should be reintroduced slowly to the malnourished patient while medical and metabolic status is closely monitored. Careful estimation of energy requirements should be made through a complete nutritional assessment (see Chapter 15). Care should also be taken to minimize fluid retention (weight gain >1 kg/wk can be assumed to be fluid retention and should be avoided) and provide adequate repletion of phosphorus, potassium, and magnesium on a daily basis. Weight and fluid balance should be monitored daily to assess the rate of weight regain. Refeeding formulas (whether enteral or parenteral) must also contain adequate amounts of other essential nutrients such as vitamins and minerals. Greater than routine amounts are not necessary, but their absence may be lethal. After one week, intake of kcalories, fluid, and sodium can be liberalized without fear of consequences because the various metabolic equilibrations should have taken place.

hypophosphatemia
low serum phosphorus levels

cardiac decompensation
impaired cardiac output (reasons not entirely understood)

hypoxia
lack of oxygen to the cells

hyporeflexia
a neurologic condition characterized by weakened reflex reactions

Reference: Solomon SM, Kirby DF: The refeeding syndrome: a review, J Parenteral Enteral Nutr 14:90, 1990; and Apovian CM, McMahon MM, Bistrian BR: Guidelines for refeeding the marasmic patient, Crit Care Med 18:1030, 1990.

It is important to determine whether marasmus or kwashiorkor is predominant so appropriate medical nutrition therapy can be initiated. The undernourished, unstressed (hypometabolic) patient is at risk of complications such as those observed in refeeding syndrome, and the stressed patient at risk for kwashiorkor is more likely to suffer from underfeeding.[6]

Nurses can be key players in the recognition and prevention of any of the different forms of PEM. By being alert to clinical signs and laboratory values seen in kwashiorkor and marasmus, further deterioration of the patient's nutritional status can be prevented.

MULTIPLE ORGAN DYSFUNCTION SYNDROME

multiple organ dysfunction syndrome (MODS)
the progressive failure of two or more organ systems at the same time (e.g., the renal, hepatic, cardiac, or respiratory systems)

Multiple organ dysfunction syndrome (MODS) involves the progressive failure of two or more organ systems at the same time (e.g., the renal, hepatic, cardiac, or respiratory systems).[14,15] It may occur following trauma, severe burns, infection, or shock, usually results from an uncontrolled inflammatory response, and can progress to organ failure and death.[14,16] MODS commonly begins with lung failure followed by failure of the liver, intestine, and kidney.[16] Myocardial failure generally manifests later, but central nervous system changes can occur at any time.[16] The pathogenesis of MODS is complex but usually results in the initiation of the stress response and release of catecholamines,[14] producing a hypermetabolic state in the patient.[16] Higher levels of kcalories and protein are necessary to meet increased metabolic demands. How patients are fed is also important. Early enteral feedings (Chapter 14) appear to maintain gut mucosal mass and barrier function and promote normal enterocytic growth in the gut.[13,17] This is not possible with parenteral feedings (Table 15-4).

Table 15-4
Nutritional Concerns in Multiple Organ Dysfunction Syndrome

Pulmonary	Adult respiratory distress syndrome (ARDS): patients requiring ventilator support may need higher lipid content in their diet (even with cardiac failure)	**Central Nervous System**	Lethargy Altered level of consciousness Fever: increased energy needs Hepatic encephalopathy
Gastrointestinal	Abdominal distention and ascites Intolerance to internal feedings Paralytic ileus Diarrhea Ischemic colitis Mucosal ulceration Bacterial overgrowth in stool	**Immune**	Infection: increased energy needs Decreased lymphocyte count Anergy
Liver	Increased serum ammonia level		
Hypermetabolism	Decreased lean body mass Muscle wasting Severe weight loss Negative nitrogen balance Hyperglycemia	**Gallbladder**	Abdominal distention Unexplained fever: increased kcalorie needs Decreased bowel sounds

From Baldwin KM et al.: Shock, multiple organ dysfunction syndrome, and burns in adults. In McCance KL, Huether SE, eds.: Pathophysiology: the biologic basis for diseases in adults and children, ed 3, St Louis, 1998, Mosby; and Escott-Stump S: Nutrition and diagnosis-related care, ed 4, Baltimore, 1997, Williams & Wilkins.

SURGERY

In a perfect world, all patients undergoing surgery would be at optimal nutritional status to help them tolerate the physiologic stress of the surgery and temporary starvation that follows. But, all too often, surgical patients may be malnourished secondary to the medical condition causing the need for surgery. Additionally, they may experience anorexia, nausea, or vomiting, which decrease their ability to eat. Fever may increase their metabolic rate. Or nutritional needs may not be met because of malabsorption. For surgery to be successful, patients who are malnourished or in danger of malnutrition must be identified so corrective action may be arranged. Before surgery, patients are typically limited to NPO to prevent aspiration. Oral intake is generally resumed when bowel sounds return, usually 24 to 48 hours after surgery. The postoperative diet usually progresses from clear liquid to solid foods as tolerated.

🌀 BURNS (THERMAL INJURY)

Burns are customarily defined as tissue destruction that results in circulatory and metabolic alterations that require the compensatory response to injury (Table 15-5).[18] Actual cause of burns may be thermal or nonthermal, such as chemical, electrical, or radioactive sources. Thermal burns are usually characterized as contact (hot solid object), flame (direct contact with flames), or scald injuries (heated liquid).[14] These events have significant effects on nutritional status.

Burns are generally classified by physical appearance and symptoms associated with the affected skin[14] and are often described in terms of percent of body surface burned. *First-degree burns* (or *partial thickness injury*) involve only the epidermis, resulting in simple reddening of the area with no injury to underlying dermal or subcutaneous tissue.[14,15] Sunburns are an example of first-degree burns caused by ultraviolet radiation damage to skin. First-degree burns heal within 3 to 5 days without scarring.[14] *Second-degree burns (superficial partial-thickness injury* and *deep partial-thickness injury)* involve two categories of burn depth with distinctly different characteristics.[14] Superficial partial-thickness burns are characterized by redness and blistering that affect epidermis and some dermis.[14,15] Deep partial-thickness burns are characterized by destruction of epidermis and dermis (resulting in a waxy, white, mottled appearance),

Table 15-5 Nutritional Goals for Burned Patients	
Goal	**Action**
Minimize metabolic response	Control environmental temperature
	Monitor fluid and electrolyte balance
	Control pain and anxiety
	Cover wounds early
Meet nutritional needs	Provide adequate kcalories to prevent weight loss >10% of usual body weight
	Provide adequate protein for positive nitrogen balance and maintenance or repletion of visceral protein stores
Prevent Curling's ulcer	Provide antacids or continuous enteral feedings

Modified from Winkler MF, Manchester S: Nutritional care in metabolic stress: sepsis, trauma, burns, and surgery. In Mahan LK, Escott-Stump S: Krause's food, nutrition, and diet therapy, ed 9, Philadelphia, 1996, WB Saunders.

leaving only skin appendages such as hair follicles and sweat glands.[14] Second-degree burns take weeks to months to heal. *Third-degree burns (full-thickness injury)* are characterized by destruction of the entire epidermis, dermis, and frequently the underlying subcutaneous tissue. Occasionally, muscle or bone tissue may be destroyed.[14] Third-degree burns do not heal and require skin grafts[14] (Box 15-3).

Box 15-3 Love Greg & Lauren

On September 11, 2001, at 8:48 AM, Lauren Manning, a senior vice president, partner, and director of global data sales for Cantor Fitzgerald, was entering the lobby of 1 World Trade Center in New York City. As the first of two planes drove into the World Trade Center buildings, an explosive fireball ran through the lobby. Lauren was burned on more than 82.5% of her body. Below is an excerpt from her husband's day-by-day e-mail account of Lauren's struggle to heal and survive for her son, Tyler, and her husband, Greg. Consider the effect of serious injuries on patients, their families, and the medical personnel who assist in the healing process.

From: Greg
To: Everyone
Date: Saturday, September 29, 2001, 12:40 AM
Subject: Lauren Update for September 28 (Friday)

Today was a stable day. Lauren still has the septic infection, which they are fighting with antibiotics, but her lungs are functioning well, as is her stomach, two very important factors. The oxygen and the protein intake she is receiving through a feeding tube are needed to build new tissue and for her skin to heal.

I have a better understanding now of something the doctor told me about doing Lauren's grafts. He said he would "mesh 3-1" when doing autografts. Basically, a special machine is used to create a mesh pattern in the donor skin—her own skin—that permits it to cover an area three times as large as the site from which it was taken. The homograft, or skin-bank skin, is then placed over this mesh, creating a layer that enables the autograft beneath to heal better. The goal is for the mesh to take and for healing to occur in the open spots. More than one graft is often necessary to finish each site.

The grafts already done look good, which means the majority have probably taken. Unfortunately, the infection does have an adverse effect on the healing process, both of the grafts, and of the donor sites. That is why Lauren's time in the burn ICU is such a balancing act. Negative factors have to be controlled so that positive factors can win out. The good aspect for Lauren is that she was strong and healthy going in, so she has managed to keep herself mostly stable, a word that has become very important for the families of all the burn patients.

Her nurse explained to me tonight how Lauren's various systems were adjusting on their own to maintain stability. For example, her heart was pumping faster to maintain her blood pressure despite a slight dilation of blood vessels due to infection. A glass-half-full type of sign.

I put two pictures—of Lauren and of Lauren, Tyler, and my dad—up on her wall. The pictures are an important way for the nursing staff to make a connection to her. They are all looking forward to meeting her when she is more awake, later in her treatment course.

That alone should tell you how difficult the work is that these nurses do; the patients arrive gravely injured, frequently unable to communicate, and highly critical. The medical and nursing staffs often fight for weeks to keep the patient improving; this is well before they have a chance to encounter the patient's personality. The staff first gets to know the patient through the family visitors, and the photographs help the staff connect with the life they are trying to help the patient return to.

The WTC disaster families have been there for seventeen days now and we know each other well.

This bonding between families is due to the utter stress of the situation; we have all spent days, now weeks, and hopefully will spend months, worrying minute to minute about a loved one's condition. It is the same as if a surgical procedure were to last for weeks on end. We learn to read the facial expressions and voices of doctors and nurses.

So we, the waiting, speak to each other, and to the staff psychologists and chaplain and the Red Cross volunteers who wander through, and we are visited by Good Samaritans of all types, who provide food…And in the end, we alone understand what we are going through: we are the loved ones of critically injured patients from a massive tragedy in which most victims either died or walked out under their own power.

We, the waiting, are therefore at somewhat of a disconnect from the world at large, which is pursuing closure (not my favorite word), whether coping with loss of a family member; coming to terms with having one's life saved by something so trivial as arriving late for work; or honoring the heroism of lost firefighters, and police.

Most of the world is already viewing the attacks from a distance, but we are pretty much still there at Time Zero, with the outcome unknown.

However, we are all making it through, with the help of the huge support networks that have sprung up all around us. Including y'all…It really does help us, me and Lauren, to know how many people care.

Love,
Greg & Lauren
Lauren Manning left home for work on September 11, 2001, and returned home on March 15, 2002. She continues to work to regain the life she had.

In addition to pain management, wound care, and infection control, nutrition support is recognized as one of the most significant considerations of patient care.[14,16] The first 24 to 48 hours of treatment for burn patients are dedicated to replacement of fluid and electrolytes. Fluid needs are based on the patient's age, weight, and extent of the burn.[19] *Total body surface area (TBSA),* used to estimate the extent of the burn, can be estimated using the "rule of nines" (Figure 15-4). Thermal injury wounds will heal *only* if the patient is in an anabolic state. Therefore, feeding should be initiated as soon as the patient has been hydrated.[19] Very early enteral feeding (within 4 to 12 hours of hospitalization) has been shown to be successful in decreasing the hypercatabolic response, decreasing the release of catecholamines and glucagon, reducing weight loss, and shortening the length of the hospital stay.[20]

Nutritional goals for patients with burns are outlined in Table 15-5. Several methods may be used to estimate energy and protein needs in burn patients. Energy needs vary according to the size of the burn.[16] One of the simplest and easiest to use is the Curreri formula (adults):[21]

$$\text{kcal needed per day} \times [25 \text{ kcal} \times \text{kg } \textit{usual} \text{ body weight (kg)}] +$$
$$[40 \text{ kcal} \times \% \text{ TBSA burned}]$$

Estimates using the Curreri formula may exceed actual energy needs,[15,19] but it is not uncommon for a patient to need 4000 to 5000 kcalories.[15] Another method is to calculate BEE (Harris-Benedict) and multiply by a factor of 1.5 to 2.0.[15]

Protein lost through urine and wounds, increased protein use for gluconeogenesis, and wound healing increase protein needs in burned patients.[16] It is therefore important that kcalories from protein are not calculated into total energy needs.[5] Carbohydrates and fats are good for protein sparing (nonprotein energy sources).[5,16] Whether a patient receives adequate amounts of energy or protein is best evaluated by wound healing, graft take, and basic nutritional assessment parameters.[16]

In conjunction with increased energy demands, vitamin and mineral needs are generally increased in burn patients, but exact requirements are not known.[16] Most patients will receive vitamins in excess of the recommended intake because of their

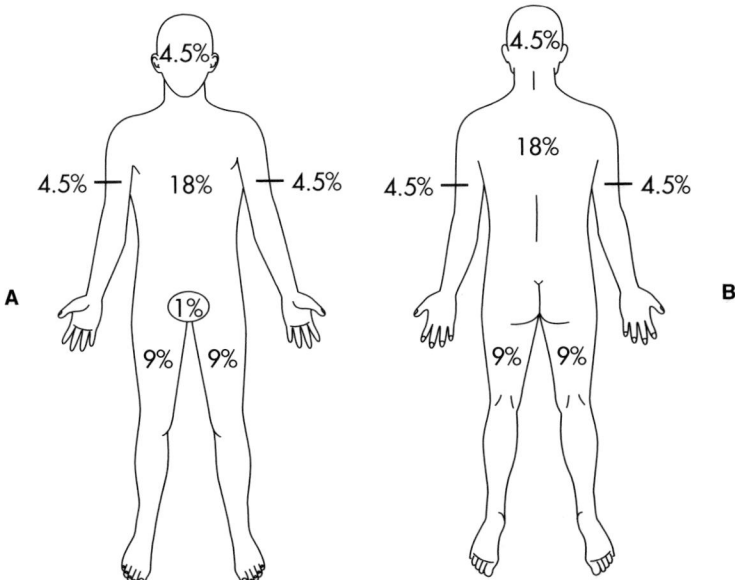

Figure 15-4 Rule of nines—a commonly used assessment tool with estimates of the percentages (in multiples of 9) of the total body surface area burned. **A,** Adults (anterior view). **B,** Adults (posterior view). (From Thompson JM et al.: *Mosby's clinical nursing,* ed 5, St Louis, 2002, Mosby.)

high kcaloric intakes, but special consideration should be given to vitamin C (collagen synthesis, immune function) and vitamin A (immune function and epithelialization). Supplements are commonly recommended.[16]

SUMMARY

The stress response of the body also affects nutritional status. Whether the stress response is caused by physiologic or psychologic determinants, the entire body is affected. Metabolic changes take place in reaction to stress. This includes changes caused by uncomplicated stress that is present when patients are at nutritional risk and severe stress caused by trauma or disease. The functioning of the immune system is also affected by the hormonal and metabolic changes that occur when metabolic stress develops. The immune system's ability to protect the body is further depressed if impaired nutritional status accompanies the metabolic stress.

THE NURSING APPROACH
Caring for a Burned Client

Martin, age 49, was involved in an explosion on his job site and received burns to nearly 40% of his body. He was hospitalized for 8 weeks for care and multiple skin grafts at a burn center. His condition is now considered stable and he was discharged home but will need further rehabilitation and physical therapy. His family has been supportive while at home and home health nurses visit everyday to change his wound dressings. Before the accident, Martin enjoyed cooking and eating the Sunday dinner for his family.

In addition to the nutritional needs, the multiple nursing diagnoses for Martin include the following:
- Impaired skin integrity related to injury and treatment
- Risk for infection related to altered skin integrity
- Impaired physical mobility related to open burn wounds, pain, and scar and contracture
- Body image disturbance related to change in physical appearance, change in lifestyle, and alterations in sensory and motor functions

ASSESSMENT

Subjective
- Continues to feel pain when wound dressings changed
- Feels depressed and states, "Life is not the same anymore," but looks forward to returning to work
- Currently eats one to two meals a day after returning home from the burn center

Objective
- Wounds are healing
- Height: 5'10"
- Weight: 142 lbs
- Laboratory results:
  - Urea nitrogen 17 mg/dl (normal 5-15 mg/dl)
  - Glucose 120 mg/dl (normal 60-120 mg/dl)
  - Electrolytes
  - Sodium 130 mEq/L (normal 136-145 mEq/L)
  - Potassium 5.9 mEq/L (normal 3.5-5.0 mEq/L)
  - Chloride 110 mE/L (normal 96-106 mEq/L)
  - Total protein 5 g/dl (normal 6-8.0 g/dl)
  - Albumin 3 g/dl (normal 3.5-5.0 g/dl)

THE NURSING APPROACH–cont'd
Caring for a Burned Client

NURSING DIAGNOSIS

Altered nutrition, less than body requirements related to increase metabolic rate, reduced caloric intake, altered glucose, fat and protein metabolism, and increased urinary nitrogen losses

PLANNING

Goal

Martin will maintain adequate nutrition intake for meeting the body's caloric requirement as evidenced by maintaining body weight, normal serum protein levels, and wound healing.

IMPLEMENTATION

1. Calculate the client's caloric needs and sources of protein for wound healing by consulting with a dietitian.
2. Encourage Martin to verbalize about his not eating and contributing factors such as depression and pain.
   a. Discuss with the family and Martin the foods he enjoys and calculate the daily source of calories and protein served during his meals.
   b. Serve meals before his dressing changes and times when he feels like eating.
   c. Provide foods that Martin can ingest as well as supplemental nutrition between meals.
   d. Record the foods and fluids eaten daily.

EVALUATION

The goal will be achieved as evidenced by the following:
- Eating a high-caloric and high-protein diet after 1 week at home.
- Able to discuss and identify his concerns, which contribute to his lack of eating an adequate diet.

CRITICAL THINKING
Clinical Applications

Kristin, age 19, is a member of her college's cheerleading team and was involved in a serious motor vehicle accident when the team was returning from a game. She was admitted through the emergency room of your hospital suffering from multiple fractures and contusions. Kristin is 5'5" tall and weighed 120 lbs before the accident. Because she is young, looked healthy, and is somewhat muscular from being a cheerleader, the physician did not request a consult for the dietitian to evaluate Kristin's nutritional status. After 2 weeks in intensive care, she developed pneumonia. The nurse learned that before the automobile accident, Kristin had been using a commercial weight-loss product and was consuming approximately 400 kcal/day for 3 months before the accident in an attempt to "make weight" so that she could remain on the cheerleading team.

1. How did the very low-calorie diet (VLCD) affect Kristin's nutritional status?
2. Why did Kristin develop pneumonia?
3. Describe the variety of stresses Kristin experienced.
4. Could the pneumonia have been prevented? How?

Web Sites of Interest

Burnsurgery.org

www.burnsurgery.org/

This site provides up-to-date educational tools for health professionals who focus on burn care by providing dissemination of the most recent advances in burn treatment.

KidSource OnLine!

www.kidsource.com/kidsource/content2/ecoli/anna.1.html

This online community of parents presents support and resources on many topics related to parenting. The particular page cited above is a parent's personal account of her daughter's experience with MODS caused by an *Escherichia coli* infection.

References

1. Myrvik QN: Immunology and nutrition. In Shils ME et al., eds.: *Modern nutrition in health and disease,* ed 9, Philadelphia, 1999, Williams & Wilkins.
2. Gould BE: *Pathophysiology for the health-related professions,* ed 2, Philadelphia, 2002, WB Saunders.
3. Cahill GF: Starvation: some biological aspects. In Kinney JM et al., eds.: *Nutrition and metabolism in patient care,* Philadelphia, 1988, WB Saunders.
4. Wolfe BM: Nutrition in hypermetabolic conditions. In Zeman FJ, ed.: *Clinical nutrition and dietetics,* ed 2, New York, 1991, Macmillan.
5. Bessey PQ, Wilmore DW: The burned patient. In Kinney JM et al., eds.: *Nutrition and metabolism in patient care,* Philadelphia, 1988, WB Saunders.
6. Morgan SL, Weinsier RL: *Fundamentals of clinical nutrition,* ed 2, St Louis, 1998, Mosby.
7. American Dietetic Association: *Manual of clinical dietetics,* ed 6, Chicago, 2000, American Dietetic Association.
8. Long CL: The energy and protein requirements of the critically ill patient. In Wright RA, Heymsfield SB, McManus CB III, eds.: *Nutritional assessment,* Boston, 1984, Blackwell Scientific Publications.
9. Souba WB, Wilmore DW: Diet and nutrition in the care of the patient with surgery, trauma and sepsis. In Shils ME et al., eds.: *Modern nutrition in health and disease,* ed 9, Philadelphia, 1999, Williams & Wilkins.
10. Silverman D: Trauma/sepsis. In Lysen LK, ed.: *Quick reference to clinical dietetics,* Gaithersburg, Md, 1997, Aspen.
11. Heimburger DC, Weinsier RL: *Handbook of clinical nutrition,* ed 3, St Louis, 1997, Mosby.
12. Moore MC: *Mosby's pocket guide to nutritional care,* ed 4, St Louis, 2000, Mosby.
13. Speath G et al.: Food without fiber promotes bacterial translocation from the gut, *Surgery* 108(2):240, 1990.
14. Baldwin KM et al.: Shock, multiple organ dysfunction syndrome, and burns in adults. In McCance KL, Huether SE, eds.: *Pathophysiology: the biologic basis for diseases in adults and children,* ed 3, St Louis, 1998, Mosby.
15. Escott-Stump S: *Nutrition and diagnosis-related care,* ed 4, Baltimore, 1997, Williams & Wilkins.
16. Winkler MF, Manchester S: Nutritional care in metabolic stress: sepsis, trauma, burns and surgery. In Mahan LK, Escott-Stump S, eds.: *Krause's food, nutrition, and diet therapy,* ed 10, Philadelphia, 2000, WB Saunders.
17. Wilmore DW et al.: The gut: a central organ after surgical stress, *Surgery* 104(5):917, 1988.
18. Gottschlick MM: Nutrition management for specific medical conditions. In Lysen LK, ed.: *Quick references to clinical dietetics,* Gaithersburg, Md, 1997, Aspen.
19. Saffle JR, Larson CM, Sullivan J: A randomized trial of indirect calorimetry-based feedings in thermal injury, *J Trauma* 30:776, 1990.
20. Chiarelli A et al.: Very early nutrition supplementation in burned patients, *Am J Clin Nutr* 51:1035, 1990.
21. Currei PW: Supportive therapy in burn care. Nutritional replacement modalities, *J Trauma* 19(11 Suppl):906, 1979.

CHAPTER 16

Interactions: Complementary and Alternative Medicine, Dietary Supplements, and Medications

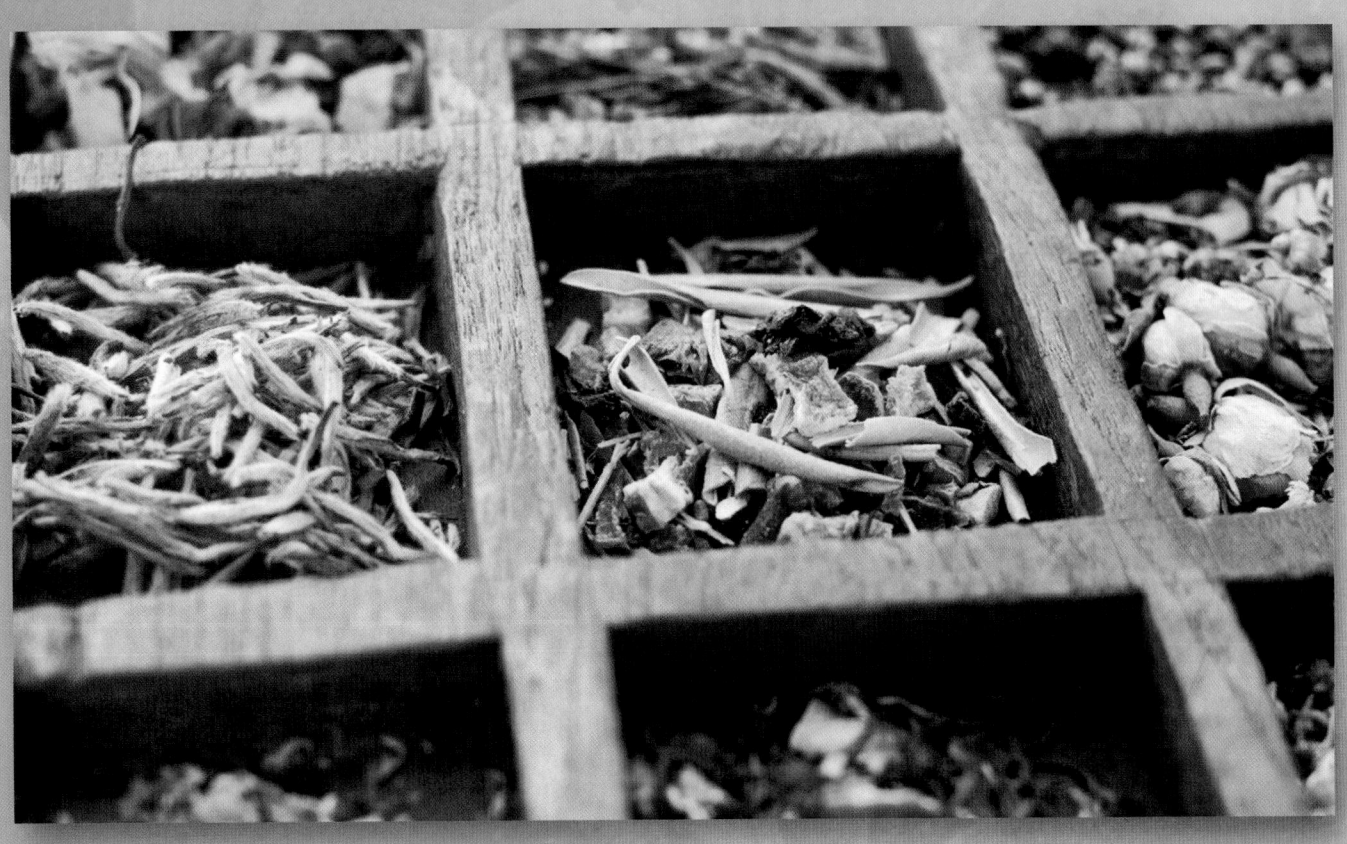

Herbs are not innocuous but can have significant effects on the bioavailability of foods, nutrients, and drugs.

ROLE IN WELLNESS

This chapter first discusses the roles of complementary and alternative medicine (CAM) as they interact with conventional medicine. Dietary supplements, a component of CAM, have become an everyday part of life for many Americans. Because supplement use has substantially grown, part of this chapter discusses supplements as an influence that interacts with health status. This chapter closes with consideration of the interactions that occur among medications, food, nutrients, and herbs. These interactions can limit the bioavailability of medications or nutrients and can even cause serious symptoms that affect blood clotting and blood pressure.

The five dimensions of health provide additional perspectives as CAM, dietary supplements, and medications interact with health. The physical health dimension can be impacted when dietary supplements interact with medications and inadvertently alter the effects of medications. Intellectual health becomes valuable because critical thinking skills are required to assess the efficacy and appropriateness of incorporating alternative medicine therapies. Emotional health may be enhanced as complementary approaches address stress and anxiety that sometimes occur when dealing with chronic disorders. Social health can be supported by several alternative modalities, such as yoga and tai chi, which often involve classes that provide a social support group. The last dimension, spiritual health, can evolve by adopting modalities such as meditation and biofeedback, which provide physical and spiritual benefits by using the body to heal itself.

COMPLEMENTARY AND ALTERNATIVE MEDICINE

CAM has become a significant component of healthcare in the United States. Consider that in 1997, 42% of Americans used CAM therapies at a cost of $2.7 billion per year.[1] To address this increased interest in CAM, the National Institutes of Health created the National Center for Complementary and Alternative Medicine (NCCAM) in 1998. For this discussion, the categories of CAM as outlined by NCCAM will be used. The CAM categories simplify the distinctions between the systems of healing and the related modalities but provide an adequate overview of the methods of application. (See Appendix I for a more complete list of CAM systems and modalities.)

complementary and alternative medicine
a cluster of medical and healthcare approaches, methods, and items not associated with conventional medicine

According to NCCAM, *complementary and alternative medicine* consists of a cluster of medical and healthcare approaches, methods, and items not associated with conventional medicine.[2] Medical doctors and doctors of osteopathy practice conventional medicine, which is also called *allopathy*, and Western medicine as do other allied health professionals such as registered nurses, nurse practitioners, registered dietitians, and physician assistants. Some conventional physicians may also incorporate CAM in their practices. Studies of CAM therapies are being conducted; previously the efficacy of these therapies tended to be anecdotal based on the self-reported experiences of individuals. Some CAM systems such as Ayurveda, which includes the modality of yoga, and Traditional Chinese Medicine, which encompasses acupuncture, have been used for healing for thousands of years, thereby precluding the immediate need for "proof." Nonetheless, well-designed studies are needed to continue to identify the efficacy of particular modalities for specific disorders (see the Cultural Considerations box, "Global Strategies on Traditional and Alternative Medicine"). Providing support for such studies is part of the mission of NCCAM.

complementary medicine
non-Western healing approaches used at the same time as conventional medicine

To continue with definitions, *complementary medicine* refers to non-Western healing approaches used at the same time as conventional medicine.[2] For instance, a patient who attempts to lower hypertension takes prescription medications (conventional) but also attends yoga classes (complementary) for physical and psycho-

CULTURAL CONSIDERATIONS
Global Strategies on Traditional and Alternative Medicine

In May 2002 the World Health Organization (WHO) released a global plan that provided guidelines for countries to develop national policies to evaluate and regulate traditional or complementary/alternative medicine (TM/CAM) to ensure its availability to populations throughout the world. The concern is twofold: (1) to keep traditional medicine available and economical and (2) to assess in a formal way the efficacy, safety, and standardization of these methods.

For example, about 80% of Africans turn to traditional medicine for health maintenance. This traditional practice has not been formalized and could be institutionalized to become part of the healthcare systems of African nations. China, North and South Korea, and Vietnam have already integrated TM/CAM into their health systems. In developing countries, TM/CAM can provide healthcare availability whereas a third of the populations currently do not have access to medical personnel or facilities.

In Western nations, the use of CAM has increased substantially. Complementary medicine has been used by 75% of the French. Acupuncture is available at 77% of the pain clinics in Germany. CAM expenditures in the United Kingdom have reached $230 million dollars (US) per year. As TM/CAM gains global acceptance, concern is to limit commercialization to maintain its affordability in all nations because TM is the only accessible mode of medicine for many.

Application to Nursing: An additional concern is that TM/CAM may be inappropriately used as its benefits are translated from one culture to another. Nurses working with diverse cultural groups can be aware of the TM/CAM practices of patients' culture of origin. A prime example is the herb *ma huang* (ephedra). In China, ma huang is used for a short period to reduce respiratory congestion. In the United States ma huang was marketed as a dietary aid to reduce weight and to increase energy potential. When used long term, the herb caused strokes, heart attacks, and over 10 deaths among young, otherwise healthy adults. Consequently, encouraging the creation of policies to regulate TM/CAM will lead to positive use of traditional knowledge by all.

Reference: World Health Organization: WHO launches the first global strategy on traditional and alternative medicine, *Press Release/38, May 16, 2002; www.who.int/inf/en/pr-2002-38.html.*

---

logic benefits. In contrast, alternative medicine replaces conventional medical treatment.[2] An example is the use of herbal supplements to treat cancer instead of surgical intervention or chemotherapy. Integrative medicine merges conventional medical therapies with CAM modalities for which safety and efficacy, based on scientific data, have been demonstrated.[2]

Integrative medical centers are available that are hospital-based and under the direction of physicians and other conventional health professionals. Advanced practice nurses with Masters of Science degrees in holistic health are often at the forefront of the integrative care provided. For example, a patient recovering from heart bypass surgery can be referred to a center for integrative medicine. Once there, a board-certified physician evaluates the patient and may recommend complementary approaches of therapeutic massage for stress-reduction and yoga for exercise to assist recovery. All services are provided within the same healthcare facility. Insurance companies have slowly but steadily increased coverage for such treatments.

According to NCCAM, CAM therapies can be divided into five categories: alternative medical systems; mind-body interventions; biologically based therapies; manipulative and body-based methods; and energy therapies.[2]

alternative medicine
healing practices that replace conventional medical treatment

integrative medicine
merging of conventional medical therapies with CAM modalities for which safety and efficacy, based on scientific data, have been demonstrated

Alternative Medical Systems

Alternative medical systems develop outside mainstream Western medical approaches. These systems are based on holistic structures that incorporate distinctive philosophies and applications. Alternative medical systems evolving from Eastern cultures include *Traditional Chinese Medicine (TCM)* and *Ayurveda* (Asian Indian derivation). Western cultures have produced *naturopathic medicine* and *homeopathic medicine.*[2]

The Eastern practice of TCM is a system based on the forces of nature understood through the fundamental concept of *yin* and *yang.* Illness is viewed as an imbalance of these two forces that are opposites of each other. Yin is dark, night, feminine, and

acupuncture
the use of fine needles to open blockages of the flow of Qi or life force and thus restore balance

ayurveda
a system of healing focusing on diet and herbal remedies that emphasizes the use of body, mind, and spirit to prevent and treat disorders

naturopathic medicine
the use of the body's natural healing forces to recover from disease and to achieve wellness; it incorporates techniques from Eastern and Western traditions

homeopathic medicine
an alternative medical system through which a small amount of a diluted substance is prescribed to relieve symptoms for which the same substance, given in larger amounts, will cause the same symptoms

meditation
a self-directed technique of relaxing the body and calming the mind

faith healing
healing by invoking divine intervention without the use of conventional or surgical therapy

biofeedback
the use of special devices to convey physiologic information to enable a person to learn how to consciously control medically important functions

dietary supplements
substances consumed orally as an addition to dietary intake

contracting; yang is light, day, masculine, and expanding. The imbalance of these two forces affects *Qi,* (pronounced chi), the life force. Therapeutic modalities, such as acupuncture, massage, meditation, incense, diet, herbs, and tai chi (exercise of slow movements), aim to reduce symptoms and restore energy balance. For example, acupuncture is the use of fine needles placed in the 2000 specific acupuncture points on the body to open blockages of the flow of Qi or life force and thus restore balance.

The Eastern ancient practice of Ayurveda is 5000 years old, evolving from the Indian subcontinent. As an alternative medical system, Ayurveda focuses on diet and herbal remedies that emphasize the use of body, mind, and spirit to prevent and treat disorders.[2]

The Western approach of naturopathic medicine is based on the use of the body's natural healing forces to recover from disease and to achieve wellness.[2] This system incorporates techniques from Eastern and Western traditions. Techniques may include acupuncture, exercise, massage, and dietary alterations.

Homeopathic medicine is an alternative medical system through which a small amount of a diluted substance is prescribed to relieve symptoms for which the same substance, given in larger amounts, will cause the same symptoms. This theory is called *"like cures like."*[2]

Training in homeopathic medicine is necessary for practitioners to be able to diagnose and treat disorders appropriately. Individuals with the same illness may each receive different treatments because homeopathic practitioners focus on the needs of the specific individual, not on the disorder. Although the amounts of medications prescribed will usually not interfere with conventional medications, patients should reveal the use of homeopathic treatments to their healthcare providers.

Mind-Body Interventions

The focus of mind-body intervention is to expand the mind's ability to influence physical functions. These modalities include meditation, faith healing or prayer, biofeedback, and such therapies that influence behavior through creative approaches of music, dance, and art therapy.[2]

Several of these modalities are commonly recommended and are used not only for physical healing but also for stress reduction and other concerns related to contemporary life. Meditation is a self-directed technique of relaxing the body and calming the mind. Based in Eastern religions, meditation evolved from religious practice. Meditation calms the mind and body through guided imagery and rhythmic breathing. Faith healing is healing by invoking divine intervention without the use of conventional or surgical therapy. Faith healing is a form of prayer that is either practiced individually or as a group; the practice is often associated with religious institutions or communities. Biofeedback involves the use of special devices to convey information about heart rate, blood pressure, skin temperature, and muscle relaxation to enable a person to learn how to consciously control these medically important functions. Patients need several training sessions to become able to produce the desired responses on their own.

Biologically Based Therapies

Biologically based therapies encompass materials found in nature. These materials include nutrients, food, and herbs. This category incorporates dietary supplements, alternative dietary patterns, aromatherapy, and other alternative natural treatments such as shark cartilage for cancer treatment.[2]

Dietary supplements are substances consumed orally as an addition to dietary intake. The ingredients of dietary supplements may include one or more of the following: minerals, vitamins, amino acids, herbs, plant extracts, enzymes, metabolites, and organ tissues.[3] Dietary supplements are processed into various forms, including tablets, liquids, capsules, extracts, powders, concentrates, gel caps, liquids, and powders. There are special requirements for supplement labeling. Under the Dietary Supplement Act of 1994, dietary supplements are considered foods, not drugs.[3] Because of the popularity of use, extensive range of supplements available, and connections to nutrition, the next section of this chapter explores supplements.

An alternative dietary pattern is the macrobiotic diet. The macrobiotic dietary pattern evolves from the yin–yang philosophy of opposing forces. By consuming a balance of foods that contain yin and yang characteristics, health can be maintained, disease prevented, and treatment achieved. Although macrobiotic diet was originally intended for general good health, it has recently become most associated with treatment for cancer. This has occurred because the Japanese philosopher who originated this concept views cancer as an imbalance caused by dietary, environmental, and social and personal factors that affect an individual. Locations of cancer are even tied to yin–yang, with yin cancers in the upper parts of the body and in hollow organs and yang cancer in the lower body and in more dense organs.

Because all foods are categorized as yin or yang, dietary recommendations would, for example, support consumption of yang foods to offset a yin cancer. Also considered are the person's age, sex, activity levels, and climate. Although the original macrobiotic diet consisted of a rigid 10-step program, the current version is not as restrictive and is health promoting. The core diet focuses on consumption of whole cereals and grains as 50% to 60% of intake with 40% to 50% from other foods, preferably organically grown, with minimal intake of animal foods except for small amounts of white fish. Consequently, intake of fatty foods, milk products, processed foods, and eggs is to be avoided because the belief is that such foods contain toxins that cause illness. Because this diet is low in fat and high in fiber and plant foods, it appears to support the health and recovery of individuals with cancer when used in conjunction with conventional treatments for cancer. The safety of the macrobiotic diet depends on the implementation to support sufficient intake of calories and nutrients. This requires substantial commitment to food preparation with planning to ensure nutrient adequacy.[4]

aromatherapy
using extracts or essences of herbs, flowers, and trees in the form of essential oils to support health and well-being

Aromatherapy is using extracts or essences of herbs, flowers, and trees in the form of essential oils to support health and well-being.[2] The essential oils are added to candles, oils, and lotions through which the aroma is dispersed and inhaled with subsequent physiologic responses. Often, the essential oils are an integral part of massage therapy. Applications of aromatherapy continue to increase. Pillows can be purchased that have a special pocket in which to place essential oils to provide aromatherapy while one sleeps. A dental practice in New York City now offers aromatherapy along with foot massages to decrease stress while dental procedures are conducted.[5] In a number of breast cancer treatment centers, nurses use essential oils and massage to reduce anxiety and discomfort of patients during chemotherapy treatments.

Manipulative and Body-Based Methods

Manipulative and body-based methods involve manipulation or movements of body parts. These methods include osteopathic or chiropractic manipulation, massage, and bodywork.

Osteopathic manipulation is a part of osteopathic medicine. Although osteopathic medicine is considered part of conventional medicine, it differs in its view of disease as stemming from the musculoskeletal system.[2] This approach is based on the assumption that the systems of the body function together. Therefore disturbances in one system may affect other systems. Some osteopathic physicians conduct osteopathic manipulation, which is a method of hands-on actions to reduce pain, reinstate function, and promote health and well-being.[2]

osteopathic medicine
an approach based on the assumption that the systems of the body function together with disease stemming from the musculoskeletal system

chiropractic manipulation
a manipulation modality addressing the ties between body structure (particularly of the spine) and function and how those ties impact the maintenance and return to health

Chiropractic manipulation addresses the ties between body structure (particularly of the spine) and function and how those ties impact the maintenance and return to health.[2] Manipulative therapy is the foundation of treatment.[2]

Massage therapy is the manipulation of muscle and connective tissue to improve function and to enhance relaxation and well-being; trained massage therapists conduct manipulation. Massage therapists do not diagnose and treat disorders, as do practitioners of osteopathy or chiropractic. Instead, their treatment is adjunct to other medical interventions or may be used to generally enhance physical and psychologic health.

Health benefits occur because massage strengthens and loosens the muscles and connective tissue. This in turn allows better blood flow through the body, increases the removal of metabolic waste products, and stimulates the release of endorphins and serotonins in the brain and nervous system.

Several types of massage therapy exist; each form addresses different aspects of body muscularity. These massage therapies may include Swedish massage that focuses deeply on muscles, sports massage that kneads deeply into muscles most affected by athletic pursuits, and Trager massage that through gentle massage along with rhythmic rocking of body parts creates physical and psychologic relaxation. Massage therapies continue to emerge as acceptance of massage as a health-promoting technique gains more popularity.

Energy Therapies

Energy therapies manipulate energy fields. Two kinds of energy therapies are biofield therapies and bioelectromagnetic-based therapies. Biofield therapies influence energy fields that encircle and go through the body. Whether these energy fields exist has not been determined based on Western scientific research. Nonetheless, these therapies manipulate body biofields by placing hands around or on the body thereby changing the movement of energy.

Biofield therapies include Qi gong, reiki, and therapeutic touch. Qi gong is a modality of TCM that merges breathing regulation, movement, and meditation to increase the flow of Qi or life force in the body. This practice of Qi gong enhances circulatory and immune function.[2] Reiki means Universal Life Energy in Japanese. The energy therapy bearing the name "reiki" is based on the belief that by healing the patient's spirit, the physical body will also heal. Spirits are healed when a reiki practitioner channels spiritual energy, or Universal Life Force, through to the patient.[2] Therapeutic touch, developed in the 1970s by Dr. Dolores Krieger, a nursing professor at New York University, is an updated version of the ancient technique called *laying-on of hands*. Therapeutic touch is based on the blockage of energy flow in and around the body. The therapist proceeds to identify and undo blockages to promote healing. Therapists, while in a meditative state, move their hands above patients to determine blockages in energy fields and then clear blockages by the downward motions of their hands around the patients' bodies. The healing energy powers of therapists are transferred to patients to restore energy balance within their bodies.[2,6]

Bioelectromagnetic-based therapies consist of the unusual use of electromagnetic fields. These fields include magnetic fields, pulsed fields, and direct or alternating current fields.[2] Although magnets have been used for a long time as healing tools, the efficacy of their use has not, as yet, been validated.

Application to Nursing

Familiarity with these CAM modalities is valuable. Although some do not directly impact nutrition status, many indirectly do by increasing awareness of the holistic nature of healing of which nourishing the body is fundamental (see the Cultural Considerations box, "Treating Chronic Illness: New Approaches Using Old Methods"). Acceptance without judgment of alternative healing approaches provides a more secure environment for patients to feel supported in their quest for health. Referrals can be made to nutritionists who have special training in integrating CAM therapies with dietary recommendations.

Qi gong
a modality of Traditional Chinese Medicine that merges breathing regulation, movement, and meditation to increase the flow of Qi or life force in the body

reiki
an energy therapy based on the belief that by healing the patient's spirit, the physical body will also heal

therapeutic touch
an energy system based on the blockage of energy flow in and around the body

CULTURAL CONSIDERATIONS
Treating Chronic Illness: New Approaches Using Old Methods

Chronic physical illness can be difficult to treat using conventional medicinal approaches. To bridge cultures by increasing interactions between Native American traditional healers and non-Natives, a study was conducted to compare persistent benefits of an intensive treatment program using traditional healing practices. The program created with traditional healers, which lasted 7 to 10 days, was significantly more successful in terms of health benefits and cost-effectiveness in treating chronic physical illness. The process appears to use a dynamic energy system that addresses spiritual, mental, and physical dimensions treated with counseling and ceremonies. Treating one of the dimensions interacts with the other dimensions.

Application to Nursing: Aspects of the Native American traditional healing practices could be adapted in consultation with the healers for use with the general population.

Reference: *Mehl-Madrona LE: Native American medicine in the treatment of chronic illness: developing an integrated program and evaluation and effectiveness,* Altern Ther Health Med 5(1):36, Jan 1999.

DIETARY SUPPLEMENTS

Knowledge of nutrients began to be discovered at the beginning of the twentieth century. First, the role of vitamins in preventing deficiency diseases was revealed. More recently, other nutrient-related substances like concentrated garlic, fish oils, and psyllium came into use for believed health benefits. The concept of dietary supplements evolved because of the growing body of knowledge resulting in the availability of substances in the form of pills, powder, and liquid to enhance the quality of dietary intakes.[5] As the effects of nutrients on health continued to be learned, knowledge of the inappropriate eating habits of Americans increased. Consequently, the value of dietary supplements to rectify poor eating habits caught the attention of the American public as an easier way to improve health than by changing eating behavior.

Throughout this time, physicians tended to discount the value of dietary supplements, including vitamin supplementation. Instead, physicians and dietitians strongly recommended that all nutrients be consumed through food rather than supplements.[7] The view of supplementation of essential nutrients has changed somewhat during the past few years. Supplements may be recommended as a safety net for poor dietary intake. As a safety net, vitamin/mineral supplements at 100% or less of the Dietary Reference Intake (DRI) are appropriate. Additional vitamin/mineral supplements are also recommended for some specific nutrients for certain subgroups within the population. For example, calcium and vitamin D supplementation is suggested for adults older than 70 years because the new DRI for calcium and vitamin D for this age group is higher than what most individuals can generally consume.

Regulation and Labeling

The range of dietary supplements, though, has expanded from vitamins and minerals to a diverse selection of substances including herbs, protein powders, fatty acid capsules, natural and synthetic energy, and growth enhancers. Regulation to control the identity, potency, contents, and labeling of these substances is currently under the Dietary Supplement Health and Education Act (DSHEA) of 1994.

DSHEA establishes a definition of dietary supplements as products that supplement dietary intake and contain one or more of the following:[3]

- A vitamin or a mineral
- An herb or other botanical
- An amino acid
- A dietary substance for use by man to supplement the diet by increasing the total dietary intake
- A concentrate, metabolite, constituent, extract, or a combination of the preceding ingredients

Based on this definition, dietary supplements are to be considered foods; they are not drugs or food additives. This distinction affects the way they are regulated and actually eases the approval process. Drugs require more strident testing for safety and efficacy and food additives must also meet more stringent criteria. Consequently, dietary supplements can enter the marketplace much quicker with less data confirming their function.

The Food and Drug Administration (FDA) oversees the regulation of dietary supplements. If a manufacturer distributes a product containing a new dietary ingredient, the manufacturer must notify the FDA 75 days before the product is to be released. In addition, the manufacturer must also provide data regarding the safety and efficacy of the product. Supplements already on the market or supplement ingredients previously used are considered generally safe and do not need reapproval.[3]

Labeling of dietary supplements must follow the format used for nutrition labels (see Chapter 2). This means that the label needs to identify the product as a dietary supplement and must include the name and amount of each item contained in the product. Labels may also include approved statements of health claims such as are allowable on food product labels. For example, a claim may be made that a diet containing soluble fiber from whole oats and psyllium may reduce the risk of coronary heart disease. Other health-related claims may also be made about the effect of the supplement on the "structure or function" of the body as well as on "general well-being." Claims related to reducing the risk of nutrition deficiency diseases are also acceptable. In addition, if claims are made, the label must include the statement, "This statement has not been evaluated by the Food and Drug Administration. This product is not intended to diagnose, treat, cure, or prevent any disease."[3]

Supplement Use

In the past, use of supplements was limited to a small group of individuals and supplements were available in an equally small number of locations such as health food stores and specialty shops. Currently, supplements are available through numerous outlets including supermarkets, drug stores, mail order companies, and Internet Web sites. Sales of dietary supplements have increased tremendously from about $8 billion in 1994 to an estimated $17 billion in 2000 (Figure 16-1).[8] These numbers represent the purchases of more than 158 million consumers.[8] According

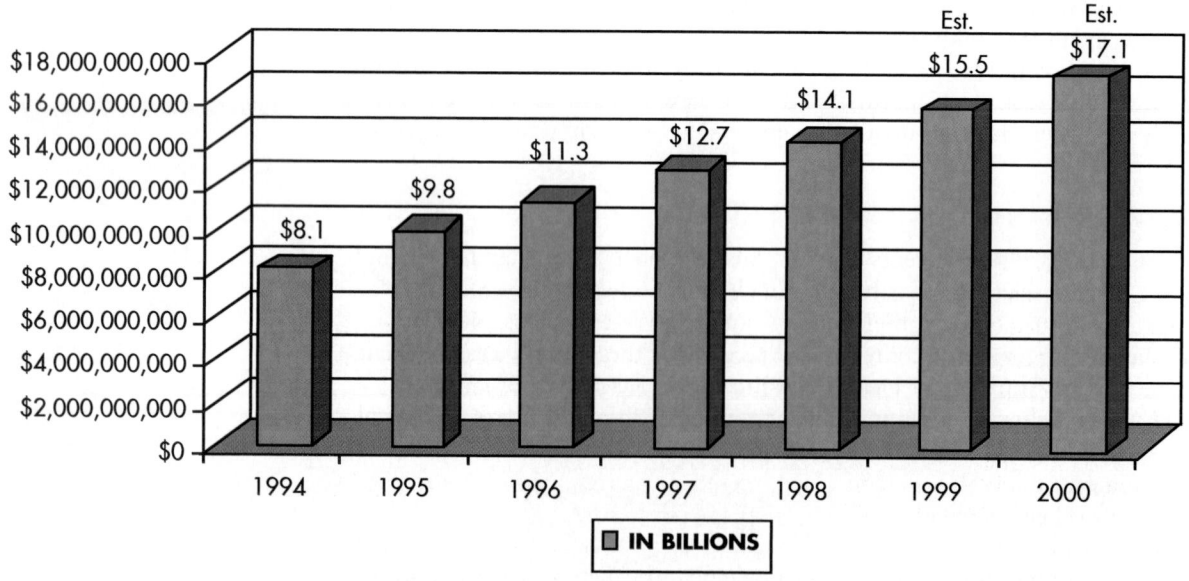

Figure 16-1 Dietary supplement sales, 1994 through 2000. (From US Dietary Supplements Market Size Expressed as Dollar Sales by Top Six Product Categories for 1994 to 1998 and Forecast for 1999 and 2000, *Nutrition Business Journal*, 2000, Dialog File No. 93, San Francisco: The Dialog Corporation, 2000.)

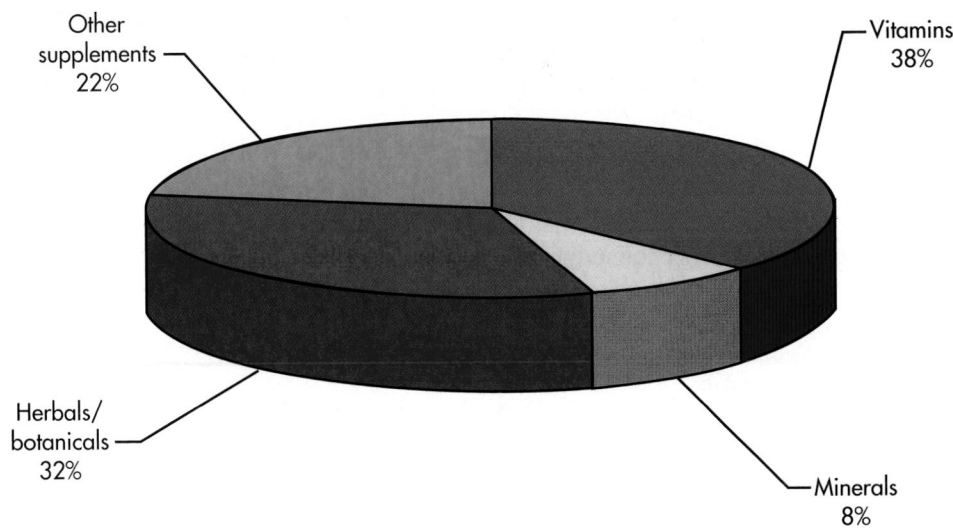

Figure 16-2 Dietary supplement estimated sales breakdown of $17.1 billion market, 2000. (From Nutrition Business Journal 2000: *Dialog file No. 93*, San Francisco, 2000, The Dialog Corp; accessed at www.cfsan.fda.gov/~dms/ds-stra2.html.)

to survey results, 115.3 million consumers purchase vitamin and minerals for their own use whereas about 56 million buy these nutrient supplements for other members of their families.[8] Sales are divided as follows: vitamins, 38%; herbals/botanicals, 32%; other supplements, 22%; and minerals, 8%[9] (Figure 16-2).

Survey results also suggest that the reason for the increased use of dietary supplements is that consumers have self-care goals for which dietary supplements provide perceived value. Concurrently, such self-care goals may reflect consumers experiencing alienation from conventional healthcare systems.[3] This alienation from conventional healthcare systems may be why patients do not reveal their use of dietary supplements.

About 22.8 million consumers use herbal supplements rather than prescription drugs, and 19.6 million use herbs with prescription medications.[3] These consumers may view the dietary supplements either as not "medicine" or that their self-care goals would not be approved of by their healthcare providers. Not revealing supplement use may result in misuse of substances or interaction with prescription and over-the-counter (OTC) drugs (Table 16-1). Consequently, it is most important to question patients in detail to ascertain use of supplements beyond prescription medications.

Looking to the Future

The consumption of dietary supplements as part of American dietary patterns will continue to evolve. Physiologically active substances have been added to food products resulting in a category of foods called *functional foods*. Functional foods are generally regarded as foods that provide good health by containing physiologically active food components. This may include foods that have been modified to increase nutrient density including fortified, enriched, or enhanced foods.

Some functional food components are marketed as dietary supplements, such as herb-enriched beverages. Care must be taken though because the amounts and sources of herb and other phytochemical ingredients are not sufficiently regulated.[10] A fruit juice beverage may contain the herb St. John's wort. St. John's wort may be effective to treat mild depression but must be taken regularly for several months for a response to occur. Consuming a small amount in a juice beverage is ineffective for depression treatment and pointless for any other purpose.

Health professionals can be aware of the range of products available and advise patients accordingly based on basic principles of good health. As the public becomes

Text continued on p. 471.

Table 16-1
Herb-Drug Interactions

Herb	Drug(s)	Interaction
Arnica (*Arnica Montana*)	Antihypertensives	May reduce effectiveness of drugs
Belladonna (*Atropa belladonna*)	Additive anticholinergic effects with drugs such as tricyclic antidepressants, some antihistamines, phenothiazines, and quinidine	Symptoms of excessive anticholinergic activity (e.g., sedation, dry mouth, difficult urination) may occur
Betel nut (*Areca catechu*)	Antipsychotics Bronchodilators	Rigidity, bradykinesia, jaw tremor Inadequate control of asthma
Black cohosh (*Cimicifuga racemosa*)	Antihypertensives	May potentiate activity and increase risk of hypotension
Blue cohosh (*Caulophyllum thalictroides*)	Nicotine patches	May increase side effects or potentiate patches; use together cautiously
Chili pepper (*Capsicum*)	ACE inhibitor Theophylline	Cough Increased absorption and bioavailability
Coenzyme Q_{10} (ubiquinone, Co-Q_{10})	Warfarin (Coumadin)	Decreased warfarin effects; Co-Q_{10} may act similarly to vitamin K
Danshen (*Salvia miltiorrhiza*)	Warfarin (Coumadin) Pentobarbital, barbital Caffeine, amphetamines	Increased INR and prolonged prothrombin time/partial thromboplastin time Use cautiously together; may increase sedation May antagonize CNS stimulating effect
Devil's claw (*Harpagophytum procumbens*)	Warfarin (Coumadin)	Pupura
Dong quai (*Angelica sinensis*)	Warfarin (Coumadin) Estrogen	Increased INR, widespread bruising Unknown effect; should not be used together
Echinacea (*Echinacea* species)	Corticosteroids Cyclosporine Warfarin (Coumadin)	May offset immunosuppressive effects of corticosteroids May offset immunosuppressive effects of corticosteroids Additive effect with warfarin
Ephedra or ma huang (*Ephedra sinica*)	Caffeine, decongestants, stimulants Digoxin, halothane Hypoglycemic agents MAOIs Antihypertensives Oxytocin	Increased CNS stimulation and possible increase in heart rate and blood pressure Combination can cause arrhythmias Increased blood glucose levels Increased blood pressure and heart rate Antagonistic effects Can cause severe hypertension

References: Fugh-Berman A: Herb-drug interactions, Lancet 355:134, 2000; Cupp MJ: Herbal remedies: adverse effects and drug interactions, Am Fam Physician 59(5):1239, 1999; Lambrecht JE et al.: A review of herb-drug interactions: documented and theoretical, US Pharmacist 25:8, 2000; www.uspharmacist.com/NewLook/Display/Article.cfm?item_num=566, accessed June 7, 2002; Miller LG: Herbal medicinals, Arch Intern Med 158:2200, 1998; Kuhn MA: Herbal remedies: drug-herbal interactions, Crit Care Nurse 22(2):22, 2002; Riddle SM: Drug interactions: examining the impact of botanicals and dietary supplements, Renal Nutrition Forum 20(3):1, 2001.

ACE, Angiotensin-converting enzyme; CNS, central nervous system; GI, gastrointestinal; INR, International Normalized Ratio; MAOI, monoamine oxidase inhibitor; NSAIDS, nonsteroidal antiinflammatory drugs; SSRI, selective serotonin reuptake inhibitor.

Table 16-1—cont'd
Herb-Drug Interactions

Herb	Drug(s)	Interaction
Evening primrose oil (Oenothera biennis)	Phenothiazines	Increases likelihood of seizures
Feverfew (Tanacetum parthenium)	Warfarin (Coumadin)	Inhibits platelet activity
Flaxseed (Linum usitatissimum)	Niacin	Increases flushing
	Laxatives	Potentiate laxative effect
Garlic (Allium sativum)	Warfarin (Coumadin)	Increased INR
Ginger (Zingiber officinale)	Warfarin (Coumadin)	Decreased platelet aggregation; may increase risk of bleeding
	Antihypertensive drugs	May cause unpredictable blood pressure responses (increase or decrease)
	Hypoglycemic drugs	Additive effects may decrease blood glucose
Ginkgo (Ginkgo biloba)	Aspirin	Increases inhibition of platelet aggregation
	Acetaminophen and ergotamine/caffeine	Bilateral subdural hematoma
	Warfarin (Coumadin)	Intracerebral hemorrhage
	Thiazide diuretic	Hypertension
Ginseng (Panax quinquefolius, Panax ginseng, Eleutherococcus senticosus)	Warfarin (Coumadin)	Decreased INR
	MAOIs	Headache and tremor; mania
	Corticosteroids	May potentiate medications or increase side effects
	Digoxin	Increased likelihood of toxic effects or may interfere with effectiveness
	Insulin, oral hypoglycemics	Fluctuations in blood glucose
	Alcohol	Increase alcohol clearance
	Hormones, steroids,	Can exaggerate responses to medications
	coffee, tea, cola	Increases stimulation, tachycardia, hypertension
Guarana (Paullinia cupana)	Respiratory drugs	Increases likelihood of adverse effects because guarana contains theophylline; should not be used concurrently
	Caffeine products along with oral contraceptives, cimetidine, verapamil, and some quinolone antibiotics	Lowers caffeine clearance by 30%-50%; should not be used concurrently
	Lithium	May inhibit clearance of lithium; should not be used concurrently
	Adenosine	May lower response; should not be used concurrently
	Benzodiazepines	Drugs may be less effective; should not be used concurrently
Guar gum (Cyamopsis tetragonolobus)	Oral hypoglycemic agents	Slows absorption of digoxin, paracetamol, and bumetaride; decreases absorption of metformin, phenoxymethylpenicillin, and some formulations of glibenclamide

ACE, Angiotensin-converting enzyme; CNS, central nervous system; GI, gastrointestinal; INR, International Normalized Ratio; MAOI, monoamine oxidase inhibitor; NSAIDS, nonsteroidal antiinflammatory drugs; SSRI, selective serotonin reuptake inhibitor.

Continued

Table 16-1—cont'd
Herb-Drug Interactions

Herb	Drug(s)	Interaction
Hawthorn (*Crataegus oxyacantha*)	Digoxin, ACE inhibitors, most cardiovascular medications	May potentiate effects of drugs
Indian snakeroot	Digoxin	Arrhythmias (especially bradycardia) and angina
	Barbiturates	Increased sedation
	Levodopa	Decreased levodopa effectiveness with increased extrapyramidal symptoms
	Sympathomimetics (e.g., albuterol, pseudoephedrine)	Increases in blood pressure
	Antihypertensives	Increased effect of both drugs and herb (e.g., decreased blood pressure)
	MAOIs	CNS excitation and increased blood pressure
	Beta-blockers	Enhanced beta blockade, with decreased heart rate and blood pressure
	Tranquilizers	Increased effects
Karela or bitter melon (*Momordica charantia*)	Chlorpropamide	Less glycosuria
Kava (*Piper methysticum*)	Antianxiety	Increases sedation, leading to coma
	Levodopa	Increases dyskinesias (tremor)
	Tricyclic antidepressants	Decreases effectiveness; potentiates, increases adverse effects
	CNS stimulants	Possible antagonistic effects; results unpredictable
	Benzodiazepines	Severe CNS effects; cases of comatose states have been reported
	Alcohol	Additive CNS depressant effects
Licorice (*Glycyrrhiza glabra*)	Prednisone	Decreases plasma clearance, increases area under the concentration/time curve, increases plasma concentrations of prednisone
	Hydrocortisone	Potentiates cutaneous vasoconstrictor response
	Antihypertensive medications	Increased sodium and water retention may offset effects of drugs and increase blood pressure
	Thiazide and loop diuretics	Offset effects of diuretics by increasing sodium and water retention; potentiates risks of hypokalemia
	Digoxin	May interfere with both monitoring and pharmacodynamic activity
	Oral contraceptives	Hypertension, edema, hypokalemia
Papaya (*Carica papaya*)	Warfarin (Coumadin)	Increased INR
Psyllium (*Plantago psyllium*)	Lithium	Decreased lithium concentrations
St. John's wort (*Hypericum perforatum*)	Antidepressant (SSRIs, MAOIs)	Lethargy/incoherence, mild serotonin syndrome
	Amitriptyline	Worsens depression
	Indinavir	Decreases indinavir drug levels
	Theophylline	Decreases theophylline concentrations
	Digoxin	Decreases digoxin drug levels

ACE, Angiotensin-converting enzyme; CNS, central nervous system; GI, gastrointestinal; INR, International Normalized Ratio; MAOI, monoamine oxidase inhibitor; NSAIDS, nonsteroidal antiinflammatory drugs; SSRI, selective serotonin reuptake inhibitor.

Table 16-1—cont'd
Herb-Drug Interactions

Herb	Drug(s)	Interaction
St. John's wort—cont'd (*Hypericum perforatum*)	Cyclosporine	Decreased concentrations in serum and increases risk of rejection
	Chlorpromazine, tetracycline	Increased photosensitivity
	Alcohol, barbiturates, benzodiazepines	Synergistic effect and increases sedative effect; may result in coma
	Combined oral contraceptive (ethinyloestradiol and desogestrel)	Breakthrough bleeding; decreased effectiveness of oral contraceptive therapy possible
	Warfarin (Coumadin)	Increased warfarin metabolism with resulting decrease in INR values
Saw palmetto (*Serenoa repens*)	Finasteride	Additive or antagonistic effects possible
	Testosterone	Antiandrogenic effects
	Oral contraceptives and hormone replacement therapy	Antiestrogenic effects
Turmeric	NSAIDs	May increase bleeding and increase GI bleeding
Valerian (*Valeriana officinalis*)	Alcohol	Mixture of valepotriates reduces adverse effect of alcohol on concentration
	Sedatives	May intensify effects
	Metronidazole, sleeping pills of any kind	Causes person to wake up feeling hungover and groggy
Yohimbine (*Pausinystalia yohimbe*)	Tricyclic antidepressants	Hypertension
	MAOIs	Additive effects possible
	Stimulants, appetite suppressants, decongestants	Additive stimulative effects, MAOI interaction possible
	Antihypertensives	Antagonistic effects
	Clonidine	Antagonism of clonidine can precipitate hypertensive crisis or withdrawal symptoms

ACE, Angiotensin-converting enzyme; CNS, central nervous system; GI, gastrointestinal; INR, International Normalized Ratio; MAOI, monoamine oxidase inhibitor; NSAIDS, nonsteroidal antiinflammatory drugs; SSRI, selective serotonin reuptake inhibitor.

more educated about phytochemicals as a natural component of whole foods, perhaps the perception of dietary supplements will change. For example, tomatoes naturally contain lycopene, a phytochemical. Instead of taking a supplement containing lycopene, consumption of tomatoes would provide the same benefit. Nonetheless, the development of functional foods will continue because of several factors. These factors include (1) an aging population; (2) increased cost of healthcare; (3) growth of self-care regarding health; (4) continued evidence of the effect of dietary intake on disease prevention and treatment; and (5) changes in food regulation that appear to support the expanded growth of dietary supplements and functional foods.[10]

Application to Nursing

Nurses can understand the appeal of dietary supplements as an aspect of self-care. Compliance with conventional medications and recommended dietary and lifestyle changes can also be suggested as an aspect of self-care to decrease risk or to alleviate a disorder. It is also possible that patients may use supplements instead of conventional medications because of high prescription costs. If this is the case, patients can be referred to social services that may be able to assist financially. Information on dietary supplements when appropriate can be offered to patients, and they can then discuss this with their primary healthcare providers. An example would be to provide information on a dietary supplement such as the herb chamomile *(Matricaria recutita or chamomilla),* which seems to stimulate digestion and may decrease inflammation and spasms of the gastrointestinal (GI) tract. Chamomile may also be calming. However, if an individual has ragweed allergy, allergic reactions can occur. Consequently, a patient can discuss dietary supplement use with a primary healthcare provider.

Referral to registered dietitians for medical nutrition therapy involving dietary supplements or for general nutrition counseling is always an option. Registered dietitians are trained to consider several factors when advising on nutrient and other dietary supplements. Factors considered include the level of scientific evidence available on the substance, demographics (i.e., age, gender), disease states, clinical parameters (e.g., blood pressure and weight), medications (prescribed and OTC) currently used, and risks or benefits of the substance. Dietary supplements should always be complementary to a sound diet. Dietary intake should first be adjusted to fulfill nutrient gaps before dietary supplements are used.[11]

MEDICATIONS

Drug-Nutrient Interactions

Drug-nutrient interactions become more of a concern as the use of dietary supplements increases along with continued use of OTC medication and the plethora of prescription drugs. In essence, dietary supplements may act as drugs, particularly when patients take many medications. The rule of eights may apply. If a patient takes eight or more medications and/or supplements, there are bound to be some drug-drug or nutrient-drug interactions.

All drugs produce physiologic effects; some of these effects are unintended (side effects) and constitute the risks of medication use. The amount and rate of drug absorption can be affected by the composition and timing of food intake. Conversely, food intake, absorption, and metabolism can be altered by medication. Drug-nutrient interactions have the potential to reduce drug efficacy, interfere with disease control, foster nutritional deficiencies, influence food intake, or provoke a toxic reaction.[12] The Joint Commission on Accreditation of Healthcare Organizations (JCAHO) strongly recommends evaluation of drug and diet combinations. Documentation of these interactions, which may be done by the registered dietitian or nurse, is essential in complying with JCAHO standards. In addition to medications, use of alcohol and street drugs also affect nutritional status and nutrient requirements (see the Social Issue box).

Risk Factors of Drug-Nutrient Interactions

Determination of risk for drug-nutrient reactions depends on characteristics of the individual, including age, physiologic status, multiple drug intake, hepatic and renal function, and typical dietary intake.[13]

◄▸► SOCIAL ISSUE
Nutritional Effects of Street Drugs

References denoting drug-nutrient interactions or a prescription drug's effect on nutritional status are plentiful. Literature on the effects of alcohol on nutritional status is also available. However, nursing personnel may also be faced with caring for patients who use street drugs. Use of nicotine and other addictive drugs can be common, and these drugs also have an impact on nutritional status. Marijuana, heroin, and cocaine can alter food, water, and salt intakes, weight maintenance, and the metabolism and status of other nutrients. The nutritional impact of these drugs can produce unfavorable and sometimes pernicious health effects.

SOCIAL ISSUE–cont'd
Nutritional Effects of Street Drugs

MARIJUANA

Marijuana increases appetite and food intake in some individuals. This effect occurs also when it is administered orally. This can lead to increased kcaloric intake and increased body weight. Studies have indicated that although kcaloric intake increases with marijuana use, quality of dietary intake may be decreased, especially when marijuana use is coupled with alcohol use.

HEROIN

Heroin abuse can alter glucose tolerance and metabolism. It can cause destruction of skeletal muscle (rhabdomyolysis) accompanied by a decrease of myoglobin in the blood to below normal levels and presence of myoglobin in urine, which can lead to acute kidney failure. Animal studies have shown depressed water intake, preference for salty solutions, and increased consumption of alcohol, which could have important implications for humans. These studies also demonstrated a dose-dependent ability of heroin to raise levels of insulin, cortisol, glucagon, and epinephrine and to induce hypoglycemia and hyperglycemia—findings that could have important consequences for persons with diabetes. Animal subjects also developed hypercholesterolemia (serum cholesterol levels above normal).

COCAINE

Cocaine abuse has been found to lead to diminished intake of meals per day, increased alcohol and coffee consumption, and increased intake of fatty foods. There is also an increased prevalence of anorexia nervosa and bulimia among cocaine users when compared with nonaddicts.

NICOTINE

Nicotine, the focal point of smoking research, was designated as an addictive drug in 1988 by the U.S. Surgeon General. Nicotine alone, or in combination with smoking, changes food selections based on taste. Smokers tend to show the least preference for sweet foods when offered a choice of bland, salty, and sweet foods; but those who stop smoking show preference for sweet-tasting foods. Smokers also tend to have higher fat intakes than nonsmokers. This effect appears to be dose-dependent; persons smoking more than 20 cigarettes per day consumed more fat than those smoking fewer cigarettes. Women who smoke during pregnancy deliver significantly smaller babies although maternal weight gain and daily dietary intake during pregnancy are adequate. Research studies have also shown what smokers have been attesting to for years—weight gain occurs after smoking cessation. This phenomenon may be caused by increased consumption of sweet/sugary foods and fatty foods, but there is some indication that nicotine increases metabolism; thus lowered metabolism after smoking cessation may be the reason for weight gain.

CAFFEINE

Although not really a street drug, caffeine is probably the most widely used drug in the United States. It can be ingested in large enough quantities to alter metabolism. Caffeine is one of the compounds categorized as a methylxanthine, along with theophylline and theobromine. These chemicals are found naturally in coffee, tea, cocoa, and cola beverages. Methylxanthines stimulate the central nervous system (keep us awake and alert), produce diuresis, stimulate the cardiac muscle (potential problems for cardiac patients), relax smooth muscle (especially the bronchial muscle, potential benefit for patients with asthma), and increase gastric secretions (potential problems for individuals with gastrointestinal problems). Although moderate amounts of caffeine are probably not harmful in healthy individuals, the safety of its use during pregnancy is inconclusive.

To the extent that these drugs affect nutritional status or food intake, a balanced eating pattern may help renourish individuals and prevent any negative effects of inadequate nutrient intake.

methylxanthine
caffeine, theobromine, and theophylline; found in beverages such as coffee, tea, cocoa, and cola drinks, and having pharmacologic properties that stimulate the central nervous system

Reference: Mohs ME, Watson RR, Leonard-Green T: Nutritional effects of marijuana, heroin, cocaine, and nicotine, J Am Dietetic Assoc 90:1261, 1990; and Gold M: Eating disorders are linked to chemical dependency, Alcoholism Addiction 8:13, May-June 1988.

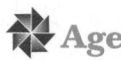 ## Age

Older adults are more at risk for drug-nutrient reactions because of the greater variety of medications used and reduced physiologic functioning affecting drug use. Older patients often experience several different disorders simultaneously, each with complications and medications that may interact. Nutritional status may be compromised because of physical and social dimensions that affect their ability to procure and prepare nutritious meals. The high rate of drug reactions noted among older adults may also be caused by a combination of these factors, including drug misuse or overuse.[13]

Young children can also be affected by drug-nutrient interactions. Use of vitamins/minerals, dietary supplements, and OTC medications intended for adults can result in drug-nutrient reactions because the substances will be metabolized differently by the developing body systems of children.

Physiologic Status

Impaired ability to absorb, metabolize, or excrete nutrients and medications because of disorders of the GI tract and reduced hepatic and renal functioning increases the risk of drug-nutrient reactions. Postoperative trauma or injury may also trigger atypical physiologic responses to drug-nutrient interactions. Age alters physiologic status as the body matures. Drug doses can vary depending on weight and metabolic function as an aspect of age-related physiologic status. Use of medications during pregnancy requires caution because of the multiple effects on the fetus and on the nutritional status of the mother.

Polypharmacy (Multiple Drug Intake)

Certain types of illness or disease groups tend to require combinations of therapeutic drugs plus other medications, including OTC drugs, for relief of symptoms. The resulting drug-nutrient reactions may be related to the disease itself or be a reaction to medications.[13] For example, intestinal bleeding often causes iron deficiency anemia among patients with arthritis. This intestinal bleeding is a common side effect of long-term use of nonsteroidal antiinflammatory drugs (NSAIDs), either prescribed or OTC, taken to reduce the symptoms of arthritis. Other chronic conditions such as hypertension and diabetes may result in similar drug-nutrient interactions.[12] If other acute disorders develop, the combination of medications may affect nutrient availability or function.

Influence of Typical Dietary Intake

The basis of a person's nutritional status depends on foods regularly consumed; the nutritional content of these foods impacts body functions. A well-nourished individual is better able to withstand a medical regimen that may affect nutrient functioning. In contrast, individuals who are malnourished or marginally deficient in nutrient intake are more at risk for complications of drug-nutrient reactions as the body's stores of nutrients are diminished. For example, individuals who excessively consume alcohol tend to be marginally deficient in a number of nutrients either because of inadequate food intake (alcohol is an appetite depressant) or because of drug (alcohol)-nutrient interactions. If illness necessitates therapeutic drug intervention, nutritional status may be further compromised, increasing the likelihood of drug-nutrient interactions.

Prescription and Over-the-Counter Medications

We receive an avalanche of messages to use medications to cure every ailment we experience. Knowledge of medications is not confined to healthcare providers because television, radio, and print media present advertisements about prescription drugs. Often, the descriptions of the disorders seem to apply to most of the audience—so much so that patients now approach primary healthcare providers requesting prescriptions for conditions for which they have not yet been diagnosed.

Although the public has become more educated about prescription drugs, OTC medications may be viewed as harmless because prescriptions are not required. Harmless they are not. A number of OTC medications that were originally prescription medications are now available without prescriptions. Although the directions for use tend to be lower doses than when used as a prescription drug, interactions with other medications, foods, nutrients, and supplements such as herbs may occur (Table 16-2). For example, antiulcer agents or histamine blockers such as ranitidine (Zantac) and famotidine (Pepcid) are available OTC. Originally prescription drugs for ulcer treatment, ads suggest their use for ordinary indigestion caused by overeating or eating spicy, high-fat foods. Both are dietary distress situations that can be remedied by dietary behavior change rather than medication. Regular use of these histamine blockers can decrease absorption of vitamin B_{12}, which is a problem for older adults who are often the target audience for these medications.

✿ Effects of Drugs on Food and Nutrients

Most drug absorption occurs through the GI mucosa, predominately in the small intestine. Before drugs can be absorbed they must first be metabolized and dissolved in gastric juices of the stomach. The speed with which the drug leaves the stomach depends on the gastric emptying time, which affects the rate of drug absorption. The rate of drug absorption may either increase or decrease based on the amount of food in the GI tract. In the fasting state, the medication leaves the empty stomach quickly and is absorbed from the small intestine. For some drugs that is too quick because time is needed for disintegration into absorbable particles. For those drugs, it is better to take the medication in the fed state in which the stomach, containing food, empties more slowly, especially after consuming large meals, heated food, and meals with fat, all of which slow emptying time.

Drugs can alter food intake, nutrient absorption, metabolism, and excretion. These drugs include prescription medications, OTC drugs, and even alcohol. If a nutrient binds with a medication, decreased solubility of both the nutrient and drug can result. Drugs used to lower serum cholesterol levels bind with fat-soluble vitamins and bile salts. As a result, both the bile salts and vitamins are excreted. Some drugs can decrease the amount of digestive enzymes available and thereby decrease nutrient absorption. Drugs that decrease transit time in the GI tract will also decrease nutrient absorption. The tables in this chapter provide information on selected drug-nutrient interactions.

Mineral status can be affected by drugs, resulting in either depletion or overload. Depletion may occur from the simultaneous use of several medications of which each has the side effect of mineral depletion. A common source of mineral depletion is the use of potassium-depleting diuretics in addition to the use of laxatives that may also cause potassium loss. Older adults often use these products; their dietary intake may be marginal in mineral content as well.[13] Overload may occur in instances in which renal function is compromised and potassium-sparing diuretics (e.g., spironolactone) and potassium supplements are used. Patient education is vital regarding the use of potassium supplements. Clear information is essential; patients should be taught about the kind of diuretic they are taking and potential side effects to reduce inappropriate supplementation.

Medications can also alter food intake by acting as appetite depressants or stimulants (Box 16-1), altering taste sensations (Box 16-2), or producing nausea and vomiting, which further decrease appetite. Suggestions for minimizing drug side effects are presented in the Teaching Tool box. *Text continued on p. 480.*

Table 16-2
Medications that Affect Food and/or Nutrients

Drug Class	Examples	Use	Action	Nutrients Affected	How to Avoid
Alcohol, particularly excessive use	Beer, wine, spirits		Increases turnover of some vitamins, decreases food intake	B$_{12}$, folate, magnesium	Do not use excessively
Analgesics, NSAIDs	Salicylates (aspirin)	Pain, fever		Increases loss of vitamin C, competes with folate and vitamin K	Increase intake of foods high in vitamin C, folate, and vitamin K; take with 8-oz glass of water
Antacids		Stomach upset	Inactivates thiamine, decreases absorption of some nutrients	Foods containing thiamine (B$_1$) should be consumed at a different time. Depends on antacid, possibly magnesium, phosphorus, iron, vitamin A, folate	
Antiulcer agents (histamine blockers)	Ranitidine (Zantac®), cimetidine (Tagamet®), famotidine (Pepcid®)	Ulcers	Decrease vitamin absorption	B$_{12}$	Consult physician or dietitian regarding B$_{12}$ supplementation
Antibiotics	Tetracycline, ciprofloxacin (Cipro®)	Infection	Chelation of minerals; taking with caffeine may increase excitability and nervousness	Calcium, magnesium, iron, zinc, caffeine	Take tetracycline at least 1 hr before or 2 hrs after a meal; do not take with caffeine-containing products
Antineoplastic drugs	Methotrexate	Cancer	Causes mucosal damage, which may cause decreased nutrient absorption	Folate, B$_{12}$; see also Antibiotics	Consult physician or dietitian regarding supplementation
Anticholinergics	Amitriptyline (Elavil®), chlorpromazine (Thorazine®)		Saliva thickens and loses ability to prevent tooth decay	Fluids	
Anticonvulsants	Phenobarbital, phenytoin (Dilantin®)	Seizures, epilepsy	Increases metabolism of folate (possibly leading to megaloblastic anemia), vitamins D (especially in children) and K	Folate, vitamins D and K	
Antidepressants	Lithium carbonate, lithium (Lithane, Lithonate, Lithotabs, Eskalith), lithobid	Depression, anxiety	May cause metallic taste, nausea, vomiting, dry mouth, anorexia, weight gain, and increased thirst		Water (2-3 qts/d); take with food

Drug category	Drug	Use	Effect	Nutrients affected	Recommendation
Antiinflammatory agents		Fever, infection	Decreases absorption	Folate	
Antihyperlipemics	Cholestyramine (Questran®), colestipol (Colestid®)	High serum cholesterol	Binds bile salts and nutrients	Fat-soluble vitamins (A, D, E, K), folate, B_{12}, iron	Include rich sources of these vitamins and minerals in diet
Antituberculosis	Isoniazid (INH®)	Tuberculosis	Inhibits conversion of B_6 to active form		B_6 supplementation is necessary to prevent deficiency and peripheral neuropathy
Corticosteroids	Prednisone®, methylprednisolone (Solu-Medrol®), hydrocortisone		Increases excretion	Protein, potassium, calcium, magnesium, zinc, vitamin C, vitamin B_6	
Loop diuretics	Furosemide (Lasix®)	Water retention, hypertension	Increases mineral excretion in urine	Potassium, calcium, magnesium, zinc, sodium, chloride	Include fresh fruits and vegetables in diet
Thiazide diuretics	Hydrochlorothiazide (HCTZ®)	Water retention, hypertension	Increases excretion of most electrolytes, but enhances reabsorption of calcium	Potassium, calcium, magnesium, zinc, sodium, chloride, calcium	
Potassium-sparing diuretics	Triamterene (Dyrenium®)	Water retention, hypertension	Hyperkalemia	Potassium	Avoid potassium-based salt substitutes
Laxatives	FiberCon®, Mitrolan®	Constipation	Decreases nutrient absorption	Vitamins, minerals	Consult physician or dietitian regarding supplementation
Sedatives	Barbiturates		Increases metabolism of vitamins	Folate, vitamin D, vitamin B_{12}, thiamine, vitamin C	
Mineral oil		Laxative	Decreases absorption	Fat-soluble vitamins (A, D, E, K), beta-carotene, calcium, phosphorus, potassium	
Oral contraceptives		Birth control	May cause selective malabsorption, or increased metabolism and turnover	B_6, folate	

Modified from Anderson SL: Drug-nutrient interactions. In Williams SR, Schlenker ED: Essentials of nutrition and diet therapy, ed 8, St Louis, 2003, Mosby.

References: Anderson J, Hart H: Nutrient-drug interactions and food, Colorado State University Cooperative Extension; www.ext.colostate.edu/pubs/foodnut/09361.html, accessed June 3, 2002; Bland SE: Drug-food interactions, J Pharm Society Wisconsin, 28(Nov/Dec), 1998; Bobrof LB, Lentz A, Turner RE: Food/drug and drug/nutrient interactions: what you should know about your medications, University of Florida Cooperative Extension Service, Institute of Food and Agricultural Science; http://edis.ufl.edu/BODY_HE776, accessed June 3, 2002; Brown CH: Overview of drug interactions, US Pharmacist 25(5); www.uspharmacist.com/NewLook/DisplayArticle.cfm?item_num=522, accessed June 3, 2002; Crownsville Hospital Center Pharmacy Department: Food/drug interactions, 2001; www.dhmh.state.md.us/crownsville/Pharmacy/Interactions.htm, accessed June 9, 2002; Kuhn MA: Drug interactions with medications and food, Nursing Spectrum; www.nsweb.nursingspectrum.com/ce/ce174.htm, accessed June 9, 2002; National Consumers League: Food and drug interactions; www.ncbnet.org/Food%20&%20Drug.pdf, accessed June 9, 2002.

Box 16-1 Selected Drugs that Affect Appetite

APPETITE STIMULANTS

ANTIDEPRESSANTS

Amitriptyline (Elavil, Endep)
Clomipramine HCl (Anafranil)
MAOI
   Tranylcypromine sulfate (Parnate)

ANTIHISTAMINES

Astemizole (Hismanal)
Cyproheptadine HCl (Periactin)

BRONCHODILATOR

Albuterol sulfate (Proventil, Ventolin)

STEROIDS

Anabolic steroids
   Oxandrolone (Anavar)
Corticosteroids
   Hydrocortisone (Cortef)
Glucocorticoids
   Dexamethasone (Decadron)
   Methylprednisolone (Medrol)

TRANQUILIZERS

Lithium carbonate (Lithane)
Benzodiazipines
   Chlordiazepoxide HCl (Librium)
   Diazepam (Valium)
   Prazepam (Centrax)
Phenothiazines
   Chlorpromazine HCl (Thorazine)
   Promethazine HCl (Phenergan)

APPETITE DEPRESSANTS

AMPHETAMINES

Benzphetamine HCl (Didrex)
Fenfluramine HCl (Pondimin)
Phenylpropanolamine (Dexatrim,
   Dimetapp, Triaminic)

ANTIARRHYTHMICS

Digitalis
Digitoxin (Crystodigin, Digitoxin)
Digoxin (Digoxin, Lanoxin)

ANTIBIOTICS

Amphotericin B (Fungizone)
Gentamicin (Garamycin)
Metronidozale (Flagyl)
Zidovudine (AZT)

ANTIDEPRESSANT

Fluoxetine HCl (Prozac)

ANTIHISTAMINE

Azatadine maleate (Optimine)

ANTIHYPERTENSIVE

Amiloride and hydrochlorothiazide
   (Moduretic)
Captopril (Capoten)
Chlorthalidone (Hygroton)

MUSCLE RELAXANT

Dantrolene sodium (Dantrium)

STIMULANT/AntiADD

Methylphenidate HCl (Ritalin)

Reference: Pronsky ZM, et al: Food medication interactions, ed 12, Pottstown, Penn, 2001, Food-Medication Interactions.

Box 16-2 Selected Drugs that Alter Taste

ANTIARRHYTHMIC

Amiodarone (Cordarone)

ANTIARTHRITIC/CHELATING AGENT

Penicillamine (Cuprimine, Depen)

ANTIBIOTICS

Ampicillin
Clarithromycin (Biaxin)

ANTICONVULSANT

Phenytoin (Dilantin)

ANTIDEPRESSANTS

Clomipramine HCl (Anafranil)
Fluoxetine HCl (Prozac)

ANTIFUNGAL

Griseofulvin (Fulvicin, Grifulvin V,
   Grisacrin)

ANTIGOUT

Allopurinol (Zyloprim)

ANTIHYPERTENSIVES

Captopril (Capoten)
Labetalol HCl (Normodyne, Trandate)

ANTIMANICS

Lithium carbonate (Eskalith, Lithane,
   Lithobid)
Lithium citrate (Cibalith-S)

ANTI-PARKINSON

Levodopa (Dopar, Larodopa)

ANTIVIRAL/ANTI-HIV

Didanosine (Videx)

MUSCLE RELAXANT

Dantrolene sodium (Dantrium)

MUSCLE RELAXANT/ANTISPASMODIC

Baclofen (Lioresal)

STIMULANT/AMPHETAMINE

Dextroamphetamine sulfate (Tar-
   razine, Dexedrine)

Reference: Pronsky ZM: Food medication interactions, ed 12, Pottstown, Penn, 2001, Food-Medication Interactions.

TEACHING TOOL
Minimizing Drug Side Effects

A number of drugs have side effects—symptoms not caused by the illness for which the drugs have been prescribed but as physiologic responses of the body to the drug itself. The side effects may be mild or quite bothersome. Some may be serious enough to warrant a change in medication. Before using these strategies as education tools, consult the client's primary healthcare provider to ascertain if additional medical intervention is required.

SIDE EFFECT: DIMINISHED APPETITE

- Consider eating several small meals or snacks throughout the day.
- Describe a setting and atmosphere for meal times that enhances appetite. Assist the client in exploring approaches to encourage an optimum eating environment.
- Discuss client's favorite foods. Brainstorm about how recipes can be adapted to comply with dietary therapeutic plans.

SIDE EFFECT: MODIFIED TASTE SENSATIONS

- Visit a dentist regularly to maintain oral hygiene.
- Mask the taste of medications, if needed, with fruit sauces such as applesauce, crushed pineapple, or milk products. First determine if combinations are acceptable and not contraindicated.

SIDE EFFECT: INCREASED APPETITE

- Alert client to the appetite (and craving sweets) stimulant effect of certain medications.
- Evaluate client's typical dietary intake. Suggest high-fiber foods to provide a quick sense of feeling full.
- Advise limiting availability to high kcalorie foods and drinks to minimize excess kcaloric intake.
- Increase activity.

SIDE EFFECT: GI TRACT IRRITATION AND DISCOMFORT

- Advise client to sit up or stand after taking medications that have the potential to cause heartburn or indigestion.
- Reduce intake of fat, greasy, and/or highly acidic foods, including citrus juices and tomato products.
- Limit food intake in the evening to prevent reflux.
- Control consumption of spicy foods, peppermint, colas, chocolate, alcohol, pepper, decaffeinated coffee, and caffeine if these produce gastric discomfort.

SIDE EFFECT: NAUSEA

- Control liquid intake by serving after meals or drink only small quantities with meals.
- Sustain adequate fluid volume; cold, carbonated, or clear liquids are easier to tolerate.

SIDE EFFECT: DRY OR SORE MOUTH

- Consume softer, moist foods such as applesauce, puddings, pureed foods, and mashed potatoes.
- Include iced and cold foods throughout the day; consider ice pops, frozen yogurt, ice cream, sorbets, and cooled melons.
- Encourage oral hygiene before and after eating.
- Avoid mouthwashes, which can further dry the oral mucosa.

Reference: Pronsky ZM: Food medication interactions, ed 12, Pottstown, Penn, 2001, Food-Medication Interactions.

Drugs may cause additional nutrition problems by affecting GI tract motility (which can change nutrient absorption) or GI tract pH. Drugs may also cause injury of GI mucosa, development of drug-nutrient compounds, decreased bile acid function, and depressed nutrient transport mechanisms (Table 16-3). Nutrient metabolism and excretion may be modified by drug therapy in a mechanism similar to that of nutrient absorption with the addition of effects caused by physical characteristics of solubility and stability of the drug.

The metabolic and excretion rate of the drug itself may also interfere with nutrient metabolism and excretion. Nutrient metabolism can be affected by vitamin analogs that compete metabolically with the vitamin. Certain medications act as vitamin antagonists, preventing vitamins from completing metabolic functions. Warfarin (Coumadin), the anticoagulant, is a vitamin K antagonist that prevents the activation of the storage form of vitamin K; blood clotting, for which vitamin K is a factor, is then reduced. Other drugs, such as oral contraceptives, may cause marginal deficiencies of B vitamins and vitamin C by causing increased use of these vitamins. Excretion of nutrients may be altered if a medication results in retention of a drug normally excreted. As described in relation to mineral depletion, some diuretics are potassium sparing, causing the body to conserve more potassium than usual; other diuretics are potassium depleting. Depending on the type of diuretic, dietary support of additional food sources of potassium may be warranted.

Table 16-2 presents information on how various drug classes affect food intake, nutrient absorption, metabolism, and excretion.

Conversely, foods and nutrients may affect drug action, producing uncomfortable side effects. Most noteworthy are the adverse side effects associated with monoamine oxidase (MAO) inhibitors. MAO inhibitors, such as phenelzine (Nardil) and tranylcypromine (Parnate), may be prescribed to treat depression. These drugs inhibit the enzyme monoamine oxidase. The function of monoamine oxidase is to inactivate tyramine, a compound found in some foods. Without monoamine oxidase, the level of tyramine increases the release of norepinephrine. Elevated levels of norepinephrine may cause increased blood pressure, headache, pallor, and heart palpitations. Life-threatening severe hypertension can develop. Patients who take MAO inhibitors should avoid foods and drugs that contain tyramine. OTC medications list warnings when appropriate, but foods are not so labeled. An important component of patient education is for patients who take MAO inhibitors to know which foods contain significant levels of tyramine (Box 16-3).

Effects of Food and Nutrients on Drugs

Medications must be absorbed to have a therapeutic effect. Food intake, or lack thereof, in addition to composition of the food may affect drug absorption. The timing of drug administration and meals also has clinical significance. If absorption is increased by the presence of food, medication should be taken with a meal or a snack. If drug absorption is depressed by the presence of food in the stomach, optimum absorption occurs if medication is taken at least 1 hour before or 2 hours after eating or tube feeding. Table 16-4 lists some common drug classes whose absorption is affected by food. A specific food example is grapefruit juice. Grapefruit juice, sometimes used to take medications, can affect the bioavailability of certain drugs (Box 16-4).

The established drug administration schedules in healthcare facilities often conflict with the optimal bioavailability of the drug. Absorption response can be altered in 77% to 93% of drugs by the presence of food in the digestive tract.[14] Concomitant food intake with drug administration usually delays absorption of the drug, but this may or may not decrease the amount of drug absorbed. As a general guideline,

Text continued on p. 487.

Table 16-3
Drugs that May Cause Nutritional Problems

Nutritional Problem	Drugs	Use
May cause depression that results in weight fluctuation	Barbidopa/levodopa	Antiparkinson
	Beta blockers	Antihypertensive
	Clonidine	Antihypertensive
	Benzodiazepines	Antianxiety
	Barbiturates	Antianxiety
	Anticonvulsants	Epilepsy
	Histamine H_2 blockers	Peptic ulcer disease
	Calcium channel blockers	Antihypertensive
	Thiazide diuretics	Antihypertensive
	Digoxin	Antiarrhythmic
May delay gastric emptying time	Anesthetic agents	Anesthesia
	Opiates	Narcotic
	Tricyclic antidepressants	Antidepressant
	Clonidine	Antihypertensive
	Calcium channel blockers	Antihypertensive
	Nitrates	Antianginal
	Meperidine	Analgesic
	Theophylline	Bronchodilator
	Caffeine	Stimulant
May increase gastric emptying time	Metclopramide	Antiemetic
	Cisapride	Cholinergic enhancer
	Bethanechol	Cholinergic
	Erythromycin	Antibacterial
Can cause folate deficiency	Phenytoin	Seizures
	Methotrexate	Antimetabolites
	Trimethoprim	Antibacterial
Can cause drowsiness, may cause missed meals	Antihistamines	Allergies
	Beta blockers	Antihypertensive
	Skeletal muscle relaxants	Relieve stiffness, pain, discomfort
	Antiemetics	Nausea and vomiting
	Benzodiazepines	Antianxiety
	Antipsychotics	Psychotic disorders
	Antidepressants	Depression
May cause nausea and vomiting	Selective serotonin reuptake inhibitors (SSRIs)	Antidepressants
	Antibiotics	Antibacterial
	Antineoplastic agents	Chemotherapy
	Digitalis	Antiarrhythmic
	General anesthetics	Anesthesia
	Theophylline	Bronchodilator
	Opioid derivatives	Narcotics

References: Losben N: Dietitians and consultant pharmacists: a team approach to improved quality care, The Consultant Pharmacist, 1997; www.ascp.com/public/pubs/tcp/1997/dec/dietitians.html, accessed July 13, 2002; MEDLINEPlus Health Information; http://medlineplus.gov/, accessed July 13, 2002.

Box 16-3 Tyramine-Containing Foods

AVOID: CONTAIN HIGH TYRAMINE LEVELS

AGED FOODS

Hard (aged) cheeses and meats,
salami or mortadella,
air-dried sausage

PICKLED/SMOKED FOODS

Smoked or pickled fish,
herring in brine,
sauerkraut,
kim chee

BEVERAGES

Malt beverages (beer and ale),
Chianti and vermouth wines,
alcohol-free beer

FERMENTED

Fermented bean curd,
miso,
broad beans,
fava beans

EXTRACTS

Hydrolyzed protein extracts
(in many processed foods),
concentrated yeast extracts,
brewer's yeast

USE WITH CAUTION IN SMALL SERVINGS ($\frac{1}{4}$-$\frac{1}{2}$ CUP; 2-4 OZ)

AGED FOODS

Bologna,
pepperoni,
aged kielbasa sausage,
liverwurst

PICKLED/SMOKED FOODS

Smoked meats and fish,
Schmaltz herring in oil,
pate,
lumpfish roe

BEVERAGES

Red and white wines,
port wines,
distilled spirits,
coffee,*
cola*

FERMENTED FOODS

Soy sauce,
yogurt and cream from unpasteurized milk

FRESH FOODS

Fresh liver,
avocado,
figs,
bananas,
raspberries,
chocolate,*
peanuts

*Reference: McCabe BJ: Dietary tyramine and other pressor amines in MAOI regimens: a review, J Am Dietetic Assoc 86:1059, 1986; and Pronsky ZM, Food medication interactions, ed 12, Pottstown, Penn, 2001, Food-Medication Interactions. *Caffeine in amounts >500 mg may intensify reactions.*

Box 16-4 Grapefruit "Juices" Certain Medications

Almost all oral drugs are subject to first-pass metabolism. That is, any substance the body views as a toxin (e.g., drugs, alcohol) goes through the liver via hepatic portal circulation thus removing some of the active substance from blood before it enters general circulation. This causes a fraction of the original dose of the drug to not be "available" to systemic circulation because it has undergone biotransformation. In other words, bioavailability of the drug has been altered—or lowered. One mechanism responsible for this is an enzyme system found in the intestinal wall and liver. The *cytochrome P-450 3A4 system* (specifically CYP3A4-mediated drug metabolism) is responsible for first-pass metabolism of many medications. Most medications are lipid-soluble and readily absorbed. To eliminate toxins (i.e., drugs) from the body, however, the cytochrome P-450 system either breaks them down in the gut or changes the drug into a more water-soluble version in the liver, allowing it to be eliminated via urine.

Where does grapefruit juice come into play? Grapefruit juice blocks CYP3A4 enzyme in the wall of the small intestine, thus increasing bioavailability of the drug. This means a higher serum drug level occurs that may cause unpleasant consequences, including side effects or toxicity.

Box 16-4 Grapefruit "Juices" Certain Medications—cont'd

What is in grapefruit juice that does this? The precise chemical nature of the substance responsible for inhibiting gut wall CYP3A4 enzyme is unknown, but it is believed that more than one component present in grapefruit juice may contribute to the inhibitory effect on CYP3A4.

One 8-oz glass of grapefruit juice has the potential to increase bioavailability and enhance beneficial or adverse effects of a broad range of medications. These effects can persist up to 72 hours after grapefruit juice consumption, until more CYP3A4 has been metabolized. Interactions have been found between grapefruit juice and the following drugs:

Category	Generic Name	Trade Name	Effect
Antihypertensive (calcium channel blockers)	Felodipine	Plendil®	Flushing, headache, tachycardia, decreased blood pressure
	Nifedipine	Procardia®, Adalat®	
	Nimodipine	Nimotop®	
	Nisoldipine	Sular®	
	Nicardipine	Cardene®	
	Isradipine	DynaCirc®	
	Verapamil	Calan®, Isoptin®	Same as above + bradycardia and atrioventricular block
Nonsedating antihistamines	Astemizole	Hismanal®	
Immunosuppressants	Cyclosporine	Neoral®, Sandimmune®, SangCya®	Kidney toxicity, increased susceptibility to infections
	Tacrolimus	Prograf®	
Statins (HMG-CoA reductase inhibitors)	Atorvastatin	Lipitor®	Headache, GI complaints, muscle pain, increased risk of myopathy
	Lovastatin	Mevacor®	
	Simvastatin	Zocor®	
Caffeine			Nervousness, over stimulation
Antianxiety, insomnia, or depression	Buspirone	BuSpar®	
	Diazepam	Valium®	
	Alprazolam	Xanax®	
	Midazolam	Versed®	Increased sedation
	Triazolam	Halcion®	
	Zaleplon	Sonata®	
	Carbamazepine	Tegretol®	
	Clomipramine	Anafranil®	
	Trazodone	Desyrel®	
Protease inhibitors	Saquinavir	Fortovase®, Invirase®	Doubles bioavailability, resulting in increased efficacy or toxicity depending on dose and patient variability
Sexual dysfunction	Sildenafil	Viagra®	Delayed absorption (takes longer to become effective)

Medications considered safe for use with grapefruit

Cetirizine (Zyrtec®, Reactine®)   Fluvastatin (Lescol®)   Pravastatin (Pravachol®)
Fexofenadine (Allegra®)   Loratadine (Claritin®)

From Anderson SL: Drug-nutrient interactions. In Williams SR, Schlenker ED: Essentials of nutrition and diety therapy, *ed 8, St Louis, 2003, Mosby.*
Sources: Bailey DG et al.: Grapefruit juice–drug interactions, Br J Clin Pharmacol 46(2):101, 1998; *Kane GC, Lipsky JJ: Drug–grapefruit juice interactions,* Mayo Clin Proc 75:933, 2000; *Guo L et al.: Role of furanocoumarin derivatives on grapefruit juice-mediated inhibition of human CYP3A4 activity,* Drug Met Disposition 28:766, 2000; *Ho P et al.: Inhibition of human CYP3A4 activity by grapefruit flavonoids, furanocoumarins and related compounds,* J Pharm Pharmaceut Sci 4(3):217, 2001; *Hyland R et al.: Identification of the cytochrome P450 enzymes involved in the N-demethylation of sildenafil,* Clin Pharmacol 51:239, 2000; *Jetter A et al.: Effects of grapefruit juice on the pharmacokinetics of sildenafil,* Clin Pharmacol Ther 71(1):21, 2002; *Muirhead GJ et al.: Pharmacokinetic interactions between sildenafil and saquinavir/ritonavir,* Br J Clin Pharmacol 50:99, 2000; *Pronsky ZM:* Food medication interactions, *ed 12, Birchrunville, Penn, Food-Medication Interactions, 2002; Schmiedlin-Ren P et al.: Mechanisms of enhanced oral availability of CYP3A4 substrates by grapefruit constituents,* Drug Met Disposition 25(1):1228, 1997; *University of Illinois–Chicago, College of Pharmacy, Drug Information Center: Grapefruit juice interactions; www.uic.edu/pharmacy/services/di/grapefru.htm, accessed June 10, 2002; University of Michigan Health System Drug Information Service, 936-8200,* Selected drugs interacting with grapefruit juice, *Ann Arbor, 1999, University of Michigan.*

Table 16-4
Foods and/or Nutrients that Affect Medications

Drug Class	Examples	Use	Action	Food/Nutrients	How to Avoid
Alcohol, particularly excessive use	Beer, wine, spirits		Slows absorption	Food	Consume alcohol with food or meals
Analgesics, NSAIDs	Salicylates (aspirin), ibuprofen (Motrin®, Advil®), naproxen (Anaprox®, Aleve®, Naprosyn®)	Pain, fever	Alcohol ingestion increases hepatotoxicity	Alcohol	Limit alcohol intake to ≤3 drinks/d
Analgesics	Acetaminophen (Tylenol®)	Pain, fever	Liver damage or stomach bleeding	Alcohol	Limit alcohol intake to ≤3 drinks/d
Antacids		Stomach upset			
Antiulcer agents (histamine blockers)	Cimetidine (Tagamet®)	Ulcers	Increased blood alcohol levels; reduced caffeine clearance	Alcohol; caffeine-containing foods and beverages	
Antibiotics	Ciprofloxacin (Cipro®)	Infection	Decreases absorption	Dairy products	Avoid dairy products
Anticoagulant	Warfarin (Coumadin®)	Blood clots	Reduced efficacy; increased anticoagulation	Vitamins K and E (supplements) may reduce efficacy; alcohol and garlic may increase anticoagulation; high doses of vitamin C can increase risk of bleeding	Limit foods high in vitamin K: broccoli, spinach, kale, turnip greens, cauliflower, brussels sprouts; avoid high does of vitamin E (400 IU or more); avoid vitamin C supplements
Antineoplastic drugs	Methotrexate	Cancer	Increased hepatotoxicity with chronic alcohol use	Alcohol	
Antiemetic	Amitriptyline HCl (Elavil®), chlorpromazine HCl (Thorazine®)	Antidepressant; antipsychotic/antiemetic	Increased sedation	Alcohol	
Anticonvulsants	Phenobarbital	Seizures, epilepsy	Increased sedation	Alcohol	
Antidepressants: Monoamine oxidase (MAO) inhibitors	Phenelzine (Nardil®), Tranylcypromine (Parnate®)	Depression, anxiety	Rapid, potentially fatal increase in blood pressure	Foods or alcoholic beverages containing tyramine (beer, red wine, cheese [American processed, cheddar, bleu,	

Drug category	Examples	Use	Effect	Food/nutrient	Comments
				brie, mozzarella, Parmesan]; yogurt, sour cream; beef or chicken liver; cured meats such as sausage and salami; game meats; caviar; dried fish; avocados, bananas, yeast extracts, raisins, sauerkraut, soy sauce, miso soup; broad (fava) beans, ginseng, caffeine-containing products (colas, chocolate, coffee, tea)	
Antihistamine	Fexofenadine (Allegra®), loratadine (Claritin®), cetirizine (Zyrtec®), astemizole (Hismanal®)	Allergies	Increases drowsiness and slows mental and motor performance	Alcohol	Use caution when operating machinery or driving
Antihypertensives		Hypertension	Reduced effectiveness	Natural licorice and tyramine-rich foods	Avoid these foods
Antihyperlipemics (HMG-CoA reductase inhibitors) or statins	Atorvastatin (Lipitor®), lovastatin (Mevacor®), pravastatin (Pravachol®), simvastatin (Zocor®)	High serum LDL cholesterol	Enhance absorption; increase risk of liver damage	Food/meals; alcohol	Lovastatin should be taken with evening meal to enhance absorption; avoid large amounts of alcohol
Antiparkinson	Levodopa (Dopar®, Larodopa®)	Parkinson's disease	Decreased absorption	High-protein foods (e.g., eggs, meat, protein supplements); vitamin B_6	Spread protein intake equally in 3-6 meals/d to minimize reaction; avoid B_6 supplements or multivitamin supplement in doses >10 mg

Continued

From Anderson SL: Drug-nutrient interactions. In Williams SR, Schlenker ED: Essentials of nutrition and diet therapy, ed 8, St Louis, 2003, Mosby.
References: Anderson J, Hart H: Nutrient-drug interactions and food, Colorado State University Cooperative Extension; www.ext.colostate.edu/pubs/foodnut/09361.html, accessed June 3, 2002; Bland SE: Drug-food interactions, J Pharm Society Wisconsin 28(Nov/Dec), 1998; Bobrof LB, Lentz A, Turner RE: Food/drug and drug/nutrient interactions: what you should know about your medications, University of Florida Cooperative Extension Service, Institute of Food and Agricultural Science; http://edis.ufl.edu/BODY_HE776, accessed June 3, 2002. Brown CH: Overview of drug interactions, US Pharmacist 25(5); www.uspharmacist.com/NewLook/DisplayArticle.cfm?Item_num=522, accessed June 3, 2002; Crownsville Hospital Center Pharmacy Department: Food/drug interactions. 2001; www.dhmh.state.md.us/crownsville/Pharmacy/Interactions.htm, accessed June 9, 2002; Kuhn MA: Drug interactions with medications and food, Nursing Spectrum; www.nsweb.nursingspectrum.com/ce/ce174.htm, accessed June 9, 2002; Food and Drug Administration/National Consumers League: Food and drug interactions; www.nclnet.org/Food%208%20Drug.pdf, accessed June 9, 2002.
CNS, Central nervous system; LDL, low-density lipoproteins; NSAIDS, nonsteroidal antiinflammatory drugs.

Table 16-4—cont'd
Foods and/or Nutrients that Affect Medications

Drug Class	Examples	Use	Action	Food/Nutrients	How to Avoid
Antituberculosis	Isoniazid (INH®)	Tuberculosis	Reduced absorption with foods; increased hepatotoxicity and reduced INH levels with alcohol	Alcohol	Take on empty stomach; avoid alcohol
Bronchodilators	Theophylline (Slo-bid®, Theo-Dur®)	Asthma, chronic bronchitis, emphysema	Increased stimulation of CNS; alcohol can increase nausea, vomiting, headache, and irritability; charcoal-broiled foods can speed theophylline through body, reducing effectiveness	Caffeine, alcohol, charcoal-broiled foods	Avoid caffeine-containing foods/beverages (e.g., chocolate, colas, teas, coffee); avoid alcohol if taking theophylline medications; avoid charcoal-broiled foods
Corticosteroids	Prednisone (Pediapred®, Preline®), methylprednisolone (Solu-Medrol®), hydrocortisone	Inflammation and itching	Stomach irritation	Food	Take with food or milk to decrease stomach upset
Hypoglycemic agents	Sulfonylurea (Diabinese®); metformin (Glucophage®)	Diabetes	Severe nausea and vomiting	Alcohol	Avoid alcohol

CNS, Central nervous system; LDL, low-density lipoproteins; NSAIDS, nonsteroidal antiinflammatory drugs.
From Anderson SL: Drug-nutrient interactions. In Williams SR, Schlenker ED: Essentials of nutrition and diet therapy, ed 8, St. Louis, 2003, Mosby.

drugs should be given at least 1 hour before or 2 hours after a meal unless the medication causes GI distress when taken on an empty stomach. Such timing should enhance drug absorption and decrease hindrance of nutrient absorption.

Tube feedings present other issues of drug-nutrient interactions (Box 16-5).

Box 16-5 Tube Feedings and Drug-Nutrient Interactions

Drug-nutrient interactions can compromise pharmacologic and nutritional therapeutic objectives of safety, efficacy, and quality of care. Moreover, these interactions can affect cost-effectiveness of healthcare. Before administering an oral drug through a gastric or nasogastric feeding tube, ask yourself the following questions:

1. Is the feeding tube placed correctly?
2. Can the medication be crushed and delivered through a feeding tube?
3. Will there be an interaction between the medication and the feeding solution?
   - If so, will the interaction degrade the nutritional components of the feeding solution?
   - Or alter the medication's availability?
   - Or clog the tube?

4. Will the medication change the osmolality or pH in the feeding system?
   - Or cause nausea, vomiting, cramping, or diarrhea?

Pharmacists have valuable expertise in optimizing prescriptions. The number of potential drug-feeding formula interactions is nearly endless, and new medications and feeding formulas are becoming available almost daily. Consultation with pharmacy services is recommended to detect possible incompatibilities and recommendations for appropriate alternative forms of medications if necessary. Questions regarding specific feeding formulas and adverse drug reactions can be directed to the dietitian.

These general guidelines will help nurses avoid common problems when administering oral drugs through a feeding tube.

POTENTIAL PROBLEM	SOLUTION
Should I administer the tablet or liquid form of the medication?	Whenever possible, use the liquid form of a drug because it bypassed the dissolution process. But, be aware that many liquid medications are formulated for pediatric patients, therefore large volumes must be dispensed to meet the required dose for adults. This often results in diarrhea as a result of excessive amounts of sorbitol in the adjusted dose.
Okay, I checked and the only form of the medication available is a tablet. What should I do?	If a tablet is the only preparation available, consultation with the pharmacist is mandatory. Some tablets can be crushed if they are simple, compressed tablets designed to dissolve immediately in the GI tract. Keep in mind that crushing the tablet allows it to enter the bloodstream faster. The difference may or may not be clinically significant. Always confirm the type of coating on the tablet with the pharmacy.
I've checked with the pharmacy and was told the tablet could be crushed. How do I do that?	Ideally, medication(s) should be crushed in the pharmacy. But if you must do it yourself, the best technique is to position a unit-dose tablet in a mortar without removing it from the package. Then, crush the tablet by tapping it through the package with a pestle (to avoid tearing the package, don't grind). If the medication isn't packaged as a unit-dose, place it between two paper medicine cups and pulverize the tablet with the mortar and pestle. Mix the crushed tablet thoroughly with 15-30 ml water (5-10 ml for children), and administer through the feeding tube. Tubing *must* be flushed with a minimum of 30 ml of room temperature sterile water before *and* after administration of each medication.
It seems like it would be easier to add the medication to the feeding formula.	*Never* add medications directly to the feeding formula. This can alter the medication's therapeutic effect and disrupt the integrity of the feeding formula, causing it to resemble curdled milk.
The pharmacy has the prescribed medications in liquid form. Is there anything special I need to do?	Check whether dilution of the medication formulation before administration is required. Hypertonic, irritating, or viscous medications should be diluted in at least 30 ml of water immediately before infusion to avoid gastric irritation and diarrhea. In some cases, 90 ml of water may be necessary for dilution. Adjust water amounts appropriately for pediatric patients and patients on fluid restrictions. Document amount of water used on patient's intake and output records.

Sources: *Lehmann S, Barber JR: Giving medications by feeding tube,* Nursing 91:58, November 1991; *Lourenco R: Enteral feedings: drug/nutrient interaction,* Clin Nutr 20(2):187, 2001; *Belknap DC et al.: Administration of medications through enteral feeding catheters,* Am J Crit Care 6(5):382, 1997.

Continued

Box 16-5 Tube Feedings and Drug-Nutrient Interactions—cont'd

POTENTIAL PROBLEM—cont'd	SOLUTION—cont'd

If sugar-coated tablets can be crushed, are there tablets that cannot be crushed?

Some types of tablets *must not be crushed*. These include:

Buccal or *sublingual tablets* (e.g., nitroglycerin or isosorbide) are intended to be absorbed by veins under the tongue or in the cheek therefore bypassing the liver (avoiding first-pass effect) and protecting the medication from contact with other drugs, foods, and GI secretions that could affect the medication's potency or bioavailability.

Enteric-coated tablets (e.g., bisacodyl [Dulcolax] and ferrous sulfate [Feosol]) are formulated to inhibit release of the active drug until after the tablet has passed from the stomach into the small intestine. Moreover, the tablet's coating protects the stomach from irritation from the medication. Crushing the tablet would put an end to the protective coating.

Uncoated gastric irritants (including aspirin) remain effective following crushing, but they are more apt to trigger undesirable GI reactions such as cramping or bleeding. Ask for an alternative form or different medication.

Sustained-release or *effervescent tablets* (e.g., Slow-L, Procan SR, Theolair-SR, Inderal LA) were designed to dissolve and release medication gradually (they contain 2-3 doses of the medication). As a result, if crushed, the patient would get an overdose of the medication. In addition, the planned beneficial effects would not be maintained throughout the dosing interval.

The prescribed medication is in the form of a capsule. Can't I just place it in the tube and flush it down with some water?

Capsules should not be crushed, but you can open some and mix the contents with water:

Hard gelatin capsules (e.g., ampicillin and doxycycline) contain a medication in a powdered form. The capsule can be opened (it's designed to separate in the middle) and the powder mixed thoroughly with water.

Sustained-release capsules (e.g., Slo-bid and Feosol Spansules) release the active medication slowly, over time, through coated beads or pellets inside the capsules. They are designed to dissolve in the GI tract at different rates, lengthening the medication's duration of action. Obviously, crushing capsules or their contents would damage the timed-release coatings. A better alternative would be a liquid form or a simple compressed tablet that can be crushed (ascertain dosage frequency is increased appropriately).

Soft gel capsules (e.g., chloral hydrate, some vitamin preparations) can be dispensed through a feeding tube by poking a pinhole in one end and squeezing out the liquid contents. The liquid contents can also be drawn up in a syringe. Neither method should be used if delivering an exact dose is important. Some of the drug will always remain inside the capsule. Dissolve the capsule in 15-30 ml of warm water (5-10 ml for pediatric patients), then administer. The drug–water mixture will also work if you plan ahead—dissolving the capsule can take as long as 1 hour.

HERBS TO CONSIDER BEFORE SURGERY

Affect blood clotting:

ginkgo biloba   ginseng
feverfew   dong quai
garlic   danshen
ginger

Prolong narcotic and anesthesia drug effects:

valerian

kava kava (may also cause liver damage)

St. John's wort

Effects of Herbs on Food, Nutrients, and Drugs

As discussed earlier, herbs are not innocuous but can have significant effects on the bioavailability of foods, nutrients, and drugs. Rather than support health, the interactions may cause additional health problems. Table 16-1 lists numerous herbs and potential drug interactions that may result. For example, taking the herb feverfew for migraines may interfere with warfarin by further inhibiting blood platelet formation. Even taken alone, feverfew decreases blood clotting and should be discontinued 2 weeks before surgery (see the margin note).

Application to Nursing

Regulation of herbs and the need for education of the public and healthcare professionals is revealed by Table 16-5, which describes herbal products patients may use to treat selected conditions. Herbs when used medicinally should be prescribed

Text continued on p. 495.

Table 16-5
Commonly Used Herbal Products and Nutraceuticals that May Be Used to Treat Selected Conditions*

Condition	Herb	Use	Associated Adverse Effects
Asthma	Tylophora indica, Tylophora asthmatica	Inhibits histamine release	Sore mouth, loss of taste for salt, morning nausea and vomiting
	Adhatoda vasica	Bronchodilator	Vomiting and diarrhea; lack of conclusive efficacy data
	Picrorhiza kurroa	Bronchodilator	Vomiting, cutaneous rash, anorexia, diarrhea, itching, giddiness, headache, abdominal pain, increased dyspnea
	Khellin	Bronchodilator	Delirium, tachycardia, nausea, high incidence of GI side effects
	Onion extract (Allium cepa)	May inhibit leukotriene and thromboxane	Clinical efficacy unproven
	Ginkgo (Ginkgo biloba)	Smooth muscle relaxant	
Anxiety and depression	Chamomile (Chamaemelium nobile, Matricaria chemomilla, Matricaria recutita)	GI spasm or irritation, sedative	Therapeutic amounts may vary depending on effect chamomile has on an individual; side effects infrequent
	Valerian (Valeriana officinalis)	Insomnia, mild to moderate anxiety, stress and tension, premenstrual tension, hyperactivity, depression, insomnia, migraine headaches	Side effects not reported, but if used in too large a dose initially, it may cause excitability
	Passion flower (Passiflora incarnata)	Relaxation and sleep	Not recommended for children <2 years; use of decreased initial dose recommended for those >65 years
	Kava (Piper methysticum)	Sedation, anticonvulsive, antispasmodic, central muscular relaxant	Prolonged use causes a temporary yellow coloring of skin, hair, and nails; may interact with other CNS depressant agents; not recommended for use with other CNS depressants, including alcohol
	Hops (Humulus lupulus)	Insomnia, digestive aid, treatment of intestinal ailments	

References: Miller LG, Murray WJ, eds,: Herbal medicinals: a clinician's guide, New York, 1998, Pharmaceutical Products Press, an imprint of The Haworth Press, Inc.; Tyler VE: The honest herbal, ed 3, New York, 1993, Pharmaceutical Products Press, an imprint of The Haworth Press, Inc.

AIDS, Acquired immunodeficiency syndrome; CHD, coronary heart disease; CNS, central nervous system; GI, gastrointestinal; HDL, high-density lipoprotein; LDL, low-density lipoprotein; LES, lower esophageal sphincter; NSAIDS, nonsteroidal antiinflammatory drugs.

*It is not the intent of this table to provide information on how to use herbs, nor to be exhaustive in every herbal product that may be used. Rather, the intent is to provide information regarding herbal products that your patients may use.

Continued

Table 16-5–cont'd
Commonly Used Herbal Products and Nutraceuticals that May Be Used to Treat Selected Conditions

Condition	Herb	Use	Associated Adverse Effects
Anxiety and depression—cont'd	Ginseng (Panax quinquefolius, Panax ginseng, Eleutherococcus senticosus)	Increase energy, improve stamina, enhance memory	Typically mild and dose related; most commonly observed are nervousness, sleeplessness, nausea, and occasionally headache
	St. John's wort (Hypericum perforatum)	Depression	Fatigue, pruritus, weight gain, emotional vulnerability; photosensitivity; decreased effectiveness of oral contraceptive therapy possible
	Black cohosh (Cimicifuga racemosa)	Sedative, relaxant	Not for use in pregnancy
	California poppy (Reschschotzia california)	Hypnotic, tranquilizer	
	Damask rose (Rosa damascena)	Antidepressant	Use only good quality of damask rose.
	Lemon balm (Melissa officinalis)		
	Neroli oil (Citrus aurantium)		
	Jamaican dogwood (Piscidia erythrina)	Insomnia, migraine	
	Linden (Tifia europaea)	Reduces nervous tension	
	Gotu kola (Centella asiatica)	Relaxant	Gotu kola may cause rash; avoid while pregnant and breastfeeding
	Mugwort (Artemisia vulgaris)		
	Skullcap (Scutellaria lateriflora)		
	Vervain (Verbena officinalis)		
	Pasque flower (Anemone pulsatilla)	Sedative action	Use only dried plant
	Lavender (Lavandula species)	Sedative	Avoid high doses of lavender in pregnancy. Excess amounts of wild lettuce can lead to insomnia. Large doses of wood betony can cause vomiting; avoid high doses in pregnancy
	Wild lettuce (Lactuca virosa)		
	Wood betony (Stachys officinalis)		

AIDS, *Acquired immunodeficiency syndrome;* CHD, *coronary heart disease;* CNS, *central nervous system;* GI, *gastrointestinal;* HDL, *high-density lipoprotein;* LDL, *low-density lipoprotein;* LES, *lower esophageal;* NSAIDS, *nonsteroidal antiinflammatory drugs.*

Table 16-5—cont'd
Commonly Used Herbal Products and Nutraceuticals that May Be Used to Treat Selected Conditions

Condition	Herb	Use	Associated Adverse Effects
Cancer prevention and treatment	Shark cartilage	Antiangiogenic effect	Doubtful oral bioavailability of biologically active components
	Aloe vera	May stimulate macrophage function (antitumor activity)	May have deleterious effects in patients with AIDS
	Echinacea (Echinacea augustifolia, E. pallida)	Immunostimulatory activity	Unknown whether effective orally
	Mistletoe (Phoradendron species and Viscum species)	Potent inducer of cytokines stimulating release of TNF-alpha and interleukin-1	
	Antioxidant vitamins A and E	May reduce risk of lung cancer by reducing formation of free radicals	Vitamin A can be toxic
	Garlic and onion (Allium sativum and Allium cepa)	May decrease nitrosamine formation	
	Green tea	Antioxidant properties, inhibits nucleoside transport	Contradictory epidemiologic studies regarding efficacy in cancer
	Chaparral (Larrea tridentate, L. divaricata, L. mexicana)	Antioxidant properties	Hepatoxic; unproven and dangerous
	Ginseng (Panax quinquefolius, Panax ginseng, Eleutherococcus senticosus)	Antiestrogen properties	More data needed
	Laetrile	May have tumor static activity	Unproven
	Goldenseal (Hydrastis canadensis), Oregon grape root (Mahonia aquifolium, M. nervosa), Barberry root (Berberis vulgaris)	May prevent carcinogenesis	Use may be limited by toxicity
	Pineapple	May cause tumor regression	More study needed
	Sweet and red clover (Trifolium pratense)	Stimulates macrophage activity	
	Cloud fungus	Immunostimulatory activity	

AIDS, *Acquired immunodeficiency syndrome;* CHD, *coronary heart disease;* CNS, *central nervous system;* GI, *gastrointestinal;* HDL, *high-density lipoprotein;* LDL, *low-density lipoprotein;* LES, *lower esophageal;* NSAIDS, *nonsteroidal antiinflammatory drugs.*

Continued

Table 16-5–cont'd
Commonly Used Herbal Products and Nutraceuticals that May Be Used to Treat Selected Conditions

Condition	Herb	Use	Associated Adverse Effects
Colds and flu	Anise (Pimpinella anisum)	Expectorant action	May cause contact dermatitis; avoid use while pregnant or breastfeeding
	Boneset (Eupatorium perfoliatum)	Antipyretic; influenza	Individuals with hypersensitivity to the Asteraceae family (e.g., chamomile, feverfew) should avoid use
	Coltsfoot (Tussilago farfara)	Antitussive	Possible hepatotoxicity; has abortifacient effects, should not be taken while pregnant or breastfeeding
	Echinacea (Echinacea augustifolia, E. Pallida) Purple coneflower (E. purpurea) is a different species with similar properties	Prophylaxis and treatment of cold and flu symptoms	Continuous use (>6-8 weeks) may lead to immunosuppression; contraindicated in autoimmune diseases
	Horehound (Marrubium vulgare)	Controversial use as expectorant, antitussive, cough suppressant, digestive aid, appetite stimulant	Large doses have produced cardiac irregularities
	Slippery elm (Ulmus rubra)	Demulcent and emollient to treat sore throats	Pollen can be an allergen; may cause contact dermatitis
	Zinc lozenges	Reduces duration and severity of cold symptoms	Possible nausea, unpleasant taste
Diabetes	Karela (Momordica charantia)	Hypoglycemic	May sufficiently lower blood glucose to merit decrease in insulin or oral medications to avoid or minimize incidence of hypoglycemia; karela juice will cause greater decrease in blood glucose than when slices of karela are fried
	Ginseng (Panax quinquefolius, Panax ginseng, Eleutherococcus senticosus)	Hypoglycemic	Korean or Chinese ginseng may exert greater hypoglycemic effect than Japanese ginseng
	Brewer's yeast	Hypoglycemic	May cause unfavorable variability in blood glucose control if medical staff is unaware of concomitant use with chromium

AIDS, Acquired immunodeficiency syndrome; CHD, coronary heart disease; CNS, central nervous system; GI, gastrointestinal; HDL, high-density lipoprotein; LDL, low-density lipoprotein; LES, lower esophageal; NSAIDS, nonsteroidal antiinflammatory drugs.

Table 16-5—cont'd
Commonly Used Herbal Products and Nutraceuticals that May Be Used to Treat Selected Conditions

Condition	Herb	Use	Associated Adverse Effects
Diabetes—cont'd	GS₄ (Gymnema sylvestre)	Hypoglycemic	May decrease insulin and glyburide requirements but should not be relied on for blood glucose control
	Devil's claw (Harpagophytum procumbens)		May cause hyperglycemia
	Ginseng (Panax quinquefolius, Panax ginseng, Eleutherococcus senticosus)		
	Hydrocotyle (Centella asiatica)		
	Licorice (Glycyrrhiza glabra; G. uralensis)		
	Ephedra or ma huang (Ephedra sinica)		
Dyslipidemia and atherosclerosis	Nicotinic acid (niacin)	Reduces total serum cholesterol, LDL cholesterol, and triglycerides; increases HDL cholesterol	Should be used only under physician's supervision; may elevate blood glucose levels; severe heptotoxicity may occur, especially with SR nicotinic acid products
	Soluble fiber products (oat bran, guar gum, psyllium, and other dietary sources)	Can lower total serum cholesterol and LDL cholesterol depending on product and amount consumed	Flatulence, cramping, bloating, nausea, diarrhea, indigestion, heartburn
	Fish oils (omega-3 fatty acids)	Inhibit platelet aggregation, lower triglyceride levels when consumed in high doses (20-30 g/d)	Triglyceride-lowering effect may diminish with continued use; produces variable effects (decreases and increases) on blood cholesterol levels; may increase bleeding risk
	Vitamin E	200 IU or more per day *may* reduce risk of CHD	
	Garlic (Allium sativum)	Standardized powdered garlic products may produce modest reduction in total cholesterol	
	Nuts	Lower plasma lipoprotein levels	

AIDS, *Acquired immunodeficiency syndrome;* CHD, *coronary heart disease;* CNS, *central nervous system;* GI, *gastrointestinal;* HDL, *high-density lipoprotein;* LDL, *low-density lipoprotein;* LES, *lower esophageal;* NSAIDS, *nonsteroidal antiinflammatory drugs.*

Continued

Table 16-5—cont'd
Commonly Used Herbal Products and Nutraceuticals that May Be Used to Treat Selected Conditions

Condition	Herb	Use	Associated Adverse Effects
Dyslipidemia and atherosclerosis—cont'd	Beta-sitosterol	May produce modest reductions in total and LDL cholesterol	
	Alfalfa seed (*Medicago sativa*)	May produce modest reduction in cholesterol	Potential toxic effects outweigh any advantages that might be obtained
	Chromium	May produce modest cholesterol reductions; administration as picolinate salt seems to increase bioavailability	
GI problems	Aloes (*Aloe barbadensis, A. ferox, A africana, A. spicate*)	Orally a powerful carthartic and not generally recommended	A harsh purgative; less toxic laxatives are available. Contraindicated with hemorrhoids, kidney disease, intestinal obstruction, abdominal pain, nausea, or vomiting
	Bilberry fruit (*Vaccinium myrtillus*)	Treatment of diarrhea	No known side effects or interactions
	Cascara (*Rhamnus purshiana*)	Stimulant laxative	Do not take while pregnant or breastfeeding. Fresh bark may cause severe vomiting. Electrolyte imbalance with misuse; potentiates toxicities of cardiac glycosides and thiazide diuretics
	Ginger (*Zingiber officinate*)	Treatment of motion sickness and nausea	May cause prolonged bleeding times; caution in patients on anticoagulant therapy. Reported to be an abortifacient, so avoid while pregnant or breastfeeding
	Licorice (*Glycyrrhiza glabra; G. uralensis*)	Treatment of peptic ulcer, expectorant	Considered unsafe. Contraindicated in patients taking cardiac glycosides or thiazide diuretics
	Peppermint (*Mentha piperita*)	Decreases muscle spasms of the GI tract. Treatment of abdominal pain. Enteric-coated capsules used to treat irritable bowel syndrome	Should not be used by infants or small children; tea from leaves can cause laryngeal and bronchial spasms. Overuse can lead to heartburn and relaxation of LES
	Psyllium (*Plantago arenaria, P. psyllium, P. indica, P. ovata*)	Bulk-forming laxative for constipation, irritable bowel syndrome	Can possibly interfere with absorption of other drugs. Bezoars may occur if liquid intake is inadequate

AIDS, Acquired immunodeficiency syndrome; CHD, coronary heart disease; CNS, central nervous system; GI, gastrointestinal; HDL, high-density lipoprotein; LDL, low-density lipoprotein; LES, lower esophageal; NSAIDS, nonsteroidal antiinflammatory drugs.

Table 16-5—cont'd
Commonly Used Herbal Products and Nutraceuticals that May Be Used to Treat Selected Conditions

Condition	Herb	Use	Associated Adverse Effects
GI problems—cont'd	Senna (Cassia acutifolia; C. angustifolia, Senna. alexandrina)	Cathartic; used to treat constipation	Chronic use can result in electrolyte imbalance and potassium loss. May increase toxicity of cardiac glycosides and thiazide diuretics
Hypertension	Garlic (Allium sativum)	Antihypertensive	Routine use not recommended. Avoid use of garlic with NSAIDs, anticoagulants, and drugs that inhibit liver metabolism (e.g., cimetidine) and drugs that may be affected by liver inhibition (e.g., propranolol, diazepam)
	Grapefruit juice		May cause significant decrease in blood pressure if taken with nifedipine
	Licorice (Glycyrrhiza glabra; G. uralensis)		May induce hypertension accompanied by hypokalemia. Patients taking oral contraceptives or thiazide diuretics may be predisposed to licorice toxicity if taken concomitantly
	Yohimbine (Pausinystalia yohimbe)	May be used to treat impotence secondary to antihypertensive medications	May increase blood pressure. Should not be co-administered with tricyclic antidepressants or clonidine

AIDS, Acquired immunodeficiency syndrome; CHD, coronary heart disease; CNS, central nervous system; GI, gastrointestinal; HDL, high-density lipoprotein; LDL, low-density lipoprotein; LES, lower esophageal; NSAIDS, nonsteroidal antiinflammatory drugs.

by healthcare professionals who have knowledge of the herbal actions so that the desired benefits are produced without the negative side effects. Because herbs are easily available, many individuals self-diagnose and treat themselves without consultation with trained healthcare professionals.

Because herbs are not considered medications, patients often do not volunteer information regarding their use when they are asked, "What medications do you regularly take?" Consequently, nurses can assist this process by asking more detailed questions about supplement intake.

Questions to ask patients who may take herbal products:
- Do you use any dietary supplements? (Direct patient to include in the answer vitamins, minerals, botanicals, amino acids, concentrates, and extracts.)
- If so, what dosage do you take? What other directions do you follow such as taking with meals or at bedtime?
- What is the purpose of taking the dietary supplement? (Avoid questions like, "What is that supposed to do?" because such implied skepticism can embarrass the patient and discourage honest reporting of supplement use.)
- Have you experienced any side effects?
- Do you take an herbal product, herbal supplement, or other "natural remedy"?

- If so, do you take any prescription or nonprescription medications for the same purpose as the herbal product?
- Have you used this herbal product before?
- Are you allergic to any plant products?
- Are you pregnant or breastfeeding?
- Are you seeing an herbalist, acupuncturist, naturopathic practitioner, nutritionist, or natural healer?
- Is your physician or primary healthcare provider aware that you take these supplements (in addition to any prescribed medications)?

Keep an open mind about alternative supplements and medications, and remain current with new findings in this quickly changing area.

SUMMARY

Complementary and alternative medicine (CAM) is becoming a significant component of healthcare in the United States. CAM consists of a cluster of medical and healthcare approaches, methods, and items not associated with conventional medicine. Complementary medicine refers to non-Western healing approaches used at the same time as conventional medicine. In contrast, alternative medicine replaces conventional medical treatment. Integrative medicine merges conventional medical therapies with CAM modalities for which safety and efficacy, based on scientific data, have been demonstrated. CAM therapies can be divided into five categories: alternative medical systems; mind-body interventions; biologically based therapies; manipulative and body-based methods; and energy therapies. Familiarity with CAM modalities will promote a secure environment for patients.

Dietary supplements are substances consumed orally as an addition to dietary intake. The Dietary Supplement Health and Education Act (DSHEA) of 1994 regulates supplement identity, potency, contents, and labeling under the supervision of the FDA. Supplement use has grown substantially and may interact with other medications and treatments.

Drug-nutrient interactions may occur. Nutrients and foods may interact with drug function; drugs may affect use of food and nutrients. Use of herbs as dietary supplements or as natural medications can interact with bioavailability of foods, nutrients, and drugs. Knowledge of potential interactions assists nurses to provide more comprehensive patient care.

THE NURSING APPROACH
Providing Herbal Supplement Advice

Nurses are often approached for medical advice. As the use of CAM modalities increases, patients (and their friends and family) will probably pose more questions toward nurses. In particular, concerns about herbs will arise as individuals consider replacing conventional medication with herbal substitutes. The following are examples of questions that may be asked and an appropriate nursing response:

- *My neighbor takes an herbal supplement for depression and he feels better. I think I am depressed, too. Should I take the supplement, too? What do you think?*

   Although it is useful to hear that others benefit from herbal supplements, keep in mind that there are people who are not helped by the same supplements. Some medical conditions are self-limiting and other serious conditions may wax and wane. Although your neighbor is doing better, that herbal supplement may not be appropriate for you. Consult your primary care provider about your condition or problem.

- *My doctor has prescribed medications for my hypertension and I know there are natural herbs that can do the same thing. Should I switch to the natural herbs and stop taking my prescribed medications?*

   First, it is important to tell your primary care provider that you are considering taking a natural herb for your condition *before* you stop any medication. Second, you

THE NURSING APPROACH–cont'd
Providing Herbal Supplement Advice

need to weigh the benefits and side effects of medications vs. the benefits and side effects of the herbal supplement. Your primary care healthcare provider can be of help.

- *I am having surgery next month and I've heard that some herbs can cause problems. Are there any herbs that I should avoid?*

  Be sure to inform your doctor of the various herbal supplements you have been taking. Ginkgo biloba and feverfew may reduce the number of platelets in the blood and interfere with blood clotting. Other herbs reported to inhibit clotting include garlic, ginger, ginseng, dong quai, and danshen. Some herbs such as valerian, kava kava, and St. John's wort may prolong the effects of narcotic drugs and anesthesia.

- *I have been taking herbal supplements for many years and have difficulty bringing this up to my doctor. He states that they are all useless. What should I do?*

  Research shows that some herbal supplements interact with prescribed medications and treatments. Additionally, many doctors aren't trained in CAM. On your next doctor's visit, explain why you are bringing up the subject and bring copies of the articles about the supplements. Request that this information be placed in your medical record because you understand that herbal supplements combined with certain prescribed medications and treatments may pose serious risks.

- *What are reliable sources of information on herbs and supplements?*

  The Internet provides thousands of sites that pertain to herbs and other dietary supplements; however, only a limited number are credible. Generally, Web sites that end with ".gov" (U.S. government sites) or ".edu" (educational institution sites) are valid sources of information on medical concerns. (The Web sites listed in the Web Sites of Interest in this chapter are respectable sites.)

CRITICAL THINKING
Clinical Applications

Faye, a 20-year-old student from Germany, seeks medical attention at the urging of her roommates, who report that her mood has become increasingly depressed during the past two semesters. She has become withdrawn and moody— a significant change from her affect since first coming to the United States to attend college. She is otherwise healthy. Faye reports a 5-lb weight loss during the past 3 months. She takes oral contraceptives for regulation of menses. Her mother has been treated for depression with *Hypericum perforatum* (St. John's wort) by the family physician for the past 10 years. She reports smoking a pack of cigarettes per day. Plans are to treat her with 50 mg sertraline (Zoloft) per day and to provide counseling therapy. During the diet history, the dietitian asks Faye if she uses any over-the-counter vitamins, minerals, or herbal supplements. She tells the dietitian that her mother suggested she try *Hypericum perforatum* because in Germany it is prescribed to treat depression. Faye did as her mother suggested because it is available without prescription in the United States.

1. Faye's depression will be treated with sertraline, a selective serotonin reuptake inhibitor (SSRI). How do SSRIs work?
2. What is St. John's wort?
3. How is St. John's wort used in the United States.? How is it regulated?
4. How does St. John's wort work as an antidepressant?
5. Does St. John's wort have any side effects?
6. How is St. John's wort used in Europe?
7. Why do you think people are interested in alternative medicine and herbal treatments?
8. What is your immediate concern regarding Faye's use of St. John's wort?

Revised with permission from Nelms MN, Anderson SL: Medical nutrition therapy: a case study approach, *Belmont, Calif, 2002, Wadsworth Group/ Thomson Learning.*

Web Sites of Interest

American Botanical Council

www.herbalgram.org

The American Botanical Council is a nonprofit education and research organization that disperses information and research findings to encourage appropriate use of phytomedicines and medicinal plants.

The Dietary Supplement

www.TheDietarySupplement.com

This online version of a reputable newsletter provides information on supplemental use of vitamins, minerals, botanicals, and related products.

An FDA Guide to Choosing Medical Treatments

www.fda.gov/oashi/aids/fdaguide.html

This guide for consumers from the FDA explains how to assess the validity and effectiveness of medical treatments.

National Center for Complementary and Alternative Medicine,
National Institutes of Health

www.nccam.nih.gov/

The NCCAM is part of the NIH. Its mission is to promote scientific research on CAM, to prepare CAM researchers, and to distribute information to the public and health professionals on the efficacy of CAM modalities

Office of Dietary Supplements, National Institutes of Health

dietary-supplements.info.nih.gov/

The Office of Dietary Supplements (ODS) is the part of the NIH that promotes research and distributes research findings about dietary supplements. The ODS is a resource to other federal agencies concerning dietary supplement research findings.

References

1. National Center for Complementary and Alternative Medicine (NCCAM), National Institutes of Health: Exploring the scientific basis of complementary and alternative medicine, *NIH News Release*, March 8, 2002.
2. National Center for Complementary and Alternative Medicine (NCCAM), National Institutes of Health: *What is complementary and alternative medicine (CAM)?*; nccam.nih.gov/health/whatiscam/.
3. Crawford LM: *Dietary supplement strategic plan cost out*, US Food and Drug Administration, Center for Food Safety and Applied Nutrition, May 29, 2002; www.cfsan.fda.gov/~dms/ds-stra2.html
4. Center for the Study of Alternative and Complementary Medicine, University of Medicine and Dentistry of New Jersey: *Biological based system: macrobiotic diet*, July 20, 2002; www.umdnj.educsacmweb/modalities/biological/macrobiotic.htm.
5. Rapp E: Massage, aromatherapy, oils and a root canal, *The New York Times*, NJ sec 10:1, July 21, 2002.
6. Nurse Healers Professional Associates: *Therapeutic touch*, October 18, 2002; www.therapeutic-touch.org/content/ttouch.asp.
7. Thomas P: The regulation of dietary supplements, part 1: the 20th century through 1994, *The Dietary Supplement*, Jan/Mar 2000.
8. *Prevention* magazine's survey of consumer use of dietary supplements, *Prevention*, 2000, p. 4; www.cfsan.fda.gov/~dms/ds-stra2.html, accessed July 24, 2002.9. National Business Journal 2000: *Dialog file No. 93*, San Francisco, 2000, The Dialog Corporation.
10. American Dietetic Association: Functional foods—position of ADA, *J Am Dietetic Assoc* 99:1278, 1999.
11. Thomson C et al.: Guidelines regarding the recommendation and sale of dietary supplements, *J Am Dietetic Assoc* 102(8):1158, 2002.
12. Baldwin KM et al.: Shock, multiple organ dysfunction syndrome, and burns in adults. In McCance KL, Huether SE, eds.: *Pathophysiology: the biologic basis for diseases in adults and children*, ed 3, St Louis, 1998, Mosby.
13. Barrocas A: Complementary and alternative medicine: friend, foe, or OWA? *J Am Dietetic Assoc* 97:1373, 1997.
14. National Center for Complementary and Alternative Medicine, Clearinghouse, National Institutes of Health; nccam.nih.gov/health/clearinghouse/.

CHAPTER 17

Nutrition for Disorders of the Gastrointestinal Tract

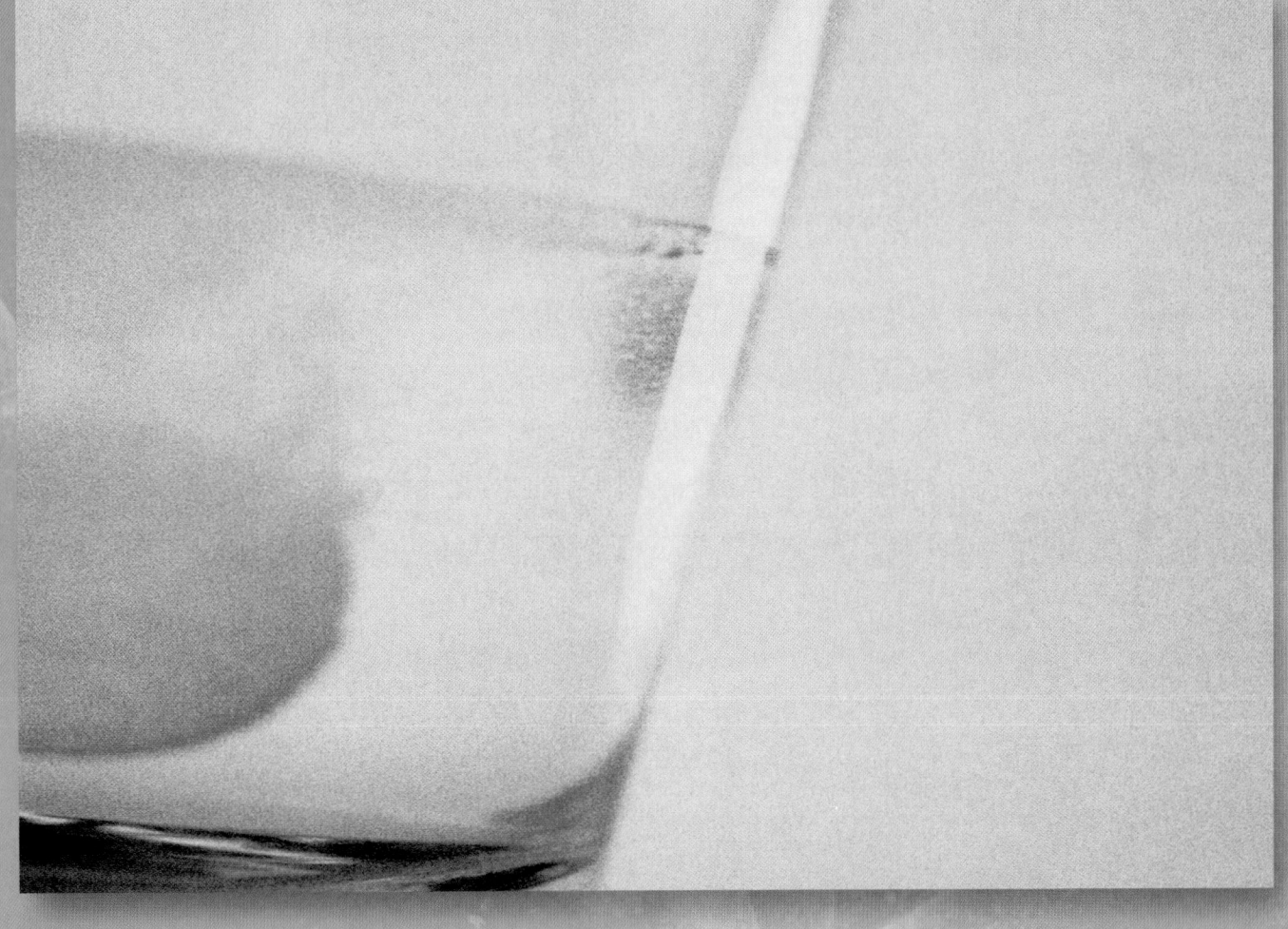

The ability to chew, swallow, digest, and absorb nutrients, while passing fiber and other substances on for elimination, may be compromised by disorders of the gastrointestinal tract.

ROLE IN WELLNESS

Almost everyone experiences intermittent gastrointestinal (GI) complaints from time to time. Indigestion, gas, bloating, nausea, abdominal pain or cramping, diarrhea, and esophageal reflux are some of the symptoms occasionally experienced by healthy people. Most of these complaints are often simply related to consumption of usual or unusual types of foods or amounts of specific foods.[1]

Many GI disorders produce significant nutritional implications and, in many situations, diet is the cornerstone of therapy for GI complaints. Evaluation of a patient's GI symptoms requires a team effort to separate GI symptoms associated with dietary practices from those associated with GI disease or dysfunction. The registered dietitian's role is to help identify unusual dietary practices, nutritional inadequacies, or food intolerances through the use of an in-depth diet history.[1]

The simple act of eating an apple may no longer be easy for individuals with disorders of the GI tract. The ability to chew, swallow, digest, and absorb nutrients, while passing fiber and other substances on for elimination, may be compromised by disorders of the GI tract (Figure 17-1). These disorders affect provision of nutrients to all other organs and systems of the body, thereby influencing overall health.

Consider disorders of the GI tract through the five dimensions of health. The physical health dimension is most affected if the disorder is chronic and intensifies over time; eventually weight loss and nutrient deficiencies pose other health risks in addition to the primary GI tract disorder. Intellectual health is tested as the patient, caregivers, and dietetic and nursing staff work together to devise food combinations and textures that are physically and anesthetically acceptable to the patient;

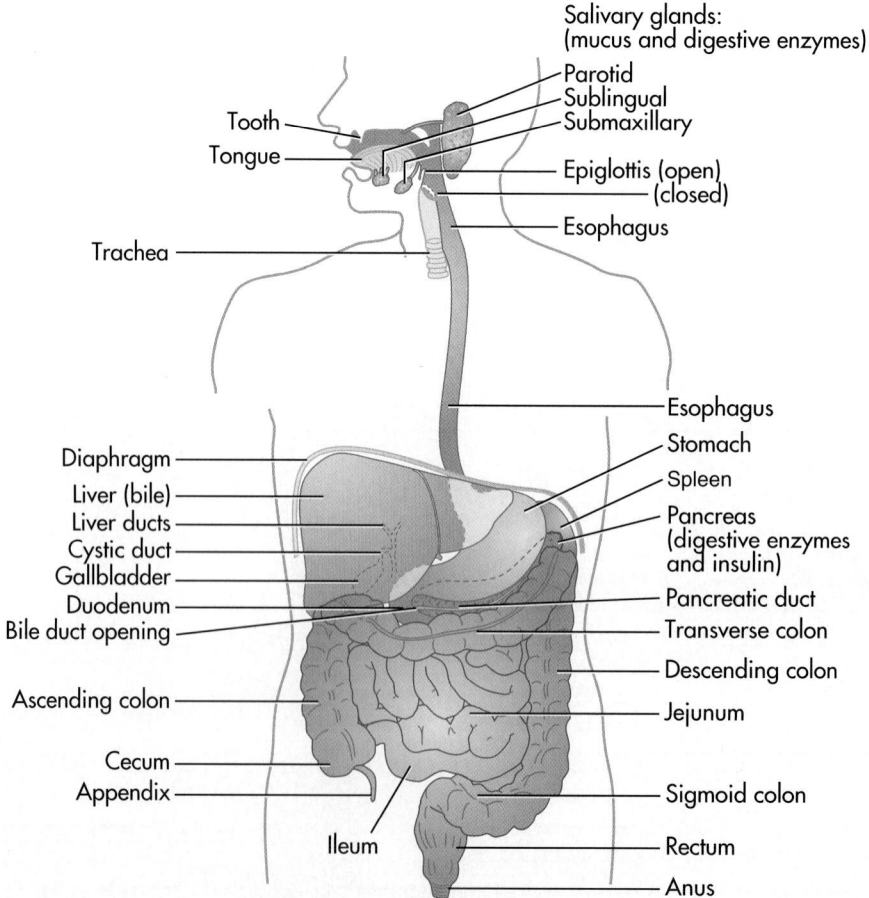

Figure 17-1 The gastrointestinal tract. (From Mahan LK, Escott-Stump S: *Krause's food, nutrition, and diet therapy,* ed 10, Philadelphia, 2000, WB Saunders.)

other disorders require constant vigilance to restrict inadvertent consumption of problematic foods (e.g., gluten for patients with celiac disease). Emotional health may be taxed when patients struggle with acceptance of dietary or physical limitations; nurses can refer patients to disorder support groups as an additional therapeutic strategy. Some disorders may affect social health functioning. Nurses can provide patients with social strategies to deal with the physical ramifications of colostomies, dumping syndrome, and other disorders. Spiritual and physical health including health of the GI tract may be enhanced by the practices of yoga and meditation, which are tied to teachings related to both mind and body.

DYSPHAGIA

The main focus of medical nutrition therapy for dysphagia is to provide nutrition in a form that fits specific anatomic and functional needs of the patient while maintaining or improving nutritional status and avoiding aspiration.[2] For patients with chewing or swallowing difficulties, diets must be devised to meet nutritional needs and prevent aspiration. Patients may also experience changes in consistency tolerance. Thickening agents provide varying levels of consistency to accommodate individual needs because thin liquids are usually more difficult to swallow.

We rarely think about swallowing, just as we don't think about breathing or our heart beating. Swallowing takes place in three stages, as outlined in Figure 17-2:

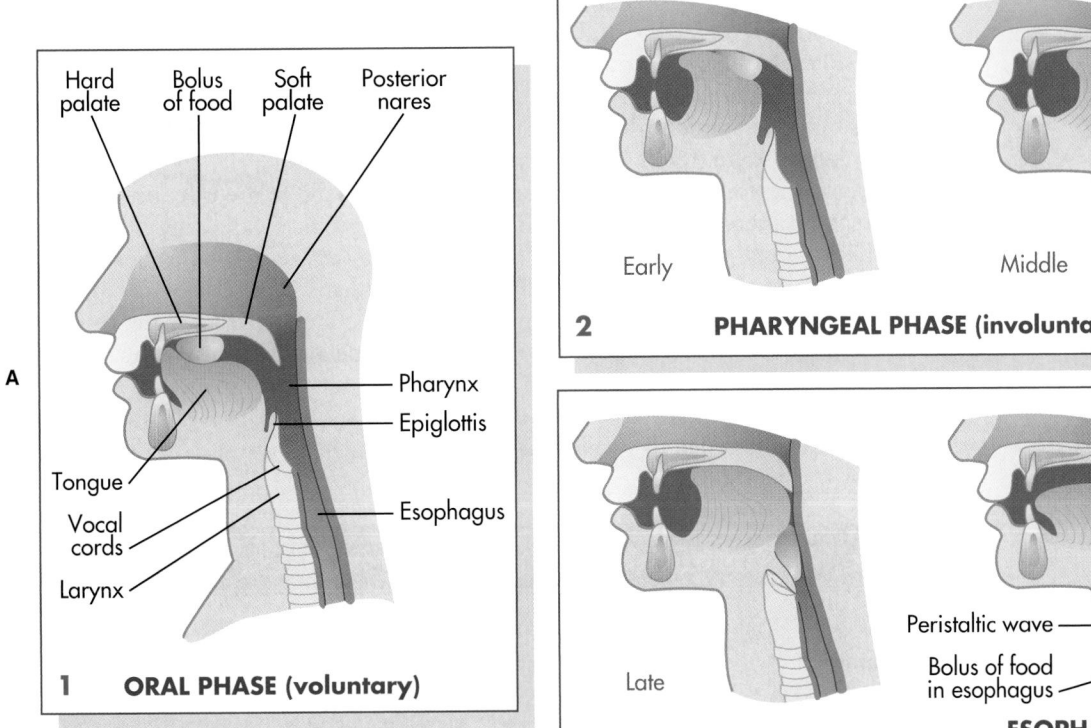

Figure 17-2 Swallowing occurs in three phases: **A,** Voluntary or oral phase. The tongue presses food against the hard palate, forcing it toward the pharynx. **B,** Involuntary, pharyngeal phase. *Early:* wave of peristalsis forces a bolus between the tonsillar pillars. *Middle:* soft palate draws upward to close posterior nares and respirations cease momentarily. *Late:* vocal cords approximate and the larynx pulls upward, covering the airway and stretching the esophagus open. **C,** Involuntary, esophageal phase. Relaxation of the upper esophageal (hypopharyngeal) sphincter allows the peristaltic wave to move the bolus down the esophagus. (From Mahan LK, Escott-Stump S: *Krause's food, nutrition, and diet therapy,* ed 10, Philadelphia, 2000, WB Saunders.)

oral preparation and transit, pharyngeal transit, and esophageal transit. A disorder affecting any of these stages may require medical nutrition therapy.

Patients sometimes give warning signs that they are at risk for swallowing problems.[3,4] Some of these signs include the following:
- Collecting food under the tongue, in the cheeks, or on the hard palate
- Spitting food out of the mouth, or tongue thrusting
- Inability to control tongue
- Excessively moving tongue
- Decreasing oral transit time
- Experiencing delay or absence of elevation of larynx while swallowing
- Coughing before or after swallowing
- Choking
- Drooling
- Experiencing gargled voice after eating or drinking
- Regurgitating food or liquid through nose, mouth, or tracheostomy tube
- Not taking in adequate amounts of food or fluids, resulting in weight loss
- Increasing time required to eat
- Resisting food, such as clenching teeth, pushing food away, clutching throat
    Box 17-1 presents conditions that may cause dysphagia.

Medical Nutrition Therapy

No two patients with dysphagia are alike. Therefore one's diet must be individualized based on the swallowing ability of the patient and, of course, the patient's personal food preferences. Solid foods and liquids should be evaluated separately and modified based on texture, cohesiveness, density, viscosity, consistency, temperature, and taste. A nutritionally adequate diet for dysphagia involves considering these characteristics, along with careful planning to ensure nutritional adequacy.[2] A four-stage dysphagia diet is outlined in Table 17-1.

When caring for patients with dysphagia, several aspects are of concern: bolus consistency, patient positioning, feeding rate, and specific swallowing techniques. Videofluoroscopy swallow study (VFSS) determines the level of bolus consistency the patient can tolerate. Different physiologic problems dictate necessity for different consistencies of food. For example, the most common swallowing disorder in older adults who have experienced stroke is a delayed or absent pharyngeal swallow.[5]

Patients with this type of disorder need puréed foods to provide stimulation that provokes the reflex to swallow. If the pharyngeal swallow is reduced (but not

---

Box 17-1 Conditions that Cause Dysphagia

AIDS, such as with oral or esophageal thrush	Head or neck cancer or surgery
Alzheimer's disease/dementia	Multiple sclerosis (MS)
Amyotrophic lateral sclerosis (ALS)	Muscular dystrophy (MD)
Cerebral palsy (CP)	Myasthenia gravis
Cerebrovascular accident (CVA)/stroke	Myotonic dystrophy
Closed head trauma	Parkinson's disease
Dermatomyositis	Poliomyelitis
Dysautonomia	Reflux esophagitis
Guillain-Barré syndrome	Stricture or inflammation of pharynx or esophagus
Huntington's chorea	Tumor or obstruction of throat

From American Dietetic Association: Manual of clinical dietetics, *ed 6, Chicago, 2000, American Dietetic Association.*

Table 17-1
Four-Stage Dysphagia Diet

Stage	Rationale	Description	Adequacy
Stage 1: Puréed Diet	Suitable for persons with severely reduced oral preparatory stage abilities, impaired lip and tongue control, delayed swallow reflex triggering, oral hypersensitivity, reduced pharyngeal peristalsis, and/or cricopharyngeal dysfunction	Thick homogeneous textures are emphasized. Puréed foods should be "spoon-thick" or "puddinglike" consistency. No coarse textures, nuts, raw fruits, or raw vegetables allowed. Liquid or crushed medications (refer to physician or pharmacist for pharmo-efficacy of medications) are required and may be mixed with puréed fruits. Liquids and water are thickened with commercial thickening agent as needed to recommended consistency.	Intake may be limited because of decreased appetite or increased time required to eat. If this is the case, supplementation to meet the Dietary Reference Intakes (DRI) and recommended dietary allowances (RDA) may be necessary. Additional enteral feeding could be necessary; fluid intake should be monitored.
Stage 2: Ground/ Minced Diet	Intended for patients who can tolerate a minimum amount of easily chewed foods. May be suitable for persons with moderately impaired oral preparatory stage abilities, edentulous oral cavity, decreased pharyngeal peristalsis, and/or cricopharyngeal muscle dysfunction.	No coarse textures, nuts, raw fruits (except ripe or mashed bananas), or vegetables, except as noted. Puréed or slurried bread, if necessary. Liquid or crushed medications may still be required (refer to physician or pharmacist for pharmo-efficacy of medications). Liquids and water thickened as needed with commercial thickening agent to recommended consistency.	Diet designed to provide adequate quantities of nutrients as indicated by the DRI/RDA. Individual selection and amounts consumed will determine whether supplementation is necessary. Feedings that are more frequent are recommended; fluid intake should be monitored.
Stage 3: Soft/Easy-to-Chew Diet	For patients who may have difficulty chewing, manipulating, and swallowing certain foods. Based on a mechanical diet; consists of soft food items prepared without blenderizing or puréeing. May be appropriate for persons beginning to chew or with mild oral preparatory state deficits.	Textures are soft with no tough skins. No nuts or dry, crispy, raw, or stringy foods allowed. Meats should be minced or cut in small pieces (diced pieces should be cubes of 1 cm (0.4 in) or less). Liquid or crushed medications may still be required (refer to physician or pharmacist for pharmo-efficacy of medications). Liquids and water thickened as needed with commercial thickening agent to recommended consistency.	Contingent on individual selection and amounts consumed, this diet is designed to provide adequate quantity of nutrients as indicated by the DRI/RDA. Monitor fluid intake.
Stage 4: Modified General Diet	Designed for patients who chew soft textures. Based on a soft diet; may be appropriate for persons with mild oral preparatory stage deficits.	Soft textures not requiring grinding or chopping used. No nuts or crisp, deep-fried foods allowed. All liquids and medications used as tolerated. Liquids and water thickened as needed with commercial thickening agent to recommended consistency.	Contingent on individual selection and amounts consumed, this diet is designed to provide adequate quantity of nutrients as indicated by the DRI/RDA. Monitor fluid intake. Nutritional supplementation may be needed.

Reference: *American Dietetic Association: Manual of clinical dietetics, ed 6, Chicago, 2000, American Dietetic Association.*

delayed or absent), liquids tend to be the most difficult consistency with which to deal. Thickening agents can be used to acquire the appropriate consistency. For patients who have lost coordination of the upper esophageal sphincter (cricopharyngeal dysfunction), thin liquids are the most appropriate.[6]

One of the safest eating positions for patients who have trouble swallowing is the upright position. If patients cannot sit up by themselves, the head of the bed should be raised to provide support, and pillows and wedges should be used to support arms, head, neck, or trunk when necessary. The upright position allows gravity to assist with the passage of food along the esophagus and helps prevent choking and aspiration.[7,8]

Sometimes patients eat too quickly or stuff their mouths too full of food and then choke when trying to swallow. Staff can observe and supervise patients while they eat to remind them to complete the swallowing sequence before taking their next bite of food.

Enlisting the aid of a speech therapist is usually necessary to teach the patient various techniques to compensate for swallowing problems. Techniques include the supraglottic swallow and the Mendelson maneuver. The supraglottic swallow is appropriate for patients with reduced laryngeal function. This method requires teaching the patient to take a breath before swallowing, consciously hold the breath during the swallow, exhale forcefully or cough gently after the swallow, and reswallow to clear the mouth. The Mendelson maneuver is helpful for individuals with cricopharyngeal dysfunction. The patient is taught to elevate the larynx voluntarily to the maximum level during a swallow to allow food to pass. In cases where lubrication is a problem, nursing personnel can also use several techniques to assist the patient. Encouraging the patient to think or talk about food before mealtime can help stimulate the flow of saliva, which aids in the formation of a bolus and the chewing and swallowing process. Tart or sour foods can stimulate saliva production. Having the patient lick jelly from the lips, pucker them, hum, or whistle helps strengthen mouth muscles, which may help the patient learn to close the lips around a fork or spoon.[9]

Feeding patients with swallowing difficulty is usually the responsibility of nursing personnel. The following safe procedures are recommended.[2,8,10]

1. Position patient upright.
2. Eliminate distractions so patient can focus all attention on the meal.
3. The person feeding should sit at or below patient's eye level while feeding.
4. Avoid asking patient to talk while eating.
5. Instruct patient not to use liquids to clear mouth of foods; in fact, they should only be used after the patient has cleared the food from the mouth. Encourage frequent dry swallows or coughing to help clear food from the mouth between bites.
6. Encourage small bites ($\frac{1}{2}$ to 1 tsp solid food or about 10- to 15-ml liquid), especially if patient's ability to manage food is impaired.
7. Allow adequate time to feed.
8. Use spoons rather than cups because patients have less difficulty taking food/ and liquid this way.
9. While patient eats, check for voice quality. A wet or gurgled voice indicates food may be resting on the vocal cords.

During the early stages of feeding, nursing supervision is necessary at meals to prevent or minimize swallowing problems. Patients should be reevaluated on a regular basis to determine whether any changes need to be made in the consistency of fluids or food. Evaluating and documenting the patient's food intake are also prudent to ensure adequate nutritional intake and status. If the patient's nutritional needs are not or cannot be met orally, alternative methods should be considered.[8]

For patients with dysphagia, mealtime can be made safe and nutritious, but it may be difficult to make eating the pleasure it once was. The one thing nursing personnel can do to make sure meals are as relaxing as possible is to let patients eat at their own pace. Patience on the part of nursing staff may be rewarded with patients who eat with minimal difficulty while maintaining their nutritional status.

✺ GASTROESOPHAGEAL REFLUX DISEASE, HIATAL HERNIA, AND ESOPHAGITIS

More commonly known as *heartburn*, gastroesophageal reflux disease (GERD) is a common experience for some people. In fact, some consider it a normal state of being and never report the symptoms to their physicians. The reflux usually takes place within 1 to 4 hours after a meal.[11,12]

Normally, the lower esophageal sphincter (LES) prevents stomach contents from entering the esophagus, but various factors often decrease sphincter pressure (Box 17-2 and Figure 17-3). Unlike gastric mucosa, esophageal mucosa can be damaged when exposed to gastric contents. If not treated, GERD can result in esophagitis. The reflux is thought to be aggravated by reclining after eating, stress, and increased intraabdominal pressure. Increased intraabdominal pressure can occur with coughing, straining, bending, vomiting, obesity, pregnancy, trauma, ascites, tightly fitting clothing around the waist, lifting heavy objects, and exercising strenuously.[13] Older patients often experience respiratory symptoms of GERD, such as pneumonitis,[13] chronic bronchitis, or asthma.[14,15]

GERD is treated medically by reducing intraabdominal pressure and gastric acid production. Medical management can be divided into five stages (Box 17-3). Stages 1 to 4 entail medical management, and stage 5 involves surgical intervention.[16]

gastroesophageal reflux disease (GERD)
return of gastric contents into the esophagus that results in a severe burning sensation under the sternum

esophagitis
inflammation of the lower esophagus

✺ Box 17-2 Causes of Lowered Esophageal Sphincter (LES) Pressure

- Increased levels of progesterone caused by pregnancy, oral contraceptives containing progesterone, late stages of the menstrual cycle
- Hiatal hernia (see Figure 17-3)
- Foods: chocolate, alcohol, mint, carbonated beverages, citrus fruits and juices, tomato-based products, caffeinated products, peppermint
- Smoking

---

hiatal hernia
herniation of a portion of the stomach into the chest through the esophageal hiatus of the diaphragm

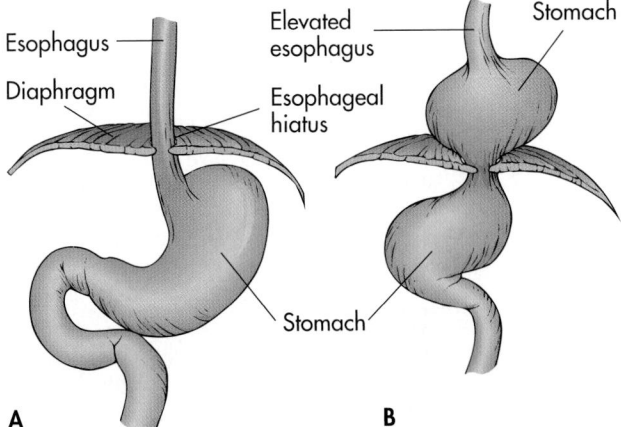

Figure 17-3 **A,** Normal stomach placement, compared with, **B,** hiatal hernia. (From Rolin Graphics).

Medical Nutrition Therapy

Because eating habits as well as the type of foods eaten can contribute to excess gas production, a thorough appraisal of the patient's usual eating pattern and habits is necessary. Specific treatment depends on the source of the gas. Gas-forming foods can be avoided on a trial basis to determine if they are a source of discomfort. Remaining upright for 30 minutes after meals may also be beneficial.

✳ CONSTIPATION

Constipation is a symptom, not a disease.[34] There can be many different causes of constipation. Organic causes include intestinal obstruction, spasms of the sigmoid colon, diverticulitis, and tumors. The most common cause of functional constipation is failure to respond to the urge to defecate. Other functional causes include lack of fiber or fluid, prolonged bed rest or lack of regular exercise, or habitual use of laxatives or enemas. When these conditions are untreated, the colon becomes atonic.[25] Many women experience constipation during the last trimester of pregnancy as the growing fetus impairs the passage of feces.

atonic
lacking normal muscle tone

If constipation becomes severe, bowel movements may diminish in frequency to only once every week or so. This allows tremendous quantities of fecal material to accumulate in the colon, causing its diameter to distend to a diameter as great as 3 to 4 inches. This condition, megacolon, can occur because of a number of reasons. Congenital megacolon (also called *Hirschsprung's disease*) is the result of lack or deficiency of autonomic ganglion cells in the smooth muscle wall of the colon.[25,35] Consequently, neither defecation reflexes nor peristaltic motility can occur through this area of the large intestine.[25] Toxic megacolon is a complication of ulcerative colitis and may result in perforation of the colon, leading to septicemia and death. The most common treatment for congenital and toxic megacolon is surgery.[35] Acquired megacolon results from chronic refusal to defecate, with the colon becoming dilated and impacted with feces. Laxatives and enemas are often the necessary treatment.[35]

megacolon
massive, abnormal dilation of the colon that may be congenital, toxic, or acquired in nature

Medical Nutrition Therapy

Although laxatives are commonly chosen for self-treatment, diet is usually the treatment of choice for constipation. Recommendations include consuming adequate fluids and a wide variety of foods that contain ample amounts of fiber (see Table 17-4). Fiber is important in providing bulk in the diet, which stimulates peristalsis. Care should be taken to increase fiber in the diet gradually to avoid any potential adverse reactions. Although dietary fiber cannot be digested by humans, it can be broken down by bacteria that live in our intestine. Therefore flatulence and osmotic diarrhea may result.

osmotic diarrhea
diarrhea-associated water retention in the large intestine resulting from an accumulation of nonabsorbable water-soluble solutes

Some foods high in fiber are also high in phytates and oxalate, which decrease the bioavailability of certain vitamins and minerals, namely calcium, copper, selenium, zinc, iron, and magnesium.[2] However, nutrient deficiencies are unlikely to occur if an adequate balanced diet from a variety of foods is consumed. The body may adjust to the decreased availability of nutrients by increased absorption of those that are available.[2]

Corpulent amounts of fiber, particularly wheat bran, may result in the formation of bezoars in some persons. This tends to occur more commonly in persons who have diabetes and who suffer from gastroparesis.[2] (See Chapter 19 for more information about gastroparesis.)

bezoars
physical obstacles created by tangles of fibrous material in the GI tract that may cause dangerous GI obstructions

DIARRHEA

Diarrhea (like constipation) is a symptom, not a disease. It is usually categorized in one of two ways: acute or chronic. Treatment is determined by cause. Acute diarrhea is typically of short duration and is usually the result of enteritis. Box 2-6 lists

enteritis
infection of the small intestine caused by a virus, bacteria, or protozoa

common food-borne pathogens that may cause diarrhea. Other causes of acute diarrhea include the intended effect or side effects of medications, change in dietary habits or intake, or emotional stress. Diarrhea that lasts longer than 2 weeks is considered chronic. Long-term diarrhea is usually the result of GI irritation or malabsorption. Both may necessitate permanent dietary changes. Chronic, persistent diarrhea may signify a more serious disease and should be evaluated by a physician.

Medical Nutrition Therapy

Medical nutrition therapy is based on the cause of diarrhea. In severe cases, the patient may be restricted to nothing by mouth to allow the GI tract to rest; however, it is usually unnecessary to withhold all feedings. Administration of fluids to achieve or maintain hydration is a primary concern. This may be done with enteral or parenteral fluids (carbohydrate and electrolytes). Enteral therapy may consist of oral rehydration solutions or a clear liquid diet for 1 or 2 days before progressing to a low-fat, low-fiber, or low-lactose diet. Small, frequent meals are often better tolerated than three larger meals. After 2 or 3 days, progression to a general or normal diet is usually tolerated.[18] It is also important to educate the patient regarding cause and prevention of subsequent incidences of diarrhea.[18]

SUMMARY

Disorders of the GI tract include those that affect the esophagus, stomach, small intestine, and large intestine. Some disorders affect the muscular action of these sections of the GI tract, thereby affecting flow of sustenance through the GI tract; these include dysphagia and hiatal hernia. Other disorders, such as peptic ulcer and diverticulitis, lead to site-specific tissue inflammation and pain. Several disorders may be caused by inability of the body to produce necessary digestive enzymes (e.g., lactase in lactose intolerance) or inability to metabolize nutrient substances (e.g., gliadin, resulting in severe reactions caused by celiac disease). Most disorders are also influenced by lifestyle behaviors that affect stress levels and alter dietary patterns. All GI disorders require some level of medical nutritional therapy that is individualized to meet the needs of each patient.

THE NURSING APPROACH
Impaired Swallowing and Weight Loss

Mark, age 62, suffered a stroke 3 months ago. Currently, he has difficulty swallowing foods. He also experienced weakness of the upper arms that progressed to the legs. Now restricted to a bed or chair, he is beginning to have speech difficulties and some respiratory problems. Family members care for Mark and a home health nurse visits three times a week.

ASSESSMENT

Subjective
- Increase in episodes of choking and regurgitation while being fed (recently about two episodes every day)
- Amount of time to chew and swallow food increasing over the past month (increased to 1 hour/meal)

Objective
- Fluid intake: about 800 ml per day
- Height: 5'10"
- Weight: 130 lb with weight loss about 2 lb per month

THE NURSING APPROACH–cont'd
Impaired Swallowing and Weight Loss

NURSING DIAGNOSIS #1

Impaired swallowing related to cranial nerve deficits and weakness of the muscles necessary for swallowing as evidenced by increase in time necessary to chew and swallow and increase in choking episodes

PLANNING

Goal

Mark will experience a decrease in the number of choking episodes to less than one per day within the next 2 weeks.

IMPLEMENTATION

Recommend consultation with speech and swallowing therapist for formal swallowing evaluation. Based on that evaluation, teach Mark and his caregivers the following:
1. Assess his ability to swallow by testing the gag reflex every morning.
2. Position Mark in an upright position (high Fowler's) and maintain position 30 minutes after meals.
3. Provide mouth care before and after meals.
4. Offer foods he prefers and offer a soft diet.
5. Avoid thin fluids; thicken juices and water with gelatin; put ice cream in milk.
6. Do not use liquids to clear solid food from the mouth; remind Mark to swallow food when it remains.
7. Have Mark take a breath before swallowing, hold breath during swallowing, and exhale forcefully after swallowing.
8. Provide reassurance when he experiences choking episodes.

EVALUATION

The achievement of the goal will be evidenced by (depending on swallowing evaluation):
• Fewer choking episodes in the next 2 weeks
• Decreased time (less than 1 hour) to finish his meal

NURSING DIAGNOSIS #2

Altered nutrition, less than body requirements, of fluid and kcalories, related to difficulty swallowing, as evidenced by weight loss and insufficient intake of fluids

PLANNING

Goals

1. Mark will maintain weight at current level.
2. Mark will increase fluid intake to 1000 ml within 2 weeks.

IMPLEMENTATION

1. Use custard, gelatin, and liquid nutritional supplements (two per day) to increase fluid and kcaloric intake between meals.
2. Distribute the fluid intake pattern so that 200 ml is provided with each meal, with the remaining 400 ml between meals and after dinner.
3. Record daily intake and output.
4. Weigh once a week on Mondays at 9 AM on the chair scale.

EVALUATION

The achievement of the goal will be evidenced by:
• A record of 1000 ml daily fluid after 2 weeks
• Weight of 130 lb each week

NOTE: *Periodic swallowing reevaluation recommended; swallowing dysfunction is different for every patient, and appropriate dietary modifications are determined by speech pathologists and dietetic specialists.*

CRITICAL THINKING
Clinical Applications

Theresa, age 35, is admitted with microcytic anemia. Her medical history indicates that she underwent a total gastrectomy 2 years ago to treat bleeding ulcers. On admission she weighs 120 lb and she is 5'9" tall. She has lost 30 lb since the surgery. She has been taking ferrous sulfate and monthly injections of vitamin B_{12}. On admission her laboratory findings are as follows: hemoglobin 8.0 gm/dl; hematocrit 26%; serum albumin 2.7 gm/dl. Her typical dietary intake is as follows:

BREAKFAST

1 egg scrambled in 1 tsp margarine
½ cup cream of wheat with 1 tsp margarine
1 slice white toast with 1 tsp margarine
1 cup black coffee

10 AM

6 saltine crackers
12-oz can diet cola

LUNCH

2 baked chicken wings
1 cup cooked carrots
1 medium boiled red potato
1 medium banana
12-oz diet lemon/lime soda

3 PM

½ bagel with 1 tbsp cream cheese
8-oz chocolate milk

DINNER

1 broiled chicken breast
½ cup steamed broccoli
1 cup hot tea with artificial sweetener

9 PM

6 saltine crackers
1 tbsp peanut butter
1 cup black coffee

1. What are common nutrition problems found in patients who have gastrectomies?
2. Which of these problems were experienced by Theresa?
3. What factors explain iron deficiency anemia that develops after a gastrectomy? What is used to treat this anemia?
4. How do Theresa's laboratory values compare with normal values? What do these values indicate?
5. Why is Theresa receiving monthly injections of vitamin B_{12}? Would you advise her to eat more foods high in B_{12}? Explain your rationale.
6. After reviewing Theresa's usual dietary intake, what food groups and/or nutrients are lacking in her diet?
7. What suggestions would you offer Theresa concerning her dietary habits?
8. Should Theresa continue to consume six smaller meals and snacks? Why or why not?

Web Sites of Interest

Crohn's Disease/Ulcerative Colitis Site
http://qurlyjoe.bu.edu/cduchome.html
This site for individuals, their families, and friends provides information on several digestive diseases including ulcerative bowel disease. The site includes chat rooms, resources, retail items, and pharmaceutical links.

National Digestive Diseases Information Clearinghouse (NDDIC)
www.niddk.nih.gov/health/digest/nddic.htm
This database is sponsored by the National Institute of Digestive Diseases, a division of the NIH's National Institute of Diabetes and Digestive and Kidney Diseases. The health promotion and education materials listed here include many that are not indexed on other databases.

National Institute of Diabetes and Digestive and Kidney Diseases (NIDDK)
www.niddk.nih.gov
Through the NIH, the NIDDK provides this site for patients, the public, health professionals, and researchers that contains information, resources, and related links on digestive diseases, diabetes, kidney and urologic diseases, and nutrition.

References

1. Beyer PL: Gastrointestinal disorders: roles of nutrition and the dietetics practitioner, *J Am Diet Assoc* 98:272, 1998.
2. American Dietetic Association: *Manual of clinical dietetics*, ed 6, Chicago, 2000, American Dietetic Association.
3. Palmer JB, Drennan JC, Baba M: Evaluation and treatment of swallowing impairments, *Am Fam Physician* 61(8):2453, 2000.
4. Spieker MR: Evaluating dysphagia, *Am Fam Physician* 61(12):3639, 2000.
5. Agency for Health Care Policy and Research (AHCPR): *Diagnosis and treatment of swallowing disorders (dysphagia) in acute-care stroke patients,* AHCPR Pub No 99-E023, 1999; http://hstat.nlm.nih.gov/hq/Hquest/screen/DirectAccess/db/14, accessed June 24, 2002.
6. Milazzo LS, Buchard J, Lund DA: The swallowing process: effects of aging and stroke. In Erickson RV, ed.: Medical management of the elderly stroke patient, *Phys Med Rehab* 3:489, 1989.
7. Galvin TJ: Dysphagia: going down and staying down, *Am J Nurs* 101(1):37, 20001.
8. Joanna Brigs Institute for Evidence Based Nursing: Identification and nursing management of dysphagia in adults and neurological impairment, *Best Practice,* Evidence Based Practice Information Sheets for Health Professionals, 4(2):1, 2000.
9. Loustau A, Lee KA: Dealing with the dangers of dysphagia, *Nursing* 15:47, 1985.
10. Kuthlemeier KV, Palmer JB, Rosenberg D: Effect of liquid bolus consistency and delivery method on aspiration and pharyngeal retention in dysphagia patients, *Dysphagia* 16:119, 2001.
11. Orland RC: The pathogenesis of gastroesophageal reflux disease: the relationship between epithelial defense, dysmotility, and acid exposure, *Am J Gastroenterol* 92(suppl4):3S, 1997.
12. Isolauri J et al.: Natural course of gastroesophageal reflux disease: 17-22 year follow-up of 60 patients, *Am J Gastroenterol* 92(1):37, 1997.
13. Swearingen PL, Ross DG: *Manual of medical-surgical nursing,* ed 4, St Louis, 1999, Mosby.
14. Sontag SJ et al.: Effect of positions, eating and bronchodilators on gastroesophageal reflux in asthmatics, *Dig Dis Sci* 35:849, 1990.
15. Mansfield LE: Gastroesophageal reflux and respiratory disorders: a review, *Ann Allergy* 62:158, 1989.
16. Scott M, Gelhot AR: Gastroesophageal reflux disease: diagnosis and management, *Am Fam Physician* 59(5):1161, 1999.
17. McCance KL, Huether SE: *Pathophysiology: the biological basis for diseases in adults and children,* ed 4, St Louis, 2002, Mosby.
18. *Merck Manual*; www.merck.com/pubs/mmanual, accessed June 23, 2002.
19. Walling AD: Antibiotic treatment of patients with *H. pylori, Am Fam Physician* 61(12):3682, 2000.
20. Meurer LN, Bower DJ: Management of *Helicobacter pylori* infection, *Am Fam Physician* 65(7):1327, 2002.
21. American Gastroenterology Association: *Peptic ulcer disease*; www.gastro.org/public/ulcers.html, accessed June 26, 2002.
22. Kritz FL: Ulcers: what really causes ulcers? *Am Gastroenterol Assoc, Dig Health Nutr*; www.dhn-online.org/free_month_issues/02/ulcers.html, accessed June 26, 2002.
23. Willis J: Gastrointestinal diseases. In Carey CF, Lee HH, Woeltje KF: *The Washington manual of medical therapeutics,* ed 29, Philadelphia, 1998, Lippincott, Williams & Wilkins.
24. Beyer PL: Medical nutrition therapy for upper gastrointestinal tract disorders. In Mahan LK, Escott-Stump S: *Krause's food, nutrition, and diet therapy,* ed 10, Philadelphia, 2000, WB Saunders.
25. Guyton AC: *Textbook of medical physiology,* ed 8, Philadelphia, 1991, WB Saunders.
26. Vecht J, Masclee AA, Lamers CB: The dumping syndrome: current insights into pathophysiology, diagnosis, and treatment, *Scand J Gastroenterol* Suppl 223:21, 1997.
27. Beyer PL: Medical nutrition therapy for lower gastrointestinal tract disorders. In Mahan LK, Escott-Stump S: *Krause's food, nutrition, and diet therapy,* ed 11, Philadelphia, 2003, WB Saunders.
28. Fasano A, Catassi C: Current approaches to diagnosis and treatment of celiac disease: an evolving spectrum. *Gastroenterology* 120:636, 2001.

29. Kuroki F et al.: Multiple vitamin status in Crohn's disease: correlation with disease activity, *Dig Dis Sci* 38(9):1614, 1993.

30. Vogelsang H et al.: Bone disease in vitamin D-deficient patients with Crohn's disease, *Dig Dis Sci* 34(7):1094, 1989.

31. Lashner BA: Red blood cell folate is associated with the development of dysplasia and cancer in ulcerative colitis, *J Cancer Res Clin Oncol* 119(9):549, 1993.

32. Escott-Stump S: *Nutrition and diagnosis related care*, ed 4, Baltimore, 1997, Williams & Wilkins.

33. Wang-Cheng RM: Diverticulosis vs. diverticulitis, *MCW Health Link, 2002*; http://healthlink.mcw.edu/article/1013634026.html, accessed June 24, 2002.

34. Stollman NH, Raskin JB: Diagnosis and management of diverticular disease of the colon in adults, *Am J Gastroenterol* 94(11):3110, 1999.

35. American Gastroenterological Association: *Constipation*; www.gastro/org/public/constipation.html, accessed June 26, 2002.

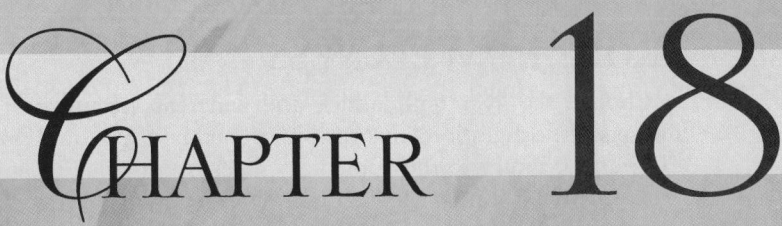

CHAPTER 18

Nutrition for Disorders of the Liver, Gallbladder, and Pancreas

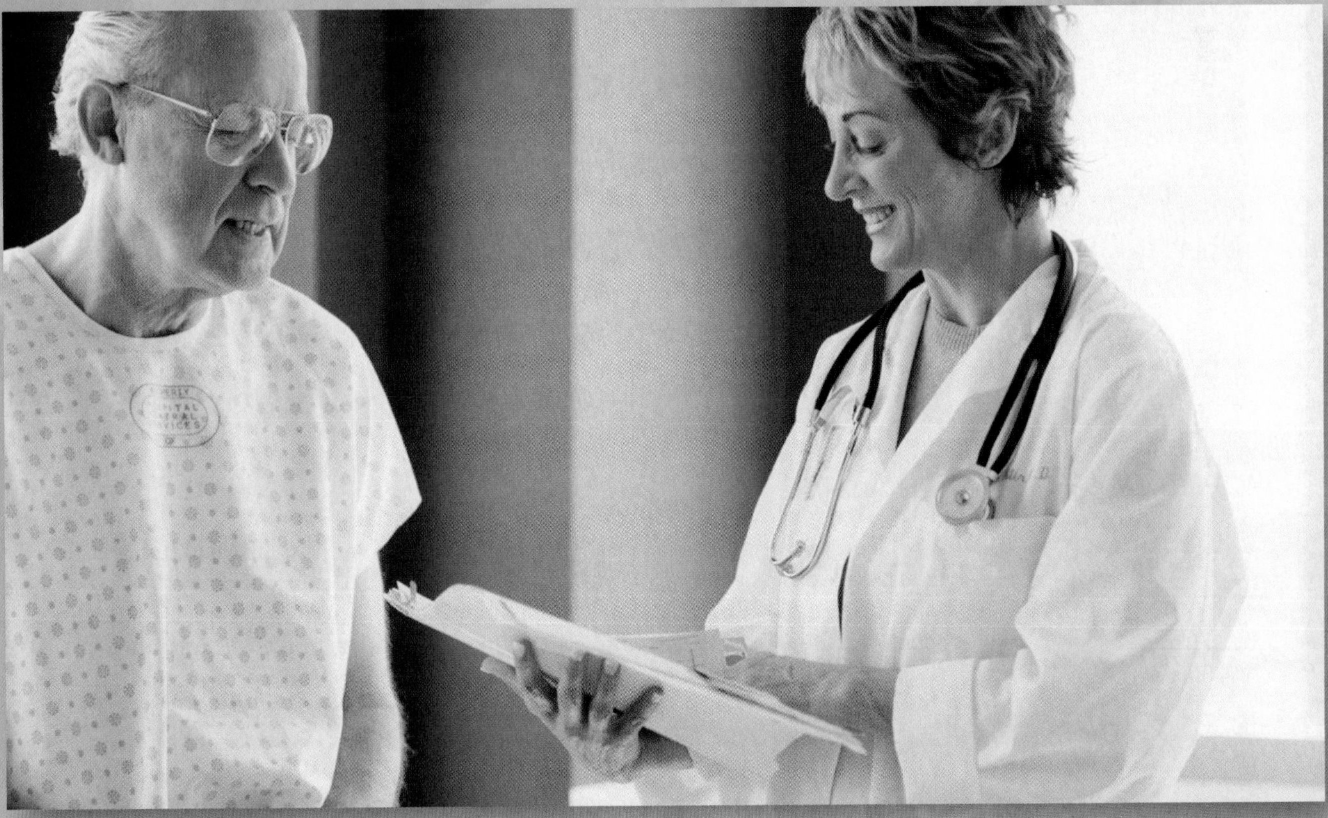

Although the liver, gallbladder, and pancreas are not part of the digestive tract proper, little digestion, absorption, or metabolism would take place without them.

ROLE IN WELLNESS

Although the liver, gallbladder, and pancreas are not part of the digestive tract proper, little digestion, absorption, or metabolism would take place without them. Disease or injury to these ancillary digestive organs can have a devastating effect on nutritional status. Medical nutrition therapy is part of the treatment for disorders of the liver, gallbladder, and pancreas. It is also necessary to prevent nutritional deficiencies because of the role these organs have on digestive functioning.

Wellness requires well-functioning body organs for health to occur. In particular, consider how disorders of the liver, gallbladder, and pancreas affect the five dimensions of health. The physical health dimension is crucially dependent on these organs. As ancillary digestive organs, their malfunctioning can devastate nutritional status. Reasoning skills, an aspect of intellectual health, are required to make lifestyle decisions related to levels of alcohol and fat intake if a person is at risk for cirrhosis or pancreatic disorders. The strain in dealing with chronic life-threatening illness, such as cystic fibrosis (CF), challenges emotional health. Because of the relationship of these disorders to digestive functioning, restrictive dietary guidelines may inhibit the ability to easily socialize with others, thereby limiting social health. The spiritual dimension of health, through religious beliefs, may provide patients with comforting perspectives for coping with serious physical disorders.

LIVER DISORDERS

The liver, the largest organ in the body, lies beneath the diaphragm in the right upper quadrant of the abdomen (Figure 18-1) and is responsible for the majority of biochemical functions that take place in the body. The liver's management of bile production and its role in intermediary metabolism of carbohydrates, protein, lipids, and vitamins influence nutritional status. Thus it is easy to understand that impaired liver function can result in major imbalances in metabolism and nutritional status. As with many other diseases, progressive decline of nutritional status can further impair liver function.[1] Figure 18-1 summarizes only a few of the liver's many roles in metabolism and nutritional status.

Fatty Liver

Fatty liver (also called *hepatic steatosis*) is typically a symptom of an underlying problem. Although it is the earliest form of alcoholic liver disease, it can also be caused by excessive kcaloric intake, obesity, complications of drug therapy (e.g., corticosteroids, tetracyclines), total parenteral nutrition (TPN), pregnancy, diabetes mellitus, inadequate intake of protein (e.g., kwashiorkor), infection, or malignancy.[2-4] Fatty infiltration of the liver develops when triglycerides build up in the liver tissue, which may eventually produce an enlarged liver. This infiltration is a function of improper fat metabolism. It can be reversed if the causative agent is removed.[2] Therefore, if alcohol abuse occurs, then abstinence from alcohol is necessary as part of the treatment and may lead to reversal of the infiltration and prevent further fibrosis or necrosis. Whatever the cause, proper nutrition in the form of a well-balanced diet is important in reversing fatty infiltration.

❋ Viral Hepatitis

Defined as inflammation of the liver, acute hepatitis can occur as the result of infectious mononucleosis, cirrhosis, toxic chemicals, or viral infection. There are five types of hepatitis that have been characterized, and although symptomatology, clinical signs, and presentation are similar, immunologic and epidemiologic characteristics are different (Table 18-1).

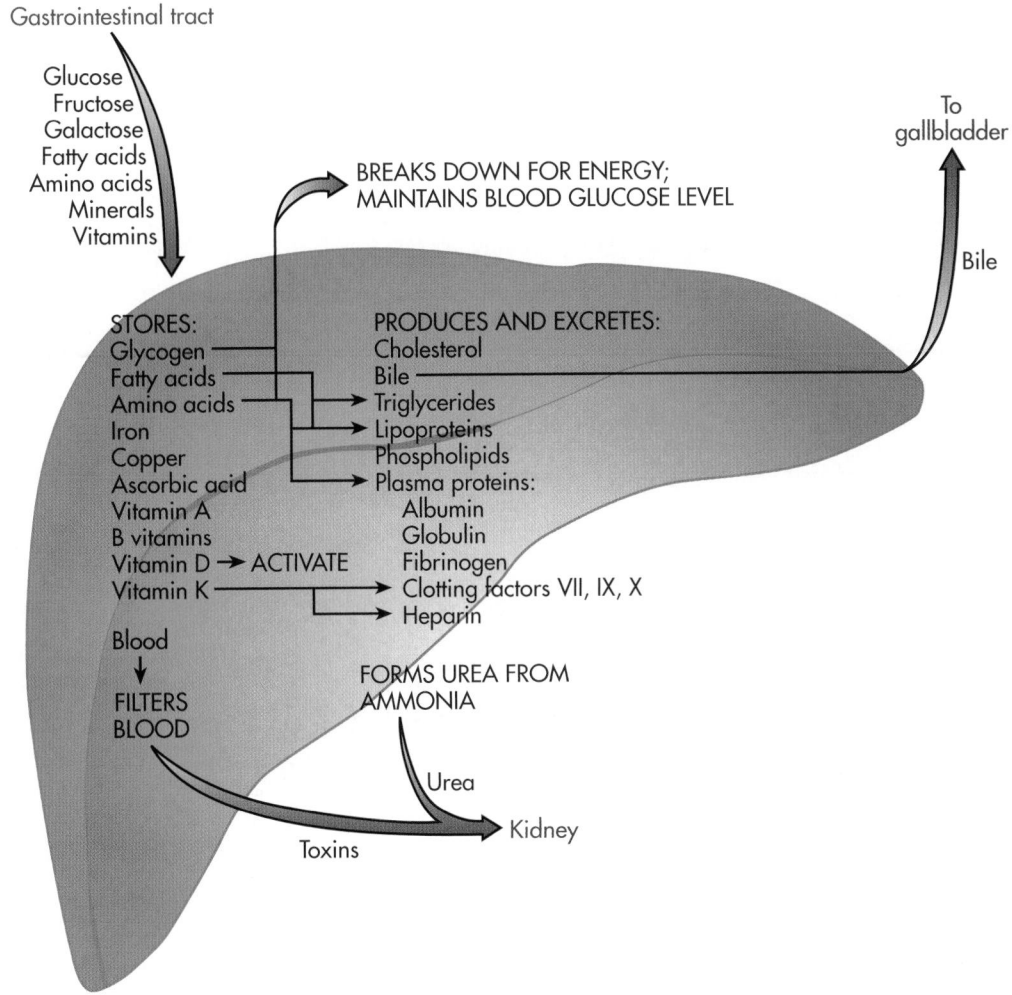

Figure 18-1 Role of the liver in metabolism and nutrition. Any damage to the liver may affect nutritional status. (From Rolin Graphics. Modified from Davis J, Sherer K: *Applied nutrition and diet therapy for nurses*, ed 2, Philadelphia, 1994, WB Saunders.)

Hepatitis A virus (HAV) is typically transmitted through the fecal-oral route (contaminated food or water) but occasionally can be spread by transfusion of infected blood.[5,6] It is frequently the result of poor hand washing or stool precautions and is widespread in overcrowded areas with poor sanitation. Vaccination is recommended for persons at risk for HAV.[7] Onset of HAV is rapid—typically within 4 to 6 weeks[5]—and time to onset of symptoms may be dose related.[8] Occurrence of disease manifestations and severity of symptoms directly correlate with the patient's age.[8] Treatment of acute HAV is generally supportive—usually consisting of bed rest—because no antiviral therapy is available. Hospitalization and intravenous (IV) fluids may be necessary for dehydration caused by nausea and vomiting.[8,9] An adequate diet that excludes alcohol is recommended.[8]

Hepatitis B virus (HBV) is an exceptionally resistant virus capable of surviving extreme temperatures and humidity.[9,10] HBV is transmitted via blood and sexual contact.[9,10] Globally, the vast majority of cases are transmitted perinatally.[9] (See the Cultural Considerations box for information about the prevalence of HBV among ethnic groups.) HBV transmits more easily than the human immunodeficiency virus (HIV) or hepatitis C, with the virus readily found in serum, semen, vaginal mucus, saliva, and tears. IV drug users, patients with hemophilia, those on renal dialysis, and those who have undergone organ transplants are at increased risk for

RISK FACTORS FOR HEPATITIS A VIRUS[7]

- Travelers to areas where HAV is common

- Homosexual men

- Sexual contact with infected persons

- Use of injectable and noninjectable drugs

- Household contact with infected persons

- Healthcare and public safety workers

- Persons, especially children, living in regions of the United States that have consistently increased rates of HAV

Table 18-1
Comparison of Hepatitis Viruses

	Hepatitis A (HAV)	Hepatitis B (HBV)	Hepatitis C (HCV)	Hepatitis D (HDV)	Hepatitis E (HEV)
Likely mode of transmission	Fecal-oral, foodborne, sexual, ingestion of contaminated food or water, parenteral (rare)	Parenteral, sexual, perinatal (rare)	Blood or serum; sharing of contaminated needles, razors, toothbrushes, nail files, barber's scissors, tattooing equipment, body piercing, or acupuncture needles	Develops in those coinfected with both HBV and HDV; parenteral, sexual	Fecal-oral, food-borne, waterborne (contaminated drinking water)
Symptoms	Jaundice, low-grade fever (<101° F), malaise, anorexia, dark urine, diarrhea, pale stools	Same symptoms as HAV plus presence of HbsAg in serum	Same as HAV and HBV; majority are asymptomatic	Same as HBV; many infected individuals are asymptomatic	Jaundice, flulike aches and pains
Population most often affected	Can affect anyone. Children; those living in or traveling to areas with poor sanitation	Persons who inject drugs, healthcare and public safety workers exposed to blood, homosexual men, persons with multiple sexual partners, hemodialysis patients, staff of institutions for the developmentally disabled	Persons who inject drugs, those who have received blood products before 1991, potential risk for healthcare and public safety workers exposed to blood, persons with high-risk sexual activity, perinatal	Drug addicts, hemophiliacs, persons living in developing countries, persons with HBV	People living in or traveling to parts of Asia, Africa, or Mexico where sanitation is poor
Means to reduce exposure	Hand washing, good personal hygiene, sanitation, appropriate infection control measures	Hand washing, good personal hygiene, appropriate infection control measures, safe-sex practices	Same as HBV	HBV-HDV coinfection; pre- or postexposure prophylaxis; education to reduce risk behaviors	Same as HAV; avoid drinking water of unknown purity, avoid uncooked shellfish
Treatment	Antipyretics; most recover without treatment	Interferon, ribavirin, liver transplant	Interferon alfa, ribavirin, liver transplant	Interferon alfa	None available

Modified from Nelms MN, Anderson SL: Medical nutrition therapy: a case study approach, Belmont, Calif, 2002, Wadsworth/Thomson Learning.

HBV. As a result, routine HBV vaccination is recommended for risk groups of all ages and for children up to age 18.[11] Average incubation time of HBV is approximately 12 weeks.[9,10] As with HAV, the majority of patients are asymptomatic.[10] Those who acquire chronic HBV infection (determined by biopsy) can be healthy, asymptomatic carriers but remain infectious to others through parenteral or sexual transmission.[9] As with acute HAV, no well-established antiviral treatment is available for acute HBV infection.[9] Chronic HBV is treated with interferon alfa and lamivudine to reduce symptoms and prevent or delay progression of chronic hepatitis to cirrhosis or hepatocellular carcinoma (HCC).[9,10] An adequate diet that excludes alcohol is recommended for patients with acute and chronic HBV without cirrhosis.[10]

Hepatitis C virus (HCV) (previously called *non-A, non-B hepatitis*) infection is increasing worldwide and is the major cause of hepatitis in the United States.[12] It is transmitted through contaminated blood, saliva, or semen, although HCV is predominately associated with blood exposure (e.g., transfusion, IV drug use,[4] acupuncture, tattooing, and sharing razors).[13] Onset is usually slow (i.e., approximately 8 weeks), can develop into some form of chronic liver disease,[6,9,12] and is a risk factor for liver cancer.[5,9] Most cases of acute HCV are asymptomatic; therefore, it is infrequently detected.[7] Chronic infection develops in 70% to 80% of persons infected with HCV.[10] Progression from HCV to cirrhosis may take 10 to 40 years.[9,12] A more rapid disease progression is observed in those infected with HIV or HBV, persons with alcoholism, men, and those who acquired the infection at an older age.[12] Treatment goals include the following:

1. Decrease viral replication or eradicate HCV.
2. Delay fibrosis and progression to cirrhosis.
3. Decrease incidence of HCC.
4. Ameliorate symptoms such as fatigue and joint pain.
5. Prevent hepatic decompensation and obviate liver transplantation.[9,12]

Chronic HCV is treated with a combination therapy of interferon alfa and ribavirin.[9,12] No special diet is recommended.

Hepatitis D virus (HDV) can only occur if an individual with HBV is subsequently exposed to HDV (coinfection or superinfection).[5,6,13] The incubation period is 21 to 45 days but may be shorter in cases of superinfection.[13] Clinical course varies, ranging from acute, self-limiting infection to acute fulminant liver failure.[13] HDV is found throughout the world but is prevalent in the Mediterranean basin,

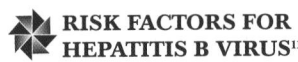

RISK FACTORS FOR HEPATITIS B VIRUS[11]

- Persons with multiple sex partners or partners diagnosed with a sexually transmitted disease
- Homosexual men
- Sexual contact with infected persons
- Use of injectable drugs
- Household contact with chronically infected persons
- Infants born to infected mothers
- Infants and children of immigrants from areas with high rates of HBV infection
- Healthcare and public safety workers
- Patients receiving hemodialysis treatments

CULTURAL CONSIDERATIONS
Hepatitis B Virus Prevalence Rates

Hepatitis B virus (HBV) prevalence rates among Asian/Pacific Islanders are the highest of any racial or ethnic group. In China, 90% of people are exposed to the hepatitis virus and 10% are carriers of HBV.

About 50% of women who deliver infants who carry HBV in the United States are foreign-born Asian/Pacific Islanders. Similarly, 85% of men and 60% of women in Korea are exposed to HBV. HBV is a major risk factor for chronic cirrhosis and liver cancer and accounts for up to 80% of liver cancers. The mortality from liver cancer is five times higher among Chinese Americans.

Currently, there are two medications used for immunoprophylaxis against HBV: hepatitis B immunoglobulin (HBIG), which provides passive immunization, and the hepatitis B vaccine. *Healthy People 2010* recommends that by 2010 HBV transmission be reduced through the implementation of vaccination programs targeted to adolescents and adults of high-risk groups.

Application to nursing: Nurses working with clients who are at high risk for HBV can advocate for hepatitis B vaccinations for these individuals. These clients may include foreign-born individuals, individuals with alternative sexual orientation, persons with histories of current or past drug abuse, and persons exposed to or already diagnosed with HIV.

Reference: Tong M: The impact of hepatitis B infection in Asian Americans, Asian Am Pac Islander J Health 4(1-3):125, 1996.

fatty infiltration
accumulation of fat (triglycerides) in the liver

alcoholic cirrhosis
associated with chronic alcohol abuse; accounts for 50% of all cases; also called Laënnec's cirrhosis

postnecrotic cirrhosis
associated with history of viral hepatitis, improperly treated hepatitis, or hepatic damage from toxic chemicals; accounts for about 20% of all cases

biliary cirrhosis
associated with obstruction of biliary drainage or biliary disorders; accounts for 15% of all cases

Wilson's disease
a rare, inherited disorder of copper metabolism in which copper accumulates slowly in the liver and is then released and taken up in other parts of the body; as copper accumulates in red blood cells, hemolysis and hemolytic anemia occur

hemochromatosis
a rare disease of iron metabolism characterized by excess iron deposits throughout the body

hepatotoxic
potentially destructive to liver cells

portal hypertension
increased blood pressure in the portal circulation caused by compression or occlusion in the portal or hepatic vascular system

esophageal varices
large and swollen veins at the lower end of the esophagus that are especially vulnerable to ulceration and hemorrhage, usually the result of portal hypertension

Middle East, Amazon Basin, Samoa, China, Japan, Taiwan, and Myanmar (formerly Burma).[5,6,13] Of those infected with HDV, 90% are likely to be asymptomatic.[13] Parenteral transmission is understood to be the most common means of infection,[9,13] making IV drug use a risk factor.[13] Treatment is composed of support for the most part.[13] Patients coinfected with HBV and HDV are less responsive to interferon therapy than patients infected with HBV alone.[9] Diet does not need to be restricted.[13]

Hepatitis E virus (HEV) is an enterically transmitted (oral-fecal route), self-limiting infection.[9,14] Prevalence of HEV in the United States is generally attributed to travel in endemic areas[14] (e.g., South, Southeast, and Central Asia; Africa; Mexico;[9] and India[14]). Predominating factors for transmission include tropical climates, inadequate sanitation, and poor personal hygiene. The incubation period ranges from 15 to 60 days, and symptoms include myalgia, anorexia, nausea/vomiting, weight loss (typically 5 to 10 lbs), dehydration, jaundice, dark urine, and light-colored stools.[14] Therapy should be predominantly preventive. Travelers to endemic areas should avoid drinking water or other beverages that may be contaminated. Uncooked fruits or vegetables should not be eaten. No vaccines are available for HEV.[14] Once infection occurs, therapy is limited to support.[9,14] Patients should receive adequate hydration and electrolyte repletion. Hospitalization may be necessary for those unable to maintain an adequate oral intake.[14]

Medical Nutrition Therapy

Treatment for all types of hepatitis is similar. Because there are no medications to treat hepatitis, bed rest and proper nutrition are the major constituents of therapy. During periods of nausea and vomiting, hydration via IV fluids may be necessary.

Oral feedings should be initiated as soon as possible, beginning with a liquid diet then progressing to small, frequent feedings that are high in kcalories and in high-quality protein, as tolerated. Carbohydrates should provide at least 40% of the kcalories to promote glycogen synthesis and spare protein. Dietary fats should not be limited unless they are not well tolerated (e.g., steatorrhea). Fat plays an important role in providing concentrated kcalories and making food taste better, which is important when trying to get a lot of kcalories into a patient who probably doesn't have an appetite. Fluid intake should be high (2500 to 3000 ml/day) to accommodate the high protein intake unless otherwise contraindicated. Supplementation with a multivitamin that includes vitamin B complex (especially thiamine and vitamin B_{12} because of decreased absorption and hepatic uptake of these vitamins), vitamin K (to normalize bleeding tendency), vitamin C, and zinc for poor appetite is recommended.[15]

Cirrhosis

Cirrhosis is a chronic degenerative disease in which liver cells are replaced by the buildup of fibrous connective tissue and fat infiltration (fatty infiltration) (Figure 18-2). This damage can be the result of a variety of reasons, including the following:
- Alcoholic cirrhosis (see Health Debate box)
- Hepatitis (postnecrotic cirrhosis)
- Biliary cirrhosis disorders
- Chronic autoimmune disease
- Metabolic disorders (Wilson's disease or hemochromatosis)
- Chronic hepatotoxic drug use

Such conditions may cause liver cells to die, and the formation of new cells results in scarring that can cause congestion of hepatic circulation (blood backing up in the portal vein), which results in further decline of liver function, portal hypertension, and esophageal varices.

Esophageal varices are usually the result of collateral circulation that develops around the esophagus when normal blood flow through the liver is blocked

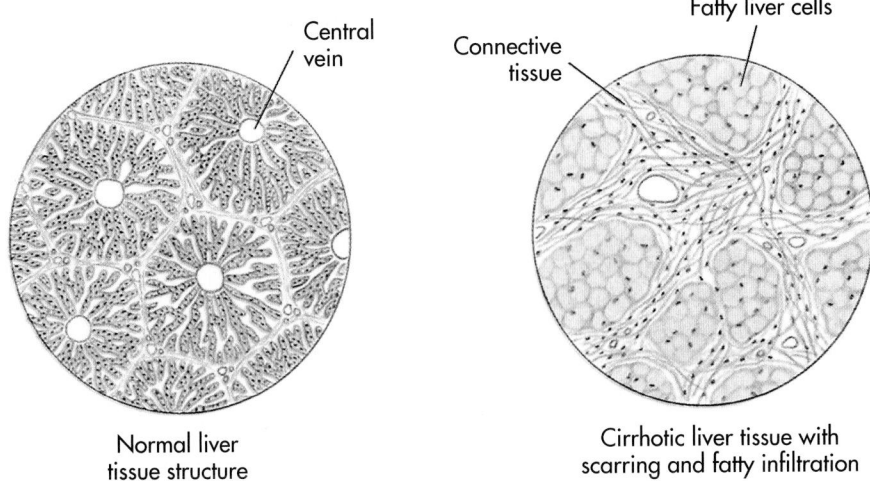

Central
vein

Connective
tissue

Fatty liver cells

Normal liver
tissue structure

Cirrhotic liver tissue with
scarring and fatty infiltration

Figure 18-2 Comparison of normal liver tissue structure with cirrhotic liver tissue changes. (Medical and Scientific Illustration. From Williams SR: *Nutrition and diet therapy*, ed 8, St Louis, 1997, Mosby.)

HEALTH DEBATE
Alcohol: Proscribe or Prescribe?

Alcohol is probably the most commonly used hepatotoxic drug. Next to caffeine, it is probably the most socially acceptable drug in the United States. It is legal, but sales are regulated by state-controlled establishments, and advertising on television is limited. The advertisements we see give us the message that if we would just drink a specific brand of beer or wine we would: (1) be more athletic, (2) learn to "speak Australian," (3) become irresistible to a gorgeous man/woman, (4) hike through the Rocky Mountains, (5) fulfill a deep desire to become an English bulldog with an attitude, and/or (6) pretend we're jet-setters by drinking imported or microbrewed beer.

However, we get negative messages too, and rightly so. Alcohol's link to birth defects and traffic accidents is well recognized. Heavy alcohol intake (three or more drinks* daily) causes damage to the liver (e.g., fatty liver and cirrhosis), brain, and heart and increases the risk of cancer. Could any possible good come from such a drug? The answer seems to be yes.

Current research indicates that alcohol may decrease the risk of heart disease. Several population studies have found a lower coronary artery disease mortality risk among moderate drinkers (defined as one to two drinks daily) as compared with nondrinkers. At first it looked as if red wine was the magic elixir, but white wine, beer, and hard liquor seem to be just as beneficial. On the other hand, it appears the more one drinks, the greater the risk of developing certain cancers. Chronic, heavy drinking is associated with cancers of the mouth, throat, larynx, and liver. Moderate alcohol consumption has been linked to cancers of the breast, colon, and rectum.

So what's a person to do? Don't drink if you: do not currently drink, are pregnant or trying to conceive, are taking medication, driving, or unable to control your drinking. The dangers outweigh any possible benefits. If you're concerned about heart disease and drink small quantities of alcohol every day or every other day, you're probably okay. Remember that alcohol is a drug. And like any drug, it is most effective when administered at the appropriate dosage. It may be beneficial to discuss this matter with your personal physician.

Reference: Goldberg IJ: *To drink or not to drink?* N Engl J Med 348(2): 163, Jan 9, 2003; Mukamal KJ et al.: *Roles of drinking pattern and type of alcohol consumed in coronary heart disease in men.* N Engl J Med 348(2): 109, Jan 9, 2003.
*One drink equals 12 oz of beer, 5 oz of wine, or 1½ oz of hard liquor.

ascites
abnormal intraperitoneal accumulation of fluid containing large amounts of protein and electrolytes, usually resulting in abdominal swelling, hemodilution, edema, or decreased urinary output

third space (or third spacing)
a condition in which fluid shifts from the blood into a body cavity or tissue where it is no longer available as circulating fluid

hepatic encephalopathy
a type of brain damage caused by liver disease and consequent ammonia intoxication

hepatic coma
neuropsychiatric symptom of extensive liver damage caused by chronic or acute liver disease

(Figure 18-3). Blood vessels tend to enlarge and bulge into the lumen of the esophagus where they may rupture. This bleeding tends to recur and can eventually be fatal. Patients with esophageal varices should eat soft, low-fiber foods. Another complication of cirrhosis, ascites, is the accumulation of fluid in the peritoneal cavity. Body fluid is trapped in a "third space" from which it cannot escape.[5] This causes the characteristic swollen or distended abdomen often seen in patients with cirrhosis.

To treat patients with ascites, a dietary sodium restriction (2000 mg) is used, sometimes along with a fluid restriction.[13] If diuretics are used, attention should be given to whether the drug depletes or spares potassium. If a potassium-depleting diuretic is used, potassium levels should be monitored.

As liver disease continues to progress, blood is shunted from portal circulation to systemic circulation. This causes blood to bypass the liver and could result in hepatic encephalopathy, which if left untreated can lead to hepatic coma. Hepatic encephalopathy may be best described as a form of "cerebral intoxication" caused by intestinal contents that have not been metabolized by the liver.[6] This results in toxins (e.g., ammonia) not being eliminated from the body, and nutrient metabolism may be compromised. Patients with hepatic encephalopathy

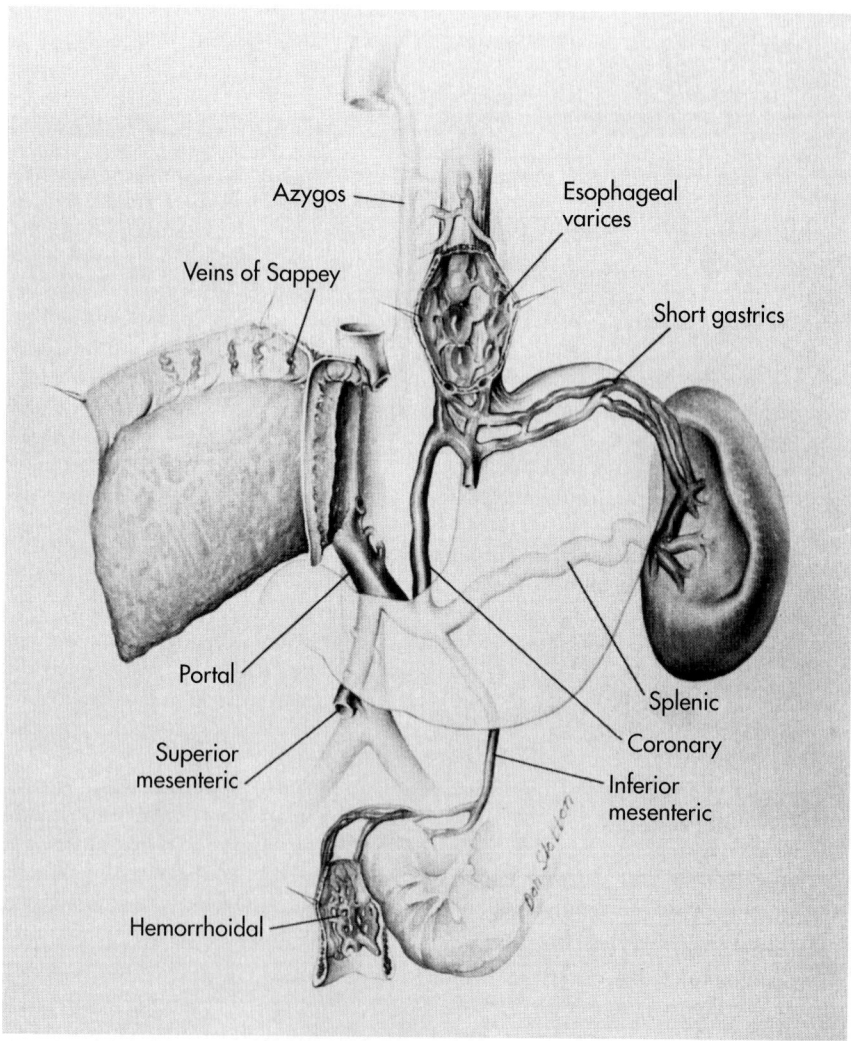

Figure 18-3 Esophageal varices related to portal hypertension. Portal vein, its major tributaries, and the most important shunts (collateral veins) between the portal and caval systems. (From Kissane JM, ed.: *Anderson's pathology,* ed 9, St Louis, 1990, Mosby.)

have been reported to experience changes in consciousness, changes in behavior, loss of concentration and memory, confusion, apathy, personality changes, and other psychiatric symptoms.[2,5,6,16] Neurologic changes include spasticity, muscle spasms, asterixis or flapping (involuntary jerky movements, especially of the hands), **athetoid** postures, and rigidity of the limbs with flexion withdrawal of the lower limbs.[2,15]

Exact cause of encephalopathy has not been identified with certainty,[6] but it probably results from a combination of biochemical alterations that affect neurotransmission.[5] The most hazardous substances appear to be end products of protein metabolism, particularly ammonia.[5]

Several methods are used to lower ammonia levels, but each has potential side effects. Neomycin is an antibiotic used to sterilize the bowel by reducing the numbers of bacteria in the gastrointestinal (GI) tract, thus decreasing the amount of urea that can be converted to ammonia.[5] Neomycin treatment allows more protein to be included in the diet for tissue regeneration. One disadvantage of neomycin use is that it contributes to malabsorption of most nutrients and can cause nausea, vomiting, diarrhea, and nephrotoxicity.[5] Another method is use of lactulose, a nonabsorbable disaccharide that is metabolized by intestinal bacteria resulting in a lower pH stool.[6] The lowered pH traps ammonia in the colon; the ammonia is then excreted. It has a laxative action and diarrhea is common.

Medical Nutrition Therapy

The most important aspect of medical nutrition therapy to keep in mind is that each patient has individual nutritional needs that must be addressed. Protein and energy malnutrition is commonplace in patients with end-stage liver disease who have cirrhosis. A minimum of 0.8 g protein per kg body weight per day is essential. To promote positive nitrogen balance and avert breakdown of endogenous protein stores, 1.2 to 1.5 g protein per kg body weight are recommended. Protein restriction should be avoided, because it could possibly worsen malnutrition.[17-19] If a patient appears to be protein sensitive (e.g., increased occurrence of encephalopathy), branched-chain amino acid-based formulas with restricted aromatic amino acids can be used to ensure a sustained level of protein intake.[17,18] A protein restriction of less than 0.5-g/kg body weight/day may result in endogenous protein breakdown and further nutritional decline.[17]

Energy intake should be high enough to prevent protein (muscle) catabolism and spare dietary protein that might otherwise be used for anabolism. Most patients' protein requirements will be met by 25 to 35 kcal/kg dry weight.[17] However, adjustments must be made for catabolic stress factors such as infection, trauma, surgery, or loss of nutrients (steatorrhea).[17]

Sodium may need to be restricted to 2000 mg if edema or ascites are present.[17,18] Sometimes it is necessary to restrict sodium to as little as 1000 mg per day for patients whose edema and ascites are resistant to diuretic therapy. Diets this low in sodium are restrictive, unpalatable, difficult to comply with, and possibly deficient in calcium.[17]

Fluids are given in relation to input/output records, daily weights, and electrolyte values.[17] Fluid restrictions are often necessary to prevent or decrease ascites formation.[12] Fluid restrictions usually begin at 1500 ml/day and may decrease to 1000 to 1200 ml/day depending on the patient's response. The nurse may provide suggestions on how to cope with thirst in an effort to improve compliance with these kinds of fluid restrictions. Sample suggestions are listed in the Teaching Tool box, "Suggestions for Coping with Fluid Restriction."

Vitamin deficiencies in patients with cirrhosis are common, and often nutrition intake was poor before the onset of liver disorders. If clinical evaluation reveals the presence of deficiencies, water-soluble supplements with emphasis on folate, vitamin B_{12}, and thiamin may be necessary. In addition, fat-soluble vitamins should be given in water-soluble form if steatorrhea is present.[17]

athetoid
purposeless weaving motions of the body or extremities

TEACHING TOOL
Suggestions for Coping with Fluid Restriction

$\mathcal{T}$hese simple yet effective suggestions may help patients cope with fluid restrictions while maintaining personal comfort.

1. Drink to quench thirst only. Avoiding high-sodium foods will result in less thirst. (See Table 8-5 for a list of high-sodium foods.)
2. Try to avoid drinking from habit or to be sociable.
3. Eat ice-cold fruit between meals.
4. Sliced lemon wedges can stimulate saliva and moisten a dry mouth.
5. Keep the mouth clean by brushing teeth frequently and rinsing mouth with water (do not swallow rinse water).
6. Chew gum, suck hard candy (tart or sour is best), or use mints to stimulate saliva flow.
7. Try sucking on ice; most people find it more satisfying than the same amount of water since it stays in the mouth longer.
8. Limit fluids at meal time; when appropriate, take medications with meal time liquids or soft foods like applesauce.
9. Take medications at one time to decrease amount of total fluid needed.
10. Add lemon juice to ice cubes to suck on; you will use fewer because the tartness of the lemon will make your mouth water. Use about half of a lemon per tray of water. Or freeze lemonade into small, individualized popsicles in an ice cube tray.
11. Take small amounts of fluid at one time.
12. If allowable, use high-fat foods to help decrease the desire for fluid with a meal. (Gravies and margarine will moisten foods and make them easier to swallow.)

Modified from Dunning S: Ideas to control fluid, *Bio-Medical Applications of Carbondale, Dialysis Services Division, Carbondale, Ill., 1995, Fresenius Medical Care.*

Liver Transplantation

Once considered experimental, liver transplantation is regarded as an appropriate treatment for end-stage liver disease. Nutritional goals for those awaiting organ transplantation depend on the individual's weight history and current status.[18] Most patients in this condition show some indications of compromised nutritional status and therefore require special attention to nutritional needs.[17,18] It is often difficult to assess nutritional status in patients with liver disorders because many assessment parameters (e.g., body weight, nitrogen balance studies, total lymphocyte count, serum protein levels) are affected by edema, ascites, and hepatic necrosis seen in end-stage liver failure.[17,20-22] Therefore it may be more appropriate to use subjective parameters such as weight changes, appetite, satiety level, taste changes, diet history, and GI symptoms.[17,18] Weight change, however, is more often a reflection of fluid shifts rather than true weight loss. Physical examination findings such as temporal wasting of muscle and wasting of the upper extremities can be helpful to estimate the degree of malnutrition.

Medical Nutrition Therapy

Each phase of the transplant procedure dictates specific nutritional requirements (Table 18-2). The primary objective in pretransplant medical nutrition therapy is to provide enough kcalories and protein to decrease protein catabolism and correct any nutritional deficiencies. The 4 to 8 weeks following surgery—the immediate posttransplant period—require individualization of medical nutrition therapy according to the needs of the patient.[17] Ascites, edema, or excess fluid make using the patient's actual weight unreliable for determining kcalories and protein needs. Ideal (desirable) weight is a better reference point. Adequate kcalories and protein are necessary for the hypercatabolic (but not necessarily hypermetabolic) stresses

Table 18-2
Nutrition Care Guidelines for Liver Transplant

	Pretransplant	Posttransplant	Long-Term Management
Energy	27-30 kcal/kg or 1.1-1.3 x BEE (if stable) 35-40 kcal/kg or 1.5-1.75 x BEE (if malnourished)	30-35 kcal/kg or 1.2-1.5 x BEE (based on dry weight)	Adjust to maintain desired body weight
Protein	1.0-1.2 g/kg to 1.5 g/kg	1.2-2 g/kg	1 g/kg
Vitamins		400-800 IU vitamin D	400 IU vitamin D
Minerals		Calcium supplementation in form of carbonate or citrate salt should begin immediately posttransplant with daily goals of 1500-2000 mg/d (food and supplements)	1000-1500 mg

Reference: American Dietetic Association: Manual of clinical dietetics, ed 6, Chicago, 2000, American Dietetic Association.
BEE, Basal energy expenditure; IU, International Units.

that result from surgery and high doses of glucocorticoids.[17] Total parenteral nutrition may be necessary if nutritional needs cannot be met enterally (feeding by mouth and/or with nasoenteric feeding).[17] When oral intake is initiated, early satiety and altered tastes may prevent adequate intake. In such cases, between-meal feedings or supplements should be used to meet kcalorie and protein goals.

For the long-term posttransplant patient, a healthy, well-balanced diet is the nutrition goal. Because of common posttransplantation complications (e.g., excessive weight gain, hypertension, hyperlipidemia, diabetes), adjustments in kcalories, fat, and concentrated carbohydrates may be necessary.[17]

❊ GALLBLADDER DISORDERS

The gallbladder lies directly beneath the right lobe of the liver, and, along with the hepatic, cystic, and common bile ducts, composes the biliary system (Figure 18-4). Bile is transported from the liver to the gallbladder via the common hepatic duct system where it is concentrated and stored until released into the duodenum to expedite absorption of fats, fat-soluble vitamins, and certain minerals and to activate release of pancreatic enzymes. The most common disorders of the gallbladder include cholelithiasis, choledocholithiasis, and cholecystitis.

One of the main constituents of bile is cholesterol, which is also a major constituent of gallstones. The amount of cholesterol in bile is determined in part by the amount of dietary fat consumed.[2,3] As might be expected, chronic intake of high-fat foods increases risk of developing cholelithiasis (Figure 18-5). Gallstones are commonly found in women who are multiparous, on estrogen therapy, or use oral contraceptives; obese individuals; those with sedentary lifestyles; those who have experienced rapid weight loss; and the aged.[23] Other predisposing conditions

cholelithiasis
presence of stones in the gallbladder

choledocholithiasis
gallstones in the common bile duct

cholecystitis
acute inflammation of the gallbladder associated with pain, tenderness, and fever

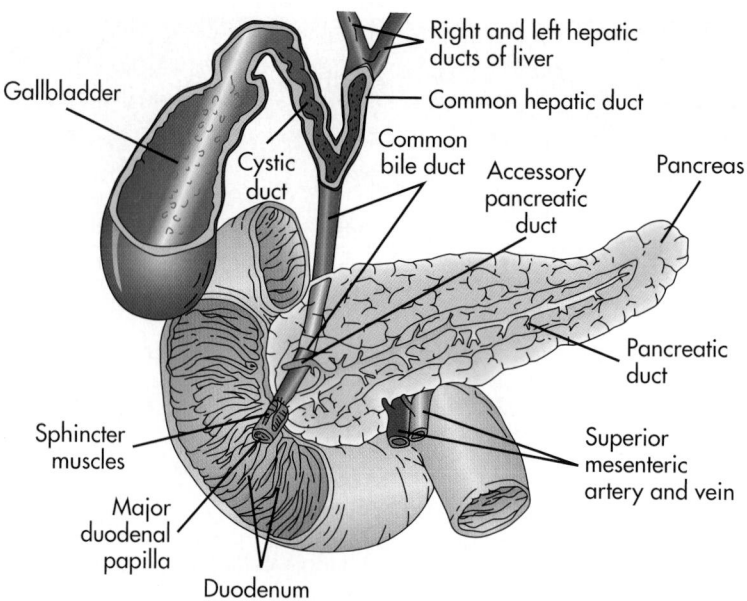

Figure 18-4 Gallbladder and bile ducts. Obstruction of either the hepatic or the common bile duct by stone or spasm prevents bile from being ejected into the duodenum. (From Rolin Graphics.)

very low-calorie diets (VLCDs)
usually defined as diets containing 800 kcalories per day or less

colic
sharp visceral pain

to the development of gallstones are diabetes mellitus, regional enteritis, and familial tendencies[6] (Box 18-1).

An interesting phenomenon is that people who lose a great deal of weight rapidly (e.g., through very low-calorie diets [VLCDs] and some commercial weight-loss programs) are at a greater risk for developing gallstones than obese persons. In fact, gallstones are one of the most medically significant complications of voluntary weight loss.[20,21] Dieting may cause a shift in the balance of bile salts and cholesterol in the gallbladder. Cholesterol level is increased and the amount of bile salts is decreased. Following a diet too low in fat or going for long periods without eating (e.g., skipping breakfast), a common practice among dieters, may also decrease gallbladder contractions. If the gallbladder does not contract often enough to empty out the bile, gallstones may form.[24] Persons considering losing a significant amount of weight should see a physician to evaluate their medical history, individual circumstances, and the proposed method of weight loss.

If cholelithiasis is asymptomatic, no specific therapy is necessary.[25] Symptoms usually manifest after eating, especially a high-fat meal, and include a mild, aching pain in the midepigastrium that may increase in intensity during a colic attack. The pain may radiate to the right upper quadrant and right subscapular region. Nausea, vomiting, tachycardia, and diaphoresis may also be present.[26]

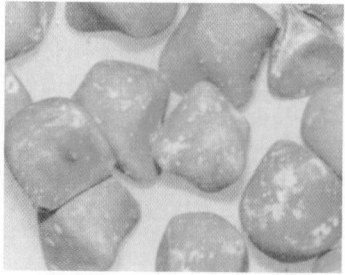

Figure 18-5 Gallstones. (From Stevens A, Lowe J: *Pathology*, London, 1995, Mosby.)

Box 18-1 Suggested Risk Factors in Gallbladder Disease

Advanced age
Gender (female)
Obesity with high-fat intake
Hormonal imbalance (estrogen, progestin, insulin)

Certain drugs (oral contraceptives, clofibrate, cholestyramine)
Enzyme defects
Very low-kcalorie diets (medically supervised VLCDs used for weight loss)

Reference: Escott-Stump S: Nutrition and diagnosis-related care, ed 4, Baltimore, 1998, Lippincott Williams & Wilkins.

Cholecystitis occurs when gallstones block the cystic duct or as the result of stasis, bacterial infection, or ischemia of the gallbladder. This inflammation is associated with pain, tenderness, and fever. Fat intolerance may manifest as regurgitation, flatulence, belching, epigastric heaviness, indigestion, heartburn, chronic upper abdominal pain, and nausea. Jaundice and steatorrhea may also be present.[5] Recommended therapy for symptomatic cholelithiasis and cholecystitis is surgical removal of the gallbladder (cholecystectomy).

cholecystectomy
surgical removal of the gallbladder, performed to treat cholelithiasis and cholecystitis

Medical Nutrition Therapy

Because cholelithiasis and cholecystitis usually produce rather painful symptoms, the main objective of nutritional care is to decrease the patient's discomfort. Most patients become acutely aware of foods that cause discomfort and thus avoid these foods. Low-fat diets are traditionally used to treat cholecystitis. During an acute attack, the hospitalized patient may receive IV fluids with nothing orally. Avoidance of fatty foods is often advised, but no good evidence supports this recommendation.[27]

Chronic cholecystitis with inflammation is usually treated with a fat-restricted diet. Individual food intolerances vary widely, but many complain of foods that cause flatulence and bloating.[25]

Following cholecystectomy, bile enters the small intestine continually rather than in response to food in the GI tract. Immediately after an open laparotomy cholecystectomy, patients may receive nothing orally or receive clear liquids until they can tolerate a regular diet. Some patients need to follow a low-fat diet for several weeks after surgery. Total amount of fat in the diet is more important than the type of fat consumed. Following a laparoscopic cholecystectomy, patients may be on a regular diet immediately after surgery.

PANCREATITIS

In addition to hormonal functions, the pancreas secretes enzymes necessary for protein, carbohydrate, and fat digestion. The pancreas also secretes sodium bicarbonate to neutralize acidic gastric contents as they enter the duodenum, which provides the optimal pH for the activation of these enzymes.

Pancreatitis is an inflammatory process characterized by decreased production of digestive enzymes and bicarbonate and malabsorption of fats and proteins. This acute inflammation causes blood vessels that supply the pancreas to become exceptionally permeable and leak fluid and plasma proteins into spaces between pancreatic cells, causing localized edema and damage. Pancreatic enzymes are ordinarily secreted into the intestinal lumen where they are activated. However, if the pancreas is damaged, the enzymes are retained and activated within the pancreas, resulting in autodigestion and severe pain.[5,6] When the enzymes amylase and lipase cannot be secreted into the intestine, they enter the bloodstream and levels can become high. In fact, elevated levels of serum amylase are an indication of pancreatitis. In addition to severe pain, patients with pancreatitis often experience nausea and vomiting.[6]

Acute pancreatitis is most commonly caused by excessive alcohol consumption and gallbladder disease.[3] Chronic pancreatitis is usually associated with chronic alcohol consumption and is characterized by chronic pain and exocrine and endocrine insufficiency.[3] Diabetes mellitus can occur as the result of chronic pancreatitis if beta cells are damaged, thus decreasing insulin production.[5]

pancreatitis
inflammation of the pancreas; may be acute or chronic

beta cells
insulin-producing cells situated in the islets of Langerhans of the pancreas

Medical Nutrition Therapy

The primary goal is to provide for the patient's nutritional needs while minimizing pancreatic secretions.[28,29] This may be accomplished with either enteral or parenteral nutrition, although enteral nutrition is generally not used until pain is controlled, GI symptoms have abated, and inflammation has resolved.[28,29] Because malabsorption of fats and protein and severe weight loss are benchmarks of chronic pancreatitis, most patients are malnourished when diagnosed. This factor is the reason to initiate nutritional support as soon as possible.

When enteral feeding is appropriate, low-fat, elemental formulas are recommended because they tend to reduce pancreatic stimulation.[28] Feeding into the lower small bowel, in the jejunum distal to the ligament of Treitz, allows for areas associated with pancreatic stimulation to be bypassed.[25] Patients receiving enteral feedings should be closely monitored for increases in pancreatic enzymes, abdominal pain, or discomfort. Enteral feedings should be terminated if any of these symptoms occur.[28]

The American Society of Parenteral and Enteral Nutrition (ASPEN) guidelines recommend use of parenteral support when enteral feedings exacerbate abdominal pain.[30] Peripheral parenteral nutrition can be used for nonstressed patients who are expected to receive nothing by mouth for less than 10 days. Central parenteral nutrition may be necessary if the patient will receive nothing by mouth for longer than 5 to 7 days.[28]

Whatever feeding route is chosen, the patient must receive adequate energy and nutrients based on the severity of the pancreatitis. Restricting fat to less than 50 grams per day typically prevents symptoms of steatorrhea. A medium-chain triglyceride product such as MCT oil may be used to increase kcalories if needed. The rest of the kcalories should come from protein (at least 1.5 g protein/day) and carbohydrates. Because patients are usually anorectic, providing meals in six feedings daily may facilitate adequate nutritional intake. In some cases, replacement pancreatic enzymes are taken orally with meals to control maldigestion and malabsorption. Complete abstinence from alcohol is essential but often difficult to achieve.

✦ CYSTIC FIBROSIS

Cystic fibrosis (CF) is an autosomal recessive inherited disease of the mucus-producing exocrine glands that is characterized by high levels of sodium and chloride in saliva and tears; high levels of electrolytes in sweat; and highly viscous secretions in the pancreas, bronchi, bile ducts, and small intestine that may be obstructive.[5] CF occurs in about 1 of every 3300 live births of Caucasian infants and 1 in every 15,300 non-Caucasian births.[31] Average life span has been increasing from approximately 24 years up to 30 to 40 years.[31] Physical signs such as growth retardation, failure to gain weight, abdominal protuberance, lack of subcutaneous fat, and poor muscle tone are common findings.[32,33] Frequent pulmonary infections, pancreatic insufficiency, and GI malabsorption put individuals with CF at great nutritional risk.[33] Death most often results from malnutrition, bronchopneumonia, lung collapse, and cor pulmonale.[15] Box 18-2 presents one patient's method of coping with CF.

cor pulmonale
an abnormal cardiac condition characterized by hypertrophy of the right ventricle as a result of hypertension of the pulmonary circulation

Medical Nutrition Therapy

Nutrition is of prime importance in the treatment of CF.[34] Nutritional requirements vary depending on the age of the patient and severity of disease.[35] Poor nutritional status because of undernutrition contributes to poor growth, pulmonary complications, and susceptibility to infection. The primary goal of nutritional therapy for patients with CF is to exceed the Dietary Reference Intakes (DRI) for kcalories and all other nutrients.[36] Dietitians estimate individual energy requirements based on basal metabolic rate, activity level, lung function, and fat absorption. Improvements in pancreatic enzyme replacement therapy now allow higher amounts of dietary fats, which were previously prohibited.[35] Because fat provides such a concentrated source of energy, it does not need to be restricted below 30% to 40% of total kcalories, and pancreatic enzyme replacement therapy can be in-

Box 18-2 Ways of Coping

There are many Web sites for specific disorders. These sites can often reveal another perspective of dealing with illness—the perspective of the patient. By exploring Web sites, we can read about the experiences of patients and their families and sometimes even enter chat rooms. Below is an Internet essay written in 1995 for a college English course by Jeffrey Mason, a person with cystic fibrosis, whose Web site first appeared on Cystic Fibrosis 101 (www3.nbnet.nb.ca/normap/CF.htm). Jeffrey, who was 23 years old, died in 1997 shortly after receiving a double lung transplant, but his words and love of humor live on.

SICK HUMOR AS A METHOD OF COPING

As one who lives daily with the reality of a chronic illness, I have found that seemingly "sick" humor may serve as a means of coping with the spectre of death which looms in my own life. Many professionals also agree that "sick" humor is a natural mechanism in helping people cope with tragedy.

Although many people find it offensive and distasteful, "sick" humor is often an essential part of the coping mechanism when one is faced with situations beyond one's control.

During the winter of 1994, I was very ill, and many of the doctors wondered if I would pull through or not. Several months before, in the fall of 1993, I had had to have what is known as a gastrostomy tube, or G-tube, placed in my stomach. This tube went from the outside of my body, through my abdomen wall and into my stomach. Its purpose was to provide extra nutrition by infusing a formula of high calorie liquid nutrition through the tube at night as I slept.

This was still fairly new to me in February, and I was having a hard time adjusting to it. I was hospitalized for nearly the entire month of February. While I was hospitalized and my parents and friends came to visit me, we decided to come up with a "Top 10" style list of the Top 10 Reasons Why Having Cystic Fibrosis Is Great. We proceeded to come up with more than ten reasons, one of the best being the ability to throw up (through the G-Tube) without opening my mouth! This, indeed, would be considered vulgar or "sick" by many, but for me, it was a real way of helping me deal with the new appendage which was protruding from my stomach.

Another personal example of "sick" humor as a coping mechanism involves the life expectancy of a patient in my condition. Having a relatively "severe" case of the disease, it is known that without a lung transplant in the near future, this disease will progressively choke the life out of me. To cope with such a reality of death, my family and I participate in what we refer to as Dead Jeff Jokes. These basically take the form of, "Jeff, when you die, can I have your. . . ?" where various possessions of mine such as my cassette and compact disc collection or my car are inserted at the end of the sentence. Although this sounds downright mean and nasty, it is, for us, a legitimate way for our family to cope with the gravity of my illness. We have often said, "If you can't laugh at it, what can you do?"

One final personal example of the use of "sick" humor to cope with fears involves a friend of mine named Dottie. Dottie and I were at a meeting of Cystic Fibrosis patients at the home of another friend and patient. During the meeting, we watched a brief segment of the local news in which several Cystic Fibrosis patients, including Dottie, were interviewed. At one point in the segment, the reporter stated, "The average life expectancy of a patient with Cystic Fibrosis is twenty nine. Dottie is twenty six." Immediately following this statement, another patient, a good friend of Dottie's, shouted, "Bye, Dottie!" as if to say that the reporter had just stated that she had but three years left to live. The room burst with laughter, and we still joke about it today. By joking about the reality of the death which surrounds us, we are able to better cope with it and feel we have some semblance of control over it.

Although many people find it outrageous and offensive, "sick" humor offers a very effective and legitimate means of coping with situations that are beyond one's control. Anthropologists, psychologists, and psychiatrists have come to recognize this as a natural means of dealing with tragic and uncontrollable events. In my own life, the "sick" humor which abounds has been an essential element by which I am able to continue to fight the disease which surely seeks to destroy me.

From Mason J: Sick humor as a method of coping, July 6, 1998. (Used with permission of Leon and Diana Mason.)

---

dividualized according to the patient's intake.[35] Although the sodium requirement may be considerably higher for patients with CF, routine sodium supplementation appears unnecessary because the average American diet contains an overabundance of sodium.[35] Multivitamin supplements should be prescribed for all patients with CF.[33] Additional fat-soluble vitamins may be prescribed as well in a water-miscible form if fat malabsorption is severe.

Infants

Pancreatic enzyme replacement therapy should be used along with all types of milk products, including breast milk.[36] Supplemental fat or carbohydrate may be necessary for some infants to increase kcaloric density to more than 20 kcal/oz. Introduction of **beikost** is not different for infants with CF.[36]

beikost (BYE-cost)
supplemental or weaning foods

✿ Children and Adolescents

Nutritional adequacy of the diet, compliance with pancreatic enzymes, and growth patterns should be closely monitored because as the child becomes older and more independent, compliance may become questionable.[33]

Reevaluation of the patient's diet is important to ascertain whether recommendations are adequate to support growth and maintain nutritional status. As changes occur in the disease process and growth continues, nutritional needs will also change. Weight gain, linear growth, and level of pancreatic enzyme replacement therapy should also be closely monitored and assessed during this time.

SUMMARY

The liver, gallbladder, and pancreas are important ancillary digestive organs. Disorders of the liver include hepatitis, an inflammation of the liver, and cirrhosis, a chronic degenerative disease that causes fibrous connective tissue and fat infiltration of the liver. Medical nutrition therapy includes bed rest and proper nutrition for hepatitis and individual nutrition plans for cirrhosis that often restricts protein to ease liver function. Meeting medical nutrition therapy needs while still providing for adequate energy and RDA nutrient levels is challenging. Liver transplants occur as treatment for end-stage liver disease. Medical nutrition therapy involves a variety of dietary plans specific to each phase of the procedure.

Gallbladder disorders include cholelithiasis, choledocholithiasis, and cholecystitis; these disorders are characterized by the formation of gallstones within the gallbladder. Medical nutrition therapy may require low-fat diets, but not all individuals may respond. Chronic cholecystitis with inflammation is usually treated with fat- and kcalorie-controlled diets until surgery. Moderation of fat is often indicated postoperatively.

Pancreatitis affects production of digestive secretions, resulting in malabsorption of dietary fats and protein. In serious cases, medical nutritional therapy tends to require enteral or parenteral nutrition. Regardless of the feeding route, fat intake is restricted.

Cystic fibrosis is an inherited disease of the mucus-producing exocrine glands. Medical nutrition therapy is of prime importance, with the goal to exceed the RDA for kcalories and all other nutrients, necessitating the use of vitamin supplementation.

THE NURSING APPROACH
Case Study: Cirrhosis of the Liver

Henry is seriously ill with cirrhosis of the liver related to chronic hepatitis as a result of contracting hepatitis B. The liver damage is progressive. He has developed severe ascites and mild encephalopathy. He is being treated with diuretics (spironolactone) and lactulose to reduce ammonia levels. His fluids are restricted to 1200 ml per day, and he is to consume a daily diet of 2000 calories, 20 grams of protein, and 1 gram of sodium. However, it is becoming difficult to get Henry to eat all his food.

ASSESSMENT

Subjective

- General malaise
- Weakness
- Muscle pain
- Irritability
- Anorexia
- Thirst
- Nausea and vomiting
- Premorbid weight: 205 lb

THE NURSING APPROACH–cont'd
Case Study: Cirrhosis of the Liver

Objective
- Abdominal distention, ascites
- Peripheral edema, ankles and lower legs
- Jaundice of skin and sclera
- Muscle wasting of upper extremities and thigh
- Body weight: 210 lb
- Dark amber urine
- Laboratory results:
  - *Blood urea nitrogen:* 7 (normal 8-25 mg/dl)
  - *Hematocrit:* 40% (normal 45%-52%)
  - *Albumin:* 3.0 (normal 3.5- 5.0 gm/dL)
  - *Serum liver enzymes:* elevated
- Radiographs show enlargement of the liver

NURSING DIAGNOSIS #1

Altered nutrition, less than body requirements related to anorexia, nausea, and vomiting as evidenced by muscle wasting and loss of true body weight

PLANNING

Goals

1. Provide optimal intake of nutrients and calories to promote liver tissue healing.
2. Experience no further weight loss other than that accounted for by fluid loss (NOTE: every 500 ml of excess fluid loss is equivalent to 1 lb weight loss).

IMPLEMENTATION

1. Plan a diet high in carbohydrates and calories with moderate amounts of fat and protein. Small, frequent meals that the client likes are often preferred.
2. Include high-caloric snacks in consultation with the dietitian.
3. The nurse may ask the family to prepare foods from home. Fried, fatty, dried, and salty foods are to be avoided.
4. Provide supplemental vitamins and liquid feedings, such as Ensure or Ensure Plus.
5. Administer antiemetic medications as prescribed.
6. Remove noxious odors or move unpleasant objects or substances.
7. Record intake and output of foods and fluids.

EVALUATION

The achievement of the goal will be evidenced by the following:
- Henry will comply with increased nutritional intake and maintenance of body weight.

NURSING DIAGNOSIS #2

Fluid volume excess related to increased intraheptic pressure and decreased colloidal osmotic pressure as evidenced by ascites and peripheral edema

PLANNING

Goal

Reduce fluid excess in the body by 1000 ml of fluid.

IMPLEMENTATION

1. Maintain sodium restriction.
2. Restrict fluids to 1200 ml per day (i.e., 300 ml with each meal and 300 ml total between meals).
3. Give ice, hard candy, and lemon wedges as tolerated for thirst.
4. Weigh and measure fluid intake and output.
5. Administer diuretics as prescribed, and monitor side effects.
6. Measure abdominal girth in supine position daily at 10 AM.
7. Teach family members the importance of maintaining fluid restriction.

EVALUATION

The achievement of the goal will be evidenced by the following:
- Henry will lose more than 1000 ml fluid (1 lb) in 1 week

CRITICAL THINKING
Clinical Applications   **?**

Chronic alcohol abuse is usually the cause of chronic liver disease (cirrhosis and hepatic encephalopathy) and chronic pancreatitis. One way to evaluate the risk of alcohol-related liver disease is to assess the pattern, quantity, and duration of alcohol intake; usual dietary intake; and socioeconomic factors affecting eating habits. Data can be collected from the patient or reliable friend or family member and evaluated to determine amount (grams) and the kcaloric value of alcohol consumed. When consumed in large quantities, alcohol can provide the majority of the day's kcaloric intake.

To assess this information, we should review a few basics. Alcohol provides 7 kcalories per gram. The average percent alcohol content (based on weight per volume) of various forms of alcoholic beverages is as follows:

Beer = 4% to 6%
Wine = 9% to 12%
Distilled alcohol (whiskey, rum, gin, or brandy) = 35% to 50%

The concentration of alcohol in distilled beverages (hard liquor) is usually referred to as *proof*. One proof equals 0.5% alcohol, which means that 80-proof tequila contains 40% alcohol. Hard liquor is routinely measured in a jigger or shot, which is 1½ oz or 45 ml.

1. How many grams of alcohol and kcalories would 2 shots of 80-proof tequila provide?
2. What is the best way to obtain information from an individual about his/her alcohol consumption?
3. You obtain the following information from the alcohol intake questionnaire and diet history: Alcohol is consumed 7 days/week at home, work, and bars. A typical day's intake consists of a Bloody Mary (1 cup tomato juice, 2 shots 80-proof vodka) first thing in the morning, followed by 5 cups of black coffee (some at home, some at work). Three more shots of 80-proof vodka are consumed at work. Lunch is usually fast-food double cheeseburger, small fries, and a cup of black coffee. After work, four 12-oz bottles of beer (4% alcohol) and pretzels (about 30) are consumed at the local pub with friends. Dinner at home consists of a lunchmeat sandwich (usually 2 slices white bread, 2 oz bologna, 1 tsp mustard), 10 potato chips, and 2 more 12-oz beers. Total kcalorie intake for the day is approximately 3200 kcal.

How many grams of alcohol are consumed? _____ grams alcohol
How many kcalories are provided by the alcohol? _____ kcal from alcohol
What percent of the kcalories are provided by alcohol? _____ % energy from alcohol

ALCOHOL INTAKE ASSESSMENT TOOL

1. How many days a week do you drink alcoholic beverages?

   Circle number of days:
   0   1   2   3   4   5   6   7

2. Where do you drink?

   Circle all that apply:
   a. at home
   b. at a friend's
   c. at a bar
   d. at work
   e. in the car
   f. other (specify)

From Zeman FJ, Ney DM: Applications of clinical nutrition, Englewood Cliffs, NJ, 1988, Prentice Hall.
*Any beverages used as mixers should be included in the estimated kcalorie intake.

CRITICAL THINKING–cont'd
Clinical Applications

ALCOHOL INTAKE ASSESSMENT TOOL–cont'd

3. Which alcoholic beverages do you consume?

Circle all that apply:
a. beer
b. white, red, or rosé wine
c. sherry or port
d. gin
e. whiskey
f. vodka
g. rum
h. other (specify)

4. How do you determine how much you drink?

Circle all that apply:
a. Count the number of beer cans
b. Count the number of wine glasses
c. Count the number of shots poured
d. Count the number of bottles of wine
e. Count the number of bottles of liquor used a day or week
f. I don't know exactly how much I drink
g. Other method of deciding alcohol intake (specify)

5. On any drinking day, how many drinks do you usually have?

Circle letter(s) indicating drinks consumed and number within each category consumed to indicate number of drinks per day:

a. beer	1	2	3	4	>5
b. white, red, or rosé wine	1	2	3	4	>5
c. sherry or port	1	2	3	4	>5
d. gin	1	2	3	4	>5
e. whiskey	1	2	3	4	>5
f. vodka	1	2	3	4	>5
g. rum	1	2	3	4	>5
h. other (specify)	1	2	3	4	>5

6. For how long have you been drinking this quantity?

7. Do you drink this amount on a regular basis?

Professionals working with individuals who consume excessive amounts of alcohol advise that self-reported intakes may constitute about half of what is actually consumed. Therefore double-checking any information obtained from a patient about alcohol intake with a reliable family member or friend is recommended.

Web Sites of Interest

Alcoholics Anonymous

www.alcoholics-anonymous.org

This official Web site of Alcoholics Anonymous (AA) is dedicated to the self-help approach for overcoming alcoholism. It includes links for teenagers, newcomers, health professionals, and the AA Grapevine.

American Liver Foundation
www.liverfoundation.org/
This organization is a national nonprofit health agency devoted to research, education, and support groups related to hepatitis and all liver diseases. The site focuses extensively on documents and links that are new or important. It provides a wealth of information, including publications and video resources on liver disease.

Welcome to Cystic Fibrosis 101
www3.nbnet.nb.ca/normap/CF.htm
This site provides more than 240 links to sites related to cystic fibrosis (CF). The home page graphically categorizes links of support groups, chat rooms, associations, books, and home pages of people with CF as well as memorials to those who have died from CF.

References

1. Morgan SL, Weinsier RL: *Fundamentals of clinical nutrition,* ed 2, St Louis, 1999, Mosby.
2. Lee SP: Diseases of the liver and biliary tract. In Kinney JM et al., eds.: *Nutrition and metabolism in patient care,* Philadelphia, 1988, WB Saunders.
3. Guyton AC: *Textbook of medical physiology,* ed 8, Philadelphia, 1991, WB Saunders.
4. Ismail MK, Riely C: Alcoholic fatty liver, *eMedicine Journal* 3(1):January 29, 2002; www.emedicine.com/med/topic99.htm, accessed June 27, 2002.
5. McCance KL, Huether SE: *Pathophysiology: the biological basis for disease in adults and children,* ed 3, St Louis, 1998, Mosby.
6. Price SA, Wilson LM: *Pathophysiology: clinical concepts of disease processes,* ed 6, St Louis, 2002, Mosby.
7. Centers for Disease Control and Prevention: *Hepatitis A fact sheet;* www.cdc.gov/hepatitis, accessed August 24, 2002.
8. Gilroy R, Mukherjee S: Hepatitis A, *eMedicine Journal* 3(2):February 11, 2002; www.emedicine.com/med/topic99.htm, accessed June 27, 2002.
9. Wolf DC: Hepatitis, viral, *eMedicine Journal* 3(5):May 10, 2002; www.emedicine.com/med/topic99.htm, accessed June 27, 2002.
10. Pyrsopoulos NT, Reddy KR: Hepatitis B, *eMedicine Journal* 3(5):May 22, 2002; www.emedicine.com/med/topic99.htm, accessed June 27, 2002.
11. Centers for Disease Control and Prevention: *Hepatitis B fact sheet;* www.cdc.gov/hepatitis, accessed August 24, 2002.
12. Dhawan VK: Hepatitis C, *eMedicine Journal* 3(4):April 5, 2002; www.emedicine.com/med/topic99.htm, accessed June 27, 2002.
13. Lacey SR: Hepatitis D, *eMedicine Journal* 2(9):September 6, 2001; www.emedicine.com/med/topic99.htm, accessed June 27, 2002.
14. Flora KD: Hepatitis E, *eMedicine Journal* 2(9):September 20, 2001; www.emedicine.com/med/topic99.htm, accessed June 27, 2002.
15. Escott-Stump S: *Nutrition and diagnosis-related care,* ed 4, Baltimore, 1998, Williams & Wilkins.
16. Fischer JE, Baldesarini RJ: False neurotransmitters and hepatic failure, *Lancet* 2:75, 1971.
17. American Dietetic Association: *Manual of clinical dietetics,* ed 6, Chicago, 2000, American Dietetic Association.
18. Weseman RA, Mukherjee S: Nutritional requirements of adults before transplantation, *eMedicine Journal* 3(1):January 7, 2002; www.emedicine.com/med/topic99.htm, accessed June 29, 2002.
19. Wolf DC: Cirrhosis, *eMedicine Journal* 2(9):September 6, 2001; www.emedicine.com/med/topic99.htm, accessed June 27, 2002.
20. DiCecco SR et al.: Assessment of nutritional status of patients with end-stage liver disease undergoing liver transplantation, *Mayo Clinic Proc* 64:95, 1989.
21. Hehir DJ et al.: Nutrition in patients undergoing orthotopic liver transplant, *J Parenteral Enteral Nutr* 9:695, 1985.

22. Hasse JM: Nutritional implications of liver transplantation, *Henry Ford Hospital Medical Journal* 38:235, 1990.

23. Gladden D, Migala AF: Cholecystitis, *eMedicine Journal* 3(4):April 5, 2002; www.emedicine.com/med/topic99.htm, accessed June 27, 2002.

24. Public Health Service, National Institutes of Health, and National Institute of Diabetes and Digestive and Kidney Diseases: *Dieting and gallstones*, NIH Pub No 02-3677, Washington, DC, 2002, National Institutes of Health.

25. Willis J: Gastrointestinal diseases. In Carey CF, Lee HH, Woeltje KF, eds.: *The Washington manual of medical therapeutics*, ed 29, Philadelphia, 1998, Lippincott Williams & Wilkins.

26. Allen J, Cuschieri A: Cholelithiasis, *eMedicine Journal* 3(2):February 4, 2002; www.emedicine.com/med/topic99.htm, accessed June 27, 2002.

27. Hasse JM, Matarese LE: Medical nutrition therapy for liver, biliary system, and exocrine pancreas disorders. In Mahan LK, Escott-Stump S, eds.: *Krause's food, nutrition, and diet therapy*, ed 10, Philadelphia, 2000, WB Saunders.

28. Hurst J, Gallagher AL: Pathophysiology and nutritional management in acute pancreatitis, *Support Line* 16:6, 1994.

29. Havala T, Shronts E, Cerra F: Nutritional support in acute pancreatitis, *Gastroenterol Clin North Am* 18:525, 1989.

30. American Society of Parenteral and Enteral Nutrition (ASPEN) Board of Directors: Nutrition support for adults with specific diseases and conditions, *J Parenteral Enteral Nutr* 17(suppl):16SA, 1993.

31. The Merck Manual: *Cystic fibrosis*; www.merck.com/pubs/mmanual/section19/chapter267/267a.htm, accessed June 23, 2002.

32. Public Health Service, National Institutes of Health, and National Institute of Diabetes and Digestive and Kidney Diseases: *Facts about cystic fibrosis*, NIH Pub No 95-3650, Washington, DC, 1995, National Institutes of Health.

33. Wilson-Goodman V et al.: Factors affecting the dietary habits of adolescents with cystic fibrosis, *J Am Dietetic Assoc* 90:429, 1990.

34. Dowsett J: Nutrition in the management of cystic fibrosis, *Nutr Rev* 54(1):31, 1996.

35. Farrell PM, Lai H: Nutrition and cystic fibrosis. In Coulston AM, Rock CL, Monsen ER: *Nutrition in the prevention and treatment of disease*, San Diego, 2001, Academic Press.

36. Ramsey BS, Farrel PM, Pincharz P: Nutritional assessment and management in cystic fibrosis: a consensus report, *Am J Clin Nutr* 55:108, 1992.

CHAPTER 19

Nutrition for Diabetes Mellitus

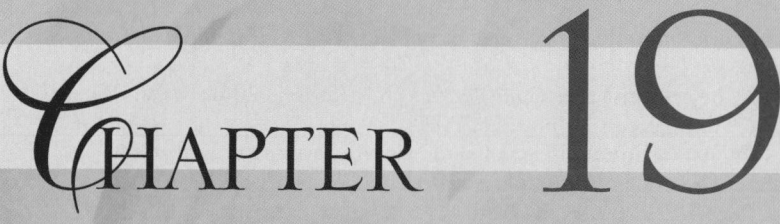

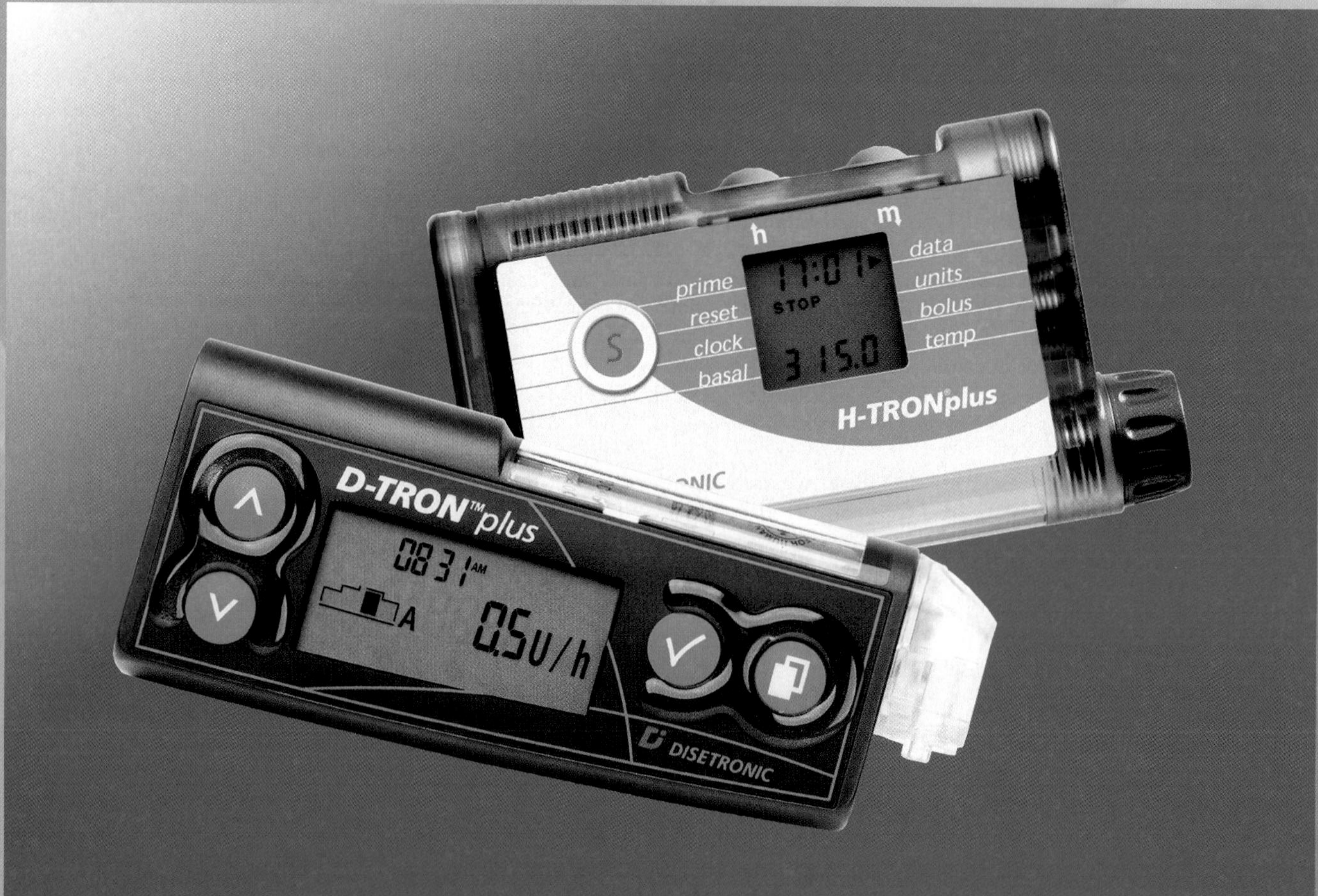

Courtesy Disetronic Medical Systems, Inc., St. Paul, Minn.

Diabetes mellitus is a group of conditions characterized by either a relative or complete lack of insulin secretion by the beta cells of the pancreas or by defects of cell insulin receptors, which result in disturbances of carbohydrate, protein, and lipid metabolism.

ROLE IN WELLNESS

The number of persons diagnosed with diabetes is at epidemic proportions in the United States,[1-3] and it is estimated that more than 5 million people with the disease have not been diagnosed.[4] As a chronic disorder, diabetes mellitus requires long-term lifestyle changes of both dietary intake and physical activity. Approaching this disorder in a proactive manner by maintaining blood glucose levels as near normal as possible can lessen the negative impact of diabetes and achieve a higher level of wellness.

A way to achieve a proactive approach is to consider diabetes through the five dimensions of health. Long-term serious physical health complications may be avoided if hyperglycemia is controlled through dietary and lifestyle modifications to maintain the physical dimension of health. The ability of the individual to understand the condition; to be compliant on a regular basis regarding insulin injections, if required; and to follow dietary and exercise recommendations may depend on the intellectual health dimension. Emotional health may be tested. Not only must the individual deal with a chronic lifelong condition but also changes in dietary intake may necessitate the loss of symbolic foods, which may be emotionally upsetting. Support, especially by family members and friends, is crucial. Social health may be pivotal in adjustment to this disorder. If one is already secure in social relationships, adaptations in social situations will be easier and more acceptable. People who eat special diets based on their religious or spiritual beliefs may need special adaptations of the diabetic diet to sustain their spiritual dimension of health.

DIABETES MELLITUS

Diabetes mellitus is a group of conditions characterized by either a relative or complete lack of insulin secretion by the beta cells of the pancreas or by defects of cell insulin receptors, which result in disturbances of carbohydrate, protein, and lipid metabolism and elevated blood glucose.[5] Diabetes is usually diagnosed and characterized by elevated fasting blood glucose (>126 mg/dl if found on at least two occasions) or hyperglycemia. The main goal of treatment is maintenance of insulin/glucose homeostasis.

In addition to everyday maintenance necessary to control blood glucose levels, diabetes mellitus is associated with disability and premature death because of the disease's effect on structural and functional alterations in many body systems, especially macrovascular and microvascular damage. Ranked as one of the most costly health problems in America,[6] diabetes mellitus is often called a *"silent killer."*[7] All persons with diabetes mellitus are vulnerable to long-term complications (Table 19-1) and premature death, which is associated with all types of diabetes. Manifestation of these complications may be preempted with control of hyperglycemia.[6-11] Macrovascular complications increase risk of coronary artery disease, peripheral vascular disease, and cerebrovascular accidents. Microvascular effects include nephropathy (kidney disorder) and retinopathy (eye disorder from blood vessel changes). As a result of nephropathy, approximately half of all individuals with type 1 diabetes mellitus (type 1 DM) develop chronic renal failure and end-stage renal disease (ESRD). Retinopathy is the leading cause of blindness in North America. In addition, neuropathy complications affect peripheral circulation, causing decreased sensations in extremities that may result in injury without the patient's knowledge. Healing is impaired because of the effects of diabetes on the circulatory system; gangrene may develop, and amputation may be necessary. Autonomic effects of diabetes may include orthostatic hypotension, persistent tachycardia, gastroparesis, neurogenic bladder (urinary bladder dysfunction from neurologic damage), impotence, and impaired visceral pain sensation that can obscure symptoms of angina pectoris or myocardial infarction.

Development of these long-term complications is believed to be correlated to the level and frequency of hyperglycemia experiences throughout the life span of a per-

Table 19-1
Clinical Complications of Diabetes Mellitus

Complication	Manifestation	Incidence
Dental disease	Periodontitis	Those with diabetes are often at twice the risk of those without diabetes. Almost 30% of people with diabetes have severe periodontal diseases with loss of attachment of gums to the teeth measuring 5 mm or more.
Pregnancy	Congenital malformations	Poorly controlled diabetes before conception and during the first trimester of pregnancy can cause major birth defects in 5%-10% of pregnancies and spontaneous abortions in 15%-20% of pregnancies. Poorly controlled diabetes during second and third trimesters of pregnancy can result in excessively large newborns.
Microvascular*	Retinopathy	Leading cause of blindness in adults between 20-74 years
	Nephropathy	More than 30% of people with type 1 DM will develop kidney disease, compared with perhaps 10% of those with type 2 DM. People with type 1 DM have 15 times the risk of end-stage renal disease as those with type 2 DM.
Macrovascular†	Coronary artery disease	Patients with DM are two to four times more likely to have heart disease; heart disease deaths are also two to four times higher than in adults without DM.
	Peripheral vascular disease Cerebrovascular disease	Patients with DM are two to four times more likely to suffer stroke
Neuropathy	Peripheral	Approximately 60%-70% of people with diabetes have mild to severe forms of nerve damage. Neuropathy is a major contributing factor in foot and leg amputations among people with diabetes. Risk of leg amputation is 15-40 times greater for a person with DM.

Compiled from American Diabetes Association: Complications; www.diabetes.org/main/Type2/complications/complicationsljsp, accessed March 29, 2002; American Diabetes Association: Skin conditions; www.diabetes.org/main/application/commercewf?origin= *.jsp&event= link(D3_1, accessed March 29, 2002; National Institute of Diabetes and Digestive and Kidney Diseases (NIDDK). National Diabetes Information Clearinghouse. Diabetes Control and Complications Trial (DCCT); www.niddk.nih.gov/health/diabetes/pubs/dcct1/dcct.htm, accessed March 22, 2002; National Institute of Diabetes and Digestive and Kidney Diseases (NIDDK): National diabetes statistics: general information and national estimates on diabetes in the United States, National Institutes of Health Pub No 02-3892, Mar 2002; www.niddk.nih.gov/health/diabetes/pubs/dmstats/dmstats.htm, accessed March 29, 2002; Orland MJ: Diabetes mellitus. In Carey CF, Lee HH, Woeltje KF, eds.: The Washington manual of medical therapeutics, ed 29, Philadelphia, 1998, Lippincott Williams & Wilkins.
*Compounds effects of macrovascular problems.
†Exacerbated by concurrent hypertension, hypercholesterolemia, smoking, and aging.

intensive therapy
consists of (1) administration of insulin more than three times daily (injection or pump) with dosage adjusted according to results of self-monitoring of blood glucose performed at least four times daily, (2) dietary intake, and (3) anticipated exercise[3]

son who has diabetes. Results of the Diabetes Control and Complications Trial[6] indicate that intensive therapy is more effective than conventional therapy in delaying and slowing the progression of retinopathy by 75%, nephropathy by 50%, and neuropathy by 60% in patients with type 1 DM. Results of the U.K.'s Prospective Diabetes Study indicate that better blood glucose control reduces risk of retinopathy by 25% and nephropathy by 30% and possibly reduces neuropathy.[12]

Glucose intolerance can be classified into two primary categories: type 1 diabetes mellitus (type 1 DM)* and type 2 diabetes mellitus (type 2 DM). Other types

*According to the Report of the Expert Committee on the Diagnosis and Classification of Diabetes Mellitus,[5] the terms *insulin-dependent diabetes mellitus* and *non-insulin dependent diabetes mellitus* and their acronyms, *IDDM* and *NIDDM* should no longer be used because they are confusing and have frequently resulted in classifying patients based on treatment rather than etiology.

Table 19-1—cont'd
Clinical Complications of Diabetes Mellitus

Complication	Manifestation	Incidence
Neuropathy—cont'd	Autonomic (postural hypotension, persistent tachycardia, neurogenic bladder, incontinence, gastroparesis, impotence)	Impotence occurs in approximately 13% of men who have type 1 DM and 8% of men with type 2 DM. Some reports indicate men older than 50 years have impotence rates as high as 50%-60%.
Skin conditions	Atherosclerosis	As blood vessels narrow, the skin changes. It becomes hairless, thin, cool, and shiny. Toes become cold. Toenails thicken and discolor.
	Fungal infections (usually *Candida albicans*)	Common fungal infections are "jock itch," "athlete's foot," ringworm, and vaginal infection that cause itching.
	Bullosis diabeticorum (diabetic blisters)	Rare condition that can occur on backs of hands, fingers, toes, feet, and sometimes legs or forearms. They look like burn blisters, are painless, and have no redness. Often occur in people with neuropathy; only treatment is to bring blood glucose levels under control.
	Diabetic dermopathy	Light brown scaly skin patches often mistaken for age spots; occurs most often on the front of both legs. Patches do not hurt, open up, or itch.
	Necrobiosis lipoidica diabeticorum (NLD)	Rare condition. Similar to diabetic dermopathy, however, spots are fewer but larger and deeper. Often start as dull, red raised area. Sometimes itchy and painful; spots may crack open.
	Eruptive xanthomatosis	Firm, yellow, pealike enlargements in the skin. Occurs most often on backs of hands, feet, arms, legs, and buttocks. Usually occurs in young men with type 1 DM who have high levels of cholesterol and lipids in their blood. Usually disappear when glucose levels are controlled.
	Digital sclerosis	Tight, thick, waxy skin on backs of hands. Finger joints become stiff. Occurs in about 30% of those with type 1 DM. Only treatment is to control blood glucose levels.
	Disseminated granuloma annular	Sharply defined ring-shaped or arc-shaped raised areas on skin that can be red, red-brown, or skin-colored. Occurs most often on distal parts of the body.
	Acanthosis nigricans	Tan or brown raised areas on sides of the neck, axilla, and groin. May sometimes occur on hands, elbows, and knees. Usually manifests in the obese.

include gestational diabetes mellitus (GDM), impaired glucose tolerance (IGT), and other forms of diabetes.[1] These classifications, based on etiology, treatment needs, and their symptoms, are summarized in Table 19-2. The majority (more than 90%) of persons with diabetes have type 2 DM, whereas 5% to 10% have type 1 DM.[4]

Type 1 Diabetes Mellitus

Onset of type 1 DM is usually sudden. Cells use glucose for energy, and without endogenous insulin, cells literally start starving. The body responds by sending signals to eat because cells are hungry, but because the end product of digestion (glucose) cannot enter cells, glucose builds up in the bloodstream (Table 19-3). It is common for the person to experience weight loss while consuming large

conventional therapy consists of (1) one or two daily injections of insulin, including mixed intermediate and rapid-acting insulins; (2) daily self-monitoring of urine or blood glucose; and (3) education about diet and exercise.[3]

Table 19-2
Criteria for Diagnosing Diabetes

Diabetes Type	Former Term	Etiology	Criteria
Type 1 diabetes*: immune mediated or idiopathic	Insulin-dependent diabetes mellitus (IDDM), type I diabetes, juvenile-onset diabetes, ketosis-prone diabetes, brittle diabetes	Beta cell destruction, usually leading to absolute insulin deficiency	Symptoms† of DM and casual plasma glucose ≥200 mg/dl (casual is defined as any time of day without regard to last meal) OR FPG ≥126 mg/dl (fasting is defined as no kcaloric intake for at least 8 hrs) OR
Type 2 diabetes (adults)	Non–insulin-dependent diabetes mellitus (NIDDM), type II diabetes, adult-onset diabetes, maturity-onset diabetes, ketosis-resistant diabetes, stable diabetes	Insulin resistance with insulin secretory defect	2-hr PG ≥200 mg/dl during OGTT (performed as described by WHO using glucose load containing the equivalent of 75 g anhydrous glucose dissolved in water)
Type 2 diabetes (children)			Overweight (BMI >85th percentile for age and gender, weight for height >85th percentile, or weight >120% of ideal for height) PLUS Any two of the following: • Family history of type 2 DM in first- or second-degree relative • Native American, African American, Hispanic American, Asian-American/Pacific Islander • Signs of insulin resistance or conditions associated with insulin resistance (acanthosis nigricans, HTN, dyslipidemia, or PCOS)
Gestational diabetes (GDM)	Gestational diabetes, Type III diabetes		*One-step approach:* Diagnostic OGTT *Two-step approach:* Initial screening to measure plasma or serum glucose concentration 1 hr after 50 g oral glucose load (GCT) and perform diagnostic OGTT on those women exceeding glucose threshold value on GCT. Glucose threshold ≥140 mg/dl identifies about 80% of women with GDM.
Impaired glucose tolerance (IGT)	Borderline diabetes, chemical diabetes		2-hr PG ≥140 mg/dl and <200 mg/dl or 2-hr PG 140 mg/dl to 199 mg/dl

Copyright © 2002 American Diabetes Association. Modified from Diabetes Care, Vol 25, Supplement 1, 2002, S33-S49. Reprinted with permission from The American Diabetes Association. In Anderson SL: Diabetes mellitus. In Williams SR, Schlenker ED: Essentials of nutrition and diet therapy, ed 8, St Louis, 2003, Mosby.
*Patients with any form of diabetes may require insulin treatment at some stage of their disease. Such use of insulin does not classify the patient as having type 1 DM.
†Symptoms include polyuria, polydipsia, and unexplained weight loss.
BMI, Body mass index; GCT, glucose challenge test; PCOS, polycystic ovarian syndrome; WHO, World Health Organization; FPG, fasting plasma glucose; HTN, hypertension; OGTT, oral glucose tolerance test; PG, plasma glucose.

quantities of food (polyphagia). Because glucose cannot enter cells and builds up in the bloodstream, blood becomes hypertonic and the body tries to get rid of the excess glucose by increasing urine output (polyuria). In reaction to increased excretion of urine, the body again responds by increasing thirst (polydipsia) to replace lost fluids.

Type 1 DM results from destruction of pancreatic beta cells. Destruction of the insulin-producing beta cells is thought to result from a progressive autoimmune response believed to be caused by a combination of genetic predisposition, viral infections, and environmental or unknown stimuli.[13]

Type 2 Diabetes Mellitus

Type 2 DM is an insidious disease. Persons with type 2 DM rarely have the classic symptoms of diabetes (i.e., polyuria, polyphagia, polydipsia). In fact, some of the first symptoms that cause persons to seek medical attention are the complications (e.g., heart attack, stroke, neuropathic problems) associated with diabetes. It is not uncommon for a person to have type 2 DM years before diagnosis.

Unlike type 1 DM, the primary metabolic problem in type 2 DM is insulin resistance or failure of cells to respond to insulin produced by the body. Family history and obesity are the two strongest risk factors for type 2 DM. In fact, obesity by itself produces an insulin-resistant state that causes beta cells to produce excessive amounts of insulin. Because not all obese persons develop diabetes, there seems to be a genetic tendency for diabetes that leads to beta cell exhaustion and hyperglycemia in some obese persons.[13] Additionally, upper body obesity has been recognized as an even greater risk factor for diabetes than degree of obesity.[14] Upper body obesity, defined as a waist-to-hip ratio greater than 0.8 for women and 0.95 to 1.0 for men, is a risk factor not only for diabetes but also for heart disease and hypertension[7] (see also the Cultural Considerations box for more about rates of diabetes).

polyphagia
excessive hunger and eating

polyuria
excessive urination

polydipsia
excessive thirst

SYMPTOMS AND CLINICAL SIGNS OF TYPE 1 DIABETES MELLITUS
Sudden onset of polyphagia, polyuria, polydipsia, and weight loss

SYMPTOMS AND CLINICAL SIGNS OF TYPE 2 DIABETES MELLITUS
Gradual onset of polyuria and polydipsia; easily fatigued; frequent infections (especially of the urinary tract)

Table 19-3
Metabolic Goals in Diabetes Management

Indicator	Normal Value	Goal	Additional Action Suggested*
Plasma values (mg/dl)			
Average preprandial glucose	<110	90-130	<90/>150
Average bedtime glucose	<120	110-150	<110/>180
Whole blood values† (mg/dl)			
Average preprandial glucose	<100	80-120	<80/>140
Average bedtime glucose	<110	100-140	<100/>160
HgbA$_{1c}$ (%)	<6	<7	>8
LDL-cholesterol		<100 mg/dl	
HDL-cholesterol		>55 mg/dl	
Triglycerides		<150 mg/dl	
Blood pressure		<130/80	

Copyright © 2002 American Diabetes Association. Modified from Diabetes Care, Vol. 25, Supplement 1, 2002; 533-549. Reprinted with permission from The American Diabetes Association. In Anderson SL: Diabetes mellitus. In Williams SR, Schlenker ED: Essentials of nutrition and diet therapy, ed 8, St Louis, 2003, Mosby.
*Depends on individual patient circumstances.
†Measurement of capillary blood glucose.

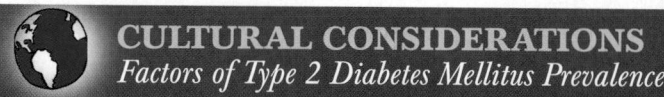

Insulin

All persons with type 1 DM require exogenous insulin to maintain normal blood glucose levels. Some individuals with type 2 DM may require insulin to optimize blood glucose control. Regardless of the type of diabetes, the goal of insulin therapy is to mimic physiologic insulin delivery.[15] This is usually accomplished by a variety of methods: split-dose regimen, multidose therapy, or insulin pumps.

The following factors are usually considered by the physician when deciding when to begin insulin therapy[16]:

- Severity of the diabetes (e.g., degree of hyperglycemia) and presence or absence of clinical symptoms
- Presence or absence of concurrent diseases and conditions
- Preferences of the patient after being informed about use, expected therapeutic effects, and possible side effects of oral glucose-lowering medications or insulin
- Motivation of the patient

Oral Glucose-Lowering Medications

Oral glucose-lowering medications are used to treat type 2 DM when diet and physical activity cannot control hyperglycemia. Effectiveness of medications varies with each individual and is closely associated to residual beta cell function.[16] The variety of new drugs for treatment of diabetes has greatly expanded during the past several years.[17] To complement insulin and sulfonylurea drugs, several other classes of medications have become available: thiazolidinediones, alpha-glucosidase inhibitors, biguanides, and meglintinides.[18,19] Table 19-4 provides a brief review of these drugs.

Exercise

Along with medical nutrition therapy (discussed later in this chapter) and insulin, exercise is the third component used to treat diabetes. Exercise, like insulin, lowers blood glucose levels, assists in maintaining normal lipid levels, and increases circulation. For most individuals, consistent and individualized exercise helps reduce the therapeutic dose of insulin. Patients should be instructed not to perform exercise at the time insulin is at its peak. Ideally, they should exercise when blood glucose levels are between 100 and 200 mg/dl or about 30 to 60 minutes after meals. They should avoid exercising when blood glucose is above 250 mg/dl[20] and ketones are present in the urine.[16] Figure 19-1 describes metabolic effects of

Type 1 DM

Insulin	Hepatic Glucose Output	Peripheral Glucose Use	Counter-regulatory Hormones		Blood Glucose
Adequate	⇩	⇩	⇩	➡	⇩
Inadequate	⇧	⇧	⇧	➡	⇧

Type 2 DM

Hepatic Glucose Output	Peripheral Glucose Use	Counter-regulatory Hormones	Insulin Sensitivity		Blood Glucose Control
⇩	⇧	⇩	⇧	➡	Improved

Figure 19-1 Metabolic effects of exercise in type 1 and type 2 DM. (Copyright © 1994, American Diabetes Association. From Maximizing the Role of Nutrition in Diabetes Management. Reprinted and adapted with permission from *The American Diabetes Association*.)

exercise on type 1 and type 2 DM. In the case of type 1 DM, glucose control can be compromised if proper adjustments are not made in food intake or insulin administration. Patients with type 2 DM who take oral hypoglycemic agents may be at risk of postexercise hypoglycemia.[21]

General guidelines that may assist in regulating the glycemic response to exercise in persons with type 1 DM are summarized as follows[20]:
- *Metabolic control before exercise:* Avoid exercise if fasting glucose levels are greater than 250 mg/dl and ketosis is present or if glucose levels are greater than 300 mg/dl, regardless of whether ketosis is present. Ingest added carbohydrate if glucose levels are less than 100 mg/dl.
- *Blood glucose monitoring before and after exercise:* Identify when changes in insulin or food intake are necessary. Learn the blood glucose response to different exercise conditions.
- *Food intake:* Consume added carbohydrate as needed to avoid hypoglycemia. Carbohydrate-based foods should be readily available during and after exercise (Box 19-1).

Box 19-1 Strategies for Metabolic Control (Type 2 Diabetes Mellitus)

- Nutritionally adequate meal plan with a reduction of total fat, especially saturated fats
- Meals spaced throughout the day
- Mild to moderate weight loss (5-10 kg [10-20 lb]) even if desirable body weight is not achieved (moderate decrease in energy intake + increase in kcalorie expenditure)
- Regular exercise
- Monitoring of blood glucose levels, glycosylated hemoglobin, lipids, and blood pressure
- Oral hypoglycemic or insulin if above does not work

Table 19-4
Medications Used to Treat Diabetes

Drug Class	Drug Name(s)	Action	Target Organ(s)	Side Effects	How Taken
Alpha-glucosidase inhibitor	acarbose (Precose, Glucobay, Prandase, Glucor) miglitol (Glyset, Miglibay, Bayglitol)	Delays absorption of glucose from gastrointestinal tract	Small intestine	Excess flatulence, diarrhea (particularly after high-carbohydrate meal), abdominal pain, may interfere with iron absorption	Must be taken with meals
Biguanides	metformin (Glucophage) metformin + glibenclamide (Glucovance, Glucophage + Glyburide)	Decrease hepatic glucose production and intestinal glucose absorption; improves insulin sensitivity	Liver, small intestine, peripheral tissues	Less likely to gain weight; may lose weight; anorexia, nausea, diarrhea, metallic taste; may reduce absorption of vitamin B_{12} and folic acid; rarely suitable for adults >80 years	Take with first main meal
Insulin and related agents	*Insulin mixtures:* Humulin 50/50, Humulin 70/30, Novolin 70/30	Exogenous insulin preparations		Hypoglycemia, fatigue, hunger, nausea, muscular weakness or trembling, headache, sweating, blurred vision, fainting, weight gain, skin irritation	Subcutaneous injection
	Intermediate acting: Humulin L, Humulin N, Lente Iletin II, Iletin II NPH, Novolin L, Novolin N	Same as above		Same as above	Same as above
	Long-acting: Humulin U, Lantus (insulin glargine)	Same as above		Same as above	Same as above

Class	Examples	Action	Site of Action	Side Effects / Precautions	Administration
	Rapid-acting: Humalog, Insulin Lispro, Insulin Aspart	Same as above		Same as above	Same as above; intramuscular or intravenous in special situations
	Short-acting: Humulin R, Regular Iletin II, Novolin R, Novolin BR	Same as above		Same as above	Same as above
Meglitinides (nonsulfonylurea insulin releasers)	nateglinide (Starlix) repaglinide (Prandin, Aculin)	Stimulates secretion of insulin	Pancreatic beta cells	Hypoglycemia, weight gain; repaglinide has slightly increased risk for cardiac events	Take with meals
Sulfonylureas	acetohexamide (Dymelor) tolazamide (Tolinase) tolbutamide (Orinase) chlorpropamide (Diabenese) glimepiride (Amaryl) glyburide (DiaBeta, Micronase, Glynase PresTabs)	Stimulates secretion of insulin	Pancreatic beta cells	Hypoglycemia, weight gain; tolbutamide may be associated with cardiovascular complications; chlorpropamide can cause hyponatremia; should not be used by women who are pregnant or nursing, or by individuals allergic to sulfa drugs; sulfonylureas interact with many other drugs (prescription, over-the-counter, alternative); chlorpropamide: avoid alcohol	Take before or with meals
Thiazolidinediones (TZDs)	pioglitazone (Actos) rosiglitazone (Avandia)	Improves insulin sensitivity	Activates genes involved with fat synthesis and carbohydrate metabolism	Possible liver damage, weight gain, mild anemia	Once or twice daily

From Anderson SL: Diabetes mellitus. In Williams SR, Schlenker ED: Essentials of nutrition and diet therapy, ed 8, St Louis, 2003, Mosby. Compiled from Setter SM: New drug therapies for treatment of diabetes, On the Cutting Edge Diabetes Care and Education Newsletter 19(2):3, 1998; Sharp AR: Nutritional implications of new medications to treat diabetes, On the Cutting Edge Diabetes Care and Education Newsletter 19(2):1998; White JR, Campbell RK: Recent developments in the pharmacological reduction of blood glucose in patients with Type 2 diabetes, Clinical Diabetes 19:153, 2001: http://clinical.diabetesjournals.org/cgi/content/full/19/4/153, accessed March 30, 2002; Rosen ED: Drug classes for diabetes, Veritas Medicine for Patients; www.veritasmedicine.com, accessed July 27, 2001.

People with type 1 DM who do not have complications and are in good blood glucose control can perform all levels of exercise, including leisure activities, recreational sports, and competitive sports.[20] To do this safely, the patient must possess the ability to collect self-monitored blood glucose data (during exercise) and then use these data to adjust the therapeutic regimen (insulin and medical nutrition therapy).[20]

Exercise can increase the risk for hypoglycemia in persons with type 1 DM. Hypoglycemia during exercise of 40 minutes or less is rare. Onset is more likely to occur after exercise, often between 4 and 10 hours afterward.[10] Blood glucose levels should be monitored at 1- or 2-hour intervals after exercise to assess response to the exercise and allow for adjustments in insulin and food intake.[16]

Blood Glucose Monitoring

fasting blood glucose
level of glucose circulating in blood serum after an 8-hour fast; also called *fasting blood sugar*

glycosylated hemoglobin (HgbA$_{1c}$)
a substance (glycohemoglobin) formed when hemoglobin combines with some of the glucose in the bloodstream

Blood glucose levels are the cornerstone of diabetes management.[22] Blood glucose levels can be monitored several ways: (1) fasting blood glucose, (2) glycosylated hemoglobin, and (3) self-monitoring.

Fasting blood glucose, also called *fasting blood sugar,* is the level of glucose in the blood after an 8-hour fast. Normal values range from 70 to 110 mg/dl depending on the standards set by individual laboratories. Fasting levels of blood glucose are elevated in uncontrolled diabetes.

Glycosylated hemoglobin (HgbA$_{1c}$) is formed through an irreversible process. As red blood cells (RBCs) circulate in the bloodstream, hemoglobin combines with glucose, forming glycohemoglobin. The amount of glycohemoglobin formed depends on the amount of glucose in the bloodstream circulation over the RBCs' 120-day life span. Therefore the amount of HgbA$_{1c}$ is a reflection of average blood glucose level for the 100- to 120-day period before the test; the more glucose the RBC was exposed to, the greater the value. This value is not affected by short-term factors such as food intake, exercise, or stress, therefore the blood sample can be drawn at any time; this is an easier sample to obtain than the fasting blood glucose test.

Self-monitoring can be performed in the patient's home with blood glucose meters (sometimes called *glucometers*), which can be purchased at pharmacies. A droplet of blood is obtained through a finger prick on a regular basis to monitor glucose levels before and after meals and at bedtime. Self-monitoring and charting is particularly useful in evaluating glycemic control, physical activity, and effectiveness of the meal plan in meeting the goals of medical nutrition therapy.

Records should be kept of self-monitored blood glucose levels for review by the healthcare team to determine food, insulin, and exercise needs. This allows for individualized treatment, especially with meal plans, and makes indiscriminate, general dietary advice or tear-off diet sheets unjustified. The frequency of monitoring depends on the type of diabetes and therapy prescribed. For some, monitoring up to seven times a day may be appropriate: before and after (1 to 2 hours after) breakfast, lunch, and dinner and at bedtime.[21]

Hypoglycemia

SYMPTOMS OF HYPOGLYCEMIA

Hunger; erratic behavior; confusion; trembling, shaking; cool, clammy, pale skin

Hypoglycemia (below normal values of blood glucose levels) usually results from too much insulin, skipping meals, or too much exercise without a concomitant increase in food intake. Onset is sudden and can be fatal if left untreated. Usually, hypoglycemia occurs at a time when plasma insulin (or oral hypoglycemic agents) levels peak or during the night when the patient sleeps (fasting).

Symptoms usually occur when blood glucose drops below 50 mg/dl or there is a relatively significant drop in blood glucose. For example, if a patient is in a consistent state of hyperglycemia (e.g., 180 to 200 mg/dl) and blood glucose levels are brought down to 90 mg/dl, the patient may experience hypoglycemia although the blood glucose level is in the normal range. The key is that, for this patient, the normal blood glucose is low.

Diabetic Ketoacidosis

Diabetic ketoacidosis (DKA) is a life-threatening condition caused by insulin deficiency. When glucose cannot be used by cells, or when endogenous sources of energy are unavailable, the body breaks down fats and proteins for energy, which can cause ketosis. Ketosis is an abnormal accumulation of ketones caused by metabolism of fatty acids for energy with little carbohydrate metabolism occurring; ketoacidosis may then result. This condition results in hyperglycemia that causes osmotic diuresis, leads to dehydration, and precipitates lactic acidosis. Lowered pH, resulting from the acidosis, stimulates the respiratory center and produces deep, rapid respirations known as Kussmaul's respirations. Large amounts of ketone bodies in the body also produce a fruity or acetone odor on the breath (a person suffering from DKA could be mistaken for someone who is inebriated). If this condition is not recognized and treated promptly, the acidosis and dehydration may lead to loss of consciousness and possibly coma and death.[20] Common conditions that precipitate DKA include insufficient or interrupted insulin therapy, too much food, infection, or other stresses (e.g., trauma, surgery, emotional stress, myocardial infarction).[15]

Hyperosmolar Hyperglycemic Nonketotic Syndrome

Hyperosmolar hyperglycemic nonketotic syndrome (HHNK), like DKA, is a life-threatening emergency caused by a relative or actual insulin deficiency resulting in severe hyperglycemia. Most often HHNK is triggered by stress (trauma, infection) that increases the body's demand for insulin. Although enough insulin may be present in the plasma to prevent formation of ketones, thus preventing acidosis, there may not be enough to prevent hyperglycemia. If hyperglycemia is left untreated, serum becomes hyperosmolar and produces osmotic diuresis and simultaneous significant loss of electrolytes via urine. Mortality for HHNK is 10% to 25%.[14]

✿ MEDICAL NUTRITION THERAPY

In 2002 the American Diabetes Association (ADA) published its seventh set of recommendations[22] since 1950 (Table 19-5). These new recommendations are categorized into goals of medical nutrition therapy that apply to all persons with diabetes or goals that apply to specific situations (see Table 19-5 for a comparison of the new recommendations against earlier ones). General goals that apply to all persons with DM include the following:
1. Attain and maintain optimal metabolic outcomes including the following:
   a. Blood glucose levels in the normal (or near normal) range
   b. Lipid and lipoprotein profiles that reduce risk for macrovascular diseases
   c. Blood pressure levels that reduce risk for vascular disease
2. Prevent and treat chronic complications.
3. Improve health through healthy food choices and physical activity.
4. Address *individual* nutritional needs taking into consideration personal and cultural preferences and lifestyle while respecting *individual's wishes and willingness to change* (emphasis is author's).
Goals that apply to specific situations include:
1. Youth with type 1 DM:
   a. Provide adequate energy to ensure normal growth and development.
   b. Integrate insulin regimens into usual eating and physical activity habits.
2. Youth with type 2 DM:
   a. Facilitate changes in eating and physical activity habits that reduce insulin resistance and improve metabolic status.

SYMPTOMS AND CLINICAL SIGNS OF DKA

Polyuria; polyphagia; weight loss; nausea; dry, flushed skin and mucous membranes; dehydration and metabolic acidosis; polydipsia; fruity (acetone) breath; generalized weakness; vomiting; weakness, fatigue

SYMPTOMS AND CLINICAL SIGNS OF HHNK

Polyuria; polyphagia; weight loss; nausea; dry, flushed skin and mucous membranes; dehydration secondary to osmotic diuresis; polydipsia; possible seizures and tremors; generalized weakness; vomiting; fatigue

Table 19-5
Historical Perspective of Nutrition Recommendations for Diabetes Mellitus

Year	Percent of Carbohydrate	Percent of Fat	Percent of Protein
Pre-1921			Starvation diets
1921	20	70	10
1950	40	40	20
1971	45	35	20
1986	≤60	<30	12-20
1994	Based on nutrition assessment and treatment goal	Based on nutrition assessment and treatment goals; less than 10% of energy from saturated fats	10-20
2002	Carbohydrates and monounsaturated fat should together provide 60%-70% of energy intake; individual metabolic profile and need for weight loss should be considered when determining monounsaturated fat content. Whole grains, fruits, vegetables, and low-fat milk are important and should be included in a healthy diet. Total amount of carbohydrates in meals or snacks is more important than source or type. Sucrose and sucrose-containing foods do not need to be restricted; however, they should be substituted for other carbohydrate sources or, if added, be covered with insulin or other glucose-lowering medication. Less than 10% of energy intake should be from saturated fats. Dietary cholesterol intake should be less than 300 mg/d.		15%-20% (In individuals with controlled type 2 DM, ingested protein does not increase plasma glucose concentrations, although ingested protein influences insulin secretion the same as carbohydrate.)

Reference: American Dietetic Association: Nutrition recommendations and principles for people with diabetes mellitus, J Am Dietetic Assoc 94:504, 1994; Franz MJ et al.: Evidence-based nutrition principles and recommendations for the treatment and prevention of diabetes and related complications, Diabetes Care 25:148, 2002.

3. Pregnant and lactating women:
   a. Provide adequate energy and nutrients necessary for optimal pregnancy outcome.
4. Older adults:
   a. Provide for nutritional and psychosocial needs of an aging individual.
5. Individuals treated with insulin or insulin secretagogues:
   a. Provide self-management education for treatment (and prevention) of hypoglycemia, acute illnesses, and exercise-related blood glucose problems.
6. Individuals at risk for diabetes (Box 19-2):
   a. Decrease risk by encouraging physical activity.
   b. Promote food choices that facilitate moderate weight loss or at least prevent weight gain.

Owing to the complexity of nutrition issues, the ADA[23] recommends that a registered dietitian who is knowledgeable and skilled in implementing nutrition therapy into diabetes management and education be the medical team member responsible for providing medical nutrition therapy (see the Myth box for more about common nutrition myths and diabetes). It is also essential that all healthcare team members be knowledgeable about nutrition therapy and supportive of the patient with diabetes who needs to make these important lifestyle changes.

Medical Nutrition Therapy for Type 1 and Type 2 Diabetes Mellitus

Medical nutrition therapy is an integral component of diabetes management and diabetes self-management education.[24] It involves conducting a nutrition assessment to evaluate a patient's food intake, metabolic status, lifestyle, and willingness to

Box 19-2 Individuals at Risk for Diabetes Mellitus

*G*enerally, persons with type 1 DM display acute symptoms and noticeably elevated blood glucose levels. However, type 2 DM is often not diagnosed until complications develop. Roughly one third of all persons with type 2 DM may be undiagnosed. According to the American Diabetes Association, there is sufficient indirect evidence to justify opportunistic screening of individuals at high risk of developing DM. Criteria for testing asymptomatic, undiagnosed adults and children at risk for occurrence or development of type 2 DM are listed below.

Adults ≥45 years of age	All
Adults <45 years of age	Overweight (BMI ≥25 kg/m²) First-degree relative has diabetes Member of a high-risk population (e.g., African American, Hispanic American, Native American, Asian/Pacific Islander) Delivered an infant weighing >9 lbs or previously diagnosed with GDM Hypertensive (≥140/90 mmHg) HDL cholesterol level ≤35 mg/dl and/or a triglyceride level ≥250 mg/dl On previous testing, had IGT Other clinical conditions associated with insulin resistance (e.g., PCOS or acanthosis nigricans)
Children (10 years of age or at onset of puberty, if puberty occurs at a younger age)	Overweight (≥85th percentile for age and gender, >85th percentile weight for height, or weight >120% of ideal for height) *Plus any two of the following:* • Family history of type 2 DM in first- or second-degree relative • Race/ethnicity (e.g., African American, Hispanic American, Native American, Asian-American/Pacific Islander • Signs of insulin resistance or conditions associated with insulin resistance (acanthosis nigricans, hypertension, dyslipidemia, or PCOS)

Modified from Copyright © 2002. American Diabetes Association. From Diabetes Care, Vol. 2, Supplement 1, 2002; S33-S49. Reprinted with permission from The American Diabetes Association.

BMI, *Body mass index;* GDM, *gestational diabetes mellitus;* IGT, *impaired glucose tolerance;* PCOS, *polycystic ovarian syndrome.*

make changes; goal setting; nutrition education; and evaluation.[24] To enhance compliance, the medical nutrition therapy plan should be individualized and take into consideration patients' lifestyle, cultural background, and financial situation.[24]

The ADA's recommendations are outlined as follows:[23]

Carbohydrate

• Terms such as *simple sugars, complex carbohydrates,* and *fast-acting carbohydrates* are not well-defined and use of these terms should be avoided. Preferred terms are *sugars, starch,* and *fiber.*
• Foods containing carbohydrate from whole grains, fruits, vegetables, and low-fat milk should be included in a healthy diet.
• Total amount of carbohydrate in meals or snacks is more important than source or type.
• Sucrose does not increase glycemia to a greater extent than isocaloric amounts of starch. Sucrose and sucrose-containing foods do not need to be restricted, but if used, should be substituted for other carbohydrate sources.

MYTH
Diabetes Myths: Setting the Record Straight

*D*iabetes is a serious condition that affects millions of Americans. The importance of quality nutrition for diabetes prevention and for improving quality of life for individuls with diabetes has been accepted for years. However, the relationship between food and diabetes continues to be misunderstood.

To help clear the confusion, Hope Warshaw, MMSc, RD, CDE, author of *Diabetes Meal Planning Made Easy* and *Guide to Healthy Restaurant Eating*, offers the following comments about the most common myths surrounding diet and diabetes.

The guidelines about what and when (those with diabetes) should eat if (they) have diabetes have changed dramatically in the last decade or so. That's because new medications are available, new research findings have punched holes in old dogmas and the goals for managing diabetes have changed. Here are a few common myths and facts about what and when the person with diabetes should eat.

Myth: *If you have diabetes you can't eat any sugar or sweets and you need to avoid starchy foods.*

Fact: In the old days, at least before 1994, this was the rule of thumb. Through much research, begun in the 1970s, holes have been punched in this theory. Due to the findings from many research studies the American Diabetes Association now notes that it is the total amount of carbohydrate that is eaten that raises blood glucose levels, not the specific type of carbohydrate. Thus, people can fit occasional sugary foods and sweets into their food choices as long as they substitute them for other carbohydrate-containing foods or adjust their diabetes medication to compensate. Sugary foods and sweets should be eaten in moderation—that's the same message as for the general public.

Myth: *Starchy foods, such as bread, cereal, and pasta, are the only foods that contain carbohydrate and are the only foods that will make blood glucose levels rise.*

Fact: This was never correct. Foods that contain carbohydrates are: starches, including cereal, pasta, beans and peas, crackers, bread and others; dairy foods; fruits; vegetables; and sugary foods. All these foods raise blood glucose levels. That's OK. That's how the body gets energy. Most of these carbohydrate-containing foods are some of the healthiest foods that can be eaten—whole grains, fruits, vegetables, and low-fat dairy foods. These foods should not be overly restricted. What is important is that similar portions of these foods are eaten at similar times each day to keep blood glucose levels in control.

Myth: *People with diabetes should buy foods in the "diet section" of the supermarket and make sure foods say "sugar-free."*

Fact: There is truly no need to march directly to the "diet section" of the supermarket and purchase "sugar-free" foods. Often these foods are sweetened with "sugar alcohols." They are just another source of carbohydrate. People with diabetes do not need to buy special foods. They need to follow the guidelines for healthy eating.

Myth: *The first place someone with diabetes should look on the Nutrition Facts label is the "sugars."*

Fact: The Sugars line on Nutrition Facts labels is indented from Total Carbohydrates. Also, Total Carbohydrate is in bold and Sugars is in regular type. The Sugars are counted in the Total Carbohydrate. Also, these are not just added sugars, like corn sweeteners or brown sugar; they are also the naturally occurring sugars, such as the sugar in milk—lactose—or the sugar in fruit—sucrose. Again, look at the grams of Total Carbohydrate to determine if that particular food item should be chosen. Also, look at the ingredients to see if there are a lot of added sugars.

Myth: *Everyone with diabetes must eat every few hours, or three meals and three snacks a day.*

Fact: Today this is simply not true. The frequency of meals and snacks (if the person needs to eat any) should depend on a number of factors: whether diabetes medication is taken and the type and dose. Some of the newer diabetes medications do not even cause hypoglycemia. And avoiding hypoglycemia was the main reason for eating snacks. The frequency of meals and snacks should be most dependent on individual food habits and needs.

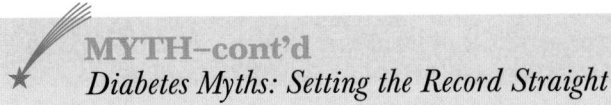

- Nonnutritive sweeteners are safe when consumed within acceptable daily intake levels established by the Food and Drug Administration.
- Individuals using intensive insulin therapy should adjust their before-meal insulin doses based on carbohydrate content of meals.
- As with the general public, consumption of dietary fiber should be encouraged.
- Individuals using daily insulin injections should be consistent in day-to-day carbohydrate intake (Box 19-3).

Protein
- Although protein stimulates insulin secretion as potently as carbohydrate, ingested protein does not increase plasma glucose levels in *controlled* type 2 DM.
- For patients not in optimal glucose control, protein needs may be greater (but not greater than usual intake) than the recommended dietary allowances (RDA).
- Protein intake of 15% to 20% of total daily energy does not need to be modified if renal function is normal.
- Long-term effects of high-protein, low-carbohydrate diets are unknown. Although they generate short-term weight loss and improved glucose levels, there is no evidence that weight loss is maintained.

Dietary Fat
- Less than 10% of energy intake should come from saturated fats.
- Dietary cholesterol intake should be less than 300 mg/day.
- To lower low-density lipoprotein (LDL)-cholesterol, saturated fat intake can be reduced if weight loss is desired. If weight loss is not a goal, saturated fat can be replaced with either carbohydrate or monounsaturated fat.
- Intake of *trans*-unsaturated fatty acids should be minimized.
- Reduced-fat diets contribute to modest weight loss and improvement of dyslipidemia when maintained.
- Polyunsaturated fat intake should be approximately 10% of total energy intake.

Energy Balance and Obesity
- In insulin-resistant patients, reduced energy intake and modest weight loss improve short-term insulin resistance and glucose control.
- Long-term weight loss is best facilitated by structured programs that emphasize lifestyle changes that include (1) education, (2) reduced fat (<30% total kcalories) and energy intake, (3) regular physical activity, and (4) regular personal contact.
- Exercise and behavior modification are most useful as adjuncts to other weight-loss strategies.
- Standard weight-reduction diets, when used alone, are unlikely to produce long-term weight loss.

Box 19-3 Carbohydrate Counting

Carbohydrate counting is one of the meal planning approaches used in the Diabetes Control and Complications Trial (DCCT) and allows for greater focus on consistency in food consumption. The proposition of carbohydrate counting gives priority to the total amount of carbohydrates consumed—regardless of whether monosaccharides, disaccharides, or polysaccharides—rather than the source. Scientific evidence indicates that all forms of carbohydrate basically affect blood glucose levels similarly when eaten in the same gram amount: "A carbohydrate is a carbohydrate is a carbohydrate."

One carbohydrate choice = 15 grams carbohydrate
1 starch
1 fruit
1 milk

Carbohydrate counting can be used for all types of diabetes and in clients of all age groups. The challenges and advantages of carbohydrate counting are outlined below. Three levels of carbohydrate counting based on increasing levels of complexity and required skills have been jointly developed, organized, and published by the American Dietetic Association and the American Diabetes Association.

Level 1: *Getting Started* is the basic booklet that introduces the goal of carbohydrate consistency and flexible food choices. This level works well with clients who have type 1 DM, type 2 DM, and gestational diabetes. It is recommended that one to three client contacts of 30 to 90 minutes each with a registered dietitian or certified diabetes educator be used when teaching Level 1.

Level 2: *Moving On* is the intermediate booklet that assumes basic understanding and knowledge for the client to adjust medication, food, and activities based on patterns from daily records. This level works well with persons using diet only, oral hypoglycemic agents, or insulin to control their diabetes and who have mastered the basics of carbohydrate counting (Level 1). Level 2 takes one to three client contacts of 30 to 60 minutes each with a registered dietitian or certified diabetes educator.

Level 3: *Using Carbohydrate/Insulin Ratios* is an advanced booklet for which clients need understanding and knowledge at the intermediate level to adjust insulin doses based on the client's individual responses to food, medication, and activity. Level 3 is intended for persons on intensive insulin therapy and who have mastered insulin adjustment and supplementation. Level 3 takes one to three contacts of 30 to 60 minutes each with a registered dietitian or certified diabetes educator.

CARBOHYDRATE COUNTING

ADVANTAGES

- Focuses on a single nutrient
- Flexibility in food choices
- Potential for improved blood glucose levels
- Clients feel more empowered
- More precise matching of food and insulin

CHALLENGES

- Weighing/measuring foods
- Maintaining food records (initially and periodically)
- Recording blood glucose levels (before/after eating)
- Dealing with numbers and calculations
- Weight management
- Maintenance of healthy eating pattern

Compiled from Diabetes Control and Complications Trial Research Group: The effect of intensive treatment of diabetes on the development and progression of long-term complications in insulin-dependent diabetes mellitus, N Engl J Med 329:977, *1993; Holler HJ, Pastors JG:* Diabetes medical nutrition therapy: a professional guide to management and nutrition education resources, *Chicago, 1997, American Dietetic Association; American Diabetes Association:* Nutrition recommendations and principles for people with diabetes mellitus *(position statement); www.diabetes.org/diabetescare/supplement198/S32.htm, accessed Nov 28, 1998; American Diabetes Association, American Dietetic Association:* Carbohydrate counting series: getting started (level 1), moving on (level 2), using carbohydrate/insulin ratios (level 3), information for the health professional, *Chicago, 1995, American Dietetic Association.*

Micronutrients
- There is no benefit from vitamin or mineral supplementation when there are no underlying deficiencies. Exceptions include folate for prevention of birth defects and calcium for prevention of osteoporosis.
- Routine supplementation of the diet with antioxidants is not advised because of uncertainties related to long-term efficacy and safety.

Alcohol
- If individuals choose to drink alcohol, daily intake should be limited to two drinks for men and one drink for women. One drink is defined as 12 oz of beer, 5 oz of wine, or 1.5 oz of spirits (approximately 80 proof).
- Alcohol should be consumed with food to reduce risk of hypoglycemia.
- Alcohol should never be mixed with chlorpropamide (Diabinese).

- Abstention from alcohol is recommended for women during pregnancy and those with other medical problems such as pancreatitis, advanced neuropathy, severe hypertriglyceridemia, or alcohol abuse.

Individualized Recommendations

Medical nutrition therapy for diabetes is complex. Physicians and nurses can no longer depend on preprinted diet sheets or formulated meal patterns to provide nutrition care to patients with diabetes.[24] There is no one diabetic diet or "ADA diet." Although the term *"ADA diet"* has never been clearly defined, in the past it usually meant a physician-determined kcalorie level with specific percentages of carbohydrate, protein, and fat based on the exchange lists.[25] The ADA recommends that the term *"ADA diet"* not be used because the ADA no longer sanctions any single meal plan or specified percentages of nutrients.[26] Patients with diabetes require an assessment by a registered dietitian to determine an appropriate nutrition prescription and plan for self-management education.[24,26] Diet orders such as "no concentrated sweets," "no sugar added," "low sugar," and "liberal diabetic" are not considered suitable because they do not reflect diabetes nutrition recommendations and pointlessly restrict sucrose. Such meal plans propagate the false notion that merely restricting sucrose-sweetened foods will improve blood glucose control[26] (see the Teaching Tool, "Better than Sugar? Is Stevia a Good Sugar Substitute?").

Medical nutrition therapy should be individualized, taking into consideration a person's usual eating habits and other lifestyle factors.[27] Consistency within an eating pattern will result in lower glycosylated hemoglobin levels rather than following an arbitrary eating style.[28] Nutrition recommendations for total fat, saturated fat, cholesterol, fiber, vitamins, and minerals are the same for individuals with diabetes as for the general population. Recommendations are modified for protein, carbohydrates, sucrose, and alcohol because of the nature of diabetes in relation to carbohydrate metabolism or the effects of diabetic complications. Protein intake can range from 15% to 20% of daily kcalories from animal and vegetable protein sources. If the patient has nephropathy, lower intakes of protein (about 10% of daily energy intake) may be warranted. Protein restrictions and other modifications necessary for renal disease should be designed by a registered dietitian familiar with

TEACHING TOOL
Better than Sugar? Is Stevia a Good Sugar Substitute?

Stevia (pronounced *STEE-vee-uh*) is a plant native to South America whose leaves have been used for centuries by native peoples in Paraguay and Brazil to sweeten foods. Stevioside (the main ingredient in stevia) is almost kcalorie-free and hundreds of times sweeter than sucrose (regular table sugar). As such, it appeals to many as a natural alternative to artificial sweeteners.

A liquid or powdered form of stevia is used to sweeten a variety of foods available in Japan, Brazil, and Korea. Although it cannot be purchased in the supermarket as a sweetener or added to foods (the FDA has not approved stevia as a safe food) in the United States, it can be purchased in health food stores (at a hefty price) as a dietary supplement (the FDA has little control over supplements). Canada and the European Union also do not allow stevia to be added to foods.

There is no evidence that stevia is harmful in small doses, but likewise, there is no scientific proof that it is safe in large doses.

Reference: Columbus M: The cultivation of stevia, "nature's sweetener." Ministry of Agriculture and Food, Ontario, Canada. Available at www.gov.on.ca/OMAFRA/english/crops/facts/stevia.htm.accessed April 27, 2002.

medical nutrition therapy for diabetes.[23] Carbohydrate recommendations are individualized based on the person's eating habits and blood glucose and lipid goals. Blood glucose control is not impaired by the use of sucrose in the meal plan, but sucrose-containing foods are substituted for other carbohydrates and foods and are not eaten in addition to a meal plan. Blood glucose levels are not affected by moderate alcohol use *if* diabetes is well controlled. Alcohol kcalories should be considered an addition to regular food or meals, and no food should be omitted.[23]

Other related nutrient issues include use of fructose and other nutritive and nonnutritive sweeteners. Although fructose creates a smaller rise in plasma glucose than sucrose and other carbohydrates, large amounts of fructose (up to 20% of daily kcalorie intake) provide no advantage as a sweetener based on its negative effects on serum cholesterol and LDL-cholesterol levels. Other nutritive sweeteners such as corn sweeteners, fruit juice or juice concentrate, honey, molasses, dextrose, and maltose affect glycemic response and caloric content in a manner similar to that of sucrose. The sugar alcohols (sorbitol, mannitol, and xylitol) result in lower glycemic responses than other simple and complex carbohydrates, and ingesting large amounts may have a laxative effect. Nonnutritive sweeteners approved for use by the Food and Drug Administration (FDA), such as saccharin, aspartame, and acesulfame K, are considered safe for consumption by individuals with diabetes. Each product has undergone rigorous testing and scrutiny before approval. All were shown to be safe when consumed by the public, including people with diabetes, and during pregnancy.[23] Table 19-6 summarizes nutrition therapy recommendations.

Table 19-6
Summary of 2002 Medical Nutrition Therapy Recommendations for Diabetes Mellitus

Nutrition principles and recommendations are classified into the following four categories according to levels of supporting evidence:

A—Strong supporting evidence
B—Some supporting evidence
C—Limited supporting evidence
D—Based on expert consensus

Nutrition Recommendation	Grading
Carbohydrates	
• Whole grains, fruits, vegetables, and low-fat milk should be included.	A
• Total amount of carbohydrates in meals and snacks is more important than the source or type of carbohydrate.	A
• Individuals receiving intensive insulin therapy should adjust their before-meal insulin doses based on the carbohydrate content of the meal.	A
• Individuals receiving fixed daily insulin doses should try to be consistent in day-to-day carbohydrate intake.	B
• There is not sufficient evidence of long-term benefit to recommend or use low-glycemic index diets as a primary strategy in food/meal planning for individuals with type 1 DM.	B
• As for the general public, consumption of fiber should be encouraged.	B
• Percentages of carbohydrates should be based on individual nutrition assessment.	B
• Carbohydrate and monounsaturated fat together should provide 60%-70% of energy intake.	D

Copyright © 2002 American Diabetes Association. Modified from Diabetes Care Vol. 25, 2002; 148-198. Reprinted with permission from The American Diabetes Association. In Anderson SL: Diabetes mellitus. In Williams SR, Schlenker ED: Essentials of nutrition and diet therapy, ed 8, St Louis, 2003, Mosby.

Table 19-6–cont'd
Summary of 2002 Medical Nutrition Therapy Recommendations for Diabetes Mellitus

Nutrition Recommendation	Grading
Nutritive Sweeteners	
• Sucrose does not increase glycemia to a greater extent than isocaloric amounts of starch.	A
• Sucrose and sucrose-containing foods do not need to be restricted; however, if included in the food/meal plan, they should be substituted for other carbohydrate sources or, if added, be adequately covered with insulin or other glucose-lowering medication.	A
• Fructose reduces postprandial glycemia when it replaces sucrose or starch.	B
• Consumption of fructose in large amounts may have adverse effects on plasma lipids.	B
• Use of sugar alcohols as sweetening agents appears to be safe.	B
• Sugar alcohols may cause diarrhea, especially in children.	B
• Use of added fructose as a sweetening agent is not recommended.	C
• Sucrose and sucrose-containing foods should be eaten in the context of a healthy diet, and the intake of other nutrients ingested with sucrose, such as fat, should be taken into account.	D
• There is no reason to recommend avoidance of naturally occurring fructose in fruits, vegetables, and other food.	D
• It is unlikely that sugar alcohols in amounts ingested in individual food servings or meals will contribute to a significant reduction in total energy or carbohydrate intake (although no studies have been conducted to support this).	D
Resistant Starches	
• Resistant starches (nondigestible) have no established benefit.	C
Nonnutritive Sweeteners	
• Nonnutritive sweeteners are safe when consumed within the acceptable daily intake established by the FDA.	A
• It is unknown if use of nonnutritive sweeteners improves long-term glycemic control or assists in weight loss.	D
Dietary Protein	
• In those with controlled type 2 DM, ingested protein does not increase plasma glucose concentrations, although ingested protein is just as potent a stimulant of insulin secretion as carbohydrate.	A
• There is no evidence to suggest that usual protein intake (15%-20% of total daily energy) should be modified if renal function is normal.	B
• Protein requirements may be greater than the RDA but not greater than usual intake for those with less-than-optimal glycemic control.	B
• Dietary protein does not slow absorption of carbohydrate and dietary protein, and carbohydrates do not raise plasma glucose later than carbohydrate alone and thus do not prevent late-onset hypoglycemia.	B
• It may be prudent to avoid protein intake >20% of total daily energy.	C
• Long-term effects of diets high in protein and low in carbohydrate are unknown. Although such diets may produce short-term weight loss and improved glycemia, it has not been established that weight loss is maintained. Long-term effect of such diets on plasma LDL cholesterol is also a concern.	D
Dietary Fat	
• In all, <10% of energy intake should be derived form saturated fats. Some persons (i.e., those with LDL cholesterol ≥100 mg/dl) may benefit from lowering saturated fat intake to <7% of energy intake.	A
• Dietary cholesterol intake should be <300 mg/day. Some persons (i.e., those with LDL cholesterol ≥100 mg/dl) may benefit from lowering dietary cholesterol to <200 mg/day.	A
• Intake of transunsaturated fatty acids should be minimized.	A
• Current fat replacers/substitutes approved by the FDA are safe for use in food.	A
• To lower plasma LDL cholesterol, energy derived from saturated fat can be reduced if concurrent weight loss is desirable or replaced with carbohydrate or monounsaturated fat if weight loss is not a goal.	A

Continued

Table 19-6—cont'd
Summary of 2002 Medical Nutrition Therapy Recommendations for Diabetes Mellitus

Nutrition Recommendation	Grading
Dietary Fat—cont'd	
• Polyunsaturated fat intake should be approximately 10% of energy intake.	B
• In weight-maintaining diets, when monounsaturated fat replaces carbohydrate, it may beneficially affect postprandial glycemia and plasma triglycerides but not necessarily fasting plasma glucose of HgbA$_{1c}$.	B
• Incorporation of two or three servings of plant stanols/sterols (approximately 2 g) food per day, substituted for similar food, will lower LDL and total cholesterol.	B
• Reduced-fat diets, when maintained long term, contribute to modest loss of weight and improvement of dyslipidemia.	B
• Two or more servings of fish per week provide dietary Ω-3 polyunsaturated fat and can be recommended.	C
• Monounsaturated fat and carbohydrate together should provide 60%-70% of energy intake. However, increasing fat intake may result in increased energy intake.	D
• Fat intake should be individualized and designed to fit ethnic and cultural backgrounds.	D
• Use of low-fat food and fat replacers/substitutes may reduce total fat and energy intake and thereby facilitate weight loss.	D
Energy Balance and Obesity	
• In insulin-resistant individuals, reduced energy intake and modest weight loss improve insulin resistance and glycemia in the short term.	A
• Structured programs that emphasize lifestyle changes—including education, reduced fat (<30% daily energy) and energy intake, regular physical activity, and regular participant contact—can produce long-term weight loss of 5%-7% of starting weight.	A
• Exercise and behavior modification are most useful as adjuncts to other weight-loss strategies. Exercise is helpful in maintaining weight loss.	A
• Nutrition interventions, such as standard weight-reduction diets, when used alone are unlikely to produce long-term weight loss. Structured, intensive lifestyle programs are necessary.	A
• Optimal strategies for preventing and treating obesity long-term have yet to be defined.	A
• Currently available weight-loss drugs have modest beneficial effects. These drugs should be used only in people with BMI >27.0 kg/m².	B
• Gastric reduction surgery can be considered for patients with BMI >35 kg/m². Long-term data comparing benefits and risks of gastric reduction surgery to those of medical therapy are not available.	C

🌀 Role of the Nurse

The role of the nurse in caring for the nutritional needs of patients with diabetes varies depending on setting and age of the client. However, the general approach is to become aware of and help assess the patient's knowledge and understanding and adherence with the prescribed diet. When possible, observing meals and food choices as well as monitoring glucose levels can give important clues to the level of compliance. When compliance is faulty, the nurse needs to determine whether knowledge or motivation is the problem. Knowledge deficits can be remedied in appropriate areas by the nurse or dietitian; lack of motivation may be harder to handle. For example, (1) adolescents with diabetes may not believe long-term complications are related to diet and may be more motivated by the need to eat like their peers, or (2) older adults with diabetes may be set in long-time food intake patterns and may not want to change them as long as they take medication for hyperglycemia.

When a trusting relationship exists between the nurse and patient, discussions about motivations and concerns can take place. The nurse may then influence the patient to be more concerned about his or her long-term welfare. A care plan that

Table 19-6—cont'd
Summary of 2002 Medical Nutrition Therapy Recommendations for Diabetes Mellitus

Nutrition Recommendation	Grading
Micronutrients	
• There is no clear evidence of benefit from vitamin and mineral supplementation by those who do not have underlying deficiencies. Exceptions include folate for prevention of birth defects and calcium for prevention of bone disease.	B
• Although difficult to ascertain, if deficiencies of vitamins and minerals are identified, supplementation can be beneficial.	B
• Routine supplementation of the diet with antioxidants is not advised because of uncertainties related to long-term efficacy and safety.	B
• Select populations, such as older adults, pregnant or lactating women, strict vegetarians, and people on kcalorie-restricted diets, may benefit from supplementation with a multivitamin preparation.	D
• There is no evidence to suggest long-term benefit from herbal preparations.	D
Alcohol	
• If individuals choose to drink alcohol, daily intake should be limited to one drink for women and two drinks for men. One drink is defined as a 12-oz beer, 5-oz glass of wine, or 1.5-oz glass of distilled spirits.	A
• The type of alcoholic beverage consumed does not make a difference.	A
• When moderate amounts of alcohol are consumed with food, blood glucose levels are not affected.	A
• To reduce risk of hypoglycemia, alcohol should be consumed with food.	A
• Ingestion of light-to-moderate amounts of alcohol does not raise blood pressure; excessive, chronic ingestion of alcohol raises blood pressure and may be a risk factor for stroke.	A
• Pregnant women and people with medical problems such as pancreatitis, advanced neuropathy, severe hypertriglyceridemia, or alcohol abuse should be advised to not ingest alcohol.	A
• There are potential benefits from ingestion of moderate amounts of alcohol, such as decreased risk of type 2 DM, coronary heart disease, and stroke.	B
• Alcoholic beverages should be consumed in addition to the regular food/meal plan for all patients with diabetes. No food should be omitted.	D

meets the patient's social, psychologic, and physical needs can be developed as a result of collaboration among the nurse, physician or primary healthcare provider, dietitian, and patient (see the Teaching Tool, "Helping Clients Follow Instructions). Additional forms of support may be provided by community agencies and associations. These resources, such as the ADA, are listed in Appendix C, Nutrition and Health Organizations.

As mentioned previously, nutrition and diet are considered by both patients and health professionals to be the most difficult problems in the management of diabetes. Every day we are faced with changes in our environments that require some adaptation to the situation. We're late for work, so maybe we skip breakfast or grab something quick along the way. The kids have ball practice tonight, so dinner becomes sandwiches and fruit instead of a full-course meal. Most of us make the required changes in stride, not thinking too much about it. Why should we think life for persons with diabetes is any different? Historically, those with diabetes have been taught consistency in everything they do: eat at the same time every day, eat the same number of kcalories every day, take the same amount of insulin every day, and on and on. The new recommendations for medical nutritional therapy consider these perpetual lifestyle changes.

TEACHING TOOL
Helping Clients Follow Instructions

*D*iabetes is on the rise, particularly among ethnic groups for whom English may be a second language or whose education may be limited (e.g., reading at a fourth or fifth grade level). About 90 million adult Americans have low literacy skills that may affect their ability to understand their disease and to follow treatment instructions. Because diabetes requires long-term behavioral changes and monitoring, compliance is important. Health professionals working with individuals who have low literacy skills and diabetes mellitus can improve understanding and compliance by (1) using patient education materials that are simple and concise, (2) using culturally appropriate graphics showing step-by-step instructions, and (3) involving family members.

Reference: Mayeaux EJ Jr et al.: Improving patient education for patients with low literacy skills, Am Fam Physician 53(1):205, 1996.

Wouldn't it also be practical when encouraging dietary adherence with a person who has diabetes to discuss situations that cause the individual problems in maintaining control over his or her eating? Schlundt et al.[29] have identified seven situations that provide obstacles to adhering to a prescribed diet (Box 19-4).

Box 19-4 Obstacles to Dietary Adherence in Diabetes Mellitus

Obstacle: Extent to which social, career, recreational, and personal goals create situations within which the person must choose between making appropriate food choices and furthering another important life goal.

Assessment: Does the patient see this as a problem? To what extent? Does the patient feel frustrated about it? How has the patient dealt with it in the past? Does the patient make compromises, or give in to the competing goals? Is the conflict anticipated, or simply handled when it arises? Does time pressure have any effect on the patient's ability to make appropriate choices?

Obstacle: Tempted to overeat to cope with stress and negative emotions

Assessment: How stressful is the patient's life? How does the patient respond to frustration, stress, anxiety, and depression? Any conflicts with friends, family, supervisors, or other authorities? Is food used as an escape or avoidance strategy? If so, how much and what kinds of foods are eaten? How is boredom handled?

Obstacle: Ability to resist temptation when confronted with inappropriate foods or when experiencing specific food cravings

Assessment: Does the patient encounter inappropriate foods in the everyday environment? If so, how often? How does the patient react to seeing other people eat these foods? Does the patient experience specific food cravings? If so, what foods, how often, and how strong are the cravings? Is there family support to reduce the availability of inappropriate foods?

Obstacle: Reaction to eating at restaurants, social events, parties, special occasions, and holidays

Assessment: What are family food traditions? How often does the patient eat socially with peers? Do friends and family eat in moderation, or do they overeat at holidays and social events? How does the patient make food choices when faced with a large array of foods? Can the patient order an appropriate meal from a menu? Does the patient even try to stick to the meal plan, or simply give up?

Obstacle: Social support

Assessment: Do family and friends make it easier or harder to eat appropriately? What behaviors from family and friends create obstacles? Do others deliberately sabotage the patient? Are there any supportive behaviors that friends or family could do?

Obstacle: Assessment of patient's history of dietary adherence

Assessment: Does the patient get discouraged and give up altogether? Is there a history of taking *vacations* from appropriate diabetes care? Does the patient work out compromises, or give up entirely?

Obstacle: Assessment of whether the patient can respond assertively when being pressured to deviate from an appropriate eating pattern

Assessment: Can the patient say "No" clearly and firmly? How worried is the patient about being different from others?

Modified from Schlundt DG et al.: Situational obstacles to dietary adherence for adults with diabetes, J Am Diet Assoc 94:874, 1994.

Comprehensive education for persons with diabetes should include assessment of these obstacles and situational problem solving.[29]

SPECIAL CONSIDERATIONS

Illness

During periods of illness, blood glucose levels may become elevated and diabetes control may worsen. This is caused by an increase in hepatic production of glucose that has been stimulated by infection, illness, injury, or stress (specifically, by the release of epinephrine, norepinephrine, glucagon, and cortisol). Under such conditions, this hyperglycemia increases insulin requirements.[23]

Often, while illness causes an increased need for insulin, there is also a decreased appetite and food intake. Liquids and soft foods are usually better tolerated and also help provide some kcaloric intake while preventing dehydration. The following guidelines have been used in cases of brief illness on an emergency basis for a maximum of 3 days[23,24,30] (see also the Teaching Tool, "Sick Day Guidelines"):

1. Monitor blood glucose at least four times a day (before each meal and at bedtime).
2. Test urine for ketones (if blood glucose is greater than 240 mg/dl).
3. If regular foods are not tolerated, replace carbohydrates in the meal plan with liquid, semiliquid, or soft foods. The source of the carbohydrate is not of major concern. Sugar-containing liquids may be the only food source tolerated. More important is what the patient can tolerate. A general rule is to consume every 1 to 2 hours approximately 15 grams carbohydrate (e.g., 1/2 cup juice or 1/2 cup applesauce), or every 3 to 4 hours, 50 grams carbohydrate (e.g., 1 cup juice and 3/4 cup applesauce or 10 saltine crackers, 1 cup soup, and 1/2 cup juice). If blood glucose is greater than 240 mg/dl, the entire amount may not need to be consumed.
4. Drink 8 to 12 oz of fluid (water, broth, tea) each hour. A carbohydrate source may also be the fluid source.
5. If vomiting, diarrhea, or fever occur, consume small amounts of salted foods and liquids more frequently to replace lost electrolytes.

Gastroparesis

Approximately 20% to 30% of individuals with diabetes develop gastroparesis with delayed gastric emptying that can manifest with heartburn, nausea, abdominal pain, vomiting, early satiety, and weight loss for some persons. Gastroparesis occurs as a result of vagal autonomic neuropathy and occurs more often in type 1 DM than in type 2 DM.[31]

Dietary treatment of gastroparesis involves monitoring intake carefully. Carbohydrates should be replaced with tolerated foods. Six small meals may be better tolerated than three large meals. If constipation or diarrhea occur, fiber intake is altered according to patient needs. If the patient complains of dry mouth, fluids can be increased and food moistened with broth. A low-fat (40 grams) soft or liquid diet may be useful to prevent delay in gastric emptying. If metoclopramide (Reglan) is used to increase gastric contractions and relax the pyloric sphincter, the patient may experience side effects of dry mouth or nausea. Insulin should be matched with meals to regulate delayed absorption and glucose changes. Bezoar formation is common with oranges, coconuts, green beans, apples, figs, potato skins, brussels sprouts, and sauerkraut. If problems are severe, a temporary jejunostomy tube feeding may be indicated.[31]

🌀 Diabetes Management through the Life Span

The role of medical nutrition therapy is crucial for optimal blood glucose control. In various life stages, pregnancy outcome, and growth and development of children can be influenced by nutritional intake.

TEACHING TOOL
Sick Day Guidelines

Colds, fever, flu, nausea, vomiting, and diarrhea can cause special problems for individuals with diabetes. Teach these guidelines to clients to help them manage common illnesses and maintain control of their diabetes.

1. These guidelines apply only to mild, short-term, 1-day illnesses. Call your physician if any of the following occur:
   - You can't keep any liquids or carbohydrates down for more than 8 hours.
   - You are vomiting or have diarrhea.
   - You are spilling ketones in your urine.
   - You begin to breathe rapidly, become drowsy, or lose consciousness.
   - You have questions or concerns.
2. If you take insulin, you must continue to take your usual dose to prevent ketoacidosis. Your need for insulin continues or may increase during illness. Never omit your insulin.
3. If you take oral hypoglycemic agents (tablets), continue to take your usual dose unless you are vomiting. Resume your medication when you are able to tolerate fluids and food again. If vomiting continues, contact your physician.
4. Monitor your blood glucose and test urine for ketones at least four times per day (i.e., before each meal and at bedtime). If your blood glucose reading is greater than 240 mg/dl and there are moderate to large ketone levels in the urine, call your physician.
5. If you can't eat your regular food, replace it with carbohydrates in the form of liquids or soft foods. Eat at least 50 grams of carbohydrates every 3 to 4 hours, especially if your blood sugar is less than 240 mg/dl. If your blood sugar is greater than 240 mg/dl, continue to drink liquids, especially those that don't contain kcalories (water, broth, diet soft drinks, tea).

FOODS CONTAINING 10 GRAMS CARBOHYDRATES

½ cup regular soft drink (ginger ale, cola)
½ frozen fruit bar (twin bar)
2 tsp corn syrup or honey
2 ½ tsp granulated sugar
¼ cup regularly sweetened gelatin

FOODS CONTAINING 15 GRAMS CARBOHYDRATES

½ cup orange or grapefruit juice
⅓ cup grape or apple juice
½ cup ice cream
½ cup cooked cereal
¼ cup sherbet
⅓ cup regularly sweetened gelatin
1 cup broth-based soups (reconstituted with water)
1 cup cream soups
¾ cup regular soft drink (ginger ale, cola)
¼ cup milkshake
1 ½ cups milk
½ cup eggnog (commercial)
⅓ cup tapioca pudding
½ cup custard
1 cup plain yogurt
1 slice toast
6 saltine crackers

6. Drink a large glass of kcalorie-free liquid every hour to replace fluids. If you feel nauseous or are vomiting, take small sips (1 to 2 tablespoons) every 15 to 30 minutes. Call your physician.
7. When illness subsides, return to your regular meal plan and usual insulin schedule.

From Franz MJ, Joynes JO: Diabetes and brief illness, *Minneapolis, 1993, International Diabetes Center.*

Pregnancy

Women with preexisting diabetes who become pregnant are vulnerable to fetal complications, and maternal health can be compromised when complications of diabetes occur.[15] Occasionally, the stress of pregnancy may induce gestational diabetes mellitus (GDM), which is a form of glucose intolerance that has its onset during pregnancy and is resolved on parturition.[32] Whether the mother has preexisting diabetes or GDM, risk of fetal abnormalities and mortality are increased in the presence of hyperglycemia, so every effort should be made to control blood glucose levels.[25] All women with GDM should receive nutrition counseling by a registered dietitian when possible.[33]

Changes that take place during pregnancy greatly affect diabetes control and insulin use. Some hormones and enzymes produced by the placenta are antagonistic to insulin, thus reducing its effectiveness. Maternal insulin does not cross the placenta, but glucose does. This will cause the fetus's pancreas to increase insulin production if blood glucose levels get too high. The increased production of insulin causes the most typical characteristic of infants born to women with diabetes—macrosomia. Newborns may also have other problems such as respiratory difficulties, hypocalcemia, hypoglycemia, hypokalemia, or jaundice.[15]

macrosomia
larger body size

Individualization of medical nutrition therapy contingent on maternal weight and height is recommended.[33] Medical nutrition therapy should include provision of adequate kcalories and nutrients to meet the needs of the pregnancy and should be consistent with established maternal blood glucose goals.[33] Self-monitoring of blood glucose (SMBG) presents important information about the impact of food on blood glucose levels.[34] At the start, minimal daily SMBG should be planned four times a day (fasting and 1 or 2 hours after each meal).[34] Blood glucose goals during pregnancy are the following[35]:
- *Fasting*: less than 95 mg/dl
- *1 hour postprandial*: 140 mg/dl
- *2 hours postprandial*: less than 120 mg/dl

Frequency of SMBG may be decreased once blood glucose control is established. However, some monitoring should continue throughout pregnancy.[34]

Desired weight gains and nutrient requirements are the same as for established pregnancy guidelines: 0.9 kg to 1.8 kg (2 to 4 lb) for the first trimester and 1 lb per week for the second and third trimesters based on prepregnancy body mass index (BMI). No kcalorie adjustments are needed for the first trimester.[22,23] During the second and third trimesters, an increased energy intake of approximately 100 to 300 kcal/day is recommended.[22,23] High-quality protein should be increased by 10 g/day and can be met easily with one or two extra glasses of low-fat or skim milk or 1 to 2 oz of meat or meat substitute.[22] As with any pregnancy, 400 μg/day of folic acid is recommended for prevention of neural tube defects and other congenital abnormalities.[23] Alcohol consumption is not recommended in any amount.

Kcaloric restriction must be viewed with caution. A minimum of 1700 to 1800 kcal/day of carefully selected foods has been shown to prevent ketosis.[36] Intakes below this level are not advised.[34] Weight gain goals are based on prepregnancy BMI. Weight gain should still occur even if patients have gained considerable weight before onset of GDM.[34] Each patient with GDM should be evaluated individually by a registered dietitian, have her care plans adjusted, and be provided patient education as needed to achieve weight goals.[34]

Pregnancy in Overt Diabetes.   A successful pregnancy for a woman who has diabetes requires planning and commitment. Because most fetal malformations occur during the first trimester of pregnancy, achieving and maintaining excellent glycemic control before conception and during early pregnancy is a must. The optimal period of care for a woman with diabetes is *before* conception. Box 19-5 outlines preconception nutritional recommendations.

Ideally, preconception counseling should begin during puberty and continue through the childbearing years.[16,37,38] Insulin requirements increase during the second

Box 19-5 Preconception Nutritional Recommendations

Nutrient	Recommendation
Calories	Sufficient to achieve or maintain desired body weight
Carbohydrates	Individualized based on eating habits and clinical condition of the woman
Protein	10%-20% of total daily calories Decrease to 0.8 g/kg/day if evidence of nephropathy
Fat	<30% of total daily calories Up to 10% polyunsaturated fats <10% saturated fats Remainder from monounsaturated fats
Cholesterol	<300 mg/day
Fiber	20-35 g/day
Sodium	<3000 mg/day <2400 mg/day in mild to moderate hypertension <2000 mg/day with nephropathy, hypertension, or edema
Folate	400 μg/day
Vitamins and minerals	Assess for specific individual needs
Alcohol	Avoid
Caffeine	Limit to <300 mg/day

Reference: Preconception Diabetes Nutrient Recommendations *from Thomas, A:* Preconception counseling for the woman with diabetes. *Copyright Diabetes Care and Education, a Dietetic Practice Group of the American Dietetic Association. Reprinted by permission from On the Cutting Edge, Vol. 23; Number 2, 2002.*

and third trimesters because of increased blood glucose levels caused by increased production of pregnancy-associated hormones that are insulin antagonists.[16] Successful preconception care programs have used the following pre- and postprandial goals:[37]

- *Before meals:* capillary whole-blood glucose 70 to 100 mg/dl or capillary plasma glucose 80 to 110 mg/dl
- *2 hours postprandial:* capillary whole-blood glucose less than 140 mg/dl or capillary plasma glucose less than 155 gm/dl

Glycated hemoglobin levels should be normal or close to normal as possible before conception is attempted.[24]

Pregnancy will require greater attention to medical nutrition therapy on a day-to-day basis. Guidance during early pregnancy should include special consideration for food cravings and nausea. The meal plan should be individualized and should evolve throughout the pregnancy to meet changing nutritional needs and insulin requirements. Three meals and three snacks are usually recommended. The use of frequent home blood glucose monitoring can help the patient maintain normal fasting and postprandial glucose levels and avoid frequent or severe hypoglycemic reactions.

Gestational Diabetes. Gestational diabetes mellitus (GDM) will develop in about 2% to 5% of all pregnancies.[4] Women who develop GDM are often obese, but weight reduction should not be attempted at this time.[23] Although the specific components of an ideal diet for GDM have not been determined, good glucose control must be maintained and is usually accomplished by individualization of intake and graphing of weight gain.[21] Often, insulin may be prescribed in addition to medical nutrition therapy to reduce the risks of fetal macrosomia, neonatal hyperglycemia, and perinatal mortality.[23] Oral hypoglycemic agents are teratogenic

Box 19-6 Postpartum Recommendations

A woman who has had gestational diabetes can decrease her chances of developing type 2 DM by doing the following:
- Screening 6 or more weeks after delivery
- Having a lipid panel performed 5 months or more after delivery
- Maintaining her ideal body weight
- Eating a lower-fat diet
- Exercising regularly
- Breastfeeding, which decreases the incidence of diabetes in the first 3 months after delivery
- Screening before subsequent pregnancies

Postpartum Recommendations *from Gutierrez, VML: The emerging burden of diabetes: the intergenerational effect. Copyright Diabetes Care and Education, A Dietetic Practice Group of the American Dietetic Association. Reprinted by permission from On the Cutting Edge, Vol. 23, Number 2, 2002.*

to the fetus and therefore not recommended. Glucose levels usually revert to normal following delivery, but there is an increased risk for later development of type 1 or type 2 DM. Nearly 30% to 40% of women with GDM eventually develop type 2 DM[4] (Box 19-6).

Maturity Onset Diabetes of the Young (MODY)

Incidence and prevalence of type 2 DM in children have increased 30-fold over the past 20 years, causing the term *epidemic* to be used to describe the phenomenon.[24,39-44] This means the burden of diabetes and accompanying complications will affect many more individuals, thus causing an enormous drain on resources.[39,43] More Americans will be taking potent medications, which have side effects, for most of their lives.[39] What has accompanied this epidemic of type 2 DM in children across the United States? The answer apparently lies within another epidemic—that of childhood obesity.[39-44]

Obesity is the most prominent clinical risk factor for type 2 DM in children and adolescents. About one third of children with type 2 DM have a BMI greater than 40, indicating morbid obesity, and 17% have BMIs greater than 45 (normal BMI range for the pediatric population is 35 to 39).[41] Besides morbid obesity, other clinical signs that may indicate risk for type 2 DM include the following[39,40]:

- **Acanthosis nigricans** (hyperpigmentation and thickening of the skin into velvety irregular folds in the neck and flexural areas), which reflects chronic hyperinsulinemia
- Polycystic ovarian syndrome (PCOS), which is associated with insulin resistance and obesity
- Hypertension, which may occur in 20% to 30% of patients with type 2 DM
- Presence of acanthosis nigricans *and* hypertension, which suggests hyperinsulinemia

Girls appear to be more susceptible than boys to type 2 DM, with an overall female-to-male ratio of 1.7:1 regardless of race.[43] In addition, adolescents with type 2 DM generally have obese parents who themselves tend to have insulin resistance or overt type 2 DM.[40] Reported cases of type 2 DM showed diagnosis to occur during the usual pubertal age period (ages 12-16 years).[39,40] Although there are currently insufficient data to make definite type 2 DM screening recommendations for children or adolescents, a panel of experts on children with diabetes developed the recommendations outlined in Box 19-7.

As with type 2 DM in adults, the ideal treatment goal is normalization of blood glucose values and HgbA$_{1c}$. Successful control of associated comorbidities, such as hypertension and hyperlipidemia, is also important. The ultimate goal is to decrease risk of acute and chronic complications associated with diabetes.[39] Initial

acanthosis nigricans hyperpigmentation and thickening of the skin into velvety irregular folds in the neck and flexural areas

Box 19-7   Recommendations for Children and Adolescents with Type 2 Diabetes Mellitus (Maturity Onset Diabetes of the Young)

As with any person with diabetes, the ideal treatment goal is normalization of blood glucose values and HgbA$_{1c}$ to decrease risk of acute and chronic complications associated with diabetes. Initial treatment of type 2 DM in children varies depending on the clinical symptoms.

Treatment	Recommendation
Education	SMBG tailored to individual needs, but should probably include a combination of fasting and postprandial measurements
	Cessation of excessive weight gain with normal linear growth with near-normal HgbA$_{1c}$ (<approximately 7% in most laboratories) and near-normal fasting blood glucose values (<126 mg/dl)
Diet	Referral to a registered dietitian with knowledge and experience in nutritional management of children with diabetes
	Behavior modification strategies for changing lifestyle and decreasing high-kcaloric, high-fat food choices
Exercise	Increase kcaloric expenditure by increasing daily physical activity
	Decrease sedentary activity (e.g., TV viewing and computer use)
Emotional support	Patients may have been treated for depression or eating disorders before diagnosis, therefore careful and continuous follow-up are critical
Pharmaceutical therapy	Pharmacologic therapy indicated if treatment goals are not met with nutrition education and exercise
	Use metformin as first oral agent
	Efficacy and safety data are not available for children nor are any of these drugs FDA-approved for use in children, although it is reasonable to assume glucose-lowering oral agents will be effective in children
	Troglitazone has been associated with fatal hepatic failure; therefore its use in children is not recommended
	Begin treatment with insulin in patients with greatly elevated blood glucose levels or those who are symptomatic. Add metformin while decreasing insulin when glucose control established.
Monitoring complications	HgbA$_{1c}$ to monitor glycemic control
	SMBG
	Yearly evaluation for dyslipidemia, microalbuminuria, renal function, retinopathy
	Importance of foot examinations unknown, however they are painless, inexpensive, and provide an opportunity for education about foot care
Hypertension treatment	Careful control is critical
	Use ACE inhibitors in children with microalbuminuria
Hyperlipidemia treatment	Weight loss, increased activity, and improvement of glycemic control often result in improvement of lipid levels
	Use medications if these approaches fail
	HMG CoA reductase inhibitors ("statins") are absolutely contraindicated in women of childbearing age unless highly effective contraception is used and patient has been extensively counseled.

Modified from American Diabetes Association: Type 2 diabetes in children and adolescents, Pediatrics 105:671, 2000; American Diabetes Association: Type 2 diabetes in children and adolescents, Diabetes Care 23:381, 2000; Pinhas-Hamiel O: Type 2 diabetes: not just for grownups anymore, Contemp Pediatrics, 1:102, 2001.

ACE, *Angiotensin-converting enzyme;* FDA, *Food and Drug Administration;* SMBG, *self-monitoring of blood glucose.*

treatment will vary depending on clinical symptoms. The range of disease at diagnosis varies from asymptomatic hyperglycemia to DKA and hyperglycemic hyperosmolar nonketotic (HHNK) syndrome. Both DKA and HHNK are associated with high morbidity and mortality in children.[39] Medical nutrition therapy and exercise are obvious first-line treatments, but most children diagnosed with type 2 DM will require drug therapy.[23,39] Although insulin is the only FDA-approved drug for treatment of diabetes in children, oral agents are most often used for children with type 2 DM.[39]

All children with type 2 DM should receive comprehensive self-management education including SMBG, referral to a registered dietitian with knowledge and experience in nutritional management of children with diabetes, behavior modification strategies for lifestyle changes, increased daily physical activity, and decreased sedentary activity (e.g., TV viewing and computer use).[39]

Perhaps the relevance of this epidemic is best summed up by Levetan[43]:

> "Less than one century ago, there were no airplanes, no cars, and no fast-food restaurants. Not surprisingly, this phenomenal technologic growth has come at a price—an expanded girth that has extended not only to adults, but also to children. This has resulted in a 70% rise in diabetes among 30- to 40-year olds and a doubling in the number of children with type 2 diabetes in less than a decade."

SUMMARY

Diabetes mellitus (DM) is a group of conditions characterized by either a relative or complete lack of insulin secretion by the beta cells of the pancreas or defects of cell insulin receptors, which results in disturbances of carbohydrate, protein, and lipid metabolism and hyperglycemia. Long-term complications often lead to disability and premature death. The complications may be related to the level and frequency of hyperglycemia experiences throughout the life span in addition to genetic and environmental factors.

The two primary categories of glucose intolerance are type 1 DM and type 2 DM. Type 1 DM symptoms appear suddenly and include polyphagia, polyuria, polydipsia, and weight loss. All persons with type 1 DM require exogenous insulin to maintain normal blood glucose levels. The primary metabolic problem in type 2 DM is insulin resistance. Family history and obesity are the two strongest risk factors for type 2 DM. The gradually occurring symptoms of type 2 DM are polyuria, polydipsia, fatigue, and frequent infections. Some individuals with type 2 DM may require insulin to optimize blood glucose control. Additional types of diabetes include gestational diabetes, impaired glucose tolerance, and other less common forms of diabetes. Related conditions that may occur are hypoglycemia, diabetic ketoacidosis (DKA), and hyperosmolar hyperglycemic nonketotic syndrome (HHNK).

The main goal of treatment is maintenance of plasma insulin/glucose homeostasis. Treatment may include the use of insulin, medical nutrition therapy, and exercise. Control of blood glucose levels is the cornerstone of diabetes management and can be monitored several ways: (1) fasting blood glucose determination by reputable laboratories, (2) glycosylated hemoglobin determination by reputable laboratories, and (3) self-monitoring with standardized devices.

Medical nutrition therapy is an essential component of successful diabetes management, and the complexity involved requires a team approach to enhance the ability of the patient to obtain good metabolic control. The diabetes management team should include a registered nurse, a physician or primary healthcare provider, a registered dietitian, and the person with diabetes. Successful medical nutrition therapy involves the diabetes management team conducting a thorough assessment, encouraging the patient's role in goal setting, implementing nutrition intervention, and regularly evaluating the nutrition care plan.

The current guidelines for medical nutrition therapy for diabetes management include: (1) plan for near normal blood glucose levels and optimal lipid levels; (2) individualize diet plans; (3) reach a reasonable weight; and (4) if desired, consume some sugar and foods that contain sugar if substituted for other carbohydrate foods. Nutrition recommendations for total fat, saturated fat, cholesterol, fiber, vitamins, and minerals are the same for individuals with diabetes as for the general population. Recommendations are modified for protein, carbohydrates, sucrose, and alcohol because of the nature of diabetes in relation to carbohydrate metabolism or the effects of diabetic complications.

THE NURSING APPROACH
Case Study: Diabetes

Roberta, age 54, has had a medical diagnosis of type 2 DM for the past year. She comes to the physician's office for a finger-stick glucose test every 2 weeks because she has resisted learning how to perform home glucose monitoring. She currently takes glyburide, an oral hypoglycemic, every morning.

ASSESSMENT

Subjective

- Roberta reveals she enjoys eating fried foods, potato chips, Italian pastries, and chocolate.
- She can't remember how to use the *Exchange Lists for Meal Planning*.
- She takes her medication regularly every morning but "adjusts" by taking more when she knows she is going to lunch with her friends.
- She states her last blood glucose was 170 mg/dl (she incorrectly refers to her blood *sugar* reading).

Objective

- Blood glucose: 200 mg/dl (at the office before lunch)
- Weight: 175 lb
- Height: 5'4"

NURSING DIAGNOSIS

Difficulty in maintaining a consistent carbohydrate-diabetes meal plan evidenced by self-reporting of dietary intake

PLANNING

Goals

1. Attend two teaching sessions with a dietitian at a local diabetes clinic.
2. Use *The First Step in Diabetes Meal Planning* brochure until meeting with dietitian to determine an appropriate nutrition prescription.
3. Reduce blood glucose to 150 mg/dl by the next office visit.

IMPLEMENTATION

- Discuss importance of keeping blood glucose within normal limits to prevent complications.
- Review symptoms of hypoglycemia and hyperglycemia.
- Review *The First Step in Diabetes Meal Planning* brochure until meeting with dietitian to determine an appropriate nutrition prescription.
- Assist client in planning a meal using *The First Step in Diabetes Meal Planning* brochure in conjunction with her usual eating pattern.
- Assure client of her ability to eat a healthy diet.
- Make appointment with dietitian for individualization of an appropriate meal pattern.
- Encourage client not to adjust prescribed medications.

EVALUATION

The goals in 4 weeks have been achieved as evidenced by the following:
- Has met with the dietitian
- Reports she has modified her usual food intake to reduce high-fat foods
- Has a fasting blood glucose at or below 150 mg/dl

CRITICAL THINKING
Clinical Applications

Alan, age 75, is a Caucasian man admitted to the hospital following a cerebrovascular accident. He has a history of type 2 DM, hypertension, moderate obesity, and possible alcohol abuse. Medications on admission include furosemide (Lasix), hydrochlorothiazide, propranolol hydrochloride (Inderal), and chlorpropamide (Diabinese) 500 mg BID. Alan comes to the clinic regularly, and at his last visit complained of blurred vision, polydipsia, polyuria, and a weight loss of 8 lb in the past 2 weeks. He was admitted to the hospital with a diagnosis of urinary tract infection and hyperglycemic hyperosmolar nonketotic (HHNK) syndrome. Physical examination revealed the following:
- Height: 5'11"
- Weight: 215 lb
- Blood pressure: 160/82
- Cholesterol: 380 mg/dl
- Triglycerides: 300 mg/dl
- Blood sugar: 750 mg/dl
- Family history: Sister has had type 2 DM for 10 years

1. Explain how Alan's blood glucose level could become so high without producing ketones.
2. If this patient's HHNK was not treated, how would you expect his disease to progress?
3. What are Alan's blood glucose and lipid goals?
4. What is the purpose of the prescribed medications? Are there any possible drug-nutrient interactions?
5. How frequently should blood sugars be monitored?
6. What are possible complications?

Web Sites of Interest

American Diabetes Association (ADA)
www.diabetes.org
This official site of the ADA provides a wealth of information for health professionals and the public, which ranges from Internet resources to research updates to volunteer opportunities for members.

National Institute of Diabetes and Digestive and Kidney Diseases (NIDDK)
www.niddk.nih.gov/fund/divisions/DEM/DEMresources.htm
This division of the National Institutes of Health provides information and links to many related topics on diabetes, digestive diseases, kidney diseases, endocrine and metabolic diseases, nutrition, urologic diseases, and obesity.

References

1. Mokdad AH et al.: The continuing epidemics of obesity and diabetes in the United States, *J Am Med Assoc* 1195, 2001 http://jama.ama-assn.org/issues/v286n10/rfull/joc10856.html, accessed Mar 29, 2002.

2. Centers for Disease Prevention and Health Promotion: Diabetes press release from CDC; www.cdc.gov/diabetes/news/docs/010912.htm, accessed Mar 29, 2002.

3. Harris MI: Diabetes in America: epidemiology and scope of the problem, *Diabetes Care* 24(2):412, Feb 2001.

4. American Diabetes Association: *The impact of diabetes;* www.diabetes.org/main/application/commercewf?origin=*.jsp&event=link(B1_1), accessed Mar 23, 2002.

5. Committee Report: Report of the expert committee on the diagnosis and classification of diabetes mellitus, *Diabetes Care* 25:S5, 2002.

6. Diabetes Control and Complications Trial Research Group: The effect of intensive treatment of diabetes on the development and progression of long-term complications in insulin-dependent diabetes mellitus, *N Engl J Med* 329:977, 1993.

7. American Diabetes Association: *The dangerous toll of diabetes;* www.diabetes.org/ada/facts.asp, accessed Aug 16, 2000.

8. Oxford Center for Diabetes, Endocrinology and Metabolism Diabetes Trials Unit: *UK Prospective Diabetes Study;* www.dtu.ox.ac.uk/ukpds/results.html, accessed Mar 29, 2002.

9. American Diabetes Association: Implications of the diabetes control and complications trial (position statement), *Diabetes Care* 25:S25, 2002; http://care.diabetesjournals.org/cgi/content/full/25/suppl_1/s25, accessed Apr 20, 2002.

10. Robertson KE: What the UKPDS really says about cardiovascular disease and glycemic control, *Clinical Diabetes,* July 1999.

11. Ousman Y, Sharma M: The irrefutable importance of glycemic control, *Clinical Diabetes* 19:71, 2001.

12. American Diabetes Association: Implications of the United Kingdom Prospective Diabetes Study (position statement), *Diabetes Care* 25:S28, 2002.

13. National Institute of Diabetes and Digestive and Kidney Diseases: *Special report: diabetes mellitus: challenges and opportunities.* Final report and recommendations. Full report of participants in the Trans-NIH symposium. National Institutes of Health, 1997; www.niddk.nih.gov/federal/dwg/diabetesfinalreport/fulrepor.htm, accessed Apr 26, 2001.

14. Kissebah AH et al.: Relation of body fat distribution to metabolic complications of obesity, *J Clin Endocrinol Metab* 54:254, 1982.

15. Orland MJ: Diabetes mellitus. In Carey CF, Lee HH, Woeltje KF, eds.: *The Washington manual of medical therapeutics,* ed 29, Philadelphia, 1998, Lippincott Williams & Wilkins.

16. Holler HJ, Pastors JG: *Diabetes medical nutrition therapy: a professional guide to management and nutrition education resources,* Chicago, 1997, American Dietetic Association.

17. Setter SM: New drug therapies for the treatment of diabetes, *On the Cutting Edge Diabetes Care and Education Newsletter* 19(2):3, 1998.

18. White JR, Campbell RK: Recent developments in the pharmacological reduction of blood glucose in patients with type 2 diabetes, *Clinical Diabetes* 19:153, 2001.

19. Rosen ED: Drug classes for diabetes, *Veritas Medicine;* www.veritasmedicine.com, accessed July 27, 2001.

20. American Diabetes Association: *Diabetes mellitus and exercise* (position statement); www. diabetes.org/diabetescare/supplement198/S40.htm, accessed Nov 28, 1998.

21. Lee R, Nieman D: *Nutritional assessment,* ed 2, St Louis, 1996, Mosby.

22. American Diabetes Association (ADA): *Maximizing the role of nutrition in diabetes management.* A clinical education program of the ADA in cooperation with Diabetes Care and Education, a practice group of the American Dietetic Association, Alexandria, Va, 1994, ADA.

23. Franz MJ et al.: Evidence-based nutrition principles and recommendations for the treatment and prevention of diabetes and related complications, *Diabetes Care* 25:148, 2002.

24. American Diabetes Association: Standards of medical care for patients with diabetes mellitus, *Diabetes Care* 25(suppl):33S, 2002.

25. American Diabetes Association (ADA): *Exchange lists for meal planning,* Alexandria, Va, 1995, ADA.

26. American Diabetes Association: Translation of the diabetes nutrition recommendations for health care institutions, *Diabetes Care* 25 (suppl):61S, 2002.

27. American Dietetic Association: Nutrition recommendations and principles for people with diabetes mellitus, *J Am Diet Assoc* 94:504, 1994.

28. Delahanty LM, Halford BN: The role of diet behaviors in achieving improved glycemic control in intensively treated patients in the Diabetes Control and Complications Trial, *Diabetes Care* 16:1453, 1993.

29. Schlundt DG et al.: Situational obstacles to dietary adherence for adults with diabetes, *J Am Diet Assoc* 94:874, 1994.

30. Franz MJ, Joynes JO: *Diabetes and brief illness,* Minneapolis, 1993, International Diabetes Center.

31. Escott-Stump S: *Nutrition and diagnosis-related care,* ed 4, Baltimore, 1998, Lippincott Williams & Wilkins.

32. Metzger BE, Coustan DR, eds.: Proceedings of the fourth international workshop conference on gestational diabetes mellitus, *Diabetes Care* 21(suppl):1B, 1998.

33. American Diabetes Association: Gestational diabetes mellitus (position statement), *Diabetes Care* 25(suppl):94S, 2002.

34. Reader D, Sipe M: Key components of care for women with gestational diabetes, *Diabetes Spectrum* 14:188, 2001.

35. American Diabetes Association: Gestational diabetes mellitus (position statement), *Diabetes Care* 24(suppl):77S, 2001.

36. Rizzo T et al.: Correlations between antepartum maternal metabolism and intelligence of offspring, *N Engl J Med* 325:911, 1991.

37. American Diabetes Association: Preconception care of women with diabetes (position statement), *Diabetes Care* 25(suppl):82S, 2002.

38. Thomas A: Preconception counseling for the woman with diabetes, *On the Cutting Edge Diabetes Care and Education Newsletter* 23(2):9, 2002.

39. American Diabetes Association: Type 2 diabetes in children and adolescents, *Pediatrics* 105:671, 2000.

40. American Diabetes Association: Type 2 diabetes in children and adolescents, *Diabetes Care* 23:381, 2000.

41. Pinhas-Hamiel O: Type 2 diabetes: not just for grownups anymore, *Contemporary Pediatrics,* 1:102, 2001.

42. Sinha R et al.: Prevalence of impaired glucose tolerance among children and adolescents with marked obesity, *N Engl J Med* 346:802, 2002.

43. Levetan C: Into the mouths of babes: the diabetes epidemic in children, *Clinical Diabetes* 19:102, 2001.

44. Rosenbloom AL et al.: Emerging epidemic of type 2 diabetes in youth, *Diabetes Care* 22:345, 1999.

CHAPTER 20

Nutrition for Cardiovascular Diseases

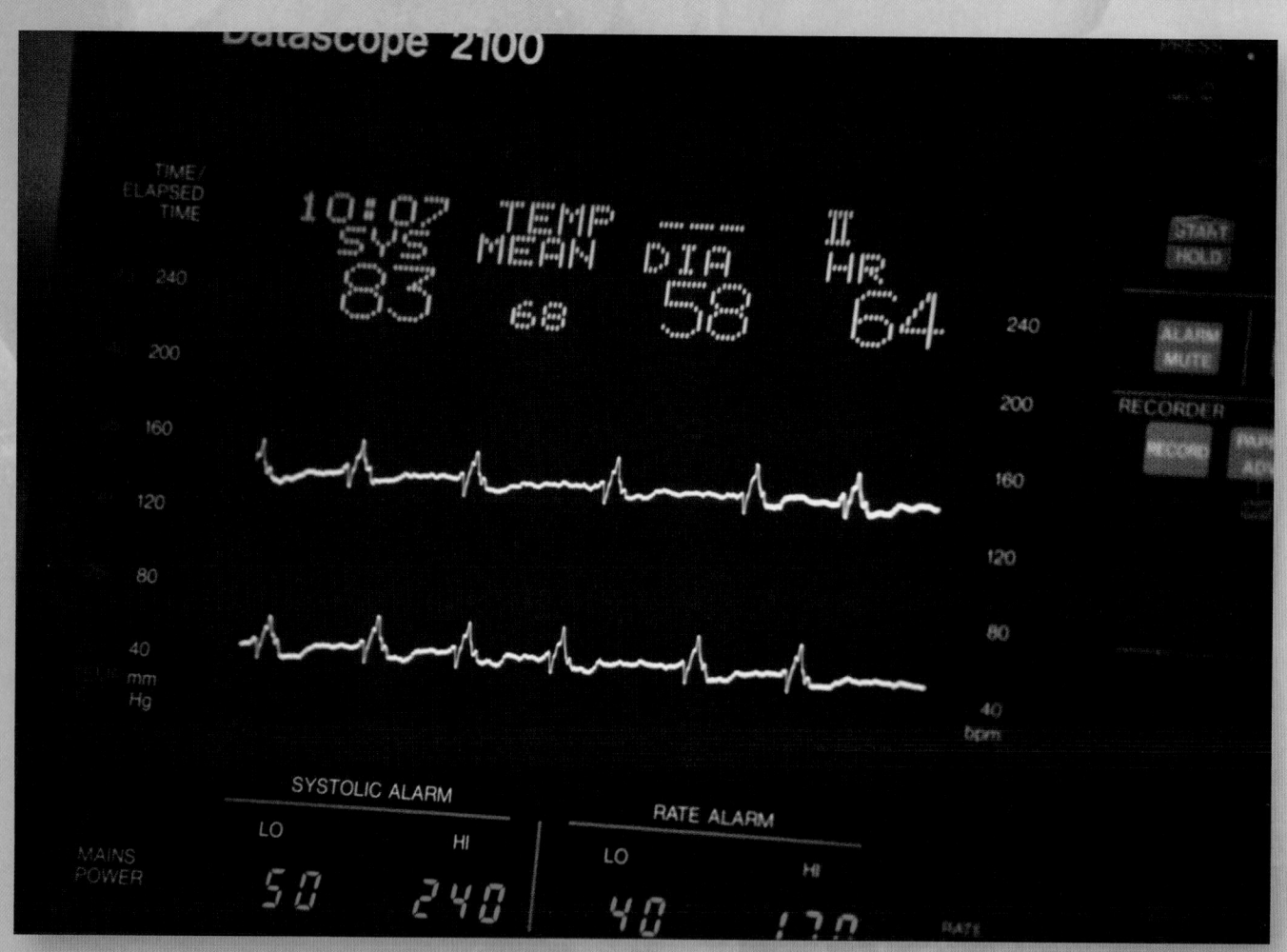

The term cardiovascular disease encompasses a group of diseases and conditions affecting the heart and blood vessels: coronary artery disease (also referred to as coronary heart disease), hypertension, peripheral vascular disease, congestive heart failure, and congenital heart disease.

ROLE IN WELLNESS

Nurses working in varied settings play a major role in teaching people how to reduce cardiovascular risk factors through lifestyle changes, including reinforcement of dietary modifications. Although dietitians are responsible for developing the medical nutrition plan and for the majority of diet education instruction, nurses reinforce that teaching and answer any additional questions of patients and their families. Therefore familiarity with diet as it affects cardiovascular disease is essential.

The term *cardiovascular disease (CVD)* encompasses a group of diseases and conditions that affect the heart and blood vessels: coronary artery disease (CAD) (also called *coronary heart disease [CHD]*), hypertension (HTN), peripheral vascular disease (PVD), congestive heart failure (CHF), and congenital heart diseases. CVD has been a public health issue since 1920 and is currently the leading cause of death in the United States for both men and women in all ethnic and racial groups. Nearly 62 million Americans have some form of CVD. More than 2600 lives are claimed each day by CVD—an average of 1 death every 33 seconds. Cardiovascular disease kills almost as many Americans each year as the next seven leading causes of death combined.[1] Most people who have heart attacks die before they ever reach a hospital for treatment, a situation that emphasizes the need for prevention of heart disease.

Although CVD has been a public health concern for decades, health professionals cannot assume that newly diagnosed CAD patients, regardless of education or socioeconomic level, are knowledgeable of the disorder and treatment approaches. Primary prevention is a public health matter. These approaches often include implementing secondary and tertiary preventive strategies. Secondary prevention behaviors reduce the effects of a disease or illness. For CVD, reducing risk factors can minimize negative health effects. The purpose of tertiary prevention is to minimize further complications or to assist in the restoration of health. For CVD, these efforts may involve significant lifestyle changes combined with medication and other medical care. Learning more about the disorder is often helpful for patients and their families.

Several risk factors for cardiovascular disease are modifiable or altogether preventable; nonetheless, more than 80% of adult Americans have at least one major risk factor.[2] Risk factors are categorized into two groups: modifiable and nonmodifiable (Table 20-1).

A way to understand the far-reaching effects of CVD is to consider this group of diseases and disorders through the five dimensions of health. Of course, the physical dimension is affected as CVD affects the heart, an essential organ; this disease impairs functioning of many body systems. Determining one's own risk factors and devising a program to reduce their effects depends on the intellectual dimension of health. The emotional dimension is stressed because client denial may occur; some individuals view heart problems as only happening to others. Mortality caused by CVD, as well as the many lifestyle modifications necessary, may be frightening; how can we reassure clients, and yet still assist them to change behaviors? Because of increased education through the work of health associations and health departments, many restaurants and resorts serve "heart healthy" entrees; with careful selections, socializing can continue unaffected thereby supporting the social dimension. The ability to cope with physical limitations because of chronic illnesses such as heart disease and diabetes may depend on the spiritual health dimension manifested through an optimistic attitude and a desire to fight back to achieve the most positive response of the body.

CORONARY ARTERY DISEASE

The underlying pathologic process responsible for coronary artery disease (CAD) is atherosclerosis (Figure 20-1). Beginning in childhood, atherosclerosis may gradually lead to arteriosclerosis.[3] The most common and serious manifestation of

peripheral vascular disease (PVD)
condition affecting blood vessels outside the heart, characterized by a variety of signs and symptoms such as numbness, pain, pallor, elevated blood pressure, and impaired arterial pulsations. Causative factors include obesity, cigarette smoking, stress, sedentary occupations, and numerous metabolic disorders

coronary artery disease
term used for several abnormal conditions that may affect the arteries of the heart and produce various pathologic effects, especially the reduced flow of oxygen and nutrients to the cardiac tissue

atherosclerosis
development of lesions (also called *fatty streaks*) in the intima of arteries; during aging, the lesions develop into fibrous plaques that project into the vessel lumen and begin to disturb blood flow

arteriosclerosis
thickening, loss of elasticity, and calcification of arterial walls, resulting in decreased blood supply

Table 20-1
Major Risk Factors in Cardiovascular Disease

| | Nonlipid Risk Factors | |
Lipid Risk Factors	Modifiable	Nonmodifiable
↑ LDL cholesterol (>100 mg/dl) ↓ HDL cholesterol (<40 mg/dl) ↑ Triglycerides (>150 mg/dl)	Tobacco smoke and exposure to tobacco smoke High serum cholesterol (>200 mg/dl) Hypertension (≥140/50 mmHg) Physical inactivity Obesity (BMI >30 kg/m²) and overweight (BMI 25-29.9 kg/m²) Diabetes mellitus Atherogenic diet (↑ intakes of saturated fats and cholesterol) Stress and coping Excessive alcohol consumption (>1 drink/day for women and >2 drinks/day for men) Individual response to stress and coping Some illegal drugs (cocaine and IV drug abuse)	Male gender Increasing age (men ≥45 yrs, women ≥55 yrs) Heredity (including race) Family history of premature CHD (MI or sudden death <55 yrs of age in father or other male first-degree relative, or <65 years of age in mother or other female first-degree relatives)

From Anderson SL: Diseases of the heart, blood vessels, and lungs. In Williams SR, Schlenker ED: Essentials of nutrition and diet therapy, ed 8, St Louis, 2003, Mosby. References: American Heart Association: Heart and stroke facts, 1992-2001; 216.185.112.5/downloadable/heart/1014833865440010/3191236985HSfacts02. pdf, accessed May 29, 2002; Grundy SM et al.: Primary prevention of coronary heart disease: guidance from Framingham, Circulation 97:1876, 1998; National Cholesterol Education Program (NCEP): Third report of the NCEP expert panel on detection, evaluation, and treatment of high blood cholesterol in adults (Adult Treatment Panel III) Executive Summary, NIH Pub No 01-3670, May 2001, Washington, DC, 2001, National Institutes of Health, National Heart, Lung, and Blood Institute; www.nhlbi.nih.gov/guidelines/cholesterol/atp3_rpt.pdf, accessed May 29, 2001; National Cholesterol Education Program (NCEP): Third report of the NCEP expert panel on detection, evaluation, and treatment of high blood cholesterol in adults (Adult Treatment Panel III), Washington, DC, 2001, National Institutes of Health, National Heart, Lung, and Blood Institute.

angina pectoris
chest pain that often radiates down the left arm and is frequently accompanied by a feeling of suffocation and impending death

thrombus
blood clot

myocardial infarction
occlusion of a coronary artery; sometimes called *heart attack*

atherosclerosis is development of lesions in coronary arteries that can cause angina pectoris if blood flow is partially occluded by a thrombus. If blood flow to the heart is completely occluded, then a myocardial infarction occurs. If thrombosis occurs in a cerebral artery, a cerebrovascular accident (CVA) or stroke occurs. Peripheral vascular disease (PVD) occurs when atherosclerosis in the abdominal aorta, iliac arteries, and femoral arteries produces temporary insufficient blood flow in the arteries upon exertion (intermittent claudication) or ischemic necrosis of the extremities, which may lead to gangrene.[4]

The most frequent approach in assessing CAD risk is to measure cholesterol and proportions of the different types of plasma lipoproteins that carry cholesterol in the blood. Cholesterol is a not actually a lipid, but it travels in the bloodstream in spherical particles called *lipoproteins*, which contain lipids and proteins. Cholesterol is an essential component of cell membranes and a precursor of bile acids and steroid hormones and is not required in the diet after weaning. Plasma lipid profile is commonly measured by analyzing the three major classes of lipoproteins in blood from a fasting individual: very low-density lipoproteins (VLDL), low-density lipoproteins

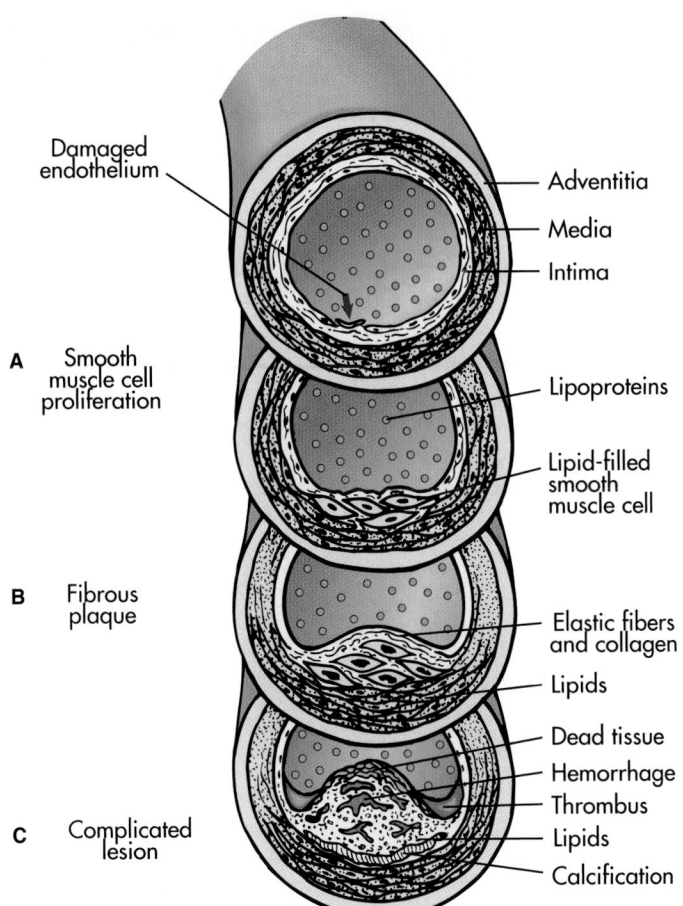

PLASMA LIPOPROTEINS
- Synthesized primarily in the liver
- Contain varying amounts of triglycerides, cholesterol, phospholipids, and proteins
- Classified according to composition and density
- Kinds of plasma lipoproteins: chylomicrons, high-density lipoproteins (HDL), low-density lipoproteins (LDL), and very low-density lipoproteins (VLDL)

Figure 20-1 The stages of development in the progression of atherosclerosis include **A,** smooth muscle cell proliferation, which creates, **B,** a raised fibrous plaque and, **C,** a complicated lesion. (From Lewis SM, Heitkemper MM, Dirksen SR: *Medical-surgical nursing: assessment and management of clinical problems,* ed 5, St Louis, 2000, Mosby.)

(LDL), and high-density lipoproteins (HDL). LDL-cholesterol contains approximately 60% to 70% of the total serum cholesterol (TC), and high serum levels are causally related to increased risk of CAD. The HDLs usually contain 20% to 30% of the total cholesterol, and serum levels are inversely correlated with risk for CAD. The VLDLs are largely composed of triglyceride, which contains 10% to 15% of the total serum cholesterol.[5,6]

The National Cholesterol Education Program (NCEP) Adult Treatment Panel III (ATP III) report[5,6] emphasizes LDL cholesterol as the primary target for cholesterol-lowering therapy. The report cites research from laboratory investigations, epidemiologic research, and clinical trials that robustly show LDL-lowering therapy reduces risk for CHD. Therefore primary goals of therapy are stated in terms of LDL cholesterol (Box 20-1).

Another risk factor for CHD is elevated triglyceride levels.[5,6] Triglyceride is the most common type of fat found in the body. The body gets triglyceride directly from foods and makes it in the liver from carbohydrates, alcohol, and some cholesterol. Serum triglyceride levels range from about 50 to 250 mg/dl.[7] There are several factors that may cause triglyceride levels to be elevated[8,9]:
- Overweight and obesity
- Physical inactivity
- Cigarette smoking

thrombosis
an abnormal vascular condition in which a blood clot (thrombus) develops within a blood vessel

ischemic
decreased blood supply to a body organ or completely blocked part

Box 20-1 Adult Treatment Panel III Classification of LDL, Total, and HDL Cholesterol (mg/dl)

LDL CHOLESTEROL		TOTAL CHOLESTEROL		HDL CHOLESTEROL	
<100	Optimal	<200	Desirable	<40	Low
100-129	Near optimal/ above optimal	200-239	Borderline high	>60	High
130-159	Borderline high	≥240	High		
160-189	High				
≥190	Very high				

From National Cholesterol Education Program (NCEP): Third report of the NCEP expert panel on detection, evaluation, and treatment of high blood cholesterol in adults (Adult Treatment Panel III) Executive Summary, NIH Pub No 01-3670, May 2001, Washington, DC, 2001, National Institutes of Health, National Heart, Lung, and Blood Institute; www.nhlbi.nih.gov/guidelines/cholesterol/atp3_rpt.pdf, accessed May 29, 2001; National Cholesterol Education Program (NCEP): Third report of the NCEP expert panel on detection, evaluation, and treatment of high blood cholesterol in adults (Adult Treatment Panel III), Washington, DC, 2001, National Institutes of Health, National Heart, Lung, and Blood Institute.

- Excess alcohol intake
- Very high carbohydrate intake (>60% of total energy)
- Other diseases (e.g., type 2 diabetes mellitus, chronic renal failure, nephritic syndrome)
- Certain drugs (e.g., corticosteroids, protease inhibitors for human immunodeficiency virus [HIV], beta-adrenergic blocking agents, estrogens)
- Genetic factors

After evaluating available research, the ATP III panel concluded that the association between serum triglyceride and CHD is stronger than previously recognized and consider elevated serum levels as a factor to identify persons at risk who are in need of intervention for risk reduction.[5,6] Classifications of triglyceride levels are outlined in Table 20-2.

The ATP III report cites convincing epidemiologic evidence identifying HDL cholesterol as a strong independent and inverse risk factor for increased CHD morbidity and mortality.[6] Low HDL cholesterol is defined as a level of less than 40 mg/dl

Table 20-2
Classification of Serum Triglycerides

Triglyceride Category	ATP III Levels
Normal	≤150 mg/dl
Borderline high	150-199 mg/dl
High	200-499 mg/dl
Very high	≥500 mg/dl

From National Cholesterol Education Program (NCEP): Third report of the NCEP expert panel on detection, evaluation, and treatment of high blood cholesterol in adults (Adult Treatment Panel III), Washington, DC, 2001, National Institutes of Health, National Heart, Lung, and Blood Institute; www.nhlbi.nih.gov/guidelines/cholesterol/atp3_rpt.pdf, accessed May 29, 2001.

in both men and women.[6] Factors contributing to low HDL cholesterol levels[8-10] include the following:

- Elevated serum triglyceride levels
- Overweight and obesity
- Physical inactivity
- Cigarette smoking
- Very high carbohydrate intake (>60% of total energy)
- Type 2 diabetes mellitus
- Certain drugs (e.g., beta blockers, anabolic steroids, progestational agents)
- Genetic factors

Often, a common form of dyslipidemia (atherogenic dyslipidemia) characterized by three lipid abnormalities (elevated triglycerides, small LDL particles, and low HDL cholesterol) is seen in persons with premature CHD.[6] Characteristics of individuals with atherogenic dyslipidemia are obesity, abdominal obesity, insulin resistance, and physical inactivity.[11,12] Because each component of atherogenic dyslipidemia is individually atherogenic, the combination is considered an independent risk factor.[6] Lifestyle modification—weight control and increased physical activity—is the treatment of choice.[6]

Nonlipid Risk Factors

Several nonlipid risk factors are associated with increased CHD risk and are targets for intervention in preventive efforts. Fixed risk factors (increasing age, male gender, and family history of premature CHD) cannot be modified, and their existence implies need for intensive lowering of LDL cholesterol.[6] Modifiable nonlipid risk factors include hypertension, cigarette smoking, diabetes, obesity, physical inactivity, and atherogenic diet. Table 20-1 summarizes CHD risk factors other than elevated LDL cholesterol.

Medical Nutrition Therapy

The ATP III report[5,6] recommends a comprehensive lifestyle approach to reducing risk for CHD called *therapeutic lifestyle changes (TLC)*, which incorporates the following components[5,6]:

- Reduced intake of saturated fats and cholesterol
- Therapeutic dietary options to enhance lowering of LDL (e.g., plant stanols/sterols and increased soluble fiber)
- Weight reduction
- Increased regular physical activity

Components of TLC are outlined in Table 20-3. ATP III also suggests ranges for other macronutrients in the TLC Diet (Table 20-4). Overall, composition of the TLC diet is consistent with recommendations of the *Dietary Guidelines for Americans* (see Chapter 2). Box 20-2 outlines the ATP III's TLC recommendations.

Components of the Therapeutic Lifestyle Changes (TLC) Diet

Saturated Fat and Cholesterol.   Reducing saturated fat (<7% of total energy intake) and cholesterol (<200 mg/d) in the diet is the foundation of the TLC diet.[5,6] The strongest nutritional influence on serum LDL cholesterol levels is saturated fats.[13] Moreover, there is a "dose response relationship" between saturated fats and LDL cholesterol levels.[6] For every 1% increase in kcalories from saturated fats as a percent of total energy, serum LDL cholesterol increases roughly 2%. Conversely, a 1% decrease in saturated fats will lower serum cholesterol by about 2%.[14,15] Although weight reduction by itself, even of a few pounds, will reduce LDL cholesterol levels,[6,11,12] weight reduction achieved using a kcalorie-controlled

Table 20-3
Essential Components of Therapeutic Lifestyle Changes (TLC)

Component	Recommendation
LDL-raising nutrients	
Saturated fats	<7% of total energy intake
Dietary cholesterol	<200 mg/d
Therapeutic options for lowering LDL	
Plant stanols/sterols	2 g/d
Soluble fiber	10-25 g/d
Total energy (kcals)	Adjust total energy intake to maintain desirable body weight and prevent weight gain
Physical activity	Include enough moderate exercise to expend at least 200 kcal/d

From Anderson SL: Diseases of the heart, blood vessels, and lungs. In Williams SR, Schlenker ED: Essentials of nutrition and diet therapy, ed 8, St Louis, 2003, Mosby. Reference: National Cholesterol Education Program (NCEP): Third report of the NCEP expert panel on detection, evaluation, and treatment of high blood cholesterol in adults (Adult Treatment Panel III), Washington, DC, 2001, National Institutes of Health, National Heart, Lung, and Blood Institute; www.nhlbi.nih.gov/guidelines/cholesterol/atp3_rpt.pdf, accessed May 29, 2001.

Table 20-4
Nutrient Composition of the Therapeutic Lifestyle Changes (TLC) Diet

Component	Recommendation
Polyunsaturated fat	Up to 10% total energy intake
Monounsaturated fat	Up to 20% total energy intake
Total fat	25%-35% total energy intake*
Carbohydrate†	50%-60% total energy intake
Dietary fiber	20-30 g/d
Protein	Approximately 15% total energy intake

From Anderson SL: Diseases of the heart, blood vessels, and lungs. In Williams SR, Schlenker ED: Essentials of nutrition and diet therapy, ed 8, St Louis, 2003, Mosby. References: National Cholesterol Education Program (NCEP): Third report of the NCEP expert panel on detection, evaluation, and treatment of high blood cholesterol in adults (Adult Treatment Panel III) executive summary, NIH Pub No 01-3670, May 2001, Washington, DC, 2001, National Institutes of Health, National Heart, Lung, and Blood Institute; www.nhlbi.nih.gov/guidelines/cholesterol/atp3_rpt.pdf, accessed May 29, 2001; National Cholesterol Education Program (NCEP): Third report of the NCEP expert panel on detection, evaluation, and treatment of high blood cholesterol in adults (Adult Treatment Panel III), Washington, DC, 2001, National Institutes of Health, National Heart, Lung, and Blood Institute.
*ATP III allows for increase of total fat to 35% total energy intake and reduction in carbohydrate to 50% for persons with the metabolic syndrome. Any increase in fat intake should be in the form of either polyunsaturated or monounsaturated fat.
†Carbohydrates should come primarily from foods rich in complex carbohydrates including grains—especially whole grains—fruits and vegetables.

Box 20-2 Guide to Therapeutic Lifestyle Changes (TLC): Healthy Lifestyle Recommendations for a Healthy Heart

FOOD ITEMS TO CHOOSE MORE OFTEN

BREADS AND CEREALS

≥6 servings per day, adjusted to caloric needs

Breads, cereals, especially whole grains; pasta; rice; potatoes; dry beans and peas; low-fat crackers and cookies

VEGETABLES

3-5 servings per day fresh, frozen, or canned without added fat, sauce, or salt

FRUITS

2-4 servings per day fresh, frozen, canned, dried

DAIRY PRODUCTS

2-3 servings per day Fat-free, ½%, 1% milk, buttermilk, yogurt, cottage cheese, fat-free and low-fat cheese

EGGS

2 egg yolks per week
Egg whites or egg substitute

MEAT, POULTRY, FISH

<5 oz. per day

Lean cuts loin, leg, round, extra lean hamburger; cold cuts made with lean meat or soy protein; skinless poultry; fish

FATS AND OILS

Amount adjusted to caloric level: unsaturated oils; soft or liquid margarines and vegetable oil spreads; salad dressings, seeds, and nuts

TLC DIET OPTIONS

Stanol/sterol-containing margarines; soluble fiber food sources: barley, oats, psyllium, apples, bananas, berries, citrus fruits, nectarines, peaches, pears, plums, prunes, broccoli, Brussels sprouts, carrots, dry beans, soy products (tofu, miso)

FOOD ITEMS TO CHOOSE LESS OFTEN

BREADS AND CEREALS

Many baked products, including doughnuts, biscuits, butter rolls, muffins, croissants, sweet rolls, Danish, cakes, pies, coffee cakes, cookies

Many grain-based snacks, including chips, cheese puffs, snack mix, regular crackers, buttered popcorn

VEGETABLES

Vegetables fried or prepared with butter, cheese, or cream sauce

FRUITS

Fruits fried or served with butter or cream

DAIRY PRODUCTS

Whole milk, 2% milk, whole-milk yogurt, ice cream, cream, cheese

EGGS

Egg yolk, whole eggs

MEAT, POULTRY, FISH

Higher fat meat cuts: ribs, t-bone steak, regular hamburger, bacon, sausage; cold cuts: salami, bologna, hot dogs; organ meats: liver, brains, sweetbreads; poultry with skin-fried meat; fried poultry; fried fish

FATS AND OILS

Butter, shortening, stick margarine, chocolate, coconut

RECOMMENDATIONS FOR WEIGHT REDUCTION

WEIGH REGULARLY

Record weight, body mass index (BMI), and waist circumferences

LOSE WEIGHT GRADUALLY

Goal: lose 10% of body weight in 6 months; Lose ½ to 1 lb per week

DEVELOP HEALTHY EATING PATTERNS

- Choose healthy foods (see Column 1)
- Reduce intake of foods in Column 2
- Limit number of eating occasions
- Avoid second helpings
- Identify and reduce hidden fat by reading food labels to choose products lower in saturated fat and calories, and ask about ingredients in ready-to-eat foods prepared away from home
- Identify and reduce sources of excess carbohydrates such as fat-free and regular crackers; cookies and other desserts; snacks; and sugar-containing beverages

RECOMMENDATIONS FOR INCREASED PHYSICAL ACTIVITY

MAKE PHYSICAL ACTIVITY PART OF DAILY ROUTINES

- Reduce sedentary time.
- Walk, wheel, or bike-ride more; drive less. Take the stairs instead of an elevator. Get off the bus a few stops early and walk the remaining distance. Mow the lawn with a push mower. Rake leaves. Garden. Push a stroller. Clean the house. Do exercises or pedal a stationary bike while watching television. Play actively with children. Take a brisk 10-minute walk or wheel before work, during your work break, and after dinner

MAKE PHYSICAL ACTIVITY PART OF EXERCISE OR RECREATIONAL ACTIVITIES

Walk, wheel, or jog. Bicycle or use an arm pedal bicycle. Swim or do water aerobics. Play basketball. Join a sport team. Play wheelchair sports. Golf (pull cart or carry clubs). Canoe. Cross-country ski. Dance. Take part in an exercise program at work, home, school, or gym.

From the National Cholesterol Education Program (NCEP): Third report of the NCEP expert panel on detection, evaluation, and treatment of high blood cholesterol in adults (Adult Treatment Panel III), Washington, DC, 2001, National Institutes of Health, National Heart, Lung, and Blood Institute.

diet low in saturated fats and cholesterol will enhance and maintain LDL cholesterol reductions.[6,15,16] Although dietary cholesterol does not have the equivalent impact of saturated fat on serum LDL cholesterol levels,[6] high cholesterol intakes increase LDL cholesterol levels.[6,17,18] Therefore reducing dietary cholesterol to less than 200 mg per day decreases serum LDL cholesterol in most persons.[6]

Monounsaturated Fat.   Substitution of monounsaturated fat for saturated fats at an intake level of up to 20% of total energy intake is recommended on the TLC diet.[5,6] Monounsaturated fats lower LDL cholesterol levels relative to saturated fats[6,14] without decreasing HDL cholesterol or triglyceride levels.[6,14,18,19] The best sources of monounsaturated fats are plant oils and nuts.[6]

Polyunsaturated Fats.   When used instead of saturated fats, polyunsaturated fats, in particular linoleic acid, reduce LDL cholesterol levels. On the other hand they can also bring about small reductions in HDL cholesterol when compared side by side with monounsaturated fats.[6,14] Liquid vegetables oils, semiliquid margarines, and other margarines low in transfatty acids are recommended by the TLC diet as the best sources of polyunsaturated fats. Recommended intakes can range up to 10% of total energy intake.[5,6]

Total Fat.   Saturated fats and transfatty acids increase LDL cholesterol levels,[20] whereas serum levels of LDL cholesterol do not appear to be affected by total fat intake.[6] For that reason, the ATP III suggests it is not essential to limit total fat intake for the particular goal of reducing LDL cholesterol levels, provided saturated fats are decreased to goal levels.[5,6]

Carbohydrate.   When saturated fats are replaced with carbohydrates, LDL cholesterol decreases. Then again, very high intakes of carbohydrates (>60% total energy intake) are associated with a reduction in HDL cholesterol and increase in serum triglyceride.[6,14,19,21,22] Increasing soluble fiber intake can sometimes reduce these responses.[6,23-25] Generally, increasing soluble fiber to 5 to 10 grams per day is accompanied by a roughly 5% reduction in LDL cholesterol.[26,27]

Protein.   Although dietary protein, as a rule, has a negligible effect on serum LDL cholesterol level, substituting plant-based proteins for animal proteins appears to decrease LDL cholesterol.[6,28] This may be caused by the lack of cholesterol and lower saturated fat content of plant-based protein foods (e.g., legumes, dry beans, nuts, whole grains, and vegetables). This is not to say all animal proteins are high in saturated fat and cholesterol. Fat-free and low-fat dairy products, egg whites, fish, skinless poultry, and lean cuts of beef and pork are low in saturated fat and cholesterol. All foods of animal origin will contain cholesterol.

Further Dietary Options to Reduce LDL Cholesterol.   When 5 to 10 g of soluble fiber (e.g., oats, barley, psyllium, pectin-rich fruit, and beans) is added to the daily diet, there is a roughly 5% reduction in LDL cholesterol.[26,27] This is considered a therapeutic alternative to augment reduction of LDL cholesterol.[6] Daily intakes of 2 to 3 g plant sterol/sterol esters (isolated from soybean and tall pine-tree oils) present an additional therapeutic option because they have been shown to lower LDL cholesterol by 6% to 15%.[6,29-35]

General Approach to Therapeutic Lifestyle Changes (TLC)

The ATP III[5,6] recommends patients at risk for CHD or with CHD be referred to registered dietitians or other qualified nutritionists for all stages of medical nutrition therapy. LDL cholesterol should be measured at 6-week intervals to evaluate response to TLC. If the LDL cholesterol target has been realized, or if improvement in LDL lowering has occurred, medical nutrition therapy should be continued. If the goal has not been achieved, several alternatives are available. First, medical nutrition therapy can be reexplained and reinforced. Next, therapeutic dietary options (outlined earlier) can be integrated into TLC. Response to medical nutrition therapy should be assessed in another 6 weeks. Achievement of the LDL cholesterol target indicates that the current intensity of medical nutrition therapy should be continued indefinitely. Thought should be given to continuing medical nutrition therapy before adding LDL-lowering medications. If it seems unlikely the LDL target will be realized with medical nutrition therapy, medications should be considered.[5,6]

Drug Therapy

Use of TLC will attain the LDL cholesterol target goal for many; LDL-lowering medications will be necessary for a segment of the population to achieve the prescribed goal for LDL cholesterol.[5,6] If treatment with TLC alone is unsuccessful after 3 months, the ATP III recommends initiation of drug treatment. Use of LDL-lowering medications does not negate continued use or need for medical nutrition therapy. Medical nutrition therapy affords further CHD risk reduction beyond drug efficacy.[6] Suggestions for combined use of TLC and LDL-lowering medications include the following[6]:

- Intensive LDL-lowering with TLC including therapeutic dietary options
  - May prevent need for drugs
  - Can augment LDL-lowering medications
  - May allow for lower doses of medications
- Weight control plus increased physical activity
  - Reduces risk beyond LDL-cholesterol lowering
  - Constitutes principal management of metabolic syndrome
  - Raises HDL cholesterol
- Initiating TLC before medication consideration
  - For most people, a trial of medical nutrition therapy of about 3 months is advised before initiating drug therapy
  - Ineffective trials of medical nutrition therapy exclusive of medications should not be protracted for an indefinite period if goals of therapy are not approached in a reasonable period; medications should not be withheld if they are needed to reach targets in persons with a short-term and/or long-term CHD risk that is high
- Initiating drug therapy simultaneously with TLC
  - For severe hypercholesterolemia in which medical nutrition therapy alone cannot attain LDL cholesterol targets
  - For those with CHD or CHD risk equivalents in whom medical nutrition therapy alone will not attain LDL cholesterol targets

The general strategy for initiation and progression of drug therapy is outlined in Figure 20-2. Major drugs used to treat hypercholesterolemia are outlined in Table 20-5.

hypercholesterolemia
total blood cholesterol levels greater than 200 mg/dl; greater than normal amounts of cholesterol in the blood; may be reduced or prevented by avoiding saturated fats

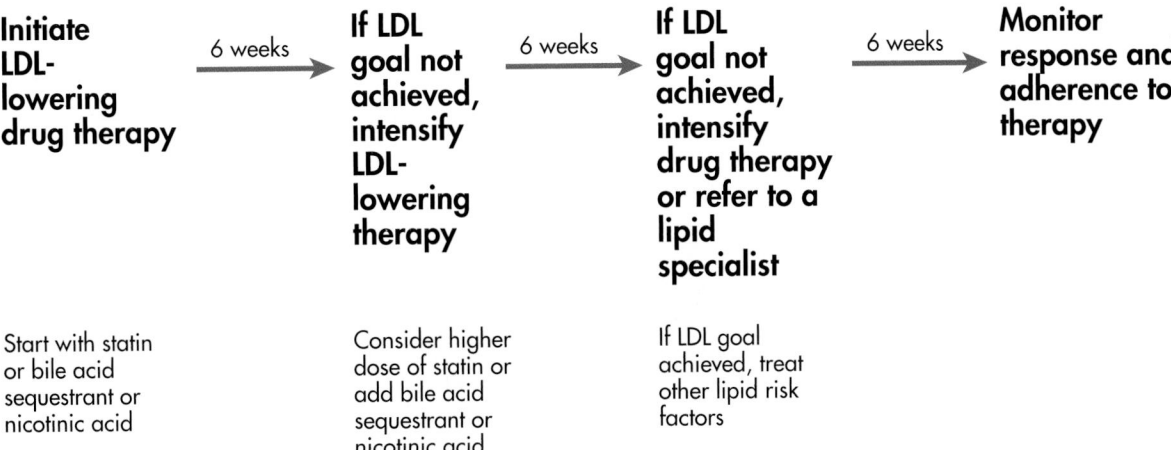

Figure 20-2 Progression of drug therapy. (From National Cholesterol Education Program (NCEP): *Third report of the NCEP expert panel on detection, evaluation, and treatment of high blood cholesterol in adults [Adult Treatment Panel III]*, Washington, DC, 2001, National Institutes of Health, National Heart, Lung, and Blood Institute.)

Table 20-5
Major Drugs Used to Treat Hypercholesterolemia

Drug Class	Available Drugs	Lipid/Lipoprotein Effects	Major Side Effects	ATP III Recommendation
HMG CoA reductase inhibitors (statins)	lovastatin, pravastatin, simvastatin, fluvastatin, atorvastatin	↓ LDL cholesterol 18%-55% ↑ HDL cholesterol 5%-15% ↓ Triglycerides 7%-30%	Myopathy, increased liver transaminases	Should be considered as the drug of choice when LDL-lowering medications are indicated to achieve LDL treatment goals
Bile acid sequestrants	cholestyramine, colestipol, colesevelam	↓ LDL cholesterol 15%-30% ↑ HDL cholesterol 3%-5% Triglycerides no effect or ↑	Upper and lower GI complaints common. Decreased absorption of other drugs	Should be considered as LDL-lowering therapy for persons with moderate elevations in LDL cholesterol, younger persons with elevated LDL cholesterol, women with elevated LDL cholesterol who are considering pregnancy, persons needing only modest reductions in LDL cholesterol, and combination therapy with statins in persons with very high LDL cholesterol
Nicotinic acid (niacin)	Crystalline nicotinic acid Sustained-release (or timed-release) nicotinic acid Extended-release nicotinic acid (Niaspan®)	↓ LDL cholesterol 5%-25% ↑ HDL cholesterol 15%-35% ↓ Triglycerides 20%-50%	Flushing, hyperglycemia, hyperuricemia or gout, upper GI distress, hepatotoxicity, especially for sustained-release form	Should be considered as a single agent in higher-risk persons with atherogenic dyslipidemia who do not have a substantial increase in LDL cholesterol levels, and in combination therapy with other cholesterol-lowering medications in higher-risk persons with atherogenic dyslipidemia combined with elevated LDL cholesterol levels. Should be used with caution in those with active liver disease, recent peptic ulcer, hyperuricemia and gout, and type 2 diabetes. High doses (>3 g/dl) generally should be avoided in persons with type 2 diabetes, although lower doses may effectively treat diabetic dyslipidemia without significantly worsening hyperglycemia.
Fibric acid derivatives (fibrates)	Gemfibrozil, fenofibrated, clofibrate	↓ LDL cholesterol 5%-20% (in nonhypertriglyceridemic persons; may be increased in hypertriglyceridemic persons) ↑ HDL cholesterol 10%-35% (more in severe hypertriglyceridemia) ↓ Triglycerides 20%-50%	Dyspepsia, various upper GI complaints, cholesterol gallstones, myopathy	Can be recommended for persons with very high triglycerides to reduce risk for acute pancreatitis. Can also be recommended for persons with elevated beta-VLDL. Should be considered an option for treatment of those with established CHD who have low levels of LDL cholesterol and atherogenic dyslipidemia. Also should be considered in combination with statin therapy in those with elevated LDL cholesterol and atherogenic dyslipidemia.

From Anderson SL: Diseases of the heart, blood vessels, and lungs. In Williams SR, Schlenker ED: Essentials of nutrition and diet therapy, ed 8, St Louis, 2003, Mosby. Reference: National Cholesterol Education Program (NCEP): Third report of the NCEP expert panel on detection, evaluation, and treatment of high blood cholesterol in adults (Adult Treatment Panel III), Washington, DC, 2001, National Institutes of Health, National Heart, Lung, and Blood Institute.

HYPERTENSION

As many as 50 million Americans age 6 and older have hypertension (HTN) (including one in every four adults).[1] Not only is it a cardiovascular disease itself but HTN is also a risk factor for CAD. According to the American Heart Association, the incidence of HTN is higher in the following groups[1]:

- Until age 55, a higher percentage of men than women have HTN.
- From ages 55 to 74, the percentage of women with HTN is higher.
- For those older than 75, a higher percentage of women have HTN.
- African Americans, Puerto Ricans, Cuban Americans, and Mexican Americans are more likely to have HTN than Caucasian Americans.
- African Americans and Caucasian Americans living in the southeastern United States have a greater prevalence of HTN than those from other regions of the country.

In about 95% of cases of HTN, the cause is not known and is called primary or essential hypertension.[3] Secondary hypertension is the term used when a cause for elevated blood pressure can be identified. Conditions that are possible causes of secondary HTN include renal insufficiency, renovascular diseases, Cushing's syndrome, and primary aldosteronism.[19] Although sometimes called a silent killer, HTN is easily detected and usually controllable. Classifications of blood pressure are outlined in Table 20-6.

hypertension (HTN)
an average systolic blood pressure ≥140 mmHg and/or a diastolic pressure ≥90 mmHg (or both)

primary or essential hypertension
elevated blood pressure for which the cause is unknown

secondary hypertension
elevated blood pressure for which the cause can be identified

Medical Nutrition Therapy

Prescribed treatment regimens for HTN are individualized and vary because the disease differs in its degree of severity. The first line of treatment is usually nonpharmacologic or focused on lifestyle modifications. Modifying dietary intake is a predominate element of nonpharmacologic treatment of existing HTN. Weight loss is the most effective means of lowering blood pressure. Other lifestyle modifications include possible beneficial effects of reducing weight if overweight, decreasing alcohol consumption, increasing physical activity if sedentary, terminating cigarette smoking, decreasing sodium intake, and increasing dietary intake of other minerals

Table 20-6
Classification of Blood Pressure for Adults

Category	Systolic (mm Hg)		Diastolic (mm Hg)
Optimal*	<120	and	<80
Normal	<130	and	<85
High-normal	130-139	or	85-89
Hypertension†			
Stage 1	140-159	or	90-99
Stage 2	160-179	or	100-109
Stage 3	≥180	or	≥110

From Anderson SL: Diseases of the heart, blood vessels, and lungs. In Williams SR, Schlenker ED: Essentials of nutrition and diet therapy, ed 8, St Louis, 2003, Mosby. Reference: The Sixth Report of the Joint National Committee on Prevention, Detection, Evaluation, and Treatment of High Blood Pressure, NIH Pub No 98-4080, Washington, DC, Nov 1997, National Institutes of Health, National Heart, Lung, and Blood Institute.

*Optimal blood pressure with respect to cardiovascular risk is below 120/80 mm Hg. However, unusually low readings should be evaluated for clinical significance.

†Based on the average of two or more readings taken at each of two or more visits after initial screening.

Box 20-3 Lifestyle Modifications for Hypertension Prevention and Management

- Lose weight if overweight.
- Limit alcohol intake to no more than 1 oz (30 ml) ethanol (e.g., 24 oz [720 ml] beer, 10 oz [300 ml] wine, or 2 oz [60 ml] 100-proof whiskey) per day or 0.5 oz (15 ml) ethanol per day for women and lighter weight people.
- Increase aerobic physical activity (30-45 minutes most days of the week).

- Reduce sodium intake to no more than 100 mmol per day (2.4 g sodium or 6 g sodium chloride).
- Maintain adequate intake of dietary potassium (approximately 90 mmol per day).
- Maintain adequate intake of dietary calcium and magnesium for general health.
- Stop smoking and reduce intake of dietary saturated fat and cholesterol for overall cardiovascular health.

Reprinted from The Sixth Report of the Joint National Committee on Prevention, Detection, Evaluation, and Treatment of High Blood Pressure, *NIH Pub No 98-4080, Washington, DC, Nov 1997, National Institutes of Health, National Heart, Lung, and Blood Institute.*

such as potassium, magnesium, and calcium. Box 20-3 summarizes these lifestyle modifications that help reduce high blood pressure and overall cardiovascular risk.

In addition to being primary treatments for hypertension, weight reduction and sodium restriction augment antihypertensive medications. Weight reduction facilitates lowered blood pressure even when it is only a loss of 10 lbs to 15 lbs.[19] Diet for weight loss and control should include a specific kcalorie restriction and exercise (aerobic) prescription. Weight loss may be difficult to maintain without a subsequent increase in physical activity (see Appendix F on kcalorie-controlled diets). Average daily sodium intake in America has been estimated to be approximately 4 to 6 grams (175 to 265 mEq). Most comes from sodium added during processing and manufacturing[36] (see Table 8-5). The other main source of dietary sodium is the discretionary use of table salt (sodium chloride). A small portion of dietary sodium also comes from natural sodium content of foods.

The U.S. National High Blood Pressure Education Program recommends trying lifestyle modifications for 3 to 6 months in cases of mild to moderate HTN[19] (see the Cultural Considerations box). A diet rich in fruits, vegetables, and low-fat dairy products along with reduced saturated and total fats has been found to significantly lower blood pressure.[37] The DASH (Dietary Approaches to Stop Hypertension) diet is recommended for prevention and management of HTN.[38] The DASH eating plan described in Table 20-7 is based on 2000 kcal/day. The

CULTURAL CONSIDERATIONS
Hypertension among Vietnamese Americans

Cardiovascular disease is the leading cause of death for all Americans including ethnic minority groups such as Vietnamese Americans. A descriptive study of about 200 Vietnamese Americans living on the West Coast found that the surveyed participants lacked knowledge of hypertension (HTN) and of related risk factors such as diet, exercise, and smoking. The survey tool used assessed information on health status, medications, dietary habits, smoking, and knowledge of hypertension.

Nearly 44% of the participants were considered hypertensive with blood pressures higher than 139/88. Most significant was the lack of knowledge the participants had regarding HTN. Responses also revealed their lack of information about the prevention and treatment of HTN.

Application to nursing: The implications for nurses are twofold: (1) culture is an important influence on blood pressure control, and (2) community-based health information on HTN risk factors such as diet, smoking, and exercise needs to be provided in a culturally appropriate format.

Reference: Duong D, Bohannon A, Ross MC: A descriptive study of hypertension in Vietnamese Americans, J Comm Health Nurs 18(1):1, 2000.

Table 20-7
DASH Diet Pattern

The DASH diet is based on 2000 kcal/day. The following table indicates the number of recommended daily servings from each food group with examples of food choices. The number of servings may increase or decrease, depending on individual calorie needs.

Food Group	Daily Serving (except where noted)	Serving Sizes	Examples and Notes	Significance to the DASH Diet Pattern
Grains and grain products	7-8	1 slice bread 1 oz dry cereal* ½ c cooked rice, pasta, or cereal	Whole wheat bread, English muffin, pita bread, bagel; cereals; grits; oatmeal	Major source of energy and fiber
Vegetables	4-5	1 c raw, leafy vegetable ½ c cooked vegetables 6 oz vegetable juice	Tomatoes, potatoes, carrots, peas, squash, broccoli, turnip greens, collards, kale, spinach, artichokes, beans, sweet potatoes	Rich sources of potassium, magnesium, and fiber
Fruits	4-5	6 oz fruit juice 1 medium fruit ¼ c dried fruit ½ c fresh, frozen, or canned fruit	Apricots, bananas, dates, grapes, oranges, orange juice, tangerines, strawberries, mangoes, melons, peaches, pineapple, prunes, raisins	Important sources of potassium, magnesium, and fiber
Low-fat or nonfat dairy foods	2-3	8 oz milk 1 c yogurt 1.5 oz cheese	Fat-free or 1% milk, fat-free or low-fat buttermilk; nonfat or low-fat yogurt; part-nonfat mozzarella cheese, nonfat cheese	Major sources of calcium and protein
Meats, poultry, and fish	≤2	3 oz cooked meats, poultry, or fish	Select only lean meats; trim away visible fats; broil, roast, or boil, instead of frying; remove skin from chicken	Rich sources of protein and magnesium
Nuts, seeds, and legumes	4-5/week	1.5 oz or ½ c nuts 0.5 oz or 2 T seeds ½ c cooked legumes	Almonds, filberts, mixed nuts, peanuts, walnuts, sunflower seeds, kidney beans, lentils	Rich sources of energy, magnesium, potassium, protein, and fiber
Fats and oils†	2-3	1 tsp soft margarine 1 T low-fat mayonnaise or salad dressing 2 T light salad dressing 1 tsp vegetable oil	Soft margarine, low-fat mayonnaise, light salad dressing, vegetable oil (e.g., olive, corn, canola, or safflower)	DASH has 27% of calories as fat, including that in or added to foods.
Sweets	5/week	1 T sugar 1 T jelly or jam ½ oz jelly beans 8 oz lemonade	Maple syrup, sugar, jelly, jam; fruit-flavored gelatin, jelly beans, fruit punch, sorbet, ices, hard candy	Sweets should be low in fat

Reprinted from U.S. Department of Health and Human Services, Public Health Service: The DASH diet, NIH Pub No 01-4082, revised May 2001, Bethesda, Md, National Institutes of Health, National Heart, Lung, and Blood Institute.
*Equals ½ - 1¼ c depending on cereal type. Check the product's nutrition label.
†Fat content changes serving counts for fats and oils. For example, 1 T of regular salad dressing equals 1 serving; 1 T of low-fat dressing equals ½ serving; 1 T of fat-free dressing equals 0 servings.

number of daily servings from each group can be modified depending on individual energy needs. See the Teaching Tool box, "Strategies for Adopting DASH."

An even larger drop in blood pressure is seen when the DASH eating plan is combined with sodium restriction.[38-40] Sodium intake levels of about 3300 mg/day (level consumed by many Americans); an intermediate intake around 2400 mg/day; and a lower intake around 1500 mg/day combined with the DASH eating plan can reduce blood pressure in those with normal blood pressure and HTN (Table 20-8). However, the largest reduction in blood pressure is seen in those using the DASH eating plan at the sodium intake level of 1500 mg/day (Box 20-4).

TEACHING TOOL
Strategies for Adopting DASH

Dietary changes are best achieved through small changes in food selections. Use this list of tips as a way to initiate discussion and dietary compliance to reduce hypertension among your clients.

TIPS ON EATING THE DASH WAY

Change gradually.

- If you now eat one or two vegetables a day, add a serving at lunch and another at dinner.
- If you don't eat fruit now or have only juice at breakfast, add a serving to your meals or have it as a snack.
- Gradually increase your use of fat-free and low-fat dairy products to three servings a day. For example, drink milk with lunch or dinner instead of soda, sugar-sweetened tea, or alcohol. Choose low-fat (1%) or fat-free (skim) dairy products to reduce your intake of saturated fat, total fat, cholesterol, and kcalories.
- Read food labels on margarines and salad dressings and choose those lowest in unsaturated fat. Some margarines are now transfat free.

Treat meat as one part of the whole meal, instead of the focus.

- Limit meat to 6 oz a day (two servings)—all that's needed. A serving of 3 to 4 ounces is about the size of a deck of cards.
- If you currently eat large portions of meat, cut portion sizes back gradually—by a half or a third at each meal.
- Include two or more vegetarian-style (meatless) meals each week.
- Increase servings of vegetables, rice, pasta, and dry beans in meals. Try casseroles, pasta, and stir-fry dishes, which have less meat and more vegetables, grains, and dry beans.

Use fruit or other foods low in saturated fat, cholesterol, and kcalories as desserts and snacks.

- Fruits and other low-fat foods offer great taste and variety. Use fruits canned in their own juice. Fresh fruits require little or no preparation. Dried fruits are a good choice to carry with you.
- Try these snacks ideas: unsalted pretzels or nuts mixed with raisins; graham crackers; low-fat, fat-free, or frozen yogurt; popcorn with no salt or butter added; and raw vegetables.

Try the following other tips.

- Choose whole grain foods to get added nutrients, such as minerals and fiber. For example, choose whole wheat bread or whole grain cereals.
- If you have trouble digesting dairy products, try taking lactase enzyme pills or drops (available at drugstores and groceries) before eating dairy foods, or buy lactose-free milk or milk with lactase enzyme added to it.
- Use fresh, frozen, or sodium-free canned vegetables.

Reprinted from U.S. Department of Health and Human Services, Public Health Service: The DASH diet, NIH Pub No 01-4082, revised May 2001, National Institutes of Health, Bethesda, Md, National Heart, Lung, and Blood Institute.

For many, a sodium intake of 1500 mg/day would be perceived as a moderately severe restriction. Additionally, maintaining sodium consumption at this level may not currently be realistic given the amount of sodium added to foods during processing and manufacturing.[36] In fact, if the U.S. food supply were lower in sodium, it would help lower blood pressure in the general population.[41] Salt not only adds its own salty flavor to foods but also seems to alter other tastes and flavors and conceals bitterness without necessarily causing the foods to taste salty. As a result, when salt is reduced or removed from a food, not only is the saltiness of that food changed but other flavors in the food are changed.[36] Although there is currently no acceptable substitute for salt that provides similar taste satisfaction,[36] a salt

---

Table 20-8
Where's the Sodium?

Only a small amount of sodium occurs naturally in foods. Most sodium is added during processing. The table below gives examples of varying amounts of sodium that occur in foods before and after processing.

Food Groups	Sodium (mg)
Grains and grain products	
Cooked cereal, rice, pasta, unsalted, ½ cup	0-5
Ready-to-eat cereal, 1 cup	100-360
Bread, 1 slice	110-175
Vegetables	
Fresh or frozen, cooked without salt, ½ cup	1-70
Canned or frozen with sauce, ½ cup	140-460
Tomato juice, canned, ¾ cup	820
Fruit	
Fresh, frozen, canned, ½ cup	0-5
Low-fat or fat-free dairy foods	
Milk, 1 cup	120
Yogurt, 8 oz	160
Natural cheeses, 1½ oz	110-450
Processed cheeses, 1½ oz	600
Nuts, seeds, and dry beans	
Peanuts, salted, ⅓ cup	120
Peanuts, unsalted, ⅓ cup	0-5
Beans, cooked from dried or frozen, without salt, ½ cup	0-5
Beans, canned, ½ cup	400
Meats, fish, and poultry	
Fresh meat, fish, poultry, 3 oz	30-90
Tuna canned, water pack, no salt added, 3 oz	35-45
Tuna canned, water pack, 3 oz	250-350
Ham, lean, roasted, 3 oz	1,020

From U.S. Department of Health and Human Services, Public Health Service: The DASH diet, NIH Pub No 01-4082, revised May 2001, National Institutes of Health, National Heart, Lung, and Blood Institute.

Box 20-4 DASHing with Less Salt: A Sample Menu

2400 MG SODIUM MENU	SODIUM (MG)	SUBSTITUTIONS TO REDUCE SODIUM TO 1500 MG	SODIUM (MG)
BREAKFAST			
²/₃ c bran cereal	161	²/₃ c shredded wheat cereal	3
1 slice whole wheat bread	149		
1 medium banana	1		
1 c fruit yogurt, fat free, no sugar added	53		
1 c fat-free milk	126		
2 tsp jelly	5		
LUNCH			
¾ c chicken salad*	201	Remove salt from recipe	127
2 slices whole wheat bread	299		
1 T Dijon mustard	372	1 T regular mustard	196
½ c fruit cocktail, juice pack	5		
SALAD:			
½ c fresh cucumber slices	8		
½ c tomato wedges	1		
2 T ranch dressing, fat free	306	2 T yogurt salad dressing†	84

This sample menu provides five fruit servings, five vegetable servings, and four dairy servings.

RECIPES

CHICKEN SALAD (MAKES 5 SERVINGS)

3¼ c chicken breast, cooked, cubed, skinless
3 T light mayonnaise
¼ c celery, chopped
1 T lemon juice
½ tsp onion powder
⅛ tsp salt

Steps:
1. Bake chicken, cut into cubes, and refrigerate.
2. Mix all ingredients in a large bowl and serve.
Serving size: ¾ cup

†YOGURT SALAD DRESSING (MAKES 5 SERVINGS)

8 oz plain yogurt, fat free
¼ c mayonnaise, fat free
2 T chives, dried
2 T dill, dried
2 T lemon juice
Mix ingredients in bowl and refrigerate.
Serving size: 2 T

substitute may be prescribed (see the Myth box). The Teaching Tool, "Seven Sneaky Sodium Stowaways," gives tips on helping patients recognize foods potentially high in sodium.

MYOCARDIAL INFARCTION

Myocardial infarctions (MIs), or heart attacks, are the single largest killer of adult men and women in the United States. An American will suffer a heart attack every 20 seconds, and someone dies from one every minute. Disability or death can result after an MI, depending on how much heart muscle is damaged.

Medical Nutrition Therapy

The purpose of medical nutrition therapy for patients suffering from an MI is to reduce the workload of the heart. This is also a good time to initiate education about modification of diet-related cardiac risk factors.

Box 20-4 DASHing with Less Salt: A Sample Menu—cont'd

2400 MG SODIUM MENU	SODIUM (MG)	SUBSTITUTIONS TO REDUCE SODIUM TO 1500 MG	SODIUM (MG)
DINNER			
3 oz spicy baked fish‡	93		
1 c green beans, cooked from frozen, without salt	12		
1 small baked potato	7		
2 T fat-free sour cream	28		
1 T chopped scallions	1		
2 T grated cheddar cheese, natural, reduced fat	86	2 T cheddar cheese, natural, reduced fat, low sodium	1
1 small whole wheat roll	148		
1 tsp soft margarine	51	1 tsp soft margarine, unsalted	1
1 medium peach	0		
1 c fat-free milk	126		
SNACK			
1 c orange juice	2		
⅓ c almonds, unsalted	5		
¼ c raisins	2		
1 c fruit yogurt, fat free with sugar	107		

RECIPES

‡SPICY BAKED COD (MAKES 4 SERVINGS)

1 lb cod, or other fish fillet, fresh or thawed from frozen
1 T olive oil
1 tsp spicy seasoning mix (see below)

Steps:
1. Preheat oven to 350° F. Spray small baking dish with cooking oil spray.
2. Wash and dry cod. Place in dish and drizzle with oil and seasoning mix.
3. Bake uncovered for 12 minutes or until fish flakes with fork.
4. Cut into four pieces and serve.

Spicy seasoning mix
Mix together the following ingredients and store in airtight container for other recipes: 1½ tsp white pepper, ½ tsp cayenne pepper, ½ tsp black pepper, 1 tsp onion powder, 1¼ tsp garlic powder, 1 T dried basil, 1½ tsp dried thyme.

From U.S. Department of Health and Human Services, Public Health Service: The DASH diet; *NIH Pub No 01-4082, revised May 2001, Bethesda, Md, National Institutes of Health, National Heart, Lung, and Blood Institute.*

TEACHING TOOL
Seven Sneaky Sodium Stowaways

*P*rovide patients with an easy way to remember categories of foods that may be potentially high in sodium. For most categories, patients on sodium-restricted diets can choose food products that are lower in sodium content; however, label reading becomes an absolute necessity. Review the sodium reduction suggestions in Chapter 8. Also consider that sodium hides in seven categories of foods in the form of salt or as part of an added ingredient. Following are the Seven Sneaky (categories of) Sodium Stowaways:
1. Snacks (corn chips, potato chips, pretzels, peanuts, certain crackers)
2. Seasonings and nonnutritive sweeteners (monosodium glutamate, sodium saccharin)
3. Soups (especially canned and dried mixes)
4. Sauces (dried mixes and bottled, includes ketchup)
5. Smoked meats and fish (smoked ham and lox)
6. Sauerkraut and other pickled foods (pickles, relishes, and pickled herring)
7. Sodium processed luncheon meats (bologna, salami, ham, corned beef)

> ## ★ MYTH
> ### Any Salt Substitute Will Do
>
> All salt substitutes are not created equal; some substitutes reduce total sodium content through the use of fillers or replace sodium with potassium, whereas others completely replace sodium with a combination of spices. Use of salt substitutes should be discussed with the patient's primary healthcare provider because they may be medically contraindicated (e.g., individuals with renal disease whose kidneys may not be able to handle additional minerals such as potassium). Some healthcare facilities may require primary healthcare providers to systematically prescribe salt substitutes when ordering sodium-restricted diets. Listed below are common types of salt substitutes and manufacturers' information to assist in locating substitutes for patients.
>
> | TYPE OF SALT SUBSTITUTE | BRAND NAME | SODIUM CONTENT | MANUFACTURER/ PHONE NUMBER |
> | --- | --- | --- | --- |
> | Herb-spice | Mrs. Dash | Sodium free | Alberto-Culver Co, (800)622-DASH |
> | Potassium chloride | Adolph's | Salt free | Union Lever (Lipton's) (800)328-7248 |
> | Reduced sodium | Morton's Lite Salt | 50% sodium (still contains salt) | Morton Salt Division, Morton Int, (312)807-2090 |
> | | Papa Dash | Low sodium | Alberto-Culver Co, (800)622-DASH |
>
> Reference: American Dietetic Association: Manual of clinical dietetics, ed 6, Chicago, 2000, American Dietetic Association.

The patient may receive a liquid diet initially (for approximately 24 hours) and progress, as tolerated, to foods of regular consistency. Smaller, frequent meals are usually better tolerated than large meals, which can increase myocardial oxygen demand by increasing splanchnic (visceral) blood flow. Caffeine-containing beverages are sometimes restricted to avoid myocardial stimulation. Foods and beverages served should be of moderate temperatures, neither too hot nor too cold. Sodium, cholesterol, fat, and kcalories (if weight loss is indicated) are controlled according to the patient's needs.

Consuming omega-3 fatty acids (see Chapter 5) appears to reduce the risk of blood clots that may cause an MI. Sources of omega-3 fatty acids include fish such as tuna, salmon, halibut, sardines, and lake trout.

CARDIAC FAILURE

congestive heart failure (CHF) circulatory congestion resulting in the heart's inability to maintain adequate blood supply to meet oxygen demands

Cardiac failure is also called **congestive heart failure (CHF)**, heart failure, and cardiac decompensation. Location of congestion depends on the ventricle involved. Left ventricle failure produces pulmonary congestion, whereas right ventricular failure results in systemic congestion that causes poor perfusion to all organ systems.[3] Right heart (ventricular) failure has also been reported to result from left heart (ventricular) failure.[4]

Medical Nutrition Therapy

To lessen the workload of the heart, medical nutrition therapy focuses on restricting dietary sodium. The more severe the heart failure, the more severe the sodium restriction to reduce extracellular fluids. Patients with mild to moderate heart failure are often prescribed a sodium restriction of 3000 mg/day. Persons unresponsive to this level or who have severe CHF are more likely to benefit from a 2000 mg/day sodium restriction.[42] Fluid restriction of 1 to 2 liters is sometimes indicated in severe heart failure, especially when hyponatremia is present. Fluid requirements depend on medical status and use of diuretics.

Energy requirements may be 20% to 30% above basal needs because of increased cardiac and pulmonary energy demands and increased metabolic rate.[43] Protein and energy intake should be sufficient to maintain body weight. Meeting these increased nutrient and energy requirements could be problematic because of early satiety, gastrointestinal congestion, shortness of breath, anorexia, and nausea.[42] If the patient has cardiac cachexia, additional kcalories and protein are needed to prevent further catabolism. Caution must be used when increasing energy, however, so as not to overfeed the patient. Kcalorie-dense (1.5 to 2.0 kcal/ml) nutritional supplements may be helpful to increase kcalories and protein intake. Enteral or parenteral nutrition (see Chapter 14) may be necessary for patients who cannot meet their nutritional needs through oral intake. If enteral nutrition support is required, continuous, rather than bolus, feedings are favored because they reduce myocardial oxygen consumption.[44] Concentrated enteral formulas are available if fluid restriction is necessary.

cachexia
general ill health and malnutrition, marked by weakness and emaciation

✿ LIFE SPAN IMPLICATIONS

CVD often seems to affect older individuals, but the illness may strike in the middle years of the 40s and 50s. With later marriages and delayed childbearing, middle years may often still be a time of parenting young children as well as teens. Dietary modifications are easier to follow when the entire family is supportive and compliant.

Dietary education should include individuals who buy and prepare meals (and snacks, too) for the patient. Lists of health associations, community hospitals and other organizations offering cooking courses, and bookstores or public libraries with available heart healthy cookbooks are excellent adjuncts to medical nutrition therapy. By including all family members in the educative process, not only is the health of the individual with CAD enhanced but primary risk factors for younger family members are also decreased. Although children may not need to follow the sometimes extreme restrictions of CAD patients, it is still easier for a 10-year-old to understand that it is heart healthy to have popcorn with little or no butter and salt than to simply blame restrictions on "Daddy's sickness." Lifelong health promotion habits develop early and benefit everyone.

OVERCOMING BARRIERS

Demystifying Labels

Label reading is an important skill for all of us but is especially so for someone with diet-related illnesses including HTN or CVD. Educating patients about the use of food label information helps demystify the process of consuming recommended levels of dietary fat and sodium. Food labels may display two types of messages about packaged food: nutrient content claims and health claims. Federal regulations formulated by the Food and Drug Administration (FDA) control how certain terms can be used in labeling. Table 20-9 defines terms related to sodium, dietary cholesterol, and fat—nutrients of concern for CVD.

SUMMARY

Cardiovascular disease consists of a group of diseases and conditions that affect the heart and blood vessels; they are coronary artery disease, hypertension, peripheral vascular disease, congestive heart failure, and congenital heart diseases.

Table 20-9
Nutrient Content Claims

Term	Fat	Saturated Fat	Cholesterol	Sodium	Kcalorie
Free ("zero," "no," "without," "trivial source of," or "dietarily insignificant source of")	<0.5 g per reference amount*	<0.5 g saturated fat and <0.5 g transfatty acids per reference amount	<2 mg per reference amount and per labeled serving	<5 mg per reference amount and per labeled amount	<5 kcal per serving
Low ("little," "few" for kcalories, "contains a small amount of," "low source of")	≤3 g per serving	≤1 g per serving	≤20 mg per serving	≤140 mg per serving	≤40 kcal per serving
Light or lite	A product has one third fewer kcalories than a comparable product or 50% of the fat found in a comparable product, or the sodium content of a low-kcalorie, low-fat food has been reduced by 50% (light may still be used to describe properties of food such as texture and color).				
Reduced/Less	A nutritionally altered product that contains 25% less of a nutrient or kcalories than the regular product (this claim cannot be made on a product if the regular food already meets the requirement for "low").				
Free	A product contains virtually none of one or more of these: fat, saturated fat, cholesterol, sodium, sugars, and kcalories				
Lean†	<10 g fat, plus	4 g saturated fat	and <95 mg of cholesterol per serving and per 100 g		
Extra lean†	<5 g fat, plus	<2 g saturated fat	and <95 mg of cholesterol per serving and per 100 g		

Data from US Department of Agriculture Center for Food Safety and Applied Nutrition: A food labeling guide; Updated June 1999; http://cfsan.fda.gov/~dms/flg-6a.html, accessed June 21, 2002.
"Reference amount" is reference amount customarily consumed.
†Used to describe the fat content of meat, poultry, seafood, and game meats.

CVD risk factors are categorized into three groups: controllable, noncontrollable, and predisposing. Controllable or lifestyle factors include tobacco use, diet, and physical inactivity. Noncontrollable factors are gender, age, and family history. Predisposing conditions may be diabetes mellitus, hypertension, obesity, and hypercholesterolemia.

CAD begins with atherosclerosis. Atherosclerosis is the development of lesions in coronary arteries that can lead to arteriosclerosis and may lead to angina pectoris or myocardial infarction. If thrombosis occurs in a cerebral artery, a cerebrovascular accident or hemorrhagic stroke occurs. CAD risk is assessed by measuring the total blood cholesterol and the proportions of the different types of lipoproteins that carry cholesterol in the blood. Lowering total cholesterol and LDL-cholesterol can be achieved by dietary intervention, including weight loss and exercise. Goals of medical nutrition therapy are to reduce total fat, saturated fat, transfatty acids, and cholesterol intake in an attempt to reduce plasma total cholesterol, LDL-cholesterol, and triglyceride levels.

HTN for which the cause is not known is called *primary* or *essential HTN*. *Secondary HTN* is the term used when the cause of elevated blood pressure can be identified. Prescribed treatment regimens for HTN are individualized and vary because the disease differs in its degree of severity. The first line of treatment is usually nonpharmacologic or focused on lifestyle modifications. Weight reduction and sodium restriction augment antihypertensive medications as well.

MIs are the single largest killer of adults in the United States. The purpose of medical nutrition therapy is to reduce the workload of the heart. The patient may receive a liquid diet initially and progress to foods of regular consistency as tolerated. Smaller, frequent meals are usually better tolerated than large meals.

CAD, lung disease, complications of hypothyroidism, or damage to the myocardial or cardiac muscle can cause cardiac failure. The condition is characterized by decreased blood flow to the kidneys and retention of sodium and fluid. Patients with congestive heart failure often experience edema of the feet and ankles and shortness of breath. To lessen the workload of the heart, medical nutrition therapy focuses on restricting dietary sodium.

THE NURSING APPROACH
Case Study: Cardiovascular Disease

Stan, age 56, has a family history of heart disease and stroke. He comes to your primary care practice office for a physical examination. He sees the physician on the first visit; on the second visit, he is referred to you, a cardiovascular clinical nurse specialist. The referral is recommended because he is diagnosed as high risk for a cardiovascular disease.

ASSESSMENT

The newest laboratory results reveal a total cholesterol of 256 mg/dl and an LDL level of 180 mg/dl. He lives a sedentary lifestyle and is overweight at 260 lbs. You ask Stan to describe some of his typical meals, and you find that he eats a lot of fried foods, some bakery pastries, and several portions of lean beef each week. When you ask him about exercise, he states he doesn't do any.

NURSING DIAGNOSIS

Knowledge deficit related to lack of understanding of relationship between fat and cholesterol as evidenced by purposeful use of some low-cholesterol foods but intake of high-fat foods

PLANNING

Goals

1. Express understanding that controlling total fat, saturated fat, and trans fatty acid intake is as important as controlling cholesterol.
2. Limit fried foods to one portion per week and eat only low-cholesterol, low-fat pastry in small amounts.
3. Increase intake of whole grain breads and cereals, fruits, and vegetables.
4. By the next office visit in 3 months, reduce total cholesterol level to 220 mg/dl, LDLs to 160 mg/dl, and weight to 255 lbs.

Continued

THE NURSING APPROACH
Case Study: Cardiovascular Disease

IMPLEMENTATION

1. Review the physiologic differences between dietary fat and cholesterol.
2. Give Stan literature on fat and cholesterol that includes foods to be limited and avoided in each category.
3. Assess Stan's understanding of the effects of high total cholesterol and LDL levels on the body.
4. In 3 months, obtain new laboratory results and have a follow-up visit with Stan.

EVALUATION

The goals will be evaluated in 3 months to see if outcomes have been achieved as evidenced by the following:

• Stan gives a simple explanation of the difference between fat and cholesterol.
• Stan's total cholesterol is 220 mg/dl or lower, LDL level is 160 mg/dl or lower, and weight is 255 lbs or lower.

Follow-up

When the previously set goals have been met, set goals to decrease weight and begin exercise.

CRITICAL THINKING
Clinical Applications

Kevin, age 69, is admitted to the coronary care unit of your hospital. He is 6' tall, medium frame, and weighs 210 lbs. He has gained 30 lbs since he retired 4 years ago, which he attributes to boredom and lack of exercise. Three months before admission, Kevin began to experience chest pain that radiated up his neck and down to his stomach. He has a history of hypertension and elevated serum cholesterol levels. After admission to the hospital, Kevin was diagnosed with having had an acute myocardial infarction.

Test results for serum lipids were as follows:
Cholesterol: 300 mg/dl
LDL-cholesterol: 200 mg/dl
HDL-cholesterol: 30 mg/dl
TG: 600 mg/dl
Medications prescribed after admission: tenormin, diltiazem (Cardizem), nitroglycerin
Diet order: therapeutic lifestyle changes (TLC) diet

1. What are the risk factors for cardiovascular disease?
2. What are Kevin's risk factors?
3. Define the term *myocardial infarction* and describe what happens when a myocardial infarction occurs.
4. What specific guidelines are included in the NCEP's TLC diet recommendations?
   While caring for Kevin you learn he snacks on high-fat cheeses, ice cream, potato chips, corn chips, peanuts, and crackers. He also drinks whole milk and eats a lot of butter on his bread at every meal. What characteristics of Kevin's intake contradict the National Cholesterol Education Program's TLC diet recommendations?
1. What are some alternative foods that are appealing to Kevin that he could eat for snacks?

Web Sites of Interest

American Heart Association (AHA)
www.americanheart.org
This official site of the AHA provides information and education about heart disease and stroke for the public and health professionals. It includes a link to a women's Web site on heart disease.

National Cholesterol Education Program (NCEP)
www.nhlbi.nih.gov/chd/
The NCEP is part of the National Heart, Lung, and Blood Institute (NHLBI) within the National Institutes of Health. This site is an entry to the wide ranges of educational and research programs of NCEP.

World Hypertension League (WHL)
www.mco.edu/whl
This organization, a division of the International Society of Hypertension, is associated with the World Health Organization. The purpose of WHL is to advocate for the detection, prevention, and treatment of HTN in populations. The site provides information for the public and health professionals along with links to other organizations devoted to control of hypertension.

References

1. American Heart Association (AHA): *American Heart Association 2002 heart and stroke statistical update*, Dallas, 2001, AHA.
2. Centers for Disease Control and Prevention: Prevalence of adults with no known major risk factors for coronary heart diseases—behavioral risk factor surveillance system, *MMWR* 43:61, 1994.
3. Price SA, Wilson LM: *Pathophysiology: clinical concepts of disease processes*, ed 6, St Louis, 2002, Mosby.
4. McCance KL, Huether SE: *Pathophysiology: the biological basis for disease in adults and children*, ed 4, St Louis, 2002, Mosby.
5. National Cholesterol Education Program (NCEP): *Third report of the NCEP expert panel on detection, evaluation, and treatment of high blood cholesterol in adults (Adult Treatment Panel III): executive summary*, NIH Pub No 01-3670, May 2001, Washington, DC, 2001, National Institutes of Health, National Heart, Lung, and Blood Institute; www.nhlbi.nih.gov/guidelines/cholesterol/atp3_rpt.pdf, accessed May 29, 2001.
6. National Cholesterol Education Program (NCEP): *Third report of the NCEP expert panel on detection, evaluation, and treatment of high blood cholesterol in adults (Adult Treatment Panel III)* NIH Pub No 02-5215, Washington, DC, 2001, National Institutes of Health, National Heart, Lung, and Blood Institute; www.nhlbi.nih.gov/guidelines/cholesterol/atp3_rpt.pdf.
7. American Heart Association: *Heart and stroke facts, 1992-2001*; 216.185.112.5/downloadable/heart/1014833865440101319123698 5HSfacts02.pdf, accessed May 29, 2002.
8. Stone NJ: Secondary causes of hyperlipidemia, *Med Clin North Am* 78:117, 1994.
9. Chait A, Brunzell JD: Acquired hyperlipidemia (secondary dyslipoproteinemias), *Endocrinol Metab Clin North Am* 19:259, 1990.
10. Krauss RM: Regulation of high-density lipoprotein levels, *Med Clin North Am* 66:403, 1982.
11. National Institutes of Health: Clinical guidelines on the identification, evaluation, and treatment of overweight and obesity in adults—the evidence report, NIH Pub No 98-4083, Bethesda, Md, 1998, National Heart, Lung, and Blood Institute.
12. National Institutes of Health: Clinical guidelines on the identification, evaluation, and treatment of overweight and obesity in adults—the evidence report, *Obesity Res* 6(suppl2)51S, 1998.
13. Grundy SM, Denke MA: Dietary influences on serum lipids and lipoproteins, *J Lipid Res* 31:1149, 1990.
14. Mensink RP, Katan MB: Effects of dietary fatty acids on serum lipids and lipoproteins: a meta-analysis of 27 trials, *Arterioscler Thromb* 12:911, 1992.

15. Caggiula AW et al.: The Multiple Risk Intervention Trial (MRFIT). IV. Intervention on blood lipids, *Prev Med* 10:443, 1981.

16. Stamler J et al.: Relation of changes in dietary lipids and weight, trial years 1-6, to change in blood lipids in the special intervention and usual care groups in the Multiple Risk Factor Intervention Trial, *Am J Clin Nutr* 65:272S, 1997.

17. Hopkins PN: Effects of dietary cholesterol on serum cholesterol: a meta-analysis and review, *Am J Clin Nutr* 55:1060, 1992.

18. Clarke R et al.: Dietary lipids and blood cholesterol: quantitative meta-analysis of metabolic ward studies, *Brit Med J* 314:112, 1997.

19. Garg A: High-monounsaturated-fat diets for patients with diabetes mellitus: a meta-analysis, *Am J Clin Nutr* 67(suppl3):577S, 1998.

20. Kris-Etherton PM et al.: High-monounsaturated fatty acid diets lower both plasma cholesterol and triacylglycerol concentrations, *Am J Clin Nutr* 70:1009, 1999.

21. National Research Council: *Diet and health: implications for reducing chronic disease risk*, Washington, DC, 1989, National Academy Press.

22. Knopp RH et al.: Long-term cholesterol-lowering effects of 4 fat-restricted diets in hypercholesterolemic and combined hyperlipidemic men. The Dietary Alternatives Study, *J Am Med Assoc* 278:1509, 1997.

23. Turely ML et al.: The effect of a low-fat, high-carbohydrate diet on serum high density lipoprotein cholesterol and triglyceride, *Eur J Clin Nutr* 52:728, 1998.

24. Jenkins DJ et al.: Effect on blood lipids of very high intakes of fiber in diets low in saturated fat and cholesterol, *N Engl J Med* 329:21, 1993.

25. Vuksan V et al.: Beneficial effects of viscous dietary fiber from Konjac-mannan in subjects with the insulin resistance syndrome: results of a controlled metabolic trial *Diabetes Care* 23:9, 2000.

26. U.S. Department of Health and Human Services, Food and Drug Administration: Food labeling: health claims; soluble fiber from certain foods and coronary heart disease. Final rule, *Federal Register* 28234, 1997.

27. U.S. Department of Health and Human Services, Food and Drug Administration. Food labeling: health claims; soluble fiber from certain foods and coronary heart disease. Final rule. *Federal Register* 8103, 1998.

28. Anderson JW: Dietary fibre, complex carbohydrate and coronary heart disease, *Can J Cardiol* 11(suppl G):55G, 1995.

29. Vuorio AF et al.: Stanol ester margarine alone and with simvastatin lowers serum cholesterol in families with familial hypercholesterolemia caused by the FH-North Karelia Mutation, *Arterio Thromb Vasc Biol* 20:500, 2000.

30. Gylling H, Miettinen TA: Cholesterol reduction by different plant stanol mixtures and with variable fat intake, *Metabolism* 48:575, 1999.

31. Gylling H et al.: Reduction of serum cholesterol in postmenopausal women with previous myocardial infarction and cholesterol malabsorption induced by dietary sitostanol ester margarine: women and dietary sitostanol, *Circulation* 96:4226, 1997.

32. Hallikainen MA, Uusitupa MI: Effects of 2 low-fat stanol ester-containing margarines on serum cholesterol concentrations as part of a low-fat diet in hypercholesterolemic subjects, *Am J Clin Nutr* 69:403, 1999.

33. Hendricks HF et al.: Spreads enriched with three different levels of vegetable oil sterols and the degree of cholesterol lowering in normocholesterolaemic and mildly hypercholesterolaemic subjects, *Eur J Clin Nutr* 53:319, 1999.

34. Miettinen TA et al.: Reduction of serum cholesterol with sitostanol-ester margarine in a mildly hypercholesterolemic population, *N Engl J Med* 333:1308, 1995.

35. Vanhanen HT et al.: Serum cholesterol, cholesterol, precursors, and plant sterols in hypercholesterolemic subjects with different apoE phenotypes during dietary sitostanol ester treatment, *J Lipid Res* 34:1535, 1993.

36. National High Blood Pressure Education Program: Implementing recommendations for dietary salt reduction, NIH Pub No 55-728N, Nov 1996, National Institutes of Health, Bethesda, Md, National Heart, Lung, and Blood Institute.

37. Sacks FM et al.: Rationale and design of the Dietary Approaches to Stop Hypertension (DASH): a multicenter controlled-feeding study of dietary patterns to lower blood pressure, *Ann Epidemiol* 5(2):108, Mar 1995.

38. National Institutes of Health: Facts about the DASH diet, NIH Pub No 01-4082, revised May 2001, Bethesda, Md, National Institutes of Health, National Heart, Lung, and Blood Institute.

39. Sacks FM et al.: Effects on blood pressure of reduced dietary sodium and the Dietary Approaches to Stop Hypertension (DASH) diet, *N Engl J Med* 344(1):3, 2001.

40. Vollmer WM et al.: Effects of diet and sodium intake on blood pressure: subgroup analysis of the DASH-sodium trial, *Ann Intern Med* 135:1019, 2001.

41. National Institutes of Health: *NIH news release: NHLBI study finds DASH diet and reduced sodium lowers blood pressure for all,* released 12/17/01; www.nih.gov/news/pr/dec2001/nhlbi-17.htm, accessed June 19, 2002.

42. American Dietetic Association: *Manual of clinical dietetics*, ed 6, Chicago, 2000, American Dietetic Association.

43. Poehlman ET et al.: Increased resting metabolic rate in patients with congestive heart failure, *Ann Intern Med* 121:860, 1994.

44. Heymsfield SB et al.: Bioenergetic and metabolic response to continuous v intermittent nasoenteric feeding, *Metabolism* 36(6):570, 1987.

CHAPTER 21

Nutrition for Diseases of the Kidneys

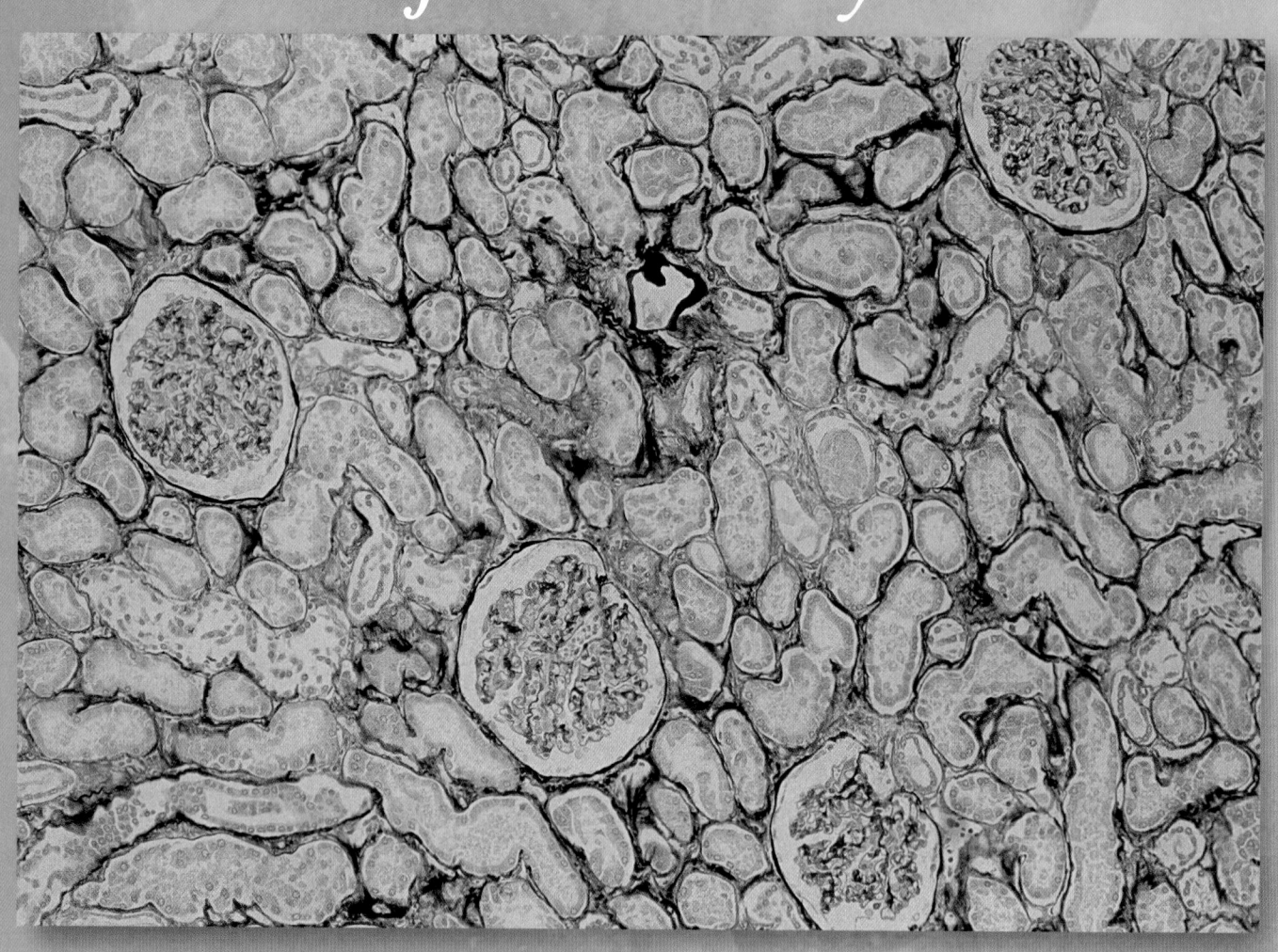

The chief, life-preserving function of the kidneys is to maintain chemical homeostasis in the body.

ROLE IN WELLNESS

Often taken for granted, kidneys filter approximately one liter of blood per minute to remove excess fluid and more than 200 waste products from the body. In addition, kidneys perform vital metabolic and hormonal functions. Because kidneys play so many roles in wellness, kidney disease has serious consequences. Nutritional needs of patients with kidney disease are complex and ever changing and require constant assessment, monitoring, and counseling. These factors present an ongoing challenge to nursing and other healthcare team members.

The dimensions of health reveal the challenges in dealing with kidney disorders. Functions of the kidneys affect total physical well-being; implementing medical nutrition therapy to aid treatment is essential for enhancing the physical health dimension. Intellectual health dimension is tested because clients need to know (or be taught) anatomy and physiology to fully understand the dysfunction processes that lead to kidney disorders and the necessity to follow a strict diet. The chronic nature and potentially life-threatening aspects of kidney disorders may be emotionally devastating; clients may benefit from psychologic counseling to deal with these illnesses to maintain emotional health. The social dimension of health may be strained by kidney disorders. Significant others may become worn down by the responsibility of caring for loved ones with renal disorders; the ever-present need for dialysis, once initiated, disrupts normal social relationships unless new ways of coping are established. Spiritual health may affect physical response to treatment. Individuals participating regularly in religious activities tend to have lower blood pressures compared with those who do not participate.

KIDNEY FUNCTION

The chief, life-preserving function of kidneys is to maintain chemical homeostasis in the body. They do this largely by processing components within blood to maintain fluid, electrolyte, and acid-base balance and by eliminating wastes in the urine. Each kidney has approximately 1 million "microscopic" workhorses called *nephrons* (Figure 21-1). Each nephron filters and resorbs essential blood constituents, secretes ions as needed for maintaining acid-base balance, and excretes fluid and other substances as urine. Other important functions of kidneys include manufacturing hormones to regulate blood pressure (renin), stimulating production of red blood cells (erythropoietin), and regulating calcium and phosphorus metabolism (final step in vitamin D synthesis). Kidneys also detoxify some drugs and poisons (Box 21-1).

Various inflammatory, obstructive, and degenerative diseases affect kidneys in different ways. These disorders interfere with normal functioning of nephrons to regulate products of body metabolism. Ultimately, kidney failure could lead to homeostatic failure and, if not relieved, death.

Box 21-1 Kidney Functions

- Maintain fluid, electrolyte, and acid-base balance
- Eliminate waste products
- Regulate blood pressure
- Stimulate red blood cell production
- Regulate calcium and phosphorus metabolism
- Eliminate many drugs

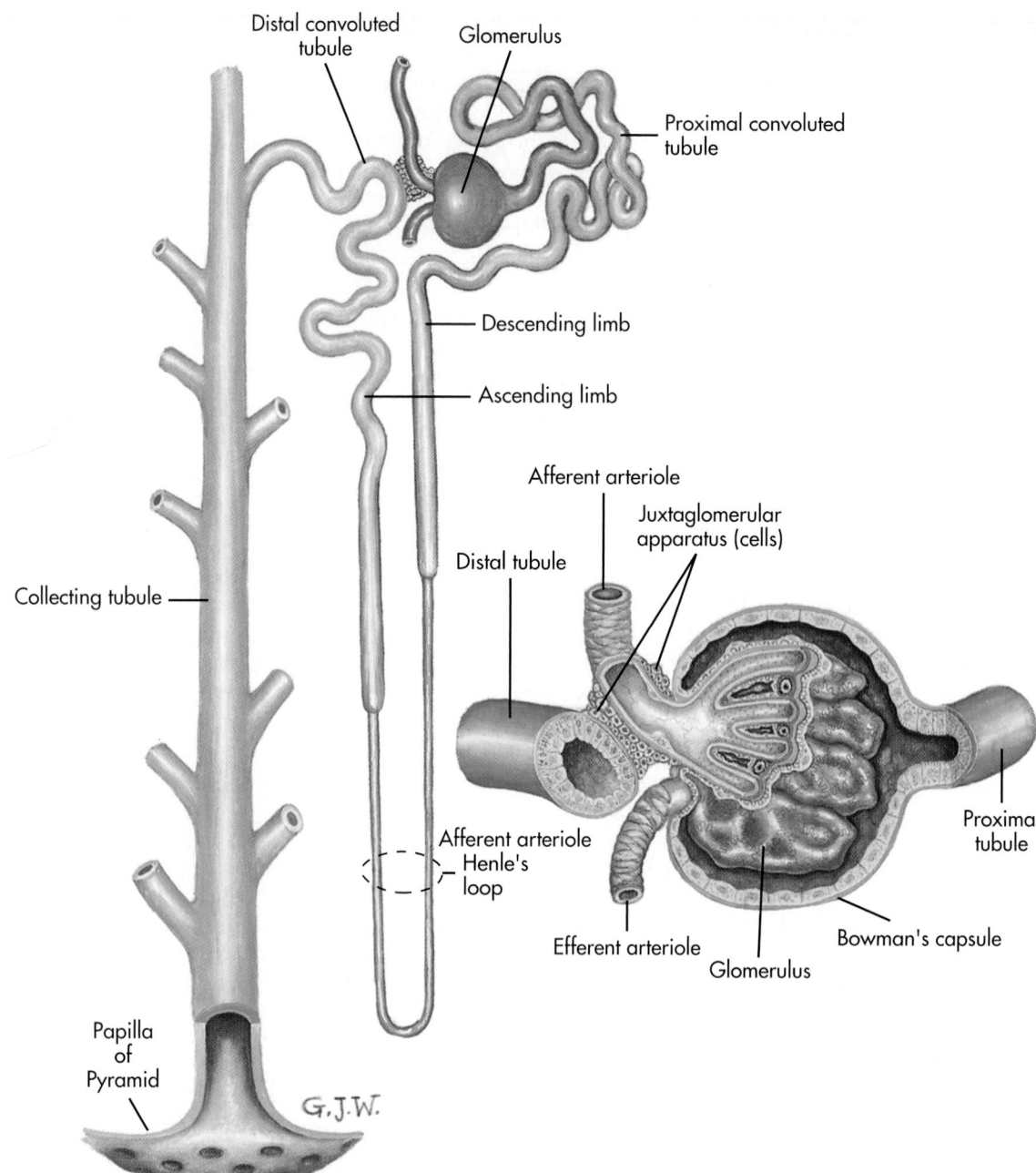

Figure 21-1 The nephron. Blood flows into the glomerulus and some of its fluid is absorbed into the tubule. Waste products are filtered and passed through the tubule into the bladder. The fluid and dissolved substances needed by the body are resorbed in vessels alongside the tubule. (From Brundage DJ: *Renal disorders, Mosby's clinical nursing series*, St Louis, 1992, Mosby.)

glomerulonephritis
inflammation of the glomerulus of the kidney, characterized by proteinuria, hematuria, decreased urine production, and edema

amyloidosis
a disorder characterized by accumulation of waxy starch-like glycoprotein (amyloid) in organs and tissues affecting function

NEPHROTIC SYNDROME

Nephrotic syndrome is a term used to describe a complex of symptoms that can occur as a result of damage to the capillary walls of the glomerulus. Glomerular damage results in increased urinary excretion of protein (proteinuria) that leads to decreased serum levels of albumin (hypoalbuminemia), hyperlipidemia, and edema.[1,2] Nephrotic syndrome is often the result of secondary disease processes: primary glomerular disease (glomerulonephritis), nephropathy secondary to amyloidosis, diabetes mellitus,

Box 21-2 Foods High in Sodium

CONDIMENTS	BREADS/ STARCHES	MEATS/MEAT SUBSTITUTES	BEVERAGES	SOUPS	VEGETABLES
Pickles, olives (black and green), salted nuts, meat tenderizers, commercial salad dressings, monosodium glutamate (MSG, Accent), steak sauce, ketchup, soy sauce, Worcestershire sauce, horseradish sauce, chili sauce, commercial mustard, salt, seasoned salts (onion, garlic, celery), butter salt	Salted crackers, potato chips, corn chips, popcorn, pretzels; dehydrated potatoes	Cured, smoked, and processed meats (ham, bacon, corned beef, chipped beef, hot dogs, luncheon meats, bologna, salt pork, canned salmon and tuna); all cheeses except low-sodium and cottage cheese; convenience foods (microwave and TV dinners); peanut butter	Commercial buttermilk, instant hot cocoa mixes	Canned soups, dehydrated soups, bouillon	Sauerkraut, hominy, pork and beans, canned tomato and vegetable juices

systemic lupus erythematosus (SLE), or infectious disease. It may be treated with corticosteroid or immunosuppressive medications, but in some patients, nephrotic syndrome is resistant to treatment and may progress to chronic renal failure (CRF).[1,2]

It is essential for nursing personnel to monitor patients' weight and intake and output closely. Intake and output should be documented in the medical record every shift.[3] The nurse and dietitian play important roles in developing a nutrition care plan for patients with CRF and in educating them regarding, for example, foods high in sodium. Box 21-2 lists foods high in sodium. For the specific sodium content of foods, see Appendix A.

Medical Nutrition Therapy

Primary goals of medical nutrition therapy are to control hypertension, minimize edema, decrease urinary albumin losses, prevent protein malnutrition and muscle catabolism, supply adequate energy, and slow the progression of renal disease.[4,5] Patients need to consume adequate amounts of protein (0.7 to 1.0 g/kg/day) and energy (35 kcal/kg/day) to prevent catabolism of lean body tissue and avoid malnutrition. Total fat intake should provide less than 30% of total energy needs. Complex carbohydrates should provide the majority of the patient's kcalories because protein, and possibly fat intake, will be limited.[5]

Limiting dietary sodium can help control hypertension and edema. Commercial preparation and processing of foods, especially convenience foods, often add substantial amounts of sodium (see Chapter 8). Patients should also be mindful of possible hidden sources of salt (e.g., water supply, medications). In addition, toothpaste and mouthwash often contain a significant amount of sodium, therefore patients should be instructed not to swallow these products (Box 21-3).

systemic lupus erythematosus (SLE)
a chronic inflammatory disease affecting many systems of the body whose cause is unknown; pathophysiology includes severe vasculitis, renal involvement, and lesions of the skin and nervous system

Box 21-3 Hidden Sources of Sodium

- Baking powder
- Drinking and cooking water
- Medications
  Antacids
  Antibiotics
  Cough medicines
  Laxatives
  Pain relievers
  Sedatives
- Mouthwash
- Toothpaste

ACUTE RENAL FAILURE

oliguria
less than 400 ml urine excretion every 24 hours

anuria
less than 250 ml urine excretion every 24 hours

acute tubular necrosis (ATN)
acute death of cells in the small tubules of the kidneys as a result of disease or injury

postischemic
injury after decreased blood supply to a body organ or part

nephrotoxic
toxic or destructive injury to a kidney

azotemia
retention of excessive amounts of nitrogenous compounds in the blood caused by the kidney's failure to remove urea from the blood; characterized by uremia

dialysis
a procedure that involves diffusion of particles from an area of high to lower concentration, osmosis of fluid across the membrane from an area of lesser to greater concentration of particles, and the ultrafiltration or movement of fluid across the membrane as a result of an artificially created pressure differential

Acute renal failure (ARF) is characterized by an abrupt loss of renal function that may or may not be accompanied by **oliguria** or **anuria**.[1,2,6,7] The most common cause of ARF is **acute tubular necrosis (ATN)**, which is generally described as **postischemic** or **nephrotoxic**.[1,7] Although a few patients do not experience any reduction in urine output, two thirds experience the following three stages[1,2,4,8]:

1. *Oliguric phase* (usually present within 24 to 48 hours after initial injury, lasting approximately 1 to 3 weeks): manifested by clinical signs of **azotemia**, acidosis, high serum potassium, high serum phosphorus, hypertension, anorexia, edema, and risk of water intoxication (indicated by low sodium levels)
2. *Diuretic phase* (usually lasts approximately 2 to 3 weeks): output of urine is gradually increased
3. *Recovery phase* (usually lasts 3 to 12 months): kidney function gradually improves, but there may be some residual permanent damage

It is important to monitor intake and output closely and document each shift. Body weight should also be taken and recorded daily. When patients do not eat, they may lose approximately 0.5 kg/day.[3] Conversely, any sudden weight gains suggest excessive fluid retention. Monitoring intake, output, and weight will help differentiate whether weight loss or gain is from fluid retention vs. lean body mass or adipose tissue. Fluid retention can mask loss of lean body mass.

Nurses and dietitians are the healthcare professionals who may be called upon to assist patients in adhering to prescribed fluid restrictions. See the Teaching Tool, "Suggestions for Coping with Fluid Restrictions," in Chapter 18 for a list of hints for helping patients with fluid restrictions. Nurses work closely with renal dietitians to coordinate meal planning and nutrition education with patients and their significant others.[3] Nutrition education may involve reduced protein, sodium, potassium, and fluid intake. Appendix A lists the specific protein, sodium, and potassium content of foods. Nurses should be watchful for constipation as a result of restricted intake of fluids and fresh fruits (most are high in potassium), bed rest, and medication side effects.[3]

Medical Nutrition Therapy

Nutritional needs are partially determined by whether **dialysis** is used for treatment. Another determinant of nutrient needs is the underlying cause of the ARF. Patients may be hypermetabolic if renal failure was caused by trauma, burns, septicemia, or infection. These conditions, other underlying medical problems, and renal failure are known to have a negative impact on the patient's appetite, thus increasing concern for nutritional status.

Energy should be provided in sufficient amounts for weight maintenance or to meet the demands of stress accompanying the ARF, usually 30 to 40 kcal/kg.[4,5] Fats, oils, simple carbohydrates, and low-protein starches should provide nonprotein kcalories. In cases where dialysis is not necessary for treatment, 0.6 g of protein per kg body weight (but not less than 40 g per day) for unstressed patients is recommended.[8] This amount can be increased as kidney function improves. When dialysis is used as part of the medical treatment, protein intake can be liberalized to 1.0 to 1.4 g/kg.[8] In either situation, use of high biologic value or high quality proteins is recommended.[8] Diets containing less than 60 g of protein per day may be deficient in niacin, riboflavin, thiamin, calcium, iron, vitamin B_{12}, and zinc,[5] and these nutrients may need to be supplemented during convalescence.

During the oliguric stage, sodium may be restricted to 1000 to 2000 mg and potassium to 1000 mg per day. Both sodium and potassium, the principal electrolytes, may be lost during the diuretic phase or during dialysis. Therefore losses

Box 21-4 **Foods High in Potassium**

Apricots	Oranges, orange juice
Avocados	Peanuts (also high in sodium)
Bananas	Potatoes, white and sweet
Cantaloupes	Prune juice
Carrots, raw	Spinach
Dried beans, peas	Swiss chard
Dried fruits	Tomatoes, tomato juice, tomato sauce
Melons	Winter squash

should be replaced as needed depending on urinary volume, serum levels, and frequency of dialysis.[5] Box 21-4 lists foods high in potassium. Fluids are usually restricted to the patient's output (urine, vomitus, and diarrhea) plus 500 ml during the oliguric phase.[5,8] During the diuretic phase, large amounts of fluid may be needed to replace losses.

CHRONIC RENAL FAILURE

Chronic renal failure (CRF) is the result of progressive, irreversible loss of kidney function.[1,2] It can develop over days, months, or years and progress to end-stage renal disease (ESRD).[2,3,7] CRF has many causes; some of the most common are glomerulonephritis, nephrosclerosis, obstructive diseases (kidney stones, tumors, congenital birth defects of kidneys and urinary tract), diabetes mellitus, systemic lupus erythematosus, and illicit use of analgesic or street drugs. Regardless of cause, results will be the same: retention of nitrogenous waste products and fluid and electrolyte imbalances that can affect all body systems.

Before ESRD, management focuses on slowing progression of CRF and minimizing complications.[3] Once CRF progresses to ESRD, management centers on reducing uremia by the use of various treatment modalities: conservative management, hemodialysis, peritoneal dialysis (PD), and renal transplantation.[3]

Medical Nutrition Therapy

Planning diets for CRF, ESRD, hemodialysis, and PD patients requires calibration by the renal dietitian of intakes of fluids, energy, protein, lipids, phosphorus, potassium, sodium, vitamins, and other minerals. It is important not only to design food combinations that include necessary nutrients but also the foods must be acceptable and enjoyable by the patient. This task can be overwhelming, but there are specialists—renal dietitians—who do this on a daily basis. The National Renal Diet is often used to develop diet guidelines and meal plans (see Appendix J).

Nurses play an important role in helping patients maintain good nutritional status, weight, morale, and appetite by working with renal dietitians to reinforce medical nutrition therapy and nutrition education. Through formal and informal teaching, nurses can help patients appreciate the need for the stringent diet and help them recognize the direct relationship between adherence to the diet and progression or lack of progression of symptoms that reduce their quality of life.

Nutritional management depends on method of treatment in addition to medical and nutritional status of the patient.[9] Table 21-1 provides a comparison of the treatment methods and primary concerns associated with each.

nephrosclerosis
necrosis of the renal arterioles, associated with hypertension

uremia
excessive amounts of urea and other nitrogenous waste products in the blood

hemodialysis
a procedure to remove impurities or wastes from the blood in treating renal insufficiency by shunting the blood from the body through a machine for diffusion and ultrafiltration and then returning it to the patient's circulation

peritoneal dialysis (PD)
a dialysis procedure performed to correct an imbalance of fluid or electrolytes in the blood or other wastes by using the peritoneum as the diffusible membrane

renal transplantation
the transfer of a kidney from one person to another

Table 21-1
Treatments and Major Concerns for Pre-ESRD, Hemodialysis, and Peritoneal Dialysis

	Pre-ESRD	Hemodialysis	Peritoneal Dialysis
Treatment Modalities	Diet + medications	Diet + medications + hemodialysis	Diet + medications + peritoneal dialysis
		Dialysis using vascular access for waste product and fluid removal	Dialysis using peritoneal membrane for waste product and fluid removal
Duration Concerns	Indefinite	3-4 hours 3 days/week	3-5 exchanges 7 days/week
	Hypertension, glycemic control in patients with diabetes mellitus	Bone disease, hypertension	Bone disease, weight gain, hyperlipidemia, glycemic control in patients with diabetes mellitus
	Glomerular hyperfiltration, rise in BUN, bone disease	Amino acid loss, interdialytic electrolyte and fluid changes	Protein loss into dialysate, glucose absorption from dialysate
	Anemia, cardiovascular disease	Anemia, cardiovascular disease	Anemia, cardiovascular disease

Reference: American Dietetic Association: National renal diet: professional guide, ed 2, Chicago, 2002, American Dietetic Association.

uremic toxicity
buildup of toxic waste products (urea and other nitrogenous waste products) in the blood; symptoms include anorexia, nausea, metallic taste in the mouth, irritability, confusion, lethargy, restlessness, and pruritus (itching)

The exact point when medical nutrition therapy should begin is highly variable, but conventional wisdom indicates dietary modifications (Table 21-2) should be initiated as early as possible to minimize uremic toxicity, delay progression of renal disease, and prevent wasting and malnutrition.[10,11] This can be accomplished by limiting foods whose metabolic byproducts add to buildup of such toxic substances and by providing adequate kcalories to prevent body tissue catabolism. Patients often find this diet difficult to follow for a long period, therefore motivation and encouragement from nursing and other health professionals are crucial.

In view of the fact that malnutrition is so clearly associated with mortality in renal failure, continuing to assess nutritional status and dietary compliance of patients with CRF is important.[12] Because patients may find that foods "don't taste like they used to," encouraging use of spices such as garlic, onions, and oregano to enhance the flavor of allowed foods can be helpful.[3] The National Renal Diet was developed by the Renal Dietitians Practice Group, American Dietetic Association, and National Kidney Foundation Council on Renal Nutrition to provide a renal diet with nationwide applicability. Diet prescription guidelines for pre-ESRD, hemodialysis, and peritoneal dialysis patients were developed over a 5-year period. Because of the national focus of these guidelines, ethnic and geographically unique foods are not currently included but can be incorporated as part of the individualized diet plan. Vegetarian choices are also not included because high biologic value proteins are the preferred protein sources for renal patients, and some foods in vegan diets are of low biologic value. Ovo-vegetarian and ovo-lacto vegetarian diets include high biologic value protein sources, but they also tend to be high in phosphorus. One point that requires emphasis is that the National Renal Diet guidelines and food lists are only a starting point for individualized meal plans and education. Patient compliance may be enhanced by designing meal plans to meet the specific needs of each patient.[9] Box 21-5 provides a sample menu for a patient with CRF.

Box 21-5 Sample Renal Diet Menu

85 g protein; 2000 mg sodium; 2000 mg potassium; 1000 mg phosphorus; 1000 ml fluid

BREAKFAST

Apple juice
Oatmeal
Blueberry muffin
Scrambled egg
Low-sodium margarine
    (2 exchanges)*
2% milk (½ cup)*
Decaffeinated coffee (½ cup)*

LUNCH

Lemonade (½ cup)*
Sirloin tips (3 oz) with noodles*
Salad with Italian dressing
Fruit cocktail

DINNER

Fruit punch (½ cup)*
Low-sodium turkey (3 oz) with parsley
    carrots*
White bread with margarine
    (2 exchanges)*
Cinnamon applesauce
Hot tea (½ cup)*

Courtesy Memorial Hospital, Carbondale, Ill.
Quantities not exact; for representation only.

HEMODIALYSIS

During hemodialysis, blood is shunted by way of a special vascular access or shunt (usually in the nondominant forearm), heparinized, cleansed of excess fluid and waste products through a semipermeable membrane, and then returned to the patient's circulation (Figure 21-2).[1,7] The dialysate is an electrolyte solution similar to the composition of normal plasma. Each constituent may be varied according to the patient's needs, the most common being potassium.[3] Average treatment lasts 3 to 6 hours and is usually performed three times per week (Figure 21-3). Hemodialysis can be performed in a dialysis unit by trained staff. Patients who have received special training may assist in their treatment.

heparinized
use of an antithrombin factor to prevent intravascular clotting

dialysate
dialysis solution

Medical Nutrition Therapy

Individual diet prescriptions (see Table 21-2) are determined by residual kidney function, dialysate components, duration of dialysis, and rate of blood flow through the artificial kidney.[8] The meal plan is designed, monitored, and reevaluated by the dietitian. Nurses and others on the medical team are crucial for providing positive reinforcement and encouragement to the patient and family members on an ongoing basis. Objectives for medical nutrition therapy are to attain or maintain good nutritional status, prevent excessive accumulation of waste products and fluid between treatments, and minimize the effects of metabolic disorders that occur as a result of ESRD.[9]

Phosphorus is routinely restricted in patients receiving hemodialysis because high levels of serum phosphorus contribute to secondary hyperparathyroidism and raise the calcium-phosphorus product in the plasma.[3,5] Although an intake of 12 mg/kg/day is the usual recommendation, it is often necessary to liberalize this restriction to meet protein needs.[9] Foods high in phosphorus, such as milk, milk products, cheese, beef liver, chocolate, nuts, and legumes, are usually limited or avoided. Medications (phosphate binders) are also used to control serum phosphorus levels. The medications of choice are calcium carbonate, calcium acetate, or sevelamer hydrochloride.[9,11] They are given at mealtimes to bind phosphate in the food.

Table 21-2
Nutrition Guidelines for Pre-ESRD, Hemodialysis, and Peritoneal Dialysis

Nutrient	Pre-ESRD	Hemodialysis	Peritoneal Dialysis	Comments
Energy	>35 kcal/kg IBW or aBW_{ef}	30-35 kcal/kg IBW or aBW_{ef} if ≥ age 60; 35 kcal/kg IBW or aBW_{ef} if < age 60	25-35 kcal/kg IBW or aBW_{ef} (includes kcal from dialysate glucose absorption)	If patient <90% or greater than 115% of medium standard weight, use aBW_{ef}
Protein	Based on creatinine clearance, GFR, urinary protein losses (0.6-1.0 g/kg IBW or aBW_{ef})	1.1-1.4 g/kg IBW or aBW_{ef}	1.2-1.3 g/kg IBW or aBW_{ef}	At least 50% from HBV animal plant sources
Fats	For lipid abnormalities: fats, cholesterol, and CHO adjusted per severity of risk factors	For lipid abnormalities: fats, cholesterol, and CHO adjusted per severity of risk factors	For lipid abnormalities: fats, cholesterol, and CHO adjusted per severity of risk factors	
Sodium	Individualized or 1-3 g/d	Individualized or 2-3 g/d	Individualized based on blood pressure and weight or 2-4 g/d	
Potassium	Individualized per laboratory values	Individualized, approximately 40 mg/kg IBW or aBW_{ef} (approximately 2-3 g/d)	Restricted only by laboratory values	
Phosphorus	Individualized or 8-12 mg/kg IBW or aBW_{ef}	Individualized, approximately ≤17 mg/kg IBW or aBW_{ef} (approximately 800-1200 mg/d)	Individualized, approximately ≤17 mg/kg IBW or aBW_{ef}	May require phosphate binder

Calcium	Individualized per calcium, phosphorus, and PTH laboratory values and use of vitamin D; approximately 1000-1500 mg/d	Individualized per calcium, phosphorus, and PTH laboratory values and use of vitamin D; approximately 1000-1500 mg/d	Individualized per calcium, phosphorus, and PTH laboratory values and use of vitamin D; approximately 1000-1500 mg/d	Supplement may be needed to maintain normal serum levels
Fluid	As desired	500-1000 ml + urine output/d	Unrestricted if weight and blood pressure controlled and residual renal function is 2-3 L/d	
Vitamin/ mineral supplementation	As appropriate	As appropriate	As appropriate	Supplements designed specially for dialysis patients are available; supplements of vitamin C should not exceed 100 mg/d to prevent hyperoxalemia; vitamin A supplementation is not recommended; in patient receiving rHuEPO, iron supplementation is almost always required; zinc supplementation may be helpful for patients with impaired taste

From National Kidney Foundation, Inc: Clinical practice guidelines for nutrition in chronic renal failure, 2000; www.kidney.org/professionals/doqi/doqi/doqi_nut.html, accessed July 2, 2002; Wiggins KL: Guidelines for nutrition care of renal patients, ed 3, Chicago, 2002, American Dietetic Association; and American Dietetic Association: Manual of clinical dietetics, ed 6, Chicago, 2000, American Dietetic Association.

aBW_{ef}, Adjusted edema-free body weight; CHO, carbohydrates; IBW, ideal body weight.

$aBW_{ef} = BW_{ef} + [(SBW - BW_{ef}) \times 0.25]$ where BW_{ef} is edema-free body weight and SBW is the standard body weight as determined from NHANES III data.

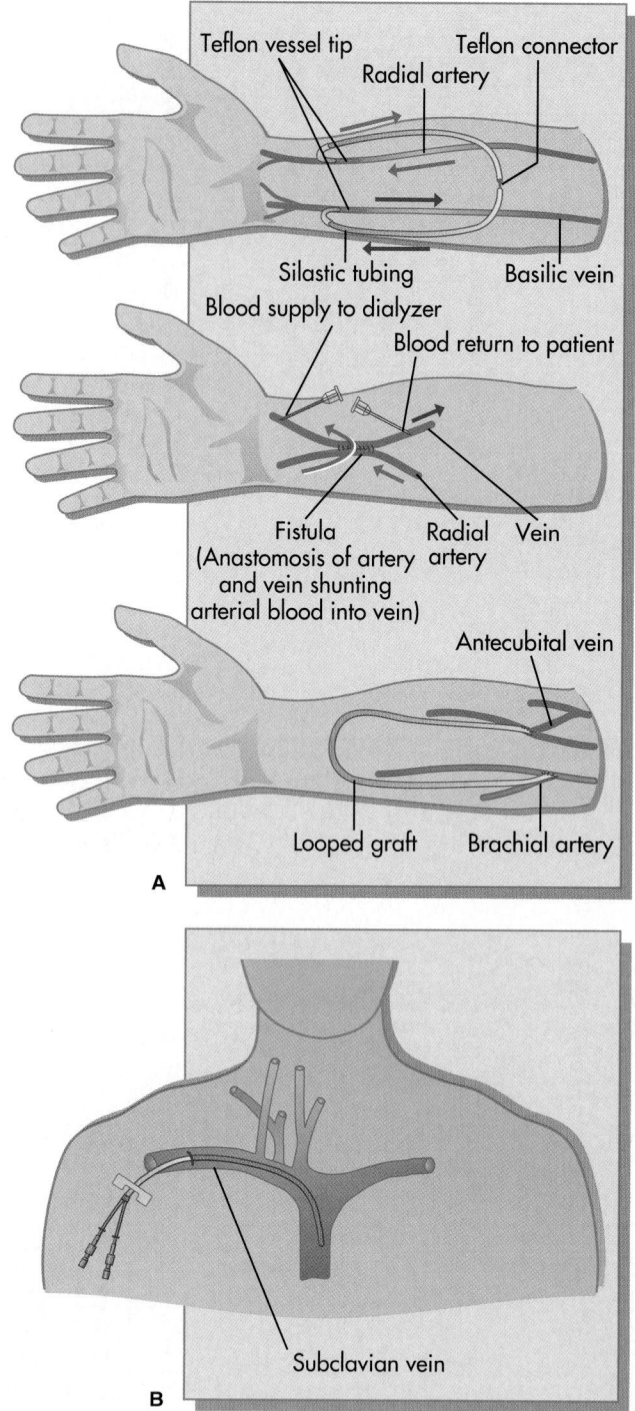

Figure 21-2 Types of access for hemodialysis. **A,** Cannula (rarely used now), AV (arteriovenous fistula), and artificial loop graft. **B,** Subclavian catheter (usually temporary). (From Mahan LK, Escott-Stump S, eds.: *Krause's food, nutrition, and diet therapy,* ed 10, Philadelphia, 2000, WB Saunders.)

In renal failure, kidneys also lose their endocrine function of producing calcitriol (the active form of vitamin D). Although many forms of vitamin D are available for supplementation, it is this active form that helps prevent bone disease.[3] The active form of vitamin D is available in oral form (e.g., Rocaltrol, doxercal-

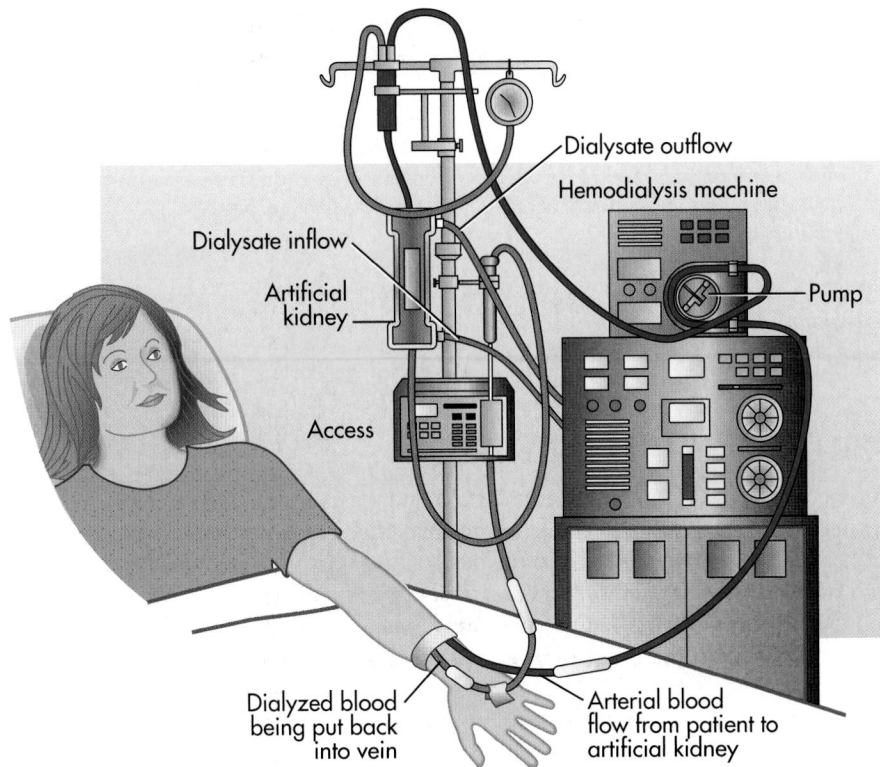

Figure 21-3 Hemodialysis. Treatment is usually for 3 to 6 hours, three times a week. (From Mahan LK, Escott-Stump S, eds.: *Krause's food, nutrition, and diet therapy,* ed 10, Philadelphia, 2000, WB Saunders.)

ciferol [Hectorol]) and intravenous (IV) form (e.g., Calcijex, paricalcitol [Zemplar], doxercalciferol [Hectoral]), which is given during hemodialysis.[11]

Anemia results from another endocrine function affected by CRF—decreased production of the hormone erythropoietin, a hormone that stimulates bone marrow to produce red blood cells. An adequate available iron supply is necessary for normal erythropoiesis to take place. Recombinant erythropoietin (EPO) (e.g., epoetin [Epogen]) can be given during dialysis (by IV) or subcutaneously just after dialysis treatment. Oral or IV iron supplementation is often necessary before administration of recombinant EPO to replenish iron stores.[3,5,11]

Patients treated with hemodialysis are also at risk for deficiencies of water-soluble vitamins, particularly vitamin B$_6$ and folic acid. The reason is twofold: poor intake and loss of the nutrients during dialysis.[9,13] Supplementation of the fat-soluble vitamins A, E, and K is usually not necessary. In fact, patients treated with hemodialysis have been reported to experience vitamin A toxicity. Supplementation of trace minerals is not necessary unless a deficiency is suspected or documented.[13]

Patients who have a poor dietary intake are at increased risk of nutrient deficiencies and poor nutritional status. Intake can be the result of poor appetite, changes in taste acuity and in food preferences (especially red meat and sweets), nausea and vomiting, or diet limitations. When patients develop changes in taste, foods with sharp, distinct flavors may be useful in stimulating appetite (Box 21-6).

Approximately one third of patients requiring hemodialysis each year have diabetes mellitus. Diets for these patients should incorporate nutritional modifications necessary for ESRD and provide consistent content and timing of meals and snacks to facilitate glycemic control.[9]

recombinant erythropoietin (EPO)

recombinant human erythropoietin; drug used to treat anemia by replacing erythropoietin for patients with CRF who do not produce this hormone in adequate amounts

---

Box 21-6 Suggestions for Patients with Altered Taste

- Brush teeth 6 to 8 times per day
- Rinse mouth with a chilled mouthwash (commercial product or water mixed with lemon juice or vinegar)
- Eat sour-ball candy
- Chew gum
- Before meals, drink water with lemon or eat a small amount of sherbet or fruit sorbet

© 1993, *American Dietetic Association.* "National Renal Diet: Professional Guide." *Used with permission.*

PERITONEAL DIALYSIS

Peritoneal dialysis (PD) removes excess fluid and waste products from blood using the peritoneal membrane as a filter. Dialysate is instilled and removed through a catheter that has been surgically placed into the peritoneal cavity. The peritoneum (i.e., the lining of the abdominal cavity) is used as the dialysis membrane (Figure 21-4). Waste products cross the membrane by passive movement from the peritoneal capillaries into the dialysate in the peritoneal cavity. The dialysate contains dextrose, which in-

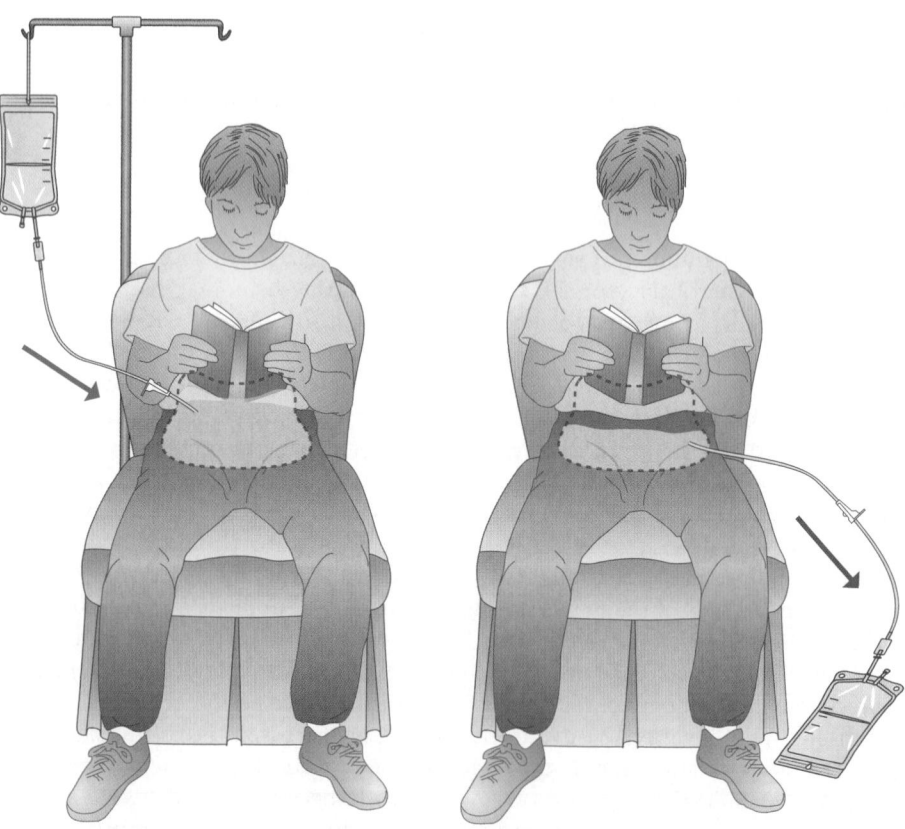

The peritoneal cavity is filled with dialysate, using gravity.

At the end of the exchange, the dialysate is drained into the bag, again using gravity.

Figure 21-4 Continuous ambulatory peritoneal dialysis; 20-minute exchanges usually are given four to five times a day, every day. (From Mahan LK, Escott-Stump S, eds.: *Krause's food, nutrition, and diet therapy,* ed 10, Philadelphia, 2000, WB Saunders.)

creases osmolality of the solution and facilitates removal of excess fluid. As the fluid moves from vascular space into the peritoneal cavity, osmolality of the solutions becomes equal. Toxins and excess fluids collected in the peritoneal cavity are then drained from the body through the catheter and discarded.[9] An advantage of PD is that it is usually performed in the home. All forms of PD require special training of the patient and caregiver.

Intermittent Peritoneal Dialysis

Intermittent peritoneal dialysis (IPD) involves infusion of approximately two liters of dialysate instilled over 20 to 30 minutes. Dialysate is then drained by gravity, and the process is repeated over an 8- to 10-hour period four to five times per week. IPD can be performed manually or mechanically. During the time of dialysis, patients are restricted to a chair or bed.[3] This method is not commonly used as a long-term treatment modality because of the time involvement.

Continuous Ambulatory Peritoneal Dialysis

Continuous ambulatory peritoneal dialysis (CAPD) entails infusion of dialysate for a 4- to 6-hour intraperitoneal dwell time during the day and an 8-hour dwell time overnight.[9] At the end of the designated time, dialysate is drained by gravity and a new exchange begins. Dialysis exchanges are done continuously, 7 days a week.[3]

Continuous Cycling Peritoneal Dialysis

Continuous cycling peritoneal dialysis (CCPD) is a combination of IPD and CAPD. At night, a cycler (mechanical) performs three dialysate exchanges. During the day, a fourth exchange is infused for the entire day.[3] At bedtime, the fourth exchange is drained and the process is started again. Although restricted to bed during nighttime infusions, patients are ambulatory during the day.

Medical Nutrition Therapy

Objectives of nutrition therapy (see Table 21-2) are to (1) maintain good nutritional status while replacing albumin lost in the dialysate, (2) minimize complications of fluid imbalance, (3) minimize symptoms of uremic toxicity, and (4) minimize metabolic disorders secondary to ESRD and PD.[9] As with hemodialysis, patients treated with PD are at risk for deficiencies of water-soluble vitamins and minerals. A daily multivitamin supplement that includes folic acid is recommended.[14] In addition, some patients may receive recombinant EPO for correction of anemia and need iron supplementation to maximize the effectiveness of the drug.[3,5]

Energy needs for patients treated with PD are usually lower than for those receiving hemodialysis because approximately 60% of the dialysate is absorbed[14] and needs to be calculated as part of the patient's energy source. Dextrose is used as an osmotic agent in PD dialysate and must be taken into consideration when energy needs are calculated.[3,9]

Protein losses during PD range from 20 to 30 g per day[4,14] and are reflected in higher dietary protein recommendations (see Table 21-2). Serum blood urea nitrogen (BUN) and creatinine levels, uremic symptoms, and weight should be monitored as indicators of sufficient protein intake, and the diet should be adjusted appropriately.[4]

During PD, sodium, potassium, and fluid are continually removed, making severe dietary restrictions unnecessary.[3,4,9] However, it is important to remember that nutrient needs vary among patients and individualized recommendations are necessary. Restriction of dietary phosphorus is critical to prevent development of osteodystrophy. Unfortunately, higher protein requirements for PD consequently

osteodystrophy
defective bone development associated with disturbances in calcium and phosphorus metabolism and renal insufficiency

provide high amounts of phosphorus. Therefore severely restricting or eliminating dairy products is necessary to control phosphorus intake, which may result in the need for calcium supplementation.[9] Phosphorus is also controlled by the use of prescribed phosphate binders.

The absorption of glucose from PD dialysate presents challenges in patients with diabetes. Blood glucose levels and hyperlipidemia become more difficult to control.[9] Weight gain caused by increased kcalorie load of the dialysate may be another common problem with PD. Another condition to watch for is dehydration, which may result from excessive fluid removal and extracellular fluid volume deficits. Careful monitoring of blood glucose, intake and output, and weight are preventive measures.

Although nutritional status is affected by various nondialysis-related causes, anorexia, nausea, and vomiting are key clinical features of uremia and inadequate dialysis. Consequently, nutritional status is an important measure of PD adequacy as well.[15] The National Kidney Foundation[15] suggests ongoing nutritional assessment of PD patients in connection with Kt/V_{urea} and C_{Cr} measurements using the Protein Equivalent of Nitrogen Appearance (PNA) and Subjective Global Assessment (SGA).

Kt/V urea
a measurement of adequacy and protein nutritional status

RENAL TRANSPLANTATION

Kidney transplants are the second most frequent transplant operation in the United States. Approximately 11,000 patients receive kidney transplants each year, and in excess of 35,000 are on waiting lists (see the Cultural Considerations box). More than 80% of kidneys transplanted from cadavers still function well 1 year after surgery. Outcomes are even better for transplants from living donors.[16] Nutritional care of renal transplant recipients involves continual reassessment of nutritional goals and efficacy of therapy during the different phases of care.[8]

Pretransplant

Nutritional status is evaluated to identify and correct deficits before surgery. Decreased visceral protein stores and decreased levels of body weight are frequently observed. Vitamin and mineral deficiencies of vitamin B_6, folic acid, vitamins C and D, and iron are common.[17] Poor nutritional status is caused by many different issues,[17] such as the following:
- Blood loss
- Loss of protein and other nutrients during dialysis

CULTURAL CONSIDERATIONS
Barriers to Organ Donations

In the United States there exists a shortage of organ donations from members of minority groups. This is a concern because successful organ transplantation requires some matching of genetic characteristics. To explain this organ shortage, a study surveyed 339 men and women. African Americans are less likely to donate organs than Caucasian Americans (38% vs. 65% respectively). Reasons for not wanting to donate organs include mistrust of doctors, mistrust of hospitals, prior negative medical experiences, and religious misconceptions. Some participants want to be buried whole as a religious concern, although some organized religions and clergy support organ donations.

Strategies can be implemented to create trust among members of minority groups who are currently less willing to donate blood and organs. The researchers suggest that the medical community develop partnerships with churches and other faith-based organizations to educate people about organ donations.

Application to nursing: Nurses know that organ transplants of kidneys and livers are life-saving medical practices. Nurses can educate minority communities by understanding that barriers to organ donations stem from historical and personal experiences with the medical and research community.

Reference: Boulware LE et al.: Understanding disparities in donor behavior: race and gender differences in willingness to donate blood and cadaveric organs, Medical Care 40(2):85, 2002.

- Catabolism caused by chronic illness
- Anorexia caused by altered taste
- Suboptimal oral intake
- Depression

Medical nutrition therapy usually involves an individualized approach as outlined in Table 21-2.[17]

Immediate and Long-Term Posttransplant

Kcalorie needs in the immediate posttransplant period are high (30 to 35 kcal/kg) because of stress from surgery and catabolism. Energy requirements decline approximately 6 to 8 weeks after transplant, and kcalories should then be provided at a level to achieve and maintain a desirable body weight.[5] Restriction of dietary protein is not necessary. In fact, protein catabolism is increased as the result of surgery and the administration of corticosteroids for immunosuppression.[5]

Steroid therapy may cause glucose intolerance and therefore necessitate restriction of simple carbohydrates.[5] Fats are used to supply energy, but may need to be limited if hypercholesterolemia or hypertriglyceridemia are present or occur.[5] Recommendations regarding sodium and potassium should be individualized for each patient.[5] Fluids are generally unrestricted and limited only by graft function. Many drugs used postoperatively and posttransplant have the potential to influence nutritional needs and status. Careful observation of the patient may prevent potential problems.

RENAL CALCULI

Renal calculi (kidney stones or urolithiasis) are a common and often recurrent urologic condition. Additionally, it is one of the oldest medical afflictions known to humans.[18] Stone formation is more common among men than women, and approximately half of those who develop renal calculi will suffer recurrence within 10 years.[19] Most calculi are composed of calcium oxalate (70% to 80%), uric acid (10%), struvite (9% to 17%), or cystine (<1%)[1] (Figure 21-5). Formation of kidney stones depends on simultaneous occurrence of the following factors: (1) low urine volume (usually the result of low or inadequate fluid intake); (2) high urine pH; (3) excessive urinary excretion of calcium, oxalate, uric acid, or a combination; and (4) decreased levels of substances in urine that normally inhibit stone formation. Dietary oxalate is another possible cause of stone formation.[19] Although calcium is the predominant component of renal calculi, dietary calcium does not appear to play a role in calcium stone formation.[20,21]

Type and cause of stone formation provide impetus for individualization of dietary modifications. A comprehensive diet history is essential to ascertain the extent of dietary modifications required. By and large, dietary interventions include combining restriction of specific dietary components associated with development of the stone in addition to generous fluid intake.[5] Patient education is important in the treatment of renal calculi. Only a motivated and informed patient can be expected to maintain any long-term preventative program.[22] The Teaching Tool box offers advice for patients on how to prevent kidney stone formation, and Box 21-7 outlines dietary recommendations for renal calculi.

Calcium Stones

Too much calcium in urine (hypercalciuria) is the most common identifiable cause of calcium renal calculi, which is responsible for approximately 70% of calcium-combining stones.[22] A variety of mechanisms can cause hypercalciuria including drugs, medical conditions, and dietary factors. The most common basis of excessive urinary calcium is absorptive hypercalciuria. Approximately 50% of persons who form calcium stones have some type of absorptive hypercalciuria, which is caused by increased gastrointestinal absorption of calcium, overly aggressive vitamin D

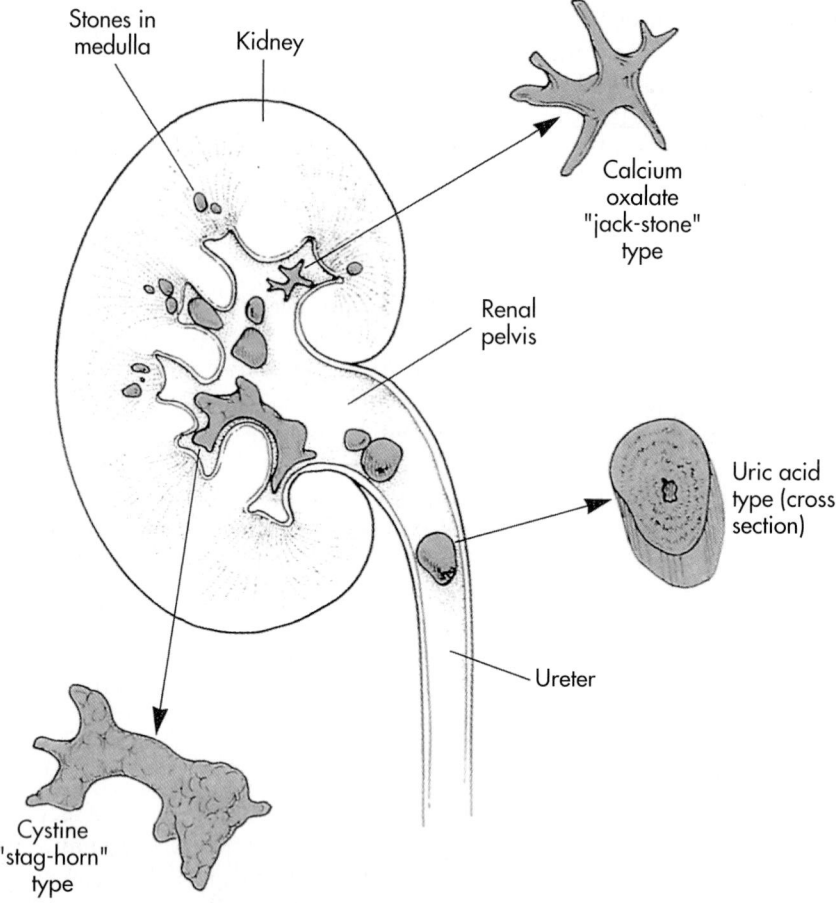

Figure 21-5 Renal calculi. (From Williams SR: *Nutrition and diet therapy*, ed 8, St Louis, 1997, Mosby.)

supplementation, or excessive ingestion of calcium-containing foods (milk-alkali syndrome).[22] Increased intestinal calcium absorption creates a subsequent increase in serum calcium levels.[22] Categories and treatment modalities of absorptive hypercalciuria are outlined in Table 21-3.

Box 21-7 Dietary Recommendations for Renal Calculi

- Tailor diet to specific metabolic disturbance and individual dietary habits (to ensure compliance).
- Calcium restriction should be avoided.
- Calcium (1000-1500 mg/d) and oxalate intakes must be in balance.
  - Limit intake of spinach, rhubarb, beets, nuts, chocolate, tea, wheat bran, and strawberries (cause significant increase in urinary oxalate excretion).
  - Do not exceed RDA for vitamin C (varies for gender and age) (causes significant increase in urinary oxalate excretion).

- Animal protein should be "restricted" to 1 g/kg body weight.
- Salt intake should be restricted to less than 100 mEq/d.
- Potassium intake should be encouraged (five or more servings of fruits and vegetables/d).
- Include a high fluid intake to produce at least 2 L of urine/day (2-3 L intake/day).

References: Borghi L et al.: Comparison of two diets for the prevention of recurrent stones in idiopathic hypercalciuria, N Engl J Med 346(2):77, 2002; Goldfarb S: Diet and nephrolithiasis, Annu Rev Med 45:235, 1994; Heilbert IP: Update on dietary recommendations and medical treatment of renal stone disease, Nephrol Dial Transplant 15:117, 2000.

TEACHING TOOL
Advice for Preventing Kidney Stones

$\mathcal{N}$o immediate "penalty" exists for failing to follow a treatment regimen to prevent formation of kidney stones. The "penalty" (the next kidney stone) may not become apparent for many months or even years.

FLUIDS

Drink fluids...a lot of fluids! Simple water is generally the best choice, but ginger ale, lemon-lime soft drinks, and fruit juices may be used.

You need to pass at least 2.5 quarts of urine a day to prevent stone formation. To do this, drink 10 to 12 (if not 16) full glasses (8 oz glasses) of water daily—more if you live in a hot, dry climate.

This is likely the single most important aspect of reducing stone formation.

CALCIUM

Do not restrict dietary calcium (dairy products and calcium-fortified orange juice)—actually don't alter calcium intake unless instructed to do so by your physician. Low-calcium intake increases risk for osteoporosis and increases risk of oxalic acid kidney stone formation. Higher intake of dietary calcium reduces risk of oxalic acid kidney stone formation. The same protection is not seen with calcium supplementation.

SODIUM

Use fresh or frozen vegetables when possible. Remove the saltshaker from the kitchen table. Other spices such as pepper or Mrs. Dash can be used instead. Use little or no salt in food preparation or cooking. When following recipes, use half the specified amount of salt. Avoid eating foods with high salt content when possible (most fast foods and packaged foods). Do not add salt to prepared or canned foods (soups, gravies, TV dinners, canned vegetables). The entire family can benefit from this advice.

PROTEIN

Keep meat (beef and pork) intake to a moderate level. Six oz of meat each day provide all the protein needed by the body. Make plans to include at least one meatless (dried beans and peas, legumes) meal per week. A diet low in animal protein and high in vegetable protein decreases the amount of red meat in the diet and increases complex carbohydrates and fiber. A diet with more plant foods is also higher in potassium.

POTASSIUM

Mom was right! Eat your veggies...and fruits. A low intake of potassium-rich foods leads to increased risk of kidney stone formation.

OXALATES

Limit foods high in oxalates. Oxalates are found primarily in plant foods, but only eight foods—*spinach, rhubarb, beets, nuts, chocolate, tea, wheat bran, and strawberries*—have been found to increase urinary oxalate levels.

CARBOHYDRATES

Increase intake of complex carbohydrates: whole grains, and fresh fruits and vegetables. (Gee, does this sound familiar?)

SUPPLEMENTS

Avoid vitamin C supplements and calcium-containing antacids (e.g., Tums). If antacids need to be used, magnesium-based antacids (Maalox) are recommended.

Sources: No need for kidney stone sufferers to curb calcium, Environmental Nutrition 16:7, 1993; Leslie SW: Hypercalciuria, eMedicine Journal 3(6), June 4, 2002; www.emedicine.com/med/topic1069.htm, accessed July 5, 2002; Mayo Clinic: What are kidney stones? Apr 17, 2002; www.mayoclinic.com/invoke.cfm?id=DS00282, accessed July 5, 2002; Rineer S: Kidney stones, eMedicine Journal 2(5), May 28, 2001; www.emedicine.com/med/topic1069.htm, accessed Jul 5, 2002.

Table 21-3
Categories and Treatment Modalities of Absorptive Hypercalciuria

Category	Occurrence	Medical Treatment
Type I	Relatively uncommon and most severe	Thiazides and orthophosphates
Type II	Most common and less severe	Thiazides may be prescribed
Type III	Also called *renal phosphate leak;* relatively rare	Oral orthophosphate therapy to correct hypophosphatemia

Reference: Leslie SW: Hypercalciuria, eMedicine Journal 3(6), June 4, 2002; www.emedicine.com/med/topic1069.htm, accessed July 5, 2002.

Conventional wisdom regarding calcium stones has been to limit foods high in calcium (milk, cheeses, yogurt, and green leafy vegetables) and sodium (2-3 g/day). But research indicates there is no need to restrict dietary calcium, and in fact a normal calcium intake combined with restricted animal protein and salt appears to protect against calcium stone development.[23] Kidney stone formation is more influenced by the amount of oxalate, not calcium, in the urinary tract. Restricting calcium seems to allow more oxalate to be absorbed and then excreted through the urinary tract. Higher levels of dietary calcium bind with oxalate so it cannot be absorbed, leading to less oxalate in the urinary tract.

In addition to calcium and oxalate, the main dietary contributors include potassium, animal protein, fluid intake,[21,22] sodium, fiber, alcohol, and caffeine.[22] Excessive animal protein (>1.7 g/kg) and high sodium intake make the body more acidic. To bring the body back into homeostasis, the body uses, in part, the body skeleton to buffer this additional acid load. This releases additional calcium into circulation, which in turn, is excreted in urine by the kidneys. Increased acid load also impedes renal calcium reabsorption, resulting in increased urinary calcium excretion. Furthermore, animal proteins are high in purines. Purines are precursors of uric acid, which can form uric acid stones, lower urinary pH, increase overall acid load, contribute to gout, and generally increase urinary calcium excretion and stone formation.[21,22] Alcohol intake also promotes urinary calcium excretion. Chronic ethanol ingestion creates low serum vitamin D levels, which lead to impaired intestinal calcium absorption and hypercalciuria. Caffeine has been shown to increase urinary calcium excretion; however, clinical significance is reasonably small unless large amounts of caffeine (34 oz of caffeine) are ingested.[22] Low fluid intake causes diminished urinary volume, increasing urine concentration and probability of stone formation even if total calcium excretion is unchanged. Low intake of potassium may be an additional risk factor for stone development. Potassium reduces urinary calcium excretion by induced transient sodium diuresis, resulting in temporary contraction of extracellular fluid volume and increased renal tubular calcium reabsorption. Potassium also increases renal phosphate absorption, thereby raising serum phosphate levels, which reduces serum vitamin D_3, resulting in decreased intestinal calcium absorption.[21,22]

Oxalate is found primarily in foods of plant origin and is the end product of ascorbic acid metabolism. Restriction of dietary oxalate intake has been used to reduce risk of recurrence of calcium oxalate kidney stones. (See Appendix L for a more complete list of oxalate content of foods.) Studies indicate that although oxalate-rich foods enhance excretion of urinary oxalate, the increase is not always proportional to oxalate content of the food.[24] Only eight foods—spinach, rhubarb, beets, nuts, chocolate, tea, wheat bran, and strawberries—caused significant increase in urinary oxalate excretion. Therefore initial medical nutrition therapy for individuals who form calcium oxalate stones can be limited to restriction of foods definitely shown to increase urinary oxalate.[25] It may also be prudent to instruct patients that vitamin C supplements (>500 mg/day) should be avoided because they may increase urinary oxalate excretion.[26]

Uric Acid Stones

Uric acid is a metabolic product of purines (a nitrogen-containing compound in protein). Uric acid stones are associated with acidic urine (hyperuricuria).[27] Other causes of hyperuricuria include gout, certain medications such as aspirin[7] and chemotherapy,[7,27] and high purine intake.[27] Acidic urine appears to be the most significant issue that affects formation of uric acid stones. For that reason, the basis of medical management, adjunct to fluid ingestion, is to increase the naturally somewhat acidic urine pH to a range of 6 to 6.5.[7] Efficacy of limiting foods high in purines (lean meats, organ meats, legumes, and whole grains) has not been proven (a more complete listing of purine content of foods can be found in Appendix L); protein intake at the level of the Recommended Dietary Allowance (RDA) (0.8 g/kg) will not be counterproductive. Sodium bicarbonate can be used to alkalinize urine, but potassium citrate is the preferred alkalinizing agent because of the availability of slow-release tablets and avoidance of a high sodium load.[19] Allopurinol (Lopurin, Zyloprim), which is effective in reducing high levels of uric acid, may also be given. In view of the fact that allopurinol reduces uric acid quickly, it may bring about an attack of gout.[28] Nonsteroidal antiinflammatory drugs (NSAIDs), except aspirin (aspirin increases uric acid levels), can be taken for 2 to 3 months to avoid this.

Cystine Stones

Cystine stones form in people with a hereditary disorder that causes the kidneys to excrete excessive amounts of the amino acid cystine (cystinuria).[27] The goal of treatment is to reduce urinary cystine concentration. To do this, urine volume should be greater than 3 L/d and urine should be alkalinized to a pH in a range of 6.5 to 7.[19,28] If urine becomes too alkaline, however, there is increased risk for calcium phosphate stone formation. Producing urine volume greater than 3 L/d requires an especially high fluid intake of approximately 4 L/d or more. If alkalinization is unsuccessful, medications such as penicillamine can be used but are often complicated by side effects such as nephrotoxicity, allergic reactions, and hematologic abnormalities.[28]

Struvite Stones

Struvite stones are caused by urinary tract infections by bacteria that split urea into ammonium in urine. The ammonium then combines with phosphate and magnesium to form stones. Treatment of the infection must be done at the same time as removal of infected stones,[27,28] and for that reason lithotripsy (Figure 21-6) or surgery is almost always performed. These stones are often large and a characteristic stag's horn shape, which can cause serious damage to the kidneys. Women are twice as likely to have struvite stones. Dietary management has no significant function in this variety of calculi formation.[7]

SUMMARY

The chief, life-preserving function of the kidneys is to help maintain chemical homeostasis in the body. Various inflammatory, obstructive, and degenerative diseases affect the kidneys in different ways. These disorders interfere with normal functioning of nephrons that regulate products of metabolism.

Because of glomerular damage, nephrotic syndrome results in increased urinary excretion of protein, decreased serum levels of albumin, hyperlipidemia, and edema. Although treated with corticosteroid or immunosuppressive medications,

lithotripsy
extracorporal shock wave lithotripsy (ESWL), a noninvasive technique whereby high-intensity shock waves cause fragmentation of stones from a device outside the body (see Figure 21-6)

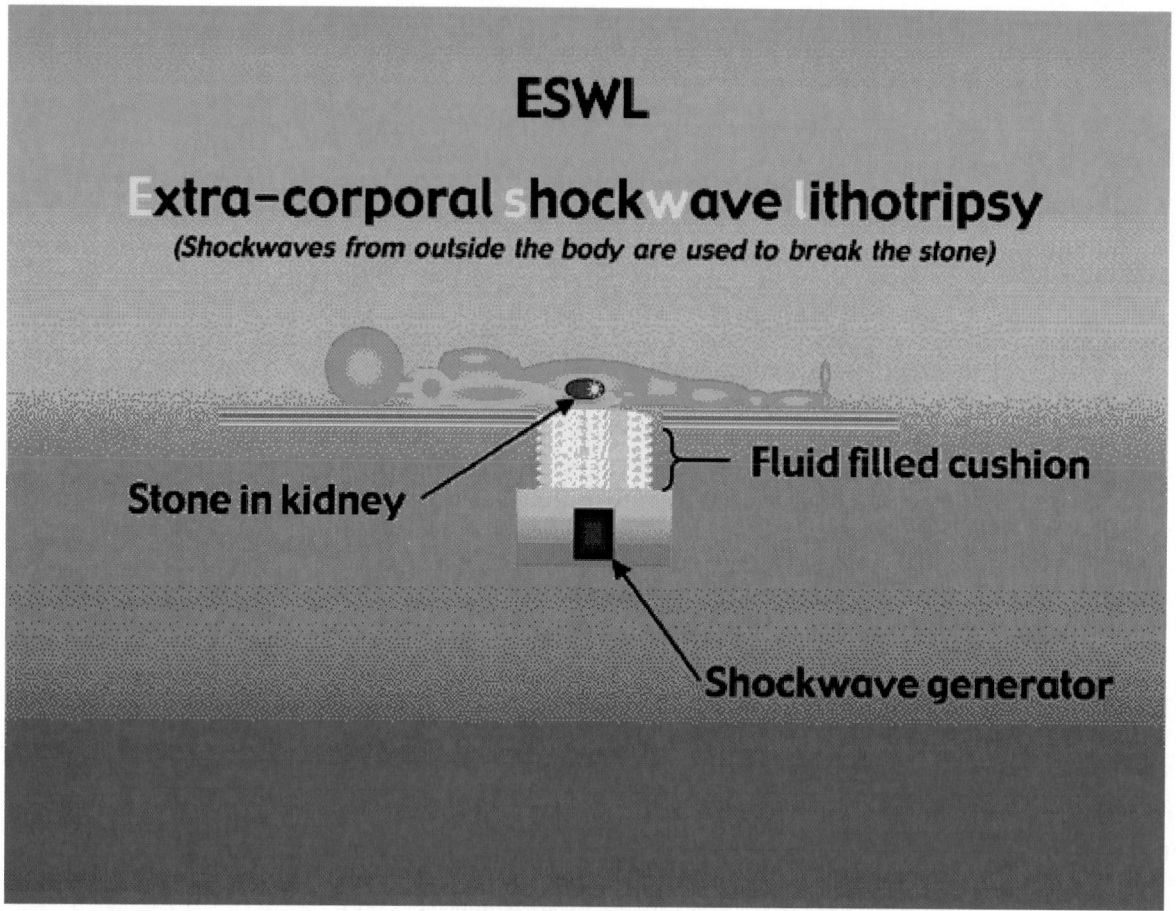

Figure 21-6 Extracorporal shockwave lithotripsy. (Reprinted with permission from Dr. Tom Shannon, www.hollywoodurology.com.)

nephrotic syndrome may resist treatment and progress to chronic renal failure (CRF). Primary goals of medical nutrition therapy are to control hypertension, minimize edema, decrease urinary albumin losses, prevent protein malnutrition and muscle catabolism, supply adequate energy, and slow the progression of renal disease.

Acute renal failure (ARF) is characterized by an abrupt loss of renal function that may or may not be accompanied by oliguria or anuria. Most common causes are trauma, hemorrhage, shock, nephrotoxic chemicals or drugs, septicemia, and streptococcal infection. Nutritional needs are determined by underlying cause of the condition and whether dialysis is used for treatment. Patients may be hypermetabolic if renal failure was caused by trauma, burns, septicemia, or infection.

CRF is the result of progressive, irreversible loss of kidney function. It can develop over days, months, or years and progress to end-stage renal disease (ESRD). Regardless of cause, results are the same: retention of nitrogenous waste products and fluid and electrolyte imbalances that affect all body systems. Before ESRD, management focuses on slowing progression of CRF and minimizing complications. Once CRF progresses to ESRD, management focuses on reducing uremia by various treatment modalities: conservative management, hemodialysis, peritoneal dialysis (PD), and renal transplantation.

Planning diets for CRF, ESRD, hemodialysis, and PD patients requires calibrating intakes of fluids, energy, protein, lipids, phosphorus, potassium, sodium, and vitamins and other minerals. Currently, the National Renal Diet is used to develop diet guidelines and meal plans. Individual diet prescriptions are based on residual kidney function, dialysate components, duration of dialysis, and rate of blood flow through the artificial kidney. Medical nutrition therapy objectives are to attain or maintain good nutritional status, prevent or minimize symptoms of uremic toxicity and fluid imbalance between treatments, and minimize effects of metabolic disorders caused by ESRD, hemodialysis, and PD. Nutritional care of renal transplant recipients involves continual reassessment of nutritional goals and efficacy of therapy during the different phases of care.

Renal calculi are a common, recurrent urologic condition. Most are composed of calcium, oxalate, or phosphorus, with a small proportion made up of cystine or uric acid. Fluid intake has the most significant impact on reducing risk of stone formation. Uric acid is a metabolic product of purines. Although limiting foods high in purines has not been proven effective, restriction of dietary protein may be effective. Kidney stone formation can be influenced by amount of oxalate in the urinary tract more than by amount of calcium. Oxalate is found primarily in plant foods and is the end product of ascorbic acid metabolism. Restriction of dietary oxalate intake is used to reduce risk of recurrence of calcium oxalate kidney stone formation.

THE NURSING APPROACH
Case Study: Renal Calculi

Tess, age 55, is a secretary who recently suffered an attack of severe flank pain found to be caused by renal calculi. Tess speaks limited English. The calculi were passed by means of forcing fluids, and Tess is now being treated with a preventive regimen because recurrence of stones occurs in the majority of cases. Based on a chemical analysis of the stones, which revealed calcium oxalate composition, the physician prescribed a low-oxalate diet. As the physician's office nurse, you are to teach Tess the preventive regimen.

NURSING DIAGNOSIS

Knowledge deficit related to prevention of renal calculi

PLANNING

Goal

Within 2 weeks, Tess will verbalize two strategies to prevent reoccurrence of renal calculi.

IMPLEMENTATION

1. Assess Tess's ability to comprehend English and obtain a professional translator if necessary.
2. Provide a teaching plan and handout of information about the etiology, diet, and understanding of renal calculi. Include drawings instead of language where possible.
3. Allow time for Tess to think about what is said and observe for nonverbal clues to confusion and lack of understanding of content.
4. Assess whether Tess wants to include family members or friends in the teaching session.

EVALUATION

Evaluate Tess's ability to verbalize two strategies to prevent recurrence of renal calculi. Determine, through questioning, whether client can verbalize foods to avoid as part of a low-oxalate diet. If client cannot, review areas and reinforce the specific information.

Continued

THE NURSING APPROACH–cont'd
Case Study: Renal Calculi

Teaching Plan

Objectives	Content	Strategy	Evaluation
Client will state the etiology of stone formation	Influence of diet, genetics, sedentary occupation	Discuss factors with client, emphasizing which ones put her at high risk	Patient will state reason for stone formation
Client will identify dietary sources of oxalate	*Foods high in oxalate:* chocolate, coffee, tea, nuts, spinach, rhubarb, beets, and strawberries	Supply a list of foods to be reduced or eliminated in the diet; discuss list and client's usual dietary intake of these foods	Patient will accurately list five or more foods that she must limit in her diet
Client will explain the importance of high fluid intake and physical activity	Approximately 3000 ml (3 qts) of fluid should be ingested per day to ensure at least 2000 ml of urine output. More fluid may be needed in hot weather or during exercise. Prolonged sitting should be avoided to prevent pooling of urine	Discussion of such factors that can help prevent future stones	When questioned, the patient will correctly explain the importance of 3000 ml fluid intake and physical activity
Client will express fears regarding diagnosis or uncertainties regarding diet	Any topic the client raises	Discussion with validation of feelings	Patient will state that any source of anxiety has been addressed

CRITICAL THINKING
Clinical Applications

Julia, age 40, works full time in an office and has a sedentary lifestyle. She is 5'6" tall, has a medium frame, and weighs 125 lb (dry weight). Her usual body weight is 132 lb. Her appetite has not been good for the past 3 months, but it is improving. She is on hemodialysis for 3 hours, three times per week. Her urine output is approximately 500 ml/24 hours.

Her predialysis laboratory results include: BUN 57 mg/dl; Na 133 mEq/l; K^+ 4.7 mEq/l; PO_4 6.3 mg/dl; Ca 9.5 mg/dl; serum albumin 3.0 g/dl; and ferritin 7 mcg/l. Her diet prescription is 2200 kcalories, 70 to 80 g protein, 2000 mg Na, 2000 mg K, 1000 mg PO_4, and 1500 ml fluid.

CRITICAL THINKING—cont'd
Clinical Applications

Julia's diet history indicates that she doesn't like meat, but does like cheese and orange juice and will occasionally overindulge on these foods. She admits to having had too much cheese and orange juice when she came in for her last dialysis. The patient is taking Nephro-Vites.

1. What is the purpose of hemodialysis?
2. How are metabolic waste products removed during dialysis?
3. Give two explanations why Julia's serum albumin levels are decreased.
4. Why is the serum ferritin often low in renal patients?
5. Why are high biologic value proteins recommended for patients with renal disease?
6. Why are water-soluble vitamin supplements (Nephro-Vites) usually prescribed for patients with renal disease?

Julia is considering trying a type of peritoneal dialysis so she won't have to go to the kidney dialysis center three times each week.

7. Explain how peritoneal dialysis works.
8. What dietary changes might need to be made if Julia switches to peritoneal dialysis?

Courtesy Kim Dittus, PhD, RD, Syracuse University, Syracuse, NY.

Web Sites of Interest

Life Options Rehabilitation Program
www.lifeoptions.org
Life Options is devoted to helping individuals live well with kidney disease. Links for patients, family members, and friends are available, including an interactive program called "kidney school," which teaches about the disorder. Part of the site is specifically for renal professionals.

National Institute of Diabetes and Digestive and Kidney Diseases (NIDDK)
www.niddk.nih.gov
This federal site of the National Institutes of Health provides information and research about kidney diseases for health professionals and the public. The site includes the National Diabetes Information Clearinghouse, which gives access to a database and online publications.

Renalnet
www.renalnet.org
Renalnet provides a clearinghouse on the cause, treatment, and management of kidney disease and end-stage renal disease (ESRD). A goal is to enhance communication among health organizations and individuals who are either patients or involved with the care of patients with kidney disease. Features available on the site include online discussion forums on related topics and a dialysis unit search.

References

1. Huether SE: Alteration of renal and urinary tract function. In McCance KL, Huether SE, eds.: *Pathophysiology: the biologic basis for disease in adults and children,* ed 4, St Louis, 2002, Mosby.
2. Guyton AC: *Textbook of medical physiology,* ed 8, Philadelphia, 1991, WB Saunders.
3. Swearingen PL, Ross DG: *Manual of medical-surgical nursing care,* ed 4, St Louis, 1999, Mosby.
4. Wilkens KG: Medical nutrition therapy for renal disorders. In Mahan LK, Escott-Stump S, eds.: *Krause's food, nutrition, and diet therapy,* ed 10, Philadelphia, 2000, WB Saunders.

5. American Dietetic Association: *Manual of clinical dietetics*, ed 6, Chicago, 2000, American Dietetic Association.

6. Morgan SL, Weinsier RL: *Fundamentals of clinical nutrition*, ed 2, St Louis, 1998, Mosby.

7. Wilson LM: Acute renal failure. In Price SA, Wilson LM, eds.: *Pathophysiology: clinical concepts of disease processes*, ed 6, St Louis, 2002, Mosby.

8. Wiggens KL: *Guidelines for nutrition care of renal patients*, ed 3, Chicago, 2002, American Dietetic Association.

9. American Dietetic Association: *National renal diet: professional guide*, ed 2, Chicago, 2002, American Dietetic Association.

10. Kopple JD: Nutritional management of nondialyzed patients with chronic renal failure. In Kopple JD, Massry SG, eds.: *Nutritional management of renal disease*, Baltimore, 1997, Lippincott Williams & Wilkins.

11. Verrelli M: Chronic renal failure, *eMedicine Journal* 3(1), Jan 23, 2002; www.emedicine.com/med/topic374.htm, accessed June 27, 2002.

12. Goldstein DJ, McQuiston B: Nutrition and renal disease. In Coulston AM, Rock CL, Monsen ER: *Nutrition in the prevention and treatment of disease*, San Diego, 2001, Academic Press.

13. Ahmed KR, Kopple JD: Nutrition in maintenance hemodialysis patients. In Kopple JD, Massry SG, eds.: *Nutritional management of renal disease*, Baltimore, 1997, Lippincott Williams & Wilkins.

14. Heimbürger O et al.: Nutritional effects and nutritional management of chronic peritoneal dialysis. In Kopple JD, Massry SG, eds.: *Nutritional management of renal disease*, Baltimore, 1997, Lippincott Williams & Wilkins.

15. National Kidney Foundation Dialysis Outcomes Quality Initiative: *Clinical practice guidelines for peritoneal dialysis adequacy*, 1997, National Kidney Foundation, Inc; www.kidney.org/professionals/doqi/doqi/doqipd.html, accessed July 3, 2002.

16. National Kidney Foundation: *About kidney disease*, Jan 1997; National Kidney Foundation, www.kidney.org/general/aboutdisease.index.cfm, accessed July 5, 2002.

17. National Kidney Foundation: *25 facts about organ donation and transplantation*, Feb 2002; National Kidney Foundation, www.kidney.org/general/news/25facts.cfm, accessed July 5, 2002.

18. Weseman RA, Mukherjee S: Nutritional requirements of adults before transplantation, *eMedicine Journal* 3(1), Jan 7, 2002; www.emedicine.com/med/topic3504.htm, accessed June 27, 2002.

19. Wolf S: Nephrolithiasis, *eMedicine Journal* 3(1), Jan 10, 2002; www.emedicine.com/med/topic1600.htm, accessed June 27, 2002.

20. Portis AJ, Sundaram CP: Diagnosis and initial management of kidney stones, *Am Fam Physician* 63(7):1329, 2001.

21. Currhan GC et al.: A prospective study of dietary calcium and other nutrients and the risk of symptomatic kidney stones, *N Engl J Med* 328(12):833, 1993.

22. Leslie SW: Hypercalciuria, *eMedicine Journal* 3(6), June 4, 2002; www.emedicine.com/med/topic1069.htm, accessed July 5, 2002.

23. Borghi L et al.: Comparison of two diets for the prevention of recurrent stones in idiopathic hypercalciuria, *N Engl J Med* 346(2):77, 2002.

24. Brinkley LJ, Gregory J, Pak CYC: A further study of oxalate bioavailability in foods, *J Urol* 144:94, 1990.

25. Massey LK, Roman-Smith H, Sutton RA: Effect of dietary calcium oxalate and calcium on urinary oxalate and risk of formation of calcium and oxalate kidney stones, *J Am Diet Assoc* 93:901, 1993.

26. National Kidney Foundation: *Family history of kidney stones? Watch those megadoses of vitamin C;* www.kidney.org/general/news/stones.cfm, accessed Jul 5, 2002.

27. Rineer S: Kidney stones, *eMedicine Journal* 2(5), May 28, 2001; www.emedicine.com/med/topic280.htm, accessed Jul 5, 2002.

28. Coyne DW: Renal diseases. In Carey CF, Lee HH, Woeltje KF, eds.: *The Washington manual of medical therapeutics*, ed 29, Philadelphia, 1998, Lippincott Williams & Wilkins.

CHAPTER 22

Nutrition in Cancer, AIDS, and Other Special Problems

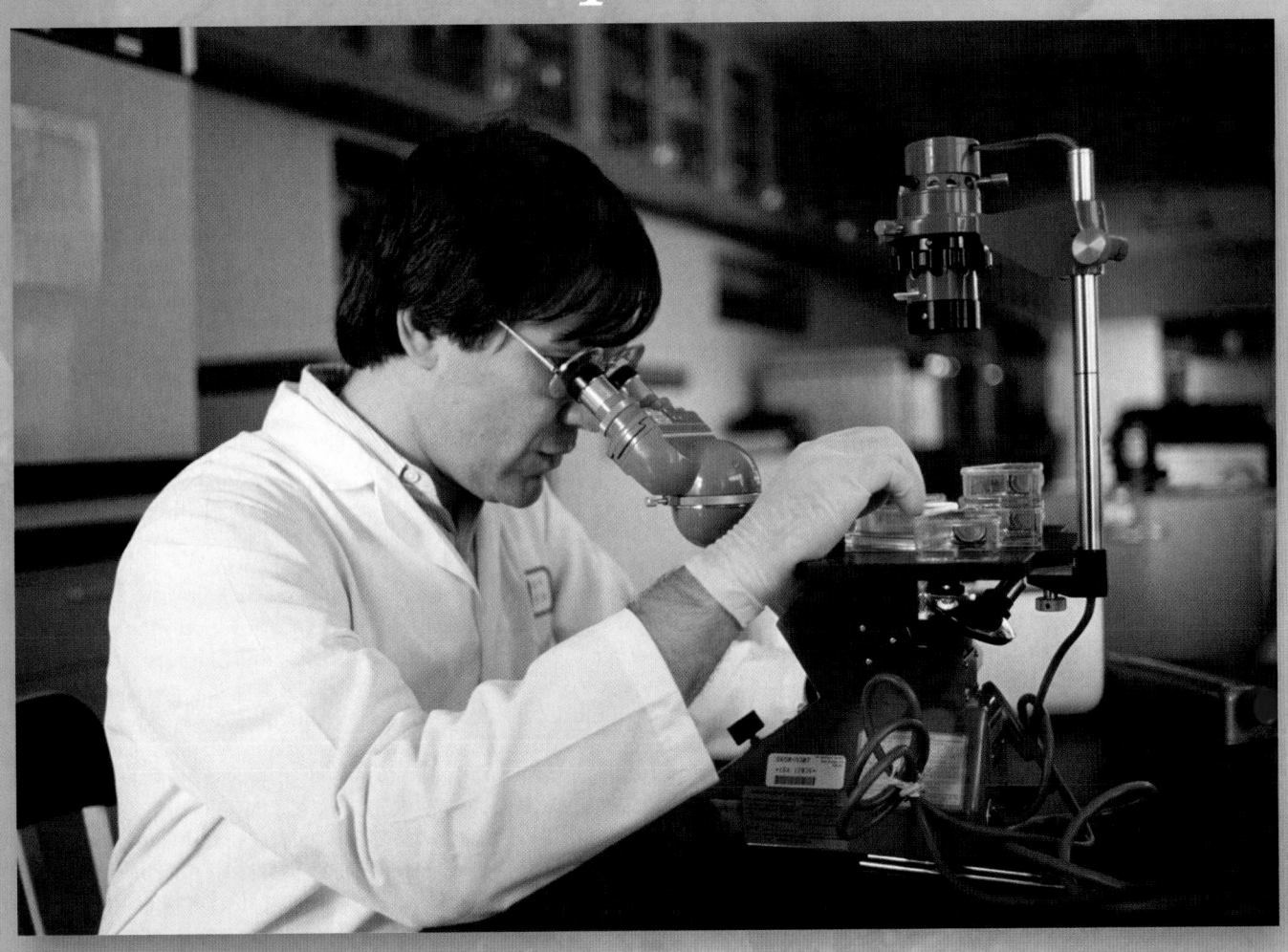

The nutritional status of patients with cancer, human immunodeficiency virus (HIV), acquired immunodeficiency syndrome (AIDS), and pulmonary disease is challenged by manifestations not only of the disease but also by the ramifications of treatment.

ROLE IN WELLNESS

Wasting and malnutrition, largely because of the effect of the disease itself or the secondary consequences of treatment, characterize the disorders of this chapter. Consequently, the nutritional status of patients with cancer, human immunodeficiency virus (HIV), acquired immunodeficiency syndrome (AIDS), and pulmonary disease is challenged by manifestations not only of the disease but also by the ramifications of treatment.

Most medical nutrition therapy prescribed focuses on reducing these effects and supporting the nutritional status of patients through the potentially debilitating side effects of treatment. Because these disorders are chronic, nursing care often continues after the patient leaves the hospital setting and returns home. The role of home care and hospice nurses is crucial for providing continued medical care, but also important are the nutritional support and food consumption strategies as patients recover and become acclimated to their conditions. The goal of maintaining good nutritional status is to improve survival rates, reduce treatment side effects, and increase the quality of life.

Consider the effects of these disorders through the health dimensions. The physical health dimension challenge is to halt or minimize malnutrition often associated with symptoms or treatments. Intellectual dimension is a factor as these disorders are marked by either their chronic or potentially life-threatening outcomes. Maintaining optimal nutrient intake while dealing with serious illness also requires intellectual abilities to comprehend the different aspects of treatment and rehabilitation. Facing death from AIDS or cancer or dealing with the chronic pulmonary diseases stresses our emotional health ability to cope; nurses need to be sensitive to the emotional burden patients and families are experiencing. Social health may be compromised as prejudice against (and fear of) clients with HIV/AIDS and cancer affects the ability of individuals to continue their social and work relations as they did in the past. Dealing with societal and emotional issues may warrant counseling support for clients and their families. Spirituality and faith can provide personal insight for gathering strength to heal.

CANCER

cancer
uncontrolled growth of cells that tend to invade surrounding tissue and metastasize to distant body sites

carcinogenesis
the process of cancer production

Cancer cells differ from normal cells in several ways. These characteristics may involve any or all of the following: (1) uncontrolled cellular reproduction where cells become independent of normal growth signals; (2) cells contain abnormal nucleus and cytoplasm; and (3) the mitosis rate generally increases. The nucleus of the cells may be an abnormal shape and have clearly abnormal chromosomes. This process that results in abnormal cell production is called carcinogenesis.[1]

The abnormalities in cell replication occur in several stages: initiation, promotion, and progression. *Initiation* of the process results in a mutation of deoxyribonucleic acid (DNA). Though exact causes are not clear for all malignancies, some factors such as physical and chemical agents or exposure to microorganisms may initially cause the mutation. The second phase is where the replication of the mutated cell is *promoted* and abnormal cell growth results. Factors that have been identified in some malignancies include estrogen, testosterone, nitrates, cigarette smoke, and alcohol. The third stage is the *progression* of the abnormal cells outside the original location of the cell.

The rate of tumor growth is dependent on characteristics of both the host and tumor. Host factors may include age, sex, nutritional status, the presence of other diseases, hormone production, and immune function. Tumor factors could include where the tumor is located and its access to adequate blood supply.[1-3]

Marcia L. Nahikian-Nelms, PhD, RD, contributed this chapter in all three editions of this text.

In the United States there are an estimated 1.2 million new cases of cancer each year. Cancer is the second leading cause of death, with more than 500,000 deaths each year. Scientists estimate that 50% to 75% of all cancer deaths can be linked to human behaviors and lifestyle factors.[4-6] Nutrition factors are considered one of the important environmental and lifestyle factors in the etiology and prevention of cancer. Nutrition and dietary factors may interact within the process of carcinogenesis in all three stages: initiation, promotion, and progression. Furthermore, nutritional factors may assist in blocking those three stages. For example, antioxidants in the diet may protect the cell from DNA mutation[4] (see the Health Debate box, "Fact or Fantasy? Food as Pharmaceuticals?"). It is important to remember that no one food causes cancer and no one food can prevent it. The National Cancer Institute encourages cancer prevention by encouraging the following guidelines:[4]

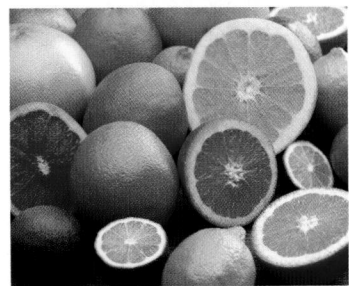

Phytochemical may play a role in preventing cancer. (From PhotoDisc.)

- Not smoking cigarettes or using other tobacco products
- Not drinking too much alcohol
- Eating five or more daily servings of fruits and vegetables
- Eating a low-fat diet
- Maintaining or reaching a healthy weight
- Being physically active
- Protecting skin from sunlight

Nutrition and the Diagnosis of Cancer

With more than 100 variations, cancer is the second leading cause of death in the United States. The physiologic response to malignancy is different for each specific tumor type, but there are general nutrition risk factors that may apply to many cancer patients. Physical impairment because of the location of the tumor or the extent of tumor involvement, metabolic changes, and the use of antineoplastic therapy all place the patient with cancer at increased risk of developing malnutrition or the wasting syndrome of cancer cachexia.[7,8]

Cancer cachexia is a complex syndrome that results in severe wasting of lean body mass and weight loss. Much research has attempted to establish an understanding of this syndrome. It is generally accepted that the etiology is multifactorial and may include the following factors: altered metabolism of carbohydrate, protein, and fat; increased energy expenditure; and anorexia.[7-10] Cachexia affects about two thirds of all cancer patients and is present even at the beginning stages of tumor development before actual weight loss is observed.

antineoplastic therapy substance, procedure, or measure that prevents the proliferation of malignant cells; usually chemotherapy, radiation therapy, surgery, biologic response modifiers, or bone marrow transplantation

Benefits of Nutritional Adequacy

Can adequate nutrition make a difference in those patients with cancer? Yes. Maintenance of nutritional status may do the following[7-14]:
- Decrease the risk of surgical complications.
- Ensure that patients are able to meet increased energy and protein requirements.
- Help to repair and rebuild normal tissues affected by antineoplastic therapy.
- Promote an increased tolerance to therapy.
- Assist in promoting an enhanced quality of life.

Nutritional Effects of Cancer Treatments

Surgery

Treatment for many malignancies (particularly, solid tumors) includes surgical resection of the tumor.[9] This route of treatment can allow for diagnosis, resect a solid tumor, prevent metastasis of the malignancy, or reduce the size of the tumor to alleviate pain. The nutritional consequences related to surgery are dependent on the type and extent of the surgical resection. Resections of any portion of the gastrointestinal

LEADING CANCER SITES

Men	Women
Prostate	Breast
Colorectal	Colorectal
Lung	Lung
Skin	Skin
Non-Hodgkin's lymphoma	

From National Cancer Institute: Cancer progress report 2001; http://progressreport.cancer. gov, accessed March 2002.

metastasis the spread of malignant cells to other sites from the original tumor location

HEALTH DEBATE
Fact or Fantasy: Food as Pharmaceuticals?

They are touted as being able to prevent cancer, heart disease, and depression. Some say they can even boost our immune system. There is some opinion that they can even slow down the aging process. They are the foods our mothers tried to make us eat when we were kids. They are fruits and vegetables. What a surprise!

Over the past 20 years, epidemiologic researchers have consistently found that people who eat greater amounts of fruits and vegetables have lower rates of cancer. Fruits and vegetables contain hundreds of compounds such as antioxidants (beta-carotene and vitamins C and E), folic acid, fiber, and at least a dozen groups of chemicals called *phytochemicals* (specific chemicals found in plants, primarily in fruits and vegetables) that are not strictly nutrients. Some families of plants have more than others, but none of the phytochemicals are found in animal foods. The list in the bottom of the box lists known phytochemicals, their action in the body, and common food sources.

Most health professionals believe that the whole plant is probably more important than the sum of its nutrients and chemical components. More benefits (some we don't even know yet) are derived from nutrients and phytochemicals by eating foods rather than swallowing supplements. Clients may question why they shouldn't just take specialized supplements of phytochemicals if we know their actions. What do you think? How will you explain your view to clients? Was Mom right? Should we all eat our vegetables?

PHYTO-CHEMICAL	ACTION	FOOD SOURCE
Limonene	Speeds up enzyme production that may dispose of potential carcinogens	Citrus fruits
Allyl sulfides	Aids potential carcinogen excretion	Garlic, onions, leeks, chives
Allium compounds	May decrease tumor cell reproduction	Garlic, onions, leeks, chives
Dithiolthiones	May block damage to cell DNA by carcinogens	Broccoli
Ellagic acid	Scavenges carcinogens, may prevent their altering cell's DNA	Grapes
Protease inhibitors	Suppresses enzyme production in cancer cells, slows tumor growth	Soybeans, dried beans
Phytosterols	Slows cell reproduction in large intestine, possibly prevents colon cancer	Soybeans, dried beans
Isoflavones	Blocks estrogen entry into cells, possibly reduces risk of breast or ovarian cancer	Soybeans, dried beans
Saponins	May prevent cancer cell multiplication	Soybeans, dried beans
Genistein	Inhibits cancer cell growth	Soybeans
Caffeic acid	May ease disposal of carcinogens from body	Fruits
Ferulic acid	May prevent nitrate conversion to carcinogenic nitrosamines, binds nitrates in stomach	Fruits
Indoles	Stimulates enzymes that make estrogen less effective, may reduce breast cancer risk	Cruciferous vegetables (bok choy, broccoli, brussels sprouts, cabbage, cauliflower, collards, kale, kohl-rabi, mustard greens, rutabaga, turnip greens, turnips)
Isothiocyanates	May block carcinogen damage to a cell's DNA	Cruciferous vegetables

Compiled from Webb D: Whole grain boast phytochemicals to fight disease, Environmental Nutrition 24:1, 2001; Peterson J, Dwyer J: Taxonomic classifications help identify flavonoid-containing foods on a semiquantitative food frequency questionnaire, J Am Dietetic Assoc 98:677, 1998.

(GI) tract can cause alterations in nutrition intake and nutrient absorption.[9] Secondly, energy and protein requirements may need to be increased to promote optimal wound healing postoperatively. Malabsorption does tend to be the primary nutritional problem with surgeries involving the GI tract; yet unless small bowel resection is extensive, the adaptability of the small intestine may prevent the occurrence of major clinical problems.[9]

Many cancer patients enter surgery already experiencing protein-calorie malnutrition that places them at higher risk for complications. Additionally, any problems associated with surgery (Table 22-1) will be further complicated if the patient receives subsequent radiation therapy and chemotherapy.

Chemotherapy

Most chemotherapy protocols include a combination of chemotherapy agents. Chemotherapy agents include alkylating drugs, antibiotics, antimetabolites, hormones, enzymes, plant alkaloids, and biologic response modifiers. These agents act by inhibiting one or more steps of DNA synthesis in rapidly proliferating cells that are characteristic of the malignant cell. Unfortunately, bone marrow and cells lining the GI tract tend to be susceptible to damage from chemotherapy because of their rapid turnover rate.[7-9] The effect on these cells account for many of the side effects that are associated with chemotherapy including nausea, vomiting, diarrhea, mucositis, hair loss, and immunosuppression.[7-10,13,14]

The severity and manifestation of the side effects depend on the particular chemotherapy agent, dosage, duration of treatment, rates of metabolism, accompanying drugs, and individual susceptibility.[7-11] These symptoms can lead to malnutrition through a variety of mechanisms: anorexia; nausea; vomiting; mucositis; stomatitis; cardiac, renal, and liver injury (toxicity); and learned food aversions.[7-10,13,14] Nutritional implications of chemotherapeutic agents are summarized in Table 22-2.

mucositis
inflammation of mucous membranes

stomatitis
inflammation of mucous membranes of the mouth

Radiation Therapy

Radiation therapy uses ionizing radiation to kill cells by altering the DNA of the malignant cell. This alteration interferes with the factors controlling replication. Radiation is used to treat tumors sensitive to radiation exposure or tumors that cannot

Table 22-1
Nutrition Side Effects of Cancer Surgery

Site of Surgery	Side Effect
Head and neck	Impaired chewing and swallowing
Esophagectomy	Diarrhea, steatorrhea, esophageal stenosis
Vagotomy	Gastric stasis, diarrhea, fat malabsorption
Gastrectomy	Dumping syndrome; hypoglycemia; malabsorption; possible deficiencies of iron, calcium, vitamin B_{12}, and fat-soluble vitamins
Pancreatectomy	Type 1 diabetes mellitus; possible malabsorption of fats, protein, fat-soluble vitamins, minerals
Small bowel resection	Possible malabsorption of many nutrients; depends on extent and site of surgery
Ileostomy	Sodium and water losses, vitamin B_{12} malabsorption, fat malabsorption, bile salt diarrhea

Reference: McCallum PD, Polisena CG, eds.: The clinical guide to oncology nutrition, Chicago, 2000, American Dietetic Association.

Table 22-2
Nutritional Implications of Chemotherapeutic Agents

Drug Classification	Selected Examples	Actions	Nutritional Implications
Alkylating agents	Cisplatin Hexamethylmelamine Dacarbazine	React with susceptible DNA sites	Anorexia, nausea, vomiting, mucositis/stomatitis
Antibiotics	Bleomycin Doxorubicin Dactinomycin	Bind to DNA and inhibit cell division, interfere with RNA transcription	Anorexia, nausea, mucositis/stomatitis, diarrhea; some may cause decreased calcium and iron absorption
Antimetabolites	Methotrexate 5-Fluorodeoxyuridine 5-Fluorouracil	Inhibit a stage of DNA synthesis	Anorexia, nausea, vomiting, diarrhea, mucositis, abdominal pain, intestinal ulceration; some may cause decreased absorption of vitamin B_{12}, fat, and xylose
Hormones	Prednisone Tamoxifen Diethylstilbestrol	Alter cell metabolism to cause unfavorable tumor growth	*Corticosteroids:* sodium and fluid retention, hyperglycemia, gastrointestinal upset, osteoporosis (calcium losses), negative nitrogen balance *Estrogens:* nausea, vomiting, anorexia, hypercalcemia
Enzymes	Asparaginase	Delay DNA and RNA synthesis by inhibiting protein synthesis (deprive cells of asparagine)	Anorexia, nausea, hyperglycemia, pancreatitis, azotemia (uremia), weight loss
Plant alkaloids	Vinblastine Vincristine	Inhibit mitosis	Nausea, vomiting, constipation, diarrhea, abdominal pain
Biologic response modifiers	Interferon Interleukin	Modify host biologic response to tumor	Nausea, vomiting, anorexia, weight change (increase or decrease)

Reference: McCallum PD, Polisena CG, eds.: The clinical guide to oncology nutrition, *Chicago, 2000, American Dietetic Association.*

fractionation
administration of radiation in smaller doses over time rather than in a single large dose; minimizes tissue damage

be surgically resected. Radiation can also be used to reduce tumor size so that a successful surgical resection can occur. Unfortunately, as with chemotherapy, normal cells within the treatment range who are also in that stage of cell replication may also be damaged. This may contribute to the physical side effects, which may include hair loss, mucositis, and vomiting and diarrhea. Nutritional problems vary according to the region or area of the body radiated, dose, **fractionation,** and whether radiation is used as combination therapy with surgery or chemotherapy.[7-10,13,14] Complications may develop only during radiation treatment or become chronic and progress even after treatment is completed.[7-10,13,14]

Primary radiation sites that result in nutrition problems include the head and neck, the abdomen and pelvis (GI tract), and the central nervous system.[13,14] Radiation at all three sites may cause anorexia, nausea, and vomiting. In the head and neck, these common effects create problems of food ingestion as stomatitis, esophageal mucositis, loss of taste sensation, and dry mouth. Side effects to the abdomen and pelvis alter the GI tract, reducing digestion and absorption of nutrients in part because of the development of diarrhea and steatorrhea, and possibly, malabsorption, ulceration, and bowel damage or obstruction.

Bone Marrow Transplantation

Bone marrow transplantation (BMT) is used to treat certain hematologic malignancies (acute and chronic leukemia and some forms of lymphoma) and, more recently, solid tumors such as in breast cancer.[7] Types of transplant include: autologous, allogeneic, and syngenic. When using bone marrow transplant as the treatment of a solid tumor, the patient's own bone marrow is harvested and saved before the initiation of chemotherapy or radiation therapy. The patient then receives high-dose chemotherapy and possibly total body irradiation to eradicate the cancer.[7-9,13] Their own bone marrow is then infused as a "rescue" from the effects of both chemotherapy or radiation. For hematologic malignancies, a patient receives bone marrow from a genetically matched donor (allogenic) or in some cases from a twin (syngenic).

The ability to maintain adequate oral intake is difficult because of the nausea, vomiting, and mucositis that is associated with such high-dose therapies. Parenteral nutrition is generally a standard component of transplantation protocols, though recent research indicates that maintaining some oral intake or providing enteral nutrition is important to maintaining the integrity of the small intestine.

Immunosuppression, as a result of the antineoplastic regimens and BMT, places the BMT patient at high risk for infections from bacterial and fungal pathogens. Pathogens are most commonly found in fresh fruits and vegetables that ordinarily do not present a hazard to healthy persons; therefore a low-bacterial diet is indicated whenever the plasma neutrophil (a type of white blood cell) count is less than 1000 mm³.[7] Standard practice varies between institutions, but in general, a low-bacterial diet includes restrictions on undercooked meats and eggs, raw vegetables (including salads and garnishes), and all fresh fruits. Frequent monitoring of nutritional intake and encouragement to take in adequate nutrition are essential in the care of these patients.[7]

A major complication that may occur with an allogenic BMT is graft vs. host disease (GVHD), which is best described as reverse rejection. In this case, the grafted tissue or organ recognizes the host's cells as foreign. GVHD may result in multiple organ damage, but the skin, GI tract, and liver are of particular concern. The nutritional management for GVHD is complicated and requires intense therapy for periods as long as 1 to 2 years posttransplant.[7-9,13]

Medical Nutrition Therapy

One of the most important steps in providing nutritional care for the cancer patient is identifying the patient who is at risk. One tool that has been developed for screening for nutritional risk in cancer patients is the Patient-generated Subjective Global Assessment (PG-SGA).[11-13,15] This screening tool allows for early identification of those patients with a nutritional deficit or who are at risk when treatment is initiated (Figure 22-1).

Cancer patients are at high risk for malnutrition.[7,10-13] This is in part because of the presence of common symptoms that cancer patients experience. Recognizing clinical signs and treating these symptoms early may assist in the prevention of protein-calorie malnutrition. Table 22-3 summarizes interventions used in treating these symptoms. As with any other disease, nutrition support of cancer patients must be individualized. Staff and patients alike should realize that nutrition is an essential component of the total management of the disease. Prognosis should be considered to appropriately adjust the aggressiveness of the nutritional intervention (supportive, adjunctive, definitive).

As mentioned previously, nutritional problems may arise as a result of the cancer itself or the method used to treat it. Nutritional interventions will be tailored

autologous
Removal of patient's own marrow when a completed remission has been induced, followed by ablative treatment of patient with hope of destruction of any residual tumor and rescue with patient's own bone marrow

allogenic
A bone marrow transplant using marrow collected from a matched healthy donor, usually a brother or sister

syngenic
Transplant from an identical twin

To destroy tap water contaminants that may cause illness, the Centers for Disease Control and Prevention recommend that individuals with weakened immune systems boil tap water before consumption. Immune system functioning may be diminished because of the effects of HIV, AIDS, chemotherapy drugs, and immunosuppressive drugs (to prevent organ-transplant rejection).
Reference: Safe Food and Water: A Guide for People with HIV and AIDS, www.cdc.gov/hiv/pubs/brochure/food.htm.

Scored Patient-Generated Subjective Global Assessment (PG-SGA)

Patient ID Information

History (Boxes 1-4 are designed to be completed by the patient.)

1. Weight (See Worksheet 1)

In summary of my current and recent weight:

I currently weigh about _____ pounds
I am about _____ feet _____ tall

One month ago I weighed about _____ pounds
Six months ago I weighed about _____ pounds

During the past two weeks my weight has:

☐ decreased (1)   ☐ not changed (0)   ☐ increased (0)

Box 1 [____]

2. Food Intake: As compared to my normal intake, I would rate my food intake during the past month as:

☐ unchanged (0)
☐ more than usual (0)
☐ less than usual (1)
   I am now taking:
   ☐ *normal food* but less than normal amount (1)
   ☐ little solid food (2)
   ☐ only liquids (3)
   ☐ only nutritional supplements (3)
   ☐ very little of anything (4)
   ☐ only tube feedings or only nutrition by vein (0)

Box 2 [____]

3. Symptoms: I have had the following problems that have kept me from eating enough during the past two weeks (check all that apply):

☐ no problems eating (0)

☐ no appetite, just did not feel like eating (3)

☐ nausea (1)   ☐ vomiting (3)
☐ constipation (1)   ☐ diarrhea (3)
☐ mouth sores (2)   ☐ dry mouth (1)
☐ things taste funny or have no taste (1)   ☐ smells bother me (1)
☐ problems swallowing (2)   ☐ feel full quickly (1)
☐ pain; where? (3) _____
☐ other** (1) _____

** Examples: depression, money, or dental problems

Box 3 [____]

4. Activities and Function: Over the past month, I would generally rate my activity as:

☐ normal with no limitations (0)

☐ not my normal self, but able to be up and about with fairly normal activities (1)

☐ not feeling up to most things, but in bed or chair less than half the day (2)

☐ able to do little activity and spend most of the day in bed or chair (3)

☐ pretty much bedridden, rarely out of bed (3)

Box 4 [____]

Additive Score of the Boxes 1-4 [____] A

The remainder of this form will be completed by your doctor, nurse, or therapist. Thank you.

(Optional for completion by clinicians)

5. Disease and its relation to nutritional requirements (See Worksheet 2)

All relevant diagnoses (specify) _____

Primary disease stage (circle if known or appropriate)   I   II   III   IV   Other _____

Age _____

Numerical score from Worksheet 2 [____] B

6. Metabolic Demand (See Worksheet 3)

Numerical score from Worksheet 3 [____] C

7. Physical (See Worksheet 4)

Numerical score from Worksheet 4 [____] D

Global Assessment (See Worksheet 5)

☐ Well-nourished or anabolic (SGA-A)
☐ Moderate or suspected malnutrition (SGA-B)
☐ Severely malnourished (SGA-C)

Total PG-SGA score

(Total numerical score of A+B+C+D above) [____]
(See triage recommendations below)

Clinician Signature _____ RD RN PA MD DO Other ___   Date _____

Nutritional Triage Recommendations: Additive score is used to define specific nutritional interventions including patient & family education, symptom management including pharmacologic intervention, and appropriate nutrient intervention (food, nutritional supplements, enteral, or parenteral triage). First line nutrition intervention includes optimal symptom management.

0-1   No intervention required at this time. Re-assessment on routine and regular basis during treatment.
2-3   Patient & family education by dietitian, nurse, or other clinician with pharmacologic intervention as indicated by symptom survey (Box 3) and laboratory values as appropriate.
4-8   Requires intervention by dietitian, in conjunction with nurse or physician as indicated by symptoms survey (Box 3).
≥ 9   Indicates a critical need for improved symptom management and/or nutrient intervention options.

© FD Ottery, 2001. Used with permission.   email: fdottery@btgc.com or noatpres1@aol.com

Figure 22-1 Patient-generated Subjective Global Assessment (PG-SGA) of nutritional status. (© FD Ottery, 2000. Used with permission.)   *Continued*

Worksheets for PG-SGA Scoring © FD Ottery, 2001. Used with permission.

Boxes 1-4 of the PG-SGA are designed to be completed by the patient. The PG-SGA numerical score is determined using
1) the parenthetical points noted in boxes 1-4 and 2) the worksheets below for items not marked with parenthetical points. Scores for
boxes 1 and 3 are additive within each box and scores for boxes 2 and 4 are based on the highest scored item checked off by the patient.

Worksheet 1 - Scoring Weight (Wt) Loss

To determine score, use 1 month weight data if available. Use 6 month data only if there is no 1 month weight data. Use points below to score weight change and add one extra point if patient has lost weight during the past 2 weeks. Enter total point score in Box 1 of the PG-SGA.

Wt loss in 1 month	Points	Wt loss in 6 months
10% or greater	4	20% or greater
5-9.9%	3	10 -19.9%
3-4.9%	2	6 - 9.9%
2-2.9%	1	2 - 5.9%
0-1.9%	0	0 - 1.9%

Score for Worksheet 1 [ ]
Record in Box 1

Worksheet 2 - Scoring Criteria for Condition

Score is derived by adding 1 point for each of the conditions listed below that pertain to the patient.

Category	Points
Cancer	1
AIDS	1
Pulmonary or cardiac cachexia	1
Presence of decubitus, open wound, or fistula	1
Presence of trauma	1
Age greater than 65 years	1

Score for Worksheet 2 = [ ]
Record in Box B

Worksheet 3 - Scoring Metabolic Stress

Score for metabolic stress is determined by a number of variables known to increase protein & calorie needs. The score is additive so that a patient who has a fever of > 102 degrees (3 points) and is on 10 mg of prednisone chronically (2 points) would have an additive score for this section of 5 points.

Stress	none (0)	low (1)	moderate (2)	high (3)
Fever	no fever	>99 and <101	≥101 and <102	≥102
Fever duration	no fever	<72 hrs	72 hrs	> 72 hrs
Corticosteroids	no corticosteroids	low dose (<10mg prednisone equivalents/day)	moderate dose (≥10 and <30 mg prednisone equivalents/day)	high dose steroids (≥30 mg prednisone equivalents/day)

Score for Worksheet 3 = [ ]
Record in Box C

Worksheet 4 - Physical Examination

Physical exam includes a subjective evaluation of 3 aspects of body composition: fat, muscle, & fluid status. Since this is subjective, each aspect of the exam is rated for degree of deficit. Muscle deficit impacts point score more than fat deficit. Definition of categories: 0 = no deficit, 1+ = mild deficit, 2+ = moderate deficit, 3+ = severe deficit. Rating of deficit in these categories are *not* additive but are used to clinically assess the degree of deficit (or presence of excess fluid).

Fat Stores:

orbital fat pads	0	1+	2+	3+
triceps skin fold	0	1+	2+	3+
fat overlying lower ribs	0	1+	2+	3+
Global fat deficit rating	**0**	**1+**	**2+**	**3+**

Muscle Status:

temples (temporalis muscle)	0	1+	2+	3+
clavicles (pectoralis & deltoids)	0	1+	2+	3+
shoulders (deltoids)	0	1+	2+	3+
interosseous muscles	0	1+	2+	3+
scapula (latissimus dorsi, trapezius, deltoids)	0	1+	2+	3+
thigh (quadriceps)	0	1+	2+	3+
calf (gastrocnemius)	0	1+	2+	3+
Global muscle status rating	**0**	**1+**	**2+**	**3+**

Fluid Status:

ankle edema	0	1+	2+	3+
sacral edema	0	1+	2+	3+
ascites	0	1+	2+	3+
Global fluid status rating	**0**	**1+**	**2+**	**3+**

Point score for the physical exam is determined by the overall subjective rating of total body deficit.

No deficit	score = 0 points
Mild deficit	score = 1 point
Moderate deficit	score = 2 points
Severe deficit	score = 3 points

Score for Worksheet 4 = [ ]
Record in Box D

Worksheet 5 - PG-SGA Global Assessment Categories

	Stage A Well-nourished	Stage B Moderately malnourished or suspected malnutrition	Stage C Severely malnourished
Category	Well-nourished	Moderately malnourished or suspected malnutrition	Severely malnourished
Weight	No wt loss **OR** Recent non-fluid wt gain	~5% wt loss within 1 month (or 10% in 6 months) **OR** No wt stabilization or wt gain (i.e., continued wt loss)	> 5% wt loss in 1 month (or >10% in 6 months) **OR** No wt stabilization or wt gain (i.e., continued wt loss)
Nutrient Intake	No deficit **OR** Significant recent improvement	Definite decrease in intake	Severe deficit in intake
Nutrition Impact Symptoms	None **OR** Significant recent improvement allowing adequate intake	Presence of nutrition impact symptoms (Box 3 of PG-SGA)	Presence of nutrition impact symptoms (Box 3 of PG-SGA)
Functioning	No deficit **OR** Significant recent improvement	Moderate functional deficit **OR** Recent deterioration	Severe functional deficit **OR** recent significant deterioration
Physical Exam	No deficit **OR** Chronic deficit but with recent clinical improvement	Evidence of mild to moderate loss of SQ fat &/or muscle mass &/or muscle tone on palpation	Obvious signs of malnutrition (e.g., severe loss of SQ tissues, possible edema)

Global PG-SGA rating (A, B, or C) = [ ]

Figure 22-1—cont'd

Table 22-3

Nutritional Approaches to Nutrition-Related Problems in Cancer and Cancer Therapy

Problem	Recommendations
Loss of appetite/ early satiety	Eat frequent small meals, increase kcal/protein content of foods, use high-protein/ high-kcalorie supplements, serve foods cool or at room temperature, avoid excess fat, exercise regularly if tolerated, limit liquids at meal time; appetite may be best in the morning
Diarrhea*	Eat frequent small meals, serve foods cool or at room temperature, increase fluid intake, eat and drink slowly, decrease fiber intake, avoid excess fat, avoid gas-forming foods, limit liquids at meal time, avoid highly seasoned foods, limit beverages containing caffeine and alcohol; trial avoidance of lactose may be helpful; take antidiarrheal medication per physician
Nausea and vomiting	Eat frequent small meals, avoid strong odors, serve foods cool or room temperature, increase fluid intake, eat and drink slowly, avoid excess fat, limit liquids at meal time, avoid highly seasoned foods, rest after meals with head elevated, take antiemetic per physician
Chewing and swallowing difficulties	Eat frequent small meals; increase kcal/protein content of foods; use high-protein/ high-kcal supplements; serve food cool or at room temperature; increase fluid intake; eat and drink slowly; add sauces and gravy to soften and moisten foods; avoid highly seasoned foods; avoid alcohol, tobacco, and commercial mouthwashes; coarse-textured and acidic foods may irritate
Constipation	Increase fluid intake, increase fiber intake, exercise regularly if tolerated; stool softener and/or laxative may be necessary
Abdominal gas	Eat and drink slowly, decrease fiber intake, avoid excess fat, avoid gas-forming foods, exercise regularly if tolerated, limit lactose if not tolerated
Dry mouth	Increase fluid intake; add sauces and gravy to soften and moisten foods; tart foods or sugar-free hard candy may be used to stimulate saliva; avoid alcohol, tobacco, and commercial mouthwash
Taste/smell alterations	Serve food cool or at room temperature, increase fluid intake, use seasonings to enhance flavors, avoid cooking odors, try alternative protein sources for meat aversion

Reference: McCallum PD, Polisena CG, eds.: The clinical guide to oncology nutrition, Chicago, 2000, American Dietetic Association.
*Diarrhea secondary to malabsorption, dumping syndrome, or other causes may require different treatment modalities.

to support the energy and protein needs of the patient so that body stores can be maintained, and then as symptoms arise, interventions can be introduced to maximize nutritional intake.

Anorexia Caused by Cancer or Its Treatment

Anorexia is best described as a loss of appetite. The etiology of anorexia is generally multifactorial in most patients. For cancer patients, this may be caused by changes in taste and smell; decreased transit time and subsequent, early satiety; opportunistic infections; therapy and other medication side effects; pain; and emotional and psychologic effects.[7,11,13]

Treatment Options

Early education of the patient on the role of nutrition is essential to promote adequate nutritional intake. Many cancer patients feel a loss of control after diagnosis of a malignancy. Often, managing their nutritional intake assists in regaining that control. It is essential that the nutrient density of food be stressed. Small, frequent meals; the use of high-calorie supplements; and a pleasant eating environment may help. Medications such as megestrol (Megace) and dronabinol (Marinol) have been used successfully to stimulate appetite in cancer patients.[11-13]

Nausea and Vomiting

Nausea and vomiting may result from (1) delayed transit time; (2) physiologic symptoms such as hypercalcemia or central nervous system (CNS) involvement; (3) medications; or (4) may even be anticipatory on the part of the patient.[11,14,16]

Treatment Options

The first line of treatment for nausea and vomiting is adequate and aggressive antiemetic therapy. It is essential to give medication 60 to 90 minutes before meals to ensure effectiveness. If nausea and vomiting can be prevented, the risk of developing anticipatory nausea and vomiting will be reduced. Cold foods without odor tend to be best tolerated when the patient experiences nausea and vomiting. Behavioral strategies such as guided imagery and relaxation techniques have also been successful in some environments.[11,14,16]

Taste Abnormalities

Many cancer patients describe alterations in their ability to taste foods.[11,14,16] These alterations may be because of the changes or destruction of the oral mucosa, the presence of tumor byproducts systemically, changes in the quantity or quality of saliva, inadequate mouth care, or drug-related taste changes.[11-13,16]

Treatment Options

It is appropriate for cancer patients to avoid those foods that taste bad to them. However it is just as important to provide cancer patients with alternate food choices for them to maintain adequate nutrient intake. Foods that are tart or spicy may enhance intake. Additionally, providing guidelines for mouth care is essential.[17]

Principles of Nutritional Care

Nutrition should be an essential component of every treatment plan for the cancer patient. Shils[9] outlines the following principles for nutritional care of the cancer patient:
- Malnutrition can result from the cancer but is further complicated by the treatment of the disease.
- Every patient should be screened regularly for nutritional risk because preventing malnutrition is much more effective than treating existing malnutrition.
- The provision of optimal nutritional care requires a multidisciplinary approach with physicians, nurses, dietitians, and pharmacists working as a team.
- Nutritional therapy, when indicated, should be initiated early.
- Nutritional therapy has the potential for difficulties as well as benefits.

✤ ACQUIRED IMMUNODEFICIENCY SYNDROME (AIDS)

In 1983 the retrovirus human immunodeficiency virus (HIV) was isolated as the cause for acquired immunodeficiency syndrome (AIDS). A retrovirus injects its ribonucleic acid (RNA) into the target cell and then transcribes the RNA into DNA using a reverse transcriptase enzyme. Target cells for HIV include the T4 or CD4 lymphocytes, B-lymphocytes, monocytes, macrophages, and other cells of the immune system.[18,19] As many as 1 billion copies of HIV can be made in one day and several generations can exist in just hours. The initial infection with HIV may

retrovirus
an RNA virus that becomes integrated into the DNA of a host cell during replication; HIV is a retrovirus

include symptoms such as fever and malaise. Antibodies are produced against the virus and are detectable within 2 to 4 months after exposure. It is at this stage that an individual can be seropositive. This presence of HIV antibodies is confirmed using two major tests: the ELISA (enzyme-linked immunosorbent assay) and the Western Blot, polymerase chain reaction (PCR).[18,19] The replication of the infected cell results in a steady depletion of the CD4+ cell count causing a severe depression of immune function and increasing the risk for opportunistic infections and malignancies (Table 22-4). The diagnosis of AIDS includes the positive antibody test for HIV; a CD4 cell count of less than 200 mm^3 or below 14% of the total

Table 22-4
Clinical and Nutritional Complications of AIDS

Opportunistic Infections	Clinical and Nutritional Presentation
Neoplasms	
Kaposi's Sarcoma	Oral, esophageal lesions
Lymphoma: Burkitt's; immunoblastic	Dependent on primary site—diarrhea and malabsorption possible if GI tract involved
Cervical cancer	Abnormal Pap smear
Protozoa/Parasites	
Cryptosporidium spp	Watery diarrhea, malabsorption, nausea, vomiting, abdominal pain, cholecystitis, pancreatitis
Pneumocystis carinii (PCP)	Pneumonia
Toxoplasmosis	Fever, headache, confusion
Entamoeba histolytica; Entamoeba coli; Giardia lamblia; Acanthamoeba	Diarrhea, nausea, vomiting, loss of appetite
Bacteria	
Mycobacterium avium complex (MAC)	Fever, diarrhea, malabsorption, anorexia
Legionella	Pneumonia
Salmonella	Fever, abdominal pain and cramping, diarrhea
Listeria	Diarrhea, abdominal pain, fever
Shigella	Bloody diarrhea, abdominal pain, fever
Fungi	
Candida albicans	Thrush, stomatitis, esophagitis
Cryptococcus	Meningitis, nausea, vomiting, fever, dementia
Aspergillosis	Pneumonia
Coccidioidomycosis	Pneumonia, fungemia
Histoplasmosis	Fever, pneumonia
Viruses	
Cytomegalovirus (CMV)	Dependent on site of infection—can involve entire GI tract with diarrhea, nausea, and vomiting
Herpes simplex	Painful blisters—symptoms dependent on site of infection

Compiled from Centers for Disease Control and Prevention: 1993 CDC HIV classification system and expanded AIDS surveillance definition for adolescents and adults, MMWR 41:RR-17, Dec. 18, 1992.

white blood cell count; and the clinical diagnosis of one of 25 AIDS-defining diseases.[20] The progression from HIV to AIDS varies for each individual and may not be evident for several years. The two major prognostic factors for HIV are the CD4 T cell count and the measurement of plasma HIV RNA (viral load for HIV).

HIV is a bloodborne and sexually transmitted infection. It is transmitted through contact with contaminated blood, semen, vaginal secretions, and breast milk. HIV also crosses the placenta from the mother to the baby. At the end of 2001, 40 million people worldwide were infected with HIV. Since the epidemic began, it is estimated that more than 60 million people have been infected. Infection in women and children has increased significantly. This is especially true in sub-Saharan Africa where AIDS is the leading cause of death.[21]

There has been significant progress for treatment of HIV and AIDS over the past decade with the use of highly active antiretroviral therapy (HAART). Up until the 1990s, treatment for HIV and AIDS focused on treatment with one or two drugs. Today, HAART uses combinations of nonnucleoside reverse transcriptase inhibitors and nucleoside analogue reverse transcriptase inhibitors with the newest class of drugs, protease inhibitors. Although there has been remarkable success in decreasing viral load with these new regimens, they have not been without complications. Adherence to these regimens is often difficult because of the number and the complexity of medications to be taken daily. Drug resistance develops easily if adherence is not maintained. Other side effects of these medications include nausea, vomiting, diarrhea, and other metabolic changes discussed later in this chapter.[22,23]

Malnutrition in HIV/AIDS

Malnutrition has been documented in all stages of HIV infection. Most nutritional problems coincide with the incidence of high viral loads, with opportunistic infections, and with the development of viral resistance. Now with the evolution of HAART, nutritional problems have shifted to include new issues such as hyperlipidemia, insulin resistance, and diabetes mellitus. It is important though to realize that much of the world does not have access to these medication regimens and that some people choose not to use these regimens. In these populations, malnutrition is still common.[21] Wasting syndrome has been included by the Centers for Disease Control and Prevention (CDC) in their classification for AIDS since 1987.[20] This classification defines wasting as an involuntary weight loss of greater than 10% in 1 month with the presence of chronic diarrhea, weakness, or fever for more than 30 days in the absence of a concurrent illness or condition.

The presence of malnutrition and weight loss is still considered an important predictor of both morbidity and mortality from the disease.[23,25] Malnutrition in HIV and AIDS is multifactorial, as shown in Figure 22-2. Altered nutrient intake, weight loss and body composition changes, physical impairment, endocrine disorders, metabolic changes, malabsorption, the presence of opportunistic infections, psychosocial issues, and economic conditions all contribute to the incidence of malnutrition (see Table 22-4).

wasting syndrome
an involuntary weight loss of more than 10% in 1 month with the presence of either chronic diarrhea, weakness, or fever for more than 30 days in the absence of a concurrent illness or condition

Altered Nutrient Intake

Anorexia or loss of appetite is a frequent symptom of altered nutrient intake. A client's lack of appetite may be caused by the HIV infection, the presence of opportunistic infections, fatigue, fever, or side effects of medications. Physical impairment from mucositis, esophagitis, pain, nausea, and vomiting affects the client's ability to ingest adequate nutrients. Depression, loneliness, fear, anxiety, or other psychosocial issues can play a significant role in the client's desire to eat. In addition, economic availability of adequate food supplies cannot be forgotten and often may be the most difficult problem to solve.

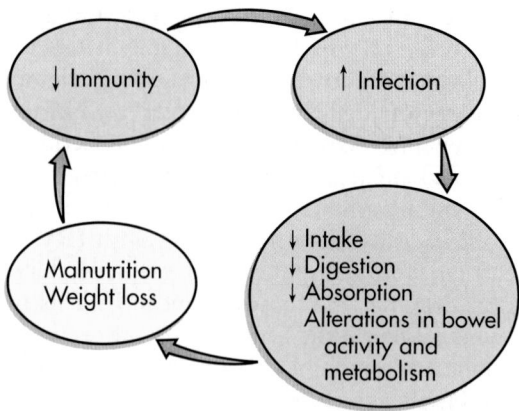

Figure 22-2 Vicious cycle of malnutrition and AIDS. (From Rolin Graphics.)

It is critical to begin interventions early. The first step should be education about the role of nutrition (see the Teaching Tool box). Nutrition should be considered a crucial element of medical care, not simply as alternative or adjunct therapy. Nutrition is one area in which clients can exert some control over their medical care. Emphasizing the benefits of maintaining nutritional status such as repair and building of tissue, preserving lean body mass and GI function, minimizing fatigue, and improving quality of life are all important components of this education.

The identification of the contributing factors to anorexia will then guide the client and practitioner in developing strategies to improve oral intake. Strategies for coping with loss of appetite are listed in Table 22-3.

Weight Loss and Body Composition Changes

Patients may experience weight loss and changes in body composition. As discussed previously, weight loss may occur from decreased nutrient intake from physical impairment or as a result of symptoms that impair appetite. Weight loss

---

 TEACHING TOOL
Maximizing Food Intake in HIV/AIDS

*C*lients dealing with the chronic effects of HIV/AIDS may have difficulty consuming enough kcalories to meet physiologic requirements. Home healthcare nurses can teach the following strategies to increase kcalories and protein without necessarily expanding the volume of food.
- Substitute kcalorie-containing and nutrient-dense foods and beverages for low- or no-kcalorie foods and beverages: milk or shakes instead of coffee or tea; regular soft drinks for sugar-free drinks.
- Increase the number or size of feedings daily. Offer five to six small meals/snacks.
- Fortify foods with kcalories and protein-containing ingredients. Add skim milk powder to milk, shakes, gravies, and hot cereals.
- Use kcalorie-containing condiments. Add butter/margarine to hot cereals, vegetables, and starches.
- Modify diet according to tolerances. Try cold or room-temperature foods, bland or salty foods; avoid greasy and sweet foods and liquids between meals.
- Add kcalorie-containing supplements as needed.

Reference: Fields-Gardner C, Thomson CA, Rhodes SS: A clinician's guide to nutrition in HIV and AIDS, Chicago, 1997, American Dietetic Association; American Dietetic Association: Manual of clinical dietetics, ed 6, Chicago, 2000, American Dietetic Association.

appears to not only occur from fat stores but also from lean body mass. This phenomenon is not as easily explained. Acute weight loss differs from chronic weight loss not only in its etiology but also in the type of energy stores that are depleted. Chronic weight loss, as seen in malnutrition, is often accompanied by a decrease in metabolic rate and a reliance on fat stores for energy. Acute weight loss, such as seen in stress, is accompanied by an increase in metabolic rate, a reliance on glucose as fuel, and a depletion of lean body mass. These changes in body composition and weight loss are commonly seen in the wasting syndrome and often coincide with increases in viral load.[22,23,25,26] Body composition changes have also been noted in lipodystrophy or the fat redistribution syndrome. These changes are discussed in detail later in this chapter.[27]

Medications are increasingly prescribed to assist with anorexia and body composition changes. Megestrol acetate (Megace),[28,29] dronabinol (Marinol), oxandrolone (Oxandrine), testosterone, dehydroepiandrosterone (DHEA), and human growth hormone (r-hGH) have all been used with this population. Dronabinol received approval from the Food and Drug Administration (FDA) in 1985 as an antiemetic for cancer patients and was approved for use as an appetite stimulant in 1992.[30-36] Studies have shown it offers improvement in appetite, mood, and nausea and has resulted in weight maintenance.[35,36] Side effects include euphoria, dizziness, and impaired thinking. The FDA initially approved oxandrolone, an oral analog of testosterone, in the 1960s. Clients have experienced an increase in lean body mass, mood elevation, and increased libido with the use of oxandrolone and with testosterone replacement.[34] Both DHEA and r-hGH have been used to increase lean body mass.[33]

Physical Impairment

Nausea, vomiting, mouth and esophageal lesions, and impaired dentition are all frequent problems for people with AIDS. These may be a result of opportunistic infections such as candidiasis and gingivitis or from side effects of antiretroviral therapy, prophylactic treatment to prevent opportunistic infections, and medication for the management of pain. Determining the causes of impaired intake is crucial to a successful intervention (see Table 22-3 for problem-solving techniques).

Endocrine and Metabolic Disorders

Hypogonadism has been identified in persons with HIV and AIDS.[37] This condition is associated with fatigue, decreased libido, loss of muscle mass, muscle weakness, impotence, and loss of body hair. The associated fatigue contributes not only to decreased appetite but also to impaired ability to prepare and consume meals. Loss of lean body mass is a prominent feature of the malnutrition and wasting syndrome of AIDS. Adrenal insufficiency may contribute to changes in appetite, loss of fuel storage, and changes in metabolism. It is unclear, though, whether any of these abnormalities are causal factors in the development of malnutrition in HIV.[37]

hypogonadism
a deficiency in the secretory activity of the ovary or testis

Fat redistribution syndrome (or lipodystrophy) has been described as a syndrome of both body composition changes and metabolic disturbances. Beginning in the late 1990s in some patients receiving antiretroviral therapy, shift in adiposity was noted. In many patients, this increase in abdominal obesity was accompanied by an increase in serum triglycerides, cholesterol, glucose, and an increase in insulin resistance. The etiology of this syndrome has not been clarified but has been associated with both protease inhibitors and nucleoside analogue therapy.[38-40]

Malabsorption

Malabsorption can be a result of (1) opportunistic infections that damage the GI tract, (2) the effects of malnutrition on villus height and enterocyte function, and (3) the disease itself. In those patients with HIV-related diarrhea, *steatorrhea* has been noted in clients without GI infections.[18,19,41] Additionally, other studies have documented abnormal D-xylose tests, which indicates the presence of malabsorption. A significant number of those subjects had diarrhea, and in almost half of those cases, no pathogen could be identified.[18,19,41]

Treatment of the underlying cause, if possible, is crucial in reversing the malnutrition caused by malabsorption. To assist with the control of malabsorptive symptoms and diarrhea, the restriction of fat and lactose is common.[18,19] The use of lactose-free supplements and those supplements containing medium-chain triglycerides such as Advera, Alitraq, Peptamen, or Lipisorb is frequently prescribed. Additionally, the use of both glutamine and arginine as part of enteral products or given separately as a supplement has been used to assist in this malabsorption syndrome and for the treatment of diarrhea.[42,43] Most information is anecdotal at this time. Careful attention must be taken to ensure adequate caloric and protein intake in the face of restricting these important calorie and protein sources. Additionally, fluid losses may be high with the presence of diarrhea. Prevention of dehydration and supplementation with vitamins and minerals are priority considerations as well.

Cycle of Malnutrition and Wasting

Malnutrition and wasting in patients with HIV and AIDS create a vicious cycle that can be fatal. It is unreasonable to expect that the treatment of malnutrition is simple when the causes are so complex. First, interventions must be integrated early. Research has shown promise concerning the efficacy of nutrition interventions. Conducting nutrition assessment and providing counseling have resulted in the ability of patients to maintain or gain weight.[18,44,45] Healthcare teams can treat the nutritional problems of HIV and AIDS by use of multiple and complementary modes of therapy (Box 22-1).

Box 22-1 Evaluation of Complementary and Alternative Therapies

Because currently there is no cure for cancer, HIV/AIDS, and chronic respiratory disease, patients are potential victims for unproven or fraudulent health and nutrition therapies. Complementary and alternative therapies are just beginning to be evaluated with long-term research studies. Until then, it is difficult to evaluate the efficacy of these treatments. For example, the yeast-free diet is commonly recommended to prevent fungal infections. This diet eliminates products containing yeast and simple sugars. Currently, there is no research to support these claims. High doses of vitamins and minerals can actually result in toxicities that potentially can be harmful. Complementary and alternative therapies may not only be extremely costly but they may also interfere with current medical treatments, putting the patient at even more risk. For example, microbial growth in herbal supplements may pose a risk of opportunistic infections in immunosuppressed patients.

Recently, the Office of Alternative Medicine (OAM) at the National Institutes of Health was organized to assist in providing the structure for the evaluation of complementary and alternative therapies. At Bastyr University in Seattle, the OAM has funded a new center for the study of HIV complementary and alternative therapies. Hopefully, in the near future we will have better sources of data to draw from to successfully provide patient recommendations.

Questionable practices or products may be reported to the following sources:

- FTC Bureau of Consumer Protection; regional FTC office; Chief Postal Inspector, US Postal Service; editor or station manager of media outlet where advertisement appeared; regional FDA office; state attorney general; state health department; local Better Business Bureau; Congressional representative; local or state professional society; local hospital (if practitioner is a staff member); state licensing board; local district attorney
- National Council Against Health Fraud (PO Box 1276, Loma Linda, CA 92340); Consumer Health Information Research Institute; local, state, or national professional or voluntary health groups

---

Compiled from Abrams D: Complementary and alternative therapies: treatment guidelines from the Journal of the American Medical Association; www.ama-assn.org/special/hiv/treatmnt/updates/alt.htm, accessed March 23, 2002; Fenton M, Silverman E: Medical nutrition therapy for human immunodeficiency virus infection and acquired immunodeficiency syndrome. In Mahan LK, Escott-Stump S, eds.: Krause's food, nutrition, and diet therapy, ed 10, Philadelphia, 2000, WB Saunders.

Nutrition Assessment

The initial step in assessing nutritional risk is to evaluate anthropometric data. Body weight compared with the client's usual body weight is much more crucial than comparison with ideal body weight. Any unexplained weight loss should be noted, but weight loss of greater than 10% in 6 months is considered to place the client at risk. Calculation of *body mass index (BMI)* also identifies nutrition risk. A calculated BMI of less than 18 is associated with malnutrition.

As discussed earlier, using only weight loss in the assessment may be misleading.[25,27] Loss of lean body mass is characteristic of the malnutrition of AIDS. Shifts in lean body mass can be noted, although weight may be initially maintained. *Bioelectrical impedance (BIA)* has been successfully used to evaluate changes in lean body mass.[46-48] If BIA is not available, a calculation of upper arm muscle area can be useful in providing a baseline measurement for which the client can be monitored over time.

Biochemical indices of serum albumin (Nl 3.5-5.0 g/dl) assess chronic losses from visceral protein stores, and prealbumin (Nl 20-50 mg/dl) can be used to monitor more acute changes. Other measures such as transferrin will not be applicable because of possible bone marrow suppression in this population.

Dietary assessment may be evaluated by 24-hour recall, food frequency, or food diary. Careful attention should be made to gut function, the presence of steatorrhea and diarrhea, and any other physical symptoms that might interfere with adequate oral intake.

Using multiple parameters will allow a more thorough evaluation of the patient's nutritional status and risk for protein-energy malnutrition. The Subjective Global Assessment tool (see Figure 22-1) would also serve as an excellent screening tool for HIV and AIDS patients to determine nutritional risk and to assess the need of referral to a registered dietitian.[11] Protocols outlining medical nutrition therapy for persons with HIV and AIDS have been established.[19]

Medical Nutrition Therapy

The following are the overall goals of nutrition management[18,19]:
- Preserve lean body mass and gut function
- Prevent development of malnutrition
- Provide adequate levels of all nutrients to maintain daily physical and mental functioning
- Minimize the symptoms of malabsorption
- Prevent nutrition-related immunosuppression
- Improve quality of life

HAART has shifted the focus of medical nutrition therapy to not only preventing malnutrition but also highlighting the need to address chronic nutrition problems, such as hyperlipidemia, hyperglycemia, and hypertension.

The objectives of the nutrition care plan need to be realistic and individualized. Interventions that are designed should be based on the nutritional assessment and the current medical treatment for that client. The first step in planning a client's medical nutrition therapy is to determine energy and protein requirements. Many clinicians use the Harris-Benedict equation to determine resting energy expenditure (REE). Using 1.3-1.5 × REE should meet most clients' energy requirements for maintenance and weight gain respectively. Protein requirements should be met with the range of 1.2-1.5 g protein/kg of actual body weight.

Vitamin and mineral status needs to be monitored closely in this population. Deficiencies may evolve not only from suppressed oral intake but also from the increased requirements for certain micronutrients. Research has studied the effects of supplementation with beta-carotene, vitamin C, vitamin E, selenium, and the amino acids glutamine and arginine but has not provided conclusive information from which to make global supplementation recommendations for the AIDS patient. It is routinely recommended, though, that persons with HIV and AIDS take a general multivitamin supplement that meets 100% of the recommended dietary allowance (RDA) for vitamins and minerals. In some individual situations, other supplements may be warranted.

Antiretroviral therapy requires specific nutrition recommendations. Many of the medications used to treat this condition result in symptoms such as nausea, vomiting, diarrhea, or anorexia that might impair oral intake. Even the number of pills that must be taken can be overwhelming to the patient. Additionally, the ingestion of food along with certain medications may affect the absorption of that drug or vice versa. Examples of these are shown below:[22]

- *Efavirenz (Sustiva):* Avoid taking with high-fat meals.
- *Lopinavir (Kaletra) + Ritonavir (Norvir):* Moderate fat meals increase availability of capsules. Should be taken with food.
- *Saquinavir (Invirase):* Take this protease inhibitor within 2 hours of a meal containing high-fat foods or a large snack containing carbohydrate, protein, or fat.
- *Ritonavir (Norvir):* If this protease inhibitor is consumed with a meal, it may decrease the abdominal cramping and diarrhea that is common when this drug is initially prescribed. These symptoms usually disappear within 8 weeks.
- *Indinavir (Crixivan):* This protease inhibitor should be taken on an empty stomach. A meal can be eaten 1 hour after the drug or 2 hours before the drug. For some, it may be necessary to eat a small snack with the drug, but fat should be avoided.

Prevention of Foodborne Illness

Prevention of foodborne illness is a crucial component of medical nutrition therapy and nutrition education for persons with HIV and AIDS. As CD4+ counts fall, clients are at higher risk for these infections from this source. Nutrition education should focus on safe methods for food purchasing, preparation, and storage. Often a low microbial diet is prescribed that recommends avoidance of undercooked meats and eggs, raw vegetables, and fruits.[18,19]

Cryptosporidium infections can be life threatening and lead to chronic, debilitating diarrhea. Infectious outbreaks have been linked to water sources. This protozoa is resistant to chlorination, and recent documentation of infections has led to recommendations for those persons with AIDS and HIV to monitor their water source.[29] Suggestions have been made to avoid all public tap water and to drink only filtered water or water that has been boiled for 1 minute. Fruits and vegetables can be cleaned with a mixture of 20 drops of 2% iodine in 1 gallon of water to prevent contamination.

Exercise Recommendations

Regular aerobic exercise and resistance training have been suggested to assist with lipid abnormalities, the fat redistribution syndrome, and other body composition changes noted in patients with HIV and AIDS. Recommendations should be individualized and initiated slowly after receiving a physician's approval. Benefits may include the following:

- Increased muscle volume, strength, functional capacity, and quality of life
- Decreased abdominal fat
- Prevention of glucose abnormalities and improved insulin sensitivity
- Improved circulation
- Improved bone metabolism[49]

Multidisciplinary Approach

Malnutrition and wasting associated with the HIV infection/AIDS are multifactorial. Many aspects are not well understood but that does not negate the fact that nutrition assessment, counseling, and support are critical components of the medical care for HIV and AIDS. Effective treatment requires a multidisciplinary approach based on collaboration of all healthcare team members including the nurse and dietitian. Early recognition and intervention for nutritional risk factors are keys to effective nutrition support and related medical therapies (see the Cultural Considerations box).

OTHER SPECIAL PROBLEMS

Disorders of the pulmonary system are classified into two categories. The first includes disorders that result in chronic long-term changes in respiratory function such as chronic obstructive pulmonary disease (COPD). COPD is a collective phrase for chronic bronchitis, asthma, and emphysema and is the second leading cause of disability in the United States.[50,51] The goal of medical nutrition therapy is to maintain respiratory muscle strength and function and to prevent or correct malnutrition. The second category includes disorders that cause acute changes in respiratory function such as respiratory distress syndrome (RDS) and acute respiratory failure (ARF). Patients who are critically ill, in shock, severely injured, or who have sepsis can develop these disorders.[50,51] For ARF and RDS, the function of medical nutrition therapy is to inhibit tissue destruction by providing the extra nutrients required for hypermetabolic conditions without contributing to declining respiratory function.

chronic obstructive pulmonary disease (COPD) a progressive and irreversible condition identified by obstruction of air flow; chronic bronchitis, asthma, and emphysema (also called *chronic obstructive lung disease*)

respiratory distress syndrome (RDS) a respiratory disorder identified by insufficient respiration and abnormally low levels of circulating oxygen in the blood

acute respiratory failure (ARF) sudden absence of respirations, with confusion or unresponsiveness caused by obstructed air flow or failure of the pulmonary gas exchange mechanism

sepsis systemic infection

Chronic Obstructive Pulmonary Disease

The energy required for breathing is something most of us often take for granted. Energy needs, however, become evident in patients with respiratory problems. Because of their weakened respiratory system, patients with advanced COPD expend

---

CULTURAL CONSIDERATIONS
AIDS, HIV, and Ethnic Issues of Healing and Medicine: Lessons from Tuskegee

As we attempt to heal those experiencing disorders such as AIDS and HIV, which are fairly "new" disorders, we need to understand history to fully comprehend the perspective of the patients with whom we work.

During the middle of the twentieth century (1932-1972), a medical study called the Tuskegee Experiment followed the course of syphilis among African American men from a poor county in Georgia. When the study began, there was no known cure for syphilis, but shortly into the study penicillin was recognized as an effective drug against the ravages of this sexually transmitted disease. Nonetheless, such treatment was withheld from the men participating in this study and most were followed to their death, which may or may not have been as a result of syphilis-related causes. The study did not end until the 1970s after the men, their wives, and their children were exposed and suffered the consequences of a serious systemic disease that could have been cured with inexpensive penicillin. Because this population was poor and African American, many view this as the reason such an unethical protocol was allowed to continue.

In 1973, a class-action lawsuit for the individuals and family members affected by the study was filed by the National Association for the Advancement of Colored People (NAACP). A $9 million settlement was awarded and distributed among those affected. In 1997 President Clinton issued a formal apology on behalf of the U.S. government.

Application to nursing: Today as we attempt to encourage and treat ethnic groups for AIDS and HIV, they may not be receptive to our treatments and medications because the shadow of deceit of the Tuskegee Experiment makes them leery of the healthcare system. Knowledge of the past treatment of subgroups provides us with an understanding of current bias toward accepting government-sponsored medical treatment. By understanding our history, we can educate about the ethical medical treatments available now.

Reference: Remembering Tuskegee: syphilis study still provokes disbelief, sadness; *www.npr.org/programs/morning/features/2002/jul/tuskegee/index.html, accessed July 25, 2002.*

a great deal of energy just breathing and, therefore, have an increased likelihood of malnutrition. It is common to see significant weight loss from both fat stores and muscle mass (Figure 22-3).[51] Muscle wasting is most evident in the diaphragm and respiratory muscles. Thus the presence of malnutrition contributes to the exacerbation of the clinical course.

Malnutrition of these individuals, as for those patients with AIDS and cancer, is multifactorial. Contributing factors include altered taste because of chronic mouth breathing and excessive sputum production, fatigue, anxiety, depression, increased energy requirements, frequent infections, and the side effects of multiple medications.

Medical Nutrition Therapy

Preventing malnutrition will not only help preserve muscle strength needed for respiratory function but will also maintain the integrity of the immune system. The first step in this prevention is to provide adequate nutrition. Unfortunately, COPD patients suffer from many of the same symptoms that inhibit adequate oral intake as those patients with cancer and AIDS. Anorexia, early satiety, nausea, and vomiting are all common. Box 22-2 discusses maximizing food intake in COPD. The same strategies as previously discussed are viable options for patients with COPD to assist in maximizing oral intake (Box 22-3).

Patients may require a range of 25 to 45 kcal/kg depending on whether they require maintenance kcalories or repletion (less than 90% ideal body weight) kcalories. Adequate but not excessive protein is known to stimulate the ventilatory drive. Patients may require 1.2 to 1.9 g protein/kg for maintenance and 1.6 to 2.5 g/kg of body weight for repletion.[50-54]

Providing nutrients in the proper combination is also important to reduce production of carbon dioxide and maintain respiratory function.[50,53,54] This is particularly

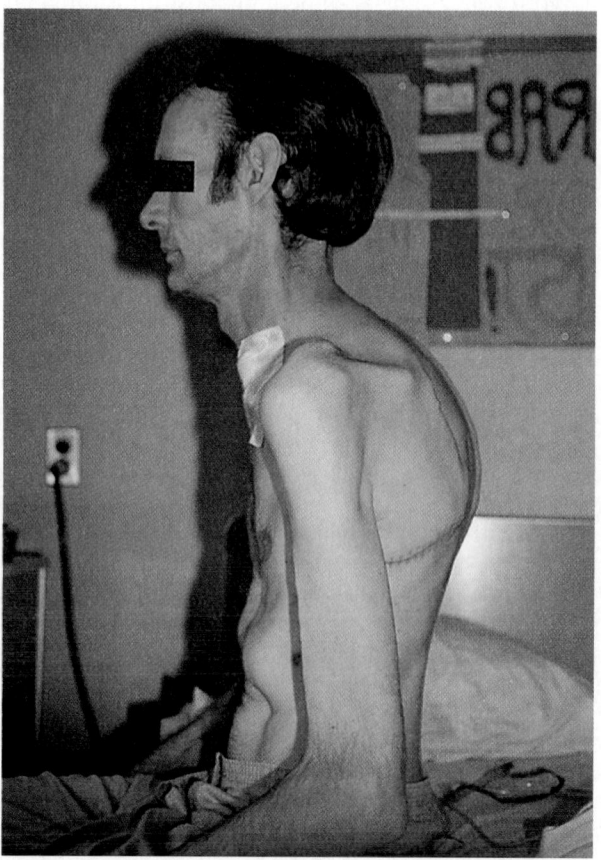

Figure 22-3 Patient with chronic obstructive pulmonary disease. (From Morgan SL, Weinsier RL: *Fundamentals of clinical nutrition,* ed 2, St Louis, 1998, Mosby.)

Box 22-2 Maximizing Food Intake in Chronic Obstructive Pulmonary Disease (COPD)

Although well-balanced, nutritionally sound meals are provided, it is sometimes difficult for patients with COPD to consume adequate amounts of nutrients, particularly in the home setting. Here are ideas to make meal times easier and more nutritious by increasing kcalorie and protein without increasing the amount of food eaten.

In clinical and home healthcare settings:
- Eat high-kcalorie foods first.
- Try more frequent meals and snacks.
- Increase kcalories by adding margarine, butter, mayonnaise, sauces, gravies, and peanut butter to foods.
- Limit liquids at meal times.
- Try cold foods, which can give a reduced sense of fullness than hot foods.
- Rest before meals.

In home healthcare settings:
- Keep favorite foods and snacks on hand.
- Keep ready-prepared meals available for periods of increased shortness of breath.
- Eat larger meals when you are not as tired.
- Avoid foods that you know cause gas.
- Add skim milk powder (2 tablespoons) to regular milk (8 oz) to add protein and kcalories.
- Use milk or half-and-half instead of water when making soups, cereals, instant puddings, cocoa, or canned soups.
- Add grated cheese to sauces, vegetables, soups, and casseroles.
- Choose dessert recipes that contain egg, such as sponge cake, angel food cake, egg custard, bread pudding, or rice pudding.

Box 22-3 Suggestions for Oral Feeding in Chronic Obstructive Pulmonary Disease (COPD)

- Suggest that patients consume small, frequent meals.
- Encourage patients to eat the most when well rested, such as the first meal of the day.
- Encourage the use of high-calorie, high-protein supplements.
- Teach patients to swallow as little air as possible when eating.
- Encourage the use of easily prepared or convenience foods to decrease any fatigue.

---

crucial for the ventilator-dependent patient. When each type of macronutrient is metabolized, carbon dioxide and water are produced. The respiratory quotient (RQ) is the ratio of carbon dioxide produced to the amount of oxygen consumed. Carbohydrate metabolism produces the greatest amount of carbon dioxide and therefore has the highest RQ. Fat metabolism produces the least amount of carbon dioxide and has the lowest RQ. An RQ greater than 1.0 is evidence of accumulating carbon dioxide, which makes respiration that much more difficult for a patient with COPD.[53,54] Nonprotein kcalories should be divided evenly between fat and carbohydrate.[53] The important issue is to provide adequate nutrition without overfeeding the patient. Overfeeding also produces an excessive amount of carbon dioxide and would be reflected in a RQ greater than 1.0.

respiratory quotient (RQ) ratio of CO_2 exhaled to O_2 inhaled; depending on the net metabolic needs of the body, the ratio ranges from 0.7 to 1.0 and averages around 0.8; carbohydrate metabolism produces an RQ = 1; protein metabolism RQ = 0.8; and fat metabolism RQ = 0.7

Acute Respiratory Failure and Respiratory Distress Syndrome

Almost half of all patients with acute respiratory failure suffer from malnutrition that impairs recovery and prolongs weaning from mechanical ventilation. A diet that minimizes carbon dioxide production while maintaining good nutrition is recommended.[54-56] Most patients in acute respiratory failure require mechanical ventilation so that in such cases, nutrition support may be provided via enteral or parenteral nutrition.

Medical Nutrition Therapy

Nutrition support should be initiated as soon as possible to help wean the patient from the ventilator[49-52] (see Box 14-2). Nutritional recommendations are similar to those for patients with COPD: high-kcalorie, high-protein, moderate to high (50% nonprotein kcalories) fat, with moderate (50% nonprotein kcalories) carbohydrate.

Enteral Nutrition.　Commercial formulas that provide 40% to 50% of total kcalories from fat are available. Higher caloric density formulas may be necessary when fluid is restricted in these patients. Low osmolality feedings are started slowly to avoid gastric retention or diarrhea. Continuous administration is recommended unless otherwise contraindicated.[50-54] Because these patients are at risk for aspiration, special precautions such as elevating the head of the bed or using a tube placed into the duodenum or jejunum are necessary.[50-54]

Parenteral Nutrition.　Parenteral nutrition may be needed in the treatment of acute respiratory failure. High glucose concentrations can lead to excess carbon dioxide production, making weaning from the ventilator more difficult; therefore this should be avoided.[49,52] The optimal parenteral solution should provide adequate protein to maintain nitrogen balance and 1 to 2 g of lipid per kg of body weight.[54-57] The remaining caloric needs can then be met by carbohydrate. It is additionally recommended to infuse nutrition support for these clients for 24 hours.

Monitoring nutrition support in the critically ill is best managed through a team approach. Using daily calorie counts, daily weights, and biochemical parameters is necessary to assess the response to nutrition support. Comparison of nutritional intake with indirect calorimetry provides useful guidance to monitor the adequacy of nutrition support.[52] Collaboration with clinical dietitians is best to monitor transition from parenteral to enteral feedings to conventional feeding.

Malnutrition and the method of refeeding have unequivocally been shown to influence the outcome in respiratory disease or respiratory failure.[52,55,57] Medical nutrition therapy is important to maintain or replenish nutritional status and can positively or negatively influence weaning from mechanical ventilation. Because a significant number of patients with respiratory disease or failure have clinically relevant malnutrition, nurses and other healthcare professionals should always be alert to alterations in nutritional status.

Summary

The disorders of cancer, acquired immunodeficiency syndrome (AIDS), and pulmonary disease are characterized by wasting and malnutrition, largely caused by the effect of the disorders or the secondary consequences of treatment on the GI tract. Medical nutrition therapy focuses on reducing these effects.

Local or systemic effects of the cancer combined with antineoplastic therapy place the patient with cancer at increased risk of developing malnutrition or cancer cachexia through a variety of mechanisms: anorexia, nausea, vomiting, mucositis, organ injury (toxicity), and learned food aversions. Nutrition support must be individualized and is an essential component of the total management of cancer. With the provision of adequate nutrition support, cancer patients may have a decreased risk of surgical complications. They will also have the nutrients needed to rebuild normal tissues that have been affected by antineoplastic therapy and have an increased tolerance to therapies. Overall, quality of life is enhanced.

AIDS, caused by the retrovirus human immunodeficiency virus (HIV), leads to the breakdown of the immune system, opportunistic infections, or enteropathy. Malnutrition, a common complication of HIV/AIDS, is multifactorial and includes decreased nutrient (food) intake, malabsorption, and altered metabolism. Goals of medical nutrition therapy are individualized, and interventions are based on nutritional status, causes of malnutrition, complications that affect nutritional status, and the ability to maintain health as long as possible. Early recognition and intervention for nutritional risk factors and indicators are keys to effective nutrition support and related medical therapies.

The two categories of pulmonary disorders cause either chronic changes in respiratory function, such as chronic obstructive pulmonary disease (COPD), or acute changes in respiratory function, such as respiratory distress syndrome (RDS) and acute respiratory failure (ARF). ARF and RDS may develop in patients who are critically ill, in shock, severely injured, or who have sepsis. The goal of medical nutrition therapy for COPD is to maintain respiratory muscle strength and function while preventing or treating existing malnutrition.

As pulmonary disorders progress, nutritional status tends to decline and malnutrition exacerbates declining respiratory muscle function and ventilatory drive. For ARF and RDS, the function of medical nutrition therapy is to inhibit tissue destruction by providing the extra nutrients required for hypermetabolic conditions. Malnutrition and the method of refeeding influence the outcome in respiratory disease or respiratory failure.

THE NURSING APPROACH
Case Study: Acquired Immunodeficiency Syndrome

Pete, age 35, has been HIV-positive for 10 years and is now suffering from AIDS. He has had multiple episodes of opportunistic infections and is currently being treated for mucositis, esophagitis, diarrhea, and wasting syndrome. In addition, Pete is taking medications, including ketoconazole (Nizoral) orally, which causes nausea and vomiting that further compromise nutritional status.

You see Pete in the clinic every 2 weeks. A dietitian also sees him every 2 weeks. On this visit, you complete the following assessment:

ASSESSMENT

Subjective
- Constant fatigue and anorexia
- Periodic lower abdominal pain (rated 3 on a pain-intensity scale from 1-10)
- Pain whenever chewing and swallowing (rated 7 on a pain-intensity scale from 1-10)

Objective
- Fluid intake: about 1200 ml/day
- Weight: 100 lbs (baseline weight 148 lbs; last visit 111 lbs)
- Height: 5'8"
- Oral and pharyngeal inflammation with scattered whitish/yellowish lesions
- Generalized muscle wasting
- Laboratory results:
  - Total serum protein: 5.1 (norm 6.6 to 7.9 g/dl; last visit 5.3 g/dl)
  - Serum albumin: 2.7 (norm 3.5 to 5.5 g/dl; last visit 3.0 g/dl)

NURSING DIAGNOSIS #1
Pain in mouth and throat related to inflammation of mucous membranes as evidenced by plaques and discomfort when eating

PLANNING

Goal
Client will experience a decrease in pain when chewing and swallowing.

IMPLEMENTATION
1. Eat cool or room-temperature foods.
2. Increase fluid intake from approximately 1200 ml to approximately 1800 ml.
3. Eat mechanically soft foods or foods with bland sauces.
4. Avoid highly seasoned foods.
5. Provide for mouth care for oral ulceration or infection (rinse with sodium bicarbonate with normal saline every 2 hours or several times/day).
6. For oral pain that interferes with the eating, suggest a prescription for analgesics. Viscous lidocaine may be necessary.
7. Encourage other methods for coping including use of distraction, prayer or other religious practices, and support from significant others.

Continued

THE NURSING APPROACH–cont'd
Case Study: Acquired Immunodeficiency Syndrome

EVALUATION

Client will state a decrease in pain experienced (on a pain intensity scale from 1-10) by the next office visit.

NURSING DIAGNOSIS #2

Altered nutrition, less than body requirements, related to diarrhea and wasting syndrome, as evidenced by weight loss and protein depletion.

PLANNING

Goal

Client will experience no further weight loss by the next office visit by eating a high-caloric diet and intake of adequate fluids.

IMPLEMENTATION

1. Eat frequent, small meals.
2. Eat favorite foods, especially foods that are high calorie, high protein, and low microbial.*
3. Drink a total of 200 ml of commercial nutritional supplement between meals.
4. Use high-caloric condiments such as butter and mayonnaise.
5. Take antidiarrheal medication prescribed by the physician.
6. Monitor intake and output and caloric count.

EVALUATION

Pete will maintain current weight and will not lose weigh by the next office visit in 2 weeks.

---

*Low-microbial diet: *any uncooked foods such as raw fruit and vegetables are eliminated because they contain a large number of microorganisms.*

CRITICAL THINKING
Clinical Applications   **?**

Minnie, age 20, is a college student with an uneventful medical history with no significant illness. After finals, she came down with the flu and has felt run-down ever since. She has also had a persistent low-grade fever and cough since the flu. With much insistence by her parents, she went to see her doctor for a physical. She was admitted to the hospital after her chest radiograph indicated a possible malignancy. Following a bone marrow biopsy, chest computerized tomography, magnetic resonance imaging, and biopsy of suspect lymph nodes, a diagnosis of non-Hodgkin's lymphoma with positive lymph nodes was made. Bone marrow, as well as other organs, indicated no presence of the disease. Minnie's physicians have determined a chemotherapy regimen using a combination of drugs to be given over 5 days every 4 weeks. Minnie complains of an overall lack of appetite, but she has no nausea, vomiting, constipation, or diarrhea. She is 5'6" tall and weighs 120 lbs on admission. Her usual weight is 130 lbs.

1. What are the possible causes of her decreased appetite?
2. What side effects from her chemotherapy might she encounter?
3. How will this affect her nutritional status?

From Marcia Nahikian-Nelms, PhD, RD.

Web Sites of Interest

American Institute for Cancer Research

www.aicr.org

This site provides excellent resources and reviews of research regarding nutrition and cancer prevention.

American Lung Association

www.lungsusa.org/

This site of the American Lung Association provides information on all aspects of lung health including asthma, air quality, and "diseases A to Z." It also includes local chapter programs and events and volunteer opportunities.

Center for AIDS Prevention Studies (CAPS)

www.caps.ucsf.edu/capsweb

CAPS is at the University of California-San Francisco. This site focuses on the prevention of HIV disease through a multidisciplinary approach and an applied and community-based approach. Fact sheets, research opportunities, prevention tools for developing and evaluating prevention programs, and other information are available.

HIV/AIDS Dietetic Practice Group

www.hivaidsdpg.org

This site is the official site for registered dietitians who provide care for patients with HIV and AIDS. There are excellent links for sites that provide information on HIV/AIDS and a list of caregivers and organizations that provide medical nutrition therapy and food outreach programs across the United States.

National Cancer Institute (NCI)

www.nci.nih.gov/ *or* www.cancer.gov

The site of the NCI, National Institutes of Health, delivers a wealth of information for health professionals, researchers, patients, and the public, especially through CancerNet. CancerNet provides information from NCI's cancer database (cancer treatment, screening, prevention, and active clinical trials), cancerTrials (clinical trials information center), and CANCERLIT (a bibliographic database).

References

1. Hansen M: *Pathophysiology: foundations of disease and clinical intervention,* Philadelphia, 1998, WB Saunders.
2. American Institute Cancer Research: *Food, nutrition and prevention of cancer;* www.aicr.org/report2.htm, accessed March 2002.
3. Tanaka T: Effect of diet on human carcinogenesis, *Critical Rev in Onc/Hem* 25:73, 1997.
4. Krenkel J, St Jeor S: Nutrition interventions for cancer prevention, *Topics in Clinical Nutrition* 9:1, 1993.
5. National Cancer Institute: *Cancer progress report 2001;* http://progressreport.cancer.gov, accessed March 2002.
6. National Cancer Institute: *Surveillance, epidemiology, and end results (SEER) program public-use data (1973-1998),* DCCPS, Surveillance Research Program, Cancer Statistics Branch, released April 2001, based on the August 2000 submission.
7. Frankmann C: Medical nutrition therapy for neoplastic disease. In Mahan LK, Escott-Stump S, eds.: *Krause's food, nutrition, and diet therapy,* ed 10, Philadelphia, 2000, WB Saunders.
8. Bloch AS, Charuhas PM: Cancer and cancer therapy. In Gottschlich M, ed.: *The science and practice of nutrition support,* Dubuque, Iowa, 2001, Kendall/Hunt.
9. Shils ME: Nutrition and diet in cancer management. In Shils ME et al., eds.: *Modern nutrition in health and disease,* ed 9, Philadelphia, 1999, Lippincott Williams & Wilkins.

10. Langer CJ, Hoffman JP, Ottery FD: Clinical significance of weight loss in cancer patients: Rationale for the use of anabolic agents in the treatment of cancer-related cachexia, *Nutrition* 17(suppl1):S1, 2001.

11. McCallum PD, Polisena CG, eds.: *The clinical guide to oncology nutrition*, Chicago, 2000, American Dietetic Association.

12. McCallum PD, Polisena CG, eds.: *Patient-generated subjective global assessment, training video*, Chicago, 2000, Oncology Nutrition Practice Group of the American Dietetic Association.

13. McMahon K, Decker G, Ottery FD: Integrating proactive nutritional assessment in clinical practices, *Semin Oncol* 25 (2suppl6):20, 1998.

14. American Dietetic Association: *Manual of clinical dietetics*, ed 6, Chicago, 2000, American Dietetic Association.

15. Society for Nutritional Oncology Adjuvant Therapy: Patient-generated subjective global assessment, *Nutritional Oncology* 1:8, 1994.

16. Nahikian-Nelms ML: General feeding problems. In Bloch A, ed.: *Nutrition management of the cancer patient*, Rockville, Md, 1990, Aspen.

17. Ottery FD: Supportive nutrition to prevent cachexia and improve quality of life, *Semin Oncol* 22(2suppl3):98, 1995.

18. Fields-Gardner C, Thomson CA, Rhodes SS: *A clinician's guide to nutrition in HIV and AIDS*, Chicago, 1997, American Dietetic Association.

19. Fenton M, Silverman E: Medical nutrition therapy for human immunodeficiency virus infection and acquired immunodeficiency syndrome. In Mahan LK, Escott-Stump S, eds.: *Krause's food, nutrition, and diet therapy*, ed 10, Philadelphia, 2000, WB Saunders.

20. Centers for Disease Control and Prevention: 1993 Revised CDC HIV classification system and expanded AIDS surveillance definition for adolescents and adults, *MMWR* 41:RR-17, Dec 18, 1992.

21. *Update 2001 and report on the global HIV/AIDS epidemic, Dec 2001*; www.unaids.org, accessed March 2002.

22. US Department of Health and Human Services: *Guidelines for the use of antiretroviral agents in HIV-infected adults and adolescents, Apr 2001*; www.medscape.com/govmt/DHHS/guidelines/HIV/pnt-HIV.html, accessed March 2002.

23. Batterham M, Brown D, Garsia R: Nutritional management of HIV/AIDS in the era of highly active antiretroviral therapy: a review, *Aust J Nutr Diet* 58: 211, 2001.

24. Wanke CA et al.: Weight loss and wasting remain common complications in individuals infected with human immunodeficiency virus in the era of highly active antiretroviral therapy, *Clin Infect Dis* 31:803, 2000

25. Wheeler DA et al.: Weight loss as a predictor of survival and disease progression in HIV infection, *J Acquir Immune Syndr Hum Retrovirol* 8:80, 1998.

26. Brown D, Batterham M: Nutritional management of HIV in the era of highly active antiretroviral therapy: a review of treatment strategies, *Aust J Nutr Diet* 58:224, 2001.

27. Gerrior J et al.: The fat redistribution syndrome in patients infected with HIV: measurements of body shape abnormalities, *J Am Diet Assoc* 101(10):1175, 2001.

28. Von Roenn JN et al.: Megesterol acetate in patients with AIDS-related cachexia, *Ann Intern Med* 121:393,1994.

29. Oster MH et al.: Megesterol acetate in patients with AIDS and cachexia, *Ann Intern Med* 121:400, 1994.

30. Struwe M et al.: Effect of dronabinol on nutritional status in HIV infection, *Ann Pharmacother* 27:827,1993.

31. Beal JE, et al.: Dronabinol as a treatment for anorexia associated with weight loss in patients with AIDS, *J Pain Sympt Manag* 10:89, 1995.

32. Fisher A, Abbaticola M: Effect of Oxandrolone on L-glutamine, on body weight, body cell mass, and body fat in patients with HIV infection—preliminary analysis, Second International Conference on Nutrition and HIV, Cannes, France, 1997.

33. Grinspoon S et al: Effects of androgen administration in men with the AIDS wasting syndrome: A randomized, double-blind, placebo controlled trial. *Ann Intern Med* 129:18, 1998.

34. Batterham MH, Garsia R: A comparison of nandrolone decanoate, megestrol acetate and dietary counseling for HIV associated weight loss, *Int J Androl* 24:232,2000.

35. Christeff N et al: Correlation between increased cortisone: DHEA ratio and malnutrition in HIV positive men, *Nutrition* 15:539, 1999.

36. Rabkin JG et al.: DHEA treatment for HIV+ patients: effects on mood, androgenic and anabolic parameters, *Psychoneuroendocrinology* 25:53, 2000.

37. Coodley GO et al.: Endocrine function in the wasting syndrome, *J AIDS* 7:46, 1994.

38. Chang ES et al.: The effects of antiretroviral protease inhibitors on serum lipid levels in HIV-infected patients, *J Am Dietetic Assoc* 101:687, 2001.

39. Gerrior J et al.: The fat redistribution syndrome in patients infected with HIV: measurements of body shape abnormalities. *J Am Dietetic Assoc* 101:1175, 2001.

40. Wanke C: Epidemiological and clinical aspects of the metabolic complications of HIV infection—the fat redistribution syndrome, *AIDS* 13:1287, 1999.

41. Ehrenpreis ED et al.: D-Xylose malabsorption: characteristic finding in patients with the AIDS wasting syndrome and chronic diarrhea, *J AIDS* 5:1047, 1992.

42. Keithley JK, Swanson B, Nerad J: HIV/AIDS. In Gottschlich M, ed.: *the science and practice of nutrition support*, Dubuque, Iowa, 2001, Kendall/Hunt.

43. Charney P: Enteral nutrition: indications, options, and formulations. In Gottschlich M, ed.: *The science and practice of nutrition support*, Dubuque, Iowa, 2001, Kendall/Hunt.

44. McKinley MJ et al.: Improved body weight status as a result of nutrition intervention in adult, HIV-positive outpatients, *J Am Dietetic Assoc* 94:1042, 1994.

45. Cimoch PJ: Nutrition health: prevention and treatment of HIV-associated malnutrition, *J Inter Ass Phys AIDS Care* 3:28, 1997.

46. Ott M et al.: Bioelectrical impedance analysis as a predictor of survival in patient with human immunodeficiency virus infection, *J AIDS* 9:20, 1995.

47. Fields-Gardner C: Using bioelectrical impedance analysis to evaluate and monitor HIV+ clients, *Positive Communication* 1:9, 1997.

48. Pebcharz PB et al.: Use of BIA measurements in the clinical management of malnutrition, *Am J Clin Nutr* 64:485S, 1995.

49. Detroyer MJ: Exercise recommendations for metabolic complications experienced with HIV/AIDS, *Positive Communication* 6:8, 2001.

50. Mueller DH: Medical nutrition therapy for pulmonary disease. In Mahan LK, Escott-Stump S, eds.: *Food, nutrition and diet therapy*, ed 10, Philadelphia, 2000, WB Saunders.

51. Confalonieri M, Rossi A: Burden of chronic obstructive pulmonary disease, *Lancet* 356:S56, 2000.

52. Schols AM: Nutrition and outcome in chronic respiratory disease, *Nutrition* 13:161, 1997.

53. Hogg JH, Klapholz A, Reid-Hector J: Pulmonary disease. In Gottschlich M, ed.: *The science and practice of nutrition support*, Dubuque, Iowa, 2001, Kendall/Hunt.

54. American Dietetic Association: Respiratory disease. In *Manual of clinical dietetics*, ed 6, Chicago, 2000, American Dietetic Association.

55. Thomsen C: Nutritional support in advanced pulmonary disease, *Respir Med* 9:249, 1997.

56. Barber JR, Miller SJ, Sacks G: Parenteral feeding formulations. In Gottschlich M, ed.: *The science and practice of nutrition support*, Dubuque, Iowa, 2001, Kendall/Hunt.

57. Matarese L: Metabolic complications of parenteral nutrition therapy. In Gottschlich M, ed.: *The science and practice of nutrition support*, Dubuque, Iowa, 2001, Kendall/Hunt.

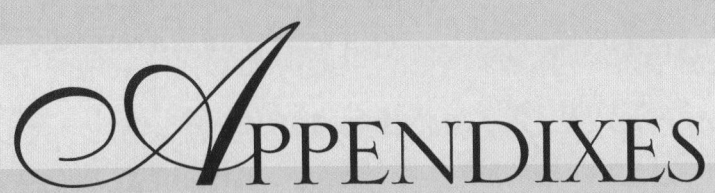

Appendixes

APPENDIX A

Food Composition Table

The following food composition table was developed by SureQuest Systems, Inc., and includes all of the foods listed in *Mosby's NutriTrac Nutrition Analysis CD-ROM, Version III*, which accompanies every copy of this text. Please note, however, that you can find some nutrient information in *Mosby's NutriTrac Nutrition Analysis CD-ROM* that is not listed here in the food composition table.

USDA ID Code / Food Name	Weight in Grams*	Quantity of Units	Unit of Measure	Protein (gm)	Fat (gm)	Carbohydrate (gm)	Kcalories	Caffeine (gm)	Fiber (gm)	Cholesterol (mg)	Saturated Fat (gm)
Baby Food											
Babyfood, Applesauce	170.0000	3.000	Ounce	0.00	0.00	17.51	62.90	0.00	2.89	0.00	0.00
Babyfood, Bananas w/ Tapioca	170.0000	3.000	Ounce	0.68	0.34	30.26	113.90	0.00	2.72	0.00	0.14
Babyfood, Barley, Ppd w/ Whole Milk	28.3500	3.000	Ounce	1.30	0.94	4.62	31.47	0.00	0.00	0.00	0.00
Babyfood, Beef	71.0000	3.000	Ounce	10.30	3.48	0.00	75.26	0.00	0.00	19.53	1.84
Babyfood, Beef and Rice	170.0000	3.000	Ounce	8.50	4.93	14.96	139.40	0.00	0.00	0.00	0.00
Babyfood, Beef Lasagna	170.0000	3.000	Ounce	7.14	3.57	17.00	130.90	0.00	0.00	0.00	0.00
Babyfood, Beef Noodle	170.0000	3.000	Ounce	4.25	3.23	12.58	96.90	0.00	1.87	13.60	1.31
Babyfood, Beef Stew	170.0000	3.000	Ounce	8.67	2.04	9.35	86.70	0.00	1.87	21.30	0.99
Babyfood, Beets	224.0000	1.000	Cup	2.91	0.22	17.25	76.16	0.00	4.26	0.00	0.04
Babyfood, Carrots	224.0000	1.000	Cup	1.79	0.45	16.13	71.68	0.00	3.81	0.00	0.09
Babyfood, Chicken	71.0000	3.000	Ounce	10.44	6.82	0.00	105.79	0.00	0.00	41.68	1.75
Babyfood, Chicken Noodle	170.0000	3.000	Ounce	4.03	2.01	14.94	93.50	0.00	1.53	15.30	0.58
Babyfood, Chicken Soup	229.0000	1.000	Cup	3.66	3.89	16.49	114.50	0.00	2.52	9.16	0.64
Babyfood, Chicken Sticks	71.0000	3.000	Ounce	10.37	10.22	0.99	133.48	0.00	0.14	55.38	2.90
Babyfood, Cookies, Arrowroot	28.3500	1.000	Ounce	2.15	4.05	20.19	125.31	0.00	0.06	0.30	0.94
Babyfood, Corn, Creamed	240.0000	1.000	Cup	3.36	0.96	39.12	156.00	0.00	5.04	2.40	0.17
Babyfood, Cottage Cheese w/ Fruit	28.3500	3.000	Ounce	0.85	0.20	4.51	22.11	0.00	0.00	0.00	0.00
Babyfood, Egg Yolks	28.3500	3.000	Ounce	2.84	4.90	0.28	57.55	0.00	0.00	208.37	1.47
Babyfood, Egg Yolks and Bacon	170.0000	3.000	Ounce	4.25	8.50	10.54	134.30	0.00	1.53	159.80	2.79
Babyfood, Fruit Dessert	170.0000	3.000	Ounce	0.51	0.00	29.24	107.10	0.00	1.02	0.00	0.00
Babyfood, Green Beans	240.0000	1.000	Cup	2.88	0.24	13.68	60.00	0.00	4.56	0.00	0.05
Babyfood, Ham	71.0000	3.000	Ounce	10.72	4.76	0.00	88.75	0.00	0.00	20.66	1.59
Babyfood, Juice, Apple	131.0000	4.200	Fl Oz	0.00	0.13	15.33	61.57	0.00	0.13	0.00	0.03
Babyfood, Juice, Mixed Fruit	127.0000	3.000	Ounce	0.13	0.13	14.73	59.69	0.00	0.13	0.00	0.03
Babyfood, Juice, Orange	127.0000	3.000	Ounce	0.76	0.38	12.95	55.88	0.00	0.13	0.00	0.05
Babyfood, Macaroni and Cheese	170.0000	3.000	Ounce	4.42	3.40	13.94	103.70	0.00	0.51	10.20	2.01
Babyfood, Macaroni and Tomato and Beef	170.0000	3.000	Ounce	4.25	1.87	15.98	100.30	0.00	1.87	6.80	0.70
Babyfood, Meat Sticks	71.0000	3.000	Ounce	9.51	10.37	0.78	130.64	0.00	0.14	49.70	4.13
Babyfood, Mixed Vegetable	170.0000	3.000	Ounce	1.70	0.00	13.43	56.10	0.00	0.00	0.00	0.00
Babyfood, Noodles and Chicken	170.0000	3.000	Ounce	2.89	3.74	15.47	108.80	0.00	1.87	0.00	0.00
Babyfood, Peach Cobbler	220.0000	3.000	Ounce	0.66	0.00	40.26	147.40	0.00	1.54	0.00	0.00
Babyfood, Peach Melba	28.3500	3.000	Ounce	0.09	0.00	4.65	17.01	0.00	0.00	0.00	0.00
Babyfood, Peaches w/ Sugar	170.0000	3.000	Ounce	0.85	0.34	32.13	120.70	0.00	2.55	0.00	0.03
Babyfood, Pears	170.0000	3.000	Ounce	0.51	0.17	19.72	73.10	0.00	6.12	0.00	0.02
Babyfood, Peas, Buttered	28.3500	3.000	Ounce	0.99	0.37	3.20	17.01	0.00	0.00	0.00	0.00

The easiest way to look for a food is to use the "Search For" feature in *Mosby's NutriTrac Nutrition Analysis CD-ROM*. However, if you do not have access to a computer or your computer time is limited, you can easily look for a food using this food composition table. The foods in the table are arranged alphabetically, within groups.

The code number before each food listing corresponds to the food data bank in *Mosby's NutriTrac Nutrition Analysis CD-ROM*. When you input your dietary intake into the CD-ROM program, you may choose to use these code numbers. Alternatively, you may choose to enter your dietary intake into *Mosby's NutriTrac Nutrition Analysis CD-ROM* by typing a food's name or partial name and using the "Search For" option.

Column heading key: *gm*, grams; *mg*, milligrams; *mcg*, micrograms; *re*, retinol equivalent.
*NOTE: The "Weight in Grams" column provides the weight in grams of the serving or of one unit of measure (e.g., if a serving is 3 oz, the "Weight in Grams" column may indicate the weight of 1 oz).

Monounsaturated Fat (gm)	Polyunsaturated Fat (gm)	Vitamin D (mg)	Vitamin K (mg)	Vitamin E (mg)	Vitamin A (re)	Vitamin C (mg)	Thiamin (mg)	Riboflavin (mg)	Niacin (mg)	Vitamin B6 (mg)	Folate (mcg)	Vitamin B12 (mcg)	Calcium (mg)	Iron (mg)	Magnesium (mg)	Phosphorus (mg)	Potassium (mg)	Sodium (mg)	Zinc (mg)
0.00	0.00	0.00	0.00	1.02	1.70	64.26	0.02	0.05	0.10	0.05	2.89	0.00	8.50	0.37	5.10	10.20	130.90	3.40	0.07
0.03	0.07	0.00	0.00	1.02	6.80	43.69	0.03	0.03	0.37	0.24	10.88	0.00	13.60	0.51	20.40	15.30	183.60	15.30	0.12
0.00	0.00	0.00	0.00	0.00	0.00	0.00	0.14	0.16	1.70	0.03	2.52	0.09	65.21	3.50	8.51	42.53	54.43	13.89	0.24
1.31	0.11	0.00	0.00	0.28	22.01	1.35	0.01	0.11	2.33	0.09	4.05	1.04	5.68	1.17	6.39	51.12	134.90	46.86	1.42
0.00	0.00	0.00	0.00	0.00	134.30	6.63	0.03	0.12	2.28	0.24	10.20	0.87	18.70	1.17	13.60	59.50	204.00	606.90	1.56
0.00	0.00	0.00	0.00	0.00	265.20	3.23	0.12	0.15	2.30	0.12	10.20	0.87	30.60	1.48	18.70	68.00	207.40	771.80	1.19
1.43	0.15	0.00	0.00	0.68	149.60	2.38	0.05	0.07	0.99	0.05	20.40	0.17	13.60	0.73	11.90	51.00	78.20	28.90	0.68
0.75	0.17	0.00	0.00	0.41	425.00	5.10	0.02	0.12	2.23	0.12	10.20	0.87	15.30	1.22	18.70	74.80	241.40	586.50	1.48
0.04	0.09	0.00	0.00	1.16	6.72	5.38	0.02	0.09	0.29	0.04	68.99	0.00	31.36	0.72	31.36	31.36	407.68	185.92	0.27
0.02	0.20	0.00	0.00	1.16	2645.44	12.32	0.04	0.09	1.12	0.18	38.75	0.00	51.52	0.87	24.64	44.80	452.48	109.76	0.40
3.07	1.65	0.00	0.00	0.28	8.52	1.07	0.01	0.11	2.43	0.13	7.88	0.28	39.05	0.70	7.81	63.90	86.62	36.21	0.72
0.80	0.46	0.00	0.00	0.31	294.10	0.17	0.05	0.07	1.19	0.09	11.90	0.02	35.70	0.65	11.90	134.30	66.30	132.60	0.68
0.98	2.06	0.00	0.00	0.55	393.88	2.29	0.05	0.07	0.66	0.09	11.91	0.27	84.73	0.62	11.45	54.96	151.14	36.64	0.50
4.45	2.12	0.00	0.00	0.28	2.13	1.21	0.01	0.14	1.43	0.07	7.88	0.28	9.94	1.11	9.94	85.91	75.26	340.09	0.72
2.55	0.24	0.00	0.00	0.00	0.00	1.56	0.14	0.12	1.63	0.01	9.92	0.02	9.07	0.85	6.24	32.89	44.23	104.90	0.15
0.29	0.43	0.00	0.00	1.25	19.20	5.28	0.02	0.12	1.20	0.10	30.48	0.05	43.20	0.65	19.20	79.20	194.40	124.80	0.55
0.00	0.00	0.00	0.00	0.17	0.57	6.75	0.00	0.01	0.01	0.00	1.45	0.02	8.79	0.04	1.13	11.06	11.91	14.46	0.05
1.96	0.64	0.00	0.00	0.22	106.60	0.40	0.02	0.08	0.01	0.05	26.11	0.44	21.55	0.78	1.98	81.36	21.83	11.06	0.54
3.76	1.09	0.00	0.00	0.46	47.60	1.53	0.09	0.14	0.46	0.05	6.97	0.15	47.60	0.80	8.50	85.00	59.50	81.60	0.46
0.00	0.00	0.00	0.00	0.39	40.80	5.10	0.03	0.02	0.24	0.05	5.95	0.00	15.30	0.36	8.50	13.60	161.50	22.10	0.09
0.00	0.12	0.00	0.00	1.25	103.20	20.16	0.05	0.24	0.77	0.10	78.48	0.00	156.00	2.59	52.80	45.60	307.20	4.80	0.46
2.26	0.65	0.00	0.00	0.28	7.10	1.49	0.10	0.13	2.02	0.14	1.49	0.07	3.55	0.72	7.81	63.19	149.10	47.57	1.21
0.00	0.04	0.00	0.00	0.79	2.62	75.85	0.01	0.03	0.10	0.04	0.13	0.00	5.24	0.75	3.93	6.55	119.21	3.93	0.04
0.01	0.05	0.00	0.00	0.25	5.08	80.77	0.03	0.01	0.15	0.05	8.51	0.00	10.16	0.43	6.35	6.35	128.27	5.08	0.04
0.06	0.08	0.00	0.00	0.76	7.62	79.38	0.06	0.04	0.30	0.06	33.53	0.00	15.24	0.22	11.43	13.97	233.68	1.27	0.08
0.90	0.22	0.00	0.00	0.41	5.10	2.21	0.10	0.10	0.94	0.03	18.70	0.05	86.70	0.51	11.90	100.30	74.80	129.20	0.54
0.77	0.14	0.00	0.00	0.41	185.30	2.55	0.09	0.10	1.28	0.09	15.30	0.41	23.80	0.61	11.90	74.80	122.40	28.90	0.61
4.60	1.13	0.00	0.00	0.28	14.91	1.70	0.04	0.12	1.05	0.06	6.32	0.21	24.14	0.98	7.81	73.13	80.94	388.37	1.35
0.00	0.00	0.00	0.00	0.00	414.80	5.61	0.02	0.03	0.70	0.14	11.39	0.00	28.90	0.53	17.00	37.40	190.40	15.30	0.41
0.00	0.00	0.00	0.00	0.00	221.00	1.36	0.07	0.07	1.16	0.03	5.78	0.15	44.20	0.83	18.70	56.10	100.30	44.20	0.54
0.00	0.00	0.00	0.00	0.51	30.80	45.10	0.02	0.04	0.57	0.02	2.42	0.00	8.80	0.22	4.40	13.20	123.20	19.80	0.07
0.00	0.00	0.00	0.00	0.00	5.67	7.37	0.00	0.01	0.09	0.00	0.54	0.00	3.12	0.09	0.57	1.42	26.37	2.55	0.08
0.12	0.15	0.00	0.00	1.02	30.60	32.13	0.02	0.05	1.11	0.03	6.63	0.00	8.50	0.46	8.50	18.70	263.50	8.50	0.10
0.03	0.03	0.00	0.00	1.02	5.10	37.40	0.02	0.02	0.32	0.02	6.46	0.00	13.60	0.43	15.30	20.40	195.50	3.40	0.14
0.00	0.00	0.00	0.00	0.00	11.62	3.60	0.02	0.02	0.39	0.00	10.26	0.00	12.76	0.29	0.00	0.00	33.17	1.42	0.00

USDA ID Code	Food Name	Weight in Grams*	Quantity of Units	Unit of Measure	Protein (gm)	Fat (gm)	Carbohydrate (gm)	Kcalories	Caffeine (gm)	Fiber (gm)	Cholesterol (mg)	Saturated Fat (gm)
	Babyfood, Plums w/ Tapioca	170.0000	3.000	Ounce	0.17	0.00	34.68	125.80	0.00	2.04	0.00	0.00
	Babyfood, Rice, Ppd w/ Whole Mil	28.3500	1.000	Ounce	1.11	1.02	4.73	32.60	0.00	0.02	3.21	0.66
	Babyfood, Rice, w/ Mixed Fruit	170.0000	3.000	Ounce	1.53	0.34	31.11	134.30	0.00	1.02	0.00	0.10
	Babyfood, Spaghetti and Tomato a	170.0000	3.000	Ounce	4.37	2.33	19.41	115.60	0.00	1.87	8.50	0.92
	Babyfood, Spinach, Creamed	28.3500	3.000	Ounce	0.85	0.40	1.81	11.91	0.00	0.51	0.00	0.00
	Babyfood, Split Pea and Ham	28.3500	3.000	Ounce	0.94	0.37	3.20	20.13	0.00	0.31	0.00	0.00
	Babyfood, Squash	224.0000	1.000	Cup	1.79	0.45	12.54	53.76	0.00	4.70	0.00	0.09
	Babyfood, Sweet potatoes	224.0000	1.000	Cup	2.46	0.22	31.14	134.40	0.00	3.36	0.00	0.04
	Babyfood, Teething Biscuits	28.3500	1.000	Ounce	3.03	1.19	21.66	111.13	0.00	0.40	0.00	0.43
	Babyfood, Tropical Fruit	113.0000	3.000	Ounce	0.23	0.00	18.53	67.80	0.00	0.00	0.00	0.00
	Babyfood, Turkey	71.0000	3.000	Ounce	10.93	5.04	0.00	91.59	0.00	0.00	37.70	1.64
	Babyfood, Turkey and Rice	170.0000	3.000	Ounce	4.03	1.56	16.27	95.20	0.00	1.70	6.80	0.41
	Babyfood, Turkey Sticks	71.0000	3.000	Ounce	9.73	10.08	0.99	129.22	0.00	0.36	46.15	2.94

Baked Goods

USDA ID Code	Food Name	Weight in Grams*	Quantity of Units	Unit of Measure	Protein (gm)	Fat (gm)	Carbohydrate (gm)	Kcalories	Caffeine (gm)	Fiber (gm)	Cholesterol (mg)	Saturated Fat (gm)
	Bagels, Blueberry	56.7000	1.000	Each	5.96	0.90	30.28	155.92	0.00	1.30	0.00	0.12
	Bagels, Cinnamon-raisin	56.7000	1.000	Each	5.56	0.96	31.30	155.36	0.00	1.30	0.00	0.16
	Bagels, Cinnamon-raisin, Toasted	56.7000	1.000	Each	6.02	1.02	33.62	166.70	0.00	1.42	0.00	0.18
	Bagels, Egg	56.7000	1.000	Each	6.02	1.20	30.06	157.62	0.00	1.30	13.60	0.24
	Bagels, Egg, Toasted	66.0000	1.000	Each	7.52	1.45	37.62	197.34	0.00	0.00	17.16	0.30
	Bagels, Oat Bran	56.7000	1.000	Each	6.06	0.68	30.22	144.58	0.00	2.04	0.00	0.10
	Bagels, Oat Bran, Toasted	66.0000	1.000	Each	7.59	0.86	37.82	180.84	0.00	0.00	0.00	0.14
	Bagels, Plain	56.7000	1.000	Each	5.96	0.90	30.28	155.92	0.00	1.30	0.00	0.12
	Bagels, Plain, Toasted	66.0000	1.000	Each	7.46	1.12	37.95	194.70	0.00	0.00	0.00	0.16
	Biscuits, Plain or Buttermilk	56.7000	1.000	Each	7.04	9.36	27.50	206.38	0.00	0.74	0.56	1.42
	Cake, Angelfood	28.3500	1.000	Slice	1.67	0.23	16.39	73.14	0.00	0.43	0.00	0.03
	Cake, Boston Cream Pie	28.3500	1.000	Slice	0.68	2.41	12.16	71.44	0.00	0.40	10.49	0.69
	Cake, Carrot, w/ Cream Cheese Frosting	111.0000	1.000	Slice	5.11	29.30	52.39	483.96	0.00	0.00	59.94	5.43
	Cake, Chocolate w/ Chocolate Fro	28.3500	1.000	Slice	1.16	4.65	15.48	104.04	0.00	0.79	11.91	1.35
124	Cake, Chocolate, Double, Layer-S	79.0000	1.000	Piece	3.00	13.00	33.00	260.00	0.00	2.00	25.00	11.00
125	Cake, Chocolate, German, Layer-S	83.0000	1.000	Piece	4.00	15.00	34.00	280.00	0.00	2.00	30.00	11.00
126	Cake, Coconut Layer-Sara Lee	81.0000	1.000	Piece	3.00	14.00	34.00	280.00	0.00	2.00	30.00	12.00
	Cake, Fruitcake	28.3500	1.000	Slice	0.82	2.58	17.46	91.85	0.00	1.05	1.42	0.30
127	Cake, Fudge Golden Layer-Sara Le	80.0000	1.000	Piece	3.00	13.00	34.00	270.00	0.00	1.00	25.00	11.00
	Cake, German Chocolate, w/ Frost	111.0000	1.000	Slice	3.89	20.65	55.17	404.04	0.00	0.00	53.28	5.26
	Cake, Gingerbread	67.0000	1.000	Slice	2.68	6.83	33.97	207.03	0.00	2.14	23.45	1.74
	Cake, Pineapple Upside-down	28.3500	1.000	Slice	0.99	3.43	14.32	90.44	0.00	0.23	6.24	0.83
	Cake, Pound	30.0000	1.000	Slice	1.65	5.97	14.64	116.40	0.00	0.15	66.30	3.47
128	Cake, Pound, All Butter, Family	76.0000	1.000	Piece	4.00	17.00	36.00	310.00	0.00	0.50	75.00	9.00
129	Cake, Pound, All Butter-Sara Lee	76.0000	1.000	Piece	4.00	16.00	38.00	320.00	0.00	0.50	85.00	9.00
130	Cake, Pound, Chocolate Swirl-Sar	83.0000	1.000	Piece	5.00	16.00	42.00	330.00	0.00	0.50	75.00	8.00
131	Cake, Pound, Reduced, Fat-Sara L	76.0000	1.000	Piece	4.00	11.00	42.00	280.00	0.00	1.00	65.00	3.00
132	Cake, Pound, Strawberry Swirl-Sa	83.0000	1.000	Piece	4.00	11.00	44.00	290.00	0.00	0.50	60.00	3.00
	Cake, Sponge	28.3500	1.000	Slice	1.53	0.77	17.32	81.93	0.00	0.16	28.92	0.23
133	Cake, Vanilla Layer-Sara Lee	80.0000	1.000	Piece	2.00	13.00	31.00	250.00	0.00	0.00	35.00	10.00
	Cake, White, w/ Coconut Frosting	28.3500	1.000	Slice	1.25	2.92	17.92	100.93	0.00	0.28	0.28	1.11
134	Cake, White, w/o Frosting	74.0000	1.000	Slice	4.00	9.18	42.33	264.18	0.00	0.00	1.48	2.42
	Cake, Yellow, w/ Chocolate Frost	28.3500	1.000	Slice	1.08	4.93	15.71	107.45	0.00	0.51	15.59	1.32
	Cake, Yellow, w/ Vanilla Frostin	28.3500	1.000	Slice	0.99	4.11	16.67	105.75	0.00	0.09	15.59	0.67
169	Cheesecake, 25% Reduced Fat, Crm	120.0000	1.000	Piece	9.00	13.00	40.00	310.00	0.00	2.00	70.00	8.00
170	Cheesecake, Cherry Cream-Sara Le	135.0000	1.000	Piece	6.00	12.00	55.00	350.00	0.00	2.00	35.00	5.00
171	Cheesecake, Chocolate Chip-Sara	120.0000	1.000	Piece	8.00	21.00	47.00	410.00	0.00	2.00	65.00	14.00
	Cheesecake, Commercially Prepare	28.3500	1.000	Slice	1.56	6.38	7.23	91.00	0.00	0.12	15.59	2.81
172	Cheesecake, French-Sara Lee	111.0000	1.000	Piece	5.00	21.00	24.00	350.00	0.00	1.00	20.00	13.00
	Cheesecake, Homemade	85.0000	1.000	Slice	0.50	22.10	21.42	303.45	0.00	0.00	102.85	12.21

Monounsaturated Fat (gm)	Polyunsaturated Fat (gm)	Vitamin D (mg)	Vitamin K (mg)	Vitamin E (mg)	Vitamin A (re)	Vitamin C (mg)	Thiamin (mg)	Riboflavin (mg)	Niacin (mg)	Vitamin B6 (mg)	Folate (mg)	Vitamin B12 (mcg)	Calcium (mg)	Iron (mg)	Magnesium (mg)	Phosphorus (mg)	Potassium (mg)	Sodium (mg)	Zinc (mg)
0.00	0.00	0.00	0.00	1.02	15.30	1.36	0.02	0.05	0.36	0.05	1.53	0.00	10.20	0.37	6.80	10.20	141.10	13.60	0.14
0.00	0.00	0.00	0.00	0.00	7.35	0.34	0.13	0.14	1.48	0.03	2.32	0.09	67.76	3.46	12.76	49.61	53.87	13.04	0.18
0.07	0.09	0.00	0.00	0.12	3.40	15.81	0.22	0.27	3.60	0.19	1.70	0.03	27.20	4.42	8.50	35.70	85.00	17.00	0.24
0.85	0.32	0.00	0.00	0.12	214.20	0.34	0.09	0.12	1.65	0.10	45.90	0.05	25.50	0.90	18.70	59.50	207.40	127.50	0.90
0.00	0.00	0.00	0.00	0.15	104.33	1.02	0.01	0.02	0.07	0.02	19.50	0.02	32.04	0.40	17.86	13.89	64.65	15.59	0.10
0.00	0.00	0.00	0.00	0.07	22.68	0.54	0.01	0.01	0.14	0.01	3.69	0.01	6.52	0.14	13.89	38.56	3.97		0.18
0.04	0.18	0.00	0.00	1.16	450.24	17.47	0.02	0.16	0.85	0.16	34.50	0.01	53.76	0.78	26.88	35.84	414.40	2.24	0.18
0.00	0.09	0.00	0.00	1.16	1487.36	21.50	0.07	0.07	0.85	0.25	23.07	0.00	35.84	0.87	26.88	53.76	544.32	49.28	0.25
0.41	0.24	0.00	0.00	0.12	3.40	2.58	0.07	0.15	1.23	0.03	13.89	0.02	74.56	1.01	9.92	46.49	91.57	102.63	0.26
0.00	0.00	0.00	0.00	0.00	2.26	21.24	0.01	0.03	0.09	0.03	3.73	0.00	11.30	0.29	5.65	9.04	65.54	7.91	0.06
1.87	1.25	0.00	0.00	0.28	7.10	1.70	0.01	0.18	2.47	0.12	8.59	0.76	19.88	0.96	8.52	67.45	127.80	51.12	1.28
0.51	0.39	0.00	0.00	0.27	319.60	0.51	0.05	0.07	1.17	0.09	13.60	0.03	40.80	0.70	15.30	62.90	146.20	136.00	0.80
3.32	2.57	0.00	0.00	0.28	4.26	1.07	0.01	0.11	1.24	0.06	8.02	0.71	51.12	0.88	11.36	73.13	64.61	342.93	1.30
0.08	0.40	0.00	0.00	0.02	0.00	0.00	0.30	0.18	2.58	0.02	49.90	0.00	41.96	2.02	16.44	54.44	57.26	302.78	0.50
0.10	0.38	0.00	0.00	0.08	0.00	0.40	0.22	0.16	1.74	0.04	51.04	0.00	10.78	2.16	15.88	56.70	83.92	182.58	0.64
0.10	0.40	0.00	0.00	0.10	3.96	0.34	0.18	0.16	1.68	0.04	43.66	0.00	11.34	2.32	13.04	47.06	92.42	196.18	0.46
0.24	0.36	0.00	0.00	0.00	18.72	0.34	0.30	0.14	1.96	0.06	49.90	0.10	7.38	2.26	14.18	47.62	38.56	286.34	0.44
0.30	0.46	0.00	0.00	0.00	21.12	0.33	0.30	0.15	2.20	0.06	11.22	0.11	9.24	2.82	17.82	59.40	48.18	358.38	0.55
0.14	0.28	0.00	0.00	0.08	0.00	0.12	0.18	0.20	1.68	0.02	45.92	0.00	6.80	1.74	17.58	62.38	65.20	287.46	0.52
0.18	0.35	0.00	0.00	0.00	0.00	0.07	0.19	0.22	1.89	0.13	23.10	0.00	8.58	2.18	40.92	116.82	144.54	359.70	1.48
0.08	0.40	0.00	0.00	0.02	0.00	0.00	0.30	0.18	2.58	0.02	49.90	0.00	41.96	2.02	16.44	54.44	57.26	302.78	0.50
0.09	0.49	0.00	0.00	0.00	0.00	0.00	0.31	0.20	2.91	0.03	11.22	0.00	12.54	2.52	20.46	67.98	71.94	378.84	0.62
3.92	3.52	0.00	0.00	1.66	0.56	0.00	0.24	0.16	1.90	0.02	33.46	0.08	27.78	1.88	9.64	243.82	127.00	596.48	0.28
0.02	0.10	0.00	0.00	0.00	0.00	0.00	0.03	0.14	0.25	0.01	9.92	0.02	39.69	0.15	3.40	9.07	26.37	212.34	0.02
1.29	0.29	0.00	0.00	0.30	6.52	0.06	0.12	0.08	0.05	0.01	4.25	0.05	6.52	0.11	1.70	13.89	11.06	40.82	0.05
7.24	15.10	0.00	0.00	0.00	426.24	1.22	0.15	0.17	1.13	0.08	13.32	0.11	27.75	1.39	19.98	78.81	124.32	273.06	0.54
2.48	0.52	0.00	0.00	0.00	7.09	0.03	0.01	0.04	0.16	0.01	4.82	0.04	12.19	0.62	9.64	34.59	56.70	94.69	0.20
0.00	0.00	0.00	0.00	0.00	20.00	0.00	0.00	0.00	0.00	0.00	0.00	0.00	40.00	1.00	0.00	0.00	0.00	180.00	0.00
0.00	0.00	0.00	0.00	0.00	20.00	0.00	0.00	0.00	0.00	0.00	0.00	0.00	40.00	0.70	0.00	0.00	0.00	160.00	0.00
0.00	0.00	0.00	0.00	0.00	0.00	0.00	0.00	0.00	0.00	0.00	0.00	0.00	40.00	1.00	0.00	0.00	0.00	170.00	0.00
1.19	0.94	0.00	0.00	0.47	1.13	0.14	0.01	0.03	0.22	0.01	5.39	0.00	9.36	0.59	4.54	14.74	43.38	76.55	0.08
0.00	0.00	0.00	0.00	0.00	20.00	0.00	0.00	0.00	0.00	0.00	0.00	0.00	40.00	0.50	0.00	0.00	0.00	130.00	0.00
8.71	5.46	0.00	0.00	0.00	23.31	0.00	0.11	0.14	1.10	0.02	4.44	0.10	53.28	1.22	18.87	173.16	150.96	368.52	0.49
3.75	0.90	0.00	0.00	0.00	10.72	0.07	0.13	0.12	1.05	0.03	6.70	0.05	46.23	2.22	10.72	112.56	161.47	306.86	0.27
1.47	0.93	0.00	0.00	0.38	18.43	0.34	0.04	0.05	0.34	0.01	7.37	0.02	34.02	0.42	3.69	23.25	31.75	90.44	0.09
1.77	0.32	0.00	0.00	0.00	46.80	0.00	0.04	0.07	0.39	0.01	12.30	0.08	10.50	0.41	3.30	41.10	35.70	119.40	0.14
0.00	0.00	0.00	0.00	0.00	80.00	0.00	0.00	0.00	0.00	0.00	0.00	0.00	20.00	1.20	0.00	0.00	0.00	310.00	0.00
0.00	0.00	0.00	0.00	0.00	80.00	0.00	0.00	0.00	0.00	0.00	0.00	0.00	20.00	0.70	0.00	0.00	0.00	280.00	0.00
0.00	0.00	0.00	0.00	0.00	40.00	0.00	0.00	0.00	0.00	0.00	0.00	0.00	60.00	1.20	0.00	0.00	0.00	350.00	0.00
0.00	0.00	0.00	0.00	0.00	60.00	0.00	0.00	0.00	0.00	0.00	0.00	0.00	20.00	1.00	0.00	0.00	0.00	350.00	0.00
0.00	0.00	0.00	0.00	0.00	20.00	0.00	0.00	0.00	0.00	0.00	0.00	0.00	40.00	0.70	0.00	0.00	0.00	140.00	0.00
0.27	0.13	0.00	0.00	0.08	13.04	0.00	0.07	0.08	0.55	0.01	11.06	0.07	19.85	0.77	3.12	38.84	28.07	69.17	0.14
0.00	0.00	0.00	0.00	0.00	0.00	0.00	0.00	0.00	0.00	0.00	0.00	0.00	20.00	0.50	0.00	0.00	0.00	140.00	0.00
1.05	0.61	0.00	0.00	0.20	3.12	0.03	0.04	0.05	0.30	0.01	6.24	0.02	25.52	0.33	3.40	19.85	28.07	80.51	0.09
3.93	2.33	0.00	0.00	0.00	11.84	0.15	0.14	0.18	1.13	0.02	5.18	0.06	96.20	1.12	8.88	68.82	70.30	241.98	0.24
2.72	0.60	0.00	0.00	0.64	9.36	0.00	0.03	0.05	0.35	0.01	6.24	0.05	10.49	0.59	8.51	45.64	50.46	95.54	0.18
1.73	1.46	0.00	0.00	0.00	5.39	0.00	0.03	0.02	0.14	0.01	7.65	0.04	17.58	0.30	1.70	40.54	15.03	97.52	0.07
0.00	0.00	0.00	0.00	0.00	60.00	0.00	0.00	0.00	0.00	0.00	0.00	0.00	100.00	1.00	0.00	0.00	0.00	310.00	0.00
0.00	0.00	0.00	0.00	0.00	20.00	15.00	0.00	0.16	0.00	0.00	0.00	0.00	40.00	0.70	0.00	0.00	0.00	320.00	0.00
0.00	0.00	0.00	0.00	0.00	60.00	1.20	0.00	0.00	0.00	0.00	0.00	0.00	60.00	1.20	0.00	0.00	0.00	300.00	0.00
2.45	0.45	0.00	0.00	0.45	41.39	0.11	0.01	0.05	0.06	0.01	5.10	0.05	14.46	0.18	3.12	26.37	25.52	58.68	0.14
0.00	0.00	0.00	0.00	0.00	20.00	1.20	0.00	0.00	0.00	0.00	0.00	0.00	40.00	0.50	0.00	0.00	0.00	280.00	0.00
6.87	1.75	0.00	0.00	0.00	272.85	0.34	0.03	0.18	0.34	0.04	10.20	0.21	49.30	1.06	6.80	81.60	86.70	240.55	0.47

USDA ID Code	Food Name	Weight in Grams*	Quantity of Units	Unit of Measure	Protein (gm)	Fat (gm)	Carbohydrate (gm)	Kcalories	Caffeine (gm)	Fiber (gm)	Cholesterol (mg)	Saturated Fat (gm)
	Cheesecake, No-bake Type	28.3500	1.000	Slice	1.56	3.60	10.06	77.68	0.00	0.54	8.22	1.90
173	Cheesecake, Original Cream-Sara	121.0000	1.000	Piece	7.00	18.00	39.00	350.00	0.00	1.00	50.00	9.00
	Cheesecake, Plain, w/ Cherry Top	90.0000	1.000	Slice	4.50	16.65	23.85	258.30	0.00	0.00	76.50	9.11
174	Cheesecake, Strawberry Cream-Sar	135.0000	1.000	Piece	6.00	12.00	49.00	330.00	0.00	2.00	40.00	5.00
175	Cheesecake, Strawberry French-Sa	123.0000	1.000	Piece	4.00	14.00	43.00	320.00	0.00	1.00	20.00	9.00
	Coffeecake	28.3500	1.000	Slice	1.93	6.61	13.24	118.50	0.00	0.57	9.07	1.64
198	Coffeecake, Butter Streusel-Sara	54.0000	1.000	Piece	4.00	12.00	25.00	220.00	0.00	0.50	35.00	6.00
	Coffeecake, Cheese	28.3500	1.000	Slice	1.98	4.31	12.56	96.11	0.00	0.28	24.10	1.53
199	Coffeecake, Cheese, Reduced Fat,	54.0000	1.000	Piece	3.00	6.00	28.00	180.00	0.00	0.50	20.00	1.50
200	Coffeecake, Crumb-Sara Lee	57.0000	1.000	Piece	3.00	9.00	32.00	220.00	0.00	0.50	15.00	1.50
	Coffeecake, Fruit	28.3500	1.000	Slice	1.47	2.89	14.60	88.17	0.00	0.71	1.98	0.71
201	Coffeecake, Pecan-Sara Lee	54.0000	1.000	Piece	4.00	12.00	24.00	230.00	0.00	0.50	25.00	4.50
202	Coffeecake, Raspberry-Sara Lee	54.0000	1.000	Piece	3.00	8.00	27.00	220.00	0.00	0.50	15.00	2.50
	Cream Puffs, Shell, w/ Custard F	28.3500	1.000	Each	1.90	4.39	6.49	73.14	0.00	0.11	37.99	1.04
	Crisp, Apple	282.0000	1.000	Cup	5.08	10.15	91.09	459.66	0.00	0.00	0.00	2.03
	Croissant, Apple	28.3500	1.000	Ounce	2.10	2.47	10.52	72.01	0.00	0.71	8.79	1.41
	Croissant, Butter	28.3500	1.000	Ounce	2.32	5.95	12.98	115.10	0.00	0.74	18.99	3.31
	Croissant, Cheese	28.3500	1.000	Ounce	2.61	5.93	13.32	117.37	0.00	0.74	16.16	3.01
	Croissant, Chocolate	56.0000	1.000	Medium	5.21	14.07	25.15	234.61	0.00	2.20	38.00	8.07
218	Croissants, Petite-Sara Lee	57.0000	2.000	Each	6.00	11.00	26.00	230.00	0.00	1.00	3.00	4.00
219	Croissants, Sara Lee	43.0000	1.000	Each	4.00	8.00	20.00	170.00	0.00	1.00	4.00	3.00
	Danish Pastry, Cheese	28.3500	1.000	Small	2.27	6.21	10.55	106.03	0.00	0.27	4.54	1.92
	Danish Pastry, Cinnamon	28.3500	1.000	Small	1.98	6.35	12.64	114.25	0.00	0.37	5.95	1.61
	Danish Pastry, Fruit	28.3500	1.000	Small	1.53	5.24	13.55	105.18	0.00	0.54	32.32	1.38
	Danish Pastry, Lemon	28.3500	1.000	Small	1.53	5.24	13.55	105.18	0.00	0.54	11.34	0.80
	Danish Pastry, Nut	28.3500	1.000	Small	2.01	7.14	12.96	121.91	0.00	0.57	13.04	1.65
	Danish Pastry, Raspberry	28.3500	1.000	Small	1.53	5.24	13.55	105.18	0.00	0.54	11.34	0.80
	Doughnuts, Chocolate, Sugared or	28.3500	1.000	Each	1.28	5.64	16.27	118.22	0.28	0.62	16.16	1.45
	Doughnuts, French Crullers, Glaz	28.3500	1.000	Each	0.88	5.19	16.87	116.80	0.00	0.34	3.12	1.32
	Doughnuts, Glazed	28.3500	1.000	Each	1.81	6.46	12.56	114.25	0.00	0.34	1.70	1.65
	Doughnuts, Plain	28.3500	1.000	Each	1.42	6.49	14.09	119.35	0.00	0.43	10.49	1.03
	Doughnuts, Plain, Chocolate-coat	28.3500	1.000	Each	1.42	8.79	13.61	134.38	0.57	0.57	17.29	2.30
	Doughnuts, Plain, Sugared or Gla	28.3500	1.000	Each	1.47	6.49	14.40	120.77	0.00	0.43	9.07	1.68
	Doughnuts, w/ Creme Filling	28.3500	1.000	Each	1.81	6.95	8.51	102.34	0.00	0.22	6.80	1.54
	Doughnuts, w/ Jelly Filling	28.3500	1.000	Each	1.67	5.30	11.06	96.39	0.00	0.24	7.37	1.37
	Doughnuts, Whole Wheat, Sugared	28.3500	1.000	Each	1.79	5.47	12.08	102.06	0.00	0.63	5.67	0.86
	Eclairs, Custard-filled w/ Choco	28.3500	1.000	Small	1.81	4.45	6.86	74.28	0.57	0.17	36.00	1.17
612	Mousse, Chocolate-Sara Lee	122.0000	1.000	Piece	5.00	25.00	37.00	400.00	0.00	2.00	30.00	20.00
	Muffins, Banana Nut	95.0000	1.000	Each	6.00	12.00	53.00	340.00	0.00	2.00	35.00	0.90
	Muffins, Blueberry	28.3500	1.000	Small	1.56	1.84	13.61	78.53	0.00	0.74	8.51	0.40
	Muffins, Corn	28.3500	1.000	Small	1.67	2.38	14.43	86.47	0.00	0.96	7.37	0.38
	Muffins, Oat Bran	28.3500	1.000	Small	1.98	2.10	13.69	76.55	0.00	1.30	0.00	0.31
	Muffins, Plain	28.3500	1.000	Small	1.96	3.23	11.74	83.92	0.00	0.77	11.06	0.61
	Muffins, Wheat Bran	65.0000	1.000	Large	4.62	7.93	27.24	183.95	0.00	0.00	21.45	1.47
	Pie, Apple	28.3500	1.000	Small Sl	0.68	3.54	10.52	75.13	0.00	0.00	0.00	0.86
641	Pie, Apple, 45% Reduced Fat-Sara	128.0000	1.000	Slice	4.00	8.00	51.00	290.00	0.00	2.00	4.00	1.50
642	Pie, Apple, Dutch, Homestyle-Sar	131.0000	1.000	Slice	3.00	15.00	53.00	350.00	0.00	2.00	0.00	3.00
643	Pie, Apple, Homestyle-Sara Lee	131.0000	1.000	Slice	3.00	16.00	46.00	340.00	0.00	1.00	0.00	3.50
	Pie, Banana Cream	28.3500	1.000	Small Sl	1.25	3.86	9.33	76.26	0.00	0.20	14.46	1.07
	Pie, Blueberry	28.3500	1.000	Small Sl	0.51	2.84	9.89	65.77	0.00	0.29	0.00	0.48
644	Pie, Blueberry, Homestyle-Sara L	131.0000	1.000	Slice	3.50	15.00	54.00	360.00	0.00	2.00	0.00	3.50
	Pie, Butterscotch Pudding	127.0000	1.000	Slice	5.97	18.16	42.29	354.33	0.00	0.00	77.47	5.09
	Pie, Cherry	28.3500	1.000	Small Sl	0.57	3.12	11.28	73.71	0.00	0.23	0.00	0.73
	Pie, Cherry, Fast Food	28.3500	1.000	Small	0.85	4.56	12.08	89.59	0.00	0.74	0.00	0.70
645	Pie, Cherry, Homestyle-Sara Lee	131.0000	1.000	Slice	3.00	16.00	42.00	320.00	0.00	2.00	0.00	3.50

Monounsaturated Fat (gm)	Polyunsaturated Fat (gm)	Vitamin D (mg)	Vitamin K (mg)	Vitamin E (mg)	Vitamin A (re)	Vitamin C (mg)	Thiamin (mg)	Riboflavin (mg)	Niacin (mg)	Vitamin B6 (mg)	Folate (mg)	Vitamin B12 (mcg)	Calcium (mg)	Iron (mg)	Magnesium (mg)	Phosphorus (mg)	Potassium (mg)	Sodium (mg)	Zinc (mg)
1.28	0.23	0.00	0.00	0.00	28.07	0.14	0.03	0.07	0.14	0.01	8.51	0.09	48.76	0.13	5.39	66.34	59.82	107.73	0.13
0.00	0.00	0.00	0.00	0.00	20.00	0.00	0.00	0.00	0.00	0.00	0.00	0.00	80.00	0.50	0.00	0.00	0.00	320.00	0.00
5.21	1.38	0.00	0.00	0.00	216.90	0.63	0.03	0.14	0.32	0.04	9.00	0.15	38.70	1.11	6.30	63.90	83.70	182.70	0.36
0.00	0.00	0.00	0.00	0.00	0.00	18.00	0.00	0.00	0.00	0.00	0.00	0.00	40.00	0.70	0.00	0.00	0.00	320.00	0.00
0.00	0.00	0.00	0.00	0.00	0.00	12.00	0.00	0.00	0.00	0.00	0.00	0.00	40.00	0.50	0.00	0.00	0.00	230.00	0.00
3.68	0.88	0.00	0.00	0.97	9.36	0.09	0.06	0.07	0.48	0.01	17.29	0.05	15.31	0.54	6.24	30.62	34.87	99.51	0.23
0.00	0.00	0.00	0.00	0.00	60.00	0.00	0.00	0.00	0.00	0.00	0.00	0.00	20.00	0.50	0.00	0.00	0.00	240.00	0.00
2.02	0.47	0.00	0.00	0.44	24.66	0.03	0.03	0.04	0.19	0.02	11.06	0.10	16.73	0.18	4.25	28.63	81.93	96.11	0.17
0.00	0.00	0.00	0.00	0.00	0.00	0.00	0.00	0.00	0.00	0.00	0.00	0.00	40.00	0.50	0.00	0.00	0.00	230.00	0.00
0.00	0.00	0.00	0.00	0.00	0.00	0.00	0.00	0.00	0.00	0.00	0.00	0.00	20.00	0.50	0.00	0.00	0.00	210.00	0.00
1.58	0.42	0.00	0.00	0.24	5.67	0.23	0.01	0.05	0.73	0.01	13.32	0.01	12.76	0.69	4.82	33.45	25.52	109.15	0.18
0.00	0.00	0.00	0.00	0.00	20.00	0.00	0.00	0.00	0.00	0.00	0.00	0.00	20.00	0.70	0.00	0.00	0.00	170.00	0.00
0.00	0.00	0.00	0.00	0.00	0.00	0.00	0.00	0.00	0.00	0.00	0.00	0.00	0.00	0.50	0.00	0.00	0.00	220.00	0.00
1.85	1.18	0.00	0.00	0.63	56.42	0.09	0.03	0.08	0.24	0.02	7.94	0.10	18.71	0.33	3.40	30.90	32.60	96.67	0.17
4.31	2.99	0.00	0.00	0.00	87.42	6.49	0.24	0.20	2.19	0.12	14.10	0.00	78.96	2.12	19.74	70.50	273.54	513.24	0.45
0.68	0.18	0.00	0.00	0.00	27.78	0.14	0.07	0.05	0.45	0.01	16.16	0.06	8.51	0.31	3.69	16.44	25.52	77.68	0.29
1.57	0.31	0.00	0.00	0.12	52.73	0.06	0.11	0.07	0.62	0.02	17.58	0.05	10.49	0.58	4.54	29.77	33.45	210.92	0.21
1.85	0.67	0.00	0.00	0.29	55.85	0.06	0.15	0.09	0.61	0.02	20.98	0.09	15.03	0.61	6.80	36.86	37.42	157.34	0.27
3.31	0.89	0.00	0.00	0.00	76.41	0.11	0.22	0.15	1.22	0.02	16.11	0.16	23.89	1.18	10.89	63.20	69.69	376.34	0.43
0.00	0.00	0.00	0.00	0.00	40.00	0.00	0.00	0.00	0.00	0.00	0.00	0.00	40.00	1.00	0.00	0.00	0.00	200.00	0.00
0.00	0.00	0.00	0.00	0.00	40.00	0.00	0.00	0.00	0.00	0.00	0.00	0.00	20.00	0.70	0.00	0.00	0.00	200.00	0.00
3.21	0.73	0.00	0.00	0.72	12.76	0.03	0.05	0.07	0.57	0.01	17.01	0.05	9.92	0.45	4.25	30.62	27.78	127.58	0.20
3.55	0.83	0.00	0.00	0.84	0.85	0.03	0.09	0.07	0.81	0.01	17.58	0.03	20.13	0.56	5.39	30.33	35.44	105.18	0.20
2.84	0.67	0.00	0.00	0.70	6.24	1.11	0.07	0.06	0.56	0.01	9.36	0.03	13.04	0.50	4.25	25.23	23.53	100.36	0.15
1.68	0.43	0.00	0.00	0.42	15.03	1.11	0.02	0.03	0.22	0.01	4.54	0.03	13.04	0.21	4.25	25.23	23.53	100.36	0.15
3.88	1.21	0.00	0.00	1.03	3.97	0.48	0.06	0.07	0.65	0.03	23.53	0.06	26.65	0.51	9.07	31.19	26.93	102.91	0.25
1.68	0.43	0.00	0.00	0.42	17.01	1.11	0.02	0.03	0.22	0.01	4.54	0.03	13.04	0.21	4.25	25.23	23.53	100.36	0.15
3.20	0.70	0.00	0.00	0.76	3.12	0.03	0.01	0.02	0.13	0.01	10.77	0.03	60.39	0.64	9.64	45.93	30.05	96.39	0.16
2.96	0.65	0.00	0.00	0.70	0.85	0.00	0.05	0.07	0.60	0.01	9.92	0.01	7.37	0.69	3.40	34.87	22.11	97.81	0.07
3.65	0.82	0.00	0.00	0.87	1.13	0.03	0.10	0.06	0.81	0.02	12.19	0.03	12.19	0.58	6.24	26.37	30.62	96.96	0.22
2.64	2.23	0.00	0.00	1.09	4.82	0.06	0.06	0.07	0.52	0.02	13.32	0.08	12.47	0.55	5.67	76.26	36.00	154.79	0.16
4.96	1.07	0.00	0.00	1.18	3.12	0.06	0.04	0.03	0.37	0.01	8.22	0.07	9.92	0.70	11.34	57.27	55.57	121.62	0.17
3.60	0.82	0.00	0.00	0.00	0.85	0.03	0.07	0.06	0.43	0.01	13.04	0.07	17.01	0.30	4.82	33.17	28.92	113.97	0.12
3.42	0.87	0.00	0.00	0.78	5.39	0.00	0.10	0.04	0.64	0.02	18.14	0.04	7.09	0.52	5.67	21.55	22.68	87.60	0.23
2.90	0.67	0.00	0.00	0.70	4.54	0.00	0.09	0.04	0.61	0.03	17.58	0.06	7.09	0.50	5.67	24.10	22.40	83.07	0.21
2.30	2.01	0.00	0.00	1.02	4.25	0.06	0.06	0.07	0.52	0.03	5.67	0.05	13.89	0.31	6.24	29.48	41.96	100.64	0.19
1.84	1.12	0.00	0.00	0.60	54.15	0.09	0.03	0.08	0.23	0.02	7.94	0.10	17.86	0.33	4.25	30.33	33.17	95.54	0.17
0.00	0.00	0.00	0.00	0.00	40.00	0.00	0.00	0.00	0.00	0.00	0.00	0.00	60.00	1.20	0.00	0.00	0.00	190.00	0.00
1.50	2.40	0.00	0.00	0.00	21.00	0.03	0.18	0.12	0.04	0.01	13.20	0.00	44.00	1.01	16.10	108.20	371.00	210.00	0.20
0.56	0.71	0.00	0.00	0.30	2.55	0.31	0.04	0.03	0.31	0.01	12.76	0.16	16.16	0.46	4.54	55.85	34.87	126.72	0.14
0.60	0.91	0.00	0.00	0.52	10.21	0.00	0.08	0.09	0.58	0.02	17.58	0.03	20.98	0.80	9.07	80.51	19.56	147.70	0.15
0.48	1.17	0.00	0.00	0.37	0.00	0.00	0.07	0.03	0.12	0.05	14.74	0.00	17.86	1.19	44.51	106.60	143.73	111.42	0.52
0.78	1.62	0.00	0.00	0.00	11.34	0.09	0.08	0.09	0.65	0.01	14.46	0.04	56.70	0.68	4.82	43.38	34.30	132.39	0.16
1.91	4.09	0.00	0.00	0.00	162.50	5.07	0.22	0.29	2.62	0.21	33.80	0.09	121.55	2.72	50.70	185.25	206.70	382.20	1.79
1.53	0.95	0.00	0.00	0.00	3.40	0.48	0.04	0.03	0.35	0.01	6.80	0.09	1.98	0.32	1.98	7.94	22.40	59.82	0.05
0.00	0.00	0.00	0.00	0.00	0.00	0.00	0.00	0.00	0.00	0.00	0.00	0.00	20.00	1.20	0.00	0.00	0.00	400.00	0.00
0.00	0.00	0.00	0.00	0.00	0.00	0.00	1.20	0.00	0.00	0.00	0.00	0.00	0.00	1.00	0.00	0.00	0.00	350.00	0.00
0.00	0.00	0.00	0.00	0.00	0.00	0.00	1.20	0.00	0.00	0.00	0.00	0.00	0.00	0.70	0.00	0.00	0.00	310.00	0.00
1.62	0.93	0.00	0.00	0.42	19.85	0.45	0.04	0.06	0.30	0.04	7.65	0.07	21.26	0.29	4.54	26.08	46.78	68.04	0.14
1.20	1.00	0.00	0.00	0.57	9.64	0.77	0.00	0.01	0.09	0.01	6.24	0.00	2.27	0.09	1.42	6.52	14.18	92.14	0.05
0.00	0.00	0.00	0.00	0.00	0.00	2.40	0.00	0.00	0.00	0.00	0.00	0.00	0.00	0.70	0.00	0.00	0.00	340.00	0.00
7.64	4.35	0.00	0.00	0.00	106.68	0.64	0.18	0.27	1.26	0.07	13.97	0.38	128.27	1.64	21.59	134.62	220.98	335.28	0.69
1.66	0.58	0.00	0.00	0.43	15.31	0.26	0.01	0.01	0.06	0.01	6.24	0.00	3.40	0.14	2.27	8.22	22.96	69.74	0.05
2.11	1.53	0.00	0.00	0.00	4.82	0.37	0.04	0.03	0.41	0.01	5.10	0.02	6.24	0.35	2.84	12.19	18.43	106.03	0.07
0.00	0.00	0.00	0.00	0.00	80.00	0.00	0.00	0.00	0.00	0.00	0.00	0.00	0.00	0.70	0.00	0.00	0.00	290.00	0.00

USDA ID Code	Food Name	Weight in Grams*	Quantity of Units	Unit of Measure	Protein (gm)	Fat (gm)	Carbohydrate (gm)	Kcalories	Caffeine (gm)	Fiber (gm)	Cholesterol (mg)	Saturated Fat (gm)
	Pie, Chocolate Creme	28.3500	1.000	Small Sl	0.74	5.50	9.53	86.18	0.00	0.57	1.42	1.41
	Pie, Chocolate Mousse	28.3500	1.000	Small Sl	0.99	4.37	8.39	73.71	0.28	0.00	9.92	2.32
646	Pie, Chocolate Silk Supreme-Sara	136.0000	1.000	Slice	4.00	32.00	49.00	500.00	0.00	2.00	4.00	16.00
647	Pie, Coconut Cream-Sara Lee	136.0000	1.000	Slice	4.00	31.00	47.00	480.00	0.00	2.00	0.00	14.00
	Pie, Coconut Creme	28.3500	1.000	Small Sl	0.60	4.71	10.55	84.48	0.00	0.37	0.00	1.98
	Pie, Coconut Custard	28.3500	1.000	Small Sl	1.67	3.74	8.56	73.71	0.00	0.51	9.92	1.66
	Pie, Egg Custard	28.3500	1.000	Small Sl	1.56	3.29	5.90	59.54	0.00	0.45	9.36	0.67
	Pie, Fruit, Fried	28.3500	1.000	Small Sl	0.85	4.56	12.08	89.59	0.00	0.74	0.00	0.70
	Pie, Lemon Meringue	28.3500	1.000	Small Sl	0.43	2.47	13.38	75.98	0.00	0.34	12.76	0.50
648	Pie, Lemon Meringue-Sara Lee	142.0000	1.000	Slice	2.00	11.00	59.00	350.00	0.00	5.00	0.00	2.50
	Pie, Lemon, Fried	28.3500	1.000	Small	0.85	4.56	12.08	89.59	0.00	0.74	0.00	0.70
	Pie, Mince Meat	28.3500	1.000	Small Sl	0.74	3.06	13.61	81.93	0.00	0.74	0.00	0.76
649	Pie, Mince, Homestyle-Sara Lee	131.0000	1.000	Slice	3.00	17.00	56.00	390.00	0.00	3.00	0.00	4.00
650	Pie, Peach, Homestyle-Sara Lee	131.0000	1.000	Slice	3.00	14.00	46.00	320.00	0.00	2.00	0.00	3.00
	Pie, Pecan	28.3500	1.000	Small Sl	1.13	5.24	16.22	113.40	0.00	0.99	9.07	1.01
651	Pie, Pecan, Homestyle-Sara Lee	121.0000	1.000	Slice	5.00	24.00	70.00	520.00	0.00	3.00	45.00	4.50
	Pie, Pumpkin	28.3500	1.000	Small Sl	1.11	2.69	7.74	59.54	0.00	0.77	5.67	0.51
652	Pie, Pumpkin, Homestyle-Sara Lee	131.0000	1.000	Slice	4.00	11.00	37.00	260.00	0.00	2.00	30.00	2.50
653	Pie, Raspberry, Homestyle-Sara L	131.0000	1.000	Slice	3.00	19.00	48.00	380.00	0.00	2.00	4.00	4.50
	Pie, Vanilla Creme	28.3500	1.000	Small Sl	1.36	4.08	9.24	78.81	0.00	0.17	17.58	1.14
696	Shortcake, Strawberry-Sara Lee	71.0000	1.000	Piece	2.00	7.00	27.00	180.00	0.00	0.50	15.00	5.00
	Strudel, Apple	28.3500	1.000	Small	0.94	3.18	11.65	77.68	0.00	0.62	1.70	0.58
	Sweet Rolls w/ Raisins and Nuts	57.0000	1.000	Each	3.76	7.30	29.58	196.08	0.00	0.00	13.11	1.35
	Sweet Rolls, Cheese	28.3500	1.000	Small	2.01	5.19	12.39	102.06	0.00	0.34	21.55	1.72
	Sweet Rolls, Cinnamon w/ Raisins	28.3500	1.000	Small	1.76	4.65	14.43	105.46	0.00	0.68	18.71	0.87
729	Sweet Rolls, Cinnamon, Deluxe-Sa	76.0000	1.000	Roll	5.00	15.00	41.00	370.00	0.00	1.00	40.00	9.00

Beverages

USDA ID Code	Food Name	Weight in Grams*	Quantity of Units	Unit of Measure	Protein (gm)	Fat (gm)	Carbohydrate (gm)	Kcalories	Caffeine (gm)	Fiber (gm)	Cholesterol (mg)	Saturated Fat (gm)
	Beef Broth and Tomato Juice, Cnd	168.0000	5.500	Fl Oz	1.01	0.17	14.28	62.16	0.00	0.17	0.00	0.05
	Beer, Dark	29.5000	12.000	Fl Oz	0.09	0.00	1.10	12.18	0.00	0.06	0.00	0.00
	Beer, Killians	29.5000	12.000	Fl Oz	0.09	0.00	1.10	12.18	0.00	0.06	0.00	0.00
	Beer, Light	354.0000	12.000	Fl Oz	0.71	0.00	4.60	99.12	0.00	0.00	0.00	0.00
	Beer, Regular	356.0000	12.000	Fl Oz	1.07	0.00	13.17	145.96	0.00	0.71	0.00	0.00
	Beverage, Strawberry Flavor	266.0000	1.000	Cup	7.98	8.25	32.72	234.08	0.00	0.00	31.92	5.08
	Bloody Mary	29.7000	1.000	Fl Oz	0.15	0.03	0.98	23.17	0.00	0.00	0.00	0.00
	Choc Mix, Hot, No Sugar-Swiss M	20.0000	1.000	Packet	3.00	1.50	13.00	70.00	4.00	0.00	0.00	0.00
	Choc Mix, Hot, No Sugar, Fat Fre	15.0000	1.000	Packet	4.00	0.00	9.00	50.00	4.00	0.00	0.00	0.00
	Coffee, Brewed	237.0000	1.000	Cup	0.24	0.00	0.95	4.74	137.46	0.00	0.00	0.00
	Coffee, Brewed, Decaf.	29.6000	6.000	Fl Oz	0.03	0.00	0.12	0.59	0.18	0.00	0.00	0.00
	Coffee, Instant, Cappuccino Flav	29.3000	6.000	Fl Oz	0.06	0.32	1.64	9.38	12.16	0.00	0.00	0.28
	Coffee, Instant, Decaffeinated	179.0000	6.000	Fl Oz	0.18	0.00	0.72	3.58	1.79	0.00	0.00	0.00
	Coffee, Instant, Mocha Flavor	29.3000	6.000	Fl Oz	0.09	0.29	1.32	7.91	6.83	0.00	0.00	0.25
	Coffee, Instant, Regular	179.0000	6.000	Fl Oz	0.18	0.00	0.72	3.58	57.28	0.00	0.00	0.00
203	Cola	369.0000	12.000	Fl Oz	0.10	0.10	38.50	151.00	7.60	0.00	0.00	0.00
	Cola, Diet	369.0000	12.000	Fl Oz	0.20	0.00	0.30	2.00	7.60	0.00	0.00	0.00
	Crystal Lite	29.5750	8.000	Fl Oz	0.00	0.00	0.00	0.63	0.00	0.00	0.00	0.00
	Gatorade Thirst Quencher	244.0000	8.000	Fl Oz	0.00	0.00	14.00	50.00	0.00	0.00	0.00	0.00
	Gatorlode High Carb, Loading Rec	354.0000	11.600	Fl Oz	0.00	0.00	71.00	280.00	0.00	0.00	0.00	0.00
	Gatorpro Sports Nutrition Sup.	336.0000	11.000	Fl Oz	17.00	6.00	59.00	360.00	0.00	0.00	0.00	0.50
	Juice Drink, Cranberry-apple, Bo	245.0000	1.000	Cup	0.25	0.00	41.90	164.15	0.00	0.25	0.00	0.00
	Juice Drink, Cranberry-apricot,	245.0000	1.000	Cup	0.49	0.00	39.69	156.80	0.00	0.25	0.00	0.00
	Juice Drink, Cranberry-grape, Bo	245.0000	1.000	Cup	0.49	0.25	34.30	137.20	0.00	0.25	0.00	0.07
	Juice Drink, Grape, Cnd	250.0000	1.000	Cup	0.25	0.00	32.25	125.00	0.00	0.25	0.00	0.00
	Juice Drink, Orange and Apricot,	250.0000	1.000	Cup	0.75	0.25	31.75	127.50	0.00	0.25	0.00	0.03
	Juice Drink, Pineapple and Grape	250.0000	1.000	Cup	0.50	0.25	29.00	117.50	0.00	0.25	0.00	0.03
	Juice Drink, Pineapple and Orang	250.0000	1.000	Cup	3.25	0.00	29.50	125.00	0.00	0.25	0.00	0.00
	Juice, Apple, Unsweetened	248.0000	1.000	Cup	0.15	0.27	28.97	116.56	0.00	0.25	0.00	0.05
	Juice, Carrot, Cnd	236.0000	1.000	Cup	2.24	0.35	21.92	94.40	0.00	1.89	0.00	0.07

Monounsaturated Fat (gm)	Polyunsaturated Fat (gm)	Vitamin D (mg)	Vitamin K (mg)	Vitamin E (mg)	Vitamin A (re)	Vitamin C (mg)	Thiamin (mg)	Riboflavin (mg)	Niacin (mg)	Vitamin B$_6$ (mg)	Folate (mg)	Vitamin B$_{12}$ (mcg)	Calcium (mg)	Iron (mg)	Magnesium (mg)	Phosphorus (mg)	Potassium (mg)	Sodium (mg)	Zinc (mg)
3.15	0.68	0.00	0.00	0.77	0.00	0.00	0.01	0.03	0.19	0.01	3.69	0.00	10.21	0.30	5.95	19.28	36.00	38.56	0.07
1.44	0.23	0.00	0.00	0.00	28.63	0.14	0.01	0.04	0.17	0.01	7.37	0.06	21.83	0.31	9.07	65.49	80.80	130.41	0.17
0.00	0.00	0.00	0.00	0.00	0.00	0.00	0.00	0.00	0.00	0.00	0.00	0.00	40.00	1.20	0.00	0.00	0.00	440.00	0.00
0.00	0.00	0.00	0.00	0.00	0.00	0.00	0.00	0.00	0.00	0.00	0.00	0.00	40.00	0.70	0.00	0.00	0.00	430.00	0.00
2.06	0.44	0.00	0.00	0.53	0.00	0.00	0.01	0.02	0.06	0.02	1.98	0.03	8.22	0.23	5.67	24.10	18.43	72.29	0.13
1.56	0.33	0.00	0.00	0.00	7.65	0.17	0.03	0.04	0.11	0.00	3.69	0.03	22.96	0.23	5.10	34.59	49.61	94.97	0.19
1.36	1.05	0.00	0.00	0.53	18.99	0.17	0.01	0.06	0.08	0.01	5.67	0.12	22.68	0.16	3.12	31.75	30.05	68.04	0.15
2.11	1.53	0.00	0.00	0.84	0.85	0.37	0.04	0.03	0.41	0.01	5.10	0.02	6.24	0.35	2.84	12.19	18.43	106.03	0.07
0.76	1.03	0.00	0.00	0.62	14.74	0.91	0.02	0.06	0.18	0.01	3.69	0.05	15.88	0.17	4.25	29.77	25.23	41.39	0.14
0.00	0.00	0.00	0.00	0.00	0.00	0.00	0.00	0.00	0.00	0.00	0.00	0.00	0.00	1.00	0.00	0.00	0.00	460.00	0.00
2.11	1.53	0.00	0.00	0.00	0.85	0.00	0.04	0.03	0.41	0.01	5.10	0.02	6.24	0.35	2.84	12.19	18.43	106.03	0.07
1.32	0.81	0.00	0.00	0.53	0.57	1.67	0.04	0.03	0.34	0.02	6.52	0.00	6.24	0.42	3.97	11.91	57.55	72.01	0.06
0.00	0.00	0.00	0.00	0.00	0.00	2.40	0.00	0.00	0.00	0.00	0.00	0.00	20.00	1.00	0.00	0.00	0.00	450.00	0.00
0.00	0.00	0.00	0.00	0.00	40.00	21.00	0.00	0.00	0.00	0.00	0.00	0.00	0.00	1.00	0.00	0.00	0.00	250.00	0.00
3.04	0.90	0.00	0.00	0.52	13.32	0.31	0.03	0.03	0.07	0.01	7.65	0.03	4.82	0.29	5.10	21.83	20.98	120.20	0.16
0.00	0.00	0.00	0.00	0.00	0.00	0.00	0.00	0.00	0.00	0.00	0.00	0.00	20.00	0.70	0.00	0.00	0.00	480.00	0.00
1.14	0.89	0.00	0.00	0.48	105.46	0.28	0.02	0.04	0.05	0.02	5.67	0.07	17.01	0.22	4.25	20.13	43.66	79.95	0.13
0.00	0.00	0.00	0.00	0.00	150.00	0.00	0.00	0.00	0.00	0.00	0.00	0.00	60.00	1.00	0.00	0.00	0.00	460.00	0.00
0.00	0.00	0.00	0.00	0.00	0.00	4.80	0.00	0.00	0.00	0.00	0.00	0.00	0.00	1.00	0.00	0.00	0.00	330.00	0.00
1.71	0.98	0.00	0.00	0.38	24.10	0.14	0.04	0.06	0.28	0.01	7.37	0.09	25.52	0.29	3.69	29.48	35.72	73.71	0.15
0.00	0.00	0.00	0.00	0.00	0.00	9.00	0.00	0.00	0.00	0.00	0.00	0.00	20.00	0.20	0.00	0.00	0.00	140.00	0.00
0.93	1.51	0.00	0.00	0.87	2.55	0.48	0.01	0.01	0.09	0.01	3.97	0.06	4.25	0.12	2.55	9.36	42.24	76.26	0.05
2.66	2.85	0.00	0.00	0.00	60.42	0.34	0.16	0.16	1.33	0.05	17.67	0.06	36.48	1.46	15.96	62.70	123.12	185.25	0.38
2.57	0.58	0.00	0.00	0.00	21.83	0.06	0.04	0.04	0.24	0.02	12.19	0.09	33.45	0.22	5.39	27.78	38.84	101.21	0.18
1.36	2.12	0.00	0.00	1.22	18.14	0.57	0.09	0.08	0.67	0.03	14.74	0.04	20.41	0.45	4.82	21.55	31.47	108.58	0.17
0.00	0.00	0.00	0.00	0.00	60.00	0.00	0.00	0.00	0.00	0.00	0.00	0.00	20.00	0.70	0.00	0.00	0.00	300.00	0.00
0.05	0.03	0.00	0.00	0.00	21.84	1.51	0.00	0.05	0.27	0.03	7.22	0.08	18.48	0.97	5.04	21.84	161.28	220.08	0.03
0.00	0.00	0.00	0.00	0.00	0.00	0.00	0.00	0.01	0.14	0.02	1.78	0.01	1.49	0.01	1.78	3.56	7.43	1.49	0.01
0.00	0.00	0.00	0.00	0.00	0.00	0.00	0.00	0.01	0.14	0.02	1.78	0.01	1.49	0.01	1.78	3.56	7.43	1.49	0.01
0.00	0.62	0.00	0.00	0.00	0.00	0.00	0.04	0.11	1.38	0.11	14.51	0.04	17.70	0.14	17.70	42.48	63.72	10.62	0.11
0.00	0.00	0.00	0.00	0.00	0.00	0.00	0.04	0.11	1.60	0.18	21.36	0.07	17.80	0.11	21.36	42.72	89.00	17.80	0.07
2.37	0.29	0.00	0.00	0.00	74.48	2.39	0.11	0.43	0.21	0.11	12.24	0.88	292.60	0.21	31.92	228.76	369.74	127.68	0.93
0.00	0.01	0.00	0.00	0.00	10.10	4.10	0.01	0.01	0.13	0.02	3.95	0.00	2.08	0.11	2.38	4.16	43.36	66.53	0.03
0.00	0.00	0.00	0.00	0.00	0.00	0.00	0.00	0.00	0.00	0.00	0.00	0.00	80.00	0.40	0.00	0.00	0.00	220.00	0.00
0.00	0.00	0.00	0.00	0.00	0.00	0.00	0.00	0.00	0.00	0.00	0.00	0.00	80.00	0.20	0.00	0.00	0.00	180.00	0.00
0.00	0.00	0.00	0.00	0.00	0.00	0.00	0.00	0.00	0.52	0.00	0.24	0.00	4.74	0.12	11.85	2.37	127.98	4.74	0.05
0.00	0.00	0.00	0.00	0.00	0.00	0.00	0.00	0.00	0.07	0.00	0.03	0.00	0.59	0.01	1.48	0.30	15.98	0.59	0.01
0.02	0.01	0.00	0.00	0.00	0.00	0.00	0.00	0.00	0.05	0.00	0.00	0.00	1.17	0.02	1.47	4.10	18.17	15.82	0.01
0.00	0.00	0.00	0.00	0.00	0.00	0.00	0.00	0.02	0.50	0.00	0.00	0.00	5.37	0.07	7.16	5.37	62.65	5.37	0.05
0.02	0.01	0.00	0.00	0.00	0.00	0.00	0.00	0.00	0.04	0.00	0.00	0.00	1.17	0.04	1.47	4.40	18.46	5.57	0.02
0.00	0.00	0.00	0.00	0.00	0.00	0.00	0.00	0.00	0.50	0.00	0.00	0.00	5.37	0.09	7.16	5.37	64.44	5.37	0.05
0.00	0.00	0.00	0.00	0.00	0.00	0.00	0.00	0.00	0.00	0.00	0.00	0.00	0.00	0.13	3.00	46.00	4.00	14.00	0.05
0.00	0.00	0.00	0.00	0.00	0.00	0.00	0.00	0.00	0.00	0.00	0.00	0.00	0.00	0.11	4.00	30.00	0.00	21.00	0.28
0.00	0.00	0.00	0.00	0.00	0.75	0.00	0.00	0.00	0.00	0.00	0.00	0.00	0.00	0.00	0.00	0.00	30.00	110.00	0.00
0.00	0.00	0.00	0.00	0.00	18.00	0.11	0.39	4.50	0.45	0.00	0.00	0.00	0.00	0.00	0.00	0.00	0.00	0.00	0.00
0.00	0.00	0.05	0.00	3.50	160.00	50.00	1.10	0.50	6.00	0.64	63.00	0.80	280.00	3.00	70.00	400.00	1310.00	300.00	3.60
0.00	0.00	0.00	0.00	0.00	0.00	78.40	0.02	0.05	0.15	0.05	0.49	0.00	17.15	0.15	4.90	7.35	66.15	4.90	0.10
0.00	0.00	0.00	0.00	0.00	112.70	0.00	0.02	0.02	0.29	0.05	1.47	0.00	22.05	0.37	7.35	12.25	149.45	4.90	0.10
0.00	0.05	0.00	0.00	0.84	0.00	78.40	0.02	0.05	0.29	0.07	1.72	0.00	19.60	0.02	7.35	9.80	58.80	7.35	0.10
0.00	0.00	0.00	0.00	0.00	0.00	40.00	0.03	0.03	0.25	0.05	2.00	0.00	7.50	0.25	10.00	10.00	87.50	2.50	0.08
0.08	0.05	0.00	0.00	0.00	145.00	50.00	0.05	0.03	0.50	0.08	14.50	0.00	12.50	0.25	10.00	20.00	−200.00	5.00	0.13
0.03	0.08	0.00	0.00	0.00	10.00	115.00	0.08	0.05	0.68	0.10	26.25	0.00	17.50	0.78	15.00	15.00	152.50	35.00	0.15
0.00	0.00	0.00	0.00	0.00	132.50	56.25	0.08	0.05	0.53	0.13	27.25	0.00	12.50	0.68	15.00	10.00	115.00	7.50	0.15
0.02	0.07	0.00	0.00	0.02	0.00	103.17	0.05	0.05	0.00	0.07	0.25	0.00	17.36	0.92	7.44	17.36	295.12	7.44	0.07
0.02	0.17	0.00	0.00	0.02	2584.20	20.06	0.21	0.14	0.92	0.52	8.97	0.00	56.64	1.09	33.04	99.12	689.12	68.44	0.42

USDA ID Code	Food Name	Weight in Grams*	Quantity of Units	Unit of Measure	Protein (gm)	Fat (gm)	Carbohydrate (gm)	Kcalories	Caffeine (gm)	Fiber (gm)	Cholesterol (mg)	Saturated Fat (gm)
	Juice, Clam and Tomato, Cnd	166.0000	5.500	Fl Oz	1.00	0.33	18.18	79.68	0.00	0.33	0.00	0.08
	Juice, Cranberry, Bottled	252.5860	0.750	Cup	0.00	0.25	36.37	143.97	0.00	0.00	0.00	0.00
	Juice, Grape, Cnd Or Bottle, Uns	253.0000	1.000	Cup	1.42	0.20	37.85	154.33	0.00	0.25	0.00	0.08
	Juice, Grapefruit, Cnd. Sweetene	250.0000	1.000	Cup	1.45	0.23	27.83	115.00	0.00	0.25	0.00	0.03
	Juice, Grapefruit, Cnd. Unsweete	247.0000	1.000	Cup	1.28	0.25	22.13	93.86	0.00	0.25	0.00	0.02
	Juice, Grapefruit, Pink, Fresh	247.0000	1.000	Cup	1.24	0.25	22.72	96.33	0.00	0.00	0.00	0.02
	Juice, Grapefruit, White, Fresh	247.0000	1.000	Cup	1.24	0.25	22.72	96.33	0.00	0.25	0.00	0.02
	Juice, Guava	239.9120	0.750	Cup	0.00	0.00	21.63	87.86	0.00	0.00	0.00	0.00
	Juice, Mango	239.9120	0.750	Cup	0.00	0.00	21.63	87.86	0.00	0.00	0.00	0.00
	Juice, Orange, Fresh	248.0000	1.000	Cup	1.74	0.50	25.79	111.60	0.00	0.50	0.00	0.05
	Juice, Orange, From Concentrate	249.0000	1.000	Cup	1.69	0.15	26.84	112.05	0.00	0.50	0.00	0.02
	Juice, Orange, w/ Added Calcium	248.5900	0.750	Cup	1.69	0.15	26.80	111.87	0.00	0.50	0.00	0.02
	Juice, Passion-fruit, Purple, Fr	247.0000	1.000	Cup	0.96	0.12	33.59	125.97	0.00	0.49	0.00	0.00
	Juice, Passion-fruit, Yellow, Fr	247.0000	1.000	Cup	1.65	0.44	35.69	148.20	0.00	0.49	0.00	0.05
	Juice, Pineapple, Cnd	250.0000	1.000	Cup	0.80	0.20	34.45	140.00	0.00	0.50	0.00	0.03
	Juice, Prune, Cnd	256.0000	1.000	Cup	1.56	0.08	44.67	181.76	0.00	2.56	0.00	0.00
	Juice, Tangerine, Cnd Sweetened	249.0000	1.000	Cup	1.25	0.50	29.88	124.50	0.00	0.50	0.00	0.02
	Juice, Tangerine, Fresh	247.0000	1.000	Cup	1.24	0.49	24.95	106.21	0.00	0.49	0.00	0.05
	Juice, Tomato, Cnd w/ Added Salt	243.0000	1.000	Cup	1.85	0.15	10.28	41.31	0.00	0.97	0.00	0.02
	Juice, Tomato, Cnd w/o Salt	243.0000	1.000	Cup	1.85	0.15	10.28	41.31	0.00	1.94	0.00	0.02
	Juice, Tropical Fruit, Blend	247.0000	1.000	Cup	0.00	0.00	28.90	113.62	0.00	0.25	0.00	0.00
558	Juice, V-8 Splash, Berry Blend	240.0000	8.000	Fl Oz	0.00	0.00	28.00	110.00	0.00	0.00	0.00	0.00
559	Juice, V-8 Splash, Strawberry Ki	240.0000	8.000	Fl Oz	0.00	0.00	28.00	110.00	0.00	0.00	0.00	0.00
560	Juice, V-8 Splash, Tropical Blen	240.0000	8.000	Fl Oz	0.00	0.00	30.00	120.00	0.00	0.00	0.00	0.00
	Juice, V-8, Low Salt	243.0000	8.000	Fl Oz	1.60	0.00	8.20	40.00	0.00	0.25	0.00	0.00
	Juice, Vegetable, Cnd.	242.0000	1.000	Cup	1.52	0.22	11.01	45.98	0.00	1.94	0.00	0.02
	Kool-Aid	236.0000	8.000	Fl Oz	0.00	0.00	25.10	98.00	0.00	0.00	0.00	0.00
	Lemonade Flavor Drink	266.0000	1.000	Cup	0.00	0.00	28.73	111.72	0.00	0.00	0.00	0.05
	Lemonade, Low Calorie	237.0000	1.000	Cup	0.00	0.00	1.19	4.74	0.00	0.00	0.00	0.00
	Lemonade, Pink	247.0000	1.000	Cup	0.25	0.00	25.94	98.80	0.00	0.00	0.00	0.02
	Lemonade, White	248.0000	1.000	Cup	0.25	0.00	26.04	99.20	0.00	0.25	0.00	0.02
	Liqueur, Coffee w/ Cream, 34 Pro	47.0000	1.500	Fl Oz	1.32	7.38	9.82	153.69	7.05	0.00	7.05	4.54
	Liqueur, Coffee, 53 Proof	52.0000	1.500	Fl Oz	0.05	0.16	24.34	174.72	13.52	0.00	0.00	0.06
	Liqueur, Coffee, 63 Proof	52.0000	1.500	Fl Oz	0.05	0.16	16.74	160.16	13.52	0.00	0.00	0.06
	Liqueur, Creme De Menthe, 72 Pro	50.0000	1.500	Fl Oz	0.00	0.15	20.80	185.50	0.00	0.00	0.00	0.01
	Liquor Drink, Bourbon and Soda	29.0000	1.000	Fl Oz	0.00	0.00	0.00	26.10	0.00	0.00	0.00	0.00
	Liquor Drink, Daiquiri	60.0000	2.000	Fl Oz	0.06	0.06	4.08	111.60	0.00	0.00	0.00	0.01
	Liquor Drink, Daiquiri, Bottled	207.0000	6.800	Fl Oz	0.00	0.00	32.50	258.75	0.00	0.00	0.00	0.00
	Liquor Drink, Gin and Tonic	30.0000	1.000	Fl Oz	0.00	0.00	2.10	22.80	0.00	0.00	0.00	0.00
	Liquor Drink, Manhattan	28.5000	6.000	Fl Oz	0.03	0.00	0.91	63.84	0.00	0.00	0.00	0.00
	Liquor Drink, Margarita	29.5750	6.000	Fl Oz	0.00	0.00	4.50	28.75	0.00	0.00	0.00	0.00
	Liquor Drink, Martini	28.2000	6.000	Fl Oz	0.00	0.00	0.08	62.89	0.00	0.00	0.00	0.00
	Liquor Drink, Pina Colada	141.0000	4.500	Fl Oz	0.56	2.68	39.90	262.26	0.00	0.85	0.00	1.23
	Liquor Drink, Screwdriver	30.4000	6.000	Fl Oz	0.15	0.00	2.61	24.93	0.00	0.00	0.00	0.00
	Liquor Drink, Tom Collins	29.6000	1.000	Fl Oz	0.00	0.00	0.38	16.28	0.00	0.00	0.00	0.00
	Liquor Drink, Whiskey Sour	29.9000	1.000	Fl Oz	0.06	0.03	1.67	40.66	0.00	0.00	0.00	0.01
	Liquor, Distilled, All 100 Proof	42.0000	1.500	Fl Oz	0.00	0.00	0.00	123.90	0.00	0.00	0.00	0.00
	Liquor, Distilled, All 80 Proof	42.0000	1.500	Fl Oz	0.00	0.00	0.00	97.02	0.00	0.00	0.00	0.00
	Liquor, Distilled, All 86 Proof	42.0000	1.500	Fl Oz	0.00	0.00	0.04	105.00	0.00	0.00	0.00	0.00
	Liquor, Distilled, All 90 Proof	42.0000	1.000	Jigger	0.00	0.00	0.00	110.46	0.00	0.00	0.00	0.00
	Liquor, Distilled, All 94 Proof	42.0000	1.500	Fl Oz	0.00	0.00	0.00	115.50	0.00	0.00	0.00	0.00
	Liquor, Vodka, 80 Proof	42.0000	1.500	Fl Oz	0.00	0.00	0.00	97.02	0.00	0.00	0.00	0.00
	Punch Drink, Fruit, Cnd	248.0000	1.000	Cup	0.00	0.00	29.51	116.56	0.00	0.25	0.00	0.00
	Shake, Chocolate	458.0000	22.000	Fl Oz	15.57	16.95	93.89	581.66	13.74	3.66	59.54	10.58
	Shake, Chocolate, Thick	300.0000	1.330	Cup	9.15	8.10	63.45	355.83	6.00	0.90	31.50	5.04

Monounsaturated Fat (gm)	Polyunsaturated Fat (gm)	Vitamin D (mg)	Vitamin K (mg)	Vitamin E (mg)	Vitamin A (re)	Vitamin C (mg)	Thiamin (mg)	Riboflavin (mg)	Niacin (mg)	Vitamin B₆ (mg)	Folate (mg)	Vitamin B₁₂ (mcg)	Calcium (mg)	Iron (mg)	Magnesium (mg)	Phosphorus (mg)	Potassium (mg)	Sodium (mg)	Zinc (mg)
0.02	0.03	0.00	0.00	0.00	36.52	6.81	0.07	0.05	0.32	0.13	26.39	50.80	19.92	1.00	36.52	129.48	149.40	600.92	1.79
0.00	0.00	0.00	0.00	0.00	0.00	89.42	0.02	0.02	0.09	0.05	0.51	0.00	7.58	0.38	5.05	5.05	45.47	5.05	0.18
0.00	0.05	0.00	0.00	0.00	2.53	0.25	0.08	0.10	0.66	0.18	6.58	0.00	22.77	0.61	25.30	27.83	333.96	7.59	0.13
0.03	0.05	0.00	0.00	0.13	0.00	67.25	0.10	0.05	0.80	0.05	26.00	0.00	20.00	0.90	25.00	27.50	405.00	5.00	0.15
0.02	0.05	0.00	0.00	0.12	2.47	72.12	0.10	0.05	0.57	0.05	25.69	0.00	17.29	0.49	24.70	27.17	377.91	2.47	0.22
0.02	0.05	0.00	0.00	0.00	108.68	93.86	0.10	0.05	0.49	0.10	25.19	0.00	22.23	0.49	29.64	37.05	400.14	2.47	0.12
0.02	0.05	0.00	0.05	0.12	2.47	93.86	0.10	0.05	0.49	0.10	25.19	0.00	22.23	0.49	29.64	37.05	400.14	2.47	0.12
0.00	0.00	0.00	0.00	0.00	0.00	40.55	0.00	0.00	0.00	0.00	0.00	0.00	0.00	0.00	0.00	0.00	0.00	23.65	0.00
0.00	0.00	0.00	0.00	0.00	0.00	40.55	0.00	0.00	0.00	0.00	0.00	0.00	0.00	0.00	0.00	0.00	0.00	23.65	0.00
0.10	0.10	0.00	0.10	0.22	49.60	124.00	0.22	0.07	0.99	0.10	75.14	0.00	27.28	0.50	27.28	42.16	496.00	2.48	0.12
0.02	0.02	0.00	0.00	0.47	19.92	96.86	0.20	0.05	0.50	0.10	109.06	0.00	22.41	0.25	24.90	39.84	473.10	2.49	0.12
0.02	0.03	0.00	0.00	0.00	19.89	96.70	0.20	0.04	0.50	0.11	108.88	0.00	298.31	0.25	24.86	39.77	472.32	2.49	0.12
0.02	0.07	0.00	0.00	0.12	177.84	73.61	0.00	0.32	3.61	0.12	17.29	0.00	9.88	0.59	41.99	32.11	686.66	14.82	0.12
0.05	0.27	0.00	0.00	0.12	595.27	44.95	0.00	0.25	5.53	0.15	19.76	0.00	9.88	0.89	41.99	61.75	686.66	14.82	0.15
0.03	0.08	0.00	0.00	0.05	0.00	26.75	0.15	0.05	0.65	0.25	57.75	0.00	42.50	0.65	32.50	20.00	335.00	2.50	0.28
0.05	0.03	0.00	0.00	0.03	0.00	10.50	0.05	0.18	2.02	0.56	1.02	0.00	30.72	3.02	35.84	64.00	706.56	10.24	0.54
0.05	0.07	0.00	0.00	0.22	104.58	54.78	0.15	0.05	0.25	0.07	11.45	0.00	44.82	0.50	19.92	34.86	443.22	2.49	0.07
0.10	0.10	0.00	0.00	0.22	103.74	76.57	0.15	0.05	0.25	0.10	11.36	0.00	44.46	0.49	19.76	34.58	439.66	2.47	0.07
0.02	0.05	0.00	0.00	2.21	136.08	44.47	0.12	0.07	1.63	0.27	48.36	0.00	21.87	1.41	26.73	46.17	534.60	877.23	0.34
0.02	0.05	0.00	0.00	2.21	136.08	44.47	0.12	0.07	1.63	0.27	48.36	0.00	21.87	1.41	26.73	46.17	534.60	24.30	0.34
0.00	0.00	0.00	0.00	0.00	2.47	108.43	0.02	0.02	0.05	0.02	2.22	0.00	9.88	0.22	4.94	2.47	32.11	9.88	0.10
0.00	0.00	0.00	0.00	0.00	0.00	0.00	0.00	0.00	0.00	0.00	0.00	0.00	0.00	0.00	0.00	0.00	0.00	25.00	0.00
0.00	0.00	0.00	0.00	0.00	0.00	0.00	0.00	0.00	0.00	0.00	0.00	0.00	0.00	0.00	0.00	0.00	0.00	10.00	0.00
0.00	0.00	0.00	0.00	0.00	0.00	0.00	0.00	0.00	0.00	0.00	0.00	0.00	0.00	0.00	0.00	0.00	0.00	20.00	0.00
0.00	0.00	0.00	0.00	0.00	62.50	39.00	0.04	0.05	0.00	0.00	0.00	0.00	31.00	1.20	0.00	0.00	439.00	41.00	0.00
0.02	0.10	0.00	0.00	0.77	283.14	67.03	0.10	0.07	1.77	0.34	51.06	0.00	26.62	1.02	26.62	41.14	467.06	653.40	0.48
0.00	0.00	0.00	0.00	0.00	0.00	6.00	0.00	0.00	0.00	0.00	0.00	0.00	15.00	0.00	0.00	8.00	1.00	8.00	0.00
0.00	0.00	0.00	0.00	0.00	0.00	34.05	0.00	0.00	0.00	0.00	0.00	0.00	29.26	0.05	2.66	2.66	2.66	18.62	0.08
0.00	0.00	0.00	0.00	0.00	0.00	5.93	0.00	0.00	0.00	0.00	0.24	0.00	49.77	0.09	2.37	23.70	0.00	7.11	0.07
0.00	0.02	0.00	0.07	0.00	0.00	9.63	0.02	0.05	0.05	0.02	5.43	0.00	7.41	0.40	4.94	4.94	37.05	7.41	0.10
0.00	0.02	0.00	0.00	0.00	4.96	9.67	0.02	0.05	0.05	0.02	5.46	0.00	7.44	0.40	4.96	4.96	37.20	7.44	0.10
2.10	0.31	0.00	0.00	0.12	20.21	0.00	0.00	0.03	0.04	0.01	0.00	0.06	7.52	0.06	0.94	23.50	15.04	43.24	0.08
0.01	0.06	0.00	0.00	0.00	0.00	0.00	0.00	0.01	0.07	0.00	0.00	0.00	0.52	0.03	1.56	3.12	15.60	4.16	0.02
0.01	0.06	0.00	0.00	0.00	0.00	0.00	0.00	0.01	0.07	0.00	0.00	0.00	0.52	0.03	1.56	3.12	15.60	4.16	0.02
0.01	0.09	0.00	0.00	0.00	0.00	0.00	0.00	0.00	0.00	0.00	0.00	0.00	0.00	0.04	0.00	0.00	0.00	2.50	0.02
0.00	0.00	0.00	0.00	0.00	0.00	0.00	0.00	0.00	0.01	0.00	0.00	0.00	0.87	0.01	0.29	0.58	0.58	4.06	0.02
0.01	0.01	0.00	0.00	0.00	0.00	0.96	0.01	0.00	0.02	0.01	1.20	0.00	1.80	0.09	1.20	3.60	12.60	3.00	0.04
0.00	0.00	0.00	0.00	0.00	0.00	2.69	0.00	0.00	0.02	0.00	1.66	0.00	0.00	0.02	2.07	4.14	22.77	82.80	0.06
0.00	0.00	0.00	0.00	0.00	0.00	0.12	0.00	0.00	0.00	0.00	0.15	0.00	0.60	0.01	0.30	0.30	1.50	1.20	0.02
0.00	0.00	0.00	0.00	0.00	0.00	0.00	0.00	0.00	0.03	0.00	0.03	0.00	0.57	0.03	0.57	2.00	7.41	0.86	0.01
0.00	0.00	0.00	0.00	0.00	0.00	0.00	0.00	0.00	0.00	0.00	0.00	0.00	0.00	0.00	0.00	0.00	0.00	11.88	0.00
0.00	0.00	0.00	0.00	0.00	0.00	0.00	0.00	0.00	0.00	0.00	0.06	0.00	0.56	0.03	0.56	0.85	5.08	0.85	0.01
0.23	0.49	0.00	0.00	0.00	0.00	6.63	0.04	0.01	0.17	0.07	14.38	0.00	11.28	0.31	11.28	9.87	100.11	8.46	0.18
0.00	0.00	0.00	0.00	0.00	1.82	9.48	0.02	0.00	0.05	0.01	10.67	0.00	2.13	0.02	2.43	4.26	46.51	0.30	0.01
0.00	0.00	0.00	0.00	0.00	0.00	0.50	0.00	0.00	0.00	0.00	0.21	0.00	1.18	0.00	0.30	0.30	2.37	5.03	0.02
0.00	0.01	0.00	0.00	0.00	0.30	3.77	0.06	0.00	0.04	0.01	1.55	0.00	1.79	0.02	1.20	2.09	15.85	3.29	0.01
0.00	0.00	0.00	0.00	0.00	0.00	0.00	0.00	0.00	0.00	0.00	0.00	0.00	0.00	0.02	0.00	1.68	0.84	0.42	0.02
0.00	0.00	0.00	0.00	0.00	0.00	0.00	0.00	0.00	0.00	0.00	0.00	0.00	0.00	0.02	0.00	1.68	0.84	0.42	0.02
0.00	0.00	0.00	0.00	0.00	0.00	0.00	0.00	0.00	0.00	0.00	0.00	0.00	0.00	0.02	0.00	1.68	0.84	0.42	0.02
0.00	0.00	0.00	0.00	0.00	0.00	0.00	0.00	0.00	0.00	0.00	0.00	0.00	0.00	0.02	0.00	1.68	0.84	0.42	0.02
0.00	0.00	0.00	0.00	0.00	0.00	0.00	0.00	0.00	0.00	0.00	0.00	0.00	0.00	0.00	0.00	2.10	0.42	0.42	0.00
0.00	0.00	0.00	0.00	0.00	2.48	73.41	0.05	0.05	0.05	0.00	3.22	0.00	19.84	0.52	4.96	2.48	62.00	54.56	0.30
4.95	0.64	1.83	0.00	0.32	105.34	1.83	0.27	1.15	0.73	0.23	16.03	1.56	517.54	1.42	77.86	467.16	916.00	444.26	1.88
2.34	0.30	0.00	0.00	0.30	63.00	0.00	0.15	0.66	0.36	0.09	14.70	0.96	396.00	0.93	48.00	378.00	672.00	333.00	1.44

USDA ID Code	Food Name	Weight in Grams*	Quantity of Units	Unit of Measure	Protein (gm)	Fat (gm)	Carbohydrate (gm)	Kcalories	Caffeine (gm)	Fiber (gm)	Cholesterol (mg)	Saturated Fat (gm)
	Shake, Strawberry	283.0000	10.000	Fl Oz	9.62	7.92	53.49	319.79	0.00	1.13	31.13	4.90
	Shake, Vanilla	458.0000	22.000	Fl Oz	16.03	13.74	81.98	508.38	0.00	1.83	50.38	8.52
	Shakes, Vanilla, Thick	313.0000	1.330	Cup	12.08	9.48	55.56	349.97	0.00	0.00	36.93	5.92
709	Snapple, cranberry raspberry	240.0000	8.000	Fl Oz	0.00	0.00	29.00	120.00	0.00	0.00	0.00	0.00
710	Snapple, cranberry raspberry, Di	30.0000	8.000	Fl Oz	0.00	0.00	2.00	10.00	0.00	0.00	0.00	0.00
711	Snapple, grape, white, Diet	30.0000	8.000	Fl Oz	0.00	0.00	2.00	10.00	0.00	0.00	0.00	0.00
712	Snapple, grapeade	240.0000	8.000	Fl Oz	0.00	0.00	29.00	120.00	0.00	0.00	0.00	0.00
713	Snapple, kiwi strawberry	240.0000	8.000	Fl Oz	0.00	0.00	26.00	100.00	0.00	0.00	0.00	0.00
714	Snapple, mango madness	240.0000	8.000	Fl Oz	0.00	0.00	29.00	120.00	0.00	0.00	0.00	0.00
715	Snapple, pink lemonade	240.0000	8.000	Fl Oz	0.00	0.00	29.00	120.00	0.00	0.00	0.00	0.00
704	Snapple, Tea, Iced, lemon	240.0000	8.000	Fl Oz	0.00	0.00	25.00	100.00	0.00	0.00	0.00	0.00
705	Snapple, Tea, Iced, peach	240.0000	8.000	Fl Oz	0.00	0.00	26.00	100.00	0.00	0.00	0.00	0.00
706	Snapple, Tea, Iced, peach, Diet	30.0000	8.000	Fl Oz	0.00	0.00	1.00	0.00	0.00	0.00	0.00	0.00
707	Snapple, Tea, Iced, raspberry	240.0000	8.000	Fl Oz	0.00	0.00	26.00	100.00	0.00	0.00	0.00	0.00
708	Snapple, Tea, Iced, raspberry, D	30.0000	8.000	Fl Oz	0.00	0.00	1.00	0.00	0.00	0.00	0.00	0.00
	Soda, Club	474.0000	16.000	Fl Oz	0.00	0.00	0.00	0.00	0.00	0.00	0.00	0.00
	Soda, Cream	494.0000	16.000	Fl Oz	0.00	0.00	65.70	251.94	0.00	0.00	0.00	0.00
	Soda, Dr. Pepper	491.0000	16.000	Fl Oz	0.00	0.49	51.06	201.31	49.10	0.00	0.00	0.34
	Soda, Ginger Ale	488.0000	16.000	Fl Oz	0.00	0.00	42.46	165.92	0.00	0.00	0.00	0.00
	Soda, Ginger Ale, Diet	366.0000	12.000	Fl Oz	0.00	0.00	0.00	0.00	0.00	0.00	0.00	0.00
	Soda, Grape	372.0000	12.000	Fl Oz	0.00	0.00	41.66	159.96	0.00	0.00	0.00	0.00
	Soda, Grape Drink, Cnd	250.0000	1.000	Cup	0.00	0.00	28.75	112.50	0.00	0.00	0.00	0.00
716	Soda, Lemon-lime	355.0000	12.000	Fl Oz	0.00	0.00	38.40	149.00	0.00	0.00	0.00	0.00
	Soda, Lemon-lime, Diet	355.0000	12.000	Fl Oz	0.00	0.00	0.00	0.00	0.00	0.00	0.00	0.00
	Soda, Mountain Dew	360.0000	12.000	Fl Oz	0.00	0.00	44.40	179.00	54.00	0.00	0.00	0.00
	Soda, Orange Drink, Cnd	248.0000	1.000	Cup	0.00	0.00	31.99	126.48	0.00	0.25	0.00	0.00
	Soda, Root Beer	493.0000	16.000	Fl Oz	0.00	0.00	52.26	202.13	0.00	0.00	0.00	0.00
	Soda, Root Beer, Diet	355.0000	12.000	Fl Oz	0.00	0.00	0.36	0.00	0.00	0.00	0.00	0.00
719	Starbucks-Caffe Americano	340.8000	12.000	Fl Oz	0.00	0.00	2.00	10.00	0.00	0.00	0.00	0.00
720	Starbucks-Caffe Latte w/nonfat m	340.8000	12.000	Fl Oz	12.00	0.50	17.00	120.00	0.00	0.00	0.00	0.00
721	Starbucks-Caffe Latte w/whole mi	340.8000	12.000	Fl Oz	11.00	11.00	17.00	210.00	0.00	0.00	0.00	0.00
722	Starbucks-Caffe Mocha w/nonfat mi	340.8000	12.000	Fl Oz	12.00	12.00	32.00	260.00	0.00	0.00	0.00	0.00
723	Starbucks-Caffe Mocha w/whole mil	340.8000	12.000	Fl Oz	12.00	21.00	31.00	340.00	0.00	0.00	0.00	0.00
724	Starbucks-Cappuccino w/nonfat mi	340.8000	12.000	Fl Oz	7.00	0.00	11.00	80.00	0.00	0.00	0.00	0.00
725	Starbucks-Cappuccino w/whole mil	340.8000	12.000	Fl Oz	7.00	7.00	11.00	140.00	0.00	0.00	0.00	0.00
726	Starbucks-Coffee Frappuccino	340.8000	12.000	Fl Oz	6.00	3.00	39.00	200.00	0.00	0.00	0.00	0.00
727	Starbucks-Coffee, Drip	340.8000	12.000	Fl Oz	1.00	0.00	1.00	10.00	0.00	0.00	0.00	0.00
	Tea, Brewed	237.0000	1.000	Cup	0.00	0.00	0.71	2.37	47.40	0.00	0.00	0.00
	Tea, Herb, Brewed	237.0000	1.000	Cup	0.00	0.00	0.47	2.37	0.00	0.00	0.00	0.00
	Tea, Iced, Bottled, All Flavors	236.6000	1.000	Cup	0.00	0.00	28.59	118.30	44.00	0.00	0.00	0.00
	Tea, Iced, Bottled, All Flavors,	236.6000	1.000	Cup	0.00	0.00	0.99	0.00	54.00	0.00	0.00	0.00
	Tea, Instant, Sweetened	259.0000	1.000	Cup	0.26	0.00	22.02	88.06	28.49	0.00	0.00	0.00
	Tea, Instant, Unsweetened	237.0000	1.000	Cup	0.00	0.00	0.47	2.37	30.81	0.00	0.00	0.00
	Tequila Sunrise	31.2000	6.000	Fl Oz	0.09	0.03	2.68	34.32	0.00	0.00	0.00	0.00
	Thirst Quencher Drink, Bottled	241.0000	1.000	Cup	0.00	0.00	15.18	60.25	0.00	0.00	0.00	0.00
	Water, Bottled, Perrier	192.0000	6.500	Fl Oz	0.00	0.00	0.00	0.00	0.00	0.00	0.00	0.00
	Water, Municipal	240.0000	8.000	Fl Oz	0.00	0.00	0.00	0.00	0.00	0.00	0.00	0.00
785	Water, Spring-Aquafina	240.0000	8.000	Fl Oz	0.00	0.00	0.00	0.00	0.00	0.00	0.00	0.00
786	Water, Spring-Avalon	240.0000	8.000	Fl Oz	0.00	0.00	0.00	0.00	0.00	0.00	0.00	0.00
787	Water, Spring-Dannon	240.0000	8.000	Fl Oz	0.00	0.00	0.00	0.00	0.00	0.00	0.00	0.00
788	Water, Spring-Deer Park	240.0000	8.000	Fl Oz	0.00	0.00	0.00	0.00	0.00	0.00	0.00	0.00
789	Water, Spring-Evian	240.0000	8.000	Fl Oz	0.00	0.00	0.00	0.00	0.00	0.00	0.00	0.00
790	Water, Spring-Naya	240.0000	8.000	Fl Oz	0.00	0.00	0.00	0.00	0.00	0.00	0.00	0.00
	Water, Tonic	488.0000	16.000	Fl Oz	0.00	0.00	42.94	165.92	0.00	0.00	0.00	0.00
	Wine, Dessert, Dry, 3.5 Oz Glass	103.0000	1.000	Glass	0.21	0.00	4.22	129.78	0.00	0.00	0.00	0.00

Monounsaturated Fat (gm)	Polyunsaturated Fat (gm)	Vitamin D (mg)	Vitamin K (mg)	Vitamin E (mg)	Vitamin A (re)	Vitamin C (mg)	Thiamin (mg)	Riboflavin (mg)	Niacin (mg)	Vitamin B_6 (mg)	Folate (mg)	Vitamin B_{12} (mcg)	Calcium (mg)	Iron (mg)	Magnesium (mg)	Phosphorus (mg)	Potassium (mg)	Sodium (mg)	Zinc (mg)
0.00	0.00	0.57	0.00	0.00	82.07	2.26	0.14	0.57	0.51	0.11	8.49	0.88	319.79	0.31	36.79	283.00	515.06	234.89	1.02
3.94	0.50	0.92	0.00	0.27	146.56	3.66	0.23	0.82	0.87	0.23	15.11	1.65	558.76	0.41	54.96	467.16	796.92	375.56	1.65
2.75	0.34	0.00	0.00	0.31	87.64	0.00	0.09	0.63	0.47	0.13	20.66	1.63	457.29	0.31	36.81	360.58	571.85	298.60	1.22
0.00	0.00	0.00	0.00	0.00	0.00	0.00	0.00	0.00	0.00	0.00	0.00	0.00	0.00	0.00	0.00	0.00	0.00	10.00	0.00
0.00	0.00	0.00	0.00	0.00	0.00	0.00	0.00	0.00	0.00	0.00	0.00	0.00	0.00	0.00	0.00	0.00	0.00	10.00	0.00
0.00	0.00	0.00	0.00	0.00	0.00	0.00	0.00	0.00	0.00	0.00	0.00	0.00	0.00	0.00	0.00	0.00	0.00	10.00	0.00
0.00	0.00	0.00	0.00	0.00	0.00	0.00	0.00	0.00	0.00	0.00	0.00	0.00	0.00	0.00	0.00	0.00	0.00	10.00	0.00
0.00	0.00	0.00	0.00	0.00	0.00	0.00	0.00	0.00	0.00	0.00	0.00	0.00	0.00	0.00	0.00	0.00	0.00	10.00	0.00
0.00	0.00	0.00	0.00	0.00	0.00	0.00	0.00	0.00	0.00	0.00	0.00	0.00	0.00	0.00	0.00	0.00	0.00	10.00	0.00
0.00	0.00	0.00	0.00	0.00	0.00	0.00	0.00	0.00	0.00	0.00	0.00	0.00	0.00	0.00	0.00	0.00	0.00	10.00	0.00
0.00	0.00	0.00	0.00	0.00	0.00	0.00	0.00	0.00	0.00	0.00	0.00	0.00	0.00	0.00	0.00	0.00	0.00	0.00	0.00
0.00	0.00	0.00	0.00	0.00	0.00	0.00	0.00	0.00	0.00	0.00	0.00	0.00	0.00	0.00	0.00	0.00	0.00	0.00	0.00
0.00	0.00	0.00	0.00	0.00	0.00	0.00	0.00	0.00	0.00	0.00	0.00	0.00	0.00	0.00	0.00	0.00	0.00	10.00	0.00
0.00	0.00	0.00	0.00	0.00	0.00	0.00	0.00	0.00	0.00	0.00	0.00	0.00	0.00	0.00	0.00	0.00	0.00	10.00	0.00
0.00	0.00	0.00	0.00	0.00	0.00	0.00	0.00	0.00	0.00	0.00	0.00	0.00	0.00	0.00	0.00	0.00	0.00	10.00	0.00
0.00	0.00	0.00	0.00	0.00	0.00	0.00	0.00	0.00	0.00	0.00	0.00	0.00	23.70	0.05	4.74	0.00	9.48	99.54	0.47
0.00	0.00	0.00	0.00	0.00	0.00	0.00	0.00	0.00	0.00	0.00	0.00	0.00	24.70	0.25	4.94	0.00	4.94	59.28	0.35
0.00	0.00	0.00	0.00	0.00	0.00	0.00	0.00	0.00	0.00	0.00	0.00	0.00	14.73	0.20	0.00	54.01	4.91	49.10	0.20
0.00	0.00	0.00	0.05	0.00	0.00	0.00	0.00	0.00	0.00	0.00	0.00	0.00	14.64	0.88	4.88	0.00	4.88	34.16	0.24
0.00	0.00	0.00	0.00	0.00	0.00	0.00	0.00	0.00	0.00	0.00	0.00	0.00	0.00	0.00	0.00	0.00	0.00	2.50	0.00
0.00	0.00	0.00	0.00	0.00	0.00	0.00	0.00	0.00	0.00	0.00	0.00	0.00	11.16	0.30	3.72	0.00	3.72	55.80	0.26
0.00	0.00	0.00	0.00	0.00	0.00	85.25	0.00	0.00	0.08	0.03	0.75	0.00	7.50	0.43	5.00	2.50	12.50	15.00	0.28
0.00	0.00	0.00	0.00	0.00	0.00	0.00	0.00	0.00	0.10	0.00	0.00	0.00	9.00	0.25	2.00	1.00	4.00	41.00	0.18
0.00	0.00	0.00	0.00	0.00	0.00	0.00	0.00	0.00	0.00	0.00	0.00	0.00	0.00	0.00	0.00	0.00	0.00	2.50	0.00
0.00	0.00	0.00	0.00	0.00	0.00	0.00	0.00	0.00	0.00	0.00	0.00	0.00	0.00	0.00	0.00	0.00	10.00	31.00	0.00
0.00	0.00	0.00	0.00	0.00	4.96	84.57	0.02	0.00	0.07	0.02	5.46	0.00	14.88	0.69	4.96	2.48	44.64	39.68	0.22
0.00	0.00	0.00	0.00	0.00	0.00	0.00	0.00	0.00	0.00	0.00	0.00	0.00	24.65	0.25	4.93	0.00	4.93	64.09	0.35
0.00	0.00	0.00	0.00	0.00	0.00	0.00	0.00	0.00	0.00	0.00	0.00	0.00	0.00	0.00	0.00	0.00	0.00	2.50	0.00
0.00	0.00	0.00	0.00	0.00	0.00	0.00	0.00	0.00	0.00	0.00	0.00	0.00	0.00	0.00	0.00	0.00	0.00	105.00	0.00
0.00	0.00	0.00	0.00	0.00	0.00	0.00	0.00	0.00	0.00	0.00	0.00	0.00	0.00	0.00	0.00	0.00	0.00	170.00	0.00
0.00	0.00	0.00	0.00	0.00	0.00	0.00	0.00	0.00	0.00	0.00	0.00	0.00	0.00	0.00	0.00	0.00	0.00	160.00	0.00
0.00	0.00	0.00	0.00	0.00	0.00	0.00	0.00	0.00	0.00	0.00	0.00	0.00	0.00	0.00	0.00	0.00	0.00	170.00	0.00
0.00	0.00	0.00	0.00	0.00	0.00	0.00	0.00	0.00	0.00	0.00	0.00	0.00	0.00	0.00	0.00	0.00	0.00	160.00	0.00
0.00	0.00	0.00	0.00	0.00	0.00	0.00	0.00	0.00	0.00	0.00	0.00	0.00	0.00	0.00	0.00	0.00	0.00	110.00	0.00
0.00	0.00	0.00	0.00	0.00	0.00	0.00	0.00	0.00	0.00	0.00	0.00	0.00	0.00	0.00	0.00	0.00	0.00	105.00	0.00
0.00	0.00	0.00	0.00	0.00	0.00	0.00	0.00	0.00	0.00	0.00	0.00	0.00	0.00	0.00	0.00	0.00	0.00	170.00	0.00
0.00	0.00	0.00	0.00	0.00	0.00	0.00	0.00	0.00	0.00	0.00	0.00	0.00	0.00	0.00	0.00	0.00	0.00	10.00	0.00
0.00	0.00	0.00	0.12	0.00	0.00	0.00	0.00	0.00	0.02	0.00	12.32	0.00	0.00	0.05	7.11	2.37	87.69	7.11	0.05
0.00	0.02	0.00	0.00	0.00	0.00	0.00	0.02	0.00	0.00	0.00	1.42	0.00	4.74	0.19	2.37	0.00	21.33	2.37	0.09
0.00	0.00	0.00	0.00	0.00	0.00	0.00	0.00	0.00	0.00	0.00	0.00	0.00	0.00	0.00	0.00	0.00	0.00	9.86	0.00
0.00	0.00	0.00	0.00	0.00	0.00	0.00	0.00	0.00	0.00	0.00	0.00	0.00	0.00	0.00	0.00	0.00	0.00	0.00	0.00
0.00	0.03	0.00	0.00	0.00	0.00	0.00	0.00	0.05	0.10	0.00	9.58	0.00	5.18	0.05	5.18	2.59	49.21	7.77	0.08
0.00	0.00	0.00	0.00	0.00	0.00	0.00	0.00	0.00	0.09	0.00	0.71	0.00	4.74	0.05	4.74	2.37	47.40	7.11	0.07
0.01	0.01	0.00	0.00	0.00	3.12	6.02	0.01	0.00	0.06	0.02	3.31	0.00	1.87	0.09	2.18	3.12	32.45	1.25	0.02
0.00	0.00	0.00	0.00	0.00	0.00	0.00	0.02	0.00	0.00	0.00	0.00	0.00	0.00	0.12	2.41	21.69	26.51	96.40	0.05
0.00	0.00	0.00	0.00	0.00	0.00	0.00	0.00	0.00	0.00	0.00	0.00	0.00	26.88	0.00	0.00	0.00	0.00	1.92	0.00
0.00	0.00	0.00	0.00	0.00	0.00	0.00	0.00	0.00	0.00	0.00	0.00	0.00	0.00	0.00	0.00	0.00	0.00	0.00	0.00
0.00	0.00	0.00	0.00	0.00	0.00	0.00	0.00	0.00	0.00	0.00	0.00	0.00	0.00	0.00	0.00	0.00	0.00	0.00	0.00
0.00	0.00	0.00	0.00	0.00	0.00	0.00	0.00	0.00	0.00	0.00	0.00	0.00	0.00	0.00	0.00	0.00	0.00	0.00	0.00
0.00	0.00	0.00	0.00	0.00	0.00	0.00	0.00	0.00	0.00	0.00	0.00	0.00	0.00	0.00	0.00	0.00	0.00	0.00	0.00
0.00	0.00	0.00	0.00	0.00	0.00	0.00	0.00	0.00	0.00	0.00	0.00	0.00	0.00	0.00	0.00	0.00	0.00	0.00	0.00
0.00	0.00	0.00	0.00	0.00	0.00	0.00	0.00	0.00	0.00	0.00	0.00	0.00	0.00	0.00	0.00	0.00	0.00	0.00	0.00
0.00	0.00	0.00	0.00	0.00	0.00	0.00	0.00	0.00	0.00	0.00	0.00	0.00	4.88	0.05	0.00	0.00	0.00	19.52	0.49
0.00	0.00	0.00	0.00	0.00	0.00	0.00	0.02	0.02	0.22	0.00	0.41	0.00	8.24	0.25	9.27	9.27	94.76	9.27	0.07

USDA ID Code	Food Name	Weight in Grams*	Quantity of Units	Unit of Measure	Protein (gm)	Fat (gm)	Carbohydrate (gm)	Kcalories	Caffeine (gm)	Fiber (gm)	Cholesterol (mg)	Saturated Fat (gm)
	Wine, Dessert, Sweet, 3.5 Oz Gla	103.0000	1.000	Glass	0.21	0.00	12.15	157.59	0.00	0.00	0.00	0.00
	Wine, Table, All, 3.5 Oz Glass	103.0000	1.000	Glass	0.21	0.00	1.44	72.10	0.00	0.00	0.00	0.00
	Wine, Table, Red, 3.5 Oz Glass	103.0000	1.000	Glass	0.21	0.00	1.75	74.16	0.00	0.00	0.00	0.00
	Wine, Table, Rose, 3.5 Oz Glass	103.0000	1.000	Glass	0.21	0.00	1.44	73.13	0.00	0.00	0.00	0.00
	Wine, Table, White, 3.5 Oz Glass	103.0000	1.000	Glass	0.10	0.00	0.82	70.04	0.00	0.00	0.00	0.00

Breads/Grains and Pasta

USDA ID Code	Food Name	Weight in Grams*	Quantity of Units	Unit of Measure	Protein (gm)	Fat (gm)	Carbohydrate (gm)	Kcalories	Caffeine (gm)	Fiber (gm)	Cholesterol (mg)	Saturated Fat (gm)
	Barley, Cooked	184.0000	1.000	Cup	22.96	4.23	135.20	651.36	0.00	31.83	0.00	0.88
61	Bread Sticks, Plain	10.0000	1.000	Stick	1.20	0.95	6.84	41.20	0.00	0.00	0.00	0.14
	Bread Stuffing, Plain	232.0000	1.000	Cup	8.82	16.70	51.50	389.76	0.00	0.00	0.00	3.39
	Bread, Banana	60.0000	1.000	Slice	2.58	7.08	33.06	202.80	0.00	0.00	25.80	1.83
	Bread, Cornbread	28.3500	1.000	Slice	1.90	2.01	12.33	75.41	0.00	0.00	11.34	0.44
	Bread, Cracked-wheat	28.3500	1.000	Slice	2.47	1.11	14.03	73.71	0.00	1.56	0.00	0.26
	Bread, Cracked-wheat, Toasted	23.0000	1.000	Slice	2.19	0.97	12.37	65.09	0.00	0.00	0.00	0.23
	Bread, Dinner Roll, Egg	28.3500	1.000	Each	2.69	1.81	14.74	87.03	0.00	1.05	14.18	0.45
	Bread, Dinner Roll, French	28.3500	1.000	Each	2.44	1.22	14.23	78.53	0.00	0.91	0.00	0.27
	Bread, Dinner Roll, Oat Bran	28.3500	1.000	Each	2.69	1.30	11.40	66.91	0.00	1.16	0.00	0.18
	Bread, Dinner Roll, Plain	86.0000	1.000	Each	7.22	6.28	43.34	258.00	0.00	2.58	0.86	1.51
	Bread, Dinner Roll, Rye	43.0000	1.000	Large	4.43	1.46	22.83	122.98	0.00	2.09	0.00	0.26
	Bread, Dinner Roll, Wheat	28.3500	1.000	Each	2.44	1.79	13.04	77.40	0.00	1.07	0.00	0.43
	Bread, Dinner Roll, Whole-wheat	43.0000	1.000	Each	3.74	2.02	21.97	114.38	0.00	3.24	0.00	0.36
	Bread, Egg	28.3500	1.000	Slice	2.69	1.70	13.55	81.36	0.00	0.65	14.46	0.45
	Bread, Egg, Toasted	28.3500	1.000	Slice	2.98	1.87	14.91	89.30	0.00	0.71	15.88	0.46
	Bread, French or Vienna	28.3500	1.000	Slice	2.49	0.85	14.71	77.68	0.00	0.85	0.00	0.18
	Bread, French or Vienna, Toasted	28.3500	1.000	Slice	2.72	0.94	15.99	84.48	0.00	0.94	0.00	0.20
	Bread, Italian	28.3500	1.000	Slice	2.49	0.99	14.18	76.83	0.00	0.77	0.00	0.24
	Bread, Italian, Toasted	27.0000	1.000	Slice	2.62	1.05	14.85	80.46	0.00	0.00	0.00	0.25
	Bread, Lo Cal, Oat Bran	28.3500	1.000	Slice	2.27	0.91	11.71	56.98	0.00	3.40	0.00	0.13
	Bread, Lo Cal, Oat Bran, Toasted	28.3500	1.000	Slice	2.69	1.08	13.95	67.76	0.00	4.05	0.00	0.15
	Bread, Lo Cal, Oatmeal	28.3500	1.000	Slice	2.15	0.99	12.28	59.54	0.00	0.00	0.00	0.17
	Bread, Lo Cal, Oatmeal, Toasted	19.0000	1.000	Slice	1.71	0.80	9.79	47.69	0.00	0.00	0.00	0.14
	Bread, Lo Cal, Rye	28.3500	1.000	Slice	2.58	0.82	11.48	57.55	0.00	3.40	0.00	0.10
	Bread, Lo Cal, Rye, Toasted	19.0000	1.000	Slice	2.05	0.65	9.16	45.79	0.00	0.00	0.19	0.08
	Bread, Lo Cal, Wheat	28.3500	1.000	Slice	2.58	0.65	12.36	56.13	0.00	3.40	0.00	0.10
	Bread, Lo Cal, Wheat, Toasted	19.0000	1.000	Slice	2.05	0.51	9.86	44.84	0.00	0.00	0.00	0.08
	Bread, Lo Cal, White	28.3500	1.000	Slice	2.47	0.71	12.56	58.68	0.00	2.75	0.00	0.16
	Bread, Lo Cal, White, Toasted	19.0000	1.000	Slice	1.96	0.57	10.01	46.93	0.00	0.00	0.00	0.12
	Bread, Mixed-grain	28.3500	1.000	Slice	2.84	1.08	13.15	70.88	0.00	1.81	0.00	0.23
	Bread, Mixed-grain, Toasted	28.3500	1.000	Slice	3.09	1.16	14.29	77.11	0.00	1.87	0.00	0.25
	Bread, Oat Bran	28.3500	1.000	Slice	2.95	1.25	11.28	66.91	0.00	1.28	0.00	0.20
	Bread, Oat Bran, Toasted	28.3500	1.000	Slice	3.23	1.36	12.39	73.43	0.00	1.39	0.00	0.22
	Bread, Oatmeal	28.3500	1.000	Slice	2.38	1.25	13.75	76.26	0.00	1.13	0.00	0.20
	Bread, Oatmeal, Toasted	28.3500	1.000	Slice	2.61	1.36	14.94	82.78	0.00	1.22	0.00	0.22
	Bread, Pita, White, Enriched	60.0000	1.000	Pita	5.46	0.72	33.42	165.00	0.00	1.32	0.00	0.10
	Bread, Pita, Whole-wheat	64.0000	1.000	Pita	6.27	1.66	35.20	170.24	0.00	4.74	0.00	0.26
	Bread, Pumpernickel	28.3500	1.000	Slice	2.47	0.88	13.47	70.88	0.00	1.84	0.00	0.12
	Bread, Pumpernickel, Toasted	28.3500	1.000	Slice	2.69	0.96	14.80	77.96	0.00	2.01	0.00	0.14
	Bread, Pumpkin	60.0000	1.000	Slice	2.40	7.68	30.72	198.60	0.00	0.00	26.40	1.23
	Bread, Raisin	28.3500	1.000	Slice	2.24	1.25	14.83	77.68	0.00	1.22	0.00	0.31
	Bread, Raisin, Toasted	28.3500	1.000	Slice	2.44	1.36	16.13	84.20	0.00	1.33	0.00	0.33
	Bread, Rice Bran	28.3500	1.000	Slice	2.52	1.30	12.33	68.89	0.00	1.39	0.00	0.20
	Bread, Rice Bran, Toasted	28.3500	1.000	Slice	2.75	1.42	13.41	74.84	0.00	1.50	0.00	0.22
	Bread, Rolls, Hard (includes Kai	28.3500	1.000	Each	2.81	1.22	14.94	83.07	0.00	0.65	0.00	0.17
	Bread, Rye	28.3500	1.000	Slice	2.41	0.94	13.69	73.43	0.00	1.64	0.00	0.18
	Bread, Rye, Toasted	28.3500	1.000	Slice	2.66	1.02	15.05	80.51	0.00	1.81	0.00	0.20
	Bread, Wheat (includes Wheat Ber	28.3500	1.000	Slice	2.58	1.16	13.38	73.71	0.00	1.22	0.00	0.25
	Bread, Wheat Bran	28.3500	1.000	Slice	2.49	0.96	13.55	70.31	0.00	1.13	0.00	0.22

Monounsaturated Fat (gm)	Polyunsaturated Fat (gm)	Vitamin D (mg)	Vitamin K (mg)	Vitamin E (mg)	Vitamin A (re)	Vitamin C (mg)	Thiamin (mg)	Riboflavin (mg)	Niacin (mg)	Vitamin B_6 (mg)	Folate (mg)	Vitamin B_{12} (mcg)	Calcium (mg)	Iron (mg)	Magnesium (mg)	Phosphorus (mg)	Potassium (mg)	Sodium (mg)	Zinc (mg)
0.00	0.00	0.00	0.00	0.00	0.00	0.00	0.02	0.02	0.22	0.00	0.41	0.00	8.24	0.25	9.27	9.27	94.76	9.27	0.07
0.00	0.00	0.00	0.00	0.00	0.00	0.00	0.00	0.02	0.07	0.02	1.13	0.01	8.24	0.42	10.30	14.42	91.67	8.24	0.07
0.00	0.00	0.00	0.00	0.00	0.00	0.00	0.01	0.03	0.08	0.03	2.06	0.01	8.24	0.44	13.39	14.42	115.36	5.15	0.09
0.00	0.00	0.00	0.00	0.00	0.00	0.00	0.00	0.02	0.07	0.02	1.13	0.01	8.24	0.39	10.30	15.45	101.97	5.15	0.06
0.00	0.00	0.00	0.00	0.00	0.00	0.00	0.00	0.01	0.07	0.01	0.21	0.00	9.27	0.33	10.30	14.42	82.40	5.15	0.07
0.55	2.04	0.00	0.00	1.10	3.68	0.00	1.20	0.53	8.46	0.59	34.96	0.00	60.72	6.62	244.72	485.76	831.68	22.08	5.10
0.37	0.36	0.00	0.00	0.00	0.00	0.00	0.06	0.06	0.53	0.01	3.00	0.00	2.20	0.43	3.20	12.10	12.40	65.70	0.09
7.40	4.89	0.00	0.00	0.00	160.08	3.94	0.39	0.33	3.69	0.12	39.44	0.00	148.48	3.80	34.80	113.68	303.92	1069.52	0.74
3.02	1.77	0.00	0.00	0.00	14.40	1.02	0.10	0.12	0.87	0.09	6.60	0.05	10.80	0.84	8.40	33.60	78.60	118.80	0.22
0.52	0.91	0.00	0.00	0.00	15.31	0.09	0.08	0.08	0.64	0.03	18.14	0.04	70.59	0.71	7.09	47.91	41.67	186.54	0.17
0.54	0.19	0.00	0.00	0.17	0.00	0.00	0.10	0.07	1.04	0.09	17.29	0.01	12.19	0.80	14.74	43.38	50.18	152.52	0.35
0.48	0.17	0.00	0.00	0.00	0.00	0.00	0.07	0.05	0.83	0.07	6.90	0.01	10.81	0.70	13.11	38.18	44.16	134.55	0.31
0.83	0.32	0.00	0.00	0.20	2.27	0.00	0.15	0.15	0.93	0.01	29.77	0.07	16.73	1.00	7.09	28.63	29.48	154.51	0.32
0.56	0.24	0.00	0.00	0.13	0.00	0.00	0.15	0.09	1.23	0.01	26.93	0.00	25.80	0.77	5.67	23.81	32.32	172.65	0.26
0.42	0.45	0.00	0.00	0.20	0.00	0.00	0.13	0.08	1.40	0.01	26.93	0.00	24.10	1.17	9.36	32.60	34.30	117.09	0.29
3.18	1.04	0.00	0.00	0.76	0.00	0.09	0.42	0.28	3.47	0.04	81.70	0.05	102.34	2.69	19.78	99.76	114.38	448.06	0.66
0.53	0.31	0.00	0.00	0.15	0.43	0.00	0.16	0.12	1.68	0.03	36.98	0.00	12.90	1.16	23.22	68.37	77.40	383.56	0.42
0.88	0.31	0.00	0.00	0.27	0.00	0.00	0.12	0.08	1.15	0.02	14.46	0.00	49.90	1.01	10.21	29.48	32.60	96.39	0.26
0.52	0.93	0.00	0.00	0.58	0.00	0.00	0.11	0.06	1.58	0.09	12.90	0.00	45.58	1.04	36.55	96.32	116.96	205.54	0.86
0.65	0.31	0.00	0.00	0.17	6.52	0.00	0.12	0.12	1.37	0.02	29.77	0.03	26.37	0.86	5.39	30.05	32.60	139.48	0.22
0.85	0.33	0.00	0.00	0.24	6.52	0.00	0.11	0.12	1.36	0.02	25.23	0.03	28.92	0.95	5.95	33.17	35.72	153.09	0.24
0.35	0.20	0.00	0.00	0.08	0.00	0.00	0.15	0.09	1.35	0.01	26.93	0.00	21.26	0.72	7.65	29.77	32.04	172.65	0.25
0.37	0.21	0.00	0.00	0.07	0.00	0.00	0.13	0.09	1.32	0.01	22.96	0.00	22.96	0.78	8.51	32.32	34.59	187.39	0.27
0.23	0.39	0.00	0.00	0.10	0.00	0.00	0.13	0.08	1.24	0.01	26.93	0.00	22.11	0.83	7.65	29.20	31.19	165.56	0.24
0.24	0.41	0.00	0.00	0.00	0.00	0.00	0.11	0.08	1.17	0.01	6.21	0.00	22.95	0.87	8.10	30.78	32.67	173.34	0.26
0.19	0.47	0.00	0.00	0.13	0.00	0.00	0.10	0.06	1.07	0.03	18.71	0.00	16.16	0.89	15.59	39.41	28.92	99.51	0.30
0.23	0.56	0.00	0.00	0.15	0.00	0.00	0.10	0.06	1.14	0.03	15.88	0.00	19.28	1.06	15.59	40.82	34.59	118.50	0.34
0.23	0.38	0.00	0.00	0.00	0.28	0.06	0.10	0.08	0.86	0.01	15.59	0.03	32.60	0.65	6.80	28.35	35.15	110.00	0.24
0.19	0.31	0.00	0.00	0.00	0.19	0.04	0.06	0.06	0.62	0.01	5.32	0.03	26.03	0.52	6.46	26.98	34.58	87.78	0.21
0.19	0.21	0.00	0.00	0.07	0.00	0.11	0.10	0.07	0.72	0.02	13.61	0.01	21.55	0.88	6.24	22.11	27.78	114.82	0.19
0.15	0.17	0.00	0.00	0.00	0.00	0.02	0.07	0.05	0.51	0.01	3.61	0.02	17.29	0.70	3.99	18.81	22.23	91.77	0.17
0.07	0.27	0.00	0.00	0.03	0.00	0.03	0.12	0.09	1.10	0.04	20.13	0.00	22.68	0.84	11.06	28.92	34.59	144.87	0.32
0.06	0.22	0.00	0.00	0.00	0.00	0.02	0.08	0.06	0.79	0.03	4.37	0.01	18.24	0.67	6.46	20.71	27.93	115.52	0.19
0.31	0.16	0.00	0.00	0.04	0.28	0.14	0.12	0.08	1.03	0.01	26.93	0.08	26.65	0.90	6.52	34.30	21.55	128.43	0.38
0.24	0.13	0.00	0.00		0.19	0.08	0.07	0.06	0.74	0.01	5.51	0.06	21.28	0.72	5.89	30.21	17.29	102.41	0.30
0.43	0.26	0.00	0.00	0.19	0.00	0.09	0.12	0.10	1.24	0.09	22.68	0.02	25.80	0.98	15.03	49.90	57.83	138.06	0.36
0.47	0.28	0.00	0.00	0.19	0.00	0.09	0.10	0.09	1.21	0.09	19.28	0.02	28.07	1.07	16.44	54.15	62.94	150.26	0.39
0.45	0.48	0.00	0.00	0.18	0.00	0.00	0.14	0.10	1.37	0.02	22.96	0.00	18.43	0.88	9.92	39.97	41.67	115.38	0.25
0.50	0.53	0.00	0.00	0.12	0.00	0.00	0.12	0.10	1.36	0.01	19.56	0.00	20.13	0.97	9.64	32.89	34.87	127.01	0.30
0.45	0.48	0.00	0.00	0.17	0.57	0.00	0.11	0.07	0.89	0.02	17.58	0.01	18.71	0.77	10.49	35.72	40.26	169.82	0.29
0.49	0.52	0.00	0.00	0.10	0.57	0.09	0.10	0.07	0.87	0.02	15.03	0.01	20.41	0.83	11.62	38.84	43.66	184.56	0.31
0.07	0.32	0.00	0.00	0.02	0.00	0.00	0.36	0.20	2.78	0.02	57.00	0.00	51.60	1.57	15.60	58.20	72.00	321.60	0.50
0.22	0.68	0.00	0.00	0.58	0.00	0.00	0.22	0.05	1.82	0.17	22.40	0.00	9.60	1.96	44.16	115.20	108.80	340.48	0.97
0.26	0.35	0.00	0.00	0.12	0.00	0.00	0.09	0.09	0.88	0.04	22.68	0.00	19.28	0.81	15.31	50.46	58.97	190.23	0.42
0.29	0.39	0.00	0.00	0.17	0.00	0.00	0.08	0.09	0.87	0.03	19.28	0.00	20.98	0.89	17.01	55.28	64.64	209.22	0.46
1.85	4.11	0.00	0.00	0.00	334.20	0.60	0.09	0.10	0.79	0.02	6.60	0.05	10.80	0.99	7.80	31.80	55.20	187.80	0.20
0.65	0.19	0.00	0.00	0.14	0.00	0.03	0.10	0.11	0.98	0.02	24.66	0.00	18.71	0.82	7.37	30.90	64.35	110.57	0.20
0.71	0.21	0.00	0.00	0.23	0.00	0.11	0.08	0.11	0.96	0.02	20.98	0.00	20.41	0.89	7.94	33.45	69.74	120.20	0.22
0.47	0.50	0.00	0.00	0.24	0.00	0.00	0.18	0.09	1.93	0.08	18.43	0.00	19.56	1.02	22.68	50.46	60.95	124.74	0.37
0.51	0.54	0.00	0.00	0.22	0.00	0.00	0.16	0.08	1.89	0.06	15.59	0.00	21.26	1.11	21.55	49.33	60.10	135.51	0.39
0.32	0.49	0.00	0.00	0.09	0.00	0.00	0.14	0.10	1.20	0.01	26.93	0.00	26.93	0.93	7.65	28.35	30.62	154.22	0.27
0.37	0.23	0.00	0.00	0.10	0.28	0.11	0.12	0.10	1.08	0.02	24.38	0.00	20.70	0.80	11.34	35.44	47.06	187.11	0.32
0.41	0.25	0.00	0.00	0.17	0.00	0.06	0.11	0.09	1.07	0.02	20.70	0.00	22.68	0.88	12.19	39.12	51.88	205.54	0.35
0.49	0.26	0.00	0.00	0.15	0.00	0.00	0.12	0.08	1.17	0.03	21.83	0.00	29.77	0.94	13.04	42.53	56.98	150.26	0.29
0.46	0.18	0.00	0.00	0.13	0.00	0.00	0.11	0.08	1.25	0.05	19.56	0.00	20.98	0.87	22.96	52.45	64.35	137.78	0.38

USDA ID Code	Food Name	Weight in Grams*	Quantity of Units	Unit of Measure	Protein (gm)	Fat (gm)	Carbohydrate (gm)	Kcalories	Caffeine (gm)	Fiber (gm)	Cholesterol (mg)	Saturated Fat (gm)
	Bread, Wheat Bran, Toasted	33.0000	1.000	Slice	3.20	1.22	17.33	90.09	0.00	0.00	0.00	0.28
	Bread, Wheat, Toasted	28.3500	1.000	Slice	2.81	1.25	14.54	79.95	0.00	1.50	0.00	0.27
62	Bread, White	25.0000	1.000	Slice	2.05	0.90	12.38	66.75	0.00	0.58	0.25	0.20
63	Bread, White, Toasted	23.0000	1.000	Slice	2.07	0.92	12.51	67.39	0.00	0.00	0.23	0.21
	Bread, Whole Wheat	28.3500	1.000	Slice	2.75	1.19	13.07	69.74	0.00	1.96	0.00	0.26
	Bread, Whole Wheat, Toasted	28.3500	1.000	Slice	2.61	1.67	15.99	86.47	0.00	1.90	0.00	0.25
	Breadsticks, Sesame Sticks, Whea	28.3500	1.000	Ounce	3.09	10.40	13.18	153.37	0.00	0.79	0.00	1.84
	Buns, Hamburger or Hot Dog, Mixe	28.3500	1.000	Each	5.44	3.40	25.25	149.12	0.00	2.16	0.00	0.78
	Buns, Hamburger or Hot Dog, Plai	28.3500	1.000	Each	4.82	2.90	28.52	162.16	0.00	1.54	0.00	0.68
	Cornstarch	128.0000	1.000	Cup	0.33	0.06	116.83	487.68	0.00	1.15	0.00	0.01
	Couscous, Cooked	157.0000	1.000	Cup	5.95	0.25	36.46	175.84	0.00	2.20	0.00	0.05
	Crackers, Cheese, Regular	62.0000	1.000	Cup	6.26	15.69	36.08	311.86	0.00	1.49	8.06	5.81
206	Crackers, Cheese, w/Peanut Butte	7.0000	1.000	Each	0.88	1.62	3.99	33.74	0.00	0.08	0.35	0.36
	Crackers, Crack Pepper, Fat Free	2.1400	7.000	Each	0.29	0.00	1.85	8.56	0.00	0.07	0.00	0.00
207	Crackers, Crispbread, Rye	10.0000	1.000	Each	0.79	0.13	8.22	36.60	0.00	1.62	0.00	0.01
	Crackers, Graham Snacks, Cinn.,	0.6700	20.000	Each	0.04	0.00	0.58	2.46	0.00	0.02	0.00	0.00
208	Crackers, Graham, Plain or Honey	7.0000	1.000	Each	0.48	0.71	5.38	29.61	0.00	0.19	0.00	0.18
	Crackers, Matzo, Egg	28.3500	1.000	Each	3.49	0.60	22.28	110.85	0.00	0.79	23.53	0.16
	Crackers, Matzo, Egg and Onion	28.3500	1.000	Each	2.84	1.11	21.86	110.85	0.00	1.42	12.76	0.27
	Crackers, Matzo, Plain	28.3500	1.000	Each	2.84	0.40	23.73	111.98	0.00	0.85	0.00	0.07
	Crackers, Matzo, Whole-wheat	28.3500	1.000	Each	3.71	0.43	22.37	99.51	0.00	3.35	0.00	0.07
	Crackers, Melba Toast, Plain	30.0000	1.000	Cup	3.63	0.96	22.98	117.00	0.00	1.89	0.00	0.14
209	Crackers, Melba Toast, Plain, w/	5.0000	1.000	Each	0.61	0.16	3.83	19.50	0.00	0.00	0.00	0.02
	Crackers, Melba Toast, Rye	14.1750	1.000	Each	1.64	0.48	10.96	55.14	0.00	1.13	0.00	0.06
	Crackers, Melba Toast, Wheat	14.1750	1.000	Each	1.83	0.33	10.83	53.01	0.00	1.05	0.00	0.05
	Crackers, Ritz	62.0000	1.000	Cup	4.59	15.69	37.82	311.24	0.00	0.99	0.00	2.34
	Crackers, Ritz, Low Sodium	62.0000	1.000	Cup	4.59	15.69	37.82	311.24	0.00	0.99	0.00	2.34
	Crackers, Rye, w/ Cheese Filling	14.1750	1.000	Each	1.30	3.16	8.62	68.18	0.00	0.51	1.28	0.85
210	Crackers, Rye, Wafers, Plain	25.0000	1.000	Each	2.40	0.23	20.10	83.50	0.00	0.00	0.00	0.03
	Crackers, Rye, Wafers, Seasoned	14.1750	1.000	Each	1.28	1.30	10.46	54.01	0.00	2.96	0.00	0.18
211	Crackers, Saltines	3.0000	1.000	Each	0.28	0.35	2.15	13.02	0.00	0.08	0.00	0.06
	Crackers, Saltines, Fat Free	3.0000	1.000	Each	0.40	0.00	2.40	12.00	0.00	0.00	0.00	0.00
212	Crackers, Saltines, Low Salt	3.0000	1.000	Each	0.28	0.35	2.15	13.02	0.00	0.00	0.00	0.06
	Crackers, w/ Cheese Filling, Sna	14.1750	1.000	Each	1.32	2.99	8.75	67.61	0.00	0.26	0.28	0.87
	Crackers, w/Peanut Butter Fillin	14.1750	1.000	Each	1.57	3.39	8.32	69.17	0.00	0.39	0.00	0.79
	Crackers, Wheat, Fat Free - Snac	3.0000	5.000	Each	0.40	0.00	2.40	12.00	0.00	0.20	0.00	0.00
213	Crackers, Wheat, Low Salt	2.0000	1.000	Each	0.17	0.41	1.30	9.46	0.00	0.00	0.00	0.07
214	Crackers, Wheat, Regular	2.0000	1.000	Each	0.17	0.41	1.30	9.46	0.00	0.11	0.00	0.07
	Crackers, Wheat, w/ Cheese Filli	14.1750	1.000	Each	1.39	3.54	8.25	70.45	0.00	0.44	0.99	0.59
	Crackers, Wheat, w/Peanut Butter	14.1750	1.000	Each	1.91	3.78	7.63	70.17	0.00	0.62	0.00	0.65
215	Crackers, Whole-wheat	4.0000	1.000	Each	0.35	0.69	2.74	17.72	0.00	0.42	0.00	0.12
216	Crackers, Whole-wheat, Low Salt	4.0000	1.000	Each	0.35	0.69	2.74	17.72	0.00	0.00	0.00	0.12
	Croutons, Plain	30.0000	1.000	Cup	3.57	1.98	22.05	122.10	0.00	1.53	0.00	0.45
	Croutons, Seasoned	40.0000	1.000	Cup	4.32	7.32	25.40	186.00	0.00	2.00	2.80	2.10
	English Muffins, Mixed-grain	56.7000	1.000	Each	5.16	1.02	26.26	133.24	0.00	1.58	0.00	0.14
	English Muffins, Mixed-grain, To	56.7000	1.000	Each	5.62	1.08	28.52	144.58	0.00	1.72	0.00	0.14
	English Muffins, Plain	56.7000	1.000	Each	4.36	1.02	26.08	133.24	0.00	1.54	0.00	0.14
	English Muffins, Plain, Toasted	56.7000	1.000	Each	4.76	1.14	28.36	144.58	0.00	1.64	0.00	0.16
	English Muffins, Raisin-cinnamon	56.7000	1.000	Each	4.26	1.44	27.62	137.78	0.00	1.64	0.00	0.22
	English Muffins, Raisin-cinnamon	56.7000	1.000	Each	4.62	1.64	30.06	149.68	0.00	1.76	0.00	0.24
	English Muffins, Wheat	56.7000	1.000	Each	4.94	1.14	25.40	126.44	0.00	2.62	0.00	0.16
	English Muffins, Wheat, Toasted	56.7000	1.000	Each	5.32	1.20	27.62	137.78	0.00	2.86	0.00	0.18
	English Muffins, Whole-wheat	56.7000	1.000	Each	4.98	1.20	22.90	115.10	0.00	3.80	0.00	0.18
	English Muffins, Whole-wheat, To	56.7000	1.000	Each	5.44	1.30	25.00	125.30	0.00	4.14	0.00	0.20
	Flour, White	125.0000	1.000	Cup	12.91	1.23	95.39	455.00	0.00	3.38	0.00	0.20

Monounsaturated Fat (gm)	Polyunsaturated Fat (gm)	Vitamin D (mg)	Vitamin K (mg)	Vitamin E (mg)	Vitamin A (re)	Vitamin C (mg)	Thiamin (mg)	Riboflavin (mg)	Niacin (mg)	Vitamin B₆ (mg)	Folate (mg)	Vitamin B₁₂ (mcg)	Calcium (mg)	Iron (mg)	Magnesium (mg)	Phosphorus (mg)	Potassium (mg)	Sodium (mg)	Zinc (mg)
0.59	0.24	0.00	0.00	0.00	0.00	0.00	0.12	0.09	1.44	0.06	6.60	0.00	26.73	1.11	29.37	67.32	82.17	176.22	0.49
0.53	0.28	0.00	0.00	0.17	0.00	0.00	0.10	0.08	1.14	0.03	18.43	0.00	32.32	1.02	14.18	46.21	61.80	163.30	0.32
0.40	0.19	0.00	0.00	0.00	0.00	0.00	0.12	0.09	0.99	0.02	8.50	0.00	27.00	0.76	6.00	23.50	29.75	134.50	0.16
0.41	0.19	0.00	0.00	0.00	0.00	0.00	0.10	0.08	0.90	0.01	5.98	0.00	27.37	0.77	5.98	23.69	30.13	136.16	0.16
0.48	0.28	0.00	0.00	0.24	0.00	0.00	0.10	0.06	1.09	0.05	14.18	0.00	20.41	0.94	24.38	64.92	71.44	149.40	0.55
0.36	0.92	0.00	0.00	0.45	0.00	0.00	0.08	0.07	1.12	0.06	16.16	0.00	10.21	0.96	25.23	58.12	97.81	108.01	0.47
3.09	4.94	0.00	0.00	1.11	2.55	0.00	0.03	0.02	0.44	0.03	6.24	0.00	48.20	0.21	12.76	39.12	50.18	421.85	0.33
1.62	0.66	0.00	0.00	0.32	0.00	0.00	0.26	0.18	2.54	0.06	53.86	0.00	53.86	2.24	24.94	69.18	90.72	259.68	0.60
0.48	1.42	0.00	0.00	0.88	0.00	0.06	0.28	0.18	2.22	0.02	53.86	0.04	78.82	1.80	11.34	49.84	79.94	317.52	0.36
0.02	0.03	0.00	0.00	0.00	0.00	0.00	0.00	0.00	0.00	0.00	0.00	0.00	2.56	0.60	3.84	16.64	3.84	11.52	0.08
0.04	0.10	0.00	0.00	0.02	0.00	0.00	0.10	0.04	1.54	0.08	23.55	0.00	12.56	0.60	12.56	34.54	91.06	7.85	0.41
7.51	1.53	0.00	0.00	1.64	18.60	0.00	0.35	0.27	2.90	0.34	49.60	0.29	93.62	2.96	22.32	135.16	89.90	616.90	0.70
0.85	0.31	0.00	0.00	0.00	0.00	0.00	0.03	0.02	0.46	0.10	1.75	0.00	5.53	0.20	4.06	22.68	17.15	69.44	0.08
0.00	0.00	0.00	0.00	0.00	0.00	0.00	0.00	0.00	0.00	0.00	0.00	0.00	3.42	0.06	0.00	0.00	0.00	21.40	0.00
0.02	0.06	0.00	0.00	0.00	0.00	0.00	0.02	0.01	0.10	0.02	2.20	0.00	3.10	0.24	7.80	26.90	31.90	26.40	0.24
0.00	0.00	0.00	0.00	0.00	0.00	0.00	0.00	0.00	0.00	0.00	0.00	0.00	0.00	0.01	0.00	0.00	0.00	2.01	0.00
0.35	0.11	0.00	0.00	0.00	0.00	0.00	0.02	0.02	0.29	0.00	1.19	0.00	1.68	0.26	2.10	7.28	9.45	42.35	0.06
0.17	0.13	0.00	0.00	0.00	3.69	0.03	0.22	0.18	1.44	0.01	33.17	0.05	11.34	0.77	6.80	41.96	42.53	5.95	0.21
0.28	0.28	0.00	0.00	0.00	1.98	0.06	0.16	0.12	1.39	0.03	44.79	0.06	10.21	1.24	8.51	25.23	23.53	80.80	0.21
0.04	0.17	0.00	0.00	0.02	0.00	0.00	0.11	0.08	1.10	0.03	33.17	0.00	3.69	0.90	7.09	25.23	31.75	0.57	0.19
0.05	0.18	0.00	0.00	0.38	0.00	0.00	0.10	0.08	1.53	0.05	9.92	0.00	6.52	1.32	37.99	86.47	89.59	0.57	0.74
0.23	0.38	0.00	0.00	0.02	0.00	0.00	0.12	0.08	1.23	0.03	37.20	0.00	27.90	1.11	17.70	58.80	60.60	248.70	0.60
0.04	0.06	0.00	0.00	0.00	0.00	0.00	0.02	0.01	0.21	0.00	1.30	0.00	4.65	0.19	2.95	9.80	10.10	0.95	0.10
0.13	0.19	0.00	0.00	0.09	0.00	0.00	0.07	0.04	0.67	0.01	12.05	0.00	11.06	0.52	5.53	25.94	27.36	127.43	0.19
0.08	0.13	0.00	0.00	0.00	0.00	0.00	0.06	0.04	0.72	0.01	18.71	0.00	6.10	0.64	7.94	23.39	20.98	118.64	0.21
6.60	5.92	0.00	0.00	2.80	0.00	0.00	0.25	0.21	2.51	0.03	47.74	0.00	74.40	2.23	16.74	141.36	82.46	525.14	0.42
6.60	5.92	0.00	0.00	2.80	0.00	0.00	0.25	0.21	2.51	0.03	47.74	0.00	74.40	2.23	16.74	141.36	220.10	231.26	0.42
1.74	0.41	0.00	0.00	0.00	5.53	0.06	0.09	0.07	0.51	0.01	11.48	0.02	31.47	0.35	5.24	48.05	48.48	147.99	0.10
0.04	0.10	0.00	0.00	0.00	0.50	0.03	0.11	0.07	0.40	0.07	11.25	0.00	10.00	1.49	30.25	83.50	123.75	198.50	0.70
0.46	0.51	0.00	0.00	0.00	0.14	0.01	0.05	0.03	0.35	0.03	7.37	0.00	6.24	0.43	15.03	43.52	64.35	125.73	0.36
0.19	0.06	0.00	0.00	0.00	0.00	0.00	0.02	0.01	0.16	0.00	0.93	0.00	3.57	0.16	0.81	3.15	3.84	39.06	0.02
0.00	0.00	0.00	0.00	0.00	0.00	0.00	0.00	0.00	0.00	0.00	0.00	0.00	0.00	0.12	0.00	0.00	25.60	36.00	0.00
0.19	0.06	0.00	0.00	0.00	0.00	0.00	0.02	0.01	0.16	0.00	0.93	0.00	3.57	0.16	0.81	3.15	21.72	19.08	0.02
1.59	0.36	0.00	0.00	0.37	2.69	0.01	0.06	0.10	0.53	0.01	11.91	0.01	36.43	0.34	5.10	57.55	60.81	198.59	0.09
1.79	0.62	0.00	0.00	0.53	0.00	0.00	0.06	0.05	0.83	0.02	11.91	0.00	13.75	0.43	7.51	34.16	31.61	133.53	0.15
0.00	0.00	0.00	0.00	0.00	0.00	0.00	0.00	0.00	0.00	0.00	0.00	0.00	4.80	0.08	0.00	0.00	9.00	34.00	0.00
0.23	0.06	0.00	0.00	0.00	0.00	0.00	0.01	0.01	0.10	0.00	0.36	0.00	0.98	0.09	1.24	4.40	4.06	5.66	0.03
0.23	0.06	0.00	0.00	0.00	0.00	0.00	0.01	0.01	0.10	0.00	0.36	0.00	0.98	0.09	1.24	4.40	3.66	15.90	0.03
1.47	1.30	0.00	0.00	0.00	1.28	0.21	0.05	0.06	0.45	0.04	9.07	0.02	28.92	0.37	7.65	54.15	43.38	129.42	0.12
1.67	1.26	0.00	0.00	0.00	0.00	0.00	0.06	0.04	0.83	0.02	9.92	0.00	24.10	0.38	5.39	49.19	42.10	114.39	0.12
0.38	0.11	0.00	0.00	0.00	0.00	0.00	0.01	0.00	0.18	0.01	1.12	0.00	2.00	0.12	3.96	11.80	11.88	26.36	0.09
0.38	0.11	0.00	0.00	0.00	0.00	0.00	0.01	0.00	0.18	0.01	1.12	0.00	2.00	0.12	3.96	11.80	11.88	9.88	0.09
0.92	0.38	0.00	0.00	0.00	0.00	0.00	0.19	0.08	1.63	0.01	39.60	0.00	22.80	1.22	9.30	34.50	37.20	209.40	0.27
3.80	0.95	0.00	0.00	0.87	4.00	0.00	0.20	0.17	1.86	0.03	35.20	0.06	38.40	1.13	16.80	56.00	72.40	495.20	0.38
0.48	0.32	0.00	0.00	0.16	0.00	0.00	0.24	0.18	2.02	0.02	45.36	0.00	111.14	1.72	23.24	45.92	88.46	235.88	0.78
0.52	0.54	0.00	0.00	0.70	0.56	0.00	0.20	0.18	2.00	0.06	37.98	0.00	120.78	1.86	27.22	91.86	95.82	256.86	0.60
0.18	0.50	0.00	0.00	0.10	0.00	0.00	0.24	0.16	2.20	0.02	45.92	0.02	98.66	1.42	11.90	75.42	74.28	263.08	0.40
0.18	0.54	0.00	0.00	0.10	0.00	0.06	0.22	0.16	2.16	0.02	41.96	0.02	107.16	1.54	12.48	82.22	81.08	285.76	0.44
0.28	0.78	0.00	0.00	0.24	0.00	0.18	0.22	0.16	2.02	0.04	45.92	0.00	83.34	1.38	8.50	39.12	117.94	253.44	0.56
0.32	0.82	0.00	0.00	0.10	0.00	0.18	0.18	0.16	3.96	0.04	39.12	0.00	90.16	1.50	9.64	47.62	128.14	275.56	0.62
0.16	0.48	0.00	0.00	0.28	0.00	0.00	0.24	0.16	1.90	0.06	31.18	0.00	100.92	1.62	20.98	60.66	105.46	216.60	0.60
0.18	0.52	0.00	0.00	0.20	0.00	0.00	0.22	0.16	1.86	0.06	26.04	0.00	109.44	1.76	23.82	70.88	114.54	235.30	0.70
0.28	0.48	0.00	0.00	0.40	0.00	0.00	0.18	0.08	1.94	0.10	27.78	0.00	150.26	1.38	40.26	159.90	119.08	361.18	0.90
0.32	0.52	0.00	0.00	0.44	0.00	0.00	0.14	0.08	1.90	0.10	20.98	0.00	163.12	1.50	43.66	174.06	129.28	392.36	0.98
0.11	0.51	0.00	0.63	0.08	0.00	0.00	0.99	0.61	7.38	0.05	192.50	0.00	18.75	5.80	27.50	135.00	133.75	2.50	0.88

USDA ID Code	Food Name	Weight in Grams*	Quantity of Units	Unit of Measure	Protein (gm)	Fat (gm)	Carbohydrate (gm)	Kcalories	Caffeine (gm)	Fiber (gm)	Cholesterol (mg)	Saturated Fat (gm)
	Flour, Whole Grain	120.0000	1.000	Cup	16.44	2.24	87.08	406.80	0.00	14.64	0.00	0.38
	Grits	165.0000	1.000	Cup	2.44	1.45	23.53	118.80	0.00	4.13	0.00	0.20
	Hominy, Cnd, Yellow	160.0000	1.000	Cup	2.37	1.41	22.82	115.20	0.00	4.00	0.00	0.19
	Hush Puppies	152.0000	1.000	Cup	11.70	20.52	69.92	512.24	0.00	4.26	68.40	3.21
	Macaroni, Ckd, Enriched	140.0000	1.000	Cup	6.68	0.94	39.68	197.40	0.00	1.82	0.00	0.14
	Macaroni, Ckd, Unenriched	140.0000	1.000	Cup	6.68	0.94	39.68	197.40	0.00	1.82	0.00	0.14
	Macaroni, Vegetable, Ckd, Enrich	134.0000	1.000	Cup	6.07	0.15	35.66	171.52	0.00	5.76	0.00	0.03
	Macaroni, Whole-wheat, Ckd	140.0000	1.000	Cup	7.46	0.76	37.16	173.60	0.00	3.92	0.00	0.14
	Noodles, Chinese, Chow Mein	45.0000	1.000	Cup	3.77	13.84	25.89	237.15	0.00	1.76	0.00	1.97
	Noodles, Egg, Ckd, Enriched	160.0000	1.000	Cup	7.60	2.35	39.74	212.80	0.00	1.76	52.80	0.50
	Noodles, Egg, Ckd, Unenriched	160.0000	1.000	Cup	7.60	2.35	39.74	212.80	0.00	0.00	52.80	0.50
	Noodles, Egg, Spinach, Ckd, Enri	160.0000	1.000	Cup	8.06	2.51	38.80	211.20	0.00	3.68	52.80	0.58
	Noodles, Japanese, Soba, Ckd	114.0000	1.000	Cup	5.77	0.11	24.44	112.86	0.00	0.00	0.00	0.02
	Noodles, Ramen	86.0000	1.000	Each	10.00	16.00	52.00	380.00	0.00	2.00	0.00	8.00
615	Noodles, Rice Stick	56.0000	2.000	Ounce	0.00	0.00	48.00	193.00	0.00	0.00	0.00	0.00
616	Noodles, Rice, dry	28.0000	0.500	Cup	2.30	3.00	21.40	121.00	0.00	0.40	0.00	0.60
	Pasta, Ckd, Enriched, w/ Added S	140.0000	1.000	Cup	6.68	0.94	39.68	197.40	0.00	2.38	0.00	0.14
	Pasta, Ckd, Enriched, w/o Added	140.0000	1.000	Cup	6.68	0.94	39.68	197.40	0.00	2.38	0.00	0.14
	Pasta, Fresh-refrigerated, Plain	57.0000	2.000	Ounce	2.94	0.60	14.21	74.67	0.00	0.00	18.81	0.09
	Pasta, Fresh-refrigerated, Spina	57.0000	2.000	Ounce	2.88	0.54	14.27	74.10	0.00	0.00	18.81	0.13
	Pasta, Homemade, Made w/ Egg, Ck	57.0000	2.000	Ounce	3.01	0.99	13.42	74.10	0.00	0.00	23.37	0.23
	Pasta, Homemade, Made w/o Egg, C	57.0000	2.000	Ounce	2.49	0.56	14.32	70.68	0.00	0.00	0.00	0.08
	Pasta, Spinach, Ckd	140.0000	1.000	Cup	6.41	0.88	36.61	182.00	0.00	0.00	0.00	0.13
	Pasta, Whole-wheat, Ckd	140.0000	1.000	Cup	7.46	0.76	37.16	173.60	0.00	6.30	0.00	0.14
690	Rice, Basmati	45.0000	0.250	Cup	3.00	0.00	34.00	150.00	0.00	0.00	0.00	0.00
	Rice, Brown, Long-grain, Ckd	195.0000	1.000	Cup	5.03	1.76	44.77	216.45	0.00	3.51	0.00	0.35
	Rice, Brown, Medium-grain, Ckd	195.0000	1.000	Cup	4.52	1.62	45.84	218.40	0.00	3.51	0.00	0.33
691	Rice, Dirty Rice, mix	38.0000	3.000	Tbsp	3.00	0.00	29.00	130.00	0.00	0.00	0.00	0.00
693	Rice, Jasmine	45.0000	0.250	Cup	3.00	0.00	34.00	150.00	0.00	0.00	0.00	0.00
	Rice, w/ Red Beans	28.3500	2.000	Ounce	3.98	0.50	19.89	94.50	0.00	3.48	0.00	0.00
	Rice, White, Long-grain, Ckd	158.0000	1.000	Cup	4.25	0.44	44.51	205.40	0.00	0.63	0.00	0.13
	Rice, White, Long-grain, Instant	165.0000	1.000	Cup	3.40	0.26	35.10	161.70	0.00	0.99	0.00	0.07
	Rice, White, Medium-grain, Ckd	186.0000	1.000	Cup	4.43	0.39	53.18	241.80	0.00	0.56	0.00	0.11
	Rice, White, Short-grain, Ckd	186.0000	1.000	Cup	4.39	0.35	53.44	241.80	0.00	0.00	0.00	0.09
	Rice, White, w/ Pasta, Ckd	202.0000	1.000	Cup	5.13	5.70	43.29	246.44	0.00	5.05	2.02	1.09
	Rice, Wild, Ckd	164.0000	1.000	Cup	6.54	0.56	35.00	165.64	0.00	2.95	0.00	0.08
	Rice, Wild, Uncle Ben's	56.0000	1.000	Cup	6.00	0.50	41.00	190.00	0.00	1.00	0.00	0.00
	Sesame Breadsticks, Wheat-based,	28.3500	1.000	Ounce	3.09	10.40	13.18	153.37	0.00	0.00	0.00	1.84
	Tabouli	28.3500	1.000	Ounce	1.00	2.00	2.00	30.00	0.00	1.00	0.00	0.00
	Taco Shells, Baked	28.3500	1.000	Ounce	2.04	6.41	17.69	132.68	0.00	2.13	0.00	0.92
	Taco Shells, Baked, w/o Added Sa	28.3500	1.000	Ounce	2.04	6.41	17.69	132.68	0.00	2.13	0.00	0.92
739	Tempeh	166.0000	1.000	Cup	31.46	12.75	28.27	330.34	0.00	0.00	0.00	1.84
	Tortillas, Corn	28.3500	1.000	Each	1.62	0.71	13.21	62.94	0.00	1.47	0.00	0.09
	Tortillas, Corn, w/o Added Salt	28.3500	1.000	Each	1.62	0.71	13.21	62.94	0.00	1.47	0.00	0.09
	Tortillas, Flour	28.3500	1.000	Each	2.47	2.01	15.76	92.14	0.00	0.94	0.00	0.50
	Tortillas, Flour, w/o Added Salt	28.3500	1.000	Each	2.47	2.01	15.76	92.14	0.00	0.94	0.00	0.50

Breakfast Foods/Cereals

USDA ID Code	Food Name	Weight in Grams*	Quantity of Units	Unit of Measure	Protein (gm)	Fat (gm)	Carbohydrate (gm)	Kcalories	Caffeine (gm)	Fiber (gm)	Cholesterol (mg)	Saturated Fat (gm)
	Biscuit	28.3500	1.000	Each	1.73	2.61	8.22	62.94	0.00	0.00	15.88	0.56
	Cereal, Bran 100%	66.0000	1.000	Cup	8.25	3.30	48.11	177.54	0.00	19.54	0.00	0.59
	Cereal, 100% Natural Cereal, Pla	48.0000	0.500	Cup	5.05	7.90	32.95	213.12	0.00	3.60	0.48	3.47
	Cereal, 100% Natural Cereal, w/	110.0000	1.000	Cup	11.22	20.35	72.38	496.10	0.00	7.26	0.00	13.68
	Cereal, 100% Natural Cereal, w/a	104.0000	1.000	Cup	10.71	19.55	69.78	477.36	0.00	6.86	0.00	15.46
	Cereal, 100% Natural Cereal, w/o	48.0000	0.500	Cup	5.05	7.90	32.95	213.12	0.00	3.60	0.48	3.47
136	Cereal, 100% Natural Crl, w/oats	51.0000	0.500	Cup	4.84	7.28	35.83	218.28	0.00	3.67	0.51	3.19
	Cereal, All-bran	30.0000	0.500	Cup	3.66	0.93	22.77	79.20	0.00	9.69	0.00	0.21
137	Cereal, All-Bran with Extra Fibe	30.0000	0.500	Cup	3.69	0.93	22.68	52.80	0.00	15.33	0.00	0.17
	Cereal, Almond Crunch	55.0000	1.000	Cup	4.35	0.83	46.92	198.00	0.00	4.62	0.00	0.17

Monounsaturated Fat (gm)	Polyunsaturated Fat (gm)	Vitamin D (mg)	Vitamin K (mg)	Vitamin E (mg)	Vitamin A (re)	Vitamin C (mg)	Thiamin (mg)	Riboflavin (mg)	Niacin (mg)	Vitamin B6 (mg)	Folate (mg)	Vitamin B12 (mcg)	Calcium (mg)	Iron (mg)	Magnesium (mg)	Phosphorus (mg)	Potassium (mg)	Sodium (mg)	Zinc (mg)
0.28	0.94	0.00	1.32	1.48	0.00	0.00	0.54	0.26	7.64	0.41	52.80	0.00	40.80	4.66	165.60	415.20	486.00	6.00	3.52
0.38	0.66	0.00	1.00	0.08	0.00	0.00	0.00	0.02	0.05	0.02	1.65	0.00	16.50	1.02	26.40	57.75	14.85	346.50	1.73
0.37	0.64	0.00	0.00	0.00	17.60	0.00	0.00	0.02	0.05	0.02	1.60	0.00	16.00	0.99	25.60	56.00	14.40	336.00	1.68
4.96	10.97	0.00	0.00	3.62	65.36	0.30	0.53	0.50	4.23	0.15	112.48	0.29	422.56	4.62	36.48	287.28	218.88	1015.36	1.00
0.11	0.38	0.00	0.00	0.04	0.00	0.00	0.28	0.14	2.34	0.06	98.00	0.00	9.80	1.96	25.20	75.60	43.40	1.40	0.74
0.11	0.38	0.00	0.00	0.04	0.00	0.00	0.03	0.03	0.56	0.06	9.80	0.00	9.80	0.70	25.20	75.60	43.40	1.40	0.74
0.01	0.05	0.00	0.00	0.05	6.70	0.00	0.15	0.08	1.43	0.03	87.10	0.00	14.74	0.66	25.46	67.00	41.54	8.04	0.59
0.11	0.29	0.00	0.00	0.14	0.00	0.00	0.15	0.07	0.99	0.11	7.00	0.00	21.00	1.48	42.00	124.60	61.60	4.20	1.13
3.46	7.80	0.00	0.00	0.07	4.05	0.00	0.26	0.19	2.68	0.05	40.50	0.00	9.00	2.13	23.40	72.45	54.00	197.55	0.63
0.69	0.66	0.00	0.00	0.00	9.60	0.00	0.30	0.13	2.38	0.06	102.40	0.14	19.20	2.54	30.40	110.40	44.80	264.00	0.99
0.69	0.66	0.00	0.00	0.00	9.60	0.00	0.05	0.03	0.64	0.06	11.20	0.14	19.20	0.96	30.40	110.40	44.80	264.00	0.99
0.78	0.56	0.00	0.00	0.08	22.40	0.00	0.40	0.19	2.35	0.18	102.40	0.22	30.40	1.74	38.40	91.20	59.20	19.20	1.01
0.03	0.03	0.00	0.00	0.00	0.00	0.00	0.10	0.03	0.58	0.05	7.98	0.00	4.56	0.55	10.26	28.50	39.90	68.40	0.14
0.00	0.00	0.00	0.00	0.00	0.00	0.00	0.00	0.00	0.00	0.00	0.00	0.00	0.00	1.60	0.00	0.00	0.00	1560.00	0.00
0.00	0.00	0.00	0.00	0.00	0.00	0.00	0.00	0.00	0.00	0.00	0.00	0.00	0.00	0.00	0.00	0.00	0.00	100.00	0.00
0.00	0.00	0.00	0.00	0.00	0.00	0.00	0.00	0.00	0.00	0.00	0.00	0.00	17.00	0.83	0.00	0.00	0.00	378.00	0.00
0.11	0.38	0.00	0.00	0.00	0.00	0.00	0.28	0.14	2.34	0.06	98.00	0.00	9.80	1.96	25.20	75.60	43.40	140.00	0.74
0.11	0.38	0.00	0.00	0.08	0.00	0.00	0.28	0.14	2.34	0.06	98.00	0.00	9.80	1.96	25.20	75.60	43.40	1.40	0.74
0.07	0.25	0.00	0.00	0.00	3.42	0.00	0.12	0.09	0.56	0.02	36.48	0.08	3.42	0.65	10.26	35.91	13.68	3.42	0.32
0.17	0.12	0.00	0.00	0.00	7.98	0.00	0.10	0.07	0.58	0.06	36.48	0.08	10.26	0.63	13.68	32.49	21.09	3.42	0.36
0.29	0.30	0.00	0.00	0.00	9.69	0.00	0.10	0.10	0.72	0.02	24.51	0.06	5.70	0.66	7.98	29.64	11.97	47.31	0.25
0.11	0.29	0.00	0.00	0.00	0.00	0.00	0.10	0.09	0.76	0.02	24.51	0.00	3.42	0.64	7.98	22.80	10.83	42.18	0.21
0.10	0.36	0.00	0.00	0.00	21.00	0.00	0.14	0.14	2.14	0.14	16.80	0.00	42.00	1.46	86.80	151.20	81.20	19.60	1.51
0.11	0.29	0.00	0.00	0.07	0.00	0.00	0.15	0.07	0.99	0.11	7.00	0.00	21.00	1.48	42.00	124.60	61.60	4.20	1.13
0.00	0.00	0.00	0.00	0.00	0.00	0.00	0.00	0.00	0.00	0.00	0.00	0.00	0.00	0.00	0.00	0.00	0.00	0.00	0.00
0.64	0.62	0.00	0.00	1.40	0.00	0.00	0.20	0.06	2.98	0.29	7.80	0.00	19.50	0.82	83.85	161.85	83.85	9.75	1.23
0.59	0.59	0.00	0.00	0.00	0.00	0.00	0.20	0.02	2.59	0.29	7.80	0.00	19.50	1.03	85.80	150.15	154.05	1.95	1.21
0.00	0.00	0.00	0.00	0.00	0.00	0.00	0.00	0.00	0.00	0.00	0.00	0.00	0.00	0.00	0.00	0.00	0.00	680.00	0.00
0.00	0.00	0.00	0.00	0.00	0.00	0.00	0.00	0.00	0.00	0.00	0.00	0.00	0.00	0.00	0.00	0.00	0.00	0.00	0.00
0.00	0.00	0.00	0.00	0.00	49.74	2.98	0.11	0.00	1.42	0.00	0.00	0.00	23.87	0.75	0.00	0.00	0.00	392.92	0.00
0.14	0.13	0.00	0.00	0.08	0.00	0.00	0.25	0.02	2.34	0.14	91.64	0.00	15.80	1.90	18.96	67.94	55.30	1.58	0.77
0.08	0.07	0.00	0.00	0.08	0.00	0.00	0.13	0.08	1.45	0.02	67.65	0.00	13.20	1.04	8.25	23.10	6.60	4.95	0.40
0.13	0.11	0.00	0.00	0.00	0.00	0.00	0.32	0.04	3.42	0.09	107.88	0.00	5.58	2.77	24.18	68.82	53.94	0.00	0.78
0.11	0.09	0.00	0.00	0.00	0.00	0.00	0.30	0.04	2.77	0.11	109.74	0.00	1.86	2.72	14.88	61.38	48.36	0.00	0.74
2.26	1.92	0.00	0.00	0.00	0.00	0.40	0.24	0.16	3.60	0.20	88.88	0.12	16.16	1.90	24.24	74.74	84.84	1147.36	0.57
0.08	0.34	0.00	0.00	0.38	0.00	0.00	0.08	0.15	2.12	0.23	42.64	0.00	4.92	0.98	52.48	134.48	165.64	4.92	2.20
0.00	0.00	0.00	0.00	0.00	0.00	2.40	0.00	0.00	0.00	0.00	0.00	0.00	24.00	1.00	0.00	0.00	0.00	620.00	0.00
3.09	4.94	0.00	0.00	0.00	2.55	0.00	0.03	0.02	0.44	0.03	6.24	0.00	48.20	0.21	12.76	39.12	50.18	8.22	0.33
0.00	0.00	0.00	0.00	0.00	100.00	12.00	0.00	0.00	0.00	0.00	0.00	0.00	0.00	0.40	0.00	0.00	0.00	75.00	0.00
2.53	2.41	0.00	0.00	1.03	0.00	0.00	0.07	0.01	0.38	0.09	29.77	0.00	45.36	0.71	29.77	70.31	50.75	104.04	0.40
2.53	2.41	0.00	0.00	1.03	0.00	0.00	0.07	0.01	0.38	0.09	29.77	0.00	45.36	0.71	29.77	70.31	50.75	4.25	0.40
2.81	7.19	0.00	0.00	0.00	114.54	0.00	0.22	0.18	7.69	0.50	86.32	1.66	154.38	3.75	116.20	341.96	609.22	9.96	3.01
0.18	0.32	0.00	0.00	0.04	0.00	0.00	0.03	0.02	0.43	0.06	32.32	0.00	49.61	0.40	18.43	89.02	43.66	45.64	0.27
0.18	0.32	0.00	0.00	0.04	0.00	0.00	0.03	0.02	0.43	0.06	32.32	0.00	49.61	0.40	18.43	89.02	43.66	3.12	0.27
1.07	0.30	0.00	0.00	0.26	0.00	0.00	0.15	0.08	1.01	0.01	34.87	0.00	35.44	0.94	7.37	35.15	37.14	135.51	0.20
1.07	0.30	0.00	0.00	0.26	0.00	0.00	0.15	0.08	1.01	0.01	34.87	0.00	11.06	0.94	7.37	35.15	37.14	135.51	0.20
0.66	1.18	0.00	0.00	0.00	14.46	0.62	0.06	0.08	0.43	0.01	10.21	0.06	58.40	0.49	4.54	42.81	39.12	116.80	0.15
0.57	1.87	0.00	0.00	1.53	0.00	62.70	1.58	1.78	20.92	2.11	46.86	6.27	46.20	8.12	312.18	801.24	652.08	457.38	5.74
3.48	1.04	0.00	0.00	0.55	0.48	0.14	0.17	0.08	0.85	0.09	12.00	0.05	46.08	1.44	50.40	148.80	210.72	12.96	1.15
3.72	1.71	0.00	0.00	0.77	6.60	0.00	0.31	0.65	2.09	0.17	45.10	0.15	159.50	3.12	124.30	347.60	537.90	47.30	2.11
1.83	1.33	0.00	0.00	0.73	6.24	1.04	0.33	0.57	1.87	0.11	16.64	0.30	157.04	2.89	71.76	350.48	513.76	52.00	2.00
3.48	1.04	0.00	0.00	0.55	0.48	0.14	0.17	0.08	0.85	0.09	12.00	0.05	46.08	1.44	50.40	148.80	210.72	12.96	1.15
3.17	0.82	0.00	0.00	0.51	0.51	0.31	0.14	0.09	0.77	0.08	11.73	0.05	38.76	1.67	47.94	149.94	213.69	11.22	1.08
0.18	0.54	0.03	0.00	0.55	225.30	15.00	0.39	0.42	5.01	0.51	90.00	1.50	105.90	4.50	128.70	294.00	341.70	60.90	3.75
0.18	0.58	0.00	0.00	0.64	259.80	17.31	0.42	0.48	5.76	0.57	120.00	1.74	115.50	5.19	119.70	287.40	300.00	126.90	4.32
0.22	0.44	0.00	0.00	3.00	47.30	0.00	0.52	0.59	7.00	0.69	99.00	2.10	26.40	5.99	48.95	129.80	170.50	284.35	1.43

USDA ID Code	Food Name	Weight in Grams*	Quantity of Units	Unit of Measure	Protein (gm)	Fat (gm)	Carbohydrate (gm)	Kcalories	Caffeine (gm)	Fiber (gm)	Cholesterol (mg)	Saturated Fat (gm)
138	Cereal, Almond Crunch w/Raisins	58.0000	1.000	Cup	5.00	2.50	46.00	210.00	0.00	5.00	0.00	0.00
	Cereal, Alpha-Bits	34.0000	1.000	Cup	2.58	0.78	29.44	133.28	0.00	1.46	0.00	0.13
139	Cereal, Apple Cinnamon Squares	55.0000	0.750	Cup	3.96	0.99	44.06	182.05	0.00	4.73	0.00	0.22
	Cereal, Apple Jacks	30.0000	1.000	Cup	1.44	0.39	26.84	115.50	0.00	0.57	0.00	0.09
	Cereal, Apple Raisin Crisp	55.0000	1.000	Cup	3.47	0.50	46.70	184.80	0.00	4.40	0.00	0.11
	Cereal, Basic 4	55.0000	1.000	Cup	4.18	2.84	41.97	200.75	0.00	3.36	0.00	0.42
	Cereal, Berry Berry-Kix	30.0000	0.750	Cup	1.31	1.16	26.13	120.00	0.00	0.18	0.00	0.20
	Cereal, Blueberry Squares	55.0000	0.750	Cup	4.18	0.99	43.78	181.50	0.00	4.84	0.00	0.22
140	Cereal, Boo Berry	30.0000	1.000	Cup	1.00	0.50	27.00	120.00	0.00	0.00	0.00	0.00
141	Cereal, Bran Buds	30.0000	0.330	Cup	2.82	0.72	23.97	82.80	0.00	11.97	0.00	0.12
	Cereal, Bran Flakes, 40%, Kello	29.0000	0.750	Cup	3.02	0.64	23.16	94.83	0.00	4.61	0.00	0.12
	Cereal, Bran Flakes, 40%, Post	47.0000	1.000	Cup	5.31	0.75	37.27	152.28	0.00	9.17	0.00	0.00
	Cereal, Bran Flakes, 40%, Ralsto	49.0000	1.000	Cup	5.64	0.69	39.10	158.76	0.00	6.91	0.00	0.00
	Cereal, Bran Flakes, Kellogg's	29.0000	0.750	Cup	3.02	0.64	23.16	94.83	0.00	4.61	0.00	0.12
	Cereal, Bran Flakes, Post	47.0000	1.000	Cup	5.31	0.75	37.27	152.28	0.00	9.17	0.00	0.12
142	Cereal, Bran, Frosted	30.0000	0.750	Cup	2.37	0.33	25.41	101.40	0.00	3.36	0.00	0.03
	Cereal, Brown Sugar Squares, Toa	55.0000	1.250	Cup	5.23	1.05	44.99	189.20	0.00	5.12	0.00	0.18
	Cereal, C.W. Post, Plain	97.0000	1.000	Cup	7.95	12.80	72.65	420.98	0.00	7.18	0.18	1.67
	Cereal, C.W. Post, w/ Raisins	103.0000	1.000	Cup	8.86	14.73	73.95	445.99	0.00	13.60	0.20	10.97
	Cereal, Cap'n Crunch	27.0000	0.750	Cup	1.35	1.37	23.04	107.19	0.00	0.86	0.00	0.37
	Cereal, Cap'n Crunch's Crunchber	26.0000	0.750	Cup	1.26	1.28	22.26	103.74	0.00	0.57	0.00	0.35
	Cereal, Cap'n Crunch's Peanut Bu	27.0000	0.750	Cup	1.95	2.32	21.51	112.32	0.00	0.78	0.00	0.52
	Cereal, Cheerios	30.0000	1.000	Cup	3.14	1.77	22.86	109.50	0.00	2.64	0.00	0.35
	Cereal, Cheerios, Apple Cinnamon	30.0000	0.750	Cup	1.86	1.63	25.05	117.90	0.00	1.59	0.00	0.30
143	Cereal, Cheerios, Frosted	30.0000	1.000	Cup	2.00	1.00	25.00	120.00	0.00	1.00	0.00	0.00
	Cereal, Cheerios, Honey Nut	30.0000	1.000	Cup	2.78	1.24	24.26	114.90	0.00	1.56	0.00	0.23
	Cereal, Cheerios, Multigrain	30.0000	1.000	Cup	2.56	1.09	24.45	111.90	0.00	1.92	0.00	0.25
	Cereal, Chex, Bran	49.0000	1.000	Cup	5.05	1.37	39.05	156.31	0.00	7.94	0.00	0.20
	Cereal, Chex, Corn	30.0000	1.000	Cup	2.18	0.37	25.61	112.80	0.00	0.54	0.00	0.07
	Cereal, Chex, Rice	31.0000	1.250	Cup	1.92	0.16	27.18	117.18	0.00	0.28	0.00	0.04
	Cereal, Chex, Wheat	30.0000	1.000	Cup	3.16	0.68	24.21	103.80	0.00	3.30	0.00	0.12
	Cereal, Cinnamon Mini Buns	30.0000	0.750	Cup	1.47	0.63	26.61	115.20	0.00	0.66	0.00	0.15
	Cereal, Cinnamon Oatmeal Squares	60.0000	1.000	Cup	7.57	2.57	47.15	231.60	0.00	4.56	0.00	0.50
	Cereal, Cinnamon Toast Crunch	30.0000	0.750	Cup	1.68	3.04	23.84	124.20	0.00	1.50	0.00	0.50
	Cereal, Cocoa Krispies	31.0000	0.750	Cup	1.55	0.81	27.25	120.28	1.24	0.40	0.00	0.59
	Cereal, Cocoa Puffs	30.0000	1.000	Cup	1.14	0.90	26.72	118.80	0.00	0.18	0.00	0.20
	Cereal, Cookie-crisp, Choc Chip	30.0000	1.000	Cup	1.53	1.08	26.25	120.00	0.60	0.42	0.00	0.60
	Cereal, Corn Bran	27.0000	0.750	Cup	1.86	0.89	22.73	89.91	0.00	4.81	0.00	0.21
144	Cereal, Corn Flakes, Country	30.0000	1.000	Cup	1.83	0.50	25.96	114.00	0.00	0.45	0.00	0.15
	Cereal, Corn Flakes, Honey and N	55.0000	1.250	Cup	4.02	2.48	45.98	222.75	0.00	0.88	0.00	0.50
145	Cereal, Corn Flakes, Honey Crunc	30.0000	0.750	Cup	5.00	1.00	44.00	190.00	0.00	5.00	0.00	0.00
	Cereal, Corn Flakes, Kellogg's	28.0000	1.000	Cup	1.84	0.20	24.22	102.20	0.00	0.78	0.00	0.06
	Cereal, Corn Flakes, Low Sodium	25.0000	1.000	Cup	1.93	0.08	22.20	99.75	0.00	0.28	0.00	0.01
	Cereal, Corn Flakes, Ralston Pur	25.0000	1.000	Cup	1.95	0.10	21.65	97.50	0.00	0.48	0.00	0.00
	Cereal, Corn Pops	31.0000	1.000	Cup	1.15	0.18	28.43	118.11	0.00	0.43	0.00	0.06
146	Cereal, Count Chocula	30.0000	1.000	Cup	1.00	1.00	26.00	120.00	0.00	0.00	0.00	0.00
	Cereal, Cracklin' Oat Bran	55.0000	0.750	Cup	4.61	6.97	40.10	224.95	0.00	6.55	0.00	2.92
	Cereal, Cream Of Rice, Ckd	244.0000	1.000	Cup	2.20	0.24	28.06	126.88	0.00	0.24	0.00	0.05
	Cereal, Cream Of Wheat, Instant	241.0000	1.000	Cup	4.34	0.48	31.57	154.24	0.00	2.89	0.00	0.07
	Cereal, Cream Of Wheat, Quick	239.0000	1.000	Cup	3.59	0.48	26.77	129.06	0.00	1.20	0.00	0.07
	Cereal, Cream Of Wheat, Regular	251.0000	1.000	Cup	3.77	0.50	27.61	133.03	0.00	1.76	0.00	0.08
	Cereal, Crisp Rice, Low Sodium	26.0000	1.000	Cup	1.43	0.08	23.66	104.52	0.00	0.36	0.00	0.09
	Cereal, Crispex	29.0000	1.000	Cup	2.15	0.29	25.00	108.46	0.00	0.64	0.00	0.09
	Cereal, Crispy Rice	28.0000	1.000	Cup	1.79	0.11	24.81	110.88	0.00	0.34	0.00	0.03
	Cereal, Crispy Wheats 'n Raisins	55.0000	1.000	Cup	4.47	0.76	44.33	191.40	0.00	3.41	0.00	0.15

Monounsaturated Fat (gm)	Polyunsaturated Fat (gm)	Vitamin D (mg)	Vitamin K (mg)	Vitamin E (mg)	Vitamin A (re)	Vitamin C (mg)	Thiamin (mg)	Riboflavin (mg)	Niacin (mg)	Vitamin B$_6$ (mg)	Folate (mg)	Vitamin B$_{12}$ (mcg)	Calcium (mg)	Iron (mg)	Magnesium (mg)	Phosphorus (mg)	Potassium (mg)	Sodium (mg)	Zinc (mg)
1.50	1.00	0.05	0.00	3.00	500.00	0.00	0.53	0.60	7.00	0.70	0.10	2.10	20.00	6.30	60.00	150.00	200.00	230.00	1.50
0.26	0.29	0.00	0.00	0.02	450.16	0.00	0.44	0.51	5.98	0.61	120.02	1.80	9.86	3.23	20.06	61.54	65.96	215.90	1.80
0.28	0.50	0.00	0.00	0.59	0.00	0.00	0.39	0.44	5.00	0.50	110.00	1.49	20.90	16.23	48.40	154.00	166.00	19.80	1.49
0.12	0.18	0.00	0.00	0.05	225.30	15.00	0.39	0.42	5.01	0.51	105.90	0.00	3.30	4.50	8.70	30.00	31.80	134.40	3.75
0.17	0.22	0.00	0.00	0.46	233.75	0.00	0.39	0.44	5.17	0.50	110.00	1.54	14.85	1.87	9.90	85.80	85.25	373.45	1.54
0.99	1.10	0.00	0.00	0.68	375.10	14.96	0.37	0.42	5.00	0.50	99.55	0.00	309.65	4.50	40.15	231.55	161.70	322.85	3.75
0.46	0.06	0.00	0.00	0.17	225.30	15.00	0.38	0.43	5.00	0.50	99.90	0.00	66.00	4.50	5.70	37.20	23.70	184.50	3.75
0.22	0.55	0.00	0.00	0.85	0.00	0.00	0.39	0.44	5.12	0.50	110.00	1.54	19.25	16.50	51.15	161.70	183.15	20.35	1.54
0.00	0.00	0.00	0.00	0.00	0.00	15.00	0.38	0.43	5.00	0.50	100.00	0.00	20.00	4.50	0.00	20.00	15.00	210.00	3.75
0.15	0.45	0.00	0.00	0.48	225.30	15.00	0.39	0.42	5.01	0.51	90.00	0.00	20.10	4.50	83.40	166.20	269.70	199.80	6.45
0.12	0.41	0.03	0.00	5.37	362.79	14.99	0.38	0.44	5.00	0.49	102.37	1.45	13.92	8.12	60.03	149.93	175.16	226.20	3.75
0.00	0.00	0.00	0.00	0.54	622.28	0.00	0.61	0.70	8.27	0.85	165.91	2.49	20.68	7.47	101.52	296.10	250.51	430.99	2.49
0.00	0.00	0.00	0.00	0.00	648.76	25.97	0.64	0.74	8.62	0.88	172.97	2.60	22.54	7.79	117.60	272.93	286.16	456.19	2.04
0.12	0.41	0.00	0.00	5.37	362.79	14.99	0.38	0.44	5.00	0.49	102.37	1.45	13.92	8.12	60.03	149.93	175.16	226.20	3.75
0.11	0.37	0.00	0.00	0.54	622.28	0.00	0.61	0.71	8.27	0.85	165.91	2.49	20.68	13.44	101.52	296.10	250.51	430.99	2.49
0.09	0.21	0.00	0.00	0.23	217.80	14.52	0.36	0.42	4.83	0.48	90.00	1.44	9.30	4.35	37.80	92.40	122.10	206.40	3.63
0.15	0.43	0.00	0.00	3.00	51.15	0.00	0.55	0.61	7.15	0.72	110.00	2.15	18.70	6.44	59.40	194.15	213.95	1.65	1.54
6.00	4.66	0.00	0.00	0.68	1284.28	0.00	1.26	1.46	17.07	1.75	342.41	5.14	46.56	15.42	66.93	224.07	197.88	166.84	1.64
1.67	1.38	0.00	0.00	0.72	1363.72	0.00	1.34	1.55	18.13	1.85	363.59	5.46	50.47	16.38	74.16	231.75	260.59	160.68	1.64
0.27	0.19	0.00	0.00	0.14	3.51	0.00	0.38	0.42	5.00	0.50	100.17	0.00	5.40	4.50	9.45	28.62	34.56	208.44	3.75
0.26	0.20	0.00	0.00	0.18	4.68	0.03	0.37	0.42	5.00	0.50	100.10	0.01	6.50	4.50	9.88	29.64	36.66	190.32	4.01
0.82	0.53	0.00	0.00	0.15	3.78	0.00	0.38	0.42	5.00	0.50	100.17	0.00	2.70	4.50	18.63	51.84	62.10	203.85	3.75
0.64	0.22	0.03	0.00	0.21	375.30	15.00	0.38	0.43	5.00	0.50	99.90	0.00	55.20	8.10	32.70	114.00	88.50	284.10	3.75
0.64	0.21	0.00	0.00	0.30	225.30	15.00	0.38	0.43	5.00	0.50	99.90	0.00	35.40	4.50	20.10	65.10	60.00	150.30	3.75
0.00	0.00	0.00	0.00	0.00	750.00	15.00	0.38	0.43	5.00	0.50	100.00	0.00	20.00	4.50	16.00	60.00	60.00	210.00	3.75
0.48	0.19	0.03	0.00	0.31	225.30	15.00	0.38	0.43	5.00	0.50	99.90	0.00	20.40	4.50	29.40	102.90	85.20	258.90	3.75
0.30	0.15	0.00	0.00	0.19	225.30	15.00	0.38	0.43	5.00	0.50	99.90	0.00	57.00	8.10	29.70	114.30	97.20	254.10	3.75
0.25	0.67	0.00	0.00	0.56	10.78	25.97	0.64	0.26	8.62	0.88	172.97	2.60	29.40	13.99	69.09	172.97	216.09	345.45	6.48
0.09	0.20	0.00	0.00	0.10	0.00	6.00	0.38	0.00	5.00	0.50	99.90	1.50	100.20	9.00	8.40	21.60	32.40	288.90	0.37
0.05	0.05	0.00	0.00	0.00	0.00	6.01	0.38	0.02	5.00	0.50	99.82	1.50	103.54	9.00	9.30	35.34	35.96	291.40	0.00
0.11	0.28	0.00	0.00	0.44	0.00	3.60	0.23	0.04	3.00	0.30	60.00	0.90	60.00	9.00	33.60	109.50	116.10	268.50	0.74
0.18	0.30	0.00	0.00	0.05	225.30	15.00	0.39	0.42	5.01	0.51	90.00	0.00	3.90	4.50	11.10	24.00	36.60	207.60	3.75
0.86	1.07	0.00	0.00	2.22	165.00	6.60	0.41	0.46	5.48	0.55	109.80	0.00	41.40	14.55	70.20	181.80	250.20	266.40	4.11
0.93	0.53	0.00	0.00	0.28	225.30	15.00	0.38	0.43	5.00	0.50	99.90	0.00	42.30	4.50	13.50	74.40	44.10	210.30	3.75
0.09	0.12	0.00	0.00	0.14	225.06	15.00	0.37	0.43	4.99	0.50	93.00	0.00	4.03	1.80	11.47	29.45	60.14	210.18	1.49
0.35	0.05	0.00	0.00	0.14	0.00	15.00	0.38	0.43	5.00	0.50	99.90	0.00	33.00	4.50	6.60	42.60	52.20	180.60	3.75
0.22	0.16	0.00	0.00	0.08	0.00	0.00	0.39	0.27	5.28	0.54	105.90	1.59	5.70	4.77	8.40	24.00	29.40	206.70	3.17
0.23	0.27	0.00	0.00	0.14	3.78	0.00	0.08	0.42	5.00	0.50	100.17	0.00	20.52	7.56	14.31	35.64	56.16	253.26	3.75
0.09	0.03	0.00	0.00	0.08	225.30	15.00	0.38	0.43	5.00	0.50	99.90	0.00	53.40	8.10	7.20	39.30	40.50	283.80	3.75
1.16	0.83	1.25	0.00	0.14	225.50	15.02	0.39	0.44	5.01	0.50	110.00	0.00	5.50	4.51	4.95	36.30	59.95	370.15	0.39
0.50	0.00	0.05	0.00	3.00	500.00	0.00	0.53	0.60	7.00	0.70	0.10	2.10	0.00	6.30	60.00	200.00	210.00	5.00	1.50
0.03	0.11	0.02	0.00	0.04	210.28	14.00	0.36	0.39	4.68	0.48	98.84	0.00	1.12	8.68	3.36	10.92	25.48	297.92	0.17
0.02	0.03	0.00	0.00	0.03	9.50	0.00	0.00	0.05	0.11	0.02	1.75	0.00	10.75	0.56	3.25	12.25	18.25	2.50	0.07
0.00	0.00	0.00	0.00	0.00	9.50	0.00	0.13	0.03	1.05	0.02	1.75	0.00	1.75	0.63	2.75	9.75	22.00	239.00	0.06
0.06	0.03	0.00	0.00	0.03	232.81	15.50	0.40	0.43	5.18	0.53	109.43	0.00	2.48	1.86	2.48	6.51	22.63	123.07	1.55
0.00	0.00	0.00	0.00	0.00	0.00	15.00	0.38	0.43	5.00	0.50	100.00	1.50	20.00	4.50	0.00	20.00	60.00	190.00	3.75
3.25	0.75	0.05	0.00	0.36	253.00	16.83	0.42	0.48	5.61	0.56	152.90	0.00	24.75	2.04	76.45	186.45	254.65	195.25	1.65
0.00	0.00	0.00	0.00	0.00	0.00	0.00	0.00	0.00	0.98	0.07	7.32	0.00	7.32	0.49	7.32	41.48	48.80	422.12	0.39
0.00	0.00	0.00	0.00	0.00	0.00	0.00	0.24	0.00	1.69	0.02	149.42	0.00	60.25	12.05	14.46	43.38	48.20	363.91	0.41
0.00	0.00	0.00	0.00	0.00	0.00	0.00	0.24	0.00	1.43	0.02	107.55	0.00	50.19	10.28	11.95	100.38	45.41	463.66	0.33
0.00	0.00	0.00	0.00	0.00	0.00	0.00	0.25	0.00	1.51	0.03	45.18	0.00	50.20	10.29	10.04	42.67	42.67	336.34	0.33
0.02	0.03	0.00	0.00	0.03	0.00	0.00	0.00	0.05	0.36	0.04	2.86	0.00	17.42	0.80	10.14	27.04	20.28	2.60	0.39
0.06	0.12	0.02	0.00	0.12	225.33	14.99	0.38	0.44	4.99	0.49	87.00	0.00	3.48	1.80	6.96	26.68	35.09	240.12	1.51
0.04	0.03	0.00	0.00	0.03	371.00	14.81	0.52	0.59	6.92	0.69	138.32	0.08	5.04	0.70	11.76	30.52	26.60	205.52	0.46
0.12	0.17	0.00	0.00	0.57	375.10	0.00	0.37	0.42	5.00	0.50	99.55	0.00	69.30	4.50	42.35	140.25	229.90	284.90	1.08

USDA ID Code	Food Name	Weight in Grams*	Quantity of Units	Unit of Measure	Protein (gm)	Fat (gm)	Carbohydrate (gm)	Kcalories	Caffeine (gm)	Fiber (gm)	Cholesterol (mg)	Saturated Fat (gm)
147	Cereal, Crunchy Pecan-Great Grai	53.0000	0.660	Cup	5.00	6.00	38.00	220.00	0.00	4.00	0.00	1.00
	Cereal, Fiber One	30.0000	0.500	Cup	2.78	0.84	24.01	61.50	0.00	14.25	0.00	0.13
	Cereal, Fortified Oat Flakes	48.0000	1.000	Cup	8.98	0.72	34.75	177.12	0.00	1.44	0.00	0.00
148	Cereal, Frankenberry	30.0000	1.000	Cup	1.00	1.00	27.00	120.00	0.00	0.00	0.00	0.00
149	Cereal, French Toast Crunch	30.0000	0.750	Cup	1.00	1.50	26.00	120.00	0.00	0.00	0.00	0.00
	Cereal, Frosted Flakes	31.0000	0.750	Cup	1.21	0.16	28.27	119.35	0.00	0.62	0.00	0.06
150	Cereal, Frosted Flakes, Cocoa-Ke	31.0000	0.750	Cup	1.00	0.00	28.00	120.00	0.00	0.00	0.00	0.00
	Cereal, Frosted Mini-Wheats	55.0000	1.000	Cup	5.17	0.88	45.38	186.45	0.00	5.89	0.00	0.17
	Cereal, Fruit Loops	30.0000	1.000	Cup	1.47	0.87	26.46	117.30	0.00	0.57	0.00	0.39
	Cereal, Fruity Pebbles	32.0000	1.000	Cup	1.28	1.66	27.55	129.60	0.00	0.42	0.00	1.37
	Cereal, Golden Grahams	30.0000	0.750	Cup	1.60	1.08	25.69	115.50	0.00	0.93	0.00	0.18
	Cereal, Graham Crackos	30.0000	1.000	Cup	2.25	0.18	25.92	108.30	0.00	1.83	0.00	0.00
151	Cereal, Granola Low Fat w/Raisin	60.0000	0.500	Cup	5.00	3.00	47.00	220.00	0.00	3.00	0.00	1.00
152	Cereal, Granola Low Fat-Kellogg'	50.0000	0.500	Cup	4.00	3.00	39.00	190.00	0.00	3.00	0.00	0.50
	Cereal, Granola w/ Almonds-Sun C	57.0000	0.500	Cup	6.71	10.27	38.30	266.19	0.00	2.96	0.00	1.27
	Cereal, Granola, Low Fat-Kellog	82.4590	1.000	Cup	7.50	4.50	64.47	314.84	0.00	4.50	0.00	1.50
	Cereal, Granola, Homemade	122.0000	1.000	Cup	17.93	30.01	64.66	569.74	0.00	12.81	0.00	5.80
	Cereal, Granola, w/ raisins, Low	55.0000	0.670	Cup	4.51	2.75	43.67	201.85	0.00	3.30	0.00	0.94
	Cereal, Granola, w/o raisins, L	55.0000	0.500	Cup	4.62	3.25	44.17	213.40	0.00	3.25	0.00	0.50
	Cereal, Granola, w/raisins&dates	31.0000	0.500	Cup	3.02	4.23	22.38	135.16	0.00	1.86	0.00	0.64
	Cereal, Granola-Nature Valley	55.0000	0.750	Cup	5.80	9.69	36.23	248.05	0.00	3.52	0.00	1.27
	Cereal, Grape-nuts	109.0000	1.000	Cup	12.75	0.44	89.38	389.13	0.00	10.90	0.00	0.06
	Cereal, Grape-nuts Flakes	39.0000	1.000	Cup	3.94	0.36	26.55	116.20	0.00	3.21	0.00	0.00
	Cereal, Great Grains	79.4600	1.000	Cup	1.13	9.00	56.97	329.84	0.00	6.00	0.00	1.50
	Cereal, Heartland Natural Cereal	115.0000	1.000	Cup	11.62	17.71	78.55	499.10	0.00	7.02	0.00	4.52
	Cereal, Heartland Natural Cereal	110.0000	1.000	Cup	10.67	15.62	75.90	467.50	0.00	6.05	0.00	3.98
	Cereal, Heartland Natural Cereal	105.0000	1.000	Cup	10.92	17.12	71.30	463.05	0.00	7.46	0.00	6.23
153	Cereal, Honey Bunches of Oats	30.0000	0.750	Cup	2.00	1.50	25.00	120.00	0.00	1.00	0.00	0.50
154	Cereal, Honey Bunches of Oats w/	31.0000	0.750	Cup	3.00	3.00	24.00	130.00	0.00	1.00	0.00	0.50
	Cereal, Honey Graham Oh!	27.0000	0.750	Cup	1.35	1.91	22.75	111.78	0.00	0.70	0.00	0.55
155	Cereal, Honey Nut Clusters	55.0000	1.000	Cup	4.00	2.50	46.00	210.00	0.00	3.00	0.00	0.00
	Cereal, Honeybran	35.0000	1.000	Cup	3.08	0.74	28.63	119.35	0.00	3.89	0.00	0.26
	Cereal, Honeycomb	22.0000	1.000	Cup	1.28	0.40	19.60	86.02	0.00	0.62	0.00	0.00
	Cereal, Just Right	55.0000	1.000	Cup	4.24	1.49	46.04	204.05	0.00	2.81	0.00	0.11
	Cereal, Just Right, Fruit & Nut	55.0000	1.000	Cup	4.13	1.60	44.28	192.50	0.00	2.75	0.00	0.28
156	Cereal, King Vitamin	31.0000	1.500	Cup	2.30	1.10	26.10	120.00	0.00	1.20	0.00	0.30
	Cereal, Kix	30.0000	1.330	Cup	1.96	0.62	25.91	114.30	0.00	0.81	0.00	0.17
	Cereal, Life	32.0000	0.750	Cup	3.15	1.28	25.18	121.28	0.00	2.05	0.00	0.24
	Cereal, Life, Cinnamon	50.0000	1.000	Cup	4.36	1.74	40.40	189.50	0.00	2.95	0.00	0.33
	Cereal, Lucky Charms	30.0000	1.000	Cup	2.15	1.08	25.17	116.10	0.00	1.20	0.00	0.22
	Cereal, Malt-o-meal, Plain and C	240.0000	1.000	Cup	3.60	0.24	25.92	122.40	2.40	0.96	0.00	0.05
	Cereal, Maypo, Ckd w/ water, w/	240.0000	1.000	Cup	5.76	2.40	31.92	170.40	0.00	5.76	0.00	0.46
	Cereal, Maypo, Ckd w/ water, w/o	240.0000	1.000	Cup	5.76	2.40	31.92	170.40	0.00	5.76	0.00	0.43
157	Cereal, Mueslix Raisin&Almond Cr	55.0000	0.660	Cup	5.00	3.00	41.00	200.00	0.00	4.00	0.00	0.00
	Cereal, Mueslix, Apple & Almond	55.0000	0.750	Cup	5.39	4.95	40.87	210.65	0.00	4.68	0.00	1.05
	Cereal, Nut & Honey Crunch	55.0000	1.250	Cup	4.02	2.48	45.98	222.75	0.00	0.88	0.00	0.50
158	Cereal, Nutri-Grain Almond Raisi	49.0000	1.250	Cup	4.00	2.50	38.00	180.00	0.00	4.00	0.00	0.00
	Cereal, Nutri-grain, Barley	41.0000	1.000	Cup	4.47	0.33	33.95	152.52	0.00	2.38	0.00	0.00
	Cereal, Nutri-grain, Corn	42.0000	1.000	Cup	3.36	0.97	35.45	160.02	0.00	2.60	0.00	0.00
	Cereal, Nutri-grain, Rye	40.0000	1.000	Cup	3.48	0.28	33.88	143.60	0.00	2.56	0.00	0.00
	Cereal, Nutri-grain, Wheat	30.0000	0.750	Cup	3.03	0.99	24.00	100.50	0.00	3.78	0.00	0.06
	Cereal, Oat Bran Cereal	57.0000	1.250	Cup	8.54	2.95	41.39	212.61	0.00	5.99	0.00	0.54
	Cereal, Oat Flakes	48.0000	1.000	Cup	7.87	0.96	36.10	180.48	0.00	1.44	0.00	0.16
	Cereal, Oatmeal Cereal, Honey Nu	49.0000	1.000	Cup	4.89	2.71	38.96	190.61	0.00	3.33	0.49	0.52
	Cereal, Oatmeal Raisin Crisp	55.0000	1.000	Cup	4.35	2.45	43.70	204.05	0.00	3.52	0.00	0.39

Monounsaturated Fat (gm)	Polyunsaturated Fat (gm)	Vitamin D (mg)	Vitamin K (mg)	Vitamin E (mg)	Vitamin A (re)	Vitamin C (mg)	Thiamin (mg)	Riboflavin (mg)	Niacin (mg)	Vitamin B_6 (mg)	Folate (mcg)	Vitamin B_{12} (mcg)	Calcium (mg)	Iron (mg)	Magnesium (mg)	Phosphorus (mg)	Potassium (mg)	Sodium (mg)	Zinc (mg)
0.00	0.00	0.00	0.00	0.00	1250.00	0.00	0.38	0.43	5.00	0.50	100.00	1.50	20.00	2.70	40.00	150.00	120.00	150.00	1.20
0.14	0.06	0.00	0.00	0.33	0.00	9.00	0.38	0.43	5.00	0.50	99.90	0.00	58.50	4.50	68.10	168.30	216.90	142.50	1.24
0.00	0.00	0.00	0.00	0.34	635.52	0.00	0.62	0.72	8.45	0.86	169.44	2.54	68.16	13.73	57.60	176.16	343.20	429.12	1.50
0.50	0.00	0.00	0.00	0.00	0.00	15.00	0.38	0.43	5.00	0.50	100.00	1.50	20.00	4.50	0.00	20.00	15.00	210.00	3.75
0.00	0.00	0.00	0.00	0.00	750.00	15.00	0.38	0.43	5.00	0.50	100.00	1.50	60.00	4.50	0.00	40.00	20.00	170.00	3.75
0.03	0.09	0.03	0.00	0.04	225.06	15.00	0.37	0.43	4.99	0.50	93.00	0.00	0.62	4.50	2.79	8.06	20.46	199.95	0.16
0.00	0.00	0.03	0.00	0.00	750.00	15.00	0.38	0.43	5.00	0.50	0.10	1.50	0.00	4.50	0.00	0.00	20.00	210.00	3.75
0.11	0.61	0.00	0.00	0.50	0.00	0.00	0.39	0.44	5.01	0.50	102.30	1.49	19.80	61.23	55.55	159.50	183.15	1.65	1.49
0.21	0.27	0.03	0.00	0.11	211.20	14.07	0.39	0.42	5.01	0.51	90.00	0.00	3.30	4.23	8.70	20.70	31.50	140.70	3.75
0.10	0.08	0.00	0.00	0.03	423.68	0.00	0.42	0.48	5.63	0.58	112.96	1.70	3.84	2.02	9.28	18.88	24.32	177.60	1.70
0.28	0.16	0.03	0.00	0.23	225.30	15.00	0.38	0.43	5.00	0.50	99.90	0.00	14.40	4.50	9.30	36.00	52.80	274.50	3.75
0.00	0.00	0.00	0.00	0.02	397.20	15.90	0.39	0.45	5.28	0.54	105.90	0.00	13.80	1.89	24.90	65.70	108.30	195.90	1.59
0.50	1.50	0.03	0.00	8.00	750.00	3.60	0.38	0.43	5.00	0.50	0.10	1.50	20.00	1.80	40.00	150.00	170.00	150.00	3.75
0.50	2.00	0.03	0.00	0.00	750.00	2.40	0.38	0.43	5.00	0.50	0.10	1.50	20.00	1.80	40.00	100.00	120.00	120.00	3.75
3.33	1.81	0.00	0.00	1.19	0.00	0.06	0.18	0.10	0.54	0.07	19.38	0.04	49.02	2.48	51.87	167.58	221.16	18.81	1.14
0.00	0.00	0.02	0.00	0.00	224.89	0.00	0.56	0.64	7.12	0.75	74.96	0.75	35.98	1.50	52.47	179.91	254.87	202.40	5.62
9.60	12.90	0.00	0.00	15.71	4.88	1.71	0.90	0.34	2.50	0.39	104.92	0.00	98.82	5.12	217.16	563.64	36.96	29.28	4.95
0.66	1.16	0.00	0.00	5.53	206.25	0.00	0.33	0.39	4.57	0.44	110.00	1.38	24.20	1.93	45.65	127.05	155.65	123.75	3.47
0.66	2.09	0.00	0.00	5.53	253.00	0.00	0.44	0.50	5.61	0.55	110.00	1.71	22.55	2.04	46.75	134.75	137.50	134.75	4.24
1.42	0.00	0.00	0.00	0.48	0.00	0.12	0.09	0.07	0.26	0.04	9.61	0.06	23.87	1.29	26.04	91.76	132.68	7.75	0.50
6.49	1.87	0.00	0.00	3.88	0.00	0.00	0.17	0.06	0.61	0.08	8.25	0.00	41.25	1.72	52.25	160.05	182.60	89.10	1.11
0.06	0.19	1.00	0.00	0.27	1443.16	0.00	1.42	1.64	19.18	1.96	384.77	5.78	10.36	31.17	73.03	273.59	364.06	757.55	2.40
0.00	0.00	0.00	0.00	0.08	429.73	0.00	0.42	0.49	5.71	0.58	114.57	1.72	12.98	9.28	35.70	96.72	112.95	183.06	0.65
0.00	0.00	0.02	0.00	0.00	374.81	0.00	0.56	0.64	7.12	0.75	74.96	0.75	35.98	2.25	52.47	179.91	179.91	224.89	1.80
4.80	7.08	0.00	0.00	0.81	6.90	1.15	0.36	0.16	1.61	0.20	64.40	0.00	74.75	4.34	147.20	416.30	385.25	293.25	3.04
4.22	6.24	0.00	0.00	0.77	6.60	1.10	0.32	0.14	1.54	0.20	44.00	0.00	66.00	4.02	140.80	376.20	414.70	225.50	2.83
3.97	5.68	0.00	0.00	0.74	6.30	1.05	0.35	0.15	1.79	0.17	56.70	0.00	66.15	5.39	137.55	380.10	384.30	213.15	2.74
0.00	0.00	0.00	0.00	0.00	1250.00	0.00	0.38	0.43	5.00	0.50	100.00	1.50	0.00	2.70	16.00	40.00	50.00	190.00	0.30
0.00	0.00	0.00	0.00	0.00	1250.00	0.00	0.38	0.43	5.00	0.50	100.00	1.50	0.00	2.70	24.00	60.00	65.00	180.00	0.30
1.06	0.28	0.00	0.00	0.11	301.32	12.04	0.38	0.47	5.02	0.50	100.44	0.00	12.42	4.51	12.69	41.85	45.09	0.00	3.76
0.00	0.00	0.00	0.00	0.00	0.00	9.00	0.38	0.43	5.00	0.50	100.00	0.00	40.00	4.50	32.00	100.00	130.00	270.00	0.60
0.08	0.26	0.00	0.00	0.81	463.40	18.55	0.46	0.53	6.16	0.63	23.45	1.86	16.10	5.57	45.85	131.95	150.50	202.30	0.90
0.00	0.00	0.02	0.00	0.09	291.28	0.00	0.29	0.33	3.87	0.40	77.66	1.17	3.74	2.09	7.48	21.78	70.40	123.86	1.17
0.28	1.05	0.00	0.00	2.24	375.65	0.00	0.39	0.44	5.01	0.50	102.30	1.49	14.30	16.23	34.10	106.15	121.00	337.70	0.88
0.77	0.55	0.00	0.00	3.00	344.30	0.00	0.33	0.39	4.57	0.44	110.00	1.38	0.00	14.85	33.00	108.90	155.65	265.65	1.05
0.40	0.30	0.00	0.00	0.00	1044.00	13.00	0.39	0.44	5.20	0.52	104.00	1.57	4.00	8.74	26.00	79.00	86.00	260.00	3.91
0.15	0.04	0.03	0.00	0.08	375.30	15.00	0.38	0.43	5.00	0.50	99.90	0.00	43.50	8.10	9.30	42.00	41.10	263.10	3.75
0.41	0.56	0.00	0.00	0.16	1.28	0.00	0.40	0.45	5.33	0.53	106.88	0.00	97.60	8.96	31.04	135.68	79.04	174.40	4.00
0.57	0.77	0.00	0.00	0.23	1.50	0.10	0.63	0.71	8.38	0.84	167.50	0.00	134.50	74.54	41.50	181.00	113.00	220.00	6.29
0.39	0.15	0.03	0.00	0.13	225.30	15.00	0.38	0.43	5.00	0.50	99.90	0.00	32.40	4.50	19.50	75.60	54.00	203.10	3.75
0.00	0.00	0.00	0.00	0.00	0.00	0.00	0.48	0.24	5.76	0.02	4.80	0.00	4.80	9.60	4.80	24.00	31.20	324.00	0.17
0.00	0.00	0.00	0.00	0.00	703.20	28.80	0.72	0.72	9.36	0.96	9.60	2.88	124.80	8.40	50.40	247.20	211.20	259.20	1.49
0.74	0.89	0.00	0.00	1.68	703.20	28.80	0.72	0.72	9.36	0.96	9.60	2.88	124.80	8.40	50.40	247.20	211.20	9.60	1.49
2.00	1.00	0.20	0.00	8.00	200.00	20.00	0.38	0.43	5.00	0.50	0.10	1.50	20.00	4.50	40.00	150.00	240.00	160.00	3.75
2.59	1.05	0.00	0.00	5.78	233.75	0.00	0.39	0.44	5.17	0.50	110.00	1.27	33.55	4.68	62.70	175.45	209.00	270.05	3.14
1.16	0.83	0.00	0.00	0.14	225.50	15.02	0.39	0.44	5.01	0.50	110.00	0.00	5.50	4.51	4.95	36.30	59.95	370.15	0.39
1.00	1.50	0.00	0.00	8.00	0.00	0.00	0.38	0.43	5.00	0.50	0.10	1.50	150.00	1.40	16.00	200.00	190.00	170.00	3.75
0.00	0.00	0.00	0.00	10.82	542.84	21.73	0.53	0.62	7.22	0.74	144.73	2.17	11.07	1.45	32.39	126.28	107.83	277.16	5.41
0.00	0.00	0.00	0.00	11.09	556.08	22.26	0.55	0.63	7.39	0.76	148.26	2.23	1.26	0.89	26.88	120.54	97.86	276.36	5.54
0.00	0.00	0.00	0.00	10.56	529.60	21.20	0.52	0.60	7.04	0.72	141.20	2.12	8.40	1.13	30.40	104.00	71.60	272.00	5.28
0.24	0.69	0.00	0.00	5.40	0.00	15.00	0.39	0.42	5.01	0.51	90.00	1.50	9.60	0.99	24.30	108.30	109.50	220.80	3.75
0.96	1.21	0.00	0.00	2.10	155.61	6.21	0.39	0.44	5.19	0.52	103.74	0.00	30.21	15.96	99.18	306.09	257.07	205.20	3.89
0.28	0.36	0.00	0.00	0.34	635.52	0.00	0.62	0.72	8.45	0.86	169.44	2.54	68.16	13.73	57.60	176.16	228.00	220.32	2.54
1.15	0.75	0.00	0.00	2.01	150.43	5.98	0.37	0.42	5.00	0.50	99.96	0.02	26.95	4.50	53.41	166.11	184.73	165.62	3.92
1.16	0.36	0.00	0.00	1.36	225.50	0.00	0.37	0.42	5.01	0.50	100.10	0.00	37.95	4.50	44.55	117.15	211.75	223.85	3.75

USDA ID Code	Food Name	Weight in Grams*	Quantity of Units	Unit of Measure	Protein (gm)	Fat (gm)	Carbohydrate (gm)	Kcalories	Caffeine (gm)	Fiber (gm)	Cholesterol (mg)	Saturated Fat (gm)
	Cereal, Oatmeal Squares	56.0000	1.000	Cup	7.27	2.59	43.32	216.16	0.00	4.26	0.00	0.48
	Cereal, Oatmeal, Dry	2.5000	1.000	Tbsp	0.34	0.20	1.73	9.95	0.00	0.17	0.00	0.03
	Cereal, Oatmeal, Prepared	28.3500	1.000	Ounce	1.42	1.16	4.34	32.89	0.00	0.31	3.21	0.64
	Cereal, Oats Granola, Toasted	55.0000	0.750	Cup	5.80	9.69	36.23	238.05	0.00	3.52	0.00	1.27
	Cereal, Oats, Instant, Plain	234.0000	1.000	Cup	5.85	2.34	23.87	138.06	0.00	3.98	0.00	0.42
	Cereal, Oats, Instant, w/ apples	149.0000	1.000	Pkt.	3.19	1.42	26.15	125.16	0.00	2.53	0.00	0.30
	Cereal, Oats, Instant, w/ bran &	195.0000	1.000	Pkt.	4.88	1.95	30.42	157.95	0.00	5.46	0.00	0.35
	Cereal, Oats, Instant, w/ cinn a	240.0000	1.000	Cup	7.20	2.88	52.32	264.00	0.00	3.84	0.00	0.53
	Cereal, Oats, Instant, w/ maple	155.0000	1.000	Pkt.	4.17	1.78	31.40	153.45	0.00	2.64	0.00	0.36
	Cereal, Oats, Instant, w/ raisin	240.0000	1.000	Cup	6.48	2.64	48.48	244.80	0.00	3.36	0.00	0.50
	Cereal, Oats, Reg and Quick and	234.0000	1.000	Cup	6.08	2.34	25.27	145.08	0.00	3.98	0.00	0.42
159	Cereal, Organic Frst Ultra Mini	55.0000	0.750	Cup	4.00	1.00	46.00	190.00	0.00	7.00	0.00	0.00
160	Cereal, Organic Mini Cr Wheat-Ba	55.0000	0.750	Cup	5.00	1.00	45.00	190.00	0.00	8.00	0.00	0.00
	Cereal, Peanut Butter Puffs-Rees	30.0000	0.750	Cup	2.57	3.20	22.98	129.30	0.00	0.39	0.00	0.64
	Cereal, Product 19	30.0000	1.000	Cup	2.67	0.39	24.96	109.80	0.00	0.99	0.00	0.03
	Cereal, Puffed Rice	14.0000	1.000	Cup	0.98	0.13	12.29	53.62	0.00	0.20	0.00	0.05
	Cereal, Puffed Wheat	15.0000	1.250	Cup	2.44	0.32	11.46	54.90	0.00	1.14	0.00	0.02
161	Cereal, Puffins-Barbara	27.0000	0.750	Cup	2.00	1.00	23.00	90.00	0.00	5.00	0.00	0.00
	Cereal, Quisp	27.0000	1.000	Cup	1.35	1.49	22.97	108.81	0.00	0.68	0.00	0.41
	Cereal, Raisin Bran, Total-Gener	55.0000	1.000	Cup	4.00	1.01	42.75	178.20	0.00	5.01	0.00	0.23
	Cereal, Raisin Bran-Kellogg's	61.0000	1.000	Cup	5.61	1.46	47.09	186.05	0.00	8.17	0.00	0.00
	Cereal, Raisin Bran-Post	56.0000	1.000	Cup	5.21	1.06	42.34	171.92	0.00	7.90	0.00	0.18
	Cereal, Raisin Bran-Ralston Puri	56.0000	1.000	Cup	4.37	0.28	46.48	178.08	0.00	7.50	0.00	0.04
	Cereal, Raisin Nut Bran	55.0000	1.000	Cup	5.16	4.40	41.45	209.00	0.00	5.06	0.00	0.72
	Cereal, Raisin Squares	55.0000	0.750	Cup	4.40	1.54	42.90	187.00	0.00	5.17	0.00	0.17
162	Cereal, Raisins, Dates & Pecans-	54.0000	0.660	Cup	4.00	5.00	39.00	210.00	0.00	4.00	0.00	0.50
	Cereal, Raisins, Rice and Rye	46.0000	1.000	Cup	2.62	0.14	39.28	154.56	0.00	2.62	0.00	0.00
	Cereal, Rice Krispies	33.0000	1.250	Cup	2.08	0.36	28.55	124.41	0.00	0.36	0.00	0.13
163	Cereal, Rice Krispies, Apple-Cin	30.0000	0.750	Cup	1.53	0.51	26.70	111.90	0.00	0.45	0.00	0.00
	Cereal, Rice, Puffed	14.0000	1.000	Cup	0.88	0.07	12.57	56.28	0.00	0.24	0.00	0.02
	Cereal, Shredded Wheat, Large	23.6000	1.000	Biscuit	2.57	0.39	19.19	84.96	0.00	2.31	0.00	0.07
	Cereal, Shredded Wheat, Small	30.0000	1.000	Cup	3.30	0.50	24.12	107.10	0.00	2.94	0.00	0.08
164	Cereal, Smacks Kellogg's	27.0000	0.750	Cup	2.00	0.50	24.00	100.00	0.00	1.00	0.00	0.00
	Cereal, S'mores Grahams	30.0000	0.750	Cup	1.68	1.20	25.59	117.00	0.00	0.84	0.00	0.18
	Cereal, Special K	31.0000	1.000	Cup	6.36	0.28	22.44	114.70	0.00	0.96	0.00	0.00
	Cereal, Super Sugar Crisp	33.0000	1.000	Cup	2.15	0.30	29.77	123.42	0.00	0.50	0.00	0.05
	Cereal, Tasteeos	24.0000	1.000	Cup	3.07	0.67	18.98	94.32	0.00	2.54	0.00	0.23
	Cereal, Team	42.0000	1.000	Cup	2.69	0.76	36.04	164.22	0.00	0.55	0.00	0.00
165	Cereal, Temptations, Fr. Vanilla	30.0000	0.750	Cup	2.13	1.65	24.72	119.40	0.00	0.78	0.00	1.05
166	Cereal, Temptations, Honey Roast	30.0000	1.000	Cup	1.80	2.25	24.42	122.40	0.00	0.69	0.00	0.51
	Cereal, Toasties	23.0000	1.000	Cup	1.84	0.05	19.73	89.01	0.00	0.78	0.00	0.01
168	Cereal, Total	30.0000	0.750	Cup	2.99	0.70	23.88	105.30	0.00	2.64	0.00	0.18
	Cereal, Triples	30.0000	1.000	Cup	2.38	1.01	24.98	116.10	0.00	0.84	0.00	0.29
	Cereal, Trix	30.0000	1.000	Cup	0.95	1.71	26.04	122.40	0.00	0.72	0.00	0.41
	Cereal, Waffelos	30.0000	1.000	Cup	1.68	1.26	25.89	121.50	0.00	0.00	0.00	0.00
167	Cereal, Weetabix	35.0000	2.000	Biscuits	4.00	1.00	28.00	120.00	0.00	4.00	0.00	0.00
	Cereal, Wheat Germ, Toasted	28.3500	1.000	Oz.	8.25	3.03	14.06	108.30	0.00	3.66	0.00	0.52
	Cereal, Wheat 'n Raisin Chex	54.0000	1.000	Cup	5.08	0.43	42.98	185.22	0.00	3.56	0.00	0.00
	Cereal, Wheatena, Ckd w/ water	243.0000	1.000	Cup	4.86	1.22	28.67	136.08	0.00	6.56	0.00	0.19
	Cereal, Wheatena, Ckd w/ water,	243.0000	1.000	Cup	4.86	1.22	28.67	136.08	0.00	6.56	0.00	0.22
	Cereal, Wheaties	30.0000	1.000	Cup	3.24	0.93	23.79	110.10	0.00	2.10	0.00	0.20
	Cereal, Whole Wheat Hot Natural	242.0000	1.000	Cup	4.84	0.97	33.15	150.04	0.00	3.87	0.00	0.15
	French Toast, Frozen, Ready-to-h	28.3500	1.000	Slice	2.10	1.73	9.10	60.39	0.00	0.31	23.25	0.43
	French Toast, Made w/ Lowfat (2%	28.3500	1.000	Slice	2.18	3.06	7.09	64.92	0.00	0.00	32.89	0.77
	French Toast, Made w/ Whole Milk	65.0000	1.000	Slice	5.01	7.35	16.19	150.80	0.00	0.00	76.05	1.95

Monounsaturated Fat (gm)	Polyunsaturated Fat (gm)	Vitamin D (mg)	Vitamin K (mg)	Vitamin E (mg)	Vitamin A (re)	Vitamin C (mg)	Thiamin (mg)	Riboflavin (mg)	Niacin (mg)	Vitamin B_6 (mg)	Folate (mg)	Vitamin B_{12} (mcg)	Calcium (mg)	Iron (mg)	Magnesium (mg)	Phosphorus (mg)	Potassium (mg)	Sodium (mg)	Zinc (mg)
0.81	1.05	0.00	0.00	2.28	169.12	6.78	0.42	0.48	5.63	0.56	112.56	0.00	35.84	15.68	70.00	185.92	227.92	263.20	4.22
0.06	0.07	0.00	0.00	0.01	0.05	0.08	0.07	0.07	0.90	0.00	0.88	0.00	18.33	1.19	3.63	12.48	11.75	0.83	0.09
0.00	0.00	0.00	0.00	0.00	7.40	0.37	0.14	0.16	1.70	0.02	2.84	0.09	62.37	3.44	9.92	45.36	57.83	13.04	0.26
6.49	1.87	0.00	0.00	3.88	0.00	0.00	0.17	0.06	0.61	0.08	8.25	0.00	41.25	1.72	52.25	160.05	182.60	189.10	1.11
0.75	0.87	0.00	0.00	0.28	599.04	0.00	0.70	0.37	7.23	0.98	128.70	0.00	215.28	8.33	56.16	175.50	131.04	376.74	1.15
0.51	0.58	0.00	0.00	0.12	305.45	0.30	0.30	0.34	4.08	0.40	93.87	0.00	104.30	3.89	29.80	113.24	105.79	210.69	0.70
0.00	0.00	0.00	0.00	0.00	479.70	0.00	0.57	0.64	8.13	0.76	156.00	0.00	173.55	7.62	56.55	206.70	235.95	247.65	1.35
0.96	1.01	0.00	0.00	0.53	705.60	0.00	0.84	0.50	8.42	1.15	228.00	0.00	256.80	9.89	76.80	216.00	156.00	417.60	1.44
0.62	0.74	0.00	0.00	0.17	302.25	0.00	0.29	0.34	4.03	0.40	80.60	0.00	105.40	3.86	38.75	131.75	111.60	234.05	0.90
0.84	0.94	0.00	0.00	0.24	669.60	0.00	0.77	0.55	8.33	1.13	228.00	0.00	252.00	10.01	55.20	201.60	228.00	343.20	1.08
0.75	0.87	0.00	0.00	0.00	4.68	0.00	0.26	0.05	0.30	0.05	9.36	0.00	18.72	1.59	56.16	177.84	131.04	374.40	1.15
0.00	0.00	0.00	0.00	0.00	0.00	0.00	0.00	0.00	0.00	0.00	0.00	0.00	0.00	0.00	0.00	0.00	0.00	200.00	0.00
0.00	0.00	0.00	0.00	0.00	0.00	0.00	0.00	0.00	0.00	0.00	0.00	0.00	0.00	0.00	0.00	0.00	0.00	240.00	0.00
1.43	0.60	0.00	0.00	0.57	225.30	15.00	0.38	0.43	5.00	0.50	99.90	0.00	21.00	4.50	15.90	43.20	61.50	177.30	3.75
0.15	0.21	0.03	0.00	22.20	225.30	60.00	1.50	1.71	20.01	2.01	390.00	6.00	2.70	18.00	12.30	33.00	40.50	216.00	15.00
0.03	0.05	0.00	0.00	0.01	0.00	0.00	0.06	0.01	0.88	0.00	1.40	0.00	1.26	0.41	4.20	16.52	16.24	0.70	0.15
0.05	0.16	0.00	0.00	0.10	0.15	0.00	0.06	0.04	1.79	0.02	5.10	0.06	3.60	0.70	19.95	49.65	54.60	0.75	0.46
0.00	0.00	0.00	0.00	0.00	0.00	0.00	0.00	0.00	0.00	0.00	0.00	0.00	0.00	0.00	0.00	0.00	0.00	190.00	0.00
0.33	0.21	0.00	0.00	0.14	3.24	0.00	0.38	0.43	5.09	0.51	101.79	0.00	5.13	4.58	13.77	42.39	36.18	194.40	3.82
0.17	0.17	0.00	0.00	29.98	375.10	0.00	1.50	1.70	20.02	2.00	399.85	6.35	238.15	18.00	44.55	258.50	287.10	239.80	15.00
0.24	0.79	0.04	0.00	0.56	250.10	0.00	0.43	0.49	5.55	0.55	122.00	1.65	35.38	5.00	89.06	214.11	436.76	353.80	4.15
0.15	0.50	0.05	0.00	1.30	741.44	0.00	0.73	0.84	9.86	1.01	197.68	2.97	26.32	8.90	95.20	234.64	344.96	365.12	2.97
0.04	0.13	0.00	0.00	1.30	556.08	1.68	0.56	0.62	7.39	0.73	148.40	2.24	26.88	27.33	84.56	247.52	287.28	486.08	1.67
1.93	0.46	0.00	0.00	2.03	0.00	0.00	0.37	0.42	5.00	0.5	99.55	0.00	73.70	4.50	53.90	162.80	218.35	245.85	1.11
0.11	0.50	0.00	0.00	0.29	0.00	0.00	0.39	0.44	5.17	0.50	110.00	1.54	18.70	16.83	47.85	159.50	259.60	3.30	1.54
0.00	0.00	0.00	0.00	0.00	1500.00	0.00	0.45	0.51	6.00	0.60	120.00	1.80	20.00	3.60	40.00	150.00	150.00	150.00	1.20
0.00	0.00	0.00	0.00	0.25	467.82	0.46	0.46	0.55	6.26	0.64	124.66	1.89	10.12	5.61	19.78	49.68	143.52	349.60	4.69
0.10	0.17	0.03	0.00	0.04	247.83	16.50	0.43	0.46	5.51	0.56	116.49	0.00	3.30	1.98	15.84	43.56	42.24	353.76	0.60
0.00	0.51	0.00	0.00	0.13	233.10	15.51	0.39	0.45	5.16	0.51	90.00	0.00	2.10	1.86	7.80	24.90	30.90	222.90	0.33
0.00	0.00	0.00	0.00	0.00	0.00	0.00	0.36	0.25	4.94	0.01	2.66	0.00	0.84	4.44	3.50	13.72	15.82	0.42	0.14
0.06	0.21	0.00	0.00	0.13	0.00	0.00	0.07	0.07	1.08	0.06	11.80	0.00	9.68	0.74	40.12	85.67	77.17	0.47	0.59
0.08	0.26	0.00	0.00	0.16	0.00	0.00	0.08	0.08	1.58	0.08	15.00	0.00	11.40	1.27	39.60	105.90	108.30	3.00	0.99
0.00	0.00	0.03	0.00	0.00	750.00	15.00	0.38	0.43	5.00	0.50	0.10	1.50	14.40	1.80	8.00	40.00	40.00	50.00	0.30
0.39	0.15	0.00	0.00	0.22	225.30	15.00	0.38	0.43	5.00	0.50	99.90	0.00	14.40	4.50	10.80	40.50	48.00	212.40	3.75
0.00	0.22	1.25	0.00	0.08	225.06	15.00	0.53	0.59	7.01	0.71	93.00	0.00	4.65	8.71	17.67	50.84	54.56	249.86	3.75
0.06	0.12	0.00	0.00	0.12	436.92	0.00	0.43	0.50	5.81	0.59	116.49	1.75	6.93	2.08	19.80	43.89	47.85	50.82	1.75
0.17	0.18	0.00	0.00	0.17	317.76	12.72	0.31	0.36	4.22	0.43	84.72	1.27	11.04	6.86	26.16	95.76	71.04	182.88	0.69
0.00	0.00	0.00	0.00	0.10	556.08	22.26	0.55	0.63	7.39	0.76	6.72	2.23	6.30	2.57	18.48	65.10	70.98	259.56	0.58
0.36	0.24	0.00	0.00	0.83	259.80	17.31	0.42	0.48	5.76	0.57	120.00	0.00	10.80	5.19	6.90	20.40	40.80	207.00	0.21
1.17	0.57	0.00	0.00	0.14	232.80	15.51	0.39	0.45	5.16	0.51	90.00	0.00	0.60	4.65	2.70	7.50	28.80	248.40	0.12
0.01	0.02	0.00	0.00	0.06	304.52	0.00	0.30	0.35	4.05	0.41	81.91	1.22	0.92	0.61	3.45	10.12	26.68	241.04	0.07
0.14	0.08	0.03	0.00	23.49	375.30	60.00	1.50	1.70	20.10	2.00	399.90	7.67	258.30	18.00	32.10	210.90	96.90	198.60	15.00
0.27	0.03	0.00	0.00	0.14	375.30	15.00	0.38	0.43	5.00	0.50	99.90	0.00	41.10	8.10	6.90	35.40	30.60	191.40	3.75
0.90	0.29	0.03	0.00	0.60	225.30	15.00	0.38	0.43	5.00	0.50	99.90	0.00	32.10	4.50	3.60	26.10	17.70	196.80	3.75
0.00	0.00	0.00	0.00	0.00	397.20	15.90	0.39	0.45	5.28	0.54	3.30	1.59	8.40	4.77	6.30	244.50	26.40	124.80	0.24
0.00	0.00	0.00	0.00	0.00	0.00	0.00	0.00	0.00	0.00	0.00	0.00	0.00	0.00	0.00	0.00	0.00	120.00	130.00	0.00
0.43	1.88	0.00	0.00	5.14	0.00	1.70	0.47	0.23	1.59	0.28	99.79	0.00	12.76	2.58	90.72	324.89	268.48	1.13	4.73
0.00	0.00	0.00	0.00	0.31	0.00	1.62	0.54	0.59	7.13	0.70	143.10	2.16	24.30	7.72	52.92	163.08	226.80	305.64	1.19
0.17	0.61	0.00	0.00	0.90	0.00	0.00	0.02	0.05	1.34	0.05	17.01	0.00	9.72	1.36	48.60	145.80	187.11	4.86	1.68
0.00	0.00	0.00	0.00	0.00	0.00	0.00	0.02	0.05	1.34	0.05	17.01	0.00	9.72	1.36	48.60	145.80	187.11	578.34	1.68
0.22	0.15	0.03	0.00	0.37	225.30	15.00	0.38	0.43	5.00	0.50	99.90	0.00	54.60	8.10	31.80	95.40	104.10	222.30	0.71
0.00	0.00	0.00	0.00	0.00	0.00	0.00	0.17	0.12	2.15	0.17	26.62	0.00	16.94	1.50	53.24	166.98	171.82	563.86	1.16
0.58	0.35	0.00	0.00	0.19	15.31	0.09	0.08	0.11	0.77	0.14	14.74	0.48	30.33	0.63	4.82	39.41	37.99	140.33	0.22
1.28	0.73	0.00	0.00	0.00	37.42	0.09	0.06	0.09	0.46	0.02	12.19	0.09	28.35	0.47	4.82	33.17	37.99	135.80	0.19
3.03	1.70	0.00	0.00	0.00	80.60	0.20	0.13	0.21	1.06	0.05	14.95	0.20	64.35	1.09	11.05	76.05	86.45	310.70	0.44

USDA ID Code	Food Name	Weight in Grams*	Quantity of Units	Unit of Measure	Protein (gm)	Fat (gm)	Carbohydrate (gm)	Kcalories	Caffeine (gm)	Fiber (gm)	Cholesterol (mg)	Saturated Fat (gm)
546	Instant Breakfast, Caffe Mocha-Ca	37.0000	1.300	Ounce	4.50	0.50	28.00	130.00	0.00	0.40	3.00	0.00
547	Instant Breakfast, Choc Malt, No	20.0000	0.700	Ounce	4.50	1.50	11.00	70.00	0.00	1.00	3.00	1.00
548	Instant Breakfast, Choc, Creamy	37.0000	1.300	Ounce	4.50	1.00	28.00	130.00	0.00	1.00	2.00	0.00
549	Instant Breakfast, Choc, No Suga	21.0000	0.720	Ounce	4.50	1.00	12.00	70.00	0.00	1.00	3.00	0.50
550	Instant Breakfast, Chocolate Mal	36.0000	1.250	Ounce	4.50	1.50	26.00	130.00	0.00	1.00	3.00	0.50
551	Instant Breakfast, Chocolate Mal	35.0000	1.200	Ounce	5.70	0.50	25.10	126.00	0.00	0.00	0.00	0.00
552	Instant Breakfast, Chocolate-Pil	35.0000	1.200	Ounce	5.70	0.50	25.70	130.00	0.00	0.00	0.00	0.00
553	Instant Breakfast, Strawberry, N	20.0000	0.700	Ounce	4.50	0.00	12.00	70.00	0.00	0.00	3.00	0.00
554	Instant Breakfast, Strawberry-Ca	36.0000	1.260	Ounce	4.50	0.00	28.00	130.00	0.00	0.00	0.00	0.00
555	Instant Breakfast, Strawberry-Pi	35.0000	1.200	Ounce	5.40	0.20	26.00	130.00	0.00	0.00	0.00	0.00
556	Instant Breakfast, Vanilla, Fren	36.0000	1.260	Ounce	4.50	0.00	27.00	130.00	0.00	0.00	3.00	0.00
557	Instant Breakfast, Vanilla-Pills	35.0000	1.200	Ounce	5.40	0.20	27.30	133.00	0.00	0.00	0.00	0.00
	Pancakes, Buttermilk	28.3500	1.000	Each	1.93	2.64	8.14	64.35	0.00	0.00	16.44	0.52
	Pancakes, Dietary	22.0000	1.000	3 In.	1.12	0.18	9.28	43.78	0.00	0.00	0.00	0.03
	Pancakes, Plain	28.3500	1.000	Each	1.81	2.75	8.02	64.35	0.00	0.00	16.73	0.60
	Pancakes, Plain, Frozen	28.3500	1.000	Each	1.47	0.94	12.36	64.92	0.00	0.51	2.55	0.22
	Pancakes, Whole-wheat	28.3500	1.000	Each	2.41	1.84	8.33	58.97	0.00	0.80	17.29	0.50
	Waffles, Buttermilk	75.0000	1.000	Each	6.23	10.20	24.75	216.75	0.00	0.00	50.25	1.88
	Waffles, Plain, Frozen, Toasted	28.3500	1.000	Each	1.76	2.32	11.54	74.84	0.00	0.65	6.80	0.41
	Waffles, Plain, Homemade	28.3500	1.000	Each	2.24	4.00	9.33	82.50	0.00	0.00	19.56	0.81

Dairy and Eggs

USDA ID Code	Food Name	Weight in Grams*	Quantity of Units	Unit of Measure	Protein (gm)	Fat (gm)	Carbohydrate (gm)	Kcalories	Caffeine (gm)	Fiber (gm)	Cholesterol (mg)	Saturated Fat (gm)
	Cheese Spread, American, Past.	28.3500	1.000	Ounce	4.65	6.02	2.47	82.35	0.00	0.00	15.65	3.78
	Cheese, American, Pasteurized Pr	28.3500	1.000	Ounce	6.28	8.86	0.45	106.44	0.00	0.00	26.76	5.58
	Cheese, Blue	28.3500	1.500	Ounce	6.07	8.15	0.66	100.09	0.00	0.00	21.32	5.29
	Cheese, Brick	132.0000	1.000	Cup	30.68	39.18	3.68	489.61	0.00	0.00	124.61	24.76
	Cheese, Brie	240.0000	1.500	Cup	49.80	66.43	1.08	800.76	0.00	0.00	240.00	41.78
	Cheese, Caraway	28.3500	1.500	Ounce	7.14	8.28	0.87	106.60	0.00	0.00	26.37	5.27
	Cheese, Cheddar	132.0000	1.000	Cup	32.87	43.74	1.69	531.41	0.00	0.00	138.47	27.84
	Cheese, Cheddar, Non-Fat	28.3500	1.500	Ounce	8.10	0.00	2.03	45.56	0.00	0.00	4.05	0.00
	Cheese, Cheddar, Reduced Fat	28.3500	1.500	Ounce	8.00	5.00	1.00	80.00	0.00	0.00	15.00	3.00
	Cheese, Colby	132.0000	1.000	Cup	31.36	42.39	3.39	519.62	0.00	0.00	125.27	26.69
	Cheese, Cottage, Creamed	113.0000	4.000	Ounce	14.11	5.10	3.03	116.79	0.00	0.00	16.84	3.22
	Cheese, Cottage, Creamed, w/ Fru	226.0000	1.000	Cup	22.37	7.68	30.06	279.40	0.00	0.00	25.31	4.86
	Cheese, Cottage, Fat Free	226.0000	0.500	Cup	26.00	0.00	0.00	140.00	0.00	0.00	20.00	0.00
	Cheese, Cottage, Lowfat, 1% Fat	226.0000	1.000	Cup	28.00	2.31	6.15	163.62	0.00	0.00	9.94	1.47
	Cheese, Cottage, Lowfat, 2% Fat	226.0000	1.000	Cup	31.05	4.36	8.20	202.68	0.00	0.00	18.98	2.76
	Cheese, Cottage, Uncreamed, Dry	145.0000	1.000	Cup	25.04	0.61	2.68	122.66	0.00	0.00	9.72	0.39
	Cheese, Cream	232.0000	1.000	Cup	17.52	80.90	6.17	809.77	0.00	0.00	254.50	50.97
	Cheese, Cream, Fat Free	17.5080	2.000	Tbsp	2.50	0.00	1.00	17.51	0.00	0.00	2.50	0.00
	Cheese, Cream, Light	16.0140	2.000	Tbsp	1.50	2.50	1.00	35.03	0.00	0.00	7.51	1.75
	Cheese, Cream, w/ Strawberry	30.0000	1.000	Ounce	4.00	0.00	2.00	35.00	0.00	0.00	3.00	0.00
	Cheese, Edam	28.3500	1.000	Ounce	7.08	7.88	0.41	101.10	0.00	0.00	25.29	4.98
	Cheese, Fat Free Slices, White	21.2630	1.000	Slice	5.00	0.00	2.00	30.00	0.00	0.00	0.00	0.00
	Cheese, Fat Free Slices, Yellow	21.2630	1.000	Slice	5.00	0.00	2.00	30.00	0.00	0.00	0.00	0.00
	Cheese, Feta	150.0000	1.000	Cup	21.32	31.92	6.14	395.34	0.00	0.00	133.50	22.43
	Cheese, Fontina	132.0000	1.000	Cup	33.79	41.10	2.05	513.52	0.00	0.00	153.12	25.34
	Cheese, Goat, Hard Type	28.3500	1.000	Ounce	8.65	10.09	0.62	128.14	0.00	0.00	29.77	6.98
	Cheese, Goat, Semisoft Type	28.3500	1.000	Ounce	6.12	8.46	0.72	103.19	0.00	0.00	22.40	5.85
	Cheese, Goat, Soft Type	28.3500	1.000	Ounce	5.25	5.98	0.25	75.98	0.00	0.00	13.04	4.13
	Cheese, Gouda	28.3500	1.500	Ounce	7.07	7.78	0.63	101.01	0.00	0.00	32.32	4.99
	Cheese, Gruyere	132.0000	1.000	Cup	39.35	42.69	0.48	545.09	0.00	0.00	145.20	24.96
	Cheese, Limburger	134.0000	1.000	Cup	26.87	36.52	0.66	438.23	0.00	0.00	120.60	22.45
	Cheese, Monterey	132.0000	1.000	Cup	32.31	39.97	0.90	492.78	0.00	0.00	117.48	25.17
	Cheese, Monterey, Reduced Fat	28.3500	1.500	Ounce	8.00	5.00	1.00	80.00	0.00	0.00	15.00	3.00
	Cheese, Mozzarella, Part Skim Mi	28.3500	1.500	Ounce	6.88	4.51	0.79	72.08	0.00	0.00	16.39	2.87
	Cheese, Mozzarella, Part Skim Mi	132.0000	1.000	Cup	36.26	22.60	4.14	369.51	0.00	0.00	71.28	14.36

Monounsaturated Fat (gm)	Polyunsaturated Fat (gm)	Vitamin D (mg)	Vitamin K (mg)	Vitamin E (mg)	Vitamin A (re)	Vitamin C (mg)	Thiamin (mg)	Riboflavin (mg)	Niacin (mg)	Vitamin B6 (mg)	Folate (mg)	Vitamin B12 (mcg)	Calcium (mg)	Iron (mg)	Magnesium (mg)	Phosphorus (mg)	Potassium (mg)	Sodium (mg)	Zinc (mg)
0.00	0.00	0.00	0.00	0.00	1750.00	27.00	0.30	0.14	5.00	0.40	100.00	0.60	350.00	4.50	80.00	250.00	340.00	100.00	3.00
0.00	0.00	0.00	0.00	0.00	1750.00	27.00	0.30	0.10	5.00	0.40	100.00	0.60	250.00	4.50	80.00	250.00	290.00	115.00	3.00
0.00	0.00	0.00	0.00	0.00	1750.00	27.00	0.30	0.14	5.00	0.40	100.00	0.60	300.00	4.50	80.00	250.00	350.00	100.00	3.00
0.00	0.00	0.00	0.00	0.00	1750.00	27.00	0.30	0.10	5.00	0.40	100.00	0.60	300.00	4.50	80.00	250.00	350.00	95.00	3.00
0.00	0.00	0.00	0.00	0.00	1750.00	27.00	0.30	0.07	5.00	0.40	100.00	0.60	250.00	4.50	80.00	250.00	250.00	130.00	3.00
0.00	0.00	0.00	0.00	0.00	1684.00	23.00	0.47	0.41	5.80	0.00	0.00	0.00	335.00	5.60	0.00	125.00	263.00	119.00	0.00
0.00	0.00	0.00	0.00	0.00	1681.00	23.00	0.46	0.35	5.80	0.00	0.00	0.00	91.00	5.64	0.00	89.00	256.00	141.00	0.00
0.00	0.00	0.00	0.00	0.00	1750.00	27.00	0.30	0.14	5.00	0.40	100.00	0.60	350.00	4.50	80.00	250.00	250.00	95.00	3.00
0.00	0.00	0.00	0.00	0.00	1750.00	27.00	0.30	0.14	5.00	0.40	100.00	0.60	350.00	4.50	80.00	250.00	250.00	160.00	3.00
0.00	0.00	0.00	0.00	0.00	1681.00	23.00	0.44	0.32	5.80	0.00	0.00	0.00	91.00	5.40	0.00	70.00	250.00	130.00	0.00
0.00	0.00	0.00	0.00	0.00	1750.00	27.00	0.30	0.14	5.00	0.40	100.00	0.60	300.00	4.50	80.00	250.00	350.00	100.00	3.00
0.00	0.00	0.00	0.00	0.00	1686.00	23.00	0.33	0.23	4.70	0.00	0.00	0.00	79.00	5.10	0.00	111.00	229.00	198.00	0.00
0.67	1.27	0.00	0.00	0.00	8.51	0.11	0.06	0.08	0.45	0.01	10.77	0.05	44.51	0.48	4.25	39.41	41.11	147.99	0.18
0.03	0.08	0.00	0.00	0.00	2.20	0.00	0.04	0.02	0.37	0.00	1.10	0.00	12.76	0.39	5.94	74.80	84.92	57.64	0.15
0.70	1.26	0.00	0.00	0.00	15.31	0.09	0.06	0.08	0.45	0.01	10.77	0.06	62.09	0.51	4.54	45.08	37.42	124.46	0.16
0.34	0.27	0.00	0.00	0.11	8.22	0.09	0.11	0.13	1.14	0.02	14.18	0.05	17.58	0.99	3.97	105.46	20.70	144.30	0.19
0.49	0.68	0.00	0.00	0.00	18.14	0.14	0.06	0.15	0.65	0.03	8.22	0.08	70.88	0.88	13.04	105.75	79.10	162.16	0.29
2.52	5.09	0.00	0.00	0.00	26.25	0.38	0.20	0.27	1.55	0.04	11.25	0.16	136.50	1.63	13.50	123.75	128.25	450.75	0.56
0.91	0.79	0.00	0.00	0.24	103.19	0.00	0.11	0.14	1.26	0.26	12.76	0.71	65.77	1.27	6.24	119.07	36.29	223.11	0.16
1.00	1.92	0.00	0.00	0.00	18.43	0.11	0.07	0.10	0.59	0.02	13.04	0.07	72.29	0.65	5.39	53.87	45.08	144.87	0.19
1.76	0.18	0.00	0.00	0.00	53.58	0.00	0.01	0.12	0.04	0.03	1.98	0.11	159.30	0.09	8.09	248.06	68.58	460.69	0.73
2.54	0.28	0.00	0.00	0.00	82.22	0.00	0.01	0.10	0.02	0.02	2.21	0.20	174.49	0.11	6.31	125.87	45.93	184.28	0.85
2.21	0.23	0.00	0.00	0.18	64.64	0.00	0.01	0.11	0.29	0.05	10.32	0.35	149.57	0.09	6.50	109.83	72.66	395.57	0.75
11.35	1.03	0.00	0.00	0.66	398.64	0.00	0.01	0.46	0.16	0.09	26.80	1.66	889.28	0.57	32.10	595.32	179.26	738.67	3.43
19.22	1.99	0.00	0.00	1.58	436.80	0.00	0.17	1.25	0.91	0.58	156.00	3.96	441.60	1.20	48.00	451.20	364.80	1510.56	5.71
2.35	0.24	0.00	0.00	0.00	81.93	0.00	0.01	0.13	0.05	0.02	5.16	0.08	190.88	0.18	6.27	138.92	26.37	195.62	0.83
12.39	1.24	0.40	0.00	0.48	366.96	0.00	0.04	0.50	0.11	0.09	24.02	1.10	952.12	0.90	36.67	675.97	129.89	819.06	4.11
0.00	0.00	0.00	0.00	0.00	60.75	0.00	0.00	0.00	0.00	0.00	0.00	0.00	243.00	0.00	0.00	0.00	0.00	283.50	0.00
0.00	0.00	0.00	0.00	0.00	60.00	0.00	0.00	0.00	0.00	0.00	0.00	0.00	240.00	0.00	0.00	0.00	23.00	180.00	0.00
12.25	1.25	0.00	0.00	0.46	363.00	0.00	0.03	0.50	0.12	0.11	24.02	1.10	903.67	1.00	34.08	602.58	166.98	797.54	4.05
1.46	0.16	0.00	0.00	0.14	54.24	0.00	0.02	0.18	0.15	0.08	13.79	0.70	67.80	0.16	5.94	148.93	95.26	457.42	0.42
2.19	0.25	0.00	0.00	0.20	81.36	0.00	0.05	0.29	0.23	0.11	21.92	1.11	107.58	0.25	9.42	236.17	151.19	914.85	0.66
0.00	0.00	0.00	0.00	0.00	0.00	0.00	0.00	0.00	0.00	0.00	0.00	0.00	240.00	0.00	0.00	0.00	0.00	840.00	0.00
0.66	0.07	0.00	0.00	0.25	24.86	0.00	0.05	0.38	0.29	0.16	28.02	1.42	137.63	0.32	12.07	302.39	193.23	917.56	0.86
1.24	0.14	0.00	0.00	0.14	45.20	0.00	0.05	0.43	0.32	0.18	29.61	1.60	154.81	0.36	13.56	340.13	217.41	917.56	0.95
0.16	0.03	0.00	0.00	0.16	11.60	0.00	0.04	0.20	0.23	0.12	21.46	1.20	45.97	0.33	5.71	150.80	46.98	18.56	0.68
22.83	2.95	0.00	0.00	2.18	886.24	0.00	0.05	0.46	0.23	0.12	30.62	0.97	185.37	2.78	14.94	242.21	277.01	685.56	1.25
0.00	0.00	0.00	0.00	0.00	50.02	0.00	0.00	0.00	0.00	0.00	0.00	0.00	60.03	0.00	0.00	0.00	0.00	90.04	0.00
0.00	0.00	0.00	0.00	0.00	40.03	0.00	0.00	0.00	0.00	0.00	0.00	0.00	24.02	0.00	0.00	0.00	0.00	75.06	0.00
0.00	0.00	0.00	0.00	0.00	10.00	0.00	0.00	0.00	0.00	0.00	0.00	0.00	24.00	0.00	0.00	0.00	0.00	200.00	0.00
2.30	0.19	0.26	0.00	0.21	71.73	0.00	0.01	0.11	0.02	0.02	4.59	0.44	207.24	0.12	8.44	151.84	53.21	273.58	1.06
0.00	0.00	0.00	0.00	0.00	40.00	0.00	0.00	0.00	0.00	0.00	0.00	0.00	120.00	0.00	0.00	0.00	18.00	310.00	0.00
6.93	0.89	0.00	0.00	0.05	192.00	0.00	0.23	1.26	1.49	0.63	48.00	2.54	738.75	0.98	28.82	505.80	92.70	1674.15	4.32
11.47	2.18	0.00	0.00	0.46	382.80	0.00	0.03	0.26	0.20	0.11	7.92	2.22	726.00	0.30	18.48	457.12	83.82	1056.00	4.62
2.30	0.24	0.00	0.00	0.22	135.23	0.00	0.04	0.34	0.68	0.02	1.13	0.03	253.73	0.53	15.31	206.67	13.61	98.09	0.45
1.93	0.20	0.00	0.00	0.18	113.40	0.00	0.02	0.19	0.33	0.02	0.57	0.06	84.48	0.46	8.22	106.31	44.79	146.00	0.19
1.36	0.14	0.00	0.00	0.13	80.23	0.00	0.02	0.11	0.12	0.07	3.40	0.05	39.69	0.54	4.54	72.58	7.37	104.33	0.26
2.20	0.19	0.00	0.00	0.10	49.33	0.00	0.01	0.09	0.02	0.02	5.93	0.44	198.39	0.07	8.22	154.88	34.16	232.27	1.11
13.25	2.28	0.00	0.00	0.46	397.32	0.00	0.08	0.37	0.15	0.11	13.73	2.11	1334.52	0.22	47.40	799.00	106.92	443.52	5.15
11.54	0.67	0.00	0.00	0.86	423.44	0.00	0.11	0.67	0.21	0.12	77.05	1.39	665.58	0.17	28.14	526.62	171.52	1072.00	2.81
11.55	1.19	0.00	0.00	0.45	333.96	0.00	0.03	0.51	0.12	0.11	24.02	1.10	985.25	0.95	35.65	586.08	106.52	707.92	3.96
0.00	0.00	0.00	0.00	0.00	60.00	0.00	0.00	0.00	0.00	0.00	0.00	0.00	240.00	0.00	0.00	0.00	18.00	180.00	0.00
1.28	0.13	0.00	0.00	0.12	50.18	0.00	0.01	0.09	0.03	0.02	2.49	0.23	183.06	0.06	6.58	131.26	23.73	132.11	0.78
6.40	0.67	0.00	0.00	0.61	252.12	0.00	0.03	0.45	0.16	0.11	13.07	1.23	965.32	0.33	34.68	691.81	125.19	696.56	4.13

USDA ID Code	Food Name	Weight in Grams*	Quantity of Units	Unit of Measure	Protein (gm)	Fat (gm)	Carbohydrate (gm)	Kcalories	Caffeine (gm)	Fiber (gm)	Cholesterol (mg)	Saturated Fat (gm)
	Cheese, Mozzarella, Stick	28.0000	1.000	Each	8.00	5.00	0.00	80.00	0.00	0.00	15.00	3.00
	Cheese, Mozzarella, Substitute	113.0000	1.000	Cup	12.96	13.81	26.75	280.24	0.00	0.00	0.00	4.19
	Cheese, Mozzarella, Whole Milk	112.0000	1.000	Cup	21.75	24.19	2.49	315.15	0.00	0.00	87.81	14.73
	Cheese, Mozzarella, Whole Milk,	28.3500	1.000	Ounce	6.12	6.99	0.70	90.26	0.00	0.00	25.34	4.41
	Cheese, Muenster	132.0000	1.000	Cup	30.90	39.65	1.48	486.22	0.00	0.00	126.19	25.23
	Cheese, Parmesan, Grated	100.0000	1.000	Cup	41.56	30.02	3.74	455.81	0.00	0.00	78.70	19.07
	Cheese, Parmesan, Grated, Fat Fr	5.0020	1.000	Tbsp	0.67	0.00	0.67	5.00	0.00	0.00	1.67	0.00
	Cheese, Parmesan, Piece	28.3500	1.000	Ounce	10.14	7.32	0.91	111.18	0.00	0.00	19.19	4.65
	Cheese, Parmesan, Shredded	5.0000	1.000	Tbsp	1.89	1.37	0.17	20.75	0.00	0.00	3.60	0.87
	Cheese, Pepper	132.0000	1.000	Cup	32.31	39.97	0.90	492.78	0.00	0.00	117.48	25.17
	Cheese, Provolone	132.0000	1.000	Cup	33.77	35.14	2.82	463.98	0.00	0.00	90.95	22.55
	Cheese, Ricotta, Part Skim Milk	246.0000	1.000	Cup	28.02	19.46	12.64	339.63	0.00	0.00	75.77	12.13
	Cheese, Ricotta, Whole Milk	246.0000	1.000	Cup	27.70	31.93	7.48	427.89	0.00	0.00	124.48	20.42
	Cheese, Romano	28.3500	1.000	Ounce	9.02	7.64	1.03	109.61	0.00	0.00	29.48	4.85
	Cheese, Roquefort	28.3500	1.000	Ounce	6.11	8.69	0.57	104.62	0.00	0.00	25.52	5.46
	Cheese, Swiss, Domestic	132.0000	1.000	Cup	37.53	36.23	4.46	496.00	0.00	0.00	121.04	23.47
	Cheese, Swiss, Pasteurized Proce	140.0000	1.000	Cup	34.62	35.01	2.94	466.98	0.00	0.00	118.72	22.47
	Cream Substitute, Non-dairy, Liq	240.0000	1.000	Cup	2.40	23.93	27.31	325.56	0.00	0.00	0.00	4.66
	Cream Substitute, Non-dairy, Pow	94.0000	1.000	Cup	4.50	33.35	51.59	513.69	0.00	0.00	0.00	30.58
	Cream, Half and Half, Cream and	242.0000	1.000	Cup	7.16	27.83	10.41	315.50	0.00	0.00	89.30	17.33
	Cream, Light, Coffee or Table	240.0000	1.000	Cup	6.48	46.34	8.78	469.03	0.00	0.00	158.64	28.85
	Cream, Medium, 25% Fat	15.0000	1.000	Tbsp	0.37	3.75	0.52	36.56	0.00	0.00	13.12	2.33
	Cream, Whipped, Pressurized	60.0000	1.000	Cup	1.92	13.33	7.49	154.39	0.00	0.00	45.60	8.30
	Cream, Whipping, Heavy	119.5000	1.000	Cup	2.45	44.22	3.33	412.01	0.00	0.00	163.83	27.52
	Cream, Whipping, Light	120.0000	1.000	Cup	2.60	37.09	3.55	350.90	0.00	0.00	133.20	23.21
	Dessert Topping, Non-dairy	75.0000	1.000	Cup	0.94	18.98	17.29	238.71	0.00	0.00	0.00	16.34
	Egg Substitute, Frozen	240.0000	1.000	Cup	27.10	26.66	7.68	383.57	0.00	0.00	4.80	4.63
	Egg Substitute, Liquid	251.0000	1.000	Cup	30.12	8.31	1.61	210.99	0.00	0.00	2.51	1.66
	Egg White Only, w/o Yolk	243.0000	1.000	Cup	25.56	0.00	2.50	121.50	0.00	0.00	0.00	0.00
	Eggnog	254.0000	1.000	Cup	9.68	19.00	34.39	341.91	0.00	0.00	149.10	11.28
	Eggnog, Reduced Fat	246.0000	1.000	Cup	12.00	8.00	48.00	320.00	0.00	0.00	90.00	5.00
	Eggs, Chicken, Whole, Ckd, Fried	46.0000	1.000	Large	6.23	6.90	0.63	91.54	0.00	0.00	211.14	1.92
	Eggs, Chicken, Whole, Ckd, Hard-	136.0000	1.000	Cup	17.11	14.43	1.52	210.80	0.00	0.00	576.64	4.45
	Eggs, Chicken, Whole, Ckd, Omele	15.2000	1.000	Tbsp	1.57	1.74	0.16	23.10	0.00	0.00	53.20	0.48
	Eggs, Chicken, Whole, Ckd, Poach	50.0000	1.000	Large	6.22	4.99	0.61	74.50	0.00	0.00	211.50	1.55
	Eggs, Chicken, Whole, Ckd, Scram	220.0000	1.000	Cup	24.40	26.86	4.84	365.20	0.00	0.00	774.40	8.10
264	Eggs, Chicken, Whole, Fresh, and	50.0000	1.000	Large	6.25	5.01	0.61	74.50	0.00	0.00	212.50	1.55
	Frozen Yogurt	148.0000	0.500	Cup	6.00	12.00	48.00	320.00	0.00	0.00	20.00	4.00
444	Frozen Yogurt Bar, Banana/Straw-	71.0000	1.000	Each	2.00	0.00	20.00	90.00	0.00	0.00	0.00	0.00
445	Frozen Yogurt Bar, Rasp/Vanilla-	71.0000	1.000	Each	2.00	0.00	20.00	90.00	0.00	0.00	0.00	0.00
446	Frozen Yogurt Bar, Straw Daiquir	70.0000	1.000	Each	2.00	1.00	18.00	90.00	0.00	0.00	15.00	0.50
447	Frozen Yogurt Bar, Toc/Cherry-Ha	71.0000	1.000	Each	3.00	0.00	21.00	100.00	0.00	0.00	0.00	0.00
448	Frozen Yogurt Bar, Toc/Vanilla-H	71.0000	1.000	Each	3.00	0.00	20.00	90.00	0.00	0.00	0.00	0.00
449	Frozen Yogurt, Capp., No Fat-Ben	95.0000	0.500	Cup	4.00	0.00	26.00	120.00	0.00	0.00	0.00	0.00
450	Frozen Yogurt, Cherry Garcia-Ben	95.0000	0.500	Cup	4.00	2.50	27.00	140.00	0.00	0.00	5.00	2.00
451	Frozen Yogurt, Cherry Vanilla-Ha	93.0000	0.500	Cup	6.00	0.00	30.00	140.00	0.00	0.00	0.00	0.00
452	Frozen Yogurt, Choc Chip Cookie	95.0000	0.500	Cup	4.00	3.00	34.00	180.00	0.00	0.00	10.00	2.00
453	Frozen Yogurt, Choc Fudge Browni	95.0000	0.500	Cup	4.00	1.00	32.00	150.00	0.00	0.00	0.00	0.00
454	Frozen Yogurt, Chocolate, No Fat	95.0000	0.500	Cup	4.00	0.00	25.00	120.00	0.00	0.00	0.00	0.00
	Frozen Yogurt, Chocolate, Soft-s	72.0000	0.500	Cup	2.88	4.32	17.93	115.20	2.16	1.58	3.60	2.61
455	Frozen Yogurt, Chocolate-Haagen-	93.0000	0.500	Cup	6.00	0.00	28.00	140.00	0.00	0.00	0.00	0.00
456	Frozen Yogurt, Coffee Fudge, No	95.0000	0.500	Cup	4.00	0.00	25.00	120.00	0.00	0.00	0.00	0.00
457	Frozen Yogurt, Coffee-Haagen-Daz	93.0000	0.500	Cup	6.00	0.00	29.00	140.00	0.00	0.00	0.00	0.00
	Frozen Yogurt, Fat Free	133.9160	0.500	Cup	7.99	0.00	43.97	199.87	0.00	0.00	0.00	0.00
	Frozen Yogurt, Low Fat	148.0000	0.500	Cup	6.00	6.00	48.00	280.00	0.00	0.00	20.00	4.00

Monounsaturated Fat (gm)	Polyunsaturated Fat (gm)	Vitamin D (mg)	Vitamin K (mg)	Vitamin E (mg)	Vitamin A (re)	Vitamin C (mg)	Thiamin (mg)	Riboflavin (mg)	Niacin (mg)	Vitamin B_6 (mg)	Folate (mg)	Vitamin B_{12} (mcg)	Calcium (mg)	Iron (mg)	Magnesium (mg)	Phosphorus (mg)	Potassium (mg)	Sodium (mg)	Zinc (mg)
0.00	0.00	0.00	0.00	0.00	40.00	0.00	0.00	0.00	0.00	0.00	0.00	0.00	240.00	0.00	0.00	0.00	0.00	170.00	0.00
7.05	1.97	0.00	0.00	2.24	493.81	0.11	0.03	0.50	0.36	0.06	12.43	0.92	689.30	0.45	46.33	658.79	514.15	774.05	2.17
7.36	0.86	0.00	0.00	0.39	269.92	0.00	0.02	0.27	0.09	0.07	7.84	0.73	579.04	0.20	20.81	415.18	75.15	417.87	2.48
1.99	0.22	0.00	0.00	0.19	77.68	0.00	0.01	0.08	0.03	0.02	2.21	0.21	162.98	0.06	5.86	116.89	21.15	117.65	0.70
11.50	0.87	0.00	0.00	0.62	417.12	0.00	0.01	0.42	0.13	0.08	15.97	1.94	946.84	0.54	36.10	617.36	177.41	828.56	3.71
8.73	0.66	0.00	0.00	0.80	173.00	0.00	0.05	0.39	0.32	0.11	8.00	1.40	1375.70	0.95	50.80	807.10	107.10	1861.50	3.19
0.00	0.00	0.00	0.00	0.00	0.00	0.00	0.00	0.00	0.00	0.00	0.00	0.00	16.01	0.00	0.00	0.00	10.00	15.01	0.00
2.13	0.16	0.20	0.00	0.23	42.24	0.00	0.01	0.09	0.08	0.03	1.96	0.34	335.52	0.23	12.39	196.86	26.14	454.03	0.78
0.44	0.03	0.00	0.00	0.00	8.65	0.00	0.00	0.02	0.01	0.01	0.40	0.07	62.65	0.04	2.54	36.75	4.85	84.80	0.16
11.55	1.19	0.00	0.00	0.45	333.96	0.00	0.03	0.51	0.12	0.11	24.02	1.10	985.25	0.95	35.65	586.08	106.52	707.92	3.96
9.75	1.02	0.00	0.00	0.46	348.48	0.00	0.03	0.42	0.21	0.09	13.73	1.93	997.79	0.69	36.41	654.85	182.56	1155.66	4.26
5.68	0.64	0.00	0.00	0.52	277.98	0.00	0.05	0.47	0.20	0.05	32.23	0.71	669.12	1.08	36.33	449.20	307.50	306.76	3.30
8.93	0.96	0.00	0.00	0.86	329.64	0.00	0.02	0.49	0.25	0.10	30.01	0.84	509.22	0.93	27.80	388.93	257.32	206.89	2.85
2.22	0.17	0.00	0.00	0.21	39.97	0.00	0.01	0.10	0.02	0.03	1.93	0.32	301.59	0.22	11.60	215.46	24.47	340.20	0.73
2.40	0.37	0.00	0.00	0.00	84.77	0.00	0.01	0.17	0.21	0.03	13.89	0.18	187.62	0.16	8.37	111.16	25.71	512.85	0.59
9.60	1.28	1.45	0.00	0.66	333.96	0.00	0.03	0.49	0.12	0.11	8.45	2.22	1268.39	0.22	47.40	798.07	146.12	343.20	5.15
9.87	0.87	0.00	0.00	0.95	320.60	0.00	0.01	0.39	0.06	0.06	8.26	1.72	1080.66	0.85	40.77	1066.10	301.70	1918.42	5.05
18.12	0.07	0.00	0.00	3.89	21.60	0.00	0.00	0.00	0.00	0.00	0.00	0.00	22.32	0.07	0.79	154.08	457.20	190.08	0.05
0.91	0.01	0.00	0.00	0.25	18.80	0.00	0.00	0.16	0.00	0.00	0.00	0.00	20.96	1.08	3.82	396.68	763.09	170.23	0.48
8.03	1.04	0.00	0.00	0.27	258.94	2.08	0.10	0.36	0.19	0.10	6.05	0.80	253.86	0.17	24.61	230.38	313.63	98.49	1.23
13.39	1.73	0.00	0.00	0.36	436.80	1.82	0.07	0.36	0.14	0.07	5.52	0.53	230.88	0.10	20.76	191.76	292.08	95.04	0.65
1.08	0.14	0.00	0.00	0.09	34.80	0.11	0.00	0.02	0.01	0.00	0.34	0.03	13.53	0.01	1.26	10.59	17.17	5.55	0.04
3.85	0.50	0.00	0.00	0.36	124.20	0.00	0.02	0.04	0.04	0.02	1.56	0.17	60.60	0.03	6.47	53.58	88.38	78.00	0.22
12.77	1.64	0.35	0.00	0.75	503.10	0.69	0.02	0.13	0.05	0.04	4.42	0.22	77.20	0.04	8.40	74.57	90.10	44.93	0.27
10.91	1.06	0.00	0.00	0.72	354.00	0.73	0.02	0.16	0.05	0.04	4.44	0.24	83.28	0.04	8.68	73.32	116.16	41.16	0.30
1.22	0.39	0.00	0.00	0.14	64.50	0.00	0.00	0.00	0.00	0.00	0.00	0.00	4.73	0.09	1.34	5.78	13.65	18.98	0.02
5.86	14.98	0.00	0.00	5.06	324.00	1.13	0.29	0.94	0.34	0.31	39.36	0.82	174.72	4.75	35.90	172.08	511.92	478.56	2.35
2.26	4.02	0.00	0.00	1.23	542.16	0.00	0.28	0.75	0.28	0.00	37.40	0.75	133.03	5.27	21.89	303.71	828.30	444.27	3.26
0.00	0.00	0.00	0.05	0.00	0.00	0.00	0.02	1.09	0.22	0.00	7.29	0.49	14.58	0.07	26.73	31.59	347.49	398.52	0.02
5.66	0.86	0.00	0.00	0.58	203.20	3.81	0.08	0.48	0.28	0.13	2.29	1.14	330.20	0.51	46.99	277.88	419.61	138.18	1.17
0.00	0.00	0.00	0.00	0.00	160.00	2.40	0.00	0.00	0.00	0.00	0.00	0.00	480.00	0.40	0.00	0.00	0.00	280.00	0.00
2.75	1.28	0.00	0.00	0.75	114.08	0.00	0.03	0.24	0.04	0.06	17.48	0.42	25.30	0.72	5.06	89.24	60.72	162.38	0.55
5.55	1.92	0.00	0.00	1.43	228.48	0.00	0.10	0.69	0.08	0.16	59.84	1.51	68.00	1.62	13.60	233.92	171.36	168.64	1.43
0.69	0.32	0.00	0.00	0.20	28.42	0.00	0.01	0.06	0.01	0.02	4.41	0.11	6.38	0.18	1.37	22.50	15.35	41.04	0.14
1.90	0.68	0.00	0.00	0.53	95.00	0.00	0.03	0.22	0.03	0.06	17.50	0.40	24.50	0.72	5.00	88.50	60.00	140.00	0.55
10.49	4.73	0.00	0.00	2.88	429.00	0.44	0.11	0.97	0.18	0.26	66.00	1.69	156.20	2.64	26.40	374.00	303.60	616.00	2.20
1.90	0.68	0.02	25.00	1.03	95.50	0.00	0.03	0.25	0.04	0.07	23.50	0.50	24.50	0.72	5.00	89.00	60.50	63.00	0.55
0.00	0.00	0.00	0.00	0.00	40.00	0.00	0.00	0.00	0.00	0.00	0.00	0.00	192.00	0.00	0.00	0.00	0.00	100.00	0.00
0.00	0.00	0.00	0.00	0.00	0.00	0.00	0.00	0.00	0.00	0.00	0.00	0.00	0.00	0.00	0.00	0.00	0.00	15.00	0.00
0.00	0.00	0.00	0.00	0.00	0.00	0.00	0.00	0.00	0.00	0.00	0.00	0.00	0.00	0.00	0.00	0.00	0.00	15.00	0.00
0.00	0.00	0.00	0.00	0.00	0.00	0.00	0.00	0.00	0.00	0.00	0.00	0.00	0.00	0.00	0.00	0.00	0.00	20.00	0.00
0.00	0.00	0.00	0.00	0.00	0.00	0.00	0.00	0.00	0.00	0.00	0.00	0.00	0.00	0.00	0.00	0.00	0.00	40.00	0.00
0.00	0.00	0.00	0.00	0.00	0.00	0.00	0.00	0.00	0.00	0.00	0.00	0.00	0.00	0.00	0.00	0.00	0.00	45.00	0.00
0.00	0.00	0.00	0.00	0.00	0.00	0.00	0.00	0.00	0.00	0.00	0.00	0.00	0.00	0.00	0.00	0.00	0.00	65.00	0.00
0.00	0.00	0.00	0.00	0.00	0.00	0.00	0.00	0.00	0.00	0.00	0.00	0.00	0.00	0.00	0.00	0.00	0.00	65.00	0.00
0.00	0.00	0.00	0.00	0.00	0.00	0.00	0.00	0.00	0.00	0.00	0.00	0.00	0.00	0.00	0.00	0.00	0.00	40.00	0.00
0.00	0.00	0.00	0.00	0.00	0.00	0.00	0.00	0.00	0.00	0.00	0.00	0.00	0.00	0.00	0.00	0.00	0.00	110.00	0.00
0.00	0.00	0.00	0.00	0.00	0.00	0.00	0.00	0.00	0.00	0.00	0.00	0.00	0.00	0.00	0.00	0.00	0.00	80.00	0.00
0.00	0.00	0.00	0.00	0.00	0.00	0.00	0.00	0.00	0.00	0.00	0.00	0.00	0.00	0.00	0.00	0.00	0.00	65.00	0.00
1.26	0.16	0.00	0.00	0.10	30.96	0.22	0.03	0.15	0.22	0.05	7.92	0.21	105.84	0.90	19.44	100.08	187.92	70.56	0.35
0.00	0.00	0.00	0.00	0.00	0.00	0.00	0.00	0.00	0.00	0.00	0.00	0.00	0.00	0.00	0.00	0.00	0.00	45.00	0.00
0.00	0.00	0.00	0.00	0.00	0.00	0.00	0.00	0.00	0.00	0.00	0.00	0.00	0.00	0.00	0.00	0.00	0.00	65.00	0.00
0.00	0.00	0.00	0.00	0.00	0.00	0.00	0.00	0.00	0.00	0.00	0.00	0.00	0.00	0.00	0.00	0.00	0.00	45.00	0.00
0.00	0.00	0.00	0.00	0.00	39.97	0.00	0.00	0.00	0.00	0.00	0.00	0.00	191.88	0.00	0.00	0.00	0.00	139.91	0.00
0.00	0.00	0.00	0.00	0.00	40.00	0.00	0.00	0.00	0.00	0.00	0.00	0.00	192.00	0.00	0.00	0.00	0.00	100.00	0.00

USDA ID Code	Food Name	Weight in Grams*	Quantity of Units	Unit of Measure	Protein (gm)	Fat (gm)	Carbohydrate (gm)	Kcalories	Caffeine (gm)	Fiber (gm)	Cholesterol (mg)	Saturated Fat (gm)
458	Frozen Yogurt, Low Fat-Ben & Jer	106.0000	0.500	Cup	4.00	3.00	31.00	170.00	0.00	0.00	10.00	2.00
459	Frozen Yogurt, Peach Melba, Tang	95.0000	0.500	Cup	3.00	0.00	29.00	130.00	0.00	0.00	0.00	0.00
460	Frozen Yogurt, Raspberry, Black,	95.0000	0.500	Cup	3.00	0.00	27.00	120.00	0.00	1.00	0.00	0.00
461	Frozen Yogurt, Vanilla Fudge, No	95.0000	0.500	Cup	4.00	0.00	31.00	140.00	0.00	1.00	0.00	0.00
462	Frozen Yogurt, Vanilla Fudge-Haa	93.0000	0.500	Cup	6.00	0.00	34.00	160.00	0.00	0.00	0.00	0.00
463	Frozen Yogurt, Vanilla Rasp Swir	96.0000	0.500	Cup	4.00	0.00	28.00	130.00	0.00	0.00	0.00	0.00
464	Frozen Yogurt, Vanilla w/ Heath	95.0000	0.500	Cup	4.00	5.00	29.00	180.00	0.00	0.00	10.00	2.50
465	Frozen Yogurt, Vanilla, No Fat-B	95.0000	0.500	Cup	4.00	0.00	26.00	120.00	0.00	0.00	0.00	0.00
	Frozen Yogurt, Vanilla, Soft-ser	72.0000	0.500	Cup	2.88	4.03	17.42	114.48	0.00	0.00	1.44	2.46
466	Frozen Yogurt, Vanilla-Haagen-Da	93.0000	0.500	Cup	6.00	0.00	29.00	140.00	0.00	0.00	0.00	0.00
	Ice Cream - fat free	72.0000	0.500	Cup	4.00	0.00	23.00	100.00	0.00	0.00	0.00	0.00
469	Ice Cream Bar, Choc/Dark Choc-Ha	102.0000	1.000	Each	5.00	24.00	28.00	350.00	0.00	2.00	85.00	15.00
470	Ice Cream Bar, Coffee/Almond Cru	106.0000	1.000	Each	5.00	26.00	27.00	360.00	0.00	1.00	100.00	15.00
471	Ice Cream Bar, Straw/White Choc-	97.0000	1.000	Each	4.00	23.00	24.00	320.00	0.00	0.00	70.00	14.00
472	Ice Cream Bar, Vanilla & Almonds	106.0000	1.000	Each	6.00	27.00	26.00	370.00	0.00	1.00	90.00	14.00
473	Ice Cream Bar, Vanilla/Dark Choc	102.0000	1.000	Each	5.00	24.00	27.00	350.00	0.00	1.00	85.00	15.00
474	Ice Cream Bar, Vanilla/Milk Choc	100.0000	1.000	Each	5.00	24.00	24.00	330.00	0.00	0.00	90.00	14.00
	Ice Cream Cones, Cake or Wafer-t	28.3500	1.000	Ounce	2.30	1.96	22.40	118.22	0.00	0.85	0.00	0.35
	Ice Cream Cones, Sugar, Rolled-t	28.3500	1.000	Ounce	2.24	1.08	23.84	113.97	0.00	0.47	0.00	0.16
	Ice Cream Sandwich	63.0000	1.000	Each	3.00	6.00	27.00	170.00	0.00	1.00	10.00	3.00
476	Ice Cream Sandwich, Vanilla/Choc	80.0000	1.000	Each	4.00	13.00	31.00	260.00	0.00	1.00	65.00	8.00
477	Ice Cream Sandwich, Vanilla/Dark	83.0000	1.000	Each	4.00	20.00	23.00	290.00	0.00	2.00	70.00	12.00
475	Ice Cream Sandwich, Vanilla-Haag	80.0000	1.000	Each	4.00	13.00	32.00	260.00	0.00	0.00	65.00	8.00
478	Ice Cream, Bailey's Irish Cream-	102.0000	0.500	Cup	5.00	17.00	23.00	270.00	0.00	0.00	115.00	10.00
479	Ice Cream, Brownies a la Mode-Ha	99.0000	0.500	Cup	4.00	18.00	26.00	280.00	0.00	0.00	100.00	11.00
480	Ice Cream, Butter Pecan-Ben & Je	106.0000	0.500	Cup	4.00	21.00	15.00	250.00	0.00	1.00	80.00	9.00
481	Ice Cream, Butter Pecan-Haagen-D	106.0000	0.500	Cup	5.00	23.00	20.00	310.00	0.00	0.00	110.00	11.00
482	Ice Cream, Cappuccino Choc Chunk	106.0000	0.500	Cup	3.00	15.00	22.00	220.00	0.00	1.00	65.00	10.00
483	Ice Cream, Cappuccino Commotion-	103.0000	0.500	Cup	5.00	21.00	25.00	310.00	0.00	1.00	100.00	12.00
484	Ice Cream, Caramel Cone Explosio	103.0000	0.500	Cup	5.00	20.00	27.00	310.00	0.00	0.00	95.00	12.00
485	Ice Cream, Cherry Garcia-Ben & J	106.0000	0.500	Cup	3.00	13.00	21.00	200.00	0.00	0.00	65.00	8.00
486	Ice Cream, Cherry Vanilla-Haagen	101.0000	0.500	Cup	4.00	15.00	23.00	240.00	0.00	0.00	100.00	9.00
487	Ice Cream, Choc Chip Cookie Doug	106.0000	0.500	Cup	4.00	14.00	27.00	230.00	0.00	0.00	65.00	8.00
488	Ice Cream, Choc Choc Chip-Haagen	106.0000	0.500	Cup	5.00	20.00	26.00	300.00	0.00	2.00	100.00	12.00
489	Ice Cream, Choc Choc, Belgian-Ha	102.0000	0.500	Cup	5.00	21.00	29.00	330.00	0.00	3.00	85.00	12.00
490	Ice Cream, Choc Fudge Brownie, L	92.0000	0.500	Cup	7.00	2.50	34.00	190.00	0.00	1.00	8.00	1.50
491	Ice Cream, Choc Fudge Brownie-Be	106.0000	0.500	Cup	4.00	11.00	27.00	220.00	0.00	2.00	40.00	7.00
492	Ice Cream, Choc Mint Chip-Haagen	106.0000	0.500	Cup	5.00	20.00	25.00	300.00	0.00	4.00	95.00	11.00
493	Ice Cream, Choc PB, Deep-Haagen-	102.0000	0.500	Cup	8.00	24.00	26.00	350.00	0.00	4.00	80.00	11.00
494	Ice Cream, Choc Peanut Butter Do	106.0000	0.500	Cup	4.00	16.00	23.00	240.00	0.00	1.00	50.00	6.00
495	Ice Cream, Choc Raspberry Swirl-	106.0000	0.500	Cup	3.00	11.00	28.00	220.00	0.00	2.00	35.00	7.00
496	Ice Cream, Choc, Deep Dark, Egg	106.0000	0.500	Cup	3.00	12.00	24.00	200.00	0.00	2.00	45.00	7.00
	Ice Cream, Chocolate	58.0000	3.500	Fl Oz	2.20	6.38	16.36	125.28	1.74	0.70	19.72	3.94
497	Ice Cream, Chocolate, Low Fat-Ha	92.0000	0.500	Cup	7.00	2.50	29.00	170.00	0.00	0.00	8.00	4.00
498	Ice Cream, Chocolate-Haagen-Daz	106.0000	0.500	Cup	5.00	18.00	22.00	270.00	0.00	1.00	115.00	11.00
499	Ice Cream, Chubby Hubby-Ben & Je	106.0000	0.500	Cup	6.00	17.00	24.00	260.00	0.00	2.00	50.00	8.00
500	Ice Cream, Chunky Monkey-Ben & J	106.0000	0.500	Cup	3.00	16.00	24.00	240.00	0.00	1.00	55.00	8.00
501	Ice Cream, Coconut Almond Fudge	106.0000	0.500	Cup	5.00	20.00	19.00	260.00	0.00	2.00	60.00	11.00
502	Ice Cream, Coffee Fudge, Low Fat	92.0000	0.500	Cup	5.00	2.50	32.00	170.00	0.00	0.00	25.00	1.50
503	Ice Cream, Coffee Mocha Chip-Haa	106.0000	0.500	Cup	4.00	19.00	25.00	290.00	0.00	0.00	110.00	12.00
504	Ice Cream, Coffee Ole-Ben & Jerr	106.0000	0.500	Cup	3.00	13.00	18.00	180.00	0.00	0.00	70.00	8.00
505	Ice Cream, Coffee w/ Heath Crunc	106.0000	0.500	Cup	3.00	16.00	24.00	240.00	0.00	0.00	60.00	9.00
506	Ice Cream, Coffee-Haagen-Daz	106.0000	0.500	Cup	5.00	18.00	21.00	270.00	0.00	0.00	120.00	11.00
507	Ice Cream, Cookie Dough Dynamo-H	103.0000	0.500	Cup	4.00	19.00	29.00	300.00	0.00	0.00	95.00	12.00
508	Ice Cream, Cookie, Sweet Cream-B	106.0000	0.500	Cup	3.00	14.00	22.00	220.00	0.00	1.00	65.00	8.00

Monounsaturated Fat (gm)	Polyunsaturated Fat (gm)	Vitamin D (mg)	Vitamin K (mg)	Vitamin E (mg)	Vitamin A (re)	Vitamin C (mg)	Thiamin (mg)	Riboflavin (mg)	Niacin (mg)	Vitamin B6 (mg)	Folate (mg)	Vitamin B12 (mcg)	Calcium (mg)	Iron (mg)	Magnesium (mg)	Phosphorus (mg)	Potassium (mg)	Sodium (mg)	Zinc (mg)
0.00	0.00	0.00	0.00	0.00	0.00	1.20	0.00	0.00	0.00	0.00	0.00	0.00	120.00	0.20	0.00	0.00	0.00	70.00	0.00
0.00	0.00	0.00	0.00	0.00	0.00	0.00	0.00	0.00	0.00	0.00	0.00	0.00	0.00	0.00	0.00	0.00	0.00	55.00	0.00
0.00	0.00	0.00	0.00	0.00	0.00	0.00	0.00	0.00	0.00	0.00	0.00	0.00	0.00	0.00	0.00	0.00	0.00	50.00	0.00
0.00	0.00	0.00	0.00	0.00	0.00	0.00	0.00	0.00	0.00	0.00	0.00	0.00	0.00	0.00	0.00	0.00	0.00	75.00	0.00
0.00	0.00	0.00	0.00	0.00	0.00	0.00	0.00	0.00	0.00	0.00	0.00	0.00	0.00	0.00	0.00	0.00	0.00	100.00	0.00
0.00	0.00	0.00	0.00	0.00	0.00	0.00	0.00	0.00	0.00	0.00	0.00	0.00	0.00	0.00	0.00	0.00	0.00	30.00	0.00
0.00	0.00	0.00	0.00	0.00	0.00	0.00	0.00	0.00	0.00	0.00	0.00	0.00	0.00	0.00	0.00	0.00	0.00	100.00	0.00
0.00	0.00	0.00	0.00	0.00	0.00	0.00	0.00	0.00	0.00	0.00	0.00	0.00	0.00	0.00	0.00	0.00	0.00	65.00	0.00
1.14	0.15	0.00	0.00	0.04	41.04	0.58	0.03	0.16	0.21	0.06	4.32	0.21	102.96	0.22	10.08	92.88	151.92	62.64	0.30
0.00	0.00	0.00	0.00	0.00	0.00	0.00	0.00	0.00	0.00	0.00	0.00	0.00	0.00	0.00	0.00	0.00	0.00	45.00	0.00
0.00	0.00	0.00	0.00	0.00	0.00	0.00	0.00	0.00	0.00	0.00	0.00	0.00	120.00	0.00	0.00	0.00	0.00	65.00	0.00
0.00	0.00	0.00	0.00	0.00	0.00	0.00	0.00	0.00	0.00	0.00	0.00	0.00	0.00	0.00	0.00	0.00	0.00	60.00	0.00
0.00	0.00	0.00	0.00	0.00	0.00	0.00	0.00	0.00	0.00	0.00	0.00	0.00	0.00	0.00	0.00	0.00	0.00	85.00	0.00
0.00	0.00	0.00	0.00	0.00	0.00	0.00	0.00	0.00	0.00	0.00	0.00	0.00	0.00	0.00	0.00	0.00	0.00	75.00	0.00
0.00	0.00	0.00	0.00	0.00	0.00	0.00	0.00	0.00	0.00	0.00	0.00	0.00	0.00	0.00	0.00	0.00	0.00	80.00	0.00
0.00	0.00	0.00	0.00	0.00	0.00	0.00	0.00	0.00	0.00	0.00	0.00	0.00	0.00	0.00	0.00	0.00	0.00	65.00	0.00
0.00	0.00	0.00	0.00	0.00	0.00	0.00	0.00	0.00	0.00	0.00	0.00	0.00	0.00	0.00	0.00	0.00	0.00	75.00	0.00
0.52	0.92	0.00	0.00	0.49	0.00	0.00	0.07	0.10	1.26	0.01	28.92	0.00	7.09	1.02	7.37	27.50	31.75	40.54	0.19
0.42	0.41	0.00	0.00	0.13	0.00	0.00	0.14	0.12	1.44	0.01	23.53	0.00	12.47	1.26	8.79	29.20	41.11	90.72	0.21
0.00	0.00	0.00	0.00	0.00	20.00	0.00	0.00	0.00	0.00	0.00	0.00	0.00	48.00	0.40	0.00	0.00	0.00	140.00	0.00
0.00	0.00	0.00	0.00	0.00	0.00	0.00	0.00	0.00	0.00	0.00	0.00	0.00	0.00	0.00	0.00	0.00	0.00	120.00	0.00
0.00	0.00	0.00	0.00	0.00	0.00	0.00	0.00	0.00	0.00	0.00	0.00	0.00	0.00	0.00	0.00	0.00	0.00	45.00	0.00
0.00	0.00	0.00	0.00	0.00	0.00	0.00	0.00	0.00	0.00	0.00	0.00	0.00	0.00	0.00	0.00	0.00	0.00	125.00	0.00
0.00	0.00	0.00	0.00	0.00	0.00	0.00	0.00	0.00	0.00	0.00	0.00	0.00	0.00	0.00	0.00	0.00	0.00	85.00	0.00
0.00	0.00	0.00	0.00	0.00	0.00	0.00	0.00	0.00	0.00	0.00	0.00	0.00	0.00	0.00	0.00	0.00	0.00	115.00	0.00
0.00	0.00	0.00	0.00	0.00	0.00	0.00	0.00	0.00	0.00	0.00	0.00	0.00	0.00	0.00	0.00	0.00	0.00	135.00	0.00
0.00	0.00	0.00	0.00	0.00	0.00	0.00	0.00	0.00	0.00	0.00	0.00	0.00	0.00	0.00	0.00	0.00	0.00	160.00	0.00
0.00	0.00	0.00	0.00	0.00	0.00	0.00	0.00	0.00	0.00	0.00	0.00	0.00	0.00	0.00	0.00	0.00	0.00	50.00	0.00
0.00	0.00	0.00	0.00	0.00	0.00	0.00	0.00	0.00	0.00	0.00	0.00	0.00	0.00	0.00	0.00	0.00	0.00	105.00	0.00
0.00	0.00	0.00	0.00	0.00	0.00	0.00	0.00	0.00	0.00	0.00	0.00	0.00	0.00	0.00	0.00	0.00	0.00	130.00	0.00
0.00	0.00	0.00	0.00	0.00	0.00	0.00	0.00	0.00	0.00	0.00	0.00	0.00	0.00	0.00	0.00	0.00	0.00	50.00	0.00
0.00	0.00	0.00	0.00	0.00	0.00	0.00	0.00	0.00	0.00	0.00	0.00	0.00	0.00	0.00	0.00	0.00	0.00	75.00	0.00
0.00	0.00	0.00	0.00	0.00	0.00	0.00	0.00	0.00	0.00	0.00	0.00	0.00	0.00	0.00	0.00	0.00	0.00	85.00	0.00
0.00	0.00	0.00	0.00	0.00	0.00	0.00	0.00	0.00	0.00	0.00	0.00	0.00	0.00	0.00	0.00	0.00	0.00	70.00	0.00
0.00	0.00	0.00	0.00	0.00	0.00	0.00	0.00	0.00	0.00	0.00	0.00	0.00	0.00	0.00	0.00	0.00	0.00	60.00	0.00
0.00	0.00	0.00	0.00	0.00	0.00	0.00	0.00	0.00	0.00	0.00	0.00	0.00	0.00	0.00	0.00	0.00	0.00	110.00	0.00
0.00	0.00	0.00	0.00	0.00	0.00	0.00	0.00	0.00	0.00	0.00	0.00	0.00	0.00	0.00	0.00	0.00	0.00	75.00	0.00
0.00	0.00	0.00	0.00	0.00	0.00	0.00	0.00	0.00	0.00	0.00	0.00	0.00	0.00	0.00	0.00	0.00	0.00	65.00	0.00
0.00	0.00	0.00	0.00	0.00	0.00	0.00	0.00	0.00	0.00	0.00	0.00	0.00	0.00	0.00	0.00	0.00	0.00	100.00	0.00
0.00	0.00	0.00	0.00	0.00	0.00	0.00	0.00	0.00	0.00	0.00	0.00	0.00	0.00	0.00	0.00	0.00	0.00	65.00	0.00
0.00	0.00	0.00	0.00	0.00	0.00	0.00	0.00	0.00	0.00	0.00	0.00	0.00	0.00	0.00	0.00	0.00	0.00	35.00	0.00
0.00	0.00	0.00	0.00	0.00	0.00	0.00	0.00	0.00	0.00	0.00	0.00	0.00	0.00	0.00	0.00	0.00	0.00	35.00	0.00
1.86	0.24	0.00	0.00	0.19	69.02	0.41	0.02	0.11	0.13	0.03	9.28	0.17	63.22	0.54	16.82	62.06	144.42	44.08	0.34
0.00	0.00	0.00	0.00	0.00	0.00	0.00	0.00	0.00	0.00	0.00	0.00	0.00	0.00	0.00	0.00	0.00	0.00	50.00	0.00
0.00	0.00	0.00	0.00	0.00	0.00	0.00	0.00	0.00	0.00	0.00	0.00	0.00	0.00	0.00	0.00	0.00	0.00	75.00	0.00
0.00	0.00	0.00	0.00	0.00	0.00	0.00	0.00	0.00	0.00	0.00	0.00	0.00	0.00	0.00	0.00	0.00	0.00	140.00	0.00
0.00	0.00	0.00	0.00	0.00	0.00	0.00	0.00	0.00	0.00	0.00	0.00	0.00	0.00	0.00	0.00	0.00	0.00	40.00	0.00
0.00	0.00	0.00	0.00	0.00	0.00	0.00	0.00	0.00	0.00	0.00	0.00	0.00	0.00	0.00	0.00	0.00	0.00	70.00	0.00
0.00	0.00	0.00	0.00	0.00	0.00	0.00	0.00	0.00	0.00	0.00	0.00	0.00	0.00	0.00	0.00	0.00	0.00	95.00	0.00
0.00	0.00	0.00	0.00	0.00	0.00	0.00	0.00	0.00	0.00	0.00	0.00	0.00	0.00	0.00	0.00	0.00	0.00	90.00	0.00
0.00	0.00	0.00	0.00	0.00	0.00	0.00	0.00	0.00	0.00	0.00	0.00	0.00	0.00	0.00	0.00	0.00	0.00	45.00	0.00
0.00	0.00	0.00	0.00	0.00	0.00	0.00	0.00	0.00	0.00	0.00	0.00	0.00	0.00	0.00	0.00	0.00	0.00	110.00	0.00
0.00	0.00	0.00	0.00	0.00	0.00	0.00	0.00	0.00	0.00	0.00	0.00	0.00	0.00	0.00	0.00	0.00	0.00	85.00	0.00
0.00	0.00	0.00	0.00	0.00	0.00	0.00	0.00	0.00	0.00	0.00	0.00	0.00	0.00	0.00	0.00	0.00	0.00	140.00	0.00
0.00	0.00	0.00	0.00	0.00	0.00	0.00	0.00	0.00	0.00	0.00	0.00	0.00	0.00	0.00	0.00	0.00	0.00	110.00	0.00

USDA ID Code	Food Name	Weight in Grams*	Quantity of Units	Unit of Measure	Protein (gm)	Fat (gm)	Carbohydrate (gm)	Kcalories	Caffeine (gm)	Fiber (gm)	Cholesterol (mg)	Saturated Fat (gm)
509	Ice Cream, Cookies & Cream, Midn	102.0000	0.500	Cup	5.00	18.00	29.00	300.00	0.00	1.00	90.00	11.00
510	Ice Cream, Cookies & Cream-Haage	102.0000	0.500	Cup	5.00	17.00	23.00	270.00	0.00	0.00	110.00	11.00
511	Ice Cream, Cool Britannia-Ben &	106.0000	0.500	Cup	3.00	12.00	23.00	200.00	0.00	0.00	55.00	8.00
512	Ice Cream, De Leche Caramel-Haag	106.0000	0.500	Cup	5.00	17.00	28.00	290.00	0.00	0.00	100.00	10.00
513	Ice Cream, DiSaronno Amaretto-Ha	103.0000	0.500	Cup	4.00	15.00	26.00	260.00	0.00	0.00	95.00	9.00
514	Ice Cream, Fudge Chunk, NY Super	106.0000	0.500	Cup	4.00	17.00	23.00	240.00	0.00	2.00	40.00	9.00
	Ice Cream, Light	67.0000	0.500	Cup	3.00	4.50	18.00	130.00	0.00	0.00	35.00	2.50
	Ice Cream, Low Fat-Haagen Daz	92.0000	0.500	Cup	7.00	2.50	29.00	170.00	0.00	0.00	0.00	0.00
	Ice Cream, Low Fat-Starbucks	99.0000	0.500	Cup	5.00	3.00	31.00	170.00	0.00	0.00	10.00	1.50
515	Ice Cream, Macadamia Nut Brittle	106.0000	0.500	Cup	4.00	20.00	25.00	300.00	0.00	0.00	110.00	11.00
516	Ice Cream, Malted Milk Ball-Ben	106.0000	0.500	Cup	3.00	14.00	22.00	220.00	0.00	0.00	65.00	9.00
517	Ice Cream, Maple Walnut-Ben & Je	106.0000	0.500	Cup	4.00	18.00	18.00	240.00	0.00	1.00	60.00	8.00
518	Ice Cream, Mint Chip-Haagen-Daz	106.0000	0.500	Cup	4.00	19.00	26.00	290.00	0.00	0.00	105.00	12.00
519	Ice Cream, Mint Choc Chunk-Ben &	106.0000	0.500	Cup	3.00	15.00	22.00	220.00	0.00	1.00	65.00	10.00
520	Ice Cream, Mint Choc Cookie-Ben	106.0000	0.500	Cup	3.00	14.00	23.00	220.00	0.00	1.00	65.00	8.00
521	Ice Cream, Mocha Fudge-Ben & Jer	106.0000	0.500	Cup	3.00	13.00	22.00	200.00	0.00	0.00	60.00	7.00
522	Ice Cream, Peanut Butter Cup-Ben	106.0000	0.500	Cup	5.00	18.00	21.00	260.00	0.00	1.00	60.00	9.00
523	Ice Cream, Pistachio Pistachio-B	106.0000	0.500	Cup	4.00	17.00	16.00	220.00	0.00	1.00	70.00	8.00
524	Ice Cream, Praline Pecan-Ben & J	106.0000	0.500	Cup	3.00	17.00	26.00	250.00	0.00	0.00	70.00	8.00
525	Ice Cream, Pralines & Cream-Haag	102.0000	0.500	Cup	4.00	18.00	27.00	290.00	0.00	0.00	95.00	9.00
526	Ice Cream, Rainforest Crunch-Ben	106.0000	0.500	Cup	4.00	18.00	19.00	240.00	0.00	0.00	70.00	9.00
527	Ice Cream, Rum Raisin-Haagen-Daz	106.0000	0.500	Cup	4.00	17.00	22.00	270.00	0.00	0.00	110.00	10.00
	Ice Cream, Strawberry	58.0000	3.500	Fl Oz	1.86	4.87	16.01	111.36	0.00	0.17	16.82	3.01
528	Ice Cream, Strawberry Cheesecake	103.0000	0.500	Cup	4.00	16.00	27.00	270.00	0.00	0.00	100.00	10.00
529	Ice Cream, Strawberry, Low Fat-H	92.0000	0.500	Cup	5.00	2.00	28.00	150.00	0.00	0.00	15.00	1.00
530	Ice Cream, Strawberry-Ben & Jerr	106.0000	0.500	Cup	2.00	10.00	19.00	170.00	0.00	1.00	55.00	6.00
531	Ice Cream, Strawberry-Haagen-Daz	106.0000	0.500	Cup	4.00	16.00	23.00	250.00	0.00	0.00	95.00	10.00
	Ice Cream, Vanilla	58.0000	3.500	Fl Oz	2.03	6.38	13.69	116.58	0.00	0.00	25.52	3.94
532	Ice Cream, Vanilla Bean-Ben & J	106.0000	0.500	Cup	3.00	13.00	18.00	190.00	0.00	0.00	75.00	8.00
533	Ice Cream, Vanilla Caramel Fudge	106.0000	0.500	Cup	2.00	12.00	24.00	180.00	0.00	0.00	70.00	7.00
534	Ice Cream, Vanilla Caramel, Low	92.0000	0.500	Cup	6.00	2.50	32.00	180.00	0.00	0.00	20.00	1.50
535	Ice Cream, Vanilla Choc Chip-Haa	106.0000	0.500	Cup	5.00	20.00	26.00	310.00	0.00	0.00	105.00	12.00
536	Ice Cream, Vanilla Choc Chunk-Be	106.0000	0.500	Cup	3.00	15.00	22.00	220.00	0.00	1.00	65.00	10.00
537	Ice Cream, Vanilla Fudge Brownie	106.0000	0.500	Cup	4.00	12.00	23.00	210.00	0.00	0.00	60.00	7.00
538	Ice Cream, Vanilla Fudge-Haagen-	106.0000	0.500	Cup	5.00	18.00	26.00	290.00	0.00	0.00	100.00	12.00
539	Ice Cream, Vanilla Swiss Almond-	106.0000	0.500	Cup	6.00	21.00	23.00	310.00	0.00	1.00	105.00	11.00
540	Ice Cream, Vanilla w/ Heath Crun	106.0000	0.500	Cup	3.00	17.00	24.00	240.00	0.00	0.00	65.00	9.00
541	Ice Cream, Vanilla, French, Coff	106.0000	0.500	Cup	5.00	18.00	21.00	270.00	0.00	0.00	120.00	11.00
	Ice Cream, Vanilla, French, Soft	86.0000	0.500	Cup	3.53	11.18	19.09	184.90	0.00	0.00	78.26	6.43
543	Ice Cream, Vanilla, Low Fat-Haag	92.0000	0.500	Cup	7.00	2.50	29.00	170.00	0.00	0.00	20.00	1.50
	Ice Cream, Vanilla, Rich	74.0000	0.500	Cup	2.59	11.99	16.58	178.34	0.00	0.00	45.14	7.38
542	Ice Cream, Vanilla-Haagen-Daz	106.0000	0.500	Cup	5.00	18.00	21.00	270.00	0.00	0.00	120.00	11.00
544	Ice Cream, Wavy Gravy-Ben & Jerr	106.0000	0.500	Cup	5.00	19.00	22.00	260.00	0.00	2.00	55.00	7.00
545	Ice Cream, White Russian-Ben & J	106.0000	0.500	Cup	3.00	13.00	18.00	190.00	0.00	0.00	70.00	8.00
	Ice Cream-Starbucks	99.0000	0.500	Cup	4.00	13.00	30.00	250.00	0.00	0.00	60.00	8.00
	Milk Substitutes, Fluid w/ hydr	244.0000	1.000	Cup	4.27	8.32	15.03	149.96	0.00	0.00	0.49	1.88
	Milk Substitutes, Fluid, w/ laur	244.0000	1.000	Cup	4.27	8.32	15.03	149.96	0.00	0.00	0.49	7.42
	Milk, Buttermilk	245.0000	1.000	Cup	8.11	2.16	11.74	99.00	0.00	0.00	8.57	1.35
	Milk, Chocolate Drink, Lowfat, 1	250.0000	1.000	Cup	8.10	2.50	26.10	157.58	5.00	1.25	7.25	1.55
	Milk, Chocolate Drink, Lowfat, 2	250.0000	1.000	Cup	8.03	5.00	26.00	178.85	5.00	1.25	17.00	3.10
	Milk, Chocolate Drink, Whole	250.0000	1.000	Cup	7.93	8.48	25.85	208.38	5.00	2.00	30.50	5.25
	Milk, Chocolate Homemade Hot Coc	250.0000	1.000	Cup	9.78	5.83	29.48	192.50	5.00	2.00	20.00	3.60
	Milk, Condensed, Sweetened, Cnd	306.0000	1.000	Cup	24.20	26.62	166.46	981.59	0.00	0.00	103.73	16.80
	Milk, Evaporated, Cnd	31.5000	1.000	Fl Oz	2.15	2.38	3.16	42.33	0.00	0.00	9.26	1.45
	Milk, Evaporated, Skim, Cnd	256.0000	1.000	Cup	19.33	0.51	29.06	199.48	0.00	0.00	9.22	0.31

Monounsaturated Fat (gm)	Polyunsaturated Fat (gm)	Vitamin D (mg)	Vitamin K (mg)	Vitamin E (mg)	Vitamin A (re)	Vitamin C (mg)	Thiamin (mg)	Riboflavin (mg)	Niacin (mg)	Vitamin B₆ (mg)	Folate (mg)	Vitamin B₁₂ (mcg)	Calcium (mg)	Iron (mg)	Magnesium (mg)	Phosphorus (mg)	Potassium (mg)	Sodium (mg)	Zinc (mg)
0.00	0.00	0.00	0.00	0.00	0.00	0.00	0.00	0.00	0.00	0.00	0.00	0.00	0.00	0.00	0.00	0.00	0.00	140.00	0.00
0.00	0.00	0.00	0.00	0.00	0.00	0.00	0.00	0.00	0.00	0.00	0.00	0.00	0.00	0.00	0.00	0.00	0.00	115.00	0.00
0.00	0.00	0.00	0.00	0.00	0.00	0.00	0.00	0.00	0.00	0.00	0.00	0.00	0.00	0.00	0.00	0.00	0.00	55.00	0.00
0.00	0.00	0.00	0.00	0.00	0.00	0.00	0.00	0.00	0.00	0.00	0.00	0.00	0.00	0.00	0.00	0.00	0.00	110.00	0.00
0.00	0.00	0.00	0.00	0.00	0.00	0.00	0.00	0.00	0.00	0.00	0.00	0.00	0.00	0.00	0.00	0.00	0.00	80.00	0.00
0.00	0.00	0.00	0.00	0.00	0.00	0.00	0.00	0.00	0.00	0.00	0.00	0.00	80.00	0.00	0.00	0.00	0.00	50.00	0.00
0.00	0.00	0.00	0.00	0.00	0.00	0.00	0.00	0.00	0.00	0.00	0.00	0.00	160.00	0.00	0.00	0.00	0.00	50.00	0.00
0.00	0.00	0.00	0.00	0.00	0.00	0.00	0.00	0.00	0.00	0.00	0.00	0.00	80.00	0.00	0.00	0.00	0.00	65.00	0.00
0.00	0.00	0.00	0.00	0.00	0.00	0.00	0.00	0.00	0.00	0.00	0.00	0.00	0.00	0.00	0.00	0.00	0.00	120.00	0.00
0.00	0.00	0.00	0.00	0.00	0.00	0.00	0.00	0.00	0.00	0.00	0.00	0.00	0.00	0.00	0.00	0.00	0.00	60.00	0.00
0.00	0.00	0.00	0.00	0.00	0.00	0.00	0.00	0.00	0.00	0.00	0.00	0.00	0.00	0.00	0.00	0.00	0.00	40.00	0.00
0.00	0.00	0.00	0.00	0.00	0.00	0.00	0.00	0.00	0.00	0.00	0.00	0.00	0.00	0.00	0.00	0.00	0.00	105.00	0.00
0.00	0.00	0.00	0.00	0.00	0.00	0.00	0.00	0.00	0.00	0.00	0.00	0.00	0.00	0.00	0.00	0.00	0.00	50.00	0.00
0.00	0.00	0.00	0.00	0.00	0.00	0.00	0.00	0.00	0.00	0.00	0.00	0.00	0.00	0.00	0.00	0.00	0.00	110.00	0.00
0.00	0.00	0.00	0.00	0.00	0.00	0.00	0.00	0.00	0.00	0.00	0.00	0.00	0.00	0.00	0.00	0.00	0.00	45.00	0.00
0.00	0.00	0.00	0.00	0.00	0.00	0.00	0.00	0.00	0.00	0.00	0.00	0.00	0.00	0.00	0.00	0.00	0.00	95.00	0.00
0.00	0.00	0.00	0.00	0.00	0.00	0.00	0.00	0.00	0.00	0.00	0.00	0.00	0.00	0.00	0.00	0.00	0.00	70.00	0.00
0.00	0.00	0.00	0.00	0.00	0.00	0.00	0.00	0.00	0.00	0.00	0.00	0.00	0.00	0.00	0.00	0.00	0.00	90.00	0.00
0.00	0.00	0.00	0.00	0.00	0.00	0.00	0.00	0.00	0.00	0.00	0.00	0.00	0.00	0.00	0.00	0.00	0.00	180.00	0.00
0.00	0.00	0.00	0.00	0.00	0.00	0.00	0.00	0.00	0.00	0.00	0.00	0.00	0.00	0.00	0.00	0.00	0.00	105.00	0.00
0.00	0.00	0.00	0.00	0.00	0.00	0.00	0.00	0.00	0.00	0.00	0.00	0.00	0.00	0.00	0.00	0.00	0.00	75.00	0.00
0.00	0.00	0.00	0.00	0.00	45.24	4.47	0.03	0.15	0.10	0.03	6.96	0.17	69.60	0.12	8.12	58.00	109.04	34.80	0.20
0.00	0.00	0.00	0.00	0.00	0.00	0.00	0.00	0.00	0.00	0.00	0.00	0.00	0.00	0.00	0.00	0.00	0.00	150.00	0.00
0.00	0.00	0.00	0.00	0.00	0.00	0.00	0.00	0.00	0.00	0.00	0.00	0.00	0.00	0.00	0.00	0.00	0.00	40.00	0.00
0.00	0.00	0.00	0.00	0.00	0.00	0.00	0.00	0.00	0.00	0.00	0.00	0.00	0.00	0.00	0.00	0.00	0.00	35.00	0.00
0.00	0.00	0.00	0.00	0.00	0.00	0.00	0.00	0.00	0.00	0.00	0.00	0.00	0.00	0.00	0.00	0.00	0.00	80.00	0.00
1.84	0.24	0.00	0.00	0.00	67.86	0.35	0.02	0.14	0.07	0.03	2.90	0.23	74.24	0.05	8.12	60.90	115.42	46.40	0.40
0.00	0.00	0.00	0.00	0.00	0.00	0.00	0.00	0.00	0.00	0.00	0.00	0.00	0.00	0.00	0.00	0.00	0.00	45.00	0.00
0.00	0.00	0.00	0.00	0.00	0.00	0.00	0.00	0.00	0.00	0.00	0.00	0.00	0.00	0.00	0.00	0.00	0.00	50.00	0.00
0.00	0.00	0.00	0.00	0.00	0.00	0.00	0.00	0.00	0.00	0.00	0.00	0.00	0.00	0.00	0.00	0.00	0.00	120.00	0.00
0.00	0.00	0.00	0.00	0.00	0.00	0.00	0.00	0.00	0.00	0.00	0.00	0.00	0.00	0.00	0.00	0.00	0.00	90.00	0.00
0.00	0.00	0.00	0.00	0.00	0.00	0.00	0.00	0.00	0.00	0.00	0.00	0.00	0.00	0.00	0.00	0.00	0.00	50.00	0.00
0.00	0.00	0.00	0.00	0.00	0.00	0.00	0.00	0.00	0.00	0.00	0.00	0.00	0.00	0.00	0.00	0.00	0.00	80.00	0.00
0.00	0.00	0.00	0.00	0.00	0.00	0.00	0.00	0.00	0.00	0.00	0.00	0.00	0.00	0.00	0.00	0.00	0.00	110.00	0.00
0.00	0.00	0.00	0.00	0.00	0.00	0.00	0.00	0.00	0.00	0.00	0.00	0.00	0.00	0.00	0.00	0.00	0.00	90.00	0.00
0.00	0.00	0.00	0.00	0.00	0.00	0.00	0.00	0.00	0.00	0.00	0.00	0.00	0.00	0.00	0.00	0.00	0.00	110.00	0.00
0.00	0.00	0.00	0.00	0.00	0.00	0.00	0.00	0.00	0.00	0.00	0.00	0.00	0.00	0.00	0.00	0.00	0.00	85.00	0.00
3.00	0.39	0.00	0.00	0.32	132.44	0.69	0.04	0.15	0.09	0.04	7.74	0.43	112.66	0.18	10.32	99.76	152.22	52.46	0.45
0.00	0.00	0.00	0.00	0.00	0.00	0.00	0.00	0.00	0.00	0.00	0.00	0.00	0.00	0.00	0.00	0.00	0.00	50.00	0.00
3.45	0.44	0.00	0.00	0.00	136.16	0.52	0.03	0.12	0.06	0.03	3.70	0.27	86.58	0.04	8.14	70.30	117.66	41.44	0.30
0.00	0.00	0.00	0.00	0.00	0.00	0.00	0.00	0.00	0.00	0.00	0.00	0.00	0.00	0.00	0.00	0.00	0.00	85.00	0.00
0.00	0.00	0.00	0.00	0.00	0.00	0.00	0.00	0.00	0.00	0.00	0.00	0.00	0.00	0.00	0.00	0.00	0.00	90.00	0.00
0.00	0.00	0.00	0.00	0.00	0.00	0.00	0.00	0.00	0.00	0.00	0.00	0.00	0.00	0.00	0.00	0.00	0.00	45.00	0.00
0.00	0.00	0.00	0.00	0.00	0.00	0.00	0.00	0.00	0.00	0.00	0.00	0.00	120.00	0.00	0.00	0.00	0.00	15.00	0.00
4.88	1.20	0.00	0.00	2.56	0.00	0.00	0.02	0.22	0.00	0.00	0.00	0.00	79.30	0.95	15.57	181.05	278.89	191.05	2.88
0.44	0.02	0.00	0.00	0.00	0.00	0.00	0.02	0.22	0.00	0.00	0.00	0.00	79.30	0.95	15.57	181.05	278.89	191.05	2.88
0.61	0.07	0.00	0.00	0.15	19.60	2.40	0.07	0.37	0.15	0.07	12.25	0.54	285.18	0.12	26.83	218.54	370.69	257.01	1.03
0.75	0.10	0.00	0.00	0.08	147.50	2.33	0.10	0.43	0.33	0.10	12.00	0.85	286.75	0.60	33.33	256.50	425.50	151.75	1.03
1.48	0.18	2.50	0.00	0.13	142.50	2.30	0.10	0.40	0.33	0.10	12.00	0.85	284.00	0.60	33.00	254.25	422.00	150.50	1.03
2.48	0.30	2.50	0.00	0.23	72.50	2.28	0.10	0.40	0.33	0.10	11.75	0.83	280.25	0.60	32.58	251.25	417.25	149.00	1.03
1.70	0.23	0.00	0.00	0.25	137.50	2.50	0.10	0.43	0.38	0.13	15.00	0.93	315.00	1.15	70.00	292.50	500.00	127.50	1.48
7.44	1.04	0.00	0.00	0.64	247.86	7.96	0.28	1.29	0.64	0.15	34.27	1.35	867.51	0.58	78.49	775.10	1136.48	388.62	2.88
0.74	0.08	0.00	0.00	0.00	17.01	0.59	0.02	0.10	0.06	0.02	2.49	0.05	82.15	0.06	7.62	63.79	95.48	33.33	0.24
0.15	0.03	5.12	0.00	0.03	299.52	3.17	0.13	0.79	0.44	0.15	22.02	0.61	741.12	0.74	69.12	498.94	848.64	294.40	2.30

USDA ID Code	Food Name	Weight in Grams*	Quantity of Units	Unit of Measure	Protein (gm)	Fat (gm)	Carbohydrate (gm)	Kcalories	Caffeine (gm)	Fiber (gm)	Cholesterol (mg)	Saturated Fat (gm)
	Milk, Light, 1% Fat	244.0000	1.000	Cup	8.03	2.59	11.66	102.14	0.00	0.00	9.76	1.61
	Milk, Malted, Beverage	265.0000	1.000	Cup	10.34	9.81	27.30	235.85	0.00	0.00	37.10	5.95
	Milk, Malted, Chocolate Flavor,	265.0000	1.000	Cup	9.01	9.01	29.95	227.90	7.95	0.00	34.45	5.53
	Milk, Non-Fat, Skim	245.0000	1.000	Cup	8.35	0.44	11.88	85.53	0.00	0.00	4.41	0.29
	Milk, Reduced, 2% Fat	244.0000	1.000	Cup	8.13	4.68	11.71	121.19	0.00	0.00	18.30	2.93
583	Milk, Rice, Enriched Brown-Rice	240.0000	8.000	Fl Oz	1.00	2.00	25.00	120.00	0.00	0.00	0.00	0.00
584	Milk, Soy	240.0000	1.000	Cup	6.60	4.58	4.34	79.00	0.00	3.12	0.00	0.51
	Milk, Whole, 3.3% Fat	244.0000	1.000	Cup	8.03	8.15	11.37	149.91	0.00	0.00	33.18	5.08
	Milk, Whole, 3.7% Fat	244.0000	1.000	Cup	8.00	8.93	11.35	156.57	0.00	0.00	34.89	5.56
	Sour Cream	230.0000	1.000	Cup	7.27	48.21	9.82	492.80	0.00	0.00	102.12	30.02
	Sour Cream, Fat Free	16.0140	1.000	Tbsp	0.50	0.00	2.50	12.51	0.00	0.00	2.50	0.00
	Sour Cream, Imitation, Non-dairy	230.0000	1.000	Cup	5.52	44.90	15.25	479.46	0.00	0.00	0.00	40.92
	Sour Cream, Light	16.0140	1.000	Tbsp	0.92	1.14	0.92	16.01	0.00	0.00	4.58	0.69
	Sour Cream, Non-Fat	16.0000	2.000	Tbsp	0.50	0.00	2.50	12.50	0.00	0.00	2.50	0.00
	Yogurt, 99% Fat Free-Dannon	227.0000	8.000	Ounce	9.00	3.00	45.00	240.00	0.00	0.00	15.00	1.50
834	Yogurt, Apl Cin., Non Fat, Chunk	170.0000	6.000	Ounce	7.00	0.00	33.00	160.00	0.00	0.00	5.00	0.00
835	Yogurt, Apple Cin, Fruit on Bott	227.0000	8.000	Ounce	9.00	3.00	46.00	240.00	0.00	1.00	15.00	1.50
836	Yogurt, Apple Cobbler, Smooth &	227.0000	8.000	Ounce	8.00	2.00	46.00	230.00	0.00	0.00	20.00	1.00
837	Yogurt, Apple Pie a la Mode, Non	227.0000	8.000	Ounce	7.00	0.00	22.00	120.00	0.00	0.00	10.00	0.00
838	Yogurt, Ban Crm/Straw, Double De	170.0000	6.000	Ounce	7.00	1.00	32.00	160.00	0.00	0.00	10.00	0.50
839	Yogurt, Banana Cream Pie, Light-	227.0000	8.000	Ounce	8.00	0.00	16.00	100.00	0.00	0.00	5.00	0.00
840	Yogurt, Bav Crm/Rasp, Double Del	170.0000	6.000	Ounce	7.00	1.00	34.00	170.00	0.00	0.00	10.00	0.50
841	Yogurt, Bavarian & Peach, Light	170.0000	6.000	Ounce	5.00	0.00	18.00	90.00	0.00	0.00	0.00	0.00
842	Yogurt, Berries, Mixed, Fruit on	227.0000	8.000	Ounce	9.00	3.00	45.00	240.00	0.00	1.00	15.00	1.50
843	Yogurt, Berry Banana Split, Non	227.0000	8.000	Ounce	8.00	0.00	21.00	120.00	0.00	0.00	10.00	0.00
844	Yogurt, Berry, Mixed, Fruit on B	125.0000	4.400	Ounce	5.00	1.50	25.00	130.00	0.00	0.00	10.00	1.00
845	Yogurt, Berry, Mixed, Lowfat-Bre	227.0000	8.000	Ounce	9.00	2.50	43.00	230.00	0.00	0.00	15.00	1.50
846	Yogurt, Berry, Tropical, Non Fat	170.0000	6.000	Ounce	7.00	0.00	32.00	160.00	0.00	0.00	5.00	0.00
847	Yogurt, Blackberry Pie, Light-Da	227.0000	8.000	Ounce	8.00	0.00	16.00	100.00	0.00	0.00	5.00	0.00
848	Yogurt, Blueberries N' Cream, No	227.0000	8.000	Ounce	8.00	0.00	23.00	120.00	0.00	0.00	10.00	0.00
849	Yogurt, Blueberries/Crm, Smooth	227.0000	8.000	Ounce	9.00	2.00	46.00	240.00	0.00	0.00	20.00	1.00
850	Yogurt, Blueberry, Blended-Breye	125.0000	4.400	Ounce	4.00	1.00	25.00	130.00	0.00	0.00	10.00	0.50
851	Yogurt, Blueberry, Danimals-Dann	125.0000	4.400	Ounce	6.00	1.00	24.00	130.00	0.00	0.00	5.00	0.50
852	Yogurt, Blueberry, Fruit on Bott	227.0000	8.000	Ounce	9.00	3.00	46.00	240.00	0.00	1.00	15.00	1.50
853	Yogurt, Blueberry, Light-Dannon	227.0000	8.000	Ounce	8.00	0.00	18.00	100.00	0.00	0.00	5.00	0.00
854	Yogurt, Blueberry, Lowfat -Breye	227.0000	8.000	Ounce	9.00	2.50	43.00	230.00	0.00	0.00	15.00	1.50
855	Yogurt, Blueberry, Non Fat, Blen	125.0000	4.400	Ounce	5.00	0.00	25.00	120.00	0.00	0.00	5.00	0.00
856	Yogurt, Blueberry, Non Fat, Chun	170.0000	6.000	Ounce	7.00	0.00	32.00	160.00	0.00	0.00	5.00	0.00
857	Yogurt, Boysenberry, Fruit on B	227.0000	8.000	Ounce	9.00	3.00	45.00	240.00	0.00	1.00	15.00	1.50
858	Yogurt, Cappuccino, Light-Dannon	227.0000	8.000	Ounce	8.00	0.00	16.00	100.00	0.00	0.00	5.00	0.00
859	Yogurt, Car Apl Cinn, Double Del	170.0000	6.000	Ounce	7.00	1.00	47.00	220.00	0.00	0.00	10.00	0.50
860	Yogurt, Car Praline, Double Deli	170.0000	6.000	Ounce	7.00	1.00	47.00	200.00	0.00	0.00	10.00	0.50
861	Yogurt, Caramel Apple Crunch, Li	227.0000	8.000	Ounce	8.00	0.00	25.00	140.00	0.00	0.00	5.00	0.00
862	Yogurt, Cheesck/Straw, Double De	170.0000	6.000	Ounce	7.00	1.00	33.00	170.00	0.00	0.00	10.00	0.50
863	Yogurt, Cheescke/Cher, Double De	170.0000	6.000	Ounce	7.00	1.00	34.00	170.00	0.00	0.00	10.00	0.50
864	Yogurt, Cheeseck & Cherry, Light	170.0000	6.000	Ounce	5.00	0.00	18.00	90.00	0.00	0.00	0.00	0.00
865	Yogurt, Cheeseck & Straw, Light	170.0000	6.000	Ounce	5.00	0.00	17.00	90.00	0.00	0.00	0.00	0.00
866	Yogurt, Cherr Van, Sprinklin' Ra	116.0000	4.000	Ounce	5.00	1.50	24.00	130.00	0.00	0.00	5.00	0.50
867	Yogurt, Cherry Bon-Bon, Non Fat-	227.0000	8.000	Ounce	8.00	0.00	22.00	120.00	0.00	0.00	10.00	0.00
868	Yogurt, Cherry Van, Non Fat, Chu	170.0000	6.000	Ounce	7.00	0.00	31.00	160.00	0.00	0.00	5.00	0.00
869	Yogurt, Cherry Vanilla Crm, Non	227.0000	8.000	Ounce	8.00	0.00	22.00	120.00	0.00	0.00	10.00	0.00
870	Yogurt, Cherry Vanilla, Light-Da	227.0000	8.000	Ounce	8.00	0.00	18.00	100.00	0.00	0.00	5.00	0.00
871	Yogurt, Cherry, Black Jubilee, N	227.0000	8.000	Ounce	8.00	0.00	23.00	120.00	0.00	0.00	10.00	0.00
872	Yogurt, Cherry, Black, Lowfat-Br	227.0000	8.000	Ounce	9.00	2.50	44.00	240.00	0.00	0.00	15.00	1.50
873	Yogurt, Cherry, Danimals-Dannon	125.0000	4.400	Ounce	6.00	1.00	23.00	120.00	0.00	0.00	5.00	0.50

Monounsaturated Fat (gm)	Polyunsaturated Fat (gm)	Vitamin D (mg)	Vitamin K (mg)	Vitamin E (mg)	Vitamin A (re)	Vitamin C (mg)	Thiamin (mg)	Riboflavin (mg)	Niacin (mg)	Vitamin B$_6$ (mg)	Folate (mg)	Vitamin B$_{12}$ (mcg)	Calcium (mg)	Iron (mg)	Magnesium (mg)	Phosphorus (mg)	Potassium (mg)	Sodium (mg)	Zinc (mg)
0.76	0.10	2.44	0.00	0.10	143.96	2.37	0.10	0.41	0.22	0.10	12.44	0.90	300.12	0.12	33.72	234.73	380.88	123.22	0.95
2.78	0.56	0.00	0.00	0.00	95.40	2.92	0.20	0.59	1.31	0.19	21.73	1.03	355.10	0.27	53.00	302.10	530.00	222.60	1.14
2.57	0.38	0.00	0.00	0.00	79.50	2.65	0.13	0.44	0.63	0.14	16.43	0.93	304.75	0.61	47.70	265.00	498.20	172.25	1.09
0.12	0.02	2.45	9.80	0.10	149.45	2.40	0.10	0.34	0.22	0.10	12.74	0.93	302.33	0.10	27.83	247.21	405.72	126.18	0.98
1.37	0.17	2.44	0.00	0.17	139.08	2.32	0.10	0.41	0.22	0.10	12.44	0.88	296.70	0.12	33.35	232.04	376.74	121.76	0.95
0.00	0.00	0.00	0.00	0.00	0.00	0.00	0.00	0.00	0.00	0.00	0.00	0.00	0.00	0.00	0.00	0.00		90.00	0.00
0.78	1.90	0.00	0.00	0.00	23.06	0.00	0.38	0.16	0.35	0.09	3.60	0.00	9.60	1.39	45.60	117.60	338.40	28.80	0.55
2.37	0.29	2.44	9.76	0.24	75.64	2.29	0.10	0.39	0.20	0.10	12.20	0.88	291.34	0.12	32.79	227.90	369.66	119.56	0.93
2.59	0.34	0.00	0.00	0.24	82.96	3.59	0.10	0.39	0.20	0.10	12.20	0.88	290.36	0.12	32.70	227.16	368.44	119.07	0.93
13.92	1.79	0.00	0.00	1.31	448.50	1.98	0.09	0.35	0.16	0.05	24.84	0.69	267.72	0.14	25.83	195.27	331.20	122.59	0.62
0.00	0.00	0.00	0.00	0.00	30.03	0.00	0.00	0.00	0.00	0.00	0.00	0.00	36.03	0.00	0.00	0.00	0.00	17.51	0.00
1.36	0.14	0.00	0.00	0.35	0.00	0.00	0.00	0.00	0.00	0.00	0.00	0.00	5.75	0.90	14.67	102.35	369.15	234.60	2.71
0.00	0.00	0.00	0.00	0.00	18.30	0.00	0.00	0.00	0.00	0.00	0.00	0.00	21.96	0.00	0.00	0.00	27.45	9.15	0.00
0.00	0.00	0.00	0.00	0.00	30.00	0.00	0.00	0.00	0.00	0.00	0.00	0.00	36.00	0.00	0.00	0.00	0.00	17.50	0.00
0.00	0.00	0.00	0.00	0.00	0.00	12.00	0.00	0.00	0.00	0.00	0.00	0.00	280.00	0.00	0.00	0.00	0.00	140.00	0.00
0.00	0.00	0.00	0.00	0.00	0.00	0.00	0.00	0.00	0.00	0.00	0.00	0.00	0.00	0.00	0.00	0.00	320.00	100.00	0.00
0.00	0.00	0.00	0.00	0.00	0.00	0.00	0.00	0.00	0.00	0.00	0.00	0.00	0.00	0.00	0.00	0.00	460.00	140.00	0.00
0.00	0.00	0.00	0.00	0.00	0.00	0.00	0.00	0.00	0.00	0.00	0.00	0.00	0.00	0.00	0.00	0.00	390.00	140.00	0.00
0.00	0.00	0.00	0.00	0.00	0.00	0.00	0.00	0.00	0.00	0.00	0.00	0.00	0.00	0.00	0.00	0.00	300.00	105.00	0.00
0.00	0.00	0.00	0.00	0.00	0.00	0.00	0.00	0.00	0.00	0.00	0.00	0.00	0.00	0.00	0.00	0.00	330.00	100.00	0.00
0.00	0.00	0.00	0.00	0.00	0.00	0.00	0.00	0.00	0.00	0.00	0.00	0.00	0.00	0.00	0.00	0.00	360.00	130.00	0.00
0.00	0.00	0.00	0.00	0.00	0.00	0.00	0.00	0.00	0.00	0.00	0.00	0.00	0.00	0.00	0.00	0.00	330.00	125.00	0.00
0.00	0.00	0.00	0.00	0.00	0.00	0.00	0.00	0.00	0.00	0.00	0.00	0.00	0.00	0.00	0.00	0.00	240.00	75.00	0.00
0.00	0.00	0.00	0.00	0.00	0.00	0.00	0.00	0.00	0.00	0.00	0.00	0.00	0.00	0.00	0.00	0.00	450.00	150.00	0.00
0.00	0.00	0.00	0.00	0.00	0.00	0.00	0.00	0.00	0.00	0.00	0.00	0.00	0.00	0.00	0.00	0.00	320.00	105.00	0.00
0.00	0.00	0.00	0.00	0.00	0.00	0.00	0.00	0.00	0.00	0.00	0.00	0.00	0.00	0.00	0.00	0.00	250.00	80.00	0.00
0.00	0.00	0.00	0.00	0.00	0.00	0.00	0.00	0.00	0.00	0.00	0.00	0.00	0.00	0.00	0.00	0.00	440.00	125.00	0.00
0.00	0.00	2.44	0.00	0.00	0.00	0.00	0.00	0.00	0.00	0.00	0.00	0.00	0.00	0.00	0.00	0.00	340.00	110.00	0.00
0.00	0.00	0.00	0.00	0.00	0.00	0.00	0.00	0.00	0.00	0.00	0.00	0.00	0.00	0.00	0.00	0.00	360.00	135.00	0.00
0.00	0.00	0.00	0.00	0.00	0.00	0.00	0.00	0.00	0.00	0.00	0.00	0.00	0.00	0.00	0.00	0.00	310.00	100.00	0.00
0.00	0.00	0.00	0.00	0.00	0.00	0.00	0.00	0.00	0.00	0.00	0.00	0.00	0.00	0.00	0.00	0.00	380.00	125.00	0.00
0.00	0.00	0.00	0.00	0.00	0.00	0.00	0.00	0.00	0.00	0.00	0.00	0.00	0.00	0.00	0.00	0.00	180.00	60.00	0.00
0.00	0.00	0.00	0.00	0.00	0.00	0.00	0.00	0.00	0.00	0.00	0.00	0.00	0.00	0.00	0.00	0.00	270.00	100.00	0.00
0.00	0.00	0.00	0.00	0.00	0.00	0.00	0.00	0.00	0.00	0.00	0.00	0.00	0.00	0.00	0.00	0.00	460.00	140.00	0.00
0.00	0.00	0.00	0.00	0.00	0.00	0.00	0.00	0.00	0.00	0.00	0.00	0.00	0.00	0.00	0.00	0.00	370.00	130.00	0.00
0.00	0.00	0.00	0.00	0.00	0.00	0.00	0.00	0.00	0.00	0.00	0.00	0.00	0.00	0.00	0.00	0.00	430.00	125.00	0.00
0.00	0.00	0.00	0.00	0.00	0.00	0.00	0.00	0.00	0.00	0.00	0.00	0.00	0.00	0.00	0.00	0.00	260.00	105.00	0.00
0.00	0.00	0.00	0.00	0.00	0.00	0.00	0.00	0.00	0.00	0.00	0.00	0.00	0.00	0.00	0.00	0.00	310.00	110.00	0.00
0.00	0.00	0.00	0.00	0.00	0.00	0.00	0.00	0.00	0.00	0.00	0.00	0.00	0.00	0.00	0.00	0.00	450.00	150.00	0.00
0.00	0.00	0.00	0.00	0.00	0.00	0.00	0.00	0.00	0.00	0.00	0.00	0.00	0.00	0.00	0.00	0.00	350.00	135.00	0.00
0.00	0.00	0.00	0.00	0.00	0.00	0.00	0.00	0.00	0.00	0.00	0.00	0.00	0.00	0.00	0.00	0.00	330.00	200.00	0.00
0.00	0.00	0.00	0.00	0.00	0.00	0.00	0.00	0.00	0.00	0.00	0.00	0.00	0.00	0.00	0.00	0.00	330.00	200.00	0.00
0.00	0.00	0.00	0.00	0.00	0.00	0.00	0.00	0.00	0.00	0.00	0.00	0.00	0.00	0.00	0.00	0.00	350.00	170.00	0.00
0.00	0.00	0.00	0.00	0.00	0.00	0.00	0.00	0.00	0.00	0.00	0.00	0.00	0.00	0.00	0.00	0.00	340.00	100.00	0.00
0.00	0.00	0.00	0.00	0.00	0.00	0.00	0.00	0.00	0.00	0.00	0.00	0.00	0.00	0.00	0.00	0.00	340.00	100.00	0.00
0.00	0.00	0.00	0.00	0.00	0.00	0.00	0.00	0.00	0.00	0.00	0.00	0.00	0.00	0.00	0.00	0.00	250.00	75.00	0.00
0.00	0.00	0.00	0.00	0.00	0.00	0.00	0.00	0.00	0.00	0.00	0.00	0.00	0.00	0.00	0.00	0.00	250.00	75.00	0.00
0.00	0.00	0.00	0.00	0.00	0.00	0.00	0.00	0.00	0.00	0.00	0.00	0.00	0.00	0.00	0.00	0.00	250.00	85.00	0.00
0.00	0.00	0.00	0.00	0.00	0.00	0.00	0.00	0.00	0.00	0.00	0.00	0.00	0.00	0.00	0.00	0.00	300.00	105.00	0.00
0.00	0.00	0.00	0.00	0.00	0.00	0.00	0.00	0.00	0.00	0.00	0.00	0.00	0.00	0.00	0.00	0.00	360.00	100.00	0.00
0.00	0.00	0.00	0.00	0.00	0.00	0.00	0.00	0.00	0.00	0.00	3.60	0.00	0.00	0.00	0.00	0.00	320.00	105.00	0.00
0.00	0.00	0.00	0.00	0.00	0.00	0.00	0.00	0.00	0.00	0.00	0.00	0.00	0.00	0.00	0.00	0.00	380.00	130.00	0.00
0.00	0.00	0.00	0.00	0.00	0.00	0.00	0.00	0.00	0.00	0.00	0.00	0.00	0.00	0.00	0.00	0.00	330.00	100.00	0.00
0.00	0.00	0.00	0.00	0.00	0.00	0.00	0.00	0.00	0.00	0.00	0.00	0.00	0.00	0.00	0.00	0.00	450.00	125.00	0.00
0.00	0.00	0.00	0.00	0.00	0.00	0.00	0.00	0.00	0.00	0.00	0.00	0.00	0.00	0.00	0.00	0.00	270.00	95.00	0.00

USDA ID Code	Food Name	Weight in Grams*	Quantity of Units	Unit of Measure	Protein (gm)	Fat (gm)	Carbohydrate (gm)	Kcalories	Caffeine (gm)	Fiber (gm)	Cholesterol (mg)	Saturated Fat (gm)
874	Yogurt, Cherry, Fruit on Bottom-	227.0000	8.000	Ounce	9.00	3.00	45.00	240.00	0.00	0.00	15.00	1.50
875	Yogurt, Cherry, Non Fat, Blended	125.0000	4.400	Ounce	5.00	0.00	23.00	110.00	0.00	0.00	5.00	0.00
877	Yogurt, Choc _clair, Double Deli	170.0000	6.000	Ounce	8.00	1.00	45.00	220.00	0.00	0.00	10.00	0.50
876	Yogurt, Choc Chscake, Double Del	170.0000	6.000	Ounce	8.00	1.00	45.00	220.00	0.00	0.00	10.00	0.50
878	Yogurt, Choc, White & Rasp, Ligh	170.0000	6.000	Ounce	5.00	0.00	17.00	90.00	0.00	0.00	0.00	0.00
879	Yogurt, Choc, White, Rasp, Light	227.0000	8.000	Ounce	8.00	0.00	16.00	100.00	0.00	0.00	5.00	0.00
880	Yogurt, Choc/Straw, Double Delig	170.0000	6.000	Ounce	8.00	1.00	45.00	210.00	0.00	0.00	10.00	0.50
881	Yogurt, Coconut Crm Pie, Light-D	227.0000	8.000	Ounce	8.00	0.00	16.00	100.00	0.00	0.00	5.00	0.00
882	Yogurt, Coffee, Lowfat-Dannon	227.0000	8.000	Ounce	10.00	3.00	36.00	210.00	0.00	0.00	15.00	2.00
883	Yogurt, Cookies 'N Cream, Light-	227.0000	8.000	Ounce	8.00	0.00	24.00	130.00	0.00	0.00	5.00	0.00
884	Yogurt, Cranberry Raspberry, Low	227.0000	8.000	Ounce	10.00	3.00	36.00	210.00	0.00	0.00	15.00	2.00
885	Yogurt, Creme Caramel, Light-Dan	227.0000	8.000	Ounce	8.00	0.00	16.00	100.00	0.00	0.00	5.00	0.00
	Yogurt, Fruit, Fat Free	247.9570	1.000	Cup	10.21	0.00	48.13	233.37	0.00	0.00	7.29	0.00
	Yogurt, Fruit, Fat Free, Light	247.9570	1.000	Cup	10.00	0.00	19.00	109.98	0.00	0.00	5.00	0.00
	Yogurt, Fruit, Lowfat, 10 Gm Pro	245.0000	1.000	Cup	10.71	2.65	46.67	249.61	0.00	0.00	10.29	1.72
	Yogurt, Fruit, Lowfat, 11 Gm Pro	227.0000	1.000	Cup	11.03	3.20	42.22	238.65	0.00	0.00	12.49	2.07
	Yogurt, Fruit, Lowfat, 9 Gm Prot	245.0000	1.000	Cup	9.75	2.82	45.67	243.14	0.00	0.00	11.03	1.81
886	Yogurt, Key Lime Pie, Non Fat-Br	227.0000	8.000	Ounce	8.00	0.00	22.00	120.00	0.00	0.00	10.00	0.00
887	Yogurt, Lem Mer Pie, Double Deli	170.0000	6.000	Ounce	6.00	1.00	37.00	180.00	0.00	0.00	10.00	0.50
888	Yogurt, Lemon Blueberry Cobbler,	227.0000	8.000	Ounce	8.00	0.00	24.00	140.00	0.00	0.00	5.00	0.00
889	Yogurt, Lemon Chiffon, Light Non	227.0000	8.000	Ounce	7.00	0.00	22.00	120.00	0.00	0.00	10.00	0.00
890	Yogurt, Lemon Chiffon, Light-Dan	227.0000	8.000	Ounce	8.00	0.00	16.00	100.00	0.00	0.00	5.00	0.00
891	Yogurt, Lemon Ice, Danimals-Dann	125.0000	4.400	Ounce	6.00	1.00	22.00	120.00	0.00	0.00	5.00	0.50
892	Yogurt, Lemon, Lowfat-Dannon	227.0000	8.000	Ounce	10.00	3.00	36.00	210.00	0.00	0.00	15.00	2.00
893	Yogurt, Light, Strawberry Kiwi-D	227.0000	8.000	Ounce	8.00	0.00	17.00	100.00	0.00	0.00	5.00	0.00
	Yogurt, Light-Dannon	227.0000	8.000	Ounce	9.00	0.00	45.00	240.00	0.00	0.00	15.00	1.50
	Yogurt, No Sugar w/ Granola, Non	227.0000	8.000	Ounce	9.00	0.00	26.00	140.00	0.00	0.00	5.00	0.00
894	Yogurt, Orange Van, Smooth & Crm	227.0000	8.000	Ounce	9.00	2.00	45.00	230.00	0.00	0.00	20.00	1.00
895	Yogurt, Orange, Fruit on Bottom-	227.0000	8.000	Ounce	9.00	3.00	45.00	240.00	0.00	0.00	15.00	1.50
896	Yogurt, Peach, Blended-Breyer's	125.0000	4.400	Ounce	4.00	1.00	26.00	130.00	0.00	0.00	10.00	0.50
897	Yogurt, Peach, Fruit on Bottom-D	227.0000	8.000	Ounce	9.00	3.00	45.00	240.00	0.00	0.00	15.00	1.50
898	Yogurt, Peach, Light-Dannon	227.0000	8.000	Ounce	8.00	0.00	18.00	100.00	0.00	0.00	5.00	0.00
901	Yogurt, Peach, Lowfat-Breyer's	227.0000	8.000	Ounce	9.00	2.50	43.00	240.00	0.00	0.00	15.00	1.50
899	Yogurt, Peach, Non Fat, Blended-	125.0000	4.400	Ounce	5.00	0.00	23.00	110.00	0.00	0.00	5.00	0.00
900	Yogurt, Peach, Non Fat, Chunky F	170.0000	6.000	Ounce	7.00	0.00	33.00	160.00	0.00	0.00	5.00	0.00
902	Yogurt, Peaches N' Crm, Light No	227.0000	8.000	Ounce	8.00	0.00	22.00	120.00	0.00	0.00	10.00	0.00
903	Yogurt, Peaches/Crm, Smooth & Cr	227.0000	8.000	Ounce	9.00	2.00	45.00	230.00	0.00	0.00	20.00	1.00
904	Yogurt, Pina Co, Non Fat, Chunky	170.0000	6.000	Ounce	7.00	0.00	32.00	160.00	0.00	0.00	5.00	0.00
905	Yogurt, Pineapple, Lowfat-Breyer	227.0000	8.000	Ounce	9.00	2.50	45.00	240.00	0.00	0.00	15.00	1.50
906	Yogurt, Plain Lowfat-Dannon	227.0000	8.000	Ounce	12.00	4.00	16.00	140.00	0.00	0.00	20.00	2.50
907	Yogurt, Plain Non Fat-Dannon	227.0000	8.000	Ounce	12.00	0.00	16.00	110.00	0.00	0.00	5.00	0.00
	Yogurt, Plain, Fat Free	247.9570	1.000	Cup	13.00	0.00	17.00	119.98	0.00	0.00	5.00	0.00
	Yogurt, Plain, Lowfat, 12 Gm Pro	245.0000	1.000	Cup	12.86	3.80	17.25	155.06	0.00	0.00	14.95	2.45
	Yogurt, Plain, Skim Milk, 13 Gm	245.0000	1.000	Cup	14.04	0.44	18.82	136.64	0.00	0.00	4.41	0.29
	Yogurt, Plain, Whole Milk, 8 Gm	245.0000	1.000	Cup	8.50	7.96	11.42	150.48	0.00	0.00	31.12	5.15
908	Yogurt, Rasp N' Cream, Light Non	227.0000	8.000	Ounce	8.00	0.00	22.00	120.00	0.00	0.00	10.00	0.00
909	Yogurt, Rasp/Cream, Smooth & Crm	227.0000	8.000	Ounce	9.00	2.00	45.00	230.00	0.00	0.00	20.00	1.00
910	Yogurt, Raspberry w/Granola, Lig	227.0000	8.000	Ounce	8.00	0.00	25.00	140.00	0.00	0.00	5.00	0.00
911	Yogurt, Raspberry, Fruit on Bott	227.0000	8.000	Ounce	9.00	3.00	45.00	240.00	0.00	1.00	15.00	1.50
912	Yogurt, Raspberry, Light-Dannon	227.0000	8.000	Ounce	8.00	0.00	17.00	100.00	0.00	0.00	5.00	0.00
913	Yogurt, Raspberry, Non Fat, Blen	125.0000	4.400	Ounce	5.00	0.00	24.00	110.00	0.00	0.00	5.00	0.00
914	Yogurt, Raspberry, Red, Lowfat-B	227.0000	8.000	Ounce	9.00	2.50	43.00	230.00	0.00	0.00	15.00	1.50
915	Yogurt, Raspberry, Wild, Danimal	125.0000	4.400	Ounce	6.00	1.00	22.00	120.00	0.00	0.00	5.00	0.50
916	Yogurt, Smooth & Crmy, Black Che	227.0000	8.000	Ounce	9.00	2.00	46.00	240.00	0.00	0.00	20.00	1.00
917	Yogurt, Straw Ban Spl, Smooth &	227.0000	8.000	Ounce	8.00	2.00	48.00	240.00	0.00	0.00	20.00	1.00

Monounsaturated Fat (gm)	Polyunsaturated Fat (gm)	Vitamin D (mg)	Vitamin K (mg)	Vitamin E (mg)	Vitamin A (re)	Vitamin C (mg)	Thiamin (mg)	Riboflavin (mg)	Niacin (mg)	Vitamin B6 (mg)	Folate (mcg)	Vitamin B12 (mcg)	Calcium (mg)	Iron (mg)	Magnesium (mg)	Phosphorus (mg)	Potassium (mg)	Sodium (mg)	Zinc (mg)
0.00	0.00	0.00	0.00	0.00	0.00	0.00	0.00	0.00	0.00	0.00	0.00	0.00	0.00	0.00	0.00	0.00	480.00	140.00	0.00
0.00	0.00	0.00	0.00	0.00	0.00	0.00	0.00	0.00	0.00	0.00	0.00	0.00	0.00	0.00	0.00	0.00	250.00	75.00	0.00
0.00	0.00	0.00	0.00	0.00	0.00	0.00	0.00	0.00	0.00	0.00	0.00	0.00	0.00	0.00	0.00	0.00	350.00	150.00	0.00
0.00	0.00	0.00	0.00	0.00	0.00	0.00	0.00	0.00	0.00	0.00	0.00	0.00	0.00	0.00	0.00	0.00	350.00	150.00	0.00
0.00	0.00	0.00	0.00	0.00	0.00	0.00	0.00	0.00	0.00	0.00	0.00	0.00	0.00	0.00	0.00	0.00	230.00	80.00	0.00
0.00	0.00	0.00	0.00	0.00	0.00	0.00	0.00	0.00	0.00	0.00	0.00	0.00	0.00	0.00	0.00	0.00	360.00	135.00	0.00
0.00	0.00	0.00	0.00	0.00	0.00	0.00	0.00	0.00	0.00	0.00	0.00	0.00	0.00	0.00	0.00	0.00	350.00	150.00	0.00
0.00	0.00	0.00	0.00	0.00	0.00	0.00	0.00	0.00	0.00	0.00	0.00	0.00	0.00	0.00	0.00	0.00	350.00	130.00	0.00
0.00	0.00	0.00	0.00	0.00	0.00	0.00	0.00	0.00	0.00	0.00	0.00	0.00	0.00	0.00	0.00	0.00	510.00	160.00	0.00
0.00	0.00	0.00	0.00	0.00	0.00	0.00	0.00	0.00	0.00	0.00	0.00	0.00	0.00	0.00	0.00	0.00	350.00	150.00	0.00
0.00	0.00	0.00	0.00	0.00	0.00	0.00	0.00	0.00	0.00	0.00	0.00	0.00	0.00	0.00	0.00	0.00	510.00	160.00	0.00
0.00	0.00	0.00	0.00	0.00	0.00	0.00	0.00	0.00	0.00	0.00	0.00	0.00	0.00	0.00	0.00	0.00	370.00	135.00	0.00
0.00	0.00	0.00	0.00	0.00	0.00	0.00	0.00	0.00	0.00	0.00	0.00	0.00	437.57	0.00	0.00	0.00	422.99	153.15	0.00
0.00	0.00	0.00	0.00	0.00	0.00	15.00	0.00	0.00	0.00	0.00	0.00	0.00	419.93	0.20	0.00	0.00	509.91	159.97	0.00
0.74	0.07	0.00	0.00	0.07	26.95	1.62	0.10	0.44	0.25	0.10	22.79	1.15	372.16	0.17	35.70	292.53	476.53	143.08	1.81
0.89	0.09	0.00	0.00	0.00	34.05	1.68	0.09	0.45	0.25	0.11	23.61	1.18	383.40	0.16	36.77	301.23	491.00	147.32	1.86
0.78	0.07	0.00	0.00	0.07	29.40	1.47	0.07	0.39	0.22	0.10	20.83	1.05	338.84	0.15	32.51	266.32	433.90	130.34	1.64
0.00	0.00	0.00	0.00	0.00	0.00	0.00	0.00	0.00	0.00	0.00	0.00	0.00	0.00	0.00	0.00	0.00	300.00	100.00	0.00
0.00	0.00	0.00	0.00	0.00	0.00	0.00	0.00	0.00	0.00	0.00	0.00	0.00	0.00	0.00	0.00	0.00	300.00	170.00	0.00
0.00	0.00	0.00	0.00	0.00	0.00	0.00	0.00	0.00	0.00	0.00	0.00	0.00	0.00	0.00	0.00	0.00	360.00	140.00	0.00
0.00	0.00	0.00	0.00	0.00	0.00	0.00	0.00	0.00	0.00	0.00	0.00	0.00	0.00	0.00	0.00	0.00	310.00	100.00	0.00
0.00	0.00	0.00	0.00	0.00	0.00	0.00	0.00	0.00	0.00	0.00	0.00	0.00	0.00	0.00	0.00	0.00	360.00	130.00	0.00
0.00	0.00	0.00	0.00	0.00	0.00	0.00	0.00	0.00	0.00	0.00	0.00	0.00	0.00	0.00	0.00	0.00	270.00	100.00	0.00
0.00	0.00	0.00	0.00	0.00	0.00	0.00	0.00	0.00	0.00	0.00	0.00	0.00	0.00	0.00	0.00	0.00	510.00	160.00	0.00
0.00	0.00	0.00	0.00	0.00	0.00	0.00	0.00	0.00	0.00	0.00	0.00	0.00	0.00	0.00	0.00	0.00	380.00	140.00	0.00
0.00	0.00	0.00	0.00	0.00	0.00	12.00	0.00	0.00	0.00	0.00	0.00	0.00	280.00	0.00	0.00	0.00	0.00	130.00	0.00
0.00	0.00	0.00	0.00	0.00	0.00	2.40	0.00	0.00	0.00	0.00	0.00	0.00	280.00	0.40	0.00	0.00	0.00	125.00	0.00
0.00	0.00	0.00	0.00	0.00	0.00	0.00	0.00	0.00	0.00	0.00	0.00	0.00	0.00	0.00	0.00	0.00	380.00	125.00	0.00
0.00	0.00	0.00	0.00	0.00	0.00	0.00	0.00	0.00	0.00	0.00	0.00	0.00	0.00	0.00	0.00	0.00	470.00	135.00	0.00
0.00	0.00	0.00	0.00	0.00	0.00	0.00	0.00	0.00	0.00	0.00	0.00	0.00	0.00	0.00	0.00	0.00	180.00	65.00	0.00
0.00	0.00	0.00	0.00	0.00	0.00	0.00	0.00	0.00	0.00	0.00	0.00	0.00	0.00	0.00	0.00	0.00	450.00	140.00	0.00
0.00	0.00	0.00	0.00	0.00	0.00	0.00	0.00	0.00	0.00	0.00	0.00	0.00	0.00	0.00	0.00	0.00	370.00	130.00	0.00
0.00	0.00	0.00	0.00	0.00	0.00	0.00	0.00	0.00	0.00	0.00	0.00	0.00	0.00	0.00	0.00	0.00	440.00	125.00	0.00
0.00	0.00	0.00	0.00	0.00	0.00	0.00	0.00	0.00	0.00	0.00	0.00	0.00	0.00	0.00	0.00	0.00	240.00	75.00	0.00
0.00	0.00	0.00	0.00	0.00	0.00	0.00	0.00	0.00	0.00	0.00	0.00	0.00	0.00	0.00	0.00	0.00	330.00	100.00	0.00
0.00	0.00	0.00	0.00	0.00	0.00	0.00	0.00	0.00	0.00	0.00	0.00	0.00	0.00	0.00	0.00	0.00	340.00	115.00	0.00
0.00	0.00	0.00	0.00	0.00	0.00	0.00	0.00	0.00	0.00	0.00	0.00	0.00	0.00	0.00	0.00	0.00	390.00	125.00	0.00
0.00	0.00	0.00	0.00	0.00	0.00	0.00	0.00	0.00	0.00	0.00	0.00	0.00	0.00	0.00	0.00	0.00	330.00	110.00	0.00
0.00	0.00	0.00	0.00	0.00	0.00	0.00	0.00	0.00	0.00	0.00	0.00	0.00	0.00	0.00	0.00	0.00	430.00	125.00	0.00
0.00	0.00	0.00	0.00	0.00	0.00	0.00	0.00	0.00	0.00	0.00	0.00	0.00	0.00	0.00	0.00	0.00	590.00	170.00	0.00
0.00	0.00	0.00	0.00	0.00	0.00	0.00	0.00	0.00	0.00	0.00	0.00	0.00	0.00	0.00	0.00	0.00	550.00	150.00	0.00
0.00	0.00	0.00	0.00	0.00	0.00	3.60	0.00	0.25	0.00	0.00	0.00	0.00	479.92	0.00	0.00	0.21	599.90	169.97	0.00
1.05	0.10	0.00	0.00	0.10	39.20	1.96	0.10	0.51	0.27	0.12	27.44	1.37	447.37	0.20	42.75	351.58	572.81	171.99	2.18
0.12	0.02	0.00	0.00	0.02	4.90	2.13	0.12	0.56	0.29	0.12	29.89	1.49	487.80	0.22	46.80	383.43	624.51	187.43	2.38
2.18	0.22	0.00	0.00	0.22	73.50	1.30	0.07	0.34	0.20	0.07	18.13	0.91	295.72	0.12	28.37	232.51	378.77	113.68	1.45
0.00	0.00	0.00	0.00	0.00	0.00	0.00	0.00	0.00	0.00	0.00	0.00	0.00	0.00	0.00	0.00	0.00	330.00	105.00	0.00
0.00	0.00	0.00	0.00	0.00	0.00	0.00	0.00	0.00	0.00	0.00	0.00	0.00	0.00	0.00	0.00	0.00	400.00	135.00	0.00
0.00	0.00	0.00	0.00	0.00	0.00	0.00	0.00	0.00	0.00	0.00	0.00	0.00	0.00	0.00	0.00	0.00	380.00	150.00	0.00
0.00	0.00	0.00	0.00	0.00	0.00	0.00	0.00	0.00	0.00	0.00	0.00	0.00	0.00	0.00	0.00	0.00	460.00	150.00	0.00
0.00	0.00	0.00	0.00	0.00	0.00	0.00	0.00	0.00	0.00	0.00	0.00	0.00	0.00	0.00	0.00	0.00	370.00	150.00	0.00
0.00	0.00	0.00	0.00	0.00	0.00	0.00	0.00	0.00	0.00	0.00	0.00	0.00	0.00	0.00	0.00	0.00	250.00	75.00	0.00
0.00	0.00	0.00	0.00	0.00	0.00	0.00	0.00	0.00	0.00	0.00	0.00	0.00	0.00	0.00	0.00	0.00	450.00	125.00	0.00
0.00	0.00	0.00	0.00	0.00	0.00	0.00	0.00	0.00	0.00	0.00	0.00	0.00	0.00	0.00	0.00	0.00	270.00	90.00	0.00
0.00	0.00	0.00	0.00	0.00	0.00	0.00	0.00	0.00	0.00	0.00	0.00	0.00	0.00	0.00	0.00	0.00	390.00	130.00	0.00
0.00	0.00	0.00	0.00	0.00	0.00	0.00	0.00	0.00	0.00	0.00	0.00	0.00	0.00	0.00	0.00	0.00	390.00	125.00	0.00

USDA ID Code	Food Name	Weight in Grams*	Quantity of Units	Unit of Measure	Protein (gm)	Fat (gm)	Carbohydrate (gm)	Kcalories	Caffeine (gm)	Fiber (gm)	Cholesterol (mg)	Saturated Fat (gm)
918	Yogurt, Straw Cheesck, Light Non	227.0000	8.000	Ounce	8.00	0.00	22.00	120.00	0.00	0.00	10.00	0.00
919	Yogurt, Straw Chscke, Smooth & C	227.0000	8.000	Ounce	9.00	2.00	46.00	240.00	0.00	0.00	20.00	1.00
920	Yogurt, Straw Sundae, Light Duet	170.0000	6.000	Ounce	5.00	0.00	17.00	90.00	0.00	0.00	0.00	0.00
924	Yogurt, Straw/Ban, Sprinklin' Ra	116.0000	4.000	Ounce	5.00	1.50	24.00	130.00	0.00	0.00	5.00	0.50
921	Yogurt, Straw-Ban, Fruit on Bot	227.0000	8.000	Ounce	9.00	3.00	43.00	240.00	0.00	1.00	15.00	1.50
922	Yogurt, Straw-Ban, Non Fat, Blen	125.0000	4.400	Ounce	5.00	0.00	23.00	110.00	0.00	0.00	5.00	0.00
923	Yogurt, Straw-Ban, Non Fat, Chun	170.0000	6.000	Ounce	7.00	0.00	32.00	160.00	0.00	0.00	5.00	0.00
925	Yogurt, Strawberry Banana, Light	227.0000	8.000	Ounce	8.00	0.00	17.00	100.00	0.00	0.00	5.00	0.00
926	Yogurt, Strawberry Banana, Lowfa	227.0000	8.000	Ounce	9.00	2.50	44.00	240.00	0.00	0.00	15.00	1.50
927	Yogurt, Strawberry, Blended-Brey	125.0000	4.400	Ounce	4.00	1.00	26.00	130.00	0.00	0.00	10.00	0.50
928	Yogurt, Strawberry, Danimals-Dan	125.0000	4.400	Ounce	6.00	1.00	24.00	130.00	0.00	0.00	5.00	0.50
929	Yogurt, Strawberry, Fruit on Bot	227.0000	8.000	Ounce	9.00	3.00	45.00	240.00	0.00	1.00	15.00	1.50
931	Yogurt, Strawberry, Light-Dannon	227.0000	8.000	Ounce	8.00	0.00	17.00	100.00	0.00	0.00	5.00	0.00
932	Yogurt, Strawberry, Lowfat-Breye	227.0000	8.000	Ounce	9.00	2.50	43.00	230.00	0.00	0.00	15.00	1.50
933	Yogurt, Strawberry, Non Fat, Ble	125.0000	4.400	Ounce	5.00	0.00	23.00	110.00	0.00	0.00	5.00	0.00
934	Yogurt, Strawberry, Non Fat, Chu	170.0000	6.000	Ounce	7.00	0.00	32.00	160.00	0.00	0.00	5.00	0.00
937	Yogurt, Strawberry, Non Fat-Brey	227.0000	8.000	Ounce	8.00	0.00	22.00	120.00	0.00	0.00	10.00	0.00
935	Yogurt, Strawberry, Smooth & Crm	227.0000	8.000	Ounce	9.00	2.00	45.00	230.00	0.00	0.00	20.00	1.00
936	Yogurt, Strawberry, Sprinklin' R	116.0000	4.000	Ounce	5.00	1.50	24.00	130.00	0.00	0.00	5.00	0.50
938	Yogurt, Tangerine Chiffon, Light	227.0000	8.000	Ounce	8.00	0.00	16.00	100.00	0.00	0.00	5.00	0.00
939	Yogurt, Tropical Punch, Danimals	125.0000	4.400	Ounce	6.00	1.00	25.00	130.00	0.00	0.00	5.00	0.50
940	Yogurt, Van/Cherry, Magic Crysta	116.0000	4.000	Ounce	5.00	1.00	21.00	110.00	0.00	0.00	5.00	0.50
941	Yogurt, Van/Orange, Magic Crysta	116.0000	4.000	Ounce	5.00	1.00	21.00	110.00	0.00	0.00	5.00	0.50
942	Yogurt, Van/Peach/Apr, Double De	170.0000	6.000	Ounce	7.00	1.00	33.00	170.00	0.00	0.00	10.00	0.50
943	Yogurt, Vanilla, Danimals-Dannon	125.0000	4.000	Ounce	6.00	1.00	23.00	120.00	0.00	0.00	5.00	0.50
944	Yogurt, Vanilla, Light-Dannon	227.0000	8.000	Ounce	8.00	0.00	16.00	100.00	0.00	0.00	5.00	0.00
	Yogurt, Vanilla, Lowfat, 11 Gm P	245.0000	1.000	Cup	12.08	3.06	33.81	209.33	0.00	0.00	12.01	1.98
945	Yogurt, Vanilla, Lowfat-Breyer's	227.0000	8.000	Ounce	10.00	3.00	38.00	220.00	0.00	0.00	20.00	2.00
946	Yogurt, Vanilla, Lowfat-Dannon	227.0000	8.000	Ounce	10.00	3.00	36.00	210.00	0.00	0.00	15.00	2.00
947	Yogurt, Vanilla/Straw, Double De	170.0000	6.000	Ounce	7.00	1.00	33.00	170.00	0.00	0.00	10.00	0.50

Fats and Oils

USDA ID Code	Food Name	Weight in Grams*	Quantity of Units	Unit of Measure	Protein (gm)	Fat (gm)	Carbohydrate (gm)	Kcalories	Caffeine (gm)	Fiber (gm)	Cholesterol (mg)	Saturated Fat (gm)
	Butter, w/ Salt	5.0000	1.000	Pat	0.05	4.06	0.01	35.85	0.00	0.00	10.95	2.53
	Butter, w/o Salt	5.0000	1.000	Pat	0.04	4.06	0.00	35.85	0.00	0.00	10.95	2.52
	Butter, Whipped	3.8000	1.000	Pat	0.03	3.08	0.00	27.24	0.00	0.00	8.32	1.92
	Lard	12.8000	1.000	Tbsp	0.00	12.80	0.00	115.46	0.00	0.00	12.16	5.02
	Margarine, Hard, Corn & soybn	4.7000	1.000	Tbsp	0.04	3.78	0.04	33.78	0.00	0.00	0.00	0.71
	Margarine, Hard, Corn (hydr)	4.7000	1.000	Tbsp	0.04	3.78	0.04	33.78	0.00	0.00	0.00	0.62
	Margarine, Imitation (appx 40% F	4.8000	1.000	Tbsp	0.02	1.86	0.02	16.57	0.00	0.00	0.00	0.37
	Margarine, Regular, w/ Salt Adde	4.7000	1.000	Tbsp	0.04	3.78	0.04	33.78	0.00	0.00	0.00	0.74
	Margarine, Regular, w/o Added Sa	4.7000	1.000	Tbsp	0.02	3.77	0.02	33.56	0.00	0.00	0.00	0.71
	Margarine, Soft, w/ Salt Added	227.0000	1.000	Cup	1.82	182.51	1.14	1626.23	0.00	0.00	0.00	31.33
	Margarine, Soft, w/o Added Salt	4.7000	1.000	Tbsp	0.04	3.77	0.04	33.67	0.00	0.00	0.00	0.65
	Mayonnaise	14.7000	1.000	Tbsp	0.13	4.91	3.51	57.29	0.00	0.00	3.82	0.72
	Mayonnaise, Fat Free	15.0070	1.000	Tbsp	0.00	0.00	3.00	10.00	0.00	0.00	0.00	0.00
	Mayonnaise, Light	15.0070	1.000	Tbsp	0.00	2.00	1.00	25.01	0.00	0.00	5.00	0.00
	Oil, Olive	13.5000	1.000	Tbsp	0.00	13.50	0.00	119.34	0.00	0.00	0.00	1.82
	Oil, Peanut	13.5000	1.000	Tbsp	0.00	13.50	0.00	119.34	0.00	0.00	0.00	2.28
	Oil, Sesame	13.6000	1.000	Tbsp	0.00	13.60	0.00	120.22	0.00	0.00	0.00	1.93
	Oil, Soybean	13.6000	1.000	Tbsp	0.00	13.60	0.00	120.22	0.00	0.00	0.00	1.96
	Oil, Soybean, (hydr)	13.6000	1.000	Tbsp	0.00	13.60	0.00	120.22	0.00	0.00	0.00	2.03
	Oil, Soybean, (hydr) & cottonsee	13.6000	1.000	Tbsp	0.00	13.60	0.00	120.22	0.00	0.00	0.00	2.45
	Oil, Vegetable Corn	13.6000	1.000	Tbsp	0.00	13.60	0.00	120.22	0.00	0.00	0.00	1.73
	Oil, Vegetable, Canola	14.0000	1.000	Tbsp	0.00	14.00	0.00	123.76	0.00	0.00	0.00	0.99
	Oil, Vegetable, Cocoa Butter	13.6000	1.000	Tbsp	0.00	13.60	0.00	120.22	0.00	0.00	0.00	8.12
	Oil, Vegetable, Cottonseed	13.6000	1.000	Tbsp	0.00	13.60	0.00	120.22	0.00	0.00	0.00	3.52
	Oil, Vegetable, Palm	13.6000	1.000	Tbsp	0.00	13.60	0.00	120.22	0.00	0.00	0.00	6.70

Monounsaturated Fat (gm)	Polyunsaturated Fat (gm)	Vitamin D (mg)	Vitamin K (mg)	Vitamin E (mg)	Vitamin A (re)	Vitamin C (mg)	Thiamin (mg)	Riboflavin (mg)	Niacin (mg)	Vitamin B6 (mg)	Folate (mg)	Vitamin B12 (mcg)	Calcium (mg)	Iron (mg)	Magnesium (mg)	Phosphorus (mg)	Potassium (mg)	Sodium (mg)	Zinc (mg)
0.00	0.00	0.00	0.00	0.00	0.00	0.00	0.00	0.00	0.00	0.00	0.00	0.00	0.00	0.00	0.00	0.00	320.00	100.00	0.00
0.00	0.00	0.00	0.00	0.00	0.00	0.00	0.00	0.00	0.00	0.00	0.00	0.00	0.00	0.00	0.00	0.00	400.00	125.00	0.00
0.00	0.00	0.00	0.00	0.00	0.00	0.00	0.00	0.00	0.00	0.00	0.00	0.00	0.00	0.00	0.00	0.00	250.00	75.00	0.00
0.00	0.00	0.00	0.00	0.00	0.00	0.00	0.00	0.00	0.00	0.00	0.00	0.00	0.00	0.00	0.00	0.00	250.00	80.00	0.00
0.00	0.00	0.00	0.00	0.00	0.00	0.00	0.00	0.00	0.00	0.00	0.00	0.00	0.00	0.00	0.00	0.00	480.00	140.00	0.00
0.00	0.00	0.00	0.00	0.00	0.00	0.00	0.00	0.00	0.00	0.00	0.00	0.00	0.00	0.00	0.00	0.00	240.00	75.00	0.00
0.00	0.00	0.00	0.00	0.00	0.00	0.00	0.00	0.00	0.00	0.00	0.00	0.00	0.00	0.00	0.00	0.00	350.00	105.00	0.00
0.00	0.00	0.00	0.00	0.00	0.00	0.00	0.00	0.00	0.00	0.00	0.00	0.00	0.00	0.00	0.00	0.00	380.00	140.00	0.00
0.00	0.00	0.00	0.00	0.00	0.00	0.00	0.00	0.00	0.00	0.00	0.00	0.00	0.00	0.00	0.00	0.00	470.00	125.00	0.00
0.00	0.00	0.00	0.00	0.00	0.00	0.00	0.00	0.00	0.00	0.00	0.00	0.00	0.00	0.00	0.00	0.00	180.00	60.00	0.00
0.00	0.00	0.00	0.00	0.00	0.00	0.00	0.00	0.00	0.00	0.00	0.00	0.00	0.00	0.00	0.00	0.00	270.00	90.00	0.00
0.00	0.00	0.00	0.00	0.00	0.00	0.00	0.00	0.00	0.00	0.00	0.00	0.00	0.00	0.00	0.00	0.00	460.00	140.00	0.00
0.00	0.00	0.00	0.00	0.00	0.00	0.00	0.00	0.00	0.00	0.00	0.00	0.00	0.00	0.00	0.00	0.00	380.00	140.00	0.00
0.00	0.00	0.00	0.00	0.00	0.00	0.00	0.00	0.00	0.00	0.00	0.00	0.00	0.00	0.00	0.00	0.00	440.00	125.00	0.00
0.00	0.00	0.00	0.00	0.00	0.00	0.00	0.00	0.00	0.00	0.00	0.00	0.00	0.00	0.00	0.00	0.00	230.00	80.00	0.00
0.00	0.00	0.00	0.00	0.00	0.00	0.00	0.00	0.00	0.00	0.00	0.00	0.00	0.00	0.00	0.00	0.00	360.00	115.00	0.00
0.00	0.00	0.00	0.00	0.00	0.00	0.00	0.00	0.00	0.00	0.00	0.00	0.00	0.00	0.00	0.00	0.00	320.00	100.00	0.00
0.00	0.00	0.00	0.00	0.00	0.00	0.00	0.00	0.00	0.00	0.00	0.00	0.00	0.00	0.00	0.00	0.00	400.00	125.00	0.00
0.00	0.00	0.00	0.00	0.00	0.00	0.00	0.00	0.00	0.00	0.00	0.00	0.00	0.00	0.00	0.00	0.00	250.00	85.00	0.00
0.00	0.00	0.00	0.00	0.00	0.00	0.00	0.00	0.00	0.00	0.00	0.00	0.00	0.00	0.00	0.00	0.00	360.00	130.00	0.00
0.00	0.00	0.00	0.00	0.00	0.00	0.00	0.00	0.00	0.00	0.00	0.00	0.00	0.00	0.00	0.00	0.00	270.00	95.00	0.00
0.00	0.00	0.00	0.00	0.00	0.00	0.00	0.00	0.00	0.00	0.00	0.00	0.00	0.00	0.00	0.00	0.00	240.00	85.00	0.00
0.00	0.00	0.00	0.00	0.00	0.00	0.00	0.00	0.00	0.00	0.00	0.00	0.00	0.00	0.00	0.00	0.00	240.00	85.00	0.00
0.00	0.00	0.00	0.00	0.00	0.00	0.00	0.00	0.00	0.00	0.00	0.00	0.00	0.00	0.00	0.00	0.00	330.00	100.00	0.00
0.00	0.00	0.00	0.00	0.00	0.00	0.00	0.00	0.00	0.00	0.00	0.00	0.00	0.00	0.00	0.00	0.00	270.00	90.00	0.00
0.00	0.00	0.00	0.00	0.00	0.00	0.00	0.00	0.00	0.00	0.00	0.00	0.00	0.00	0.00	0.00	0.00	350.00	130.00	0.00
0.83	0.10	0.00	0.00	0.07	31.85	1.84	0.10	0.49	0.27	0.12	25.73	1.30	419.69	0.17	40.25	329.77	537.29	161.21	2.03
0.00	0.00	0.00	0.00	0.00	0.00	0.00	0.00	0.00	0.00	0.00	0.00	0.00	0.00	0.00	0.00	0.00	480.00	135.00	0.00
0.00	0.00	0.00	0.00	0.00	0.00	0.00	0.00	0.00	0.00	0.00	0.00	0.00	0.00	0.00	0.00	0.00	510.00	160.00	0.00
0.00	0.00	0.00	0.00	0.00	0.00	0.00	0.00	0.00	0.00	0.00	0.00	0.00	0.00	0.00	0.00	0.00	340.00	100.00	0.00
1.17	0.15	0.00	0.00	0.08	37.70	0.00	0.00	0.00	0.00	0.00	0.15	0.01	1.20	0.01	0.10	1.15	1.30	41.30	0.00
1.17	0.15	0.00	0.00	0.08	37.70	0.00	0.00	0.00	0.00	0.00	0.14	0.01	1.18	0.01	0.10	1.14	1.30	0.55	0.00
0.89	0.11	0.00	0.00	0.06	28.65	0.00	0.00	0.00	0.00	0.00	0.11	0.00	0.89	0.01	0.08	0.87	0.99	31.41	0.00
5.77	1.43	0.00	0.00	0.15	0.00	0.00	0.00	0.00	0.00	0.00	0.06	0.00	0.01	0.00	0.00	0.00	0.00	0.00	0.01
1.73	1.18	0.00	0.00	0.52	37.55	0.01	0.00	0.00	0.00	0.00	0.06	0.00	1.41	0.00	0.12	1.08	1.99	44.34	0.00
2.15	0.85	0.00	0.00	0.55	37.55	0.01	0.00	0.00	0.00	0.00	0.06	0.00	1.41	0.00	0.12	1.08	1.99	44.34	0.00
0.75	0.66	0.00	0.00	0.11	38.35	0.00	0.00	0.00	0.00	0.00	0.03	0.00	0.85	0.00	0.07	0.66	1.21	46.06	0.00
1.68	1.19	0.00	0.00	0.60	37.55	0.01	0.00	0.00	0.00	0.00	0.06	0.00	1.41	0.00	0.12	1.08	1.99	44.34	0.00
1.72	1.18	0.00	0.00	0.60	37.55	0.00	0.00	0.00	0.00	0.00	0.03	0.00	0.82	0.00	0.07	0.63	1.16	0.10	0.00
64.69	78.54	0.00	0.00	27.24	1813.73	0.32	0.02	0.07	0.05	0.02	2.38	0.18	60.16	0.00	5.24	46.08	85.58	2448.54	0.00
1.75	1.21	0.00	0.00	0.41	37.55	0.01	0.00	0.00	0.00	0.00	0.05	0.00	1.25	0.00	0.11	0.95	1.77	1.29	0.00
1.32	2.65	0.00	0.00	0.59	12.35	0.00	0.00	0.00	0.00	0.00	0.92	0.03	2.06	0.03	0.29	3.82	1.32	104.48	0.03
0.00	0.00	0.00	0.00	0.00	0.00	0.00	0.00	0.00	0.00	0.00	0.00	0.00	0.00	0.00	0.00	0.00	10.00	105.05	0.00
0.00	0.00	0.00	0.00	0.00	0.00	0.00	0.00	0.00	0.00	0.00	0.00	0.00	0.00	0.00	0.00	0.00	5.00	130.06	0.00
9.95	1.13	0.00	7.83	1.67	0.00	0.00	0.00	0.00	0.00	0.00	0.00	0.00	0.00	0.02	0.05	0.00	0.16	0.00	0.01
6.24	4.32	0.00	0.27	1.74	0.00	0.00	0.00	0.00	0.00	0.00	0.00	0.00	0.01	0.00	0.01	0.00	0.00	0.01	0.00
5.40	5.67	0.00	1.63	0.56	0.00	0.00	0.00	0.00	0.00	0.00	0.00	0.00	0.00	0.00	0.00	0.00	0.00	0.00	0.00
3.17	7.87	0.00	0.00	2.47	0.00	0.00	0.00	0.00	0.00	0.00	0.00	0.00	0.01	0.00	0.00	0.03	0.00	0.00	0.00
5.85	5.11	0.00	0.00	2.47	0.00	0.00	0.00	0.00	0.00	0.00	0.00	0.00	0.00	0.00	0.00	0.00	0.00	0.00	0.00
4.01	6.54	0.00	0.00	3.84	0.00	0.00	0.00	0.00	0.00	0.00	0.00	0.00	0.00	0.00	0.00	0.00	0.00	0.00	0.00
3.29	7.98	0.00	0.68	2.87	0.00	0.00	0.00	0.00	0.00	0.00	0.00	0.00	0.00	0.00	0.00	0.00	0.00	0.00	0.00
8.25	4.14	0.00	116.20	2.93	0.00	0.00	0.00	0.00	0.00	0.00	0.00	0.00	0.00	0.00	0.00	0.00	0.00	0.00	0.00
4.47	0.41	0.00	0.00	0.24	0.00	0.00	0.00	0.00	0.00	0.00	0.00	0.00	0.00	0.00	0.00	0.00	0.00	0.00	0.00
2.42	7.06	0.00	0.00	5.20	0.00	0.00	0.00	0.00	0.00	0.00	0.00	0.00	0.00	0.00	0.00	0.00	0.00	0.00	0.00
5.03	1.26	0.00	1.09	2.96	0.00	0.00	0.00	0.00	0.00	0.00	0.00	0.00	0.00	0.00	0.00	0.02	0.00	0.00	0.00

USDA ID Code	Food Name	Weight in Grams*	Quantity of Units	Unit of Measure	Protein (gm)	Fat (gm)	Carbohydrate (gm)	Kcalories	Caffeine (gm)	Fiber (gm)	Cholesterol (mg)	Saturated Fat (gm)
	Oil, Vegetable, Palm Kernel	13.6000	1.000	Tbsp	0.00	13.60	0.00	117.23	0.00	0.00	0.00	11.08
	Oil, Vegetable, Safflower, Linol	13.6000	1.000	Tbsp	0.00	13.60	0.00	120.22	0.00	0.00	0.00	0.84
	Oil, Vegetable, Safflower, Oleic	13.6000	1.000	Tbsp	0.00	13.60	0.00	120.22	0.00	0.00	0.00	0.84
	Oil, Vegetable, Sunflower	14.0000	1.000	Tbsp	0.00	14.00	0.00	123.76	0.00	0.00	0.00	1.37
	Salad Dressing, Blue Cheese	16.0140	2.000	Tbsp	0.50	3.50	2.50	45.04	0.00	0.00	5.00	2.00
	Salad Dressing, Blue Cheese, Fat	17.5080	2.000	Tbsp	0.25	0.00	6.00	25.01	0.00	0.00	0.00	0.00
	Salad Dressing, Ceasar	17.1200	2.000	Tbsp	0.17	17.12	1.31	155.00	0.00	0.00	1.11	3.22
	Salad Dressing, French	12.3000	1.000	Pkt	0.07	5.04	2.15	52.85	0.00	0.00	0.00	1.17
	Salad Dressing, French, Fat Free	17.5080	2.000	Tbsp	0.00	0.00	6.00	25.01	0.00	0.00	0.00	0.00
	Salad Dressing, French, Low Fat	16.3000	1.000	Tbsp	0.03	0.95	3.54	21.87	0.00	0.00	0.00	0.13
	Salad Dressing, Honey Mustard	31.2000	2.000	Tbsp	0.05	6.33	14.22	102.11	0.00	0.23	0.00	1.33
	Salad Dressing, Italian	14.7000	1.000	Tbsp	0.10	7.10	1.50	68.69	0.00	0.00	0.00	1.03
	Salad Dressing, Italian, Creamy	29.4000	2.000	Tbsp	0.03	16.12	2.33	147.43	0.00	0.00	1.22	2.43
	Salad Dressing, Italian, Fat Fre	15.5100	2.000	Tbsp	0.00	0.00	1.00	5.00	0.00	0.00	0.00	0.00
	Salad Dressing, Italian, Low Cal	15.0000	1.000	Tbsp	0.02	1.47	0.74	15.81	0.00	0.02	0.90	0.20
	Salad Dressing, Peppercorn	26.8000	2.000	Tbsp	0.02	16.22	1.10	151.22	0.00	0.00	13.11	3.11
	Salad Dressing, Poppy Seed	29.4000	2.000	Tbsp	0.02	12.31	6.41	130.44	0.00	0.00	0.00	2.33
	Salad Dressing, Ranch	14.5190	2.000	Tbsp	0.00	9.01	1.00	85.11	0.00	0.00	2.50	1.50
	Salad Dressing, Ranch, Fat Free	17.5080	2.000	Tbsp	0.00	0.00	5.50	25.01	0.00	0.00	0.00	0.00
	Salad Dressing, Raspberry Vinegr	14.7000	2.000	Tbsp	0.10	7.10	1.50	68.69	0.00	0.00	0.00	1.03
	Salad Dressing, Russian	15.3000	1.000	Tbsp	0.24	7.77	1.59	75.58	0.00	0.00	2.75	1.12
	Salad Dressing, Russian, Low Cal	16.3000	1.000	Tbsp	0.08	0.65	4.50	23.05	0.00	0.05	0.98	0.10
	Salad Dressing, Sesame Seed	15.3000	1.000	Tbsp	0.47	6.92	1.32	67.79	0.00	0.15	0.00	0.95
	Salad Dressing, Thousand Island	15.6000	1.000	Tbsp	0.14	5.57	2.37	58.86	0.00	0.00	4.06	0.94
	Salad Dressing, Thousand Island,	17.5080	2.000	Tbsp	0.00	0.00	5.50	22.51	0.00	0.00	0.00	0.00
	Salad Dressing, Thousand Island,	15.3000	1.000	Tbsp	0.12	1.64	2.48	24.27	0.00	0.18	2.30	0.24
	Salad Dressing, Vinegar and Oil	15.6000	1.000	Tbsp	0.00	7.82	0.39	70.01	0.00	0.00	0.00	1.42

Fruits and Vegetables

USDA ID Code	Food Name	Weight in Grams*	Quantity of Units	Unit of Measure	Protein (gm)	Fat (gm)	Carbohydrate (gm)	Kcalories	Caffeine (gm)	Fiber (gm)	Cholesterol (mg)	Saturated Fat (gm)
	Apples, Cnd, Sweetened	204.0000	1.000	Cup	0.37	1.00	34.07	136.68	0.00	3.47	0.00	0.16
	Apples, Dehydrated, Sulfured	60.0000	0.250	Cup	0.79	0.35	56.12	207.60	0.00	7.44	0.00	0.06
	Apples, Fresh, w/ Skin	125.0000	1.000	Cup	0.24	0.45	19.06	73.75	0.00	3.38	0.00	0.08
	Apples, Fresh, w/o Skin	110.0000	1.000	Cup	0.17	0.34	16.32	62.70	0.00	2.09	0.00	0.06
	Applesauce, Sweetened	255.0000	1.000	Cup	0.46	0.46	50.77	193.80	0.00	3.06	0.00	0.08
	Applesauce, Unsweetened	244.0000	1.000	Cup	0.41	0.12	27.55	104.92	0.00	2.93	0.00	0.02
	Apricots, Cnd, Heavy Syrup Pack	258.0000	1.000	Cup	1.32	0.23	55.34	214.14	0.00	4.13	0.00	0.03
	Apricots, Cnd, Juice Pack	244.0000	1.000	Cup	1.54	0.10	30.11	117.12	0.00	3.90	0.00	0.00
	Apricots, Cnd, Light Syrup Pack	253.0000	1.000	Cup	1.34	0.13	41.72	159.39	0.00	4.05	0.00	0.00
	Apricots, Cnd, Water Pack	243.0000	1.000	Cup	1.73	0.39	15.53	65.61	0.00	3.89	0.00	0.02
	Apricots, Dehydrated, Sulfured	119.0000	0.500	Cup	5.83	0.74	98.64	380.80	0.00	0.00	0.00	0.05
	Apricots, Dried, Sulfured	130.0000	1.000	Cup	4.75	0.60	80.28	309.40	0.00	11.70	0.00	0.04
	Apricots, Fresh	155.0000	1.000	Cup	2.17	0.60	17.24	74.40	0.00	3.72	0.00	0.05
	Apricots, Frozen, Sweetened	242.0000	1.000	Cup	1.69	0.24	60.74	237.16	0.00	5.32	0.00	0.02
	Artichoke, Boiled, Hearts w/ Sal	84.0000	0.500	Cup	2.92	0.13	9.39	42.00	0.00	4.54	0.00	0.03
	Artichoke, Boiled, Hearts w/o Sa	84.0000	0.500	Cup	2.92	0.13	9.39	42.00	0.00	4.54	0.00	0.03
	Asparagus, Ckd	90.0000	0.500	Cup	2.33	0.28	3.81	21.60	0.00	1.89	0.00	0.06
	Asparagus, Cnd	242.0000	1.000	Cup	5.18	1.57	6.00	45.98	0.00	3.87	0.00	0.36
	Asparagus, Fresh	134.0000	1.000	Cup	3.06	0.27	6.08	30.82	0.00	2.81	0.00	0.07
	Asparagus, Frz, Ckd	180.0000	1.000	Cup	5.31	0.76	8.77	50.40	0.00	2.88	0.00	0.18
	Avocados, Fresh	150.0000	1.000	Cup	2.97	22.98	11.09	241.50	0.00	7.50	0.00	3.66
	Bamboo Shoots, Cnd	131.0000	1.000	Cup	2.25	0.52	4.22	24.89	0.00	1.83	0.00	0.12
	Bamboo Shoots, Fresh	151.0000	1.000	Cup	3.93	0.45	7.85	40.77	0.00	3.32	0.00	0.11
	Banana, Dehydrated, Chips	100.0000	1.000	Cup	3.89	1.81	88.28	346.00	0.00	7.50	0.00	0.70
	Bananas, Fresh	225.0000	1.000	Cup	2.32	1.08	52.72	207.00	0.00	5.40	0.00	0.43
	Bean Sprouts	133.3330	0.500	Cup	17.47	9.47	12.53	166.67	0.00	0.00	0.00	0.00
	Beans, Green, Cnd	135.0000	1.000	Cup	1.55	0.14	6.08	27.00	0.00	2.57	0.00	0.03
	Beans, Green, Fresh	110.0000	1.000	Cup	2.00	0.13	7.85	34.10	0.00	3.74	0.00	0.03
	Beans, Green, Fzn	135.0000	1.000	Cup	2.01	0.23	8.71	37.80	0.00	4.05	0.00	0.05
	Beans, Lima, Fzn	311.0000	1.250	Cup	20.68	0.93	60.49	326.55	0.00	18.66	0.00	0.22

Monounsaturated Fat (gm)	Polyunsaturated Fat (gm)	Vitamin D (mg)	Vitamin K (mg)	Vitamin E (mg)	Vitamin A (re)	Vitamin C (mg)	Thiamin (mg)	Riboflavin (mg)	Niacin (mg)	Vitamin B₆ (mg)	Folate (mg)	Vitamin B₁₂ (mcg)	Calcium (mg)	Iron (mg)	Magnesium (mg)	Phosphorus (mg)	Potassium (mg)	Sodium (mg)	Zinc (mg)
1.55	0.22	0.00	0.00	0.52	0.00	0.00	0.00	0.00	0.00	0.00	0.00	0.00	0.00	0.00	0.00	0.00	0.00	0.00	0.00
1.95	10.15	0.00	0.95	5.86	0.00	0.00	0.00	0.00	0.00	0.00	0.00	0.00	0.00	0.00	0.00	0.00	0.00	0.00	0.00
10.15	1.95	0.00	0.00	4.68	0.00	0.00	0.00	0.00	0.00	0.00	0.00	0.00	0.00	0.00	0.00	0.00	0.00	0.00	0.00
11.70	0.53	0.00	0.00	0.00	0.00	0.00	0.00	0.00	0.00	0.00	0.00	0.00	0.00	0.00	0.00	0.00	0.00	0.00	0.00
0.00	0.00	0.00	0.00	0.00	0.00	0.00	0.00	0.00	0.00	0.00	0.00	0.00	12.01	0.00	0.00	0.00	0.00	235.20	0.00
0.00	0.00	0.00	0.00	0.20	0.00	0.00	0.00	0.00	0.00	0.00	0.00	0.00	0.00	0.00	0.00	0.00	0.00	170.08	0.00
2.22	5.89	0.00	0.00	0.77	0.44	0.00	0.00	0.00	0.00	0.00	0.00	0.00	12.01	0.00	0.00	0.00	0.00	317.33	0.00
0.98	2.67	0.00	0.00	1.04	15.99	0.00	0.00	0.00	0.00	0.00	0.52	0.02	1.35	0.05	0.00	1.72	9.72	168.51	0.01
0.00	0.00	0.00	0.00	0.00	50.02	0.00	0.00	0.00	0.00	0.00	0.00	0.00	0.00	0.00	0.00	0.00	0.00	150.07	0.00
0.23	0.55	0.00	0.00	0.19	21.19	0.00	0.00	0.00	0.00	0.00	0.00	0.00	1.79	0.07	0.00	2.28	12.88	128.28	0.03
1.64	3.22	0.00	0.00	0.98	0.00	0.30	0.00	0.00	0.00	0.00	0.00	0.00	10.11	0.11	0.00	0.00	0.00	74.33	0.00
1.65	4.12	0.00	0.00	1.52	3.53	0.00	0.00	0.00	0.00	0.00	0.72	0.02	1.47	0.03	0.09	0.74	2.21	115.69	0.02
1.77	4.13	0.00	0.00	0.43	9.77	0.00	0.00	0.00	0.00	0.00	0.74	0.05	0.00	0.00	0.00	0.00	0.00	2.33	0.00
0.00	0.00	0.00	0.00	0.00	0.00	0.00	0.00	0.00	0.00	0.00	0.00	0.00	0.00	0.00	0.00	0.00	0.00	145.10	0.00
0.30	0.90	0.00	0.00	0.23	0.00	0.00	0.00	0.00	0.00	0.00	0.00	0.00	0.30	0.03	0.00	0.75	2.25	118.05	0.02
1.77	4.11	0.00	0.00	0.00	0.00	0.30	0.00	0.00	0.00	0.00	0.00	0.00	0.22	0.02	0.00	0.00	0.00	285.32	0.00
1.33	2.88	0.00	0.00	0.00	0.00	0.30	0.00	0.00	0.00	0.00	0.00	0.00	0.22	0.02	0.00	0.00	0.00	127.11	0.00
0.00	0.00	0.00	0.00	0.00	0.00	0.00	0.00	0.00	0.00	0.00	0.00	0.00	0.00	0.00	0.00	0.00	0.00	135.18	0.00
0.00	0.00	0.00	0.00	0.30	0.00	0.00	0.00	0.00	0.00	0.00	0.00	0.00	0.00	0.00	0.00	0.00	0.00	155.07	0.00
1.65	4.12	0.00	0.00	1.52	3.53	0.00	0.00	0.00	0.00	0.00	0.72	0.02	1.47	0.03	0.09	0.74	2.21	115.69	0.02
1.81	4.50	0.00	0.00	1.56	31.67	0.92	0.01	0.01	0.09	0.00	1.59	0.05	2.91	0.09	0.23	5.66	24.02	132.80	0.07
0.15	0.37	0.00	0.00	0.12	2.61	0.98	0.00	0.00	0.00	0.00	0.57	0.00	3.10	0.10	0.07	6.03	25.59	141.48	0.02
1.82	3.84	0.00	0.00	0.77	31.67	0.00	0.00	0.00	0.00	0.00	0.00	0.00	2.91	0.09	0.00	5.66	24.02	153.00	0.02
1.29	3.09	0.00	0.00	0.18	14.98	0.00	0.00	0.00	0.00	0.00	0.98	0.03	1.72	0.09	0.31	2.65	17.63	109.20	0.02
0.00	0.00	0.00	0.00	0.00	0.00	0.00	0.00	0.00	0.00	0.00	0.00	0.00	0.00	0.00	0.00	0.00	0.00	150.07	0.00
0.37	0.95	0.00	0.00	0.18	14.69	0.00	0.00	0.00	0.00	0.00	0.85	0.03	1.68	0.09	0.11	2.60	17.29	153.00	0.02
2.31	3.76	0.00	0.00	1.37	0.00	0.00	0.00	0.00	0.00	0.00	0.00	0.00	0.00	0.00	0.00	0.00	1.17	0.08	0.00
0.04	0.29	0.00	0.00	0.02	10.20	0.82	0.02	0.02	0.14	0.08	0.61	0.00	8.16	0.47	4.08	10.20	138.72	6.12	0.06
0.01	0.10	0.00	0.00	2.15	4.80	1.32	0.03	0.08	0.41	0.17	0.60	0.00	11.40	1.20	13.20	33.00	384.00	74.40	0.17
0.03	0.14	0.00	5.00	0.40	6.25	7.13	0.03	0.01	0.10	0.06	3.50	0.00	8.75	0.23	6.25	8.75	143.75	0.00	0.05
0.01	0.10	0.00	0.51	0.09	4.40	4.40	0.02	0.01	0.10	0.06	0.44	0.00	4.40	0.08	3.30	7.70	124.30	0.00	0.04
0.03	0.13	0.00	0.00	0.03	2.55	4.34	0.03	0.08	0.48	0.08	1.53	0.00	10.20	0.89	7.65	17.85	155.55	7.65	0.10
0.00	0.02	0.00	0.00	0.02	7.32	2.93	0.02	0.07	0.46	0.07	1.46	0.00	7.32	0.29	7.32	17.08	183.00	4.88	0.07
0.10	0.05	0.00	0.00	0.00	319.92	7.22	0.05	0.05	1.08	0.13	4.39	0.00	23.22	1.11	20.64	33.54	345.72	28.38	0.26
0.05	0.02	0.00	0.00	2.17	412.36	11.96	0.05	0.05	0.83	0.12	4.15	0.00	29.28	0.73	24.40	48.80	402.60	9.76	0.27
0.05	0.03	0.00	0.00	2.25	333.96	6.83	0.05	0.05	0.76	0.13	4.30	0.00	27.83	0.99	20.24	32.89	349.14	10.12	0.28
0.17	0.07	0.00	0.00	2.16	313.47	8.26	0.05	0.05	0.97	0.12	4.13	0.00	19.44	0.78	17.01	31.59	466.56	7.29	0.27
0.32	0.14	0.00	0.00	0.00	1507.73	11.31	0.05	0.18	4.26	0.62	5.24	0.00	72.59	7.51	74.97	186.83	2201.50	15.47	1.19
0.26	0.12	0.00	0.00	1.95	941.20	3.12	0.01	0.20	3.90	0.21	13.39	0.00	58.50	6.11	61.10	152.10	1791.40	13.00	0.96
0.26	0.12	0.00	0.00	1.38	404.55	15.50	0.05	0.06	0.93	0.08	13.33	0.00	21.70	0.84	12.40	29.45	458.80	1.55	0.40
0.10	0.05	0.00	0.00	2.15	406.56	21.78	0.05	0.10	1.94	0.15	4.11	0.00	24.20	2.18	21.78	45.98	554.18	9.68	0.24
0.00	0.06	0.00	0.00	0.16	15.12	8.40	0.06	0.06	0.84	0.09	42.84	0.00	37.80	1.08	50.40	72.24	297.36	278.04	0.41
0.00	0.06	0.00	0.00	0.16	15.12	8.40	0.06	0.06	0.84	0.09	42.84	0.00	37.80	1.08	50.40	72.24	297.36	79.80	0.41
0.01	0.13	0.00	0.00	0.00	48.60	9.72	0.11	0.12	0.97	0.11	131.40	0.00	18.00	0.66	9.00	48.60	144.00	216.00	0.38
0.05	0.68	0.00	0.00	1.04	128.26	44.53	0.15	0.24	2.30	0.27	231.35	0.00	38.72	4.43	24.20	104.06	416.24	694.54	0.97
0.01	0.12	0.00	52.26	2.68	77.72	17.69	0.19	0.17	1.57	0.17	171.52	0.00	28.14	1.17	24.12	75.04	365.82	2.68	0.62
0.02	0.32	0.00	0.00	2.25	147.60	43.92	0.13	0.18	1.87	0.04	242.46	0.00	41.40	1.15	23.00	99.00	392.40	7.20	1.01
14.42	2.94	0.00	0.00	2.01	91.50	11.85	0.17	0.18	2.88	0.42	92.85	0.00	16.50	1.53	58.50	61.50	898.50	15.00	0.63
0.01	0.24	0.00	0.00	0.50	1.31	1.44	0.04	0.04	0.18	0.18	4.19	0.00	10.48	0.42	5.24	32.75	104.80	9.17	0.85
0.02	0.20	0.00	0.00	1.51	3.02	6.04	0.23	0.11	0.91	0.36	10.72	0.00	19.63	0.76	4.53	89.09	804.83	6.04	1.66
0.15	0.34	0.00	0.00	0.00	31.00	7.00	0.18	0.24	2.80	0.44	14.00	0.00	22.00	1.15	108.00	74.00	1491.00	3.00	0.61
0.09	0.20	0.00	1.13	0.61	18.00	20.48	0.11	0.23	1.22	1.31	42.98	0.00	13.50	0.70	65.25	45.00	891.00	2.25	0.36
0.00	0.00	0.00	0.00	0.00	2.67	16.00	0.56	0.25	1.47	0.22	169.87	0.00	109.33	0.53	128.00	288.00	756.00	333.33	2.80
0.00	0.07	0.00	0.00	0.19	47.25	6.48	0.03	0.08	0.27	0.05	42.93	0.00	35.10	1.22	17.55	25.65	147.15	353.70	0.39
0.01	0.07	0.00	30.80	0.45	73.70	17.93	0.09	0.12	0.83	0.08	40.15	0.00	40.70	1.14	27.50	41.80	229.90	6.60	0.26
0.01	0.11	0.00	0.00	0.19	54.00	5.54	0.05	0.12	0.51	0.08	31.05	0.00	66.15	1.19	32.40	41.85	170.10	12.15	0.65
0.06	0.47	0.00	0.00	1.99	52.87	18.04	0.22	0.19	2.39	0.37	48.21	0.00	87.08	6.10	174.16	348.32	1278.21	90.19	1.71

USDA ID Code	Food Name	Weight in Grams*	Quantity of Units	Unit of Measure	Protein (gm)	Fat (gm)	Carbohydrate (gm)	Kcalories	Caffeine (gm)	Fiber (gm)	Cholesterol (mg)	Saturated Fat (gm)
	Beans, Yellow, Cnd	135.0000	1.000	Cup	1.55	0.14	6.08	27.00	0.00	1.76	0.00	0.03
	Beans, Yellow, Fresh	110.0000	1.000	Cup	2.00	0.13	7.85	34.10	0.00	3.74	0.00	0.03
	Beets, Ckd	85.0000	0.500	Cup	1.43	0.15	8.47	37.40	0.00	1.70	0.00	0.03
	Blueberries, Cnd, Heavy Syrup	256.0000	1.000	Cup	1.66	0.84	56.47	225.28	0.00	3.84	0.00	0.08
	Blueberries, Fresh	145.0000	1.000	Cup	0.97	0.55	20.49	81.20	0.00	3.92	0.00	0.04
	Blueberries, Frozen, Sweetened	230.0000	1.000	Cup	0.92	0.30	50.49	186.30	0.00	4.83	0.00	0.02
	Blueberries, Frozen, Unsweetened	155.0000	1.000	Cup	0.65	0.99	18.86	79.05	0.00	4.19	0.00	0.08
	Broccoli, Ckd	280.0000	1.000	Cup	8.34	0.98	14.17	78.40	0.00	8.12	0.00	0.14
	Broccoli, Flower Clusters, Fresh	71.0000	1.000	Cup	2.12	0.25	3.72	19.88	0.00	0.00	0.00	0.04
	Broccoli, Frz, Chopped, Ckd	184.0000	1.000	Cup	5.70	0.22	9.84	51.52	0.00	5.52	0.00	0.04
	Brussels Sprouts, Ckd	21.0000	1.000	Each	0.54	0.11	1.82	8.19	0.00	0.55	0.00	0.02
	Cabbage, Chinese (pak-choi)	70.0000	1.000	Cup	1.05	0.14	1.56	9.10	0.00	0.70	0.00	0.02
	Cabbage, Ckd		1.000	Head	12.87	5.43	56.29	277.64	0.00	29.03	0.00	0.63
	Cabbage, Fresh	908.0000	1.000	Head	10.99	1.63	48.76	217.92	0.00	20.88	0.00	0.18
	Carrots, Baby, Fresh	15.0000	1.000	Large	0.13	0.08	1.22	5.70	0.00	0.27	0.00	0.01
135	Carrots, Ckd	156.0000	1.000	Cup	1.70	0.28	16.35	70.20	0.00	5.15	0.00	0.05
	Carrots, Cnd, Reg Pk	228.0000	1.000	Cup	1.46	0.43	12.63	57.00	0.00	3.42	0.00	0.09
	Carrots, Fresh	128.0000	1.000	Cup	1.32	0.24	12.98	55.04	0.00	3.84	0.00	0.04
	Carrots, Frz, Ckd	146.0000	0.500	Cup	1.74	0.16	12.05	52.56	0.00	5.11	0.00	0.03
	Cauliflower, Ckd, Boiled	62.0000	0.500	Cup	1.14	0.28	2.55	14.26	0.00	1.67	0.00	0.04
	Cauliflower, Fresh	100.0000	0.500	Cup	1.98	0.21	5.20	25.00	0.00	2.50	0.00	0.03
	Cauliflower, Frz, Ckd	180.0000	1.000	Cup	2.90	0.40	6.75	34.20	0.00	4.86	0.00	0.05
	Celery, Ckd	150.0000	1.000	Cup	1.25	0.24	6.02	27.00	0.00	2.40	0.00	0.06
	Celery, Fresh	120.0000	1.000	Cup	0.90	0.17	4.38	19.20	0.00	2.04	0.00	0.05
	Cherries, Sour, Red, Cnd, Heavy	256.0000	1.000	Cup	1.87	0.26	59.57	232.96	0.00	2.82	0.00	0.05
	Cherries, Sour, Red, Cnd, Light	252.0000	1.000	Cup	1.86	0.25	48.64	189.00	0.00	2.02	0.00	0.05
	Cherries, Sour, Red, Cnd, Water	244.0000	1.000	Cup	1.88	0.24	21.81	87.84	0.00	2.68	0.00	0.05
	Cherries, Sour, Red, Cnd, X-heav	261.0000	1.000	Cup	1.85	0.23	76.29	297.54	0.00	2.09	0.00	0.05
	Cherries, Sour, Red, Fresh	155.0000	1.000	Cup	1.55	0.47	18.88	77.50	0.00	2.48	0.00	0.11
	Cherries, Sweet, Cnd, Heavy Syru	253.0000	1.000	Cup	1.52	0.38	53.81	209.99	0.00	3.80	0.00	0.08
	Cherries, Sweet, Cnd, Juice Pack	250.0000	1.000	Cup	2.28	0.05	34.53	135.00	0.00	3.75	0.00	0.00
	Cherries, Sweet, Cnd, Light Syru	252.0000	1.000	Cup	1.54	0.38	43.57	168.84	0.00	3.78	0.00	0.08
	Cherries, Sweet, Cnd, Water Pack	248.0000	1.000	Cup	1.91	0.32	29.16	114.08	0.00	3.72	0.00	0.07
	Cherries, Sweet, Cnd, X-heavy Sy	261.0000	1.000	Cup	1.54	0.39	68.46	266.22	0.00	3.92	0.00	0.08
	Cherries, Sweet, Fresh	117.0000	1.000	Cup	1.40	1.12	19.36	84.24	0.00	2.69	0.00	0.26
	Cherries, Sweet, Frozen, Sweeten	259.0000	1.000	Cup	2.98	0.34	57.91	230.51	0.00	5.44	0.00	0.08
	Chives, Raw	1.0000	1.000	Tsp	0.03	0.01	0.04	0.30	0.00	0.03	0.00	0.00
	Coleslaw	8.0000	1.000	Tbsp	0.10	0.21	0.99	5.52	0.00	0.12	0.64	0.03
	Collards, Ckd	190.0000	1.000	Cup	4.01	0.68	9.31	49.40	0.00	5.32	0.00	0.10
	Collards, Fresh	36.0000	1.000	Cup	0.88	0.15	2.05	10.80	0.00	1.30	0.00	0.02
	Collards, Frz, Chopped, Ckd	170.0000	1.000	Cup	5.05	0.70	12.09	61.20	0.00	4.76	0.00	0.10
	Corn, Ckd	140.0000	1.000	Cup	3.68	1.02	39.07	176.40	0.00	6.72	0.00	0.14
	Corn, Sweet, White, Ckd	77.0000	1.000	Cup	2.56	0.99	19.33	83.16	0.00	2.08	0.00	0.15
	Corn, Sweet, White, Cnd	164.0000	1.000	Cup	4.30	1.64	30.49	132.84	0.00	3.28	0.00	0.25
	Corn, Sweet, White, Cnd, Cream S	256.0000	1.000	Cup	4.45	1.08	46.41	184.32	0.00	3.07	0.00	0.18
	Corn, Sweet, White, Fresh	154.0000	1.000	Cup	4.96	1.82	29.29	132.44	0.00	4.16	0.00	0.28
	Corn, Sweet, Yellow, Ckd	164.0000	1.000	Cup	5.44	2.10	41.18	177.12	0.00	4.59	0.00	0.33
	Corn, Sweet, Yellow, Cnd, Brine	164.0000	1.000	Cup	4.30	1.64	30.49	132.84	0.00	3.28	0.00	0.25
	Corn, Sweet, Yellow, Cnd, Cream	256.0000	1.000	Cup	4.45	1.08	46.41	184.32	0.00	3.07	0.00	0.18
	Corn, Sweet, Yellow, Fresh	154.0000	1.000	Cup	4.96	1.82	29.29	132.44	0.00	4.16	0.00	0.28
	Crabapples, Fresh	110.0000	1.000	Cup	0.44	0.33	21.95	83.60	0.00	0.00	0.00	0.06
	Cranberries, Fresh	110.0000	1.000	Cup	0.43	0.22	13.95	53.90	0.00	4.62	0.00	0.02
	Cranberry Sauce, Cnd, Sweetened	277.0000	1.000	Cup	0.55	0.42	107.75	418.27	0.00	2.77	0.00	0.03
	Cranberry-orange Relish, Cnd	275.0000	1.000	Cup	0.83	0.28	127.05	489.50	0.00	0.00	0.00	0.03
	Cucumber, Fresh	52.0000	0.500	Cup	0.36	0.07	1.44	6.76	0.00	0.42	0.00	0.02

Monounsaturated Fat (gm)	Polyunsaturated Fat (gm)	Vitamin D (mg)	Vitamin K (mg)	Vitamin E (mg)	Vitamin A (re)	Vitamin C (mg)	Thiamin (mg)	Riboflavin (mg)	Niacin (mg)	Vitamin B6 (mg)	Folate (mg)	Vitamin B12 (mcg)	Calcium (mg)	Iron (mg)	Magnesium (mg)	Phosphorus (mg)	Potassium (mg)	Sodium (mg)	Zinc (mg)
0.00	0.07	0.00	0.00	0.39	14.85	6.48	0.03	0.08	0.27	0.05	42.93	0.00	35.10	1.22	17.55	25.65	147.15	338.85	0.39
0.01	0.07	0.00	0.00	0.00	12.10	17.93	0.09	0.12	0.83	0.08	40.15	0.00	40.70	1.14	27.50	41.80	229.90	6.60	0.26
0.03	0.05	0.00	0.00	0.26	3.40	3.06	0.03	0.03	0.28	0.06	68.00	0.00	13.60	0.67	19.55	32.30	259.25	65.45	0.30
0.13	0.36	0.00	1.28	2.56	15.36	2.82	0.08	0.13	0.28	0.10	4.10	0.00	12.80	0.84	10.24	25.60	102.40	7.68	0.18
0.07	0.25	0.00	0.00	1.45	14.50	18.85	0.07	0.07	0.52	0.06	9.28	0.00	8.70	0.25	7.25	14.50	129.05	8.70	0.16
0.05	0.14	0.00	0.00	1.63	9.20	2.30	0.05	0.12	0.58	0.14	15.41	0.00	13.80	0.90	4.60	16.10	138.00	2.30	0.14
0.14	0.43	0.00	0.00	1.55	12.40	3.88	0.05	0.06	0.81	0.09	10.39	0.00	12.40	0.28	7.75	17.05	83.70	1.55	0.11
0.06	0.48	0.00	0.00	4.73	389.20	208.88	0.17	0.31	1.60	0.39	140.00	0.00	128.80	2.35	67.20	165.20	817.60	72.80	1.06
0.01	0.12	0.00	0.00	1.18	213.00	66.17	0.05	0.09	0.45	0.11	50.41	0.00	34.08	0.62	17.75	46.86	230.75	19.17	0.28
0.02	0.11	0.00	0.00	3.04	347.76	73.78	0.11	0.15	0.85	0.24	103.78	0.00	93.84	1.12	36.80	101.20	331.20	44.16	0.55
0.01	0.05	0.00	0.00	0.18	15.12	13.02	0.02	0.02	0.13	0.04	12.60	0.00	7.56	0.25	4.20	11.76	66.57	4.41	0.07
0.01	0.07	0.00	0.00	0.08	210.00	31.50	0.03	0.05	0.35	0.14	45.99	0.00	73.50	0.56	13.30	25.90	176.40	45.50	0.13
0.38	2.52	0.00	0.00	1.39	164.06	253.66	0.76	0.76	3.53	1.39	252.40	0.00	391.22	2.15	100.96	189.30	1224.14	100.96	1.14
0.09	0.82	0.00	0.00	0.00	118.04	463.08	0.45	0.27	2.72	0.91	514.84	0.00	426.76	5.08	136.20	208.84	2233.68	163.44	1.63
0.00	0.04	0.00	0.00	0.00	225.15	1.26	0.00	0.01	0.13	0.01	4.95	0.00	3.45	0.12	1.80	5.70	41.85	5.25	0.02
0.01	0.14	0.00	0.00	0.66	3829.80	3.59	0.05	0.09	0.79	0.38	21.68	0.00	48.36	0.97	20.28	46.80	354.12	102.96	0.47
0.02	0.21	0.00	0.00	0.96	3139.56	6.16	0.05	0.07	1.25	0.25	20.98	0.00	57.00	1.46	18.24	54.72	408.12	551.76	0.59
0.01	0.10	0.00	16.64	0.59	3600.64	11.90	0.13	0.08	1.19	0.19	17.92	0.00	34.56	0.64	19.20	56.32	413.44	44.80	0.26
0.01	0.07	0.00	0.00	0.61	2584.20	4.09	0.04	0.06	0.64	0.19	15.77	0.00	40.88	0.69	14.60	37.96	230.68	86.14	0.35
0.02	0.14	0.00	0.00	0.02	1.24	27.47	0.02	0.03	0.25	0.11	27.28	0.00	9.92	0.20	5.58	19.84	88.04	9.30	0.11
0.01	0.10	0.00	191.00	0.04	2.00	46.40	0.06	0.06	0.53	0.22	57.00	0.00	22.00	0.44	15.00	44.00	303.00	30.00	0.28
0.04	0.18	0.00	0.00	0.07	3.60	56.34	0.07	0.09	0.56	0.16	73.80	0.00	30.60	0.74	16.20	43.20	250.20	32.40	0.23
0.05	0.12	0.00	0.00	0.54	19.50	9.15	0.06	0.08	0.48	0.14	33.00	0.00	63.00	0.63	18.00	37.50	426.00	136.50	0.21
0.04	0.08	0.00	0.00	0.43	15.60	8.40	0.06	0.06	0.38	0.11	33.60	0.00	48.00	0.48	13.20	30.00	344.40	104.40	0.16
0.08	0.08	0.00	0.00	0.33	181.76	5.12	0.05	0.10	0.44	0.10	19.46	0.00	25.60	3.33	15.36	25.60	238.08	17.92	0.15
0.08	0.08	0.00	0.00	0.00	183.96	5.04	0.05	0.10	0.43	0.10	19.40	0.00	25.20	3.33	15.12	25.20	239.40	17.64	0.18
0.07	0.07	0.00	0.00	0.32	183.00	5.12	0.05	0.10	0.44	0.10	19.52	0.00	26.84	3.34	14.64	24.40	239.12	17.08	0.17
0.08	0.08	0.00	0.00	0.00	182.70	4.96	0.05	0.10	0.42	0.10	19.31	0.00	26.10	3.29	13.05	23.49	237.51	18.27	0.16
0.12	0.14	0.00	0.00	0.20	198.40	15.50	0.05	0.06	0.62	0.06	11.63	0.00	24.80	0.50	13.95	23.25	268.15	4.65	0.16
0.10	0.13	0.00	0.00	0.15	37.95	9.11	0.05	0.10	1.01	0.08	10.63	0.00	22.77	0.89	22.77	45.54	366.85	7.59	0.25
0.03	0.03	0.00	0.00	0.25	32.50	6.25	0.05	0.05	1.03	0.08	10.50	0.00	35.00	1.45	30.00	55.00	327.50	7.50	0.25
0.10	0.13	0.00	0.00	0.33	40.32	9.32	0.05	0.10	1.01	0.08	10.58	0.00	22.68	0.91	22.68	45.36	372.96	7.56	0.25
0.07	0.10	0.00	0.00	0.32	39.68	5.46	0.05	0.10	1.02	0.07	10.42	0.00	27.28	0.89	22.32	37.20	324.88	2.48	0.20
0.10	0.13	0.00	0.00	0.00	39.15	9.40	0.05	0.10	1.02	0.08	10.96	0.00	23.49	0.91	20.88	44.37	370.62	7.83	0.26
0.30	0.34	0.00	0.00	0.15	24.57	8.19	0.06	0.07	0.47	0.05	4.91	0.00	17.55	0.46	12.87	22.23	262.08	0.00	0.07
0.10	0.10	0.00	0.00	0.34	49.21	2.59	0.08	0.13	0.47	0.10	10.88	0.00	31.08	0.91	25.90	41.44	515.41	2.59	0.10
0.00	0.00	0.00	0.00	0.00	4.35	0.58	0.00	0.00	0.01	0.00	1.05	0.00	0.92	0.02	0.42	0.58	2.96	0.03	0.01
0.06	0.11	0.00	0.00	0.00	6.56	2.62	0.01	0.00	0.02	0.01	2.12	0.00	3.60	0.05	0.80	2.56	14.48	1.84	0.02
0.06	0.32	0.00	0.00	1.67	594.70	34.58	0.08	0.21	1.10	0.25	176.70	0.00	226.10	0.87	32.30	49.40	494.00	17.10	0.80
0.01	0.07	0.00	0.00	0.81	137.52	12.71	0.02	0.05	0.27	0.06	59.76	0.00	52.20	0.07	3.24	3.60	60.84	7.20	0.05
0.03	0.36	0.00	0.00	0.85	1016.60	44.88	0.09	0.20	1.09	0.19	129.37	0.00	357.00	1.90	51.00	45.90	426.70	85.00	0.46
0.27	0.46	0.00	0.00	0.46	8.40	0.00	0.07	0.03	0.78	0.08	8.40	0.00	1.40	0.35	50.40	106.40	43.40	0.00	0.88
0.28	0.46	0.00	0.00	0.07	0.00	4.77	0.17	0.05	1.24	0.05	35.73	0.00	1.54	0.47	24.64	79.31	191.73	13.09	0.37
0.48	0.77	0.00	0.00	0.15	0.00	13.94	0.05	0.13	1.97	0.08	79.70	0.00	8.20	1.41	32.80	106.60	319.80	529.72	0.64
0.31	0.51	0.00	0.00	0.23	0.00	11.78	0.08	0.13	2.46	0.15	114.69	0.00	7.68	0.97	43.52	130.56	343.04	729.60	1.36
0.54	0.86	0.00	0.00	0.14	0.00	10.47	0.31	0.09	2.62	0.09	70.53	0.00	3.08	0.80	56.98	137.06	415.80	23.10	0.69
0.61	0.98	0.00	0.00	0.15	36.08	10.17	0.36	0.11	2.64	0.10	76.10	0.00	3.28	1.00	52.48	168.92	408.36	350.96	0.79
0.48	0.77	0.00	0.00	0.25	26.24	13.94	0.05	0.13	1.97	0.08	79.70	0.00	8.20	1.41	32.80	106.60	319.80	350.96	0.64
0.31	0.51	0.00	0.00	0.23	25.60	11.78	0.08	0.13	2.46	0.15	114.69	0.00	7.68	0.97	43.52	130.56	343.04	729.60	1.36
0.54	0.86	0.00	10.78	0.14	43.12	10.47	0.31	0.09	2.62	0.09	70.53	0.00	3.08	0.80	56.98	137.06	415.80	23.10	0.69
0.01	0.10	0.00	0.00	0.00	4.40	8.80	0.03	0.02	0.11	0.00	0.00	0.00	19.80	0.40	7.70	16.50	213.40	1.10	0.00
0.03	0.10	0.00	0.00	0.11	5.50	14.85	0.03	0.02	0.11	0.08	1.87	0.00	7.70	0.22	5.50	9.90	78.10	1.10	0.14
0.06	0.19	0.00	3.88	0.28	5.54	5.54	0.06	0.06	0.28	0.03	2.77	0.00	11.08	0.61	8.31	16.62	72.02	80.33	0.14
0.00	0.00	0.00	0.00	0.00	19.25	49.50	0.08	0.06	0.28	0.00	0.00	0.00	30.25	0.55	11.00	22.00	104.50	88.00	0.00
0.00	0.03	0.00	2.60	0.04	10.92	2.76	0.01	0.01	0.11	0.02	6.76	0.00	7.28	0.14	5.72	10.40	74.88	1.04	0.10

USDA ID Code / Food Name	Weight in Grams*	Quantity of Units	Unit of Measure	Protein (gm)	Fat (gm)	Carbohydrate (gm)	Kcalories	Caffeine (gm)	Fiber (gm)	Cholesterol (mg)	Saturated Fat (gm)
Dates, Domestic, Natural and Dry	178.0000	1.000	Cup	3.51	0.80	130.85	489.50	0.00	13.35	0.00	0.34
Eggplant, Ckd	99.0000	1.000	Cup	0.82	0.23	6.57	27.72	0.00	2.48	0.00	0.04
Eggplant, Fresh	82.0000	1.000	Cup	0.84	0.15	4.98	21.32	0.00	2.05	0.00	0.02
Endive, Raw	25.0000	0.500	Cup	0.31	0.05	0.84	4.25	0.00	0.78	0.00	0.01
Fruit Salad, Heavy Syrup	255.0000	1.000	Cup	0.87	0.18	48.73	186.15	0.00	2.55	0.00	0.03
Fruit Salad, Juice Pack	249.0000	1.000	Cup	1.27	0.07	32.49	124.50	0.00	2.49	0.00	0.00
Fruit Salad, Light Syrup	252.0000	1.000	Cup	0.86	0.18	38.15	146.16	0.00	2.52	0.00	0.03
Fruit Salad, Water Pack	245.0000	1.000	Cup	0.86	0.17	19.28	73.50	0.00	2.45	0.00	0.02
Fruit, Heavy Syrup	248.0000	1.000	Cup	0.97	0.17	46.90	181.04	0.00	2.48	0.00	0.02
Fruit, Juice Pack	237.0000	1.000	Cup	1.09	0.02	28.11	109.02	0.00	2.37	0.00	0.00
Fruit, Light Syrup	242.0000	1.000	Cup	0.97	0.17	36.13	137.94	0.00	2.42	0.00	0.02
Fruit, Mixed, Dried	293.0000	1.250	Cup	7.21	1.44	187.70	711.99	0.00	22.85	0.00	0.12
Fruit, Mixed, Frzn, Swtnd, Thawd	250.0000	1.000	Cup	3.55	0.45	60.58	245.00	0.00	4.75	0.00	0.08
Fruit, Mixed, Hvy Syrup	255.0000	1.000	Cup	0.94	0.26	47.84	183.60	0.00	2.55	0.00	0.03
Fruit, Water Pack	237.0000	1.000	Cup	1.00	0.12	20.17	75.84	0.00	2.37	0.00	0.02
Garlic, Raw	3.0000	1.000	Clove	0.19	0.02	0.99	4.47	0.00	0.06	0.00	0.00
Grapefruit, Fresh, Pink & Red	230.0000	1.000	Cup	1.27	0.23	17.66	69.00	0.00	0.00	0.00	0.02
Grapefruit, Fresh, White	230.0000	1.000	Cup	1.59	0.23	19.34	75.90	0.00	2.53	0.00	0.02
Grapefruit, Sections, Cnd, Juice	249.0000	1.000	Cup	1.74	0.22	22.93	92.13	0.00	1.00	0.00	0.02
Grapefruit, Sections, Cnd, Light	254.0000	1.000	Cup	1.42	0.25	39.22	152.40	0.00	1.02	0.00	0.03
Grapefruit, Sections, Cnd, Water	244.0000	1.000	Cup	1.42	0.24	22.33	87.84	0.00	0.98	0.00	0.02
Grapes, Fresh	92.0000	1.000	Cup	0.58	0.32	15.78	61.64	0.00	0.92	0.00	0.10
Kiwifruit, Fresh	177.0000	1.000	Cup	1.75	0.78	26.34	107.97	0.00	6.02	0.00	0.05
Leeks, Ckd	124.0000	1.000	Leek	1.00	0.25	9.45	38.44	0.00	1.24	0.00	0.04
Leeks, Fresh	89.0000	1.000	Cup	1.34	0.27	12.59	54.29	0.00	1.60	0.00	0.04
Lemons, Fresh, w/o Peel	212.0000	1.000	Cup	2.33	0.64	19.76	61.48	0.00	5.94	0.00	0.08
Lettuce, Butterhead, Fresh	55.0000	1.000	Cup	0.71	0.12	1.28	7.15	0.00	0.55	0.00	0.02
Lettuce, Iceberg, Fresh	55.0000	1.000	Cup	0.56	0.10	1.15	6.60	0.00	0.77	0.00	0.02
Lettuce, Looseleaf, Fresh	10.0000	1.000	Leaf	0.13	0.03	0.35	1.80	0.00	0.19	0.00	0.00
Lettuce, Romaine, Fresh	10.0000	1.000	Leaf	0.16	0.02	0.24	1.40	0.00	0.17	0.00	0.00
Lime, Raw	67.0000	1.000	Medium	0.47	0.13	7.06	20.10	0.00	1.88	0.00	0.02
Mangos, Fresh	165.0000	0.500	Cup	0.84	0.45	28.05	107.25	0.00	2.97	0.00	0.12
Melon Balls, Frozen, Unthawed	173.0000	1.000	Cup	1.45	0.43	13.74	57.09	0.00	1.21	0.00	0.10
Melons, Cantaloupe, Fresh	177.0000	1.000	Cup	1.56	0.50	14.80	61.95	0.00	1.42	0.00	0.12
Melons, Casaba, Fresh	170.0000	1.000	Cup	1.53	0.17	10.54	44.20	0.00	1.36	0.00	0.05
Melons, Honeydew, Fresh	177.0000	1.000	Cup	0.81	0.18	16.25	61.95	0.00	1.06	0.00	0.05
Mushrooms, Ckd	156.0000	1.000	Cup	3.39	0.73	8.02	42.12	0.00	3.43	0.00	0.09
Mushrooms, Cnd, Drained Solids	156.0000	1.000	Cup	2.92	0.45	7.74	37.44	0.00	3.74	0.00	0.06
Mushrooms, Enoki, Fresh	5.0000	1.000	Large	0.12	0.02	0.35	1.70	0.00	0.13	0.00	0.00
Mushrooms, Fresh	70.0000	1.000	Cup	2.03	0.23	2.86	17.50	0.00	0.84	0.00	0.04
Mushrooms, Shiitake, Ckd	145.0000	1.000	Cup	2.26	0.32	20.71	79.75	0.00	3.05	0.00	0.09
Mushrooms, Shiitake, Dried	3.6000	1.000	Medium	0.34	0.04	2.71	10.66	0.00	0.41	0.00	0.01
Nectar, Apricot, Cnd, w/ Added V	251.0000	1.000	Cup	0.93	0.23	36.12	140.56	0.00	1.51	0.00	0.03
Nectar, Apricot, Cnd, w/o Vit C	251.0000	1.000	Cup	0.93	0.23	36.12	140.56	0.00	1.51	0.00	0.03
Nectar, Papaya, Cnd.	250.0000	1.000	Cup	0.43	0.38	36.28	142.50	0.00	1.50	0.00	0.13
Nectar, Peach, Cnd, wo/ Added Vi	249.0000	1.000	Cup	0.67	0.05	34.66	134.46	0.00	1.49	0.00	0.00
Nectarine, Raw	136.0000	1.000	Medium	1.28	0.63	16.02	66.64	0.00	2.18	0.00	0.07
Okra, Ckd	80.0000	0.500	Cup	1.50	0.14	5.77	25.60	0.00	2.00	0.00	0.04
Okra, Fresh	100.0000	1.000	Cup	2.00	0.10	7.63	33.00	0.00	3.20	0.00	0.03
Okra, Frz, Ckd	255.0000	1.250	Cup	5.30	0.77	14.66	71.40	0.00	7.14	0.00	0.20
Okra, Frz, Unprepared	284.0000	1.250	Cup	4.80	0.71	18.86	85.20	0.00	6.25	0.00	0.20
Olives, Green	3.0000	5.000	Each	0.00	0.50	0.00	5.00	0.00	0.00	0.00	0.00
Olives, Ripe, Canned (jumbo-supe	8.3000	1.000	Jumbo	0.08	0.57	0.47	6.72	0.00	0.21	0.00	0.08
Olives, Ripe, Canned (small-extr	8.4000	1.000	Tbsp	0.07	0.90	0.53	9.66	0.00	0.27	0.00	0.12
Onions, Ckd	210.0000	1.000	Cup	2.86	0.40	21.32	92.40	0.00	2.94	0.00	0.06

Monounsaturated Fat (gm)	Polyunsaturated Fat (gm)	Vitamin D (mg)	Vitamin K (mg)	Vitamin E (mg)	Vitamin A (re)	Vitamin C (mg)	Thiamin (mg)	Riboflavin (mg)	Niacin (mg)	Vitamin B_6 (mg)	Folate (mcg)	Vitamin B_{12} (mcg)	Calcium (mg)	Iron (mg)	Magnesium (mg)	Phosphorus (mg)	Potassium (mg)	Sodium (mg)	Zinc (mg)
0.27	0.05	0.00	0.00	0.18	8.90	0.00	0.16	0.18	3.92	0.34	22.43	0.00	56.96	2.05	62.30	71.20	1160.56	5.34	0.52
0.02	0.09	0.00	0.00	0.03	5.94	1.29	0.08	0.02	0.59	0.09	14.26	0.00	5.94	0.35	12.87	21.78	245.52	2.97	0.15
0.02	0.07	0.00	0.00	0.02	6.56	1.39	0.04	0.02	0.49	0.07	15.58	0.00	5.74	0.22	11.48	18.04	177.94	2.46	0.11
0.00	0.02	0.00	0.00	0.11	51.25	1.63	0.02	0.02	0.10	0.01	35.50	0.00	13.00	0.21	3.75	7.00	78.50	5.50	0.20
0.03	0.08	0.00	0.00	1.17	127.50	6.12	0.05	0.05	0.89	0.08	6.38	0.00	15.30	0.71	12.75	22.95	204.00	15.30	0.18
0.02	0.02	0.00	0.00	0.00	149.40	8.22	0.02	0.02	0.90	0.07	6.47	0.00	27.39	0.62	19.92	34.86	288.84	12.45	0.35
0.03	0.08	0.00	0.00	0.00	108.36	6.30	0.03	0.02	0.93	0.08	6.55	0.00	17.64	0.73	12.60	22.68	206.64	15.12	0.18
0.02	0.07	0.00	0.00	0.00	107.80	4.66	0.05	0.05	0.91	0.07	6.37	0.00	17.15	0.74	12.25	22.05	191.10	7.35	0.20
0.02	0.07	0.00	0.00	0.72	49.60	4.71	0.05	0.05	0.92	0.12	6.45	0.00	14.88	0.72	12.40	27.28	218.24	14.88	0.20
0.00	0.00	0.00	0.00	0.47	73.47	6.40	0.02	0.05	0.95	0.12	5.93	0.00	18.96	0.50	16.59	33.18	225.15	9.48	0.21
0.02	0.07	0.00	0.00	0.70	50.82	4.60	0.05	0.05	0.92	0.12	6.53	0.00	14.52	0.70	12.10	26.62	215.38	14.52	0.22
0.67	0.32	0.00	0.00	0.00	714.92	11.13	0.12	0.47	5.65	0.47	11.43	0.00	111.34	7.94	114.27	225.61	2332.28	52.74	1.47
0.08	0.20	0.00	0.00	0.00	80.00	187.50	0.05	0.10	1.00	0.08	19.00	0.00	17.50	0.70	15.00	30.00	327.50	7.50	0.13
0.05	0.10	0.00	0.00	0.00	48.45	175.95	0.05	0.10	1.53	0.10	7.65	0.00	2.55	0.92	12.75	25.50	214.20	10.20	0.18
0.02	0.05	0.00	0.00	0.69	59.25	4.98	0.05	0.02	0.85	0.12	6.40	0.00	11.85	0.59	16.59	26.07	222.78	9.48	0.21
0.00	0.01	0.00	0.00	0.00	0.00	0.94	0.01	0.00	0.02	0.04	0.09	0.00	5.43	0.05	0.75	4.59	12.03	0.51	0.04
0.02	0.05	0.00	0.00	0.00	59.80	87.63	0.07	0.05	0.44	0.09	28.06	0.00	25.30	0.28	18.40	20.70	296.70	0.00	0.16
0.02	0.05	0.00	0.00	0.58	2.30	76.59	0.09	0.05	0.62	0.09	23.00	0.00	27.60	0.14	20.70	18.40	340.40	0.00	0.16
0.02	0.05	0.00	0.00	0.62	0.00	84.41	0.07	0.05	0.62	0.05	21.91	0.00	37.35	0.52	27.39	29.88	420.81	17.43	0.20
0.03	0.05	0.00	0.00	0.64	0.00	54.10	0.10	0.05	0.61	0.05	21.59	0.00	35.56	1.02	25.40	25.40	327.66	5.08	0.20
0.02	0.05	0.00	0.00	0.61	0.00	53.19	0.10	0.05	0.61	0.05	21.47	0.00	36.60	1.00	24.40	24.40	322.08	4.88	0.22
0.01	0.09	0.00	0.00	0.31	9.20	3.68	0.08	0.06	0.28	0.10	3.59	0.00	12.88	0.27	4.60	9.20	175.72	1.84	0.04
0.07	0.42	0.00	0.00	1.98	31.86	173.46	0.04	0.09	0.89	0.16	67.26	0.00	46.02	0.73	53.10	70.80	587.64	8.85	0.30
0.00	0.14	0.00	0.00	0.00	6.20	5.21	0.04	0.02	0.25	0.14	30.13	0.00	37.20	1.36	17.36	21.08	107.88	12.40	0.07
0.00	0.15	0.00	0.00	0.82	8.90	10.68	0.05	0.03	0.36	0.20	57.05	0.00	52.51	1.87	24.92	31.15	160.20	17.80	0.11
0.02	0.19	0.00	0.00	0.51	6.36	112.36	0.08	0.04	0.21	0.17	22.47	0.00	55.12	1.27	16.96	33.92	292.56	4.24	0.13
0.01	0.07	0.00	0.00	0.24	53.35	4.40	0.03	0.03	0.17	0.03	40.32	0.00	17.60	0.17	7.15	12.65	141.35	2.75	0.09
0.01	0.06	0.00	62.15	0.15	18.15	2.15	0.03	0.02	0.10	0.02	30.80	0.00	10.45	0.28	4.95	11.00	86.90	4.95	0.12
0.00	0.02	0.00	0.00	0.04	19.00	1.80	0.01	0.01	0.04	0.01	4.98	0.00	6.80	0.14	1.10	2.50	26.40	0.90	0.03
0.00	0.01	0.00	0.00	0.04	26.00	2.40	0.01	0.01	0.05	0.01	13.57	0.00	3.60	0.11	0.60	4.50	29.00	0.80	0.03
0.01	0.04	0.00	0.00	0.16	0.67	19.49	0.02	0.01	0.13	0.03	5.49	0.00	22.11	0.40	14.85	12.06	68.34	1.34	0.07
0.17	0.08	0.00	0.00	1.85	641.85	45.71	0.10	0.10	0.96	0.21	23.10	0.00	16.50	0.21	14.85	18.15	257.40	3.30	0.07
0.02	0.17	0.00	0.00	0.26	306.21	10.73	0.29	0.03	1.11	0.19	44.46	0.00	17.30	0.50	24.22	20.76	484.40	53.63	0.29
0.02	0.19	0.00	0.00	0.27	569.94	74.69	0.07	0.04	1.01	0.21	30.09	0.00	19.47	0.37	19.47	30.09	546.93	15.93	0.28
0.00	0.07	0.00	0.00	0.26	5.10	27.20	0.10	0.03	0.68	0.20	28.90	0.00	8.50	0.68	13.60	11.90	357.00	20.40	0.27
0.00	0.07	0.00	0.00	0.27	7.08	43.90	0.14	0.04	1.06	0.11	10.62	0.00	10.62	0.12	12.39	17.70	479.67	17.70	0.12
0.02	0.28	0.00	0.00	0.19	0.00	6.24	0.11	0.47	6.96	0.16	28.39	0.00	9.36	2.71	18.72	135.72	555.36	3.12	1.36
0.02	0.17	0.00	0.00	0.19	0.00	0.00	0.14	0.03	2.48	0.09	19.19	0.00	17.16	1.23	23.40	102.96	201.24	663.00	1.12
0.00	0.01	0.00	0.00	0.00	0.05	0.60	0.00	0.01	0.18	0.00	1.50	0.00	0.05	0.04	0.80	5.65	19.05	0.15	0.03
0.01	0.10	1.33	5.60	0.08	0.00	1.61	0.06	0.29	2.83	0.07	8.40	0.03	3.50	0.73	7.00	72.80	259.00	2.80	0.51
0.10	0.04	0.00	0.00	0.17	0.00	0.44	0.06	0.25	2.18	0.23	30.31	0.00	4.35	0.64	20.30	42.05	169.65	5.80	1.93
0.01	0.01	1.49	0.00	0.00	0.00	0.13	0.01	0.05	0.51	0.03	5.88	0.00	0.40	0.06	4.75	10.58	55.22	0.47	0.28
0.10	0.05	0.00	0.00	0.00	331.32	136.54	0.03	0.03	0.65	0.05	3.26	0.00	17.57	0.95	12.55	22.59	286.14	7.53	0.23
0.10	0.05	0.00	0.00	0.20	331.32	1.51	0.03	0.03	0.65	0.05	3.26	0.00	17.57	0.95	12.55	22.59	286.14	7.53	0.23
0.10	0.10	0.00	0.00	0.05	27.50	7.50	0.03	0.00	0.38	0.03	5.25	0.00	25.00	0.85	7.50	0.00	77.50	12.50	0.38
0.02	0.02	0.00	0.00	0.02	64.74	13.20	0.00	0.02	0.72	0.02	3.49	0.00	12.45	0.47	9.96	14.94	99.60	17.43	0.20
0.24	0.31	0.00	0.00	1.21	100.64	7.34	0.02	0.06	1.35	0.03	5.03	0.00	6.80	0.10	10.88	21.76	288.32	0.00	0.12
0.02	0.04	0.00	0.00	0.55	46.40	13.04	0.10	0.05	0.70	0.15	36.56	0.00	50.40	0.36	45.60	44.80	257.60	4.00	0.44
0.02	0.03	0.00	0.00	0.69	66.00	21.10	0.20	0.06	1.00	0.22	87.80	0.00	81.00	0.80	57.00	63.00	303.00	8.00	0.60
0.13	0.20	0.00	0.00	1.76	130.05	31.11	0.26	0.31	2.01	0.13	371.28	0.00	244.80	1.71	130.05	117.30	596.70	7.65	1.58
0.11	0.20	0.00	0.00	1.96	130.64	35.22	0.26	0.31	2.02	0.11	419.18	0.00	230.04	1.62	122.12	119.28	599.24	8.52	1.51
0.00	0.00	0.00	0.00	0.00	0.00	0.00	0.00	0.00	0.00	0.00	0.00	0.00	0.00	0.00	0.00	0.00	0.00	13.00	0.00
0.42	0.05	0.00	0.00	0.25	2.91	0.12	0.00	0.00	0.00	0.00	0.00	0.00	7.80	0.28	0.33	0.25	0.75	74.53	0.02
0.66	0.08	0.00	0.00	0.25	3.36	0.08	0.00	0.00	0.00	0.00	0.00	0.00	7.39	0.28	0.34	0.25	0.67	73.25	0.02
0.06	0.15	0.00	0.00	0.27	0.00	10.92	0.08	0.04	0.36	0.27	31.50	0.00	46.20	0.50	23.10	73.50	348.60	6.30	0.44

USDA ID Code	Food Name	Weight in Grams*	Quantity of Units	Unit of Measure	Protein (gm)	Fat (gm)	Carbohydrate (gm)	Kcalories	Caffeine (gm)	Fiber (gm)	Cholesterol (mg)	Saturated Fat (gm)
	Onions, Cnd, Solid & Liquid	63.0000	1.000	Onion	0.54	0.06	2.53	11.97	0.00	0.76	0.00	0.01
	Onions, Fresh	160.0000	1.000	Cup	1.86	0.26	13.81	60.80	0.00	2.88	0.00	0.05
	Oranges, Fresh	180.0000	1.000	Cup	1.69	0.22	21.15	84.60	0.00	4.32	0.00	0.04
	Papayas, Fresh	140.0000	1.000	Cup	0.85	0.20	13.73	54.60	0.00	2.52	0.00	0.06
	Parsnips, Ckd, w/ Salt	78.0000	0.500	Cup	1.03	0.23	15.23	63.18	0.00	3.12	0.00	0.04
	Parsnips, Ckd, w/o Salt	78.0000	0.500	Cup	1.03	0.23	15.23	63.18	0.00	3.12	0.00	0.04
	Parsnips, Fresh	133.0000	1.000	Cup	1.60	0.40	23.93	99.75	0.00	6.52	0.00	0.07
	Peaches, Cnd, Heavy Syrup Pack	262.0000	1.000	Cup	1.18	0.26	52.24	193.88	0.00	3.41	0.00	0.03
	Peaches, Cnd, Juice Pack	250.0000	1.000	Cup	1.58	0.08	28.93	110.00	0.00	3.25	0.00	0.00
	Peaches, Cnd, Light Syrup Pack	251.0000	1.000	Cup	1.13	0.08	36.52	135.54	0.00	3.26	0.00	0.00
	Peaches, Cnd, Water Pack	244.0000	1.000	Cup	1.07	0.15	14.91	58.56	0.00	3.17	0.00	0.02
	Peaches, Cnd, X-heavy Syrup Pack	262.0000	1.000	Cup	1.23	0.08	68.28	251.52	0.00	2.62	0.00	0.00
	Peaches, Cnd, X-light Syrup	247.0000	1.000	Cup	0.99	0.25	27.42	103.74	0.00	2.47	0.00	0.02
	Peaches, Dehydrated, Sulfured	116.0000	1.000	Cup	5.67	1.19	96.49	377.00	0.00	0.00	0.00	0.13
	Peaches, Dried, Sulfured	160.0000	1.000	Cup	5.78	1.22	98.13	382.40	0.00	13.12	0.00	0.13
	Peaches, Fresh	170.0000	1.000	Cup	1.19	0.15	18.87	73.10	0.00	3.40	0.00	0.02
	Peaches, Frozen, Sliced, Sweeten	250.0000	1.000	Cup	1.58	0.33	59.95	235.00	0.00	4.50	0.00	0.03
	Pears, Asian, Fresh	122.0000	1.000	Medium	0.61	0.28	12.99	51.24	0.00	4.39	0.00	0.01
	Pears, Cnd, Heavy Syrup Pack	266.0000	1.000	Cup	0.53	0.35	50.99	196.84	0.00	4.26	0.00	0.03
	Pears, Cnd, Juice Pack	248.0000	1.000	Cup	0.84	0.17	32.09	124.00	0.00	3.97	0.00	0.00
	Pears, Cnd, Light Syrup Pack	251.0000	1.000	Cup	0.48	0.08	38.08	143.07	0.00	4.02	0.00	0.00
	Pears, Cnd, Water Pack	244.0000	1.000	Cup	0.46	0.07	19.06	70.76	0.00	3.90	0.00	0.00
	Pears, Cnd, X-heavy Syrup Pack	266.0000	1.000	Cup	0.51	0.35	67.17	258.02	0.00	4.26	0.00	0.03
	Pears, Cnd, X-light Syrup Pack	247.0000	1.000	Cup	0.74	0.25	30.13	116.09	0.00	3.95	0.00	0.02
	Pears, Fresh	165.0000	1.000	Cup	0.64	0.66	24.93	97.35	0.00	3.96	0.00	0.03
	Peas and Carrots, Cnd	255.0000	1.000	Cup	5.53	0.69	21.62	96.90	0.00	5.10	0.00	0.13
	Peas and Carrots, Frz, Ckd	278.0000	1.250	Cup	8.59	1.17	28.13	133.44	0.00	8.62	0.00	0.22
	Peas and Onions, Cnd	120.0000	1.000	Cup	3.94	0.46	10.28	61.20	0.00	2.76	0.00	0.08
	Peas and Onions, Frz, Ckd	180.0000	1.000	Cup	4.57	0.36	15.53	81.00	0.00	3.96	0.00	0.07
	Peas, Edible-podded, Fresh	98.0000	1.000	Cup	2.74	0.20	7.41	41.16	0.00	2.55	0.00	0.04
	Peas, Green, Ckd	160.0000	1.000	Cup	8.58	0.35	25.02	134.40	0.00	8.80	0.00	0.06
	Peas, Green, Cnd	170.0000	1.000	Cup	7.51	0.60	21.39	117.30	0.00	6.97	0.00	0.10
	Peas, Green, Cnd, Seasoned	227.0000	1.000	Cup	7.01	0.61	21.00	113.50	0.00	4.54	0.00	0.11
	Peas, Green, Fresh	145.0000	1.000	Cup	7.86	0.58	20.97	117.45	0.00	7.40	0.00	0.10
	Peas, Green, Frz, Ckd	253.0000	1.250	Cup	13.03	0.68	36.08	197.34	0.00	13.92	0.00	0.13
	Peppers, Hot Chili, Green, Cnd	73.0000	1.000	Each	0.66	0.07	3.72	15.33	0.00	0.95	0.00	0.01
	Peppers, Hot Chili, Green, Fresh	45.0000	1.000	Each	0.90	0.09	4.26	18.00	0.00	0.68	0.00	0.01
	Peppers, Hot Chili, Red, Cnd	73.0000	1.000	Each	0.66	0.07	3.72	15.33	0.00	0.95	0.00	0.01
	Peppers, Hot Chili, Red, Fresh	45.0000	1.000	Each	0.90	0.09	4.26	18.00	0.00	0.68	0.00	0.01
	Peppers, Jalapeno, Cnd	136.0000	1.000	Cup	1.25	1.28	6.42	36.72	0.00	3.54	0.00	0.14
	Peppers, Sweet, Green, Fresh	149.0000	1.000	Cup	1.33	0.28	9.58	40.23	0.00	2.68	0.00	0.04
	Peppers, Sweet, Red, Fresh	149.0000	1.000	Cup	1.33	0.28	9.58	40.23	0.00	2.98	0.00	0.04
	Peppers, Sweet, Yellow, Fresh	186.0000	1.000	Large	1.86	0.39	11.76	50.22	0.00	1.67	0.00	0.06
	Persimmon, Japanese, Raw	168.0000	1.000	Medium	0.97	0.32	31.23	117.60	0.00	6.05	0.00	0.03
	Pickle, Cucumber ,Sour	155.0000	1.000	Cup	0.51	0.31	3.49	17.05	0.00	1.86	0.00	0.08
	Pickle, Cucumber, Dill	143.0000	1.000	Cup	0.89	0.27	5.91	25.74	0.00	1.72	0.00	0.07
	Pickle, Cucumber, Dill, Low Sodi	65.0000	1.000	Slice	0.40	0.12	2.68	11.70	0.00	0.78	0.00	0.03
	Pickle, Cucumber, Sour, Low Sodi	143.0000	1.000	Cup	0.47	0.29	3.22	15.73	0.00	1.72	0.00	0.07
	Pickle, Cucumber, Sweet	160.0000	1.000	Cup	0.59	0.42	50.90	187.20	0.00	1.76	0.00	0.11
	Pickle, Cucumber, Sweet, Low Sod	160.0000	1.000	Cup	0.59	0.42	50.90	187.20	0.00	1.76	0.00	0.11
	Pineapple, Cnd, Heavy Syrup Pack	254.0000	1.000	Cup	0.89	0.28	51.31	198.12	0.00	2.03	0.00	0.03
	Pineapple, Cnd, Juice Pack	249.0000	1.000	Cup	1.05	0.20	39.09	149.40	0.00	1.99	0.00	0.02
	Pineapple, Cnd, Light Syrup Pack	252.0000	1.000	Cup	0.91	0.30	33.89	131.04	0.00	2.02	0.00	0.03
	Pineapple, Cnd, Water Pack	246.0000	1.000	Cup	1.06	0.22	20.42	78.72	0.00	1.97	0.00	0.02
	Pineapple, Cnd, X-heavy Syrup Pa	260.0000	1.000	Cup	0.88	0.29	55.90	215.80	0.00	2.08	0.00	0.03

Monounsaturated Fat (gm)	Polyunsaturated Fat (gm)	Vitamin D (mg)	Vitamin K (mg)	Vitamin E (mg)	Vitamin A (re)	Vitamin C (mg)	Thiamin (mg)	Riboflavin (mg)	Niacin (mg)	Vitamin B6 (mg)	Folate (mcg)	Vitamin B12 (mcg)	Calcium (mg)	Iron (mg)	Magnesium (mg)	Phosphorus (mg)	Potassium (mg)	Sodium (mg)	Zinc (mg)
0.01	0.03	0.00	0.00	0.04	0.00	2.71	0.02	0.01	0.04	0.09	6.11	0.00	28.35	0.08	3.78	17.64	69.93	233.73	0.18
0.03	0.10	0.00	0.83	0.21	0.00	10.24	0.06	0.03	0.24	0.19	30.40	0.00	32.00	0.35	16.00	52.80	251.20	4.80	0.30
0.04	0.05	0.00	2.43	0.43	37.80	95.76	0.16	0.07	0.50	0.11	54.54	0.00	72.00	0.18	18.00	25.20	325.80	0.00	0.13
0.06	0.04	0.00	0.00	1.57	39.20	86.52	0.04	0.04	0.48	0.03	53.20	0.00	33.60	0.14	14.00	7.00	359.80	4.20	0.10
0.09	0.04	0.00	0.00	0.00	0.00	10.14	0.06	0.04	0.56	0.07	45.40	0.00	28.86	0.45	22.62	53.82	286.26	191.88	0.20
0.09	0.04	0.00	0.00	0.78	0.00	10.14	0.06	0.04	0.56	0.07	45.40	0.00	28.86	0.45	22.62	53.82	286.26	7.80	0.20
0.15	0.07	0.00	0.00	0.00	0.00	22.61	0.12	0.07	0.93	0.12	88.84	0.00	47.88	0.78	38.57	94.43	498.75	13.30	0.78
0.10	0.13	0.00	0.00	2.33	86.46	7.34	0.03	0.05	1.60	0.05	8.38	0.00	7.86	0.71	13.10	28.82	241.04	15.72	0.24
0.03	0.05	0.00	7.50	3.75	95.00	9.00	0.03	0.05	1.45	0.05	8.50	0.00	15.00	0.68	17.50	42.50	320.00	10.00	0.28
0.03	0.05	0.00	0.00	2.23	87.85	6.02	0.03	0.08	1.48	0.05	8.28	0.00	7.53	0.90	12.55	27.61	243.47	12.55	0.23
0.05	0.07	0.00	0.00	2.17	129.32	7.08	0.02	0.05	1.27	0.05	8.30	0.00	4.88	0.78	12.20	24.40	241.56	7.32	0.22
0.03	0.03	0.00	0.00	0.00	34.06	3.14	0.03	0.05	1.36	0.05	8.12	0.00	7.86	0.76	13.10	28.82	217.46	20.96	0.24
0.10	0.12	0.00	0.00	0.00	66.69	7.41	0.05	0.05	1.98	0.05	8.15	0.00	12.35	0.74	12.35	27.17	182.78	12.35	0.22
0.44	0.58	0.00	0.00	0.00	164.72	12.30	0.05	0.13	5.60	0.19	7.66	0.00	44.08	6.39	66.12	187.92	1567.16	11.60	0.90
0.45	0.59	0.00	0.00	0.00	345.60	7.68	0.00	0.34	7.01	0.11	0.48	0.00	44.80	6.50	67.20	190.40	1593.60	11.20	0.91
0.05	0.09	0.00	0.00	1.19	91.80	11.22	0.03	0.07	1.68	0.03	5.78	0.00	8.50	0.19	11.90	20.40	334.90	0.00	0.24
0.13	0.15	0.00	0.00	2.23	70.00	235.50	0.03	0.10	1.63	0.05	8.00	0.00	7.50	0.93	12.50	27.50	325.00	15.00	0.13
0.06	0.07	0.00	0.00	0.61	0.00	4.64	0.01	0.01	0.27	0.02	9.76	0.00	4.88	0.00	9.76	13.42	147.62	0.00	0.02
0.08	0.08	0.00	0.00	1.33		2.93	0.03	0.05	0.64	0.03	3.19	0.00	13.30	0.59	10.64	18.62	172.90	13.30	0.21
0.02	0.05	0.00	1.14	1.24	2.48	3.97	0.02	0.02	0.50	0.02	2.98	0.00	22.32	0.72	17.36	29.76	238.08	9.92	0.22
0.03	0.03	0.00	0.00	1.26	0.00	1.76	0.03	0.05	0.38	0.03	3.01	0.00	12.55	0.70	10.04	17.57	165.66	12.55	0.20
0.02	0.02	0.00	0.00	1.22	0.00	2.44	0.02	0.02	0.12	0.02	2.93	0.00	9.76	0.51	9.76	17.08	129.32	4.88	0.22
0.08	0.08	0.00	0.00	0.00	0.00	2.93	0.03	0.05	0.64	0.03	3.19	0.00	13.30	0.59	10.64	18.62	170.24	13.30	0.21
0.05	0.05	0.00	0.00	0.00	0.00	4.94	0.02	0.05	0.99	0.02	2.96	0.00	17.29	0.49	12.35	17.29	111.15	4.94	0.17
0.13	0.15	0.00	0.00	0.83	3.30	6.60	0.03	0.07	0.17	0.03	12.05	0.00	18.15	0.41	9.90	18.15	206.25	0.00	0.20
0.05	0.33	0.00	0.00	0.00	1471.35	16.83	0.18	0.13	1.48	0.23	46.67	0.00	58.65	1.91	35.70	117.30	255.00	663.00	1.48
0.11	0.56	0.00	0.00	0.89	2157.28	22.52	0.64	0.17	3.20	0.25	72.28	0.00	63.94	2.61	44.48	136.22	439.24	189.04	1.25
0.05	0.22	0.00	0.00	0.00	19.20	3.60	0.12	0.08	1.54	0.23	31.92	0.00	20.40	1.04	19.20	61.20	115.20	530.40	0.70
0.04	0.16	0.00	0.00	0.27	63.00	12.42	0.27	0.13	1.87	0.16	35.82	0.00	25.20	1.69	23.40	61.20	210.60	66.60	0.52
0.02	0.09	0.00	0.00	0.38	13.72	58.80	0.15	0.08	0.59	0.16	40.87	0.00	42.14	2.04	23.52	51.94	196.00	3.92	0.26
0.03	0.16	0.00	0.00	0.62	96.00	22.72	0.42	0.24	3.23	0.35	101.28	0.00	43.20	2.46	62.40	187.20	433.60	4.80	1.90
0.05	0.27	0.00	0.00	0.65	130.90	16.32	0.20	0.14	1.24	0.10	75.31	0.00	34.00	1.62	28.90	113.90	294.10	428.40	1.21
0.05	0.30	0.00	0.00	0.00	97.61	26.11	0.23	0.16	1.57	0.23	64.92	0.00	34.05	2.72	34.05	122.58	276.94	576.58	1.48
0.06	0.28	0.00	0.00	0.57	92.80	58.00	0.39	0.19	3.03	0.25	94.25	0.00	36.25	2.13	47.85	156.60	353.80	7.25	1.80
0.05	0.33	0.00	0.00	0.43	169.51	25.05	0.71	0.25	3.74	0.28	148.26	0.00	60.72	3.97	73.37	227.70	425.04	220.11	2.38
0.01	0.04	0.00	0.00	0.50	44.53	49.64	0.01	0.04	0.58	0.11	7.30	0.00	5.11	0.37	10.22	12.41	136.51	856.29	0.12
0.00	0.05	0.00	0.00	0.31	34.65	109.13	0.04	0.04	0.43	0.13	10.53	0.00	8.10	0.54	11.25	20.70	153.00	3.15	0.14
0.01	0.04	0.00	0.00	0.50	867.97	49.64	0.01	0.04	0.58	0.11	7.30	0.00	5.11	0.37	10.22	12.41	136.51	856.29	0.12
0.00	0.05	0.00	0.00	0.31	483.75	109.13	0.04	0.04	0.43	0.13	10.53	0.00	8.10	0.54	11.25	20.70	153.00	3.15	0.14
0.07	0.69	0.00	0.00	0.94	231.20	13.60	0.05	0.05	0.54	0.26	19.04	0.00	31.28	2.56	20.40	24.48	262.48	2272.56	0.46
0.01	0.15	0.00	0.00	1.03	93.87	133.06	0.10	0.04	0.76	0.37	32.78	0.00	13.41	0.69	14.90	28.31	263.73	2.98	0.18
0.01	0.15	0.00	0.00	1.03	849.30	283.10	0.10	0.04	0.76	0.37	32.78	0.00	13.41	0.69	14.90	28.31	263.73	2.98	0.18
0.00	0.00	0.00	0.00	0.00	44.64	341.31	0.06	0.06	1.66	0.32	48.36	0.00	20.46	0.86	22.32	44.64	394.32	3.72	0.32
0.06	0.07	0.00	0.00	0.99	364.56	12.60	0.05	0.03	0.17	0.17	12.60	0.00	13.44	0.25	15.12	28.56	270.48	1.68	0.19
0.00	0.12	0.00	0.00	0.25	23.25	1.55	0.00	0.02	0.00	0.02	1.10	0.00	0.00	0.62	6.20	21.70	35.65	1872.40	0.03
0.00	0.11	0.00	0.00	0.23	47.19	2.72	0.01	0.04	0.09	0.01	1.43	0.00	12.87	0.76	15.73	30.03	165.88	1833.26	0.20
0.00	0.05	0.00	0.00	0.00	21.45	1.24	0.01	0.02	0.04	0.01	0.65	0.00	5.85	0.34	7.15	13.65	75.40	11.70	0.09
0.00	0.11	0.00	0.00	0.07	21.45	1.43	0.00	0.01	0.00	0.01	1.02	0.00	0.00	0.57	5.72	20.02	32.89	25.74	0.03
0.00	0.18	0.00	0.00	0.26	20.80	1.92	0.02	0.05	0.27	0.03	1.60	0.00	6.40	0.94	6.40	19.20	51.20	1502.40	0.13
0.00	0.18	0.00	0.00	0.26	20.80	1.92	0.02	0.05	0.27	0.03	1.60	0.00	6.40	0.94	6.40	19.20	51.20	28.80	0.13
0.03	0.10	0.00	0.00	0.25	2.54	18.80	0.23	0.08	0.74	0.18	11.68	0.00	35.56	0.97	40.64	17.78	264.16	2.54	0.30
0.02	0.07	0.00	0.00	0.25	9.96	23.66	0.25	0.05	0.70	0.17	11.95	0.00	34.86	0.70	34.86	14.94	303.78	2.49	0.25
0.03	0.10	0.00	0.00	0.25	2.52	18.90	0.23	0.08	0.73	0.18	11.84	0.00	35.28	0.98	40.32	17.64	264.60	2.52	0.30
0.02	0.07	0.00	0.00	0.25	4.92	18.94	0.22	0.07	0.74	0.17	11.81	0.00	36.90	0.98	44.28	9.84	312.42	2.46	0.30
0.03	0.10	0.00	0.00	0.00	2.60	18.98	0.23	0.08	0.73	0.18	11.96	0.00	36.40	0.99	39.00	18.20	265.20	2.60	0.29

USDA ID Code	Food Name	Weight in Grams*	Quantity of Units	Unit of Measure	Protein (gm)	Fat (gm)	Carbohydrate (gm)	Kcalories	Caffeine (gm)	Fiber (gm)	Cholesterol (mg)	Saturated Fat (gm)
	Pineapple, Fresh	155.0000	1.000	Cup	0.60	0.67	19.20	75.95	0.00	1.86	0.00	0.05
	Plantain, Raw	179.0000	1.000	Medium	2.33	0.66	57.08	218.38	0.00	4.12	0.00	0.26
	Plums, Cnd, Purple, Heavy Syrup	258.0000	1.000	Cup	0.93	0.26	59.96	229.62	0.00	2.58	0.00	0.03
	Plums, Cnd, Purple, Juice Pack	252.0000	1.000	Cup	1.29	0.05	38.18	146.16	0.00	2.52	0.00	0.00
	Plums, Cnd, Purple, Light Syrup	252.0000	1.000	Cup	0.93	0.25	41.03	158.76	0.00	2.52	0.00	0.03
	Plums, Cnd, Purple, Water Pack	249.0000	1.000	Cup	0.97	0.02	27.46	102.09	0.00	2.49	0.00	0.00
	Plums, Cnd, Purple, X-heavy Syru	261.0000	1.000	Cup	0.94	0.26	68.67	263.61	0.00	2.61	0.00	0.03
	Plums, Fresh	165.0000	0.500	Cup	1.30	1.02	21.47	90.75	0.00	2.48	0.00	0.08
	Potato Pancakes, Home-prepared	76.0000	1.000	Each	4.68	11.58	21.77	206.72	0.00	1.52	72.96	2.31
	Potato Puffs, Frz, Prepared	128.0000	1.000	Cup	4.29	13.73	39.01	284.16	0.00	4.10	0.00	6.53
	Potato Salad	250.0000	1.000	Cup	6.70	20.50	27.93	357.50	0.00	3.25	170.00	3.58
	Potatoes, Au Gratin, Home-prepar	245.0000	1.000	Cup	12.40	18.60	27.61	323.40	0.00	4.41	36.75	8.65
	Potatoes, Baked w/o Skin	61.0000	0.500	Cup	1.20	0.06	13.15	56.73	0.00	0.92	0.00	0.02
	Potatoes, Baked, Skin only	58.0000	1.000	Each	2.49	0.06	26.72	114.84	0.00	4.58	0.00	0.02
	Potatoes, Baked, w/ Skin	202.0000	1.000	Medium	4.65	0.20	50.96	220.18	0.00	4.85	0.00	0.06
	Potatoes, Boiled, Ckd In Skin w/	78.0000	0.500	Cup	1.46	0.08	15.70	67.86	0.00	1.40	0.00	0.02
	Potatoes, Boiled, Ckd w/o Skin	78.0000	0.500	Cup	1.33	0.08	15.61	67.08	0.00	1.40	0.00	0.02
	Potatoes, Boiled, Skin only	34.0000	1.000	Each	0.97	0.03	5.85	26.52	0.00	1.12	0.00	0.01
	Potatoes, Cnd, Drained Solids	180.0000	1.000	Cup	2.54	0.38	24.50	108.00	0.00	4.14	0.00	0.09
	Potatoes, Cnd, Solids and Liquid	300.0000	1.000	Cup	3.60	0.33	29.67	132.00	0.00	4.20	0.00	0.09
	Potatoes, Hashed Brown	156.0000	1.000	Cup	3.78	21.70	33.26	326.04	0.00	3.12	0.00	8.47
	Potatoes, Mashed, Home-prepared	210.0000	1.000	Cup	4.07	1.24	36.86	161.70	0.00	4.20	4.20	0.69
	Potatoes, Mashed, Prepared From	210.0000	1.000	Cup	3.99	11.76	31.54	237.30	0.00	4.83	8.40	3.07
	Potatoes, Microwaved w/o Skin	78.0000	0.500	Cup	1.64	0.08	18.16	78.00	0.00	1.25	0.00	0.02
	Potatoes, Microwaved, Skin only	58.0000	1.000	Each	2.55	0.06	17.19	76.56	0.00	3.19	0.00	0.02
	Potatoes, Microwaved, w/ Skin	202.0000	1.000	Medium	4.93	0.20	48.74	212.10	0.00	4.65	0.00	0.06
	Potatoes, O'brien, Home-prepared	194.0000	1.000	Cup	4.56	2.48	30.01	157.14	0.00	0.00	7.76	1.55
	Potatoes, Scalloped	245.0000	1.000	Cup	7.03	9.02	26.41	210.70	0.00	4.66	14.70	3.38
	Prunes, Dehydrated	132.0000	1.000	Cup	4.88	0.96	117.57	447.48	0.00	0.00	0.00	0.08
	Prunes, Dried, Stewed, w/ Added	248.0000	1.000	Cup	2.70	0.55	81.54	307.52	0.00	9.42	0.00	0.05
	Prunes, Dried, Stewed, w/o Added	248.0000	1.000	Cup	2.90	0.57	69.64	265.36	0.00	16.37	0.00	0.05
	Prunes, Dried, Uncooked	170.0000	1.000	Cup	4.44	0.88	106.64	406.30	0.00	12.07	0.00	0.07
	Pumpkin, Ckd	245.0000	1.000	Cup	1.76	0.17	11.98	49.00	0.00	2.70	0.00	0.10
	Pumpkin, Cnd, w/o Salt	245.0000	1.000	Cup	2.70	0.69	19.80	83.30	0.00	7.11	0.00	0.37
	Radishes, Fresh	116.0000	1.000	Cup	0.70	0.63	4.16	23.20	0.00	1.86	0.00	0.03
	Radishes, Oriental, Ckd	147.0000	0.500	Cup	0.98	0.35	5.04	24.99	0.00	2.35	0.00	0.10
	Radishes, Oriental, Dried	116.0000	1.000	Cup	9.16	0.84	73.51	314.36	0.00	0.00	0.00	0.26
	Radishes, Oriental, Fresh	338.0000	1.000	Each	2.03	0.34	13.89	60.84	0.00	5.41	0.00	0.10
	Radishes, White Icicle, Fresh	50.0000	0.500	Cup	0.55	0.05	1.32	7.00	0.00	0.70	0.00	0.02
	Raisins, Golden Seedless	165.0000	1.000	Cup	5.59	0.76	131.21	498.30	0.00	6.60	0.00	0.25
	Raisins, Seeded	165.0000	1.000	Cup	4.16	0.89	129.48	488.40	0.00	11.22	0.00	0.30
	Raisins, Seedless	165.0000	1.000	Cup	5.31	0.76	130.56	495.00	0.00	6.60	0.00	0.25
	Raspberries, Cnd, Red, Heavy Syr	256.0000	1.000	Cup	2.12	0.31	59.80	232.96	0.00	8.45	0.00	0.03
	Raspberries, Fresh	123.0000	1.000	Cup	1.12	0.68	14.23	60.27	0.00	8.36	0.00	0.02
	Raspberries, Frozen, Red, Sweete	250.0000	1.000	Cup	1.75	0.40	65.40	257.50	0.00	11.00	0.00	0.03
	Sauerkraut, Cnd, Solid & Liquid	142.0000	1.000	Cup	1.29	0.20	6.08	26.98	0.00	3.55	0.00	0.06
	Shallots, Freeze-dried	0.9000	1.000	Tbsp	0.11	0.00	0.73	3.13	0.00	0.00	0.00	0.00
	Shallots, Fresh	10.0000	1.000	Tbsp	0.25	0.01	1.68	7.20	0.00	0.00	0.00	0.00
	Spinach, Ckd	180.0000	1.000	Cup	5.35	0.47	6.75	41.40	0.00	4.32	0.00	0.07
	Spinach, Cnd, Drained Solids	214.0000	1.000	Cup	6.01	1.07	7.28	49.22	0.00	5.14	0.00	0.17
	Spinach, Cnd, Reg Pk, Solid & Li	234.0000	1.000	Cup	4.94	0.87	6.83	44.46	0.00	3.74	0.00	0.14
	Spinach, Fresh	30.0000	1.000	Cup	0.86	0.11	1.05	6.60	0.00	0.81	0.00	0.02
	Spinach, Frz, Ckd	220.0000	1.250	Cup	6.91	0.46	11.75	61.60	0.00	6.60	0.00	0.07
	Spinach, Frz, Unprepared	156.0000	1.000	Cup	4.56	0.48	6.24	37.44	0.00	4.68	0.00	0.08
	Squash, Acorn, Ckd, w/o Salt	205.0000	1.000	Cup	2.30	0.29	29.89	114.80	0.00	9.02	0.00	0.06

Monounsaturated Fat (gm)	Polyunsaturated Fat (gm)	Vitamin D (mg)	Vitamin K (mg)	Vitamin E (mg)	Vitamin A (re)	Vitamin C (mg)	Thiamin (mg)	Riboflavin (mg)	Niacin (mg)	Vitamin B6 (mg)	Folate (mg)	Vitamin B12 (mcg)	Calcium (mg)	Iron (mg)	Magnesium (mg)	Phosphorus (mg)	Potassium (mg)	Sodium (mg)	Zinc (mg)
0.08	0.23	0.00	0.00	0.16	3.10	23.87	0.14	0.06	0.65	0.14	16.43	0.00	10.85	0.57	21.70	10.85	175.15	1.55	0.12
0.06	0.12	0.00	0.00	0.48	202.27	32.94	0.09	0.10	1.23	0.54	39.38	0.00	5.37	1.07	66.23	60.86	893.21	7.16	0.25
0.18	0.05	0.00	0.00	1.81	67.08	1.03	0.05	0.10	0.75	0.08	6.45	0.00	23.22	2.17	12.90	33.54	234.78	49.02	0.18
0.03	0.03	0.00	0.00	1.76	254.52	7.06	0.05	0.15	1.18	0.08	6.55	0.00	25.20	0.86	20.16	37.80	388.00	2.52	0.28
0.18	0.05	0.00	0.00	1.76	65.52	1.01	0.05	0.10	0.76	0.08	6.55	0.00	22.68	2.17	12.60	32.76	234.36	50.40	0.20
0.02	0.00	0.00	0.00	1.74	226.59	6.72	0.05	0.10	0.92	0.07	6.47	0.00	17.43	0.40	12.45	32.37	313.74	2.49	0.20
0.18	0.05	0.00	0.00	0.00	65.25	1.04	0.05	0.10	0.76	0.08	6.53	0.00	23.49	2.14	13.05	31.32	232.29	49.59	0.18
0.68	0.21	0.00	0.00	0.99	52.80	15.68	0.07	0.17	0.83	0.13	3.63	0.00	6.60	0.17	11.55	16.50	283.80	0.00	0.17
3.53	4.97	0.00	0.00	0.00	10.64	16.72	0.11	0.13	1.63	0.29	17.48	0.14	18.24	1.19	25.08	84.36	597.36	386.08	0.63
5.58	1.02	0.00	0.00	0.06	2.56	8.83	0.26	0.09	2.76	0.29	21.12	0.00	38.40	2.00	24.32	61.44	486.40	954.88	0.38
6.20	9.35	0.00	0.00	0.00	82.50	25.00	0.20	0.15	2.23	0.35	16.75	0.00	47.50	1.63	37.50	130.00	635.00	1322.50	0.78
6.35	2.65	0.00	0.00	0.00	93.10	24.26	0.15	0.29	2.43	0.42	26.95	0.00	291.55	1.57	49.00	276.85	970.20	1060.85	1.69
0.00	0.02	0.00	0.13	0.02	0.00	7.81	0.07	0.01	0.85	0.18	5.55	0.00	3.05	0.21	15.25	30.50	238.51	3.05	0.18
0.00	0.02	0.00	0.00	0.02	0.00	7.83	0.07	0.06	1.78	0.35	12.53	0.00	19.72	4.08	24.94	58.58	332.34	12.18	0.28
0.00	0.08	0.00	1.07	0.10	0.00	26.06	0.22	0.06	3.33	0.71	22.22	0.00	20.20	2.75	54.54	115.14	844.36	16.16	0.65
0.00	0.03	0.00	0.00	0.04	0.00	10.14	0.09	0.02	1.12	0.23	7.80	0.00	3.90	0.24	17.16	34.32	295.62	3.12	0.23
0.00	0.03	0.00	0.00	0.04	0.00	5.77	0.08	0.02	1.02	0.21	6.94	0.00	6.24	0.24	15.60	31.20	255.84	3.90	0.21
0.00	0.01	0.00	0.00	0.00	0.00	1.77	0.01	0.01	0.41	0.08	3.30	0.00	15.30	2.06	10.20	18.36	138.38	4.76	0.15
0.02	0.16	0.00	0.00	0.09	0.00	9.18	0.13	0.02	1.66	0.34	11.16	0.00	9.00	2.27	25.20	50.40	412.20	394.20	0.50
0.00	0.15	0.00	0.00	0.12	0.00	22.80	0.09	0.06	2.67	0.42	13.50	0.00	117.00	2.16	42.00	66.00	615.00	651.00	1.17
9.69	2.50	0.00	0.00	0.30	0.00	8.89	0.11	0.03	3.12	0.44	12.01	0.00	12.48	1.26	31.20	65.52	500.76	37.44	0.47
0.32	0.13	0.00	0.00	0.11	12.60	14.07	0.19	0.08	2.35	0.48	17.22	0.00	54.60	0.57	37.80	100.80	627.90	636.30	0.61
4.85	3.26	0.00	0.00	0.00	44.10	20.37	0.23	0.11	1.41	0.02	15.54	0.00	102.90	0.46	37.80	117.60	489.30	697.20	0.38
0.00	0.03	0.00	0.00	0.00	0.00	11.78	0.10	0.02	1.27	0.25	9.67	0.00	3.90	0.32	19.50	85.02	320.58	5.46	0.26
0.00	0.02	0.00	0.00	0.00	0.00	8.87	0.04	0.05	1.29	0.28	9.63	0.00	26.68	3.45	21.46	47.56	377.00	9.28	0.30
0.00	0.08	0.00	0.00	0.00	0.00	30.50	0.24	0.06	3.45	0.69	24.24	0.00	22.22	2.50	54.54	212.10	902.94	16.16	0.73
0.68	0.12	0.00	0.00	0.00	110.58	32.40	0.16	0.12	1.96	0.41	16.10	0.00	69.84	0.91	34.92	97.00	516.04	420.98	0.58
3.31	1.84	0.00	0.00	0.00	46.55	25.97	0.17	0.22	2.57	0.44	26.95	0.00	139.65	1.40	46.55	154.35	926.10	820.75	0.98
0.63	0.21	0.00	0.00	0.00	232.32	0.00	0.16	0.22	3.96	0.99	2.51	0.00	95.04	4.65	84.48	147.84	1396.56	6.60	0.99
0.35	0.12	0.00	0.00	0.00	71.92	6.70	0.05	0.22	1.69	0.50	0.25	0.00	52.08	2.58	47.12	81.84	773.76	4.96	0.55
0.37	0.12	0.00	0.00	0.00	76.88	7.19	0.05	0.25	1.79	0.55	0.25	0.00	57.04	2.75	49.60	86.80	828.32	4.96	0.60
0.58	0.19	0.00	0.00	2.47	338.30	5.61	0.14	0.27	3.33	0.44	6.29	0.00	86.70	4.22	76.50	134.30	1266.50	2.45	0.90
0.02	0.00	0.00	0.00	2.60	264.60	11.52	0.07	0.20	1.00	0.10	20.83	0.00	36.75	1.40	22.05	73.50	563.50	2.45	0.56
0.10	0.05	0.00	36.75	2.60	5404.70	10.29	0.05	0.12	0.91	0.15	30.14	0.00	63.70	3.41	56.35	85.75	504.70	12.25	0.42
0.02	0.06	0.00	0.00	0.00	1.16	26.45	0.01	0.06	0.35	0.08	31.32	0.00	24.36	0.34	10.44	20.88	269.12	27.84	0.35
0.06	0.16	0.00	0.00	0.00	0.00	22.20	0.00	0.03	0.22	0.06	25.58	0.00	24.99	0.22	13.23	35.28	418.95	19.11	0.19
0.14	0.38	0.00	0.00	0.00	0.00	0.00	0.31	0.79	3.94	0.72	341.85	0.00	729.64	7.81	197.20	236.64	4053.04	322.48	2.47
0.07	0.17	0.00	0.00	0.00	0.00	74.36	0.07	0.07	0.68	0.17	95.32	0.00	91.26	1.35	54.08	77.74	767.26	70.98	0.51
0.01	0.03	0.00	0.00	0.00	0.00	14.50	0.02	0.01	0.15	0.04	7.00	0.00	13.50	0.40	4.50	14.00	140.00	8.00	0.07
0.03	0.23	0.00	0.00	1.16	6.60	5.28	0.02	0.31	1.88	0.53	5.45	0.00	87.45	2.95	57.75	189.75	1230.90	19.80	0.53
0.03	0.26	0.00	0.00	1.16	0.00	8.91	0.18	0.30	1.83	0.31	5.45	0.00	46.20	4.27	49.50	123.75	1361.25	46.20	0.30
0.03	0.23	0.00	0.00	1.16	1.65	5.45	0.26	0.15	1.35	0.41	5.45	0.00	80.85	3.43	54.45	160.05	1239.15	19.80	0.45
0.03	0.18	0.00	0.00	1.15	7.68	22.27	0.05	0.08	1.13	0.10	26.88	0.00	28.16	1.08	30.72	23.04	240.64	7.68	0.41
0.06	0.38	0.00	0.00	0.55	15.99	30.75	0.04	0.11	1.11	0.07	31.98	0.00	27.06	0.70	22.14	14.76	186.96	0.00	0.57
0.05	0.23	0.00	0.00	1.13	15.00	41.25	0.05	0.13	0.58	0.08	65.00	0.00	37.50	1.63	32.50	42.50	285.00	2.50	0.45
0.01	0.09	0.00	0.00	0.14	2.84	20.87	0.03	0.03	0.20	0.18	33.65	0.00	42.60	2.09	18.46	28.40	241.40	938.62	0.27
0.00	0.00	0.00	0.00	0.00	50.49	0.35	0.00	0.00	0.01	0.02	1.05	0.00	1.65	0.05	0.94	2.66	14.85	0.53	0.02
0.00	0.00	0.00	0.00	0.00	11.90	0.80	0.01	0.00	0.02	0.04	3.42	0.00	3.70	0.12	2.10	6.00	33.40	1.20	0.04
0.02	0.20	0.00	0.00	1.73	1474.20	17.64	0.18	0.43	0.88	0.43	262.44	0.00	244.80	6.43	156.60	100.80	838.80	126.00	1.37
0.02	0.45	0.00	0.00	2.78	1878.92	30.60	0.04	0.30	0.83	0.21	209.29	0.00	271.78	4.92	162.64	94.16	740.44	57.78	0.98
0.02	0.37	0.00	0.00	2.50	1504.62	31.59	0.05	0.26	0.63	0.19	135.72	0.00	194.22	3.70	131.04	74.88	538.20	746.46	0.98
0.00	0.05	0.00	79.80	0.57	201.60	8.43	0.02	0.06	0.22	0.06	58.32	0.00	29.70	0.81	23.70	14.70	167.40	23.70	0.16
0.02	0.20	0.00	0.00	2.11	1711.60	27.06	0.13	0.37	0.92	0.33	236.50	0.00	321.20	3.34	151.80	105.60	655.60	189.20	1.54
0.02	0.20	0.00	215.28	1.50	1210.56	37.91	0.12	0.23	0.69	0.22	186.58	0.00	173.16	3.20	90.48	63.96	503.88	115.44	0.69
0.02	0.12	0.00	0.00	0.00	88.15	22.14	0.35	0.02	1.80	0.39	38.34	0.00	90.20	1.91	88.15	92.25	895.85	8.20	0.35

USDA ID Code	Food Name	Weight in Grams*	Quantity of Units	Unit of Measure	Protein (gm)	Fat (gm)	Carbohydrate (gm)	Kcalories	Caffeine (gm)	Fiber (gm)	Cholesterol (mg)	Saturated Fat (gm)
	Squash, Butternut, Ckd, w/o Salt	205.0000	1.000	Cup	1.85	0.18	21.50	82.00	0.00	0.00	0.00	0.04
	Squash, Spaghetti, Ckd. w/o Salt	155.0000	1.000	Cup	1.02	0.40	10.01	41.85	0.00	2.17	0.00	0.09
	Squash, Summer, Ckd	180.0000	0.500	Cup	1.64	0.56	7.76	36.00	0.00	2.52	0.00	0.11
	Squash, Summer, Fresh	113.0000	0.500	Cup	1.33	0.24	4.92	22.60	0.00	2.15	0.00	0.05
	Squash, Winter, Baked	205.0000	1.000	Cup	1.82	1.29	17.94	79.95	0.00	5.74	0.00	0.27
	Squash, Winter, Fresh	116.0000	1.000	Cup	1.68	0.27	10.21	42.92	0.00	1.74	0.00	0.06
	Squash, Zucchini, Baby, Fresh	16.0000	1.000	Large	0.43	0.06	0.50	3.36	0.00	0.18	0.00	0.01
	Strawberries, Fresh	152.0000	1.000	Cup	0.93	0.56	10.67	45.60	0.00	3.50	0.00	0.03
	Strawberries, Frozen, Sweetened	255.0000	1.000	Cup	1.35	0.33	66.10	244.80	0.00	4.85	0.00	0.03
	Strawberries, Frozen, Unsweetene	221.0000	1.000	Cup	0.95	0.24	20.18	77.35	0.00	4.64	0.00	0.02
	Sweet Potatoes, Baked In Skin	200.0000	1.000	Cup	3.44	0.22	48.54	206.00	0.00	6.00	0.00	0.04
	Sweet Potatoes, Boiled, w/o Skin	328.0000	1.000	Cup	5.41	0.98	79.64	344.40	0.00	5.90	0.00	0.20
	Sweet Potatoes, Candied	105.0000	1.000	Piece	0.91	3.41	29.25	143.85	0.00	2.52	8.40	1.42
	Sweet Potatoes, Mashed	255.0000	1.000	Cup	5.05	0.51	59.16	257.55	0.00	4.34	0.00	0.10
	Sweet Potatoes, Syrup Pack, Drai	196.0000	1.000	Cup	2.51	0.63	49.71	211.68	0.00	5.88	0.00	0.14
	Tangerines, Cnd, Juice Pack	249.0000	1.000	Cup	1.54	0.07	23.83	92.13	0.00	1.74	0.00	0.00
	Tangerines, Cnd, Light Syrup Pac	252.0000	1.000	Cup	1.13	0.25	40.80	153.72	0.00	1.76	0.00	0.03
	Tangerines, Fresh	195.0000	1.000	Cup	1.23	0.37	21.82	85.80	0.00	4.48	0.00	0.04
	Tator Tots	2.8350	10.000	Each	0.30	0.50	2.00	14.00	0.00	0.30	0.00	0.10
	Tomatillos, Fresh	34.0000	1.000	Slice	0.33	0.35	1.98	10.88	0.00	0.65	0.00	0.05
	Tomatoes, Cherry	149.0000	1.000	Cup	1.27	0.49	6.91	31.29	0.00	1.64	0.00	0.07
	Tomatoes, Ckd, Boiled	240.0000	1.000	Cup	2.57	0.98	13.99	64.80	0.00	2.40	0.00	0.14
	Tomatoes, Ckd, Stewed	101.0000	1.000	Cup	1.98	2.71	13.18	79.79	0.00	1.72	0.00	0.53
	Tomatoes, Cnd, Stewed	255.0000	1.000	Cup	2.42	0.33	17.29	71.40	0.00	2.55	0.00	0.05
	Tomatoes, Cnd, w/ Green Chilies	241.0000	1.000	Cup	1.66	0.19	8.72	36.15	0.00	0.00	0.00	0.02
	Tomatoes, Cnd, Wedges In Tomato	261.0000	1.000	Cup	2.06	0.42	16.47	67.86	0.00	0.00	0.00	0.05
	Tomatoes, Cnd, Whole, Reg Pk	240.0000	1.000	Cup	2.21	0.31	10.49	45.60	0.00	2.40	0.00	0.05
	Tomatoes, Fresh	149.0000	1.000	Cup	1.27	0.49	6.91	31.29	0.00	1.64	0.00	0.07
	Tomatoes, Green, Fresh	180.0000	1.000	Cup	2.16	0.36	9.18	43.20	0.00	1.98	0.00	0.05
	Tomatoes, Sun-dried	54.0000	0.250	Cup	7.62	1.60	30.11	139.32	0.00	6.64	0.00	0.23
	Tomatoes, Sun-dried, Packed In O	110.0000	1.000	Cup	5.57	15.49	25.66	234.30	0.00	6.38	0.00	2.08
	Turnips, Ckd	156.0000	1.000	Cup	1.11	0.12	7.64	32.76	0.00	3.12	0.00	0.02
	Turnips, Fresh	130.0000	1.000	Cup	1.17	0.13	8.10	35.10	0.00	2.34	0.00	0.01
	Vegetables, Mixed, Cnd	163.0000	1.000	Cup	4.22	0.41	15.09	76.61	0.00	4.89	0.00	0.08
	Vegetables, Mixed, Frz	275.0000	1.250	Cup	7.87	0.41	36.00	162.25	0.00	12.10	0.00	0.08
	Veggie Burger	90.0000	1.000	Each	18.00	4.00	8.00	140.00	0.00	5.00	0.00	1.50
	Watercress, Raw	2.5000	1.000	Sprig	0.06	0.00	0.03	0.28	0.00	0.04	0.00	0.00
	Watermelon	154.0000	1.000	Cup	0.95	0.66	11.06	49.28	0.00	0.77	0.00	0.08
	Yam, Baked	136.0000	1.000	Cup	2.03	0.19	37.54	157.76	0.00	5.30	0.00	0.04

Meats and Beans

USDA ID Code	Food Name	Weight in Grams*	Quantity of Units	Unit of Measure	Protein (gm)	Fat (gm)	Carbohydrate (gm)	Kcalories	Caffeine (gm)	Fiber (gm)	Cholesterol (mg)	Saturated Fat (gm)
	Bacon	19.0000	3.000	Slice	5.79	9.36	0.11	109.44	0.00	0.00	16.15	3.31
	Bacon, Canadian-style Bacon, Gri	46.5000	2.000	Slice	11.27	3.92	0.63	86.03	0.00	0.00	26.97	1.32
	Bacon, Turkey	14.0000	1.000	Slice	3.00	2.00	0.00	25.00	0.00	0.00	10.00	0.50
	Barbecue Loaf, Lunch Meat	23.0000	1.000	Slice	3.64	2.05	1.47	39.79	0.00	0.00	8.51	0.73
	Beans, Baked, Cnd, Vegetarian	254.0000	1.000	Cup	12.17	1.14	52.10	236.22	0.00	12.70	0.00	0.30
	Beans, Baked, Cnd, w/ Beef	266.0000	1.000	Cup	16.97	9.18	44.98	321.86	0.00	0.00	58.52	4.47
	Beans, Baked, Cnd, w/ Franks	259.0000	1.000	Cup	17.48	17.02	39.86	367.78	0.00	17.87	15.54	6.09
	Beans, Baked, Cnd, w/ Pork	253.0000	1.000	Cup	13.13	3.92	50.55	268.18	0.00	13.92	17.71	1.52
	Beans, Baked, Home Prepared	253.0000	1.000	Cup	14.02	13.03	54.12	382.03	0.00	13.92	12.65	4.93
	Beans, Black, Ckd	172.0000	1.000	Cup	15.24	0.93	40.78	227.04	0.00	14.96	0.00	0.24
	Beans, Garbanzo, Cnd	240.0000	1.000	Cup	11.88	2.74	54.29	285.60	0.00	10.56	0.00	0.29
	Beans, Kidney, Cnd	256.0000	1.000	Cup	13.31	0.79	38.09	207.36	0.00	8.96	0.00	0.13
1	Beans, Lentils	198.0000	1.000	Cup	17.87	0.74	39.87	231.00	0.00	5.46	0.00	0.11
	Beans, Lima, Cnd	241.0000	1.000	Cup	11.88	0.41	35.93	190.39	0.00	11.57	0.00	0.10
	Beans, Navy, Cnd	262.0000	1.000	Cup	19.73	1.13	53.58	296.06	0.00	13.36	0.00	0.29

Monounsaturated Fat (gm)	Polyunsaturated Fat (gm)	Vitamin D (mg)	Vitamin K (mg)	Vitamin E (mg)	Vitamin A (re)	Vitamin C (mg)	Thiamin (mg)	Riboflavin (mg)	Niacin (mg)	Vitamin B$_6$ (mg)	Folate (mcg)	Vitamin B$_{12}$ (mcg)	Calcium (mg)	Iron (mg)	Magnesium (mg)	Phosphorus (mg)	Potassium (mg)	Sodium (mg)	Zinc (mg)
0.02	0.08	0.00	0.00	0.00	1435.00	30.96	0.14	0.04	1.99	0.25	39.36	0.00	84.05	1.23	59.45	55.35	582.20	8.20	0.27
0.03	0.20	0.00	0.00	0.19	17.05	5.43	0.06	0.03	1.26	0.16	12.40	0.00	32.55	0.53	17.05	21.70	181.35	27.90	0.31
0.04	0.23	0.00	0.00	0.22	52.20	9.90	0.07	0.07	0.92	0.13	36.18	0.00	48.60	0.65	43.20	70.20	345.60	1.80	0.70
0.02	0.10	0.00	0.00	0.14	22.60	16.72	0.07	0.05	0.62	0.12	28.93	0.00	22.60	0.52	25.99	39.55	220.35	2.26	0.29
0.10	0.55	0.00	0.00	0.25	729.80	19.68	0.18	0.04	1.44	0.14	57.40	0.00	28.70	0.68	16.40	41.00	895.85	2.05	0.53
0.02	0.10	0.00	0.00	0.14	470.96	14.27	0.12	0.03	0.93	0.09	25.17	0.00	35.96	0.67	24.36	37.12	406.00	4.64	0.15
0.00	0.03	0.00	0.00	0.00	7.84	5.46	0.01	0.01	0.11	0.02	3.20	0.00	3.36	0.13	5.28	14.88	73.44	0.48	0.13
0.08	0.29	0.00	21.28	0.21	4.56	86.18	0.03	0.11	0.35	0.09	26.90	0.00	21.28	0.58	15.20	28.88	252.32	1.52	0.20
0.05	0.15	0.00	0.00	0.36	5.10	105.57	0.05	0.13	1.02	0.08	38.00	0.00	28.05	1.50	17.85	33.15	249.90	7.65	0.15
0.04	0.11	0.00	0.00	0.60	8.84	91.05	0.04	0.09	1.02	0.07	37.13	0.00	35.36	1.66	24.31	28.73	327.08	4.42	0.29
0.00	0.10	0.00	0.00	0.56	4364.00	49.20	0.14	0.26	1.20	0.48	45.20	0.00	56.00	0.90	40.00	110.00	696.00	20.00	0.58
0.03	0.43	0.00	0.00	0.92	5592.40	56.09	0.16	0.46	2.10	0.79	36.41	0.00	68.88	1.84	32.80	88.56	603.52	42.64	0.89
0.66	0.16	0.00	0.00	0.00	439.95	7.04	0.02	0.04	0.41	0.04	11.97	0.00	27.30	1.19	11.55	27.30	198.45	73.50	0.16
0.03	0.23	0.00	0.00	0.69	3858.15	13.26	0.08	0.23	2.45	0.61	27.29	0.00	76.50	3.39	61.20	132.60	535.50	191.25	0.54
0.02	0.27	0.00	0.00	0.55	1403.36	21.17	0.06	0.08	0.67	0.12	15.48	0.00	33.32	1.86	23.52	49.00	378.28	76.44	0.31
0.02	0.02	0.00	0.00	1.25	211.65	85.16	0.20	0.07	1.12	0.10	11.45	0.00	27.39	0.67	27.39	24.90	331.17	12.45	1.27
0.05	0.05	0.00	0.00	0.86	211.68	49.90	0.13	0.10	1.13	0.10	11.59	0.00	17.64	0.93	20.16	25.20	196.56	15.12	0.60
0.06	0.08	0.00	0.00	0.47	179.40	60.06	0.21	0.04	0.31	0.14	39.78	0.00	27.30	0.20	23.40	19.50	306.15	1.95	0.47
0.00	0.00	0.00	0.00	0.00	0.00	0.00	0.00	0.00	0.00	0.00	0.00	0.00	0.00	0.00	0.00	0.00	24.00	24.00	0.00
0.05	0.14	0.00	0.00	0.13	3.74	3.98	0.01	0.01	0.63	0.02	2.38	0.00	2.38	0.21	6.80	13.26	91.12	0.34	0.07
0.07	0.21	0.00	0.00	0.57	92.38	38.74	0.09	0.07	0.94	0.12	22.35	0.00	7.45	0.67	16.39	35.76	330.78	13.41	0.13
0.14	0.41	0.00	0.00	0.91	177.60	54.72	0.17	0.14	1.80	0.24	31.20	0.00	14.40	1.34	33.60	74.40	669.60	26.40	0.26
1.06	0.89	0.00	0.00	1.28	67.67	18.38	0.11	0.08	1.12	0.09	11.11	0.00	26.26	1.07	15.15	38.38	249.47	459.55	0.18
0.05	0.13	0.00	0.00	0.97	137.70	29.07	0.13	0.10	1.81	0.05	13.77	0.00	84.15	1.86	30.60	51.00	606.90	563.55	0.43
0.02	0.07	0.00	0.00	0.00	93.99	14.94	0.07	0.05	1.54	0.24	21.93	0.00	48.20	0.63	26.51	33.74	257.87	966.41	0.31
0.05	0.18	0.00	0.00	0.00	151.38	38.63	0.16	0.08	1.77	0.31	26.36	0.00	67.86	1.20	28.71	60.03	655.11	566.37	0.42
0.05	0.12	0.00	0.00	0.77	144.00	34.08	0.12	0.07	1.78	0.22	18.72	0.00	72.00	1.32	28.80	45.60	530.40	355.20	0.38
0.07	0.21	0.00	34.27	0.57	92.38	28.46	0.09	0.07	0.94	0.12	22.35	0.00	7.45	0.67	16.39	35.76	330.78	13.41	0.13
0.05	0.14	0.00	84.60	0.68	115.20	42.12	0.11	0.07	0.90	0.14	15.84	0.00	23.40	0.92	18.00	50.40	367.20	23.40	0.13
0.26	0.60	0.00	0.00	0.01	46.98	21.17	0.29	0.26	4.89	0.18	36.72	0.00	59.40	4.91	104.76	192.24	1850.58	1131.30	1.07
9.53	2.27	0.00	0.00	0.00	141.90	111.98	0.21	0.42	3.99	0.35	25.30	0.00	51.70	2.95	89.10	152.90	1721.50	292.60	0.86
0.02	0.06	0.00	0.00	0.05	0.00	18.10	0.05	0.03	0.47	0.11	14.35	0.00	34.32	0.34	12.48	29.64	210.60	78.00	0.31
0.01	0.07	0.00	0.00	0.04	0.00	27.30	0.05	0.04	0.52	0.12	18.85	0.00	39.00	0.39	14.30	35.10	248.30	87.10	0.35
0.03	0.20	0.00	0.00	0.98	1898.95	8.15	0.08	0.08	0.95	0.13	38.47	0.00	44.01	1.71	26.08	68.46	474.33	242.87	0.67
0.03	0.19	0.00	0.00	0.99	1177.00	8.80	0.19	0.33	2.34	0.19	52.25	0.00	68.75	2.26	60.50	140.25	464.75	96.25	1.35
0.00	0.50	0.00	0.00	0.00	0.00	0.00	0.25	0.00	4.00	0.00	0.00	0.00	96.00	1.50	0.00	0.00	0.00	380.00	7.50
0.00	0.00	0.00	0.00	0.03	11.75	1.08	0.00	0.00	0.01	0.00	0.23	0.00	3.00	0.01	0.53	1.50	8.25	1.03	0.00
0.17	0.23	0.00	0.00	0.23	56.98	14.78	0.12	0.03	0.31	0.22	3.39	0.00	12.32	0.26	16.94	13.86	178.64	3.08	0.11
0.01	0.08	0.00	0.00	0.22	0.00	16.46	0.14	0.04	0.75	0.31	21.76	0.00	19.04	0.71	24.48	66.64	911.20	10.88	0.27
4.50	1.10	0.00	0.00	0.10	0.00	0.00	0.13	0.06	1.39	0.05	0.95	0.33	2.28	0.31	4.56	63.84	92.34	303.24	0.62
1.88	0.38	0.00	0.00	0.12	0.00	0.00	0.38	0.09	3.22	0.21	1.86	0.36	4.65	0.38	9.77	137.64	181.35	718.89	0.79
0.00	0.00	0.00	0.00	0.00	0.00	0.00	0.00	0.00	0.00	0.00	0.00	0.00	0.00	0.00	0.00	0.00	0.00	170.00	0.00
0.95	0.19	0.21	0.00	0.00	1.61	0.00	0.08	0.06	0.52	0.06	2.07	0.39	12.65	0.27	3.91	30.36	75.67	306.82	0.57
0.10	0.48	0.00	0.00	1.35	43.18	7.87	0.38	0.15	1.09	0.33	60.71	0.00	127.00	0.74	81.28	264.16	751.84	1008.38	3.56
3.70	0.56	0.00	0.00	0.00	55.86	4.79	0.13	0.13	2.50	0.24	115.44	0.00	119.70	4.26	66.50	215.46	851.20	1263.50	3.19
7.33	2.18	0.00	0.00	1.22	38.85	5.96	0.16	0.16	2.33	0.13	77.70	0.00	124.32	4.48	72.52	269.36	608.65	1113.70	4.84
1.70	0.51	0.00	0.00	0.00	45.54	5.06	0.13	0.10	1.14	0.15	91.84	0.00	134.09	4.30	86.02	273.24	781.77	1047.42	3.69
5.39	1.87	0.00	0.00	0.00	0.00	2.78	0.35	0.13	1.04	0.23	122.45	0.00	154.33	5.03	108.79	275.77	905.74	1067.66	1.85
0.09	0.40	0.00	0.00	0.00	1.72	0.00	0.41	0.10	0.88	0.12	255.94	0.00	46.44	3.61	120.40	240.80	610.60	407.64	1.93
0.62	1.22	0.00	0.00	0.00	4.80	9.12	0.07	0.07	0.34	1.13	160.32	0.00	76.80	3.24	69.60	216.00	412.80	717.60	2.54
0.05	0.44	0.00	0.00	0.00	0.00	3.07	0.28	0.18	1.28	0.18	125.95	0.00	69.12	3.15	79.36	268.80	657.92	888.32	1.41
0.13	0.35	0.00	0.00	0.00	2.00	2.90	0.34	0.15	2.10	0.35	357.90	0.00	37.00	6.59	71.00	356.00	731.00	4.00	2.50
0.05	0.17	0.00	0.00	0.00	0.00	0.00	0.14	0.07	0.63	0.22	121.46	0.00	50.61	4.36	93.99	178.34	530.20	809.76	1.57
0.10	0.50	0.00	0.00	1.00	0.00	1.83	0.37	0.16	1.28	0.26	163.23	0.00	123.14	4.85	123.14	351.08	754.56	1173.76	2.02

USDA ID Code	Food Name	Weight in Grams*	Quantity of Units	Unit of Measure	Protein (gm)	Fat (gm)	Carbohydrate (gm)	Kcalories	Caffeine (gm)	Fiber (gm)	Cholesterol (mg)	Saturated Fat (gm)
	Beans, Pinto, Cnd	240.0000	1.000	Cup	11.66	1.94	36.60	206.40	0.00	11.04	0.00	0.41
	Beans, Refried, Cnd	15.8000	1.000	Tbsp	0.87	0.20	2.45	14.85	0.00	0.84	1.26	0.07
	Beans, Refried, Lowfat, Cnd	268.0000	0.500	Cup	16.00	0.00	42.00	240.00	0.00	14.00	0.00	0.00
2	Beans, Refried, No Fat	128.0000	0.500	Cup	7.30	0.50	19.50	92.00	0.00	6.20	0.00	0.00
	Beef, Corned, Brisket, Ckd	85.0000	3.000	Ounce	15.44	16.13	0.40	213.35	0.00	0.00	83.30	5.39
	Beef, Corned, Loaf, Jellied	28.3500	1.000	Slice	6.49	1.73	0.00	43.38	0.00	0.00	13.32	0.74
	Beef, Cured, Lunch Meat, Jellied	28.3500	1.000	Slice	5.39	0.94	0.00	31.47	0.00	0.00	9.64	0.40
	Beef, Cured, Smoked, Chopped Bee	28.3500	1.000	Slice	5.72	1.25	0.53	37.71	0.00	0.00	13.04	0.51
	Beef, Cured, Thin-sliced	21.0000	5.000	Slice	5.90	0.81	1.20	37.17	0.00	0.00	8.61	0.35
	Beef, Filet, Tnderloin, Broiled	85.0000	3.000	Ounce	23.55	9.75	0.00	188.70	0.00	0.00	70.55	3.68
	Beef, Ground, Extra Lean, Broile	85.0000	3.000	Ounce	21.59	13.88	0.00	217.60	0.00	0.00	71.40	5.46
	Beef, Ground, Extra Lean, Pan-fr	85.0000	3.000	Ounce	21.22	13.96	0.00	216.75	0.00	0.00	68.85	5.48
	Beef, Ground, Lean, Broiled	85.0000	3.000	Ounce	21.01	15.69	0.00	231.20	0.00	0.00	73.95	6.16
	Beef, Ground, Lean, Pan-fried	85.0000	3.000	Ounce	20.60	16.20	0.00	233.75	0.00	0.00	71.40	6.37
	Beef, Ground, Regular, Broiled	85.0000	3.000	Ounce	20.46	17.59	0.00	245.65	0.00	0.00	76.50	6.91
	Beef, Ground, Regular, Pan-fried	85.0000	3.000	Ounce	20.33	19.18	0.00	260.10	0.00	0.00	75.65	7.53
	Beef, Liver, Ckd, Braised	85.0000	3.000	Ounce	20.72	4.16	2.90	136.85	0.00	0.00	330.65	1.62
	Beef, Liver, Ckd, Pan-fried	85.0000	3.000	Ounce	22.71	6.80	6.67	184.45	0.00	0.00	409.70	2.27
	Beef, Loaved, Lunch Meat	28.3500	1.000	Slice	4.08	7.43	0.82	87.32	0.00	0.00	18.14	3.17
	Beef, Steaks and Roasts, Ckd, 1/	28.3500	3.000	Ounce	7.07	7.62	0.00	98.94	0.00	0.00	25.80	3.15
	Beef, Steaks and Roasts, Ckd, Fa	85.0000	3.000	Ounce	23.23	14.76	0.00	232.05	0.00	0.00	73.95	5.82
	Beef, Steaks and Roasts, Ckd., 1	85.0000	3.000	Ounce	22.05	18.31	0.00	259.25	0.00	0.00	74.80	7.26
	Beef, Thin Sliced	21.0000	5.000	Slice	5.90	0.81	1.20	37.17	0.00	0.00	8.61	0.35
	Bologna, Beef, Lunch Meat	23.0000	1.000	Slice	2.81	6.56	0.18	71.76	0.00	0.00	13.34	2.78
	Bologna, Lunch Meat	23.0000	1.000	Slice	3.52	4.57	0.17	56.81	0.00	0.00	13.57	1.58
	Bologna, Turkey	21.0000	1.000	Slice	2.88	3.19	0.20	41.79	0.00	0.00	20.79	1.06
	Buffalo (Chicken) Wings	22.7500	4.000	Each	4.50	3.00	0.50	47.50	0.00	0.00	25.00	0.75
	Chicken Roll, Light Meat	28.3500	3.000	Ounce	5.54	2.09	0.69	45.08	0.00	0.00	14.18	0.57
	Chicken Salad Sandwich Spread	28.3500	3.000	Ounce	3.30	3.83	2.10	56.70	0.00	0.00	8.51	0.98
	Chicken Spread, Cnd	28.3500	3.000	Ounce	4.37	3.32	1.53	54.43	0.00	0.00	14.74	0.96
	Chicken, Back, Meat & Skin, Ckd,	72.0000	3.000	Ounce	15.82	15.78	7.38	238.32	0.00	0.00	63.36	4.20
	Chicken, Back, Meat & Skin, Ckd,	44.0000	3.000	Ounce	12.23	9.13	2.86	145.64	0.00	0.00	39.16	2.47
	Chicken, Back, Meat & Skin, Ckd,	32.0000	3.000	Ounce	8.30	6.71	0.00	96.00	0.00	0.00	28.16	1.86
	Chicken, Back, Meat & Skin, Ckd,	36.0000	3.000	Ounce	7.98	6.53	0.00	92.88	0.00	0.00	28.08	1.81
	Chicken, Back, Meat Only, Ckd, F	35.0000	3.000	Ounce	10.50	5.36	1.99	100.80	0.00	0.00	32.55	1.44
	Chicken, Back, Meat Only, Ckd, R	24.0000	3.000	Ounce	6.77	3.16	0.00	57.36	0.00	0.00	21.60	0.86
	Chicken, Back, Meat Only, Ckd, S	26.0000	3.000	Ounce	6.58	2.91	0.00	54.34	0.00	0.00	22.10	0.79
	Chicken, Breast, Meat & Skin, Ck	84.0000	3.000	Ounce	20.87	11.09	7.55	218.40	0.00	0.25	71.40	2.96
	Chicken, Breast, Meat & Skin, Ck	59.0000	3.000	Ounce	18.79	5.23	0.97	130.98	0.00	0.06	52.51	1.45
	Chicken, Breast, Meat & Skin, Ck	58.0000	3.000	Ounce	17.28	4.51	0.00	114.26	0.00	0.00	48.72	1.27
	Chicken, Breast, Meat & Skin, Ck	66.0000	3.000	Ounce	18.08	4.90	0.00	121.44	0.00	0.00	49.50	1.37
	Chicken, Breast, Meat Only, Ckd,	52.0000	3.000	Ounce	17.39	2.45	0.27	97.24	0.00	0.00	47.32	0.67
	Chicken, Breast, Meat Only, Ckd,	52.0000	3.000	Ounce	16.13	1.86	0.00	85.80	0.00	0.00	44.20	0.53
	Chicken, Breast, Meat Only, Ckd,	57.0000	3.000	Ounce	16.52	1.73	0.00	86.07	0.00	0.00	43.89	0.48
	Chicken, Cnd	142.0000	5.000	Fl Oz	30.91	11.29	0.00	234.30	0.00	0.00	88.04	3.12
	Chicken, Dark Meat, Meat & Skin,	167.0000	3.000	Ounce	36.49	31.13	15.66	497.66	0.00	0.00	148.63	8.27
	Chicken, Dark Meat, Meat & Skin,	110.0000	3.000	Ounce	29.94	18.60	4.49	313.50	0.00	0.00	101.20	5.04
	Chicken, Dark Meat, Meat & Skin,	101.0000	3.000	Ounce	26.23	15.94	0.00	255.53	0.00	0.00	91.91	4.41
	Chicken, Dark Meat, Meat & Skin,	110.0000	3.000	Ounce	25.85	16.13	0.00	256.30	0.00	0.00	90.20	4.47
	Chicken, Dark Meat, Meat Only, C	91.0000	3.000	Ounce	26.38	10.57	2.36	217.49	0.00	0.00	87.36	2.84
	Chicken, Dark Meat, Meat Only, C	81.0000	3.000	Ounce	22.17	7.88	0.00	166.05	0.00	0.00	75.33	2.15
	Chicken, Dark Meat, Meat Only, C	86.0000	3.000	Ounce	22.33	7.72	0.00	165.12	0.00	0.00	75.68	2.11
	Chicken, Drumstick, Meat & Skin,	43.0000	3.000	Ounce	9.44	6.77	3.56	115.24	0.00	0.13	36.98	1.78
	Chicken, Drumstick, Meat & Skin,	29.0000	3.000	Ounce	7.82	3.98	0.47	71.05	0.00	0.03	26.10	1.06
	Chicken, Drumstick, Meat & Skin,	31.0000	3.000	Ounce	8.38	3.46	0.00	66.96	0.00	0.00	28.21	0.95

Monounsaturated Fat (gm)	Polyunsaturated Fat (gm)	Vitamin D (mg)	Vitamin K (mg)	Vitamin E (mg)	Vitamin A (re)	Vitamin C (mg)	Thiamin (mg)	Riboflavin (mg)	Niacin (mg)	Vitamin B6 (mg)	Folate (mg)	Vitamin B12 (mcg)	Calcium (mg)	Iron (mg)	Magnesium (mg)	Phosphorus (mg)	Potassium (mg)	Sodium (mg)	Zinc (mg)
0.38	0.70	0.00	0.00	2.26	4.80	2.16	0.24	0.14	0.70	0.17	144.48	0.00	103.20	3.50	64.80	220.80	583.20	705.60	1.66
0.09	0.02	0.00	0.00	0.00	0.00	0.95	0.00	0.00	0.05	0.02	1.74	0.00	5.53	0.26	5.21	13.59	42.19	47.24	0.18
0.00	0.00	0.00	0.00	0.00	0.00	0.00	0.00	0.00	0.00	0.00	0.00	0.00	0.00	2.00	0.00	0.00	0.00	960.00	0.00
0.00	0.00	0.00	0.00	0.00	0.00	0.00	0.00	0.00	0.00	0.00	0.00	0.00	43.00	1.92	0.00	0.00	0.00	480.00	0.00
7.84	0.57	0.00	0.00	0.14	0.00	0.00	0.03	0.14	2.58	0.20	5.10	1.39	6.80	1.58	10.20	106.25	123.25	963.90	3.89
0.76	0.09	0.00	0.00	0.05	0.00	0.00	0.00	0.03	0.50	0.03	2.27	0.36	3.12	0.58	3.12	20.70	28.63	270.18	1.16
0.41	0.05	0.00	0.00	0.00	0.00	0.00	0.04	0.08	1.37	0.07	1.98	1.46	2.84	0.98	5.10	39.41	113.97	374.79	1.01
0.52	0.07	0.00	0.00	0.00	0.00	0.00	0.02	0.05	1.30	0.10	2.27	0.49	2.27	0.81	5.95	51.31	106.88	356.64	1.11
0.35	0.04	0.00	0.00	0.03	0.00	0.00	0.02	0.04	1.11	0.07	2.31	0.54	2.31	0.57	3.99	35.28	90.09	302.19	0.84
3.81	0.44	0.00	0.00	0.00	0.00	0.00	0.09	0.26	2.90	0.25	7.65	2.30	5.95	3.13	22.95	203.15	332.35	51.85	4.07
6.08	0.52	0.00	0.00	0.15	0.00	0.00	0.05	0.23	4.22	0.23	7.65	1.84	5.95	2.00	17.85	136.85	266.05	59.50	4.63
6.11	0.52	0.00	0.00	0.15	0.00	0.00	0.05	0.22	4.00	0.23	7.65	1.70	5.95	2.01	17.85	136.00	265.20	59.50	4.61
6.87	0.59	0.00	0.00	0.17	0.00	0.00	0.04	0.18	4.39	0.22	7.65	2.00	9.35	1.79	17.85	134.30	255.85	65.45	4.56
7.09	0.60	0.00	0.00	0.17	0.00	0.00	0.04	0.19	4.07	0.24	7.65	1.93	8.50	1.85	17.00	135.15	254.15	65.45	4.42
7.70	0.65	0.00	0.00	0.20	0.00	0.00	0.03	0.16	4.90	0.23	7.65	2.49	9.35	2.07	17.00	144.50	248.20	70.55	4.40
8.40	0.71	0.00	0.00	0.20	0.00	0.00	0.03	0.17	4.96	0.20	7.65	2.30	9.35	2.08	17.00	145.35	255.00	71.40	4.31
0.55	0.91	0.00	0.00	0.00	9011.70	19.55	0.17	3.48	9.11	0.77	184.45	60.35	5.95	5.75	17.00	343.40	199.75	59.50	5.16
1.38	1.45	0.00	0.00	0.54	9119.65	19.55	0.18	3.52	12.27	1.22	187.00	95.03	9.35	5.34	19.55	391.85	309.40	90.10	4.63
3.47	0.25	0.00	0.00	0.06	0.00	0.00	0.03	0.06	1.04	0.05	1.42	1.10	3.12	0.66	3.97	33.74	58.97	376.77	0.72
3.41	0.29	0.00	0.00	0.00	0.00	0.00	0.02	0.06	0.98	0.09	1.98	0.68	2.84	0.74	5.95	54.72	81.36	16.73	1.56
6.30	0.54	0.00	0.00	0.15	0.00	0.00	0.07	0.19	3.13	0.28	5.95	2.13	7.65	2.32	19.55	179.35	274.55	52.70	5.15
7.84	0.66	0.00	0.00	0.17	0.00	0.00	0.07	0.18	3.09	0.28	5.95	2.07	8.50	2.23	18.70	172.55	266.05	52.70	4.97
0.35	0.04	0.00	0.00	0.04	0.00	0.00	0.02	0.04	1.11	0.07	2.31	0.54	2.31	0.57	3.99	35.28	90.09	302.19	0.84
3.17	0.25	0.16	0.00	0.04	0.00	0.00	0.01	0.03	0.55	0.03	1.15	0.33	2.76	0.38	2.76	20.24	36.11	225.63	0.50
2.25	0.49	0.00	0.00	0.06	0.00	8.12	0.12	0.04	0.90	0.06	1.15	0.21	2.53	0.18	3.22	31.97	64.63	272.32	0.47
1.01	0.90	0.00	0.00	0.00	0.00	0.00	0.01	0.03	0.74	0.05	1.47	0.06	17.64	0.32	2.94	27.51	41.79	184.38	0.37
0.00	0.00	0.00	0.00	0.00	15.00	0.30	0.00	0.00	0.00	0.00	0.00	0.00	6.00	0.10	0.00	0.00	0.00	225.00	0.00
0.84	0.45	0.00	0.00	0.08	6.80	0.00	0.02	0.04	1.50	0.06	0.57	0.04	12.19	0.27	5.39	44.51	64.64	165.56	0.20
0.92	1.76	0.00	0.00	0.00	11.91	0.34	0.01	0.02	0.47	0.03	1.42	0.11	2.84	0.17	2.84	9.36	51.88	106.88	0.29
1.38	0.71	0.00	0.00	0.00	7.09	0.00	0.00	0.03	0.78	0.04	0.85	0.04	35.44	0.66	3.40	25.23	30.05	109.43	0.33
6.42	3.74	0.00	0.00	0.00	25.92	0.00	0.09	0.15	4.20	0.17	14.40	0.19	18.72	1.07	13.68	98.64	129.60	228.24	1.41
3.60	2.12	0.00	0.00	0.00	16.28	0.00	0.05	0.11	3.21	0.13	6.60	0.12	10.56	0.71	10.12	73.04	99.44	39.60	1.09
2.65	1.48	0.00	0.00	0.09	31.68	0.00	0.02	0.06	2.15	0.09	1.92	0.09	6.72	0.45	6.40	49.28	67.20	27.84	0.72
2.57	1.44	0.00	0.00	0.10	31.68	0.00	0.01	0.05	1.56	0.05	1.80	0.06	6.48	0.44	5.76	43.20	52.20	23.04	0.69
2.01	1.27	0.00	0.00	0.00	10.15	0.00	0.04	0.09	2.69	0.12	3.15	0.11	9.10	0.58	8.75	61.60	87.85	34.65	0.98
1.16	0.73	0.00	0.00	0.06	6.72	0.00	0.02	0.05	1.70	0.08	1.68	0.07	5.76	0.33	5.28	39.60	56.88	23.04	0.64
1.05	0.68	0.00	0.00	0.07	7.02	0.00	0.01	0.04	1.19	0.05	1.82	0.05	5.46	0.33	4.42	33.80	41.08	17.42	0.62
4.59	2.59	0.00	0.00	0.89	16.80	0.00	0.10	0.13	8.84	0.36	12.60	0.25	16.80	1.05	20.16	155.40	168.84	231.00	0.80
2.07	1.16	0.00	0.00	0.00	8.85	0.00	0.05	0.08	8.11	0.34	3.54	0.20	9.44	0.70	17.70	137.47	152.81	44.84	0.65
1.76	0.96	0.00	0.00	0.16	15.66	0.00	0.04	0.07	7.37	0.32	2.32	0.19	8.12	0.62	15.66	124.12	142.10	41.18	0.59
1.91	1.04	0.00	0.00	0.18	15.84	0.00	0.03	0.08	5.15	0.19	1.98	0.14	8.58	0.61	14.52	102.96	117.48	40.92	0.64
0.89	0.56	0.00	0.00	0.22	3.64	0.00	0.04	0.07	7.69	0.33	2.08	0.19	8.32	0.59	16.12	127.92	143.52	41.08	0.56
0.64	0.40	0.00	0.00	0.14	3.12	0.00	0.04	0.06	7.13	0.31	2.08	0.18	7.80	0.54	15.08	118.56	133.12	38.48	0.52
0.59	0.38	0.00	0.00	0.15	3.42	0.00	0.02	0.07	4.83	0.19	1.71	0.13	7.41	0.50	13.68	94.05	106.59	35.91	0.55
4.47	2.49	0.00	0.00	0.30	48.28	2.84	0.03	0.18	8.99	0.50	5.68	0.41	19.88	2.24	17.04	157.62	195.96	714.26	2.00
12.66	7.40	0.00	0.00	0.00	51.77	0.00	0.20	0.37	9.37	0.42	30.06	0.45	35.07	2.40	33.40	242.15	308.95	492.65	3.47
7.33	4.30	0.00	0.00	0.00	34.10	0.00	0.11	0.26	7.52	0.35	12.10	0.33	18.70	1.65	26.40	193.60	253.00	97.90	2.86
6.25	3.52	0.00	0.00	0.00	58.58	0.00	0.07	0.21	6.42	0.31	7.07	0.29	15.15	1.37	22.22	169.68	222.20	87.87	2.51
6.33	3.56	0.00	0.00	0.00	59.40	0.00	0.06	0.20	4.96	0.19	6.60	0.22	15.40	1.44	19.80	146.30	182.60	77.00	2.49
3.93	2.52	0.00	0.00	0.00	21.84	0.00	0.08	0.23	6.43	0.34	8.19	0.30	16.38	1.36	22.75	170.17	230.23	88.27	2.65
2.88	1.83	0.00	0.00	0.22	17.82	0.00	0.06	0.19	5.31	0.29	6.48	0.26	12.15	1.08	18.63	144.99	194.40	75.33	2.27
2.80	1.80	0.00	0.00	0.23	18.06	0.00	0.05	0.17	4.08	0.18	6.02	0.19	12.04	1.17	17.20	122.98	155.66	63.64	2.29
2.76	1.63	0.00	0.00	0.00	11.18	0.00	0.05	0.09	2.19	0.12	7.74	0.12	7.31	0.58	8.60	63.21	79.98	115.67	1.00
1.57	0.94	0.00	0.00	0.00	7.25	0.00	0.02	0.07	1.75	0.10	2.90	0.09	3.48	0.39	6.67	51.04	66.41	25.81	0.84
1.32	0.78	0.00	0.00	0.08	9.30	0.00	0.02	0.07	1.86	0.11	2.48	0.10	3.72	0.41	7.13	54.25	70.99	27.90	0.89

USDA ID Code	Food Name	Weight in Grams*	Quantity of Units	Unit of Measure	Protein (gm)	Fat (gm)	Carbohydrate (gm)	Kcalories	Caffeine (gm)	Fiber (gm)	Cholesterol (mg)	Saturated Fat (gm)
	Chicken, Drumstick, Meat & Skin,	34.0000	3.000	Ounce	8.61	3.62	0.00	69.36	0.00	0.00	28.22	0.99
	Chicken, Drumstick, Meat Only, C	25.0000	3.000	Ounce	7.16	2.02	0.00	48.75	0.00	0.00	23.50	0.53
	Chicken, Drumstick, Meat Only, C	26.0000	3.000	Ounce	7.36	1.47	0.00	44.72	0.00	0.00	24.18	0.38
	Chicken, Drumstick, Meat Only, C	28.0000	3.000	Ounce	7.70	1.60	0.00	47.32	0.00	0.00	24.64	0.42
	Chicken, Giblets, Ckd, Fried	13.0000	3.000	Ounce	4.23	1.75	0.57	36.01	0.00	0.00	57.98	0.49
	Chicken, Giblets, Ckd, Simmered	14.0000	3.000	Ounce	3.62	0.67	0.13	21.98	0.00	0.00	55.02	0.21
	Chicken, Heart, Ckd, Simmered	1.0000	3.000	Ounce	0.26	0.08	0.00	1.85	0.00	0.00	2.42	0.02
	Chicken, Leg, Meat & Skin, Ckd,	95.0000	3.000	Ounce	20.68	15.36	8.28	259.35	0.00	0.29	85.50	4.07
	Chicken, Leg, Meat & Skin, Ckd,	67.0000	3.000	Ounce	17.98	9.67	1.68	170.18	0.00	0.07	62.98	2.61
	Chicken, Leg, Meat & Skin, Ckd,	69.0000	3.000	Ounce	17.91	9.29	0.00	160.08	0.00	0.00	63.48	2.57
	Chicken, Leg, Meat & Skin, Ckd,	75.0000	3.000	Ounce	18.13	9.69	0.00	165.00	0.00	0.00	63.00	2.68
	Chicken, Leg, Meat Only, Ckd, Fr	56.0000	3.000	Ounce	15.89	5.22	0.36	116.48	0.00	0.00	55.44	1.39
	Chicken, Leg, Meat Only, Ckd, Ro	57.0000	3.000	Ounce	15.41	4.81	0.00	108.87	0.00	0.00	53.58	1.31
	Chicken, Leg, Meat Only, Ckd, St	60.0000	3.000	Ounce	15.76	4.84	0.00	111.00	0.00	0.00	53.40	1.32
	Chicken, Liver, Ckd, Simmered	6.0000	3.000	Ounce	1.46	0.33	0.05	9.42	0.00	0.00	37.86	0.11
	Chicken, Meat Only, Ckd, Fried	140.0000	1.000	Cup	42.80	12.77	2.37	306.60	0.00	0.14	131.60	3.44
	Chicken, Meat Only, Roasted	8.7000	1.000	Tbsp	2.52	0.64	0.00	16.53	0.00	0.00	7.74	0.18
	Chicken, Meat Only, Stewed	8.7000	1.000	Tbsp	2.37	0.58	0.00	15.40	0.00	0.00	7.22	0.16
	Chicken, Thigh, Meat & Skin, Ckd	52.0000	3.000	Ounce	11.24	8.60	4.72	144.04	0.00	0.16	48.36	2.29
	Chicken, Thigh, Meat & Skin, Ckd	38.0000	3.000	Ounce	10.17	5.69	1.21	99.56	0.00	0.04	36.86	1.55
	Chicken, Thigh, Meat & Skin, Ckd	37.0000	3.000	Ounce	9.27	5.73	0.00	91.39	0.00	0.00	34.41	1.60
	Chicken, Thigh, Meat & Skin, Ckd	41.0000	3.000	Ounce	9.54	6.04	0.00	95.12	0.00	0.00	34.44	1.69
	Chicken, Thigh, Meat Only, Ckd,	31.0000	3.000	Ounce	8.74	3.19	0.37	67.58	0.00	0.00	31.62	0.86
	Chicken, Thigh, Meat Only, Ckd,	31.0000	3.000	Ounce	8.04	3.37	0.00	64.79	0.00	0.00	29.45	0.94
	Chicken, Thigh, Meat Only, Ckd,	33.0000	3.000	Ounce	8.25	3.23	0.00	64.35	0.00	0.00	29.70	0.89
	Chicken, Wing, Meat & Skin, Ckd,	29.0000	3.000	Ounce	5.76	6.32	3.17	93.96	0.00	0.09	22.91	1.69
	Chicken, Wing, Meat & Skin, Ckd,	19.0000	3.000	Ounce	4.96	4.21	0.45	60.99	0.00	0.02	15.39	1.15
	Chicken, Wing, Meat & Skin, Ckd,	21.0000	3.000	Ounce	5.64	4.09	0.00	60.90	0.00	0.00	17.64	1.14
	Chicken, Wing, Meat & Skin, Ckd,	24.0000	3.000	Ounce	5.47	4.04	0.00	59.76	0.00	0.00	16.80	1.13
	Chicken, Wing, Meat Only, Ckd, F	12.0000	3.000	Ounce	3.62	1.10	0.00	25.32	0.00	0.00	10.08	0.30
	Chicken, Wing, Meat Only, Ckd, R	13.0000	3.000	Ounce	3.96	1.06	0.00	26.39	0.00	0.00	11.05	0.29
	Chicken, Wing, Meat Only, Ckd, S	14.0000	3.000	Ounce	3.81	1.01	0.00	25.34	0.00	0.00	10.36	0.28
189	Chili w/ Beans, Cnd	255.0000	0.500	Cup	14.56	14.00	30.37	285.60	0.00	11.22	43.35	6.00
	Cornish Game Hen	110.0000	0.500	Bird	25.63	4.26	0.00	147.40	0.00	0.00	116.60	1.09
	Duck, Domesticated, Meat & Skin,	140.0000	1.000	Cup	26.59	39.69	0.00	471.80	0.00	0.00	117.60	13.54
	Duck, Domesticated, Meat Only, R	100.0000	3.000	Ounce	23.48	11.20	0.00	201.00	0.00	0.00	89.00	4.17
	Gardenburger	90.0000	1.000	Each	18.00	4.00	8.00	140.00	0.00	5.00	0.00	2.00
	Ham and Cheese Loaf(or Roll), Lu	28.3500	1.000	Slice	4.71	5.73	0.41	73.43	0.00	0.00	16.16	2.13
	Ham and Cheese Spread, Lunch Mea	15.0000	1.000	Tbsp	2.43	2.78	0.34	36.75	0.00	0.00	9.15	1.29
	Ham Salad Spread	15.0000	1.000	Tbsp	1.30	2.33	1.60	32.40	0.00	0.00	5.55	0.76
	Ham, Approx 11% Fat, Sliced	28.3500	1.000	Slice	4.98	3.00	0.88	51.60	0.00	0.00	16.16	0.96
	Ham, Chopped, Not Cnd	21.0000	1.000	Slice	3.60	3.62	0.00	48.09	0.00	0.00	10.71	1.20
	Ham, Chopped, Spiced, Cnd	21.0000	1.000	Slice	3.37	3.95	0.06	50.19	0.00	0.00	10.29	1.32
	Ham, Extra Lean, Appx 5% Fat	28.3500	1.000	Slice	5.49	1.41	0.27	37.14	0.00	0.00	13.32	0.46
	Ham, Minced	21.0000	1.000	Slice	3.42	4.34	0.39	55.23	0.00	0.00	14.70	1.51
	Hamburger Patty, Meatless	90.0000	1.000	Each	18.00	4.00	8.00	140.00	0.00	5.00	0.00	1.50
	Hot Dog, Beef	45.0000	1.000	Each	5.40	12.83	0.81	141.75	0.00	0.00	27.45	5.42
	Hot Dog, Chicken	28.3500	1.000	Ounce	3.67	5.52	1.92	72.86	0.00	0.00	28.63	1.57
	Hot Dog, Fat Free	50.0000	1.000	Each	7.00	0.00	2.00	40.00	0.00	0.00	15.00	0.00
	Hot Dog, Turkey	28.3500	1.000	Ounce	4.05	5.02	0.42	64.07	0.00	0.00	30.33	1.67
	Hummus, Fresh	15.0000	1.000	Tbsp	0.74	1.27	3.03	25.65	0.00	0.77	0.00	0.19
	Lamb, Ground, Ckd, Broiled	85.0000	3.000	Ounce	21.04	16.70	0.00	240.55	0.00	0.00	82.45	6.90
	Lamb, Leg, Shank, Meat and Fat,	85.0000	3.000	Ounce	22.45	10.58	0.00	191.25	0.00	0.00	76.50	4.33
	Lamb, Leg, Shank, Meat Only, Ckd	85.0000	3.000	Ounce	23.94	5.67	0.00	153.00	0.00	0.00	73.95	2.02
	Lamb, Leg, Sirloin, Meat and Fat	85.0000	3.000	Ounce	20.94	17.57	0.00	248.20	0.00	0.00	82.45	7.43

Monounsaturated Fat (gm)	Polyunsaturated Fat (gm)	Vitamin D (mg)	Vitamin K (mg)	Vitamin E (mg)	Vitamin A (re)	Vitamin C (mg)	Thiamin (mg)	Riboflavin (mg)	Niacin (mg)	Vitamin B6 (mg)	Folate (mg)	Vitamin B12 (mcg)	Calcium (mg)	Iron (mg)	Magnesium (mg)	Phosphorus (mg)	Potassium (mg)	Sodium (mg)	Zinc (mg)
1.38	0.81	0.00	0.00	0.09	9.18	0.00	0.02	0.06	1.43	0.06	2.38	0.07	3.74	0.45	6.80	47.94	62.56	25.84	0.90
0.74	0.49	0.00	0.00	0.12	4.50	0.00	0.02	0.06	1.54	0.10	2.25	0.09	3.00	0.33	6.00	46.50	62.25	24.00	0.81
0.49	0.36	0.00	0.00	0.07	4.68	0.00	0.02	0.06	1.58	0.10	2.34	0.09	3.12	0.34	6.24	47.84	63.96	24.70	0.83
0.54	0.38	0.00	0.00	0.08	4.76	0.00	0.01	0.06	1.20	0.06	2.24	0.07	3.08	0.38	5.88	42.00	55.72	22.40	0.85
0.57	0.44	0.00	0.00	0.00	465.27	1.13	0.01	0.20	1.43	0.08	49.27	1.73	2.34	1.34	3.25	37.18	42.90	14.69	0.82
0.17	0.15	0.00	0.00	0.18	312.06	1.12	0.01	0.13	0.57	0.05	52.64	1.42	1.68	0.90	2.80	32.06	22.12	8.12	0.64
0.02	0.02	0.00	0.00	0.00	0.09	0.02	0.00	0.01	0.03	0.00	0.80	0.07	0.19	0.09	0.20	1.99	1.32	0.48	0.07
6.25	3.66	0.00	0.00	0.00	25.65	0.00	0.11	0.21	5.16	0.26	17.10	0.27	17.10	1.33	19.00	144.40	179.55	265.05	2.06
3.81	2.23	0.00	0.00	0.00	18.76	0.00	0.06	0.16	4.39	0.23	7.37	0.21	8.71	0.96	16.08	121.94	156.11	58.96	1.80
3.62	2.07	0.00	0.00	0.19	26.91	0.00	0.05	0.14	4.28	0.23	4.83	0.21	8.28	0.92	15.87	120.06	155.25	60.03	1.79
3.78	2.15	0.00	0.00	0.20	27.00	0.00	0.04	0.14	3.44	0.14	4.50	0.15	8.25	1.01	15.00	104.25	132.00	54.75	1.82
1.92	1.24	0.00	0.00	0.00	11.20	0.00	0.04	0.14	3.75	0.22	5.04	0.19	7.28	0.78	14.00	108.08	142.24	53.76	1.67
1.74	1.12	0.00	0.00	0.15	10.83	0.00	0.05	0.13	3.60	0.21	4.56	0.18	6.84	0.75	13.68	104.31	137.94	51.87	1.63
1.76	1.13	0.00	0.00	0.16	10.80	0.00	0.04	0.13	2.88	0.13	4.80	0.14	6.60	0.84	12.60	89.40	114.00	46.80	1.67
0.08	0.05	0.00	0.00	0.09	294.78	0.95	0.01	0.11	0.27	0.03	46.20	1.16	0.84	0.51	1.26	18.72	8.40	3.06	0.26
4.69	3.01	0.00	0.00	0.64	25.20	0.00	0.13	0.28	13.52	0.67	9.80	0.48	23.80	1.89	37.80	287.00	359.80	127.40	3.14
0.23	0.15	0.00	0.00	0.02	1.39	0.00	0.01	0.02	0.80	0.04	0.52	0.03	1.31	0.11	2.18	16.97	21.14	7.48	0.18
0.21	0.13	0.00	0.00	0.02	1.31	0.00	0.00	0.01	0.53	0.02	0.52	0.02	1.22	0.10	1.83	13.05	15.66	6.09	0.17
3.48	2.03	0.00	0.00	0.00	15.08	0.00	0.06	0.12	2.97	0.14	9.88	0.15	9.36	0.75	10.92	80.60	99.84	149.76	1.06
2.23	1.30	0.00	0.00	0.00	11.02	0.00	0.03	0.09	2.64	0.13	4.56	0.11	5.32	0.57	9.50	71.06	90.06	33.44	0.96
2.28	1.27	0.00	0.00	0.10	17.76	0.00	0.03	0.08	2.36	0.11	2.59	0.11	4.44	0.50	8.14	64.38	82.14	31.08	0.87
2.39	1.33	0.00	0.00	0.11	18.04	0.00	0.02	0.08	2.00	0.07	2.46	0.08	4.51	0.56	7.79	56.99	69.70	29.11	0.92
1.18	0.75	0.00	0.00	0.00	6.51	0.00	0.03	0.08	2.21	0.12	2.79	0.10	4.03	0.45	8.06	61.69	80.29	29.45	0.86
1.29	0.77	0.00	0.00	0.08	6.20	0.00	0.02	0.07	2.02	0.11	2.48	0.10	3.72	0.41	7.44	56.73	73.78	27.28	0.80
1.22	0.74	0.00	0.00	0.09	6.27	0.00	0.02	0.07	1.72	0.07	2.31	0.07	3.63	0.47	6.93	49.17	60.39	24.75	0.85
2.60	1.47	0.00	0.00	0.00	9.86	0.00	0.03	0.04	1.53	0.09	5.22	0.07	5.80	0.37	4.64	35.09	40.02	92.80	0.40
1.69	0.94	0.00	0.00	0.00	7.22	0.00	0.01	0.03	1.27	0.08	1.14	0.05	2.85	0.24	3.61	28.50	33.63	14.63	0.33
1.60	0.87	0.00	0.00	0.06	9.87	0.00	0.01	0.03	1.40	0.09	0.63	0.06	3.15	0.27	3.99	31.71	38.64	17.22	0.38
1.58	0.86	0.00	0.00	0.06	9.60	0.00	0.01	0.02	1.11	0.05	0.72	0.04	2.88	0.27	3.84	29.04	33.36	16.08	0.39
0.37	0.25	0.00	0.00	0.00	2.16	0.00	0.01	0.02	0.87	0.07	0.48	0.04	1.80	0.14	2.52	19.68	24.96	10.92	0.25
0.34	0.23	0.00	0.00	0.04	2.34	0.00	0.01	0.02	0.95	0.08	0.52	0.04	2.08	0.15	2.73	21.58	27.30	11.96	0.28
0.32	0.22	0.00	0.00	0.04	2.24	0.00	0.01	0.02	0.73	0.04	0.42	0.03	1.82	0.16	2.52	18.76	21.42	10.22	0.28
5.95	0.92	0.00	0.00	1.87	86.70	4.34	0.12	0.27	0.91	0.34	57.89	0.00	119.85	8.75	114.75	392.70	930.75	1331.10	5.10
1.36	1.03	0.00	0.00	0.29	22.00	0.66	0.08	0.25	6.90	0.39	2.20	0.33	14.30	0.85	20.90	163.90	275.00	69.30	1.68
18.06	5.11	0.00	0.00	0.98	88.20	0.00	0.24	0.38	6.76	0.25	8.40	0.42	15.40	3.78	22.40	218.40	285.60	82.60	2.60
3.70	1.43	0.00	0.00	0.70	23.00	0.00	0.26	0.47	5.10	0.25	10.00	0.40	12.00	2.70	20.00	203.00	252.00	65.00	2.60
0.00	1.00	0.00	0.00	0.00	0.00	0.00	0.00	0.00	4.00	0.00	0.00	0.00	96.00	2.00	0.00	0.00	0.00	380.00	8.00
2.63	0.62	0.31	0.00	0.08	6.52	0.00	0.17	0.05	0.98	0.07	0.85	0.23	16.44	0.26	4.54	71.73	83.35	380.74	0.57
1.06	0.21	0.00	0.00	0.00	13.65	0.00	0.05	0.03	0.32	0.02	0.45	0.11	32.55	0.11	2.70	74.25	24.30	179.55	0.34
1.08	0.41	0.00	0.00	0.26	0.00	0.00	0.07	0.02	0.32	0.02	0.15	0.11	1.20	0.09	1.50	18.00	22.50	136.80	0.17
1.40	0.34	0.00	0.00	0.08	0.00	0.00	0.24	0.07	1.49	0.10	0.85	0.24	1.98	0.28	5.39	70.02	94.12	373.37	0.61
1.72	0.44	0.00	0.00	0.00	0.00	0.00	0.13	0.04	0.81	0.07	0.21	0.19	1.47	0.17	3.36	32.55	66.99	287.91	0.41
1.93	0.43	0.00	0.00	0.05	0.00	0.42	0.11	0.04	0.67	0.07	0.21	0.15	1.47	0.20	2.73	29.19	59.64	286.65	0.38
0.67	0.14	0.00	0.00	0.08	0.00	0.00	0.26	0.06	1.37	0.13	1.13	0.21	1.98	0.22	4.82	61.80	99.22	405.12	0.55
2.01	0.52	0.00	0.00	0.00	0.00	0.00	0.15	0.04	0.87	0.05	0.21	0.20	2.10	0.17	3.36	32.97	65.31	261.45	0.40
0.00	0.50	0.00	0.00	0.00	0.00	0.00	0.25	0.00	4.00	0.00	0.00	0.00	96.00	1.50	0.00	0.00	0.00	380.00	7.50
6.13	0.62	0.41	0.00	0.09	0.00	0.00	0.02	0.05	1.09	0.05	1.80	0.69	9.00	0.64	1.35	39.15	74.70	461.70	0.98
2.40	1.15	0.00	0.00	0.06	10.77	0.00	0.02	0.03	0.88	0.09	1.13	0.07	26.93	0.57	2.84	30.33	23.81	388.40	0.29
0.00	0.00	0.00	0.00	0.00	0.00	0.00	0.00	0.00	0.00	0.00	0.00	0.00	0.00	0.20	0.00	0.00	0.00	460.00	0.00
1.58	1.42	0.00	0.00	0.18	0.00	0.00	0.01	0.05	1.17	0.07	2.27	0.08	30.05	0.52	3.97	37.99	50.75	404.27	0.88
0.53	0.48	0.00	0.00	0.15	0.30	1.19	0.01	0.01	0.06	0.06	8.91	0.00	7.50	0.24	4.35	16.80	26.10	36.60	0.17
7.07	1.19	0.00	0.00	0.21	0.00	0.00	0.09	0.21	5.70	0.12	16.15	2.22	18.70	1.52	20.40	170.85	288.15	68.85	3.97
4.50	0.75	0.00	0.00	0.14	0.00	0.00	0.09	0.23	5.57	0.14	18.70	2.27	8.50	1.68	21.25	168.30	277.10	55.25	3.96
2.48	0.37	0.00	0.00	0.15	0.00	0.00	0.09	0.24	5.43	0.14	20.40	2.30	6.80	1.75	22.10	176.80	290.70	56.10	4.27
7.40	1.27	0.00	0.00	0.11	0.00	0.00	0.09	0.24	5.63	0.12	14.45	2.15	9.35	1.70	18.70	155.55	255.85	57.80	3.51

USDA ID Code	Food Name	Weight in Grams*	Quantity of Units	Unit of Measure	Protein (gm)	Fat (gm)	Carbohydrate (gm)	Kcalories	Caffeine (gm)	Fiber (gm)	Cholesterol (mg)	Saturated Fat (gm)
	Lamb, Leg, Sirloin, Meat Only, C	85.0000	3.000	Ounce	24.10	7.79	0.00	173.40	0.00	0.00	78.20	2.79
	Lamb, Leg, Whole, Meat and Fat,	85.0000	3.000	Ounce	21.72	14.01	0.00	219.30	0.00	0.00	79.05	5.86
	Lamb, Leg, Whole, Meat Only, Ckd	85.0000	3.000	Ounce	24.06	6.58	0.00	162.35	0.00	0.00	75.65	2.35
	Lamb, Loin, Meat and Fat, Ckd, B	64.0000	3.000	Ounce	16.11	14.77	0.00	202.24	0.00	0.00	64.00	6.29
	Lamb, Loin, Meat and Fat, Ckd, R	85.0000	3.000	Ounce	19.17	20.05	0.00	262.65	0.00	0.00	80.75	8.70
	Lamb, Loin, Meat Only, Ckd, Broi	46.0000	3.000	Ounce	13.80	4.48	0.00	99.36	0.00	0.00	43.70	1.60
	Lamb, Loin, Meat Only, Ckd, Roas	85.0000	3.000	Ounce	22.60	8.30	0.00	171.70	0.00	0.00	73.95	3.16
	Lamb, Meat and Fat, Ckd	85.0000	3.000	Ounce	20.84	17.80	0.00	249.90	0.00	0.00	82.45	7.51
	Lamb, Meat Only, Ckd	85.0000	3.000	Ounce	23.99	8.09	0.00	175.10	0.00	0.00	78.20	2.89
	Lamb, Rib, Meat and Fat, Ckd, Br	85.0000	3.000	Ounce	18.81	25.15	0.00	306.85	0.00	0.00	84.15	10.80
	Lamb, Rib, Meat and Fat, Ckd, Ro	85.0000	3.000	Ounce	17.95	25.35	0.00	305.15	0.00	0.00	82.45	10.85
	Lamb, Rib, Meat Only, Ckd, Broil	85.0000	3.000	Ounce	23.58	11.01	0.00	199.75	0.00	0.00	77.35	3.95
	Lamb, Rib, Meat Only, Ckd, Roast	85.0000	3.000	Ounce	22.24	11.31	0.00	197.20	0.00	0.00	74.80	4.05
	Lunch Meat, Dutch Brand Loaf	28.3500	1.000	Slice	3.80	5.05	1.58	68.04	0.00	0.00	13.32	1.80
	Lunch Meat, Honey Loaf	28.3500	1.000	Slice	4.47	1.27	1.51	36.29	0.00	0.00	9.64	0.41
	Lunch Meat, Olive Loaf	28.3500	1.000	Slice	3.36	4.68	2.60	66.62	0.00	0.00	10.77	1.66
	Lunch Meat, Olive Loaf, Pork	28.3500	1.000	Slice	3.35	4.68	2.61	66.62	0.00	0.00	10.77	1.66
	Lunch Meat, Pickle and Pimento L	28.3500	1.000	Slice	3.26	5.98	1.67	74.28	0.00	0.00	10.49	2.23
	Lunch Meat, Pickle and Pimiento	28.3500	1.000	Slice	3.26	5.98	1.67	74.28	0.00	0.00	10.49	2.22
	Lunch Meat, Picnic Loaf	28.3500	1.000	Slice	4.23	4.72	1.35	65.77	0.00	0.00	10.77	1.72
	Pastrami, Beef, Cured	28.3500	1.000	Slice	4.89	8.27	0.86	98.94	0.00	0.00	26.37	2.95
	Pastrami, Turkey	28.3500	1.000	Slice	5.21	1.76	0.47	39.97	0.00	0.00	15.31	0.51
	Pork, Backribs	85.0000	3.000	Ounce	20.62	25.14	0.00	314.50	0.00	0.00	100.30	9.34
	Pork, Braunschweiger	28.3500	3.000	Ounce	3.83	9.10	0.89	101.78	0.00	0.00	44.23	3.09
	Pork, Cnd, Lunch Meat	21.0000	1.000	Slice	2.63	6.36	0.44	70.14	0.00	0.00	13.02	2.27
	Pork, Ground, Ckd	85.0000	3.000	Ounce	21.84	17.65	0.00	252.45	0.00	0.00	79.90	6.56
	Pork, Ham and Cheese Loaf or Rol	28.3500	3.000	Ounce	4.71	5.73	0.41	73.43	0.00	0.00	16.16	2.13
	Pork, Ham Patties, Grilled	59.5000	3.000	Ounce	7.91	18.36	1.01	203.49	0.00	0.00	42.84	6.60
	Pork, Ham Salad Spread	28.3500	3.000	Ounce	2.46	4.40	3.02	61.24	0.00	0.00	10.49	1.43
	Pork, Ham, Chopped, Cnd	28.3500	3.000	Ounce	4.55	5.34	0.08	67.76	0.00	0.00	13.89	1.78
	Pork, Ham, Cnd, Extra Lean (appx	85.0000	3.000	Ounce	17.99	4.15	0.44	115.60	0.00	0.00	25.50	1.36
	Pork, Ham, Cnd, Extra Lean and R	85.0000	3.000	Ounce	17.80	7.17	0.42	141.95	0.00	0.00	34.85	2.39
	Pork, Ham, Cnd, Extra Lean and R	28.3500	1.000	Ounce	5.09	2.11	0.00	40.82	0.00	0.00	10.77	0.69
	Pork, Ham, Cnd, Regular (approx	85.0000	3.000	Ounce	17.45	12.92	0.36	192.10	0.00	0.00	52.70	4.28
	Pork, Ham, Extra Lean (5% Fat),	85.0000	3.000	Ounce	17.79	4.70	1.28	123.25	0.00	0.00	45.05	1.54
	Pork, Ham, Extra Lean (5% Fat),	28.3500	3.000	Ounce	5.49	1.41	0.27	37.14	0.00	0.00	13.32	0.46
	Pork, Ham, Extra Lean and Reg, R	85.0000	3.000	Ounce	18.67	6.51	0.43	140.25	0.00	0.00	48.45	2.22
	Pork, Ham, Extra Lean and Reg, U	28.3500	1.000	Slice	5.18	2.38	0.65	45.93	0.00	0.00	15.03	0.77
	Pork, Ham, Meat and Fat, Roasted	85.0000	3.000	Ounce	18.33	14.25	0.00	206.55	0.00	0.00	52.70	5.08
	Pork, Ham, Meat Only, Roasted	85.0000	3.000	Ounce	21.29	4.68	0.00	133.45	0.00	0.00	46.75	1.56
	Pork, Ham, Regular (11% Fat), Ro	85.0000	3.000	Ounce	19.23	7.67	0.00	151.30	0.00	0.00	50.15	2.65
	Pork, Ham, Regular (11% Fat), Un	28.3500	3.000	Ounce	4.98	3.00	0.88	51.60	0.00	0.00	16.16	0.96
	Pork, Spareribs, Meat and Fat, C	85.0000	3.000	Ounce	24.70	25.76	0.00	337.45	0.00	0.00	102.85	9.45
	Pork, Tenderloin, Meat and Fat,	76.0000	3.000	Ounce	22.69	6.16	0.00	152.76	0.00	0.00	71.44	2.23
	Pork, Tenderloin, Meat Only, Ckd	73.0000	3.000	Ounce	22.21	4.62	0.00	136.51	0.00	0.00	68.62	1.64
	Salami, Turkey	28.3500	1.000	Slice	4.64	3.91	0.16	55.57	0.00	0.00	23.25	1.14
	Sausage, Beerwurst, Pork	6.0000	1.000	Slice	0.85	1.13	0.12	14.28	0.00	0.00	3.54	0.38
	Sausage, Bockwurst	28.3500	1.000	Ounce	3.78	7.82	0.14	87.03	0.00	0.00	16.73	2.87
	Sausage, Bratwurst	28.3500	1.000	Ounce	3.99	7.33	0.59	85.33	0.00	0.00	17.01	2.64
	Sausage, Italian, Ckd	67.0000	1.000	Link	13.42	17.22	1.01	216.41	0.00	0.00	52.26	6.08
	Sausage, Kielbasa, Kolbassy	26.0000	1.000	Slice	3.45	7.06	0.56	80.60	0.00	0.00	17.42	2.58
	Sausage, Knockwurst	28.3500	1.000	Ounce	3.37	7.87	0.50	87.32	0.00	0.00	16.44	2.89
	Sausage, Link, Pork and Beef	16.0000	1.000	Small	2.14	4.85	0.23	53.76	0.00	0.00	11.36	1.70
	Sausage, Pepperoni	5.5000	1.000	Slice	1.15	2.42	0.16	27.34	0.00	0.00	4.35	0.89
	Sausage, Polish-style	28.3500	1.000	Ounce	4.00	8.14	0.46	92.42	0.00	0.00	19.85	2.93

Monounsaturated Fat (gm)	Polyunsaturated Fat (gm)	Vitamin D (mg)	Vitamin K (mg)	Vitamin E (mg)	Vitamin A (re)	Vitamin C (mg)	Thiamin (mg)	Riboflavin (mg)	Niacin (mg)	Vitamin B6 (mg)	Folate (mg)	Vitamin B12 (mcg)	Calcium (mg)	Iron (mg)	Magnesium (mg)	Phosphorus (mg)	Potassium (mg)	Sodium (mg)	Zinc (mg)
3.42	0.51	0.00	0.00	0.14	0.00	0.00	0.10	0.26	5.33	0.14	17.85	2.19	6.80	1.87	21.25	172.55	283.05	60.35	4.12
5.92	1.00	0.00	0.00	0.13	0.00	0.00	0.09	0.23	5.60	0.13	17.00	2.20	9.35	1.68	20.40	162.35	266.05	56.10	3.74
2.88	0.43	0.00	0.00	0.15	0.00	0.00	0.09	0.25	5.39	0.14	19.55	2.24	6.80	1.80	22.10	175.10	287.30	57.80	4.20
6.21	1.08	0.00	0.00	0.08	0.00	0.00	0.06	0.16	4.54	0.08	11.52	1.58	12.80	1.16	15.36	125.44	209.28	49.28	2.23
8.23	1.59	0.00	0.00	0.09	0.00	0.00	0.09	0.20	6.04	0.09	16.15	1.88	15.30	1.80	19.55	153.00	209.10	54.40	2.90
1.96	0.29	0.00	0.00	0.07	0.00	0.00	0.05	0.13	3.15	0.07	11.04	1.16	8.74	0.92	12.88	103.96	172.96	38.64	1.90
3.36	0.73	0.00	0.00	0.14	0.00	0.00	0.09	0.23	5.81	0.14	21.25	1.84	14.45	2.07	22.95	175.10	226.95	56.10	3.45
7.50	1.28	0.00	0.00	0.12	0.00	0.00	0.09	0.21	5.66	0.11	15.30	2.17	14.45	1.60	19.55	159.80	263.50	61.20	3.79
3.54	0.53	0.00	0.00	0.16	0.00	0.00	0.09	0.24	5.37	0.14	19.55	2.22	12.75	1.74	22.10	178.50	292.40	64.60	4.48
10.30	2.01	0.00	0.00	0.10	0.00	0.00	0.08	0.19	5.95	0.09	11.90	2.16	16.15	1.60	19.55	151.30	229.50	64.60	3.40
10.64	1.84	0.00	0.00	0.09	0.00	0.00	0.08	0.18	5.74	0.09	12.75	1.90	18.70	1.36	17.00	141.10	230.35	62.05	2.97
4.43	1.00	0.00	0.00	0.15	0.00	0.00	0.09	0.21	5.57	0.13	17.85	2.24	13.60	1.88	24.65	181.05	266.05	72.25	4.48
4.96	0.74	0.00	0.00	0.13	0.00	0.00	0.08	0.20	5.24	0.13	18.70	1.84	17.85	1.50	19.55	165.75	267.75	68.85	3.80
2.36	0.54	0.28	0.00	0.06	0.00	0.00	0.09	0.08	0.68	0.07	0.57	0.37	23.81	0.35	5.95	45.93	106.60	354.38	0.49
0.57	0.13	0.26	0.00	0.06	0.00	0.00	0.14	0.07	0.89	0.09	2.27	0.31	4.82	0.38	4.82	40.54	97.24	374.22	0.69
2.23	0.55	0.00	0.00	0.00	5.67	2.49	0.08	0.07	0.52	0.07	0.57	0.36	30.90	0.15	5.39	36.00	84.20	420.71	0.39
2.23	0.55	0.31	0.00	0.07	5.67	0.00	0.09	0.07	0.52	0.07	0.57	0.36	30.90	0.15	5.39	36.00	84.20	420.71	0.39
2.72	0.73	0.00	0.00	0.00	1.98	3.83	0.08	0.07	0.58	0.05	1.42	0.33	26.93	0.29	5.10	39.69	96.39	393.78	0.40
2.72	0.73	0.31	0.00	0.07	1.98	0.00	0.08	0.07	0.58	0.05	1.42	0.33	26.93	0.29	5.10	39.69	96.39	393.78	0.40
2.18	0.54	0.34	0.00	0.07	0.00	0.00	0.10	0.07	0.65	0.09	0.57	0.43	13.32	0.29	4.25	35.44	75.69	329.99	0.62
4.10	0.28	0.00	0.00	0.07	0.00	0.00	0.03	0.05	1.44	0.05	1.98	0.50	2.55	0.54	5.10	42.53	64.64	347.85	1.21
0.58	0.45	0.00	0.00	0.06	0.00	0.00	0.02	0.07	1.00	0.08	1.42	0.07	2.55	0.47	3.97	56.70	73.71	296.26	0.61
11.44	1.97	0.00	0.00	0.00	2.55	0.26	0.37	0.17	3.02	0.26	2.55	0.54	38.25	1.17	17.85	165.75	267.75	85.85	2.86
4.23	1.06	0.00	0.00	0.00	1196.37	2.72	0.07	0.43	2.37	0.09	12.47	5.70	2.55	2.65	3.12	47.63	56.42	324.04	0.80
3.00	0.75	0.00	0.00	0.05	0.00	0.21	0.08	0.04	0.66	0.04	1.26	0.19	1.26	0.15	2.10	17.22	45.15	270.69	0.31
7.86	1.59	0.00	0.00	0.22	1.70	0.60	0.60	0.19	3.58	0.33	5.10	0.46	18.70	1.10	20.40	192.10	307.70	62.05	2.73
2.63	0.62	0.00	0.00	0.00	6.52	7.12	0.17	0.05	0.98	0.07	0.85	0.23	16.44	0.26	4.54	71.73	83.35	380.74	0.57
8.73	1.98	0.00	0.00	0.15	0.00	0.00	0.21	0.11	1.93	0.10	1.79	0.42	5.36	0.96	5.95	60.10	145.18	632.49	1.13
2.04	0.77	0.00	0.00	0.00	0.00	1.70	0.12	0.03	0.59	0.04	0.28	0.22	2.27	0.17	2.84	34.02	42.53	258.55	0.31
2.60	0.58	0.00	0.00	0.00	0.00	0.51	0.15	0.05	0.91	0.09	0.28	0.20	1.98	0.27	3.69	39.41	80.51	386.98	0.52
2.12	0.37	0.00	0.00	0.22	0.00	0.00	0.88	0.21	4.16	0.38	4.25	0.60	5.10	0.78	17.85	177.65	295.80	964.75	1.90
3.45	0.77	0.00	0.00	0.22	0.00	0.00	0.82	0.21	4.28	0.34	4.25	0.71	5.95	0.91	17.00	187.85	298.35	907.80	1.97
1.01	0.22	0.00	0.00	0.07	0.00	0.00	0.25	0.07	1.30	0.13	1.70	0.23	1.70	0.26	4.54	58.68	94.69	361.75	0.52
6.01	1.51	0.00	0.00	0.00	0.00	11.90	0.70	0.22	4.51	0.26	4.25	0.90	6.80	1.16	14.45	206.55	303.45	799.85	2.13
2.23	0.46	0.00	0.00	0.22	0.00	0.00	0.64	0.17	3.42	0.34	2.55	0.55	6.80	1.26	11.90	166.60	243.95	1022.55	2.45
0.67	0.14	0.00	0.00	0.07	0.00	7.46	0.26	0.06	1.37	0.13	1.13	0.21	1.98	0.22	4.82	61.80	99.23	405.12	0.55
3.18	0.91	0.00	0.00	0.22	0.00	0.00	0.63	0.24	4.52	0.30	2.55	0.58	6.80	1.19	16.15	210.80	307.70	1177.25	2.24
1.12	0.26	0.00	0.00	0.07	0.00	0.00	0.25	0.07	1.44	0.11	0.85	0.23	1.98	0.26	5.10	66.91	84.20	362.31	0.58
6.70	1.54	0.00	0.00	0.22	0.00	0.00	0.51	0.19	3.79	0.32	2.55	0.54	5.95	0.74	16.15	181.90	243.10	1008.95	1.97
2.15	0.54	0.00	0.00	0.22	0.00	0.00	0.58	0.21	4.27	0.40	3.40	0.60	5.95	0.80	18.70	192.95	268.60	1127.95	2.18
3.77	1.20	0.00	0.00	0.22	0.00	0.00	0.62	0.28	5.23	0.26	2.55	0.60	6.80	1.14	18.70	238.85	347.65	1275.00	2.10
1.40	0.34	0.00	0.00	0.07	0.00	7.85	0.24	0.07	1.49	0.10	0.85	0.24	1.98	0.28	5.39	70.02	94.12	373.37	0.61
11.46	2.32	0.00	0.00	0.22	2.55	0.00	0.35	0.32	4.66	0.30	3.40	0.92	39.95	1.57	20.40	221.85	272.00	79.05	3.91
2.54	0.56	0.00	0.00	0.00	1.52	0.76	0.74	0.29	3.84	0.40	4.56	0.74	3.80	1.06	26.60	220.40	337.44	48.64	2.20
1.88	0.41	0.00	0.00	0.00	1.46	0.73	0.72	0.28	3.75	0.39	4.38	0.73	3.65	1.04	26.28	215.35	329.23	47.45	2.15
1.29	1.00	0.00	0.00	0.00	0.00	0.00	0.02	0.05	1.00	0.07	1.13	0.06	5.67	0.46	4.25	30.05	69.17	284.63	0.51
0.54	0.14	0.05	0.00	0.00	0.00	0.00	0.03	0.01	0.20	0.02	0.18	0.05	0.48	0.05	0.78	6.18	15.18	74.40	0.10
3.69	0.84	0.00	0.00	0.04	1.70	0.00	0.12	0.05	1.17	0.07	1.70	0.23	4.54	0.18	5.10	41.39	76.55	313.27	0.44
3.46	0.78	0.31	0.00	0.07	0.00	0.28	0.14	0.05	0.91	0.06	0.57	0.27	12.47	0.37	4.25	42.24	60.10	157.91	0.65
8.01	2.20	0.00	0.00	0.17	0.00	1.34	0.42	0.15	2.79	0.22	3.35	0.87	16.08	1.01	12.06	113.90	203.68	617.74	1.60
3.36	0.80	0.00	0.00	0.06	0.00	0.00	0.06	0.05	0.75	0.05	1.30	0.42	11.44	0.38	4.16	38.48	70.46	279.76	0.53
3.63	0.83	0.00	0.00	0.16	0.00	0.00	0.10	0.04	0.77	0.05	0.57	0.33	3.12	0.26	3.12	27.78	56.42	286.34	0.47
2.27	0.52	0.20	0.00	0.04	0.00	0.00	0.04	0.03	0.52	0.03	0.32	0.24	1.60	0.23	1.92	17.12	30.24	151.20	0.34
1.16	0.24	0.00	0.00	0.01	0.00	0.00	0.02	0.01	0.27	0.01	0.22	0.14	0.55	0.08	0.88	6.55	19.09	112.20	0.14
3.83	0.87	0.00	0.00	0.00	0.00	0.28	0.14	0.04	0.98	0.05	0.57	0.28	3.40	0.41	3.97	38.56	67.19	248.35	0.55

USDA ID Code	Food Name	Weight in Grams*	Quantity of Units	Unit of Measure	Protein (gm)	Fat (gm)	Carbohydrate (gm)	Kcalories	Caffeine (gm)	Fiber (gm)	Cholesterol (mg)	Saturated Fat (gm)
	Sausage, Pork, Links or Bulk, Ck	13.0000	1.000	Link	2.55	4.05	0.13	47.97	0.00	0.00	10.79	1.41
	Sausage, Pork, Smoked Link, Gril	28.3500	3.000	Ounce	6.29	9.00	0.60	110.28	0.00	0.00	19.28	3.21
	Sausage, Salami, Beef and Pork,	10.0000	1.000	Slice	2.29	3.44	0.26	41.80	0.00	0.00	7.90	1.22
	Sausage, Salami, Beef, Ckd	23.0000	1.000	Slice	3.46	4.76	0.65	60.26	0.00	0.00	14.95	2.07
	Sausage, Smoked Link, Pork	16.0000	1.000	Small	3.55	5.07	0.34	62.24	0.00	0.00	10.88	1.81
	Sausage, Smoked, Beef, Cured,	28.3500	1.000	Ounce	4.00	7.63	0.69	88.45	0.00	0.00	18.99	3.24
	Sausage, Turkey	28.3500	3.000	Ounce	4.00	2.50	1.50	45.00	0.00	0.00	15.00	1.25
743	Tofu Pups-Light Life	42.0000	1.000	Each	8.00	2.50	2.00	60.00	0.00	0.00	0.00	1.00
744	Tofu Rella, Garlic Herb	28.0000	1.000	Ounce	6.00	5.00	3.00	80.00	0.00	0.00	0.00	1.00
745	Tofu Rella, Monterey Style	28.0000	1.000	Ounce	6.00	5.00	3.00	80.00	0.00	0.00	0.00	1.00
746	Tofu Wieners-Yves	38.0000	1.000	Each	9.00	0.50	2.00	45.00	0.00	0.00	0.00	0.00
	Turkey Breast Meat	21.0000	1.000	Slice	4.73	0.33	0.00	23.10	0.00	0.00	8.61	0.10
	Turkey Burger, Breaded, Battered	28.0000	3.000	Ounce	3.92	5.04	4.40	79.24	0.00	0.14	17.36	1.31
749	Turkey Burger, Grilled	82.0000	3.000	Ounce	22.44	10.78	0.00	192.70	0.00	0.00	83.64	2.78
	Turkey Lunch Meat	28.3500	1.000	Slice	5.37	1.44	0.10	36.29	0.00	0.00	15.88	0.48
	Turkey Roast, Roasted	135.0000	1.000	Cup	28.78	7.80	4.14	209.25	0.00	0.00	71.55	2.57
	Turkey Roll, Light and Dark Meat	28.3500	3.000	Ounce	5.14	1.98	0.60	42.24	0.00	0.00	15.59	0.58
	Turkey Roll, Light Meat	28.3500	3.000	Ounce	5.30	2.05	0.15	41.67	0.00	0.00	12.19	0.57
	Turkey Sticks, Breaded, Battered	64.0000	2.250	Ounce	9.09	10.82	10.88	178.56	0.00	0.00	40.96	2.80
	Turkey Thigh, Prebasted, Meat &	314.0000	3.000	Ounce	59.03	26.82	0.00	492.98	0.00	0.00	194.68	8.32
	Turkey, Back, Meat & Skin, Ckd,	34.0000	3.000	Ounce	9.04	4.89	0.00	82.62	0.00	0.00	30.94	1.42
	Turkey, Breast, Meat & Skin, Ckd	112.0000	3.000	Ounce	32.16	8.30	0.00	211.68	0.00	0.00	82.88	2.35
	Turkey, Ckd, Roasted, Meat & Ski	260.0000	3.000	Ounce	72.75	24.57	0.18	533.00	0.00	0.00	247.00	7.20
	Turkey, Dark Meat, Ckd, Roasted	91.0000	3.000	Ounce	26.00	6.57	0.00	170.17	0.00	0.00	77.35	2.20
	Turkey, Dark Meat, Meat & Skin,	104.0000	3.000	Ounce	28.59	12.00	0.00	229.84	0.00	0.00	92.56	3.63
	Turkey, Giblets, Ckd, Simmered,	10.0000	3.000	Ounce	2.66	0.51	0.21	16.70	0.00	0.00	41.80	0.15
	Turkey, Ground, Ckd	82.0000	3.000	Ounce	22.44	10.78	0.00	192.70	0.00	0.00	83.64	2.78
	Turkey, Leg, Meat & Skin, Ckd, R	71.0000	3.000	Ounce	19.79	6.97	0.00	147.68	0.00	0.00	60.35	2.17
	Turkey, Light Meat, Ckd, Roasted	117.0000	3.000	Ounce	34.98	3.77	0.00	183.69	0.00	0.00	80.73	1.21
	Turkey, Light Meat, Meat & Skin,	136.0000	3.000	Ounce	38.86	11.33	0.00	267.92	0.00	0.00	103.36	3.18
	Turkey, Meat & Skin, Ckd, Roaste	140.0000	1.000	Cup	39.34	13.62	0.00	291.20	0.00	0.00	114.80	3.98
	Turkey, Meat Only, Ckd, Roasted	140.0000	1.000	Cup	41.05	6.96	0.00	238.00	0.00	0.00	106.40	2.30
	Turkey, Thin Sliced	28.3500	3.000	Ounce	6.38	0.45	0.00	31.19	0.00	0.00	11.62	0.14
	Turkey, Wing, Meat & Skin, Ckd,	24.0000	3.000	Ounce	6.57	2.98	0.00	54.96	0.00	0.00	19.44	0.81
	Veal, Meat and Fat, Ckd	85.0000	3.000	Ounce	25.59	9.68	0.00	196.35	0.00	0.00	96.90	3.64
	Veal, Meat Only, Ckd	85.0000	3.000	Ounce	27.12	5.59	0.00	166.60	0.00	0.00	100.30	1.56
	Venison, Ckd, Roasted	85.0000	3.000	Ounce	25.68	2.71	0.00	134.30	0.00	0.00	95.20	1.06

Nuts and Seeds

USDA ID Code	Food Name	Weight in Grams*	Quantity of Units	Unit of Measure	Protein (gm)	Fat (gm)	Carbohydrate (gm)	Kcalories	Caffeine (gm)	Fiber (gm)	Cholesterol (mg)	Saturated Fat (gm)
	Alfalfa Seeds, Sprouted, Fresh	3.0000	1.000	Tbsp	0.12	0.02	0.11	0.87	0.00	0.08	0.00	0.00
	Almond Butter, w/ salt	16.0000	1.000	Tbsp	2.43	9.46	3.40	101.28	0.00	0.59	0.00	0.90
	Almond Butter, w/o salt	16.0000	1.000	Tbsp	2.43	9.46	3.40	101.28	0.00	0.59	0.00	0.90
	Almonds, Toasted, Unblanched	141.9600	0.500	Cup	28.93	72.07	32.52	836.14	0.00	15.90	0.00	6.83
	Brazil Nuts, Dried, Unblanched	28.3500	1.000	Ounce	4.07	18.77	3.63	185.98	0.00	1.53	0.00	4.58
	Cashews, Dry Roasted	28.3500	1.000	Ounce	4.34	13.14	9.27	162.73	0.00	0.85	0.00	2.60
	Cashews, Oil Roasted	28.3500	1.000	Ounce	4.58	13.67	8.09	163.30	0.00	1.08	0.00	2.70
467	Hazelnuts, Dry Roasted	28.0000	1.000	Ounce	2.80	18.80	5.10	188.00	0.00	2.00	0.00	1.40
468	Hazelnuts, Oil Roasted	28.0000	1.000	Ounce	4.00	18.00	5.40	187.00	0.00	1.80	0.00	1.30
	Macadamias, Dried	28.3500	1.000	Ounce	2.24	21.48	3.92	203.55	0.00	2.44	0.00	3.42
	Macadamias, Oil Roasted	112.0000	0.500	Cup	9.60	83.60	15.60	769.00	0.00	10.40	0.00	13.60
	Peanut Butter, Chunk Style, w/ S	32.0000	2.000	Tbsp	7.70	15.98	6.91	188.48	0.00	2.11	0.00	3.07
	Peanut Butter, Chunk Style, w/o	32.0000	2.000	Tbsp	7.70	15.98	6.91	188.48	0.00	2.11	0.00	3.07
	Peanut Butter, Reduced Fat, Crea	18.0000	2.000	Tbsp	4.00	6.00	7.50	95.00	0.00	1.00	0.00	1.25
638	Peanut Butter, Reduced Fat, Crun	18.0000	2.000	Tbsp	4.00	6.00	7.50	95.00	0.00	1.00	0.00	1.25

Monounsaturated Fat (gm)	Polyunsaturated Fat (gm)	Vitamin D (mg)	Vitamin K (mg)	Vitamin E (mg)	Vitamin A (re)	Vitamin C (mg)	Thiamin (mg)	Riboflavin (mg)	Niacin (mg)	Vitamin B₆ (mg)	Folate (mg)	Vitamin B₁₂ (mcg)	Calcium (mg)	Iron (mg)	Magnesium (mg)	Phosphorus (mg)	Potassium (mg)	Sodium (mg)	Zinc (mg)
1.81	0.50	0.00	0.00	0.02	0.00	0.26	0.10	0.03	0.59	0.04	0.26	0.22	4.16	0.16	2.21	23.92	46.93	168.22	0.33
4.15	1.07	0.00	0.00	0.09	0.00	0.51	0.20	0.07	1.28	0.10	1.42	0.46	8.51	0.33	5.39	45.93	95.26	425.25	0.80
1.71	0.32	0.00	0.00	0.03	0.00	0.00	0.06	0.03	0.49	0.05	0.20	0.19	0.80	0.15	1.70	14.20	37.80	186.00	0.32
2.17	0.24	0.28	0.00	0.04	0.00	0.00	0.02	0.04	0.75	0.04	0.46	0.70	2.07	0.50	3.22	25.99	51.52	270.48	0.50
2.34	0.60	0.00	0.00	0.04	0.00	0.32	0.11	0.04	0.72	0.06	0.80	0.26	4.80	0.19	3.04	25.92	53.76	240.00	0.45
3.68	0.30	0.00	0.00	0.00	0.00	0.00	0.01	0.04	0.90	0.03	1.13	0.53	1.98	0.50	3.69	29.77	49.90	320.64	0.79
0.00	0.00	0.00	0.00	0.00	10.00	6.00	0.00	0.00	0.00	0.00	0.00	0.00	12.00	1.75	0.00	0.00	0.00	300.00	0.00
0.00	0.00	0.00	0.00	0.00	0.00	0.00	0.00	0.00	0.00	0.00	0.00	0.00	0.00	0.00	0.00	0.00	0.00	140.00	0.00
0.00	0.00	0.00	0.00	0.00	0.00	0.00	0.00	0.00	0.00	0.00	0.00	0.00	0.00	0.00	0.00	0.00	0.00	280.00	0.00
0.00	0.00	0.00	0.00	0.00	0.00	0.00	0.00	0.00	0.00	0.00	0.00	0.00	0.00	0.00	0.00	0.00	0.00	280.00	0.00
0.00	0.00	0.00	0.00	0.00	0.00	0.00	0.00	0.00	0.00	0.00	0.00	0.00	0.00	0.00	0.00	0.00	0.00	240.00	0.00
0.09	0.06	0.00	0.00	0.02	0.00	0.00	0.01	0.02	1.75	0.08	0.84	0.42	1.47	0.08	4.20	48.09	58.38	300.51	0.24
2.09	1.32	0.00	0.00	0.67	3.08	0.00	0.03	0.05	0.64	0.06	7.84	0.06	3.92	0.62	4.20	75.60	77.00	224.00	0.40
4.01	2.65	0.00	0.00	0.28	0.00	0.00	0.04	0.14	3.95	0.32	5.74	0.27	20.50	1.58	19.68	160.72	221.40	87.74	2.35
0.33	0.43	0.00	0.00	0.18	0.00	0.00	0.01	0.07	1.00	0.07	1.70	0.07	2.84	0.78	4.54	54.15	92.14	282.37	0.83
1.62	2.24	0.00	0.00	0.51	0.00	0.00	0.07	0.22	8.46	0.36	6.75	2.05	6.75	2.20	29.70	329.40	402.30	918.00	3.43
0.65	0.50	0.00	0.00	0.10	0.00	0.00	0.03	0.08	1.36	0.08	1.42	0.07	9.07	0.38	5.10	47.63	76.55	166.13	0.57
0.71	0.49	0.00	0.00	0.00	0.00	0.00	0.03	0.06	1.98	0.09	1.13	0.07	11.34	0.36	4.54	51.88	71.16	138.63	0.44
4.43	2.81	0.00	0.00	0.00	7.68	0.00	0.06	0.12	1.34	0.13	18.56	0.15	8.96	1.41	9.60	149.76	166.40	536.32	0.93
7.94	7.38	0.00	0.00	0.00	0.00	0.00	0.25	0.82	7.57	0.72	18.84	0.75	25.12	4.74	53.38	536.94	756.74	1372.18	12.94
1.70	1.26	0.00	0.00	0.20	0.00	0.00	0.02	0.07	1.17	0.10	2.72	0.12	11.22	0.74	7.48	64.26	88.40	24.82	1.33
2.74	2.02	0.00	0.00	0.00	0.00	0.00	0.07	0.15	7.13	0.54	6.72	0.40	23.52	1.57	30.24	235.20	322.56	70.56	2.27
7.93	6.29	0.00	0.00	0.00	176.80	0.26	0.16	0.55	12.84	1.04	52.00	3.33	67.60	5.23	62.40	520.00	707.20	174.20	8.19
1.49	1.97	0.00	0.00	0.58	0.00	0.00	0.05	0.23	3.32	0.33	8.19	0.34	29.12	2.12	21.84	185.64	263.90	71.89	4.06
3.80	3.21	0.00	0.00	0.63	0.00	0.00	0.06	0.25	3.67	0.33	9.36	0.37	34.32	2.36	23.92	203.84	284.96	79.04	4.33
0.12	0.12	0.00	0.00	0.15	179.50	0.17	0.01	0.09	0.45	0.03	34.50	2.40	1.30	0.67	1.70	20.40	20.00	5.90	0.37
4.01	2.65	0.00	0.00	0.28	0.00	0.00	0.04	0.14	3.95	0.32	5.74	0.27	20.50	1.58	19.68	160.72	221.40	87.74	2.35
2.04	1.93	0.00	0.00	0.44	0.00	0.00	0.04	0.17	2.53	0.23	6.39	0.26	22.72	1.63	16.33	141.29	198.80	54.67	3.03
0.66	1.01	0.00	0.00	0.11	0.00	0.00	0.07	0.15	8.00	0.63	7.02	0.43	22.23	1.58	32.76	256.23	356.85	74.88	2.39
3.86	2.73	0.00	0.00	0.18	0.00	0.00	0.08	0.18	8.55	0.64	8.16	0.48	28.56	1.92	35.36	282.88	387.60	85.68	2.77
4.47	3.47	0.00	0.00	0.48	0.00	0.00	0.08	0.25	7.13	0.57	9.80	0.49	36.40	2.51	35.00	284.20	392.00	95.20	4.14
1.44	2.00	0.00	0.00	0.46	0.00	0.00	0.08	0.25	7.62	0.64	9.80	0.52	35.00	2.49	36.40	298.20	417.20	98.00	4.34
0.13	0.08	0.00	0.00	0.03	0.00	0.00	0.01	0.03	2.36	0.10	1.13	0.57	1.98	0.11	5.67	64.92	78.81	405.69	0.32
1.12	0.71	0.00	0.00	0.04	0.00	0.00	0.01	0.03	1.38	0.10	1.44	0.08	5.76	0.35	6.00	47.28	63.84	14.64	0.50
3.74	0.68	0.00	0.00	0.34	0.00	0.00	0.05	0.27	6.77	0.26	12.75	1.33	18.70	0.98	22.10	203.15	276.25	73.95	4.05
2.00	0.50	0.00	0.00	0.36	0.00	0.00	0.05	0.29	7.16	0.28	13.60	1.40	20.40	0.99	23.80	212.50	287.30	75.65	4.33
0.75	0.53	0.00	0.00	0.00	0.00	0.00	0.15	0.51	5.70	0.00	0.00	0.00	5.95	3.80	20.40	192.10	284.75	45.90	2.34
0.00	0.01	0.00	0.00	0.00	0.48	0.25	0.00	0.00	0.01	0.00	1.08	0.00	0.96	0.03	0.81	2.10	2.37	0.18	0.03
6.14	1.98	0.00	0.00	3.24	0.00	0.11	0.02	0.10	0.46	0.01	10.43	0.00	43.20	0.59	48.48	83.68	121.28	72.00	0.49
6.14	1.98	0.00	0.00	3.25	0.00	0.11	0.02	0.10	0.46	0.01	10.43	0.00	43.20	0.59	48.48	83.68	121.28	1.76	0.49
46.80	15.12	0.00	0.00	22.71	0.00	0.99	0.19	0.85	4.02	0.11	91.00	0.00	401.75	6.98	432.98	780.78	1097.35	15.62	6.98
6.53	6.84	0.00	0.00	2.15	0.00	0.20	0.28	0.03	0.46	0.07	1.13	0.00	49.90	0.96	63.79	170.10	170.10	0.57	1.30
7.75	2.22	0.00	0.00	0.16	0.00	0.00	0.06	0.06	0.40	0.07	19.62	0.00	12.76	1.70	73.71	138.92	160.18	181.44	1.59
8.06	2.31	0.00	0.00	0.44	0.00	0.00	0.12	0.05	0.51	0.07	19.19	0.00	11.62	1.16	72.29	120.77	150.26	177.47	1.35
14.70	1.80	0.00	0.00	0.00	20.00	0.00	0.06	0.06	0.80	0.18	21.00	0.00	55.00	0.96	84.00	92.00	131.00	1.00	0.71
14.10	1.70	0.00	0.00	0.00	20.00	0.00	0.06	0.06	0.80	0.18	21.00	0.00	56.00	0.97	84.00	92.00	132.00	1.00	0.71
16.69	0.43	0.00	0.00	0.15	0.00	0.34	0.34	0.05	0.70	0.08	3.12	0.26	24.10	1.05	36.86	53.30	104.33	1.42	0.37
66.00	1.77	0.00	0.00	0.55	0.00		0.40	0.15	2.71	0.27	16.00	0.00	80.00	2.41	156.78	156.00	440.86	8.00	1.47
7.54	4.53	0.00	0.00	0.00	0.00	0.00	0.04	0.04	4.38	0.14	29.44	0.00	13.12	0.61	50.88	101.44	239.04	155.52	0.89
7.54	4.53	0.00	0.00	3.20	0.00	0.00	0.04	0.04	4.38	0.14	29.44	0.00	13.12	0.61	50.88	101.44	239.04	5.44	0.89
0.00	0.00	0.00	0.00	0.00	0.00	0.00	0.00	0.00	2.38	0.06	6.00	0.00	0.00	0.20	26.25	0.00	360.50	125.00	0.45
0.00	0.00	0.00	0.00	0.00	0.00	0.00	0.00	0.00	2.38	0.06	6.00	0.00	0.00	0.20	26.25	0.00	360.50	110.00	0.45

USDA ID Code / Food Name	Weight in Grams*	Quantity of Units	Unit of Measure	Protein (gm)	Fat (gm)	Carbohydrate (gm)	Kcalories	Caffeine (gm)	Fiber (gm)	Cholesterol (mg)	Saturated Fat (gm)
Peanut Butter, Smooth Style, w/	32.0000	2.000	Tbsp	8.07	16.33	6.17	189.76	0.00	1.89	0.00	3.31
Peanut Butter, Smooth Style, w/o	32.0000	2.000	Tbsp	8.07	16.33	6.17	189.76	0.00	1.89	0.00	3.31
Peanut Kernels, Oil Roasted	112.0000	0.500	Cup	37.94	70.99	27.26	836.64	0.00	12.67	0.00	9.85
Peanuts, All Types, Ckd, Boiled,	28.0000	33.000	Each	3.78	6.16	5.95	89.04	0.00	2.46	0.00	0.86
Peanuts, All Types, Dry-roasted,	1.0000	1.000	Each	0.24	0.50	0.22	5.85	0.00	0.08	0.00	0.07
Peanuts, All Types, Dry-roasted,	1.0000	1.000	Each	0.24	0.50	0.22	5.85	0.00	0.08	0.00	0.07
Peanuts, All Types, Fresh	28.3500	1.000	Ounce	7.31	13.96	4.58	160.74	0.00	2.41	0.00	1.94
Peanuts, All Types, Oil-roasted,	0.9000	1.000	Each	0.24	0.44	0.17	5.23	0.00	0.08	0.00	0.06
Peanuts, All Types, Oil-roasted,	28.0000	32.000	Each	7.38	13.80	5.30	162.68	0.00	1.93	0.00	1.92
Peanuts, Dry Roasted	28.3500	1.000	Ounce	4.90	14.59	7.19	168.40	0.00	2.55	0.00	1.96
Peanuts, Oil Roasted	28.3500	1.000	Ounce	4.40	15.92	6.31	174.35	0.00	1.56	0.00	2.58
Peanuts, Spanish, Fresh	28.3500	1.000	Ounce	7.41	14.06	4.48	161.60	0.00	2.69	0.00	2.17
Peanuts, Spanish, Oil-roasted, w	28.3500	1.000	Ounce	7.94	13.90	4.95	164.15	0.00	2.52	0.00	2.14
Peanuts, Spanish, Oil-roasted, w	28.3500	1.000	Ounce	7.94	13.90	4.95	164.15	0.00	2.52	0.00	2.14
Peanuts, Valencia, Fresh	28.3500	1.000	Ounce	7.11	13.49	5.93	161.60	0.00	2.47	0.00	2.08
Peanuts, Valencia, Oil-roasted,	28.3500	1.000	Ounce	7.67	14.53	4.62	166.98	0.00	2.52	0.00	2.24
Peanuts, Valencia, Oil-roasted,	28.3500	1.000	Ounce	7.67	14.53	4.62	166.98	0.00	2.52	0.00	2.24
Peanuts, Virginia, Fresh	28.3500	1.000	Ounce	7.14	13.82	4.69	159.61	0.00	2.41	0.00	1.80
Peanuts, Virginia, Oil-roasted,	28.3500	1.000	Ounce	7.33	13.78	5.63	163.86	0.00	2.52	0.00	1.80
Peanuts, Virginia, Oil-roasted,	28.3500	1.000	Ounce	7.33	13.78	5.63	163.86	0.00	2.52	0.00	1.80
Pecans, Dried	28.3500	1.000	Ounce	2.60	20.40	3.93	195.90	0.00	2.72	0.00	1.75
Pine Nuts	1.8000	10.000	Each	0.43	0.91	0.26	10.19	0.00	0.08	0.00	0.14
Pistachios, Dried	18.0000	30.000	Each	3.69	7.77	5.25	99.18	0.00	1.80	0.00	0.95
Pistachios, Dry Roasted	28.3500	1.000	Ounce	6.02	12.96	7.69	160.74	0.00	2.92	0.00	1.57
Sausage, Meatless	25.0000	1.000	Link	4.63	4.54	2.46	64.00	0.00	0.70	0.00	0.73
Seeds, Sesame, Toasted, w/o salt	28.3500	1.000	Ounce	4.81	13.61	7.38	160.75	0.00	4.79	0.00	1.91
Seeds, Sesame, Toasted, w/salt	28.3500	1.000	Ounce	4.81	13.61	7.38	160.75	0.00	4.79	0.00	1.91
Seeds, Sunflower, Dried	46.0000	1.000	Cup	10.48	22.80	8.63	262.20	0.00	4.83	0.00	2.39
Seeds, Sunflower, Dry Roasted, w	28.3500	1.000	Ounce	5.48	14.12	6.82	165.00	0.00	2.55	0.00	1.48
Seeds, Sunflower, Dry Roasted, w	28.3500	1.000	Ounce	5.48	14.12	6.82	165.00	0.00	3.15	0.00	1.48
Seeds, Sunflower, Oil Roasted, w	28.3500	1.000	Ounce	6.06	16.29	4.18	174.35	0.00	1.93	0.00	1.71
Seeds, Sunflower, Oil Roasted, w	28.3500	1.000	Ounce	6.06	16.29	4.18	174.35	0.00	1.93	0.00	1.71
Seeds, Sunflower, Toasted, w/ Sa	28.3500	1.000	Ounce	4.88	16.10	5.84	175.49	0.00	3.26	0.00	1.69
Seeds, Sunflower, Toasted, w/o S	28.3500	1.000	Ounce	4.88	16.10	5.84	175.49	0.00	3.26	0.00	1.69
Sesame Butter, Tahini, Toasted	15.0000	1.000	Tbsp	2.55	8.06	3.18	89.25	0.00	1.40	0.00	1.13
Soybeans, Boiled	10.7000	1.000	Tbsp	1.78	0.96	1.06	18.51	0.00	0.64	0.00	0.14
Soybeans, Dry Roasted	172.0000	1.000	Cup	68.08	37.19	56.28	774.00	0.00	13.93	0.00	5.38
Tofu, Fresh, Firm	81.0000	1.000	Ounce	6.51	3.61	2.41	62.37	0.00	0.32	0.00	0.53
Tofu, Fresh, Regular	17.6000	1.000	Ounce	1.15	0.65	0.32	10.74	0.00	0.04	0.00	0.09
Tofu, Fried	13.0000	1.000	Piece	2.23	2.62	1.37	35.23	0.00	0.51	0.00	0.38
Tofu, Fried, Prepared w/ Calcium	13.0000	1.000	Piece	2.23	2.62	1.37	35.23	0.00	0.51	0.00	0.38
Tofu, Okara	122.0000	1.000	Cup	3.93	2.11	15.30	93.94	0.00	0.00	0.00	0.23
Tofu, Salted and Fermented (fuyu	11.0000	1.000	Block	0.90	0.88	0.57	12.76	0.00	0.00	0.00	0.13
Walnuts, Black, Dried	7.8000	1.000	Tbsp	1.90	4.41	0.94	47.35	0.00	0.39	0.00	0.28
Walnuts, English, Dried	28.0000	0.500	Cup	4.26	18.26	3.84	183.12	0.00	1.88	0.00	1.72

Frozen Entrees and Packaged Foods

Apples, Escalloped-Stouffer's	170.0960	1.000	Each	0.00	4.00	41.00	200.00	0.00	0.00	0.00	0.00
Bean, Green, Mushroom Casserole-	134.6590	1.000	Each	5.00	10.00	13.00	160.00	0.00	0.00	0.00	0.00
Beef Ribs w/Barbecue Sauce, Bone	311.8430	1.000	Each	28.00	6.00	40.00	330.00	0.00	0.00	70.00	2.00
Beef Roast, Tender, Top Shelf-Ho	283.4930	1.000	Each	28.00	6.00	19.00	240.00	0.00	0.00	60.00	2.00
Beef Sirloin Tips w/ Mushroom Gr	269.3190	1.000	Each	22.00	5.00	43.00	310.00	0.00	0.00	35.00	2.00
Beef Sirloin Tips-Healthy Choice	318.9300	1.000	Each	22.00	7.00	29.00	270.00	0.00	0.00	65.00	3.00
Beef Stew, Micro Cup-Hormel	212.6200	1.000	Each	13.00	15.00	11.00	230.00	0.00	0.00	45.00	5.00
Beef Stroganoff w/ Parsley Noodl	276.4060	1.000	Each	24.00	20.00	28.00	390.00	0.00	0.00	0.00	0.00
Beef, Chipped, Creamed-Stouffer'	28.3500	1.000	Ounce	2.10	3.30	1.60	45.00	0.00	0.00	13.00	0.00
Beef, Oriental, w/ Veg., Lean Cu	244.5130	1.000	Each	20.00	9.00	31.00	290.00	0.00	0.00	40.00	2.00

Monounsaturated Fat (gm)	Polyunsaturated Fat (gm)	Vitamin D (mg)	Vitamin K (mg)	Vitamin E (mg)	Vitamin A (re)	Vitamin C (mg)	Thiamin (mg)	Riboflavin (mg)	Niacin (mg)	Vitamin B₆ (mg)	Folate (mg)	Vitamin B₁₂ (mcg)	Calcium (mg)	Iron (mg)	Magnesium (mg)	Phosphorus (mg)	Potassium (mg)	Sodium (mg)	Zinc (mg)
7.77	4.41	0.00	0.04	3.20	0.00	0.00	0.03	0.04	4.29	0.14	23.68	0.00	12.16	0.59	50.88	118.08	214.08	149.44	0.93
7.77	4.41	0.00	0.00	3.20	0.00	0.00	0.03	0.04	4.29	0.14	23.68	0.00	12.16	0.59	50.88	118.08	214.08	5.44	0.93
35.23	22.44	0.00	0.00	10.67	0.00	0.00	0.36	0.16	20.56	0.37	181.01	0.00	126.72	2.64	266.40	744.48	982.08	623.52	9.55
3.06	1.95	0.00	0.00	0.89	0.00	0.00	0.07	0.02	1.47	0.04	20.89	0.00	15.40	0.28	28.56	55.44	50.40	210.28	0.51
0.25	0.16	0.00	0.00	0.07	0.00	0.00	0.00	0.00	0.14	0.00	1.45	0.00	0.54	0.02	1.76	3.58	6.58	8.13	0.03
0.25	0.16	0.00	0.00	0.08	0.00	0.00	0.00	0.00	0.14	0.00	1.45	0.00	0.54	0.02	1.76	3.58	6.58	0.06	0.03
6.93	4.41	0.00	0.00	2.59	0.00	0.00	0.18	0.04	3.42	0.10	67.98	0.00	26.08	1.30	47.63	106.60	199.87	5.10	0.93
0.22	0.14	0.00	0.00	0.07	0.00	0.00	0.00	0.00	0.13	0.00	1.13	0.00	0.79	0.02	1.67	4.65	6.14	3.90	0.06
6.85	4.36	0.00	0.00	2.07	0.00	0.00	0.07	0.03	4.00	0.07	35.20	0.00	24.64	0.51	51.80	144.76	190.96	1.68	1.86
8.90	3.05	0.00	0.00	1.70	0.28	0.11	0.06	0.06	1.33	0.09	14.29	0.00	19.85	1.05	63.79	123.32	169.25	189.66	1.08
9.40	3.25	0.00	0.00	1.70	0.57	0.14	0.14	0.14	0.56	0.05	15.99	0.00	30.05	0.73	71.16	127.29	154.22	198.45	1.32
6.33	4.88	0.00	0.00	0.00	0.00	0.00	0.19	0.04	4.52	0.10	68.04	0.00	30.05	1.11	53.30	110.00	210.92	6.24	0.60
6.26	4.82	0.00	0.00	0.00	0.00	0.00	0.09	0.03	4.23	0.07	35.69	0.00	28.35	0.65	47.63	109.71	220.00	122.76	0.57
6.26	4.82	0.00	0.00	0.00	0.00	0.00	0.09	0.03	4.23	0.07	35.69	0.00	28.35	0.65	47.63	109.71	220.00	1.70	0.57
6.07	4.68	0.00	0.00	0.00	0.00	0.00	0.18	0.09	3.65	0.10	69.60	0.00	17.58	0.59	52.16	95.26	94.12	0.28	0.95
6.54	5.04	0.00	0.00	0.00	0.00	0.00	0.03	0.04	4.07	0.07	35.58	0.00	15.31	0.47	45.36	90.44	173.50	218.86	0.87
6.54	5.04	0.00	0.00	0.00	0.00	0.00	0.03	0.04	4.07	0.07	35.58	0.00	15.31	0.47	45.36	90.44	173.50	1.70	0.87
7.17	4.17	0.00	0.00	0.00	0.00	0.00	0.18	0.04	3.51	0.10	67.67	0.00	25.23	0.72	48.48	107.73	195.62	2.84	1.26
7.15	4.16	0.00	0.00	0.00	0.00	0.00	0.08	0.03	4.17	0.07	35.55	0.00	24.38	0.47	53.30	143.45	184.84	122.76	1.88
7.15	4.16	0.00	0.00	0.00	0.00	0.00	0.08	0.03	4.17	0.07	35.55	0.00	24.38	0.47	53.30	143.45	184.84	1.70	1.88
11.56	6.12	0.00	0.00	1.04	2.27	0.31	0.19	0.04	0.33	0.06	6.24	0.00	19.85	0.72	34.30	78.53	116.24	0.00	1.28
0.34	0.38	0.00	0.00	0.06	0.05	0.03	0.01	0.04	0.06	0.00	1.03	0.00	0.47	0.17	4.19	9.14	10.78	0.07	0.08
4.08	2.35	0.00	0.00	0.83	9.90	0.90	0.16	0.03	0.23	0.31	9.18	0.00	19.26	0.77	21.78	88.20	175.86	0.18	0.40
6.83	3.92	0.00	0.00	1.21	15.03	0.65	0.24	0.05	0.41	0.48	14.18	0.00	30.62	1.19	34.02	137.50	292.86	120.77	0.65
1.13	2.32	0.00	0.00	0.53	16.00	0.00	0.59	0.10	2.80	0.21	6.50	0.00	15.75	0.93	9.00	56.25	57.75	222.00	0.37
5.14	5.97	0.00	0.00	0.64	1.99	0.00	0.34	0.13	1.54	0.04	27.16	0.00	37.14	2.21	98.09	219.43	115.10	11.06	2.90
5.14	5.97	0.00	0.00	0.64	1.99	0.00	0.34	0.13	1.54	0.04	27.16	0.00	37.14	2.21	98.09	219.43	115.10	166.70	2.90
4.35	15.06	0.00	0.00	23.12	2.30	0.64	1.05	0.12	2.07	0.35	104.60	0.00	53.36	3.11	162.84	324.30	316.94	1.38	2.33
2.70	9.32	0.00	0.00	14.25	0.00	0.40	0.03	0.07	2.00	0.23	67.30	0.00	19.85	1.08	36.57	327.44	240.98	221.13	1.50
2.70	9.32	0.00	0.00	14.25	0.00	0.40	0.03	0.07	2.00	0.23	67.30	0.00	19.85	1.08	36.57	327.44	240.98	0.85	1.50
3.11	10.76	0.00	0.00	11.34	1.42	0.40	0.09	0.08	1.17	0.22	66.34	0.00	15.88	1.90	36.00	322.91	136.93	170.95	1.48
3.11	10.76	0.00	0.00	14.25	1.42	0.40	0.09	0.08	1.17	0.22	66.34	0.00	15.88	1.90	36.00	322.91	136.93	0.85	1.48
3.07	10.63	0.00	0.00	0.00	0.00	0.40	0.09	0.08	1.19	0.23	67.42	0.00	16.16	1.93	36.57	328.29	139.20	173.79	1.50
3.07	10.63	0.00	0.00	0.00	0.00	0.40	0.09	0.08	1.19	0.23	67.42	0.00	16.16	1.93	36.57	328.29	139.20	0.85	1.50
3.05	3.54	0.00	0.00	0.34	1.05	0.00	0.18	0.07	0.82	0.02	14.66	0.00	63.90	1.34	14.25	109.80	62.10	17.25	0.69
0.21	0.54	0.00	0.00	0.21	0.11	0.18	0.02	0.03	0.04	0.02	5.76	0.00	10.91	0.55	9.20	26.22	55.11	0.11	0.12
8.22	21.00	0.00	0.00	0.00	3.44	7.91	0.74	1.31	1.82	0.40	351.91	0.00	240.80	6.79	392.16	1116.28	2346.08	3.44	8.20
0.80	2.04	0.00	0.00	0.00	0.81	0.16	0.07	0.08	0.01	0.05	26.73	0.00	131.22	1.17	37.26	119.07	142.56	6.48	0.82
0.14	0.37	0.00	0.00	0.00	0.18	0.04	0.01	0.01	0.10	0.01	7.74	0.00	19.54	0.20	4.75	16.19	21.12	1.41	0.11
0.58	1.48	0.00	0.00	0.00	0.00	0.00	0.02	0.01	0.01	0.01	3.48	0.00	48.36	0.63	7.80	37.31	18.98	2.08	0.26
0.58	1.48	0.00	0.00	0.00	0.00	0.00	0.02	0.01	0.01	0.01	3.48	0.00	124.93	0.63	12.35	37.31	18.98	2.08	0.26
0.37	0.93	0.00	0.00	0.00	0.00	0.00	0.02	0.02	0.12	0.15	32.21	0.00	97.60	1.59	31.72	73.20	259.86	10.98	0.68
0.19	0.50	0.00	0.00	0.00	1.87	0.02	0.02	0.01	0.04	0.01	3.20	0.00	5.06	0.22	5.72	8.03	8.25	316.03	0.17
0.99	2.92	0.00	0.00	0.20	2.34	0.25	0.02	0.01	0.05	0.04	5.11	0.00	4.52	0.24	15.76	36.19	40.87	0.08	0.27
2.50	13.21	0.00	0.00	0.82	1.12	0.36	0.10	0.04	0.53	0.15	27.44	0.00	29.12	0.81	44.24	96.88	123.48	0.56	0.87
0.00	0.00	0.00	0.00	0.00	0.00	30.00	0.03	0.00	0.00	0.00	0.00	0.00	0.00	0.00	0.00	0.00	90.00	15.00	0.00
0.00	0.00	0.00	0.00	0.00	40.00	2.40	0.06	0.17	0.38	0.00	0.00	0.00	64.00	0.20	0.00	0.00	200.00	550.00	0.00
0.00	2.00	0.00	0.00	0.00	60.00	4.80	0.23	0.26	2.85	0.00	0.00	0.00	48.00	1.00	0.00	220.00	670.00	530.00	0.00
2.00	1.00	0.00	0.00	0.00	400.00	2.40	0.75	0.43	5.70	0.00	0.00	0.00	16.00	1.50	42.00	0.00	933.00	880.00	4.50
0.00	0.00	0.00	0.00	0.00	60.00	2.40	0.00	0.03	0.38	0.00	0.00	0.00	0.00	0.20	0.00	0.00	80.00	500.00	0.00
0.00	2.00	0.00	0.00	0.00	700.00	42.00	0.15	0.17	2.85	0.00	0.00	0.00	16.00	1.00	0.00	190.00	520.00	360.00	0.00
4.00	0.00	0.00	0.00	0.28	320.00	2.40	0.05	0.10	2.28	0.00	0.00	0.00	16.00	0.90	21.00	0.00	487.00	1140.00	2.40
0.00	0.00	0.00	0.00	0.00	40.00	1.20	0.12	0.34	2.85	0.00	0.00	0.00	48.00	1.50	0.00	0.00	300.00	1090.00	0.00
0.00	0.00	0.00	0.00	0.00	0.00	0.00	0.00	0.00	0.21	0.00	0.00	0.00	184.00	0.02	0.00	0.00	57.00	176.00	0.00
0.00	0.00	0.00	0.00	0.00	150.00	1.20	0.09	0.17	2.85	0.00	0.00	0.00	16.00	1.00	0.00	0.00	400.00	590.00	0.00

USDA ID Code	Food Name	Weight in Grams*	Quantity of Units	Unit of Measure	Protein (gm)	Fat (gm)	Carbohydrate (gm)	Kcalories	Caffeine (gm)	Fiber (gm)	Cholesterol (mg)	Saturated Fat (gm)
	Beef, Pot Roast, Yankee-Healthy	311.8430	1.000	Each	19.00	4.00	36.00	260.00	0.00	0.00	55.00	2.00
	Beef, Sirloin, w/ Barbecue Sauce	311.8430	1.000	Each	17.00	4.00	44.00	280.00	0.00	0.00	25.00	2.00
	Burritos, Beef and Bean (medium)	148.8340	1.000	Each	12.00	7.00	42.00	270.00	0.00	0.00	15.00	3.00
	Burritos, Beef and Bean (mild)-H	148.8340	1.000	Each	11.00	5.00	45.00	250.00	0.00	0.00	10.00	1.00
	Burritos,Chicken Con Queso (mil	148.8340	1.000	Each	15.00	8.00	40.00	280.00	0.00	0.00	20.00	2.00
	Cabbage, Stuffed, no Sauce-Stouf	28.3500	1.000	Ounce	2.00	2.10	3.10	39.00	0.00	0.00	5.00	0.00
	Cabbage, Stuffed, w/ Meat, Lean	269.3190	1.000	Each	13.00	6.00	26.00	210.00	0.00	0.00	30.00	2.00
	Cabbage, Stuffed-Stouffer's	28.3500	1.000	Ounce	1.40	1.40	2.70	29.00	0.00	0.00	4.00	0.00
	Cacciatore, Chicken, Lean Cuisin	308.2990	1.000	Each	22.00	7.00	31.00	280.00	0.00	0.00	45.00	2.00
	Cacciatore, Chicken, Top Shelf-H	283.4930	1.000	Each	21.00	3.00	25.00	210.00	0.00	0.00	50.00	0.00
	Cannelloni, Beef, w/ Sauce, Lean	272.8620	1.000	Each	14.00	3.00	28.00	200.00	0.00	0.00	25.00	1.00
	Cannelloni, Cheese, Lean Cuisine	258.6880	1.000	Each	23.00	8.00	27.00	270.00	0.00	0.00	25.00	4.00
	Chicken a la King w/ Rice-Stouff	269.3190	1.000	Each	18.00	5.00	38.00	270.00	0.00	0.00	0.00	0.00
	Chicken a la King, Top Shelf-Hor	5283.4930	1.000	Each	18.00	10.00	49.00	360.00	0.00	0.00	37.00	4.00
	Chicken a la King-Swanson	250.0000	1.000	Each	16.80	20.16	15.12	319.15	0.00	0.00	0.00	0.00
	Chicken a la Orange, Lean Cuisin	226.7950	1.000	Each	27.00	4.00	33.00	280.00	0.00	0.00	55.00	1.00
	Chicken a la Orange-Healthy Choi	255.1440	1.000	Each	20.00	2.00	36.00	240.00	0.00	0.00	45.00	2.00
	Chicken and Dumplings-Stouffer's	220.0000	1.000	Each	14.74	16.30	24.06	302.65	0.00	0.00	69.84	0.00
	Chicken and Dumplings-Swanson	200.0000	1.000	Each	10.35	10.35	17.87	206.94	0.00	0.00	0.00	0.00
	Chicken and Pasta Divan-Healthy	340.1920	1.000	Each	25.00	4.00	41.00	300.00	0.00	0.00	50.00	2.00
	Chicken and Veg. Oriental-Stouff	220.0000	1.000	Each	11.64	9.31	13.97	186.25	0.00	0.00	31.04	0.00
	Chicken and Veg. w/ Vermicelli,	333.1050	1.000	Each	18.00	5.00	30.00	240.00	0.00	0.00	30.00	1.00
	Chicken and Vegetables-Healthy C	326.0170	1.000	Each	20.00	1.00	31.00	210.00	0.00	0.00	35.00	0.00
	Chicken Classica-Stouffer's	28.3500	1.000	Ounce	1.80	0.70	2.30	22.00	0.00	0.00	5.00	0.00
	Chicken Dijon-Healthy Choice	311.8430	1.000	Each	21.00	3.00	40.00	250.00	0.00	0.00	40.00	1.00
	Chicken Divan-Stouffer's	226.7950	1.000	Each	24.00	10.00	11.00	220.00	0.00	0.00	0.00	0.00
	Chicken in BBQ Sauce, Lean Cuisi	248.0570	1.000	Each	20.00	6.00	32.00	260.00	0.00	0.00	50.00	1.00
	Chicken Italiano, Lean Cuisine-S	255.1440	1.000	Each	22.00	6.00	33.00	270.00	0.00	0.00	40.00	1.00
	Chicken Italienne-Stouffer's	28.3500	1.000	Ounce	2.20	0.90	1.20	22.00	0.00	0.00	7.00	0.00
	Chicken Oriental, Lean Cuisine-S	255.1440	1.000	Each	22.00	7.00	31.00	280.00	0.00	0.00	35.00	2.00
	Chicken Oriental-Healthy Choice	318.9300	1.000	Each	19.00	1.00	32.00	200.00	0.00	0.00	35.00	0.00
	Chicken Parmigiana-Healthy Choic	326.0170	1.000	Each	22.00	4.00	45.00	280.00	0.00	0.00	45.00	2.00
186	Chicken Piccata, Lemon Herb-Smar	238.0000	8.500	Ounce	11.00	2.00	34.00	200.00	0.00	3.00	25.00	0.50
	Chicken Stir Fry w/ Broccoli-Hea	340.1920	1.000	Each	21.00	6.00	35.00	280.00	0.00	0.00	55.00	3.00
	Chicken Tenderloins, Lean Cuisin	269.3190	1.000	Each	29.00	5.00	19.00	240.00	0.00	0.00	60.00	2.00
	Chicken w/ Barbecue Sauce-Health	361.4540	1.000	Each	24.00	6.00	65.00	410.00	0.00	0.00	55.00	2.00
	Chicken w/ Spanish Rice, Breast	283.4930	1.000	Each	27.00	15.00	38.00	400.00	0.00	0.00	75.00	7.00
	Chicken, Breast, Glazed, Top She	283.4930	1.000	Each	19.00	2.00	19.00	170.00	0.00	0.00	35.00	1.00
	Chicken, Creamed-Stouffer's	28.3500	1.000	Ounce	2.80	3.50	1.20	48.00	0.00	0.00	14.00	0.00
	Chicken, Escalloped, and Noodles	283.4930	1.000	Each	21.00	24.00	30.00	420.00	0.00	0.00	0.00	0.00
	Chicken, Fiesta -Weight Watchers	240.9750	1.000	Each	12.00	2.00	38.00	220.00	0.00	5.00	25.00	0.50
	Chicken, Glazed, w/ Veg. Lean Cu	240.9690	1.000	Each	21.00	7.00	24.00	250.00	0.00	0.00	50.00	2.00
	Chicken, Glazed-Healthy Choice	240.9690	1.000	Each	21.00	3.00	27.00	220.00	0.00	0.00	45.00	1.00
	Chicken, Glazed-Stouffer's	28.3500	1.000	Ounce	2.90	1.10	1.00	26.00	0.00	0.00	9.00	0.00
	Chicken, Herb Roasted -Healthy C	347.2790	1.000	Each	22.00	5.00	50.00	300.00	0.00	0.00	40.00	2.00
	Chicken, Honey Mustard, Lean Cui	212.6200	1.000	Each	18.00	4.00	30.00	230.00	0.00	0.00	40.00	1.00
	Chicken, Honey Mustard-Healthy C	269.3190	1.000	Each	26.00	4.00	41.00	310.00	0.00	0.00	45.00	1.00
187	Chicken, Honey Mustard-Smart One	238.0000	8.500	Ounce	11.00	2.00	37.00	200.00	0.00	3.00	30.00	0.50
	Chicken, Mandarin-Healthy Choice	311.8430	1.000	Each	23.00	2.00	39.00	260.00	0.00	0.00	50.00	0.00
	Chicken, Mexicali-Stouffer's	28.3500	1.000	Ounce	1.40	0.80	1.80	20.00	0.00	0.00	5.00	0.00
	Chicken, Oriental, w/ Spicy Pean	269.3190	1.000	Each	33.00	5.00	40.00	340.00	0.00	0.00	45.00	1.00
	Chicken, Oven Baked, Lean Cuisin	226.7950	1.000	Each	17.00	5.00	21.00	200.00	0.00	0.00	35.00	2.00
	Chicken, Salsa -Healthy Choice	318.9300	1.000	Each	20.00	2.00	36.00	240.00	0.00	0.00	50.00	1.00
	Chicken, Southwestern Style-Heal	354.3670	1.000	Each	25.00	5.00	51.00	340.00	0.00	0.00	60.00	2.00
	Chicken, Sweet and Sour-Healthy	326.0170	1.000	Each	20.00	2.00	52.00	280.00	0.00	0.00	35.00	0.00

Monounsaturated Fat (gm)	Polyunsaturated Fat (gm)	Vitamin D (mg)	Vitamin K (mg)	Vitamin E (mg)	Vitamin A (re)	Vitamin C (mg)	Thiamin (mg)	Riboflavin (mg)	Niacin (mg)	Vitamin B6 (mg)	Folate (mg)	Vitamin B12 (mcg)	Calcium (mg)	Iron (mg)	Magnesium (mg)	Phosphorus (mg)	Potassium (mg)	Sodium (mg)	Zinc (mg)
0.00	0.00	0.00	0.00	0.00	100.00	9.00	0.15	0.17	1.52	0.00	0.00	0.00	32.00	1.00	0.00	150.00	350.00	400.00	0.00
0.00	1.00	0.00	0.00	0.00	0.00	0.00	0.00	0.00	0.00	0.00	0.00	0.00	0.00	0.00	0.00	190.00	630.00	240.00	0.00
0.00	3.00	0.00	0.00	0.00	20.00	3.60	0.38	0.17	1.90	0.00	0.00	0.00	48.00	1.50	0.00	180.00	270.00	520.00	0.00
0.00	2.00	0.00	0.00	0.00	20.00	1.20	0.38	0.17	2.85	0.00	0.00	0.00	32.00	2.00	0.00	130.00	330.00	450.00	0.00
0.00	3.00	0.00	0.00	0.00	20.00	6.00	0.45	0.34	2.85	0.00	0.00	0.00	80.00	1.50	0.00	170.00	260.00	500.00	0.00
0.00	0.00	0.00	0.00	0.00	0.00	0.60	0.00	0.00	0.08	0.00	0.00	0.00	72.00	0.04	0.00	0.00	48.00	150.00	0.00
0.00	1.00	0.00	0.00	0.00	80.00	6.00	0.12	0.17	3.80	0.00	0.00	0.00	64.00	1.50	0.00	0.00	600.00	560.00	0.00
0.00	0.00	0.00	0.00	0.00	0.00	3.00	0.00	0.00	0.06	0.00	0.00	0.00	48.00	0.02	0.00	0.00	51.00	145.00	0.00
0.00	1.00	0.00	0.00	0.00	100.00	9.00	0.23	0.17	5.70	0.00	0.00	0.00	32.00	0.80	0.00	0.00	560.00	570.00	0.00
0.00	0.00	0.00	0.00	0.46	100.00	2.40	0.15	0.26	6.65	0.00	0.00	0.00	80.00	1.00	0.00	0.00	0.00	810.00	0.00
0.00	0.00	0.00	0.00	0.00	350.00	6.00	0.12	0.17	2.85	0.00	0.00	0.00	120.00	1.50	0.00	0.00	800.00	490.00	0.00
0.00	0.00	0.00	0.00	0.00	60.00	21.00	0.12	0.26	1.52	0.00	0.00	0.00	240.00	0.40	0.00	0.00	400.00	590.00	0.00
0.00	0.00	0.00	0.00	0.00	20.00	1.20	0.09	0.17	2.85	0.00	0.00	0.00	160.00	0.80	0.00	32.00	260.00	800.00	0.00
4.00	2.00	0.00	0.00	0.17	250.00	1.20	0.12	0.17	8.55	0.00	0.00	0.00	48.00	0.20	28.00	0.00	476.00	890.00	1.20
0.00	0.00	0.00	0.00	0.00	0.00	0.00	0.05	0.23	3.19	0.00	0.00	0.00	53.75	0.34	0.00	0.00	0.00	1159.01	0.00
0.00	0.00	0.00	0.00	0.00	80.00	12.00	0.23	0.17	9.50	0.00	0.00	0.00	32.00	0.40	0.00	0.00	490.00	290.00	0.00
0.00	0.00	0.00	0.00	0.00	150.00	27.00	0.15	0.10	5.70	0.00	0.00	0.00	16.00	0.80	0.00	230.00	430.00	220.00	0.00
0.00	0.00	0.00	0.00	0.00	0.00	0.00	0.00	0.01	0.44	0.00	0.00	0.00	1.06	0.16	0.00	0.00	248.33	659.63	0.00
0.00	0.00	0.00	0.00	0.00	75.25	0.00	0.03	0.10	1.79	0.00	0.00	0.00	15.05	0.38	0.00	0.00	0.00	921.83	0.00
0.00	1.00	0.00	0.00	0.00	800.00	72.00	0.38	0.26	4.75	0.00	0.00	0.00	120.00	1.00	0.00	270.00	500.00	520.00	0.00
0.00	0.00	0.00	0.00	0.00	0.00	4.66	0.00	0.00	0.59	0.00	0.00	0.00	372.49	0.08	0.00	0.00	349.21	1078.68	0.00
0.00	1.00	0.00	0.00	0.00	150.00	6.00	0.30	0.26	5.70	0.00	0.00	0.00	64.00	1.00	0.00	0.00	500.00	500.00	0.00
0.00	0.00	0.00	0.00	0.00	150.00	9.00	0.30	0.17	3.80	0.00	0.00	0.00	32.00	1.50	0.00	190.00	390.00	490.00	0.00
0.00	0.00	0.00	0.00	0.00	0.00	1.20	0.00	0.00	0.10	0.00	0.00	0.00	112.00	0.01	0.00	0.00	50.00	83.00	0.00
0.00	0.00	0.00	0.00	0.00	100.00	9.00	0.23	0.14	9.50	0.00	0.00	0.00	16.00	1.00	0.00	300.00	350.00	470.00	0.00
0.00	0.00	0.00	0.00	0.00	60.00	3.60	0.45	0.17	3.80	0.00	0.00	0.00	200.00	2.00	0.00	32.00	490.00	610.00	0.00
0.00	2.00	0.00	0.00	0.00	250.00	18.00	0.15	0.17	5.70	0.00	0.00	0.00	48.00	0.80	0.00	0.00	650.00	500.00	0.00
0.00	2.00	0.00	0.00	0.00	100.00	24.00	0.30	0.26	5.70	0.00	0.00	0.00	80.00	0.80	0.00	0.00	600.00	590.00	0.00
0.00	0.00	0.00	0.00	0.00	0.00	1.20	0.00	0.00	0.10	0.00	0.00	0.00	48.00	0.01	0.00	0.00	57.00	128.00	0.00
0.00	2.00	0.00	0.00	0.00	40.00	6.00	0.23	0.17	6.65	0.00	0.00	0.00	32.00	1.00	0.00	0.00	470.00	480.00	0.00
0.00	0.00	0.00	0.00	0.00	250.00	36.00	0.15	0.14	7.60	0.00	0.00	0.00	32.00	0.80	0.00	200.00	400.00	440.00	0.00
0.00	0.00	0.00	0.00	0.00	900.00	12.00	0.15	0.17	9.50	0.00	0.00	0.00	80.00	1.00	0.00	260.00	500.00	370.00	0.00
0.00	0.00	0.00	0.00	0.00	0.00	0.00	0.00	0.00	0.00	0.00	0.00	0.00	0.00	0.00	0.00	0.00	0.00	460.00	0.00
0.00	0.00	0.00	0.00	0.00	20.00	0.00	0.23	0.34	2.85	0.00	0.00	0.00	48.00	1.50	0.00	260.00	630.00	500.00	0.00
0.00	1.00	0.00	0.00	0.00	200.00	4.80	0.23	0.34	7.60	0.00	0.00	0.00	120.00	0.40	0.00	0.00	750.00	490.00	0.00
0.00	2.00	0.00	0.00	0.00	100.00	12.00	0.12	0.14	8.55	0.00	0.00	0.00	48.00	1.50	0.00	250.00	670.00	550.00	0.00
4.00	3.00	0.00	0.00	0.07	100.00	3.60	0.09	0.26	7.60	0.00	0.00	0.00	80.00	0.40	35.00	0.00	584.00	810.00	1.65
1.00	1.00	0.00	0.00	0.76	400.00	3.60	0.06	0.17	7.60	0.00	0.00	0.00	32.00	0.40	35.00	0.00	804.00	780.00	1.05
0.00	0.00	0.00	0.00	0.00	0.00	0.00	0.00	0.00	0.10	0.00	0.00	0.00	352.00	0.01	0.00	0.00	37.00	119.00	0.00
0.00	0.00	0.00	0.00	0.00	20.00	0.00	0.15	0.34	3.80	0.00	0.00	0.00	80.00	0.80	0.00	0.00	300.00	840.00	0.00
0.00	0.00	0.00	0.00	0.00	450.00	42.00	0.00	0.00	0.00	0.00	0.00	0.00	72.00	1.50	0.00	0.00	490.00	480.00	0.00
0.00	4.00	0.00	0.00	0.00	20.00	3.60	0.15	0.17	7.60	0.00	0.00	0.00	16.00	0.20	0.00	0.00	580.00	590.00	0.00
0.00	1.00	0.00	0.00	0.00	0.00	1.20	0.15	0.14	6.65	0.00	0.00	0.00	0.00	0.60	0.00	240.00	370.00	510.00	0.00
0.00	0.00	0.00	0.00	0.00	0.00	0.00	0.00	0.00	0.23	0.00	0.00	0.00	24.00	0.01	0.00	0.00	45.00	105.00	0.00
0.00	1.00	0.00	0.00	0.00	250.00	24.00	0.15	0.14	7.60	0.00	0.00	0.00	32.00	0.80	0.00	280.00	370.00	560.00	0.00
0.00	1.00	0.00	0.00	0.00	200.00	2.40	0.15	0.17	3.80	0.00	0.00	0.00	16.00	0.40	0.00	0.00	340.00	540.00	0.00
0.00	0.00	0.00	0.00	0.00	100.00	3.60	0.15	0.03	1.52	0.00	0.00	0.00	16.00	0.80	0.00	0.00	110.00	520.00	0.00
0.00	0.00	0.00	0.00	0.00	0.00	0.00	0.00	0.00	0.00	0.00	0.00	0.00	0.00	0.00	0.00	0.00	0.00	370.00	0.00
0.00	0.00	0.00	0.00	0.00	250.00	9.00	0.15	0.17	4.75	0.00	0.00	0.00	16.00	1.00	0.00	200.00	400.00	400.00	0.00
0.00	0.00	0.00	0.00	0.00	0.00	4.20	0.00	0.00	0.11	0.00	0.00	0.00	88.00	0.02	0.00	0.00	68.00	48.00	0.00
0.00	1.00	0.00	0.00	0.00	0.00	2.40	0.00	0.00	0.38	0.00	0.00	0.00	0.00	0.20	0.00	0.00	50.00	470.00	0.00
0.00	0.00	0.00	0.00	0.00	350.00	6.00	0.15	0.17	7.60	0.00	0.00	0.00	16.00	0.80	0.00	0.00	550.00	480.00	0.00
0.00	0.00	0.00	0.00	0.00	200.00	66.00	0.23	0.17	3.80	0.00	0.00	0.00	64.00	0.60	0.00	200.00	540.00	450.00	0.00
0.00	2.00	0.00	0.00	0.00	0.00	0.00	0.00	0.00	0.00	0.00	0.00	0.00	0.00	0.00	0.00	260.00	560.00	550.00	0.00
0.00	0.00	0.00	0.00	0.00	250.00	30.00	0.15	0.17	8.55	0.00	0.00	0.00	32.00	1.00	0.00	220.00	480.00	320.00	0.00

USDA ID Code	Food Name	Weight in Grams*	Quantity of Units	Unit of Measure	Protein (gm)	Fat (gm)	Carbohydrate (gm)	Kcalories	Caffeine (gm)	Fiber (gm)	Cholesterol (mg)	Saturated Fat (gm)
188	Chicken, Szechwan Veg, Spicy & H	252.0000	9.000	Ounce	11.00	2.00	39.00	220.00	0.00	3.00	10.00	0.50
	Chicken, Teriyaki-Healthy Choice	347.2790	1.000	Each	24.00	4.00	39.00	290.00	0.00	0.00	55.00	1.00
	Chili Beef Soup-Healthy Choice	212.6200	1.000	Each	11.00	1.00	22.00	150.00	0.00	0.00	15.00	0.00
	Chili Con Carne w/ Beans-Stouffe	248.0570	1.000	Each	20.00	10.00	28.00	280.00	0.00	0.00	0.00	0.00
	Chili Mac, Micro Cup-Hormel	212.6200	1.000	Each	10.00	9.00	18.00	192.00	0.00	0.00	22.00	4.00
	Chili no Beans, Micro Cup-Hormel	209.0760	1.000	Each	18.00	17.00	15.00	290.00	0.00	0.00	60.00	8.00
	Chili w/ Beans Soup-Stouffer's	283.9200	1.000	Cup	14.02	9.01	25.04	240.36	0.00	0.00	30.04	0.00
	Chili w/ Beans, Chunky -Hormel	253.1620	1.000	Cup	17.86	16.67	29.77	345.30	0.00	0.00	59.53	0.00
	Chili w/ Beans, Micro Cup-Hormel	209.0760	1.000	Each	15.00	11.00	23.00	250.00	0.00	0.00	49.00	4.00
	Chili w/ Beans-Hormel	253.1620	1.000	Cup	17.86	17.86	32.15	357.20	0.00	0.00	65.49	5.95
	Chili w/o Beans-Hormel	253.1620	1.000	Cup	19.05	32.15	16.67	428.64	0.00	0.00	71.44	13.10
	Chili, Fat Free	240.0000	0.500	Cup	14.00	0.00	30.00	160.00	0.00	14.00	0.00	0.00
	Chili, Hot, no Beans-Hormel	212.6200	1.000	Each	16.00	27.00	14.00	360.00	0.00	0.00	60.00	11.00
	Chili, Hot, w/ Beans, Micro Cup-	209.0760	1.000	Each	15.00	11.00	24.00	250.00	0.00	0.00	49.00	4.00
	Chili, Hot, w/ Beans-Hormel	212.6200	1.000	Each	15.00	15.00	27.00	300.00	0.00	0.00	55.00	5.00
	Chili, Three Bean-Stouffer's	283.9200	1.000	Cup	10.02	5.01	32.05	210.32	0.00	0.00	20.03	0.00
	Chow Mein w/ Rice, Chicken, Lean	255.1440	1.000	Each	14.00	5.00	34.00	240.00	0.00	0.00	30.00	1.00
	Chow Mein w/ Rice, Chicken-Stouf	304.7550	1.000	Each	13.00	5.00	39.00	250.00	0.00	0.00	0.00	0.00
	Chow Mein, Beef	247.0000	1.000	Cup	10.00	1.50	15.00	110.00	0.00	4.00	10.00	1.00
	Chow Mein, Chicken -Weight Watch	255.1500	1.000	Each	12.00	2.00	34.00	200.00	0.00	3.00	25.00	0.50
	Chow Mein, Chicken-Healthy Choic	240.9690	1.000	Each	18.00	3.00	31.00	220.00	0.00	0.00	45.00	1.00
190	Chow Mein, Chicken-Smart Ones	252.0000	9.000	Ounce	12.00	2.00	34.00	200.00	0.00	3.00	25.00	0.50
	Chow Mein, Vegetable-Stouffer's	28.3500	1.000	Ounce	0.30	0.70	1.60	14.00	0.00	0.00	0.00	0.00
	Corn Pudding-Stouffer's	28.3500	1.000	Ounce	1.20	1.70	4.50	38.00	0.00	0.00	15.00	0.00
	Corn Souffle-Stouffer's	170.0960	1.000	Each	7.00	11.00	27.00	240.00	0.00	0.00	0.00	0.00
	Corned Beef Hash-Hormel	253.1620	1.000	Cup	26.79	26.79	17.86	419.71	0.00	0.00	80.37	8.93
	Egg Roll	85.0000	1.000	Each	7.00	5.00	21.00	160.00	0.00	2.00	10.00	1.00
	Enchiladas, Beef and Bean, Lean	262.2310	1.000	Each	15.00	6.00	32.00	240.00	0.00	0.00	45.00	3.00
	Enchiladas, Beef -Healthy Choice	379.1720	1.000	Each	15.00	5.00	66.00	370.00	0.00	0.00	30.00	2.00
	Enchiladas, Cheese-Stouffer's	276.4060	1.000	Each	23.00	29.00	33.00	490.00	0.00	0.00	0.00	0.00
	Enchiladas, Chicken Suiza-Weight	255.1500	1.000	Each	15.00	8.00	28.00	250.00	0.00	4.00	25.00	3.00
	Enchiladas, Chicken, Lean Cuisin	279.9500	1.000	Each	17.00	9.00	34.00	290.00	0.00	0.00	55.00	3.00
	Enchiladas, Chicken, Nacho Grand	255.1500	1.000	Each	15.00	8.00	42.00	290.00	0.00	4.00	20.00	2.50
	Enchiladas, Chicken-Healthy Choi	269.3190	1.000	Each	14.00	9.00	44.00	310.00	0.00	0.00	35.00	3.00
	Enchiladas, Chicken-Stouffer's	283.4930	1.000	Each	21.00	31.00	31.00	490.00	0.00	0.00	35.00	3.00
	Fajitas, Chicken-Healthy Choice	198.4450	1.000	Each	17.00	3.00	25.00	200.00	0.00	0.00	35.00	1.00
442	Fettuccini Alfredo w/Broccoli-Sm	238.0000	8.500	Ounce	10.00	6.00	34.00	230.00	0.00	3.00	20.00	3.00
443	Fettuccini, Chicken-Smart Ones	280.0000	10.000	Ounce	19.00	7.00	39.00	290.00	0.00	4.00	50.00	2.00
	Fettucini Alfredo with Broccoli-	240.9750	1.000	Each	15.00	6.00	24.00	220.00	0.00	6.00	15.00	2.50
	Fettucini Alfredo, Lean Cuisine-	255.1440	1.000	Each	14.00	7.00	41.00	280.00	0.00	0.00	15.00	3.00
	Fettucini Alfredo-Stouffer's	141.7460	1.000	Each	8.00	14.00	22.00	245.00	0.00	0.00	0.00	0.00
	Fettucini Primavera, Lean Cuisin	283.4930	1.000	Each	14.00	8.00	32.00	260.00	0.00	0.00	45.00	3.00
	Fettucini Sauce (Alfredo Style)-	283.9200	1.000	Cup	14.02	67.10	11.02	701.05	0.00	0.00	180.27	0.00
	Fettucini w/ Turkey and Vegetabl	354.3670	1.000	Each	29.00	6.00	45.00	350.00	0.00	0.00	60.00	3.00
	Fettucini, Chicken -Weight Watch	233.8900	1.000	Each	22.00	9.00	25.00	280.00	0.00	2.00	40.00	3.00
	Fettucini, Chicken, Lean Cuisine	255.1440	1.000	Each	23.00	6.00	33.00	280.00	0.00	0.00	35.00	3.00
	Fettucini, Chicken-Healthy Choic	240.9690	1.000	Each	19.00	7.00	39.00	240.00	0.00	0.00	45.00	2.00
	Fish Divan, Filet of, Lean Cuisi	294.1240	1.000	Each	27.00	5.00	13.00	210.00	0.00	0.00	65.00	2.00
	Fish Florentine, Filet of, Lean	272.8620	1.000	Each	26.00	7.00	13.00	220.00	0.00	0.00	65.00	3.00
	Fish, Breaded-Healthy Choice	9.7450	1.000	Stick	1.00	0.50	1.75	15.00	0.00	0.00	2.50	0.00
	Fish, Lemon Pepper -Healthy Choi	304.7550	1.000	Each	13.00	5.00	52.00	300.00	0.00	0.00	40.00	1.00
	Ham and Asparagus Bake-Stouffer'	269.3190	1.000	Each	18.00	35.00	32.00	520.00	0.00	0.00	0.00	0.00
	Hamburger Helper, Beef Noodle	220.0000	1.000	Cup	4.00	10.50	23.00	260.00	0.00	1.00	5.00	4.00
	Hamburger Helper, Cheesy Italian	220.0000	1.000	Cup	5.00	21.00	30.00	330.00	0.00	1.00	5.00	2.00
	Hamburger Helper, Chili Mac	220.0000	1.000	Cup	3.00	16.00	30.00	290.00	0.00	1.00	4.00	4.00

Monounsaturated Fat (gm)	Polyunsaturated Fat (gm)	Vitamin D (mg)	Vitamin K (mg)	Vitamin E (mg)	Vitamin A (re)	Vitamin C (mg)	Thiamin (mg)	Riboflavin (mg)	Niacin (mg)	Vitamin B6 (mg)	Folate (mg)	Vitamin B12 (mcg)	Calcium (mg)	Iron (mg)	Magnesium (mg)	Phosphorus (mg)	Potassium (mg)	Sodium (mg)	Zinc (mg)
0.00	0.00	0.00	0.00	0.00	0.00	0.00	0.00	0.00	0.00	0.00	0.00	0.00	0.00	0.00	0.00	0.00	0.00	730.00	0.00
0.00	2.00	0.00	0.00	0.00	20.00	6.00	0.09	0.10	7.60	0.00	0.00	0.00	32.00	0.80	0.00	250.00	520.00	560.00	0.00
0.00	0.00	0.00	0.00	0.00	20.00	6.00	0.09	0.03	0.38	0.00	0.00	0.00	16.00	0.60	0.00	0.00	290.00	560.00	0.00
0.00	0.00	0.00	0.00	0.00	200.00	15.00	0.15	0.26	2.85	0.00	0.00	0.00	64.00	2.00	0.00	0.00	700.00	910.00	0.00
4.00	0.00	0.00	0.00	0.17	210.00	0.00	0.08	0.17	2.09	0.00	0.00	0.00	0.00	1.50	35.00	0.00	443.00	977.00	2.10
8.00	1.00	0.00	0.00	0.01	400.00	0.00	0.08	0.24	2.47	0.00	0.00	0.00	48.00	1.60	35.00	0.00	507.00	830.00	3.90
0.00	0.00	0.00	0.00	0.00	0.00	0.00	0.00	0.00	0.57	0.00	0.00	0.00	0.00	0.30	0.00	0.00	711.07	991.49	0.00
0.00	0.00	0.00	0.00	0.00	0.00	0.00	0.00	0.00	0.00	0.00	0.00	0.00	0.00	0.00	0.00	0.00	0.00	928.73	0.00
4.00	0.00	0.00	0.00	18.90	190.00	0.00	0.14	0.15	1.71	0.00	0.00	0.00	48.00	1.90	45.50	0.00	677.00	977.00	2.70
7.14	1.19	0.00	0.00	0.01	250.04	0.00	0.11	0.20	2.04	0.00	0.00	0.00	57.15	1.91	58.34	0.00	913.25	1226.40	2.50
15.48	1.19	0.00	0.00	0.60	785.85	0.00	0.11	0.26	2.94	0.00	0.00	0.00	47.63	1.67	41.67	0.00	591.77	1023.98	3.21
0.00	0.00	0.00	0.00	0.00	2000.00	24.00	0.00	0.00	0.00	0.00	0.00	0.00	48.00	2.00	0.00	0.00	0.00	320.00	0.00
13.00	1.00	0.00	0.00	10.56	330.00	0.00	0.05	0.22	2.47	0.00	0.00	0.00	40.00	1.40	35.00	0.00	497.00	860.00	2.70
4.00	0.00	0.00	0.00	1.95	190.00	0.00	0.14	0.15	1.71	0.00	0.00	0.00	48.00	1.90	45.50	0.00	677.00	977.00	2.70
6.00	1.00	0.00	0.00	0.00	210.00	0.00	0.09	0.17	1.71	0.00	0.00	0.00	48.00	1.80	49.00	0.00	777.00	1030.00	2.25
0.00	0.00	0.00	0.00	0.00	0.00	6.01	0.00	0.01	0.57	0.00	0.00	0.00	1.20	0.40	0.00	0.00	891.34	861.29	0.00
0.00	1.00	0.00	0.00	0.00	60.00	6.00	0.15	0.17	4.75	0.00	0.00	0.00	32.00	0.60	0.00	0.00	350.00	530.00	0.00
0.00	0.00	0.00	0.00	0.00	80.00	12.00	0.03	0.17	1.90	0.00	0.00	0.00	16.00	0.40	0.00	0.00	340.00	720.00	0.00
0.00	0.00	0.00	0.00	0.00	40.00	12.00	0.00	0.00	0.00	0.00	0.00	0.00	24.00	0.40	0.00	0.00	0.00	760.00	0.00
0.00	0.00	0.00	0.00	0.00	300.00	36.00	0.00	0.00	0.00	0.00	0.00	0.00	48.00	0.40	0.00	0.00	360.00	570.00	0.00
0.00	1.00	0.00	0.00	0.00	80.00	3.60	0.15	0.14	3.80	0.00	0.00	0.00	16.00	0.80	0.00	290.00	290.00	440.00	0.00
0.00	0.00	0.00	0.00	0.00	0.00	0.00	0.00	0.00	0.00	0.00	0.00	0.00	0.00	0.00	0.00	0.00	0.00	570.00	0.00
0.00	0.00	0.00	0.00	0.00	0.00	0.60	0.00	0.00	0.02	0.00	0.00	0.00	24.00	0.01	0.00	0.00	26.00	156.00	0.00
0.00	0.00	0.00	0.00	0.00	0.00	0.60	0.00	0.00	0.06	0.00	0.00	0.00	88.00	0.02	0.00	0.00	51.00	125.00	0.00
0.00	0.00	0.00	0.00	0.00	60.00	0.00	0.15	0.26	1.14	0.00	0.00	0.00	48.00	0.40	0.00	0.00	200.00	760.00	0.00
17.86	0.00	0.00	0.00	0.43	0.00	0.00	0.00	0.15	3.39	0.00	0.00	0.00	71.44	1.79	31.26	0.00	625.11	991.24	4.02
0.00	0.00	0.00	0.00	0.00	100.00	1.20	0.00	0.00	0.00	0.00	0.00	0.00	24.00	0.20	0.00	0.00	0.00	350.00	0.00
0.00	1.00	0.00	0.00	0.00	80.00	6.00	0.23	0.26	1.90	0.00	0.00	0.00	80.00	1.00	0.00	0.00	470.00	480.00	0.00
0.00	2.00	0.00	0.00	0.00	250.00	24.00	0.30	0.26	1.90	0.00	0.00	0.00	120.00	1.00	0.00	260.00	600.00	450.00	0.00
0.00	0.00	0.00	0.00	0.00	150.00	6.00	0.09	0.34	1.52	0.00	0.00	0.00	480.00	0.80	0.00	0.00	400.00	550.00	0.00
0.00	0.00	0.00	0.00	0.00	40.00	1.20	0.00	0.00	0.00	0.00	0.00	0.00	360.00	0.80	0.00	0.00	470.00	570.00	0.00
0.00	2.00	0.00	0.00	0.00	250.00	6.00	0.23	0.34	2.85	0.00	0.00	0.00	120.00	1.50	0.00	0.00	450.00	500.00	0.00
0.00	0.00	0.00	0.00	0.00	300.00	12.00	0.00	0.00	0.00	0.00	0.00	0.00	360.00	0.60	0.00	0.00	600.00	560.00	0.00
0.00	1.00	0.00	0.00	0.00	80.00	21.00	0.15	0.17	4.75	0.00	0.00	0.00	80.00	0.80	0.00	160.00	380.00	480.00	0.00
0.00	0.00	0.00	0.00	0.00	60.00	2.40	0.09	0.34	2.85	0.00	0.00	0.00	240.00	0.60	0.00	0.00	420.00	860.00	0.00
0.00	1.00	0.00	0.00	0.00	150.00	9.00	0.23	0.17	3.80	0.00	0.00	0.00	64.00	1.50	0.00	210.00	360.00	310.00	0.00
0.00	0.00	0.00	0.00	0.00	0.00	0.00	0.00	0.00	0.00	0.00	0.00	0.00	0.00	0.00	0.00	0.00	0.00	450.00	0.00
0.00	0.00	0.00	0.00	0.00	0.00	0.00	0.00	0.00	0.00	0.00	0.00	0.00	0.00	0.00	0.00	0.00	0.00	590.00	0.00
0.00	0.00	0.00	0.00	0.00	60.00	1.20	0.00	0.00	0.00	0.00	0.00	0.00	300.00	1.50	0.00	0.00	510.00	540.00	0.00
0.00	0.00	0.00	0.00	0.00	0.00	0.00	0.30	0.43	1.52	0.00	0.00	0.00	200.00	0.80	0.00	0.00	270.00	570.00	0.00
0.00	0.00	0.00	0.00	0.00	0.00	0.00	0.15	0.26	0.95	0.00	0.00	0.00	120.00	0.40	0.00	0.00	100.00	400.00	0.00
0.00	0.00	0.00	0.00	0.00	400.00	18.00	0.30	0.43	1.52	0.00	0.00	0.00	240.00	0.80	0.00	0.00	400.00	510.00	0.00
0.00	0.00	0.00	0.00	0.00	0.00	0.00	0.00	0.01	0.00	0.00	0.00	0.00	2.72	0.00	0.00	0.00	340.51	1812.72	0.00
0.00	2.00	0.00	0.00	0.00	150.00	0.00	0.45	0.51	3.80	0.00	0.00	0.00	120.00	1.50	0.00	310.00	450.00	480.00	0.00
0.00	0.00	0.00	0.00	0.00	40.00	0.00	0.00	0.00	0.00	0.00	0.00	0.00	240.00	1.00	0.00	0.00	730.00	590.00	0.00
0.00	0.00	0.00	0.00	0.00	0.00	0.00	0.30	0.43	5.70	0.00	0.00	0.00	120.00	0.80	0.00	0.00	420.00	500.00	0.00
0.00	2.00	0.00	0.00	0.00	0.00	0.00	0.23	0.17	2.85	0.00	0.00	0.00	64.00	1.00	0.00	210.00	190.00	370.00	0.00
0.00	1.00	0.00	0.00	0.00	20.00	27.00	0.15	0.34	1.90	0.00	0.00	0.00	120.00	0.40	0.00	0.00	800.00	490.00	0.00
0.00	2.00	0.00	0.00	0.00	500.00	1.20	0.15	0.34	1.90	0.00	0.00	0.00	120.00	0.40	0.00	0.00	780.00	590.00	0.00
0.00	0.13	0.00	0.00	0.00	0.00	0.00	0.01	0.02	0.10	0.00	0.00	0.00	0.00	0.10	0.00	0.00	20.00	31.25	0.00
0.00	2.00	0.00	0.00	0.00	80.00	48.00	0.23	0.14	1.14	0.00	0.00	0.00	32.00	0.60	0.00	180.00	410.00	370.00	0.00
0.00	0.00	0.00	0.00	0.00	60.00	36.00	0.53	0.51	2.85	0.00	0.00	0.00	160.00	0.80	0.00	0.00	360.00	1100.00	0.00
0.00	0.00	0.00	0.00	0.00	60.00	0.00	0.23	0.17	3.80	0.00	0.00	0.00	24.00	1.00	0.00	0.00	240.00	900.00	0.00
0.00	0.00	0.00	0.00	0.00	60.00	0.00	0.30	0.34	3.80	0.00	0.00	0.00	120.00	1.50	0.00	0.00	400.00	900.00	0.00
0.00	0.00	0.00	0.00	0.00	200.00	0.00	0.30	0.26	4.75	0.00	0.00	0.00	24.00	1.50	0.00	0.00	0.00	900.00	0.00

USDA ID Code	Food Name	Weight in Grams*	Quantity of Units	Unit of Measure	Protein (gm)	Fat (gm)	Carbohydrate (gm)	Kcalories	Caffeine (gm)	Fiber (gm)	Cholesterol (mg)	Saturated Fat (gm)
	Heartland Medley-Stouffer's	28.3500	1.000	Ounce	1.40	0.40	1.80	17.00	0.00	0.00	3.00	0.00
580	Lasagna Florentine-Smart Ones	280.0000	10.000	Ounce	10.00	2.00	34.00	200.00	0.00	5.00	10.00	0.00
	Lasagna Florentine-Weight Watche	283.5000	1.000	Each	13.00	2.00	37.00	210.00	0.00	5.00	10.00	0.50
	Lasagna w/ Meat Sauce, Lean Cuis	290.5810	1.000	Each	20.00	6.00	36.00	280.00	0.00	0.00	25.00	3.00
	Lasagna w/ Meat Sauce-Healthy Ch	283.4930	1.000	Each	18.00	5.00	37.00	260.00	0.00	0.00	20.00	2.00
581	Lasagna w/ Meat Sauce-Smart Ones	252.0000	9.000	Ounce	13.00	2.00	43.00	240.00	0.00	4.00	10.00	0.50
	Lasagna w/ Meat Sauce-Weight Wat	290.5910	1.000	Each	24.00	7.00	34.00	290.00	0.00	7.00	15.00	2.50
	Lasagna, Cheese, Italian -Weight	311.8500	1.000	Each	29.00	8.00	28.00	300.00	0.00	7.00	25.00	3.00
	Lasagna, Italian, Top Shelf-Horm	283.4930	1.000	Each	23.00	16.00	30.00	350.00	0.00	0.00	60.00	8.00
	Lasagna, Micro Cup-Hormel	212.6200	1.000	Each	8.00	13.00	25.00	250.00	0.00	0.00	23.00	6.00
	Lasagna, Vegetable-Stouffer's	274.0420	1.000	Each	23.00	20.00	33.00	400.00	0.00	0.00	0.00	0.00
	Lasagna, Zucchini, Lean Cuisine-	311.8430	1.000	Each	17.00	6.00	34.00	260.00	0.00	0.00	20.00	2.00
	Lasagna, Zucchini-Healthy Choice	326.0170	1.000	Each	14.00	3.00	41.00	250.00	0.00	0.00	15.00	2.00
	Lasagna-Stouffer's	283.4930	1.000	Each	18.00	12.00	40.00	340.00	0.00	0.00	0.00	0.00
	Linguini w/ Clam Sauce, Lean Cui	272.8620	1.000	Each	17.00	8.00	36.00	280.00	0.00	0.00	30.00	2.00
	Macaroni and Beef in Sauce, Lean	283.4930	1.000	Each	14.00	6.00	35.00	250.00	0.00	0.00	25.00	1.00
	Macaroni and Beef w/ Tomatoes-St	326.0170	1.000	Each	21.00	12.00	38.00	340.00	0.00	0.00	0.00	0.00
	Macaroni and Beef-Healthy Choice	240.9690	1.000	Each	12.00	3.00	32.00	200.00	0.00	0.00	15.00	1.00
	Macaroni and Cheese	111.9120	1.000	Cup	1.00	12.99	43.97	359.72	0.00	15.99	39.97	7.99
	Macaroni and Cheese, Deluxe Ligh	90.0000	1.000	Serving	14.00	4.50	48.00	290.00	0.00	0.00	15.00	2.50
	Macaroni and Cheese, Kraft	70.0000	1.000	Serving	12.00	18.50	50.00	420.00	0.00	0.00	15.00	5.00
	Macaroni and Cheese, Lean Cuisin	255.1440	1.000	Each	15.00	9.00	37.00	290.00	0.00	0.00	30.00	4.00
	Macaroni and Cheese, Micro Cup-H	212.6200	1.000	Each	12.00	11.00	28.00	260.00	0.00	0.00	45.00	6.00
	Macaroni and Cheese, Nacho-Healt	255.1440	1.000	Each	13.00	5.00	44.00	280.00	0.00	0.00	20.00	3.00
	Macaroni and Cheese-Healthy Choi	255.1440	1.000	Each	12.00	6.00	45.00	280.00	0.00	0.00	20.00	3.00
	Macaroni and Cheese-Stouffer's	170.0960	1.000	Each	11.00	13.00	23.00	250.00	0.00	0.00	0.00	0.00
	Macaroni and Cheese-Weight Watch	255.1500	1.000	Each	11.00	7.00	49.00	300.00	0.00	7.00	20.00	2.00
	Manicotti, Cheese-Healthy Choice	262.2310	1.000	Each	15.00	3.00	34.00	220.00	0.00	0.00	30.00	2.00
	Manicotti, Cheese-Stouffer's	28.3500	1.000	Ounce	1.60	1.30	2.60	29.00	0.00	0.00	4.00	0.00
	Meatballs, Swedish, w/ Pasta, Le	258.6880	1.000	Each	23.00	8.00	31.00	290.00	0.00	0.00	55.00	3.00
	Meatballs, Swedish, w/ Pasta-Sto	262.2310	1.000	Each	24.00	21.00	32.00	420.00	0.00	0.00	0.00	0.00
582	Meatballs, Swedish-Smart Ones	252.0000	9.000	Ounce	19.00	10.00	33.00	300.00	0.00	2.00	50.00	4.00
	Meatloaf w/ Mac. and Cheese, Lea	265.7750	1.000	Each	26.00	8.00	26.00	280.00	0.00	0.00	55.00	3.00
	Meatloaf-Healthy Choice	340.1920	1.000	Each	17.00	8.00	48.00	340.00	0.00	0.00	40.00	3.00
	Meatloaf-Stouffer's	28.3500	1.000	Ounce	4.40	3.40	2.10	57.00	0.00	0.00	15.00	0.00
585	Morningstar Farms- Buffalo Wings	85.0000	5.000	Each	13.00	9.00	16.00	200.00	0.00	3.00	0.00	1.50
586	Morningstar Farms- Burger, Bean,	78.0000	1.000	Each	11.00	1.00	16.00	110.00	0.00	5.00	0.00	0.00
587	Morningstar Farms- Burger, Veggi	67.0000	1.000	Each	14.00	8.00	40.00	120.00	0.00	2.00	0.00	3.50
588	Morningstar Farms- Burger/Cheese	128.0000	1.000	Each	14.00	8.00	40.00	290.00	0.00	2.00	0.00	3.50
589	Morningstar Farms- Burgers, Bett	78.0000	1.000	Each	13.00	0.00	8.00	80.00	0.00	3.00	0.00	0.00
590	Morningstar Farms- Chik Nuggets	86.0000	4.000	Each	13.00	4.00	17.00	160.00	0.00	5.00	0.00	0.50
591	Morningstar Farms- Chik Patties	71.0000	1.000	Each	9.00	6.00	15.00	150.00	0.00	2.00	0.00	1.00
592	Morningstar Farms- Corn Dogs, Me	71.0000	1.000	Each	7.00	4.00	22.00	150.00	0.00	3.00	0.00	0.50
593	Morningstar Farms- Corn Dogs, Mi	71.0000	1.000	Each	11.00	4.50	21.00	150.00	0.00	1.00	0.00	0.50
594	Morningstar Farms- Crumbles, Bur	55.0000	0.660	Cup	10.00	2.50	4.00	80.00	0.00	2.00	0.00	0.00
595	Morningstar Farms- Crumbles, Sau	55.0000	0.660	Cup	11.00	3.00	5.00	90.00	0.00	2.00	0.00	0.00
596	Morningstar Farms- Eggs, Better'	57.0000	0.250	Cup	5.00	0.00	0.00	20.00	0.00	0.00	0.00	0.00
597	Morningstar Farms- Garden Grille	71.0000	1.000	Each	6.00	2.50	18.00	120.00	0.00	4.00	0.00	1.00
598	Morningstar Farms- Grillers	64.0000	1.000	Each	15.00	6.00	5.00	140.00	0.00	2.00	0.00	1.00
599	Morningstar Farms- Ham/Cheese Sd	128.0000	1.000	Each	15.00	7.00	25.00	300.00	0.00	1.00	0.00	2.50
600	Morningstar Farms- Harvest Burge	90.0000	1.000	Each	17.00	4.50	8.00	140.00	0.00	5.00	0.00	1.50
601	Morningstar Farms- Harvest Burge	90.0000	1.000	Each	18.00	4.00	8.00	140.00	0.00	5.00	0.00	1.50
602	Morningstar Farms- Harvest Burge	90.0000	1.000	Each	16.00	4.00	9.00	140.00	0.00	5.00	0.00	1.50
603	Morningstar Farms- Links, Breakf	45.0000	2.000	Each	8.00	2.00	2.00	60.00	0.00	2.00	0.00	0.50
604	Morningstar Farms- Meatless, Gro	55.0000	0.500	Cup	10.00	0.00	4.00	60.00	0.00	2.00	0.00	0.00

Monounsaturated Fat (gm)	Polyunsaturated Fat (gm)	Vitamin D (mg)	Vitamin K (mg)	Vitamin E (mg)	Vitamin A (re)	Vitamin C (mg)	Thiamin (mg)	Riboflavin (mg)	Niacin (mg)	Vitamin B_6 (mg)	Folate (mg)	Vitamin B_{12} (mcg)	Calcium (mg)	Iron (mg)	Magnesium (mg)	Phosphorus (mg)	Potassium (mg)	Sodium (mg)	Zinc (mg)
0.00	0.00	0.00	0.00	0.00	0.00	0.60	0.00	0.00	0.06	0.00	0.00	0.00	40.00	0.02	0.00	0.00	60.00	85.00	0.00
0.00	0.00	0.00	0.00	0.00	0.00	0.00	0.00	0.00	0.00	0.00	0.00	0.00	0.00	0.00	0.00	0.00	0.00	590.00	0.00
0.00	0.00	0.00	0.00	0.00	300.00	15.00	0.00	0.00	0.00	0.00	0.00	0.00	300.00	1.50	0.00	0.00	440.00	420.00	0.00
0.00	0.00	0.00	0.00	0.00	100.00	6.00	0.15	0.26	2.85	0.00	0.00	0.00	120.00	1.00	0.00	0.00	700.00	560.00	0.00
0.00	1.00	0.00	0.00	0.00	150.00	2.40	0.30	0.26	1.90	0.00	0.00	0.00	80.00	1.50	0.00	210.00	500.00	420.00	0.00
0.00	0.00	0.00	0.00	0.00	0.00	0.00	0.00	0.00	0.00	0.00	0.00	0.00	0.00	0.00	0.00	0.00	0.00	520.00	0.00
0.00	0.00	0.00	0.00	0.00	250.00	12.00	0.00	0.00	0.00	0.00	0.00	0.00	480.00	1.50	0.00	0.00	720.00	580.00	0.00
0.00	0.00	0.00	0.00	0.00	350.00	15.00	0.00	0.00	0.00	0.00	0.00	0.00	780.00	1.50	0.00	0.00	720.00	560.00	0.00
5.00	1.00	0.00	0.00	0.70	100.00	2.40	0.30	0.51	3.80	0.00	0.00	0.00	240.00	1.50	49.00	0.00	728.00	840.00	3.15
4.00	2.00	0.00	0.00	0.00	100.00	1.80	0.12	0.20	1.90	0.00	0.00	0.00	40.00	0.80	24.50	0.00	331.00	949.00	1.05
0.00	0.00	0.00	0.00	0.00	250.00	0.00	0.12	0.43	0.76	0.00	0.00	0.00	160.00	0.60	0.00	0.00	350.00	760.00	0.00
0.00	0.00	0.00	0.00	0.00	150.00	6.00	0.15	0.26	1.90	0.00	0.00	0.00	200.00	0.80	0.00	0.00	650.00	520.00	0.00
0.00	0.00	0.00	0.00	0.00	350.00	6.00	0.38	0.26	1.90	0.00	0.00	0.00	200.00	1.50	0.00	250.00	830.00	400.00	0.00
0.00	0.00	0.00	0.00	0.00	150.00	6.00	0.15	0.34	6.65	0.00	0.00	0.00	200.00	1.00	0.00	0.00	570.00	840.00	0.00
0.00	2.00	0.00	0.00	0.00	0.00	0.00	0.30	0.17	1.90	0.00	0.00	0.00	32.00	1.50	0.00	0.00	90.00	560.00	0.00
0.00	1.00	0.00	0.00	0.00	100.00	3.60	0.15	0.17	2.85	0.00	0.00	0.00	48.00	1.50	0.00	0.00	450.00	540.00	0.00
0.00	0.00	0.00	0.00	0.00	60.00	6.00	0.06	0.10	1.90	0.00	0.00	0.00	32.00	0.80	0.00	0.00	300.00	1440.00	0.00
0.00	0.00	0.00	0.00	0.00	200.00	15.00	0.30	0.26	0.00	0.00	0.00	0.00	32.00	1.00	0.00	0.00	530.00	420.00	0.00
0.00	0.00	0.00	0.00	0.00	99.92	0.00	0.00	0.00	0.00	0.00	0.00	0.00	239.81	1.50	0.00	0.00	0.00	1029.19	0.00
0.00	0.00	0.00	0.00	0.00	0.00	0.00	0.00	0.00	0.00	0.00	0.00	0.00	160.00	1.50	0.00	0.00	0.00	810.00	0.00
0.00	0.00	0.00	0.00	0.00	0.00	0.00	0.00	0.00	0.00	0.00	0.00	0.00	120.00	1.50	0.00	0.00	0.00	760.00	0.00
0.00	0.00	0.00	0.00	0.00	0.00	0.00	0.30	0.43	1.52	0.00	0.00	0.00	200.00	0.80	0.00	0.00	160.00	550.00	0.00
3.00	1.00	0.00	0.00	0.00	80.00	6.00	0.09	0.26	1.14	0.00	0.00	0.00	80.00	0.60	24.50	0.00	209.00	650.00	1.05
0.00	0.00	0.00	0.00	0.00	0.00	0.00	0.60	0.51	0.00	0.00	0.00	0.00	160.00	0.80	0.00	0.00	420.00	560.00	0.00
0.00	1.00	0.00	0.00	0.00	0.00	0.00	0.30	0.26	1.14	0.00	0.00	0.00	120.00	1.00	0.00	230.00	220.00	520.00	0.00
0.00	0.00	0.00	0.00	0.00	20.00	0.00	0.15	0.26	0.38	0.00	0.00	0.00	160.00	0.40	0.00	0.00	140.00	640.00	0.00
0.00	0.00	0.00	0.00	0.00	100.00	0.00	0.00	0.00	0.00	0.00	0.00	0.00	300.00	1.00	0.00	0.00	410.00	570.00	0.00
0.00	0.00	0.00	0.00	0.00	250.00	6.00	0.30	0.26	1.90	0.00	0.00	0.00	120.00	1.50	0.00	210.00	590.00	310.00	0.00
0.00	0.00	0.00	0.00	0.00	0.00	2.40	0.00	0.00	0.04	0.00	0.00	0.00	296.01	0.02	0.00	0.00	45.00	108.00	0.00
0.00	1.00	0.00	0.00	0.00	20.00	0.00	0.23	0.34	3.80	0.00	0.00	0.00	48.00	1.50	0.00	0.00	450.00	550.00	0.00
0.00	0.00	0.00	0.00	0.00	20.00	1.20	0.15	0.26	2.85	0.00	0.00	0.00	48.00	1.50	0.00	0.00	350.00	740.00	0.00
0.00	0.00	0.00	0.00	0.00	0.00	0.00	0.00	0.00	0.00	0.00	0.00	0.00	0.00	0.00	0.00	0.00	0.00	510.00	0.00
0.00	1.00	0.00	0.00	0.00	60.00	9.00	0.23	0.43	3.80	0.00	0.00	0.00	120.00	2.00	0.00	0.00	550.00	540.00	0.00
0.00	1.00	0.00	0.00	0.00	0.00	0.00	0.00	0.00	0.00	0.00	0.00	0.00	0.00	0.00	0.00	240.00	690.00	560.00	0.00
0.00	0.00	0.00	0.00	0.00	0.00	0.00	0.00	0.00	0.13	0.00	0.00	0.00	48.00	0.06	0.00	0.00	4.40	193.00	0.00
2.50	5.00	0.00	0.00	0.00	0.00	0.00	1.05	0.17	3.00	0.20	0.00	1.20	40.00	2.70	0.00	0.00	390.00	730.00	0.00
0.00	0.00	0.00	0.00	0.00	0.00	0.00	0.00	0.00	0.00	0.00	0.00	0.00	40.00	1.80	0.00	0.00	350.00	470.00	0.00
3.00	1.50	0.00	0.00	0.00	0.00	0.00	0.00	0.00	0.00	0.00	0.00	0.00	100.00	1.08	0.00	0.00	130.00	400.00	0.00
3.00	1.50	0.00	0.00	0.00	0.00	0.00	0.00	0.00	0.00	0.00	0.00	0.00	60.00	1.08	0.00	0.00	130.00	400.00	0.00
0.00	0.00	0.00	0.00	0.00	0.00	0.00	0.00	0.00	0.00	0.00	0.00	0.00	20.00	1.80	0.00	0.00	390.00	360.00	0.00
1.00	2.50	0.00	0.00	0.00	0.00	0.00	0.90	0.17	2.00	0.20	0.00	1.50	20.00	1.80	0.00	0.00	330.00	670.00	0.00
1.50	3.50	0.00	0.00	0.00	0.00	0.00	0.60	0.10	0.40	0.16	0.00	0.90	0.00	0.72	0.00	0.00	150.00	570.00	0.00
1.00	2.50	0.00	0.00	0.00	0.00	0.00	0.00	0.00	0.00	0.00	0.00	0.00	0.00	1.08	0.00	0.00	60.00	500.00	0.00
2.50	1.50	0.00	0.00	0.00	0.00	0.00	0.00	0.00	0.00	0.00	0.00	0.00	0.00	1.08	0.00	0.00	90.00	580.00	0.00
0.50	2.00	0.00	0.00	0.00	0.00	0.00	0.30	0.10	4.00	0.30	0.00	1.80	20.00	1.80	0.00	0.00	120.00	210.00	0.00
0.50	2.00	0.00	0.00	0.00	0.00	0.00	1.80	0.17	4.00	0.40	0.00	1.80	20.00	1.80	0.00	0.00	80.00	370.00	0.00
0.00	0.00	0.60	0.00	1.20	225.00	0.00	0.03	0.34	0.00	0.08	0.02	0.60	20.00	0.72	0.00	0.00	75.00	90.00	0.60
1.00	0.50	0.00	0.00	0.00	0.00	0.00	0.00	0.00	0.00	0.00	0.00	0.00	60.00	1.80	0.00	0.00	130.00	280.00	0.00
2.00	3.00	0.00	0.00	0.00	0.00	0.00	1.80	0.17	2.00	0.40	0.00	2.70	40.00	1.08	0.00	0.00	130.00	260.00	0.00
3.00	1.50	0.00	0.00	0.00	0.00	0.00	0.00	0.00	0.00	0.00	0.00	0.00	60.00	1.08	0.00	0.00	100.00	520.00	0.00
0.50	0.50	0.00	0.00	0.00	0.00	0.00	0.30	0.14	4.00	0.30	0.00	1.50	80.00	2.70	0.00	0.00	440.00	370.00	6.75
0.50	0.50	0.00	0.00	0.00	0.00	0.00	0.30	0.14	4.00	0.30	0.00	1.50	80.00	2.70	0.00	0.00	430.00	370.00	7.50
0.00	0.50	0.00	0.00	0.00	0.00	0.00	0.30	0.14	4.00	0.30	0.00	1.20	80.00	2.70	0.00	0.00	450.00	370.00	6.75
0.50	1.00	0.00	0.00	0.00	0.00	0.00	1.80	0.14	2.00	0.30	0.00	3.60	0.00	1.44	0.00	0.00	60.00	340.00	0.00
0.00	0.00	0.00	0.00	0.00	0.00	0.00	0.45	0.14	3.00	0.30	0.00	1.80	20.00	1.80	0.00	0.00	100.00	260.00	0.00

USDA ID Code	Food Name	Weight in Grams*	Quantity of Units	Unit of Measure	Protein (gm)	Fat (gm)	Carbohydrate (gm)	Kcalories	Caffeine (gm)	Fiber (gm)	Cholesterol (mg)	Saturated Fat (gm)
605	Morningstar Farms- Patties, Brea	38.0000	1.000	Each	10.00	0.00	3.00	38.00	0.00	2.00	0.00	0.50
606	Morningstar Farms- Patties, Gard	67.0000	1.000	Each	10.00	2.50	9.00	100.00	0.00	4.00	0.00	0.50
607	Morningstar Farms- Pizza, Pepper	128.0000	1.000	Each	12.00	7.00	42.00	280.00	0.00	5.00	0.00	3.00
608	Morningstar Farms- Quarter Prime	96.0000	1.000	Each	24.00	2.00	6.00	140.00	0.00	3.00	0.00	0.00
609	Morningstar Farms- Scramblers	57.0000	0.250	Cup	6.00	0.00	2.00	35.00	0.00	0.00	0.00	0.00
610	Morningstar Farms- Strips, Break	16.0000	2.000	Each	2.00	4.50	2.00	60.00	0.00	1.00	0.00	0.50
611	Morningstar Farms- Veggie Dog	57.0000	1.000	Each	11.00	0.50	6.00	57.00	0.00	1.00	0.00	0.00
	Muffin, Banana Nut -Healthy Choi	70.8730	1.000	Each	3.00	6.00	32.00	180.00	0.00	0.00	0.00	0.00
	Muffin,English, Sandwich-Healthy	120.4840	1.000	Each	16.00	3.00	30.00	200.00	0.00	0.00	20.00	1.00
	Noodles and Chicken, Micro Cup-H	212.6200	1.000	Each	7.00	7.00	19.00	174.00	0.00	0.00	29.00	2.00
	Noodles Romanoff-Stouffer's	283.9200	1.000	Cup	17.03	25.04	36.05	440.66	0.00	0.00	40.06	0.00
614	Noodles, Kung Pao & Veg-Smart On	280.0000	10.000	Ounce	8.00	10.00	35.00	260.00	0.00	5.00	5.00	1.50
	Omelet, Turkey Sausage, on Engli	134.6590	1.000	Each	16.00	4.00	30.00	210.00	0.00	0.00	20.00	2.00
	Omelet, Western Style, on Englis	134.6590	1.000	Each	16.00	3.00	29.00	200.00	0.00	0.00	15.00	2.00
624	Pasta Accents, White Cheddar Sce	181.0000	1.750	Cup	9.00	9.00	37.00	270.00	0.00	3.00	10.00	2.50
625	Pasta Accents-Alfredo	160.0000	2.000	Cup	9.00	8.00	25.00	210.00	0.00	4.00	5.00	2.50
626	Pasta Accents-Crmy Cheddar	190.0000	2.330	Cup	9.00	8.00	36.00	250.00	0.00	5.00	15.00	3.00
627	Pasta Accents-Florentine	206.0000	2.000	Cup	13.00	9.00	44.00	310.00	0.00	5.00	20.00	3.00
628	Pasta Accents-Garden Herb	195.0000	2.000	Cup	9.00	7.00	32.00	230.00	0.00	7.00	15.00	4.00
629	Pasta Accents-Garlic Seasoning	188.0000	2.000	Cup	7.00	10.00	36.00	260.00	0.00	3.00	15.00	5.00
630	Pasta Accents-Lasagna Style	188.0000	2.000	Cup	9.00	10.00	33.00	260.00	0.00	4.00	10.00	3.00
631	Pasta Accents-Oriental Style	201.0000	2.500	Cup	8.00	10.00	35.00	260.00	0.00	4.00	20.00	4.00
632	Pasta Accents-Primavera	200.0000	2.250	Cup	12.00	9.00	39.00	290.00	0.00	4.00	5.00	2.50
	Pasta Accents-Primavera	175.0000	1.000	Serving	9.00	10.00	27.00	230.00	0.00	0.00	0.00	0.00
633	Pasta and Spinach Romano-Smart O	291.0000	10.400	Ounce	11.00	8.00	32.00	240.00	0.00	4.00	5.00	3.50
	Pasta Florentine-Stouffer's	283.9200	0.500	Cup	16.02	21.03	32.05	380.57	0.00	0.00	50.07	0.00
	Pasta Italiano, Vegetable-Health	283.4930	1.000	Each	7.00	1.00	46.00	220.00	0.00	0.00	0.00	0.00
	Pasta Italiano-Healthy Choice	340.1920	1.000	Each	16.00	5.00	59.00	350.00	0.00	0.00	30.00	2.00
	Pasta Roma-Stouffer's	283.9200	0.500	Cup	16.02	7.01	31.05	260.39	0.00	0.00	30.04	0.00
	Pasta Shells w/ Tomato Sauce-Hea	340.1920	1.000	Each	24.00	3.00	53.00	330.00	0.00	0.00	35.00	2.00
	Pasta Shells, Cheese w/ Sauce-St	262.2310	1.000	Each	17.00	13.00	28.00	300.00	0.00	0.00	0.00	0.00
	Pasta w/ Chicken, Cacciatore-Hea	354.3670	1.000	Each	26.00	3.00	47.00	310.00	0.00	0.00	35.00	0.00
	Pasta w/ Chicken, Teriyaki-Healt	357.9100	1.000	Each	24.00	3.00	58.00	350.00	0.00	0.00	45.00	1.00
634	Pasta w/ Tomato Basil Sauce-Smar	268.8000	9.600	Ounce	12.00	9.00	33.00	260.00	0.00	5.00	10.00	3.50
	Pasta, Angel Hair, Lean Cuisine-	283.4930	1.000	Each	10.00	5.00	38.00	240.00	0.00	5.00	10.00	1.00
635	Pasta, Bowtie & Mushroom Marsala	270.0000	9.650	Ounce	13.00	9.00	36.00	280.00	0.00	5.00	10.00	3.50
636	Pasta, Crmy Rigatoni w/ Brocc &	252.0000	9.000	Ounce	14.00	2.00	40.00	230.00	0.00	4.00	20.00	0.50
637	Pasta, Penne w/ Sun-dried Tomato	280.0000	10.000	Ounce	12.00	9.00	41.00	290.00	0.00	4.00	15.00	3.00
639	Penne Pollo-Smart Ones	280.0000	10.000	Ounce	22.00	5.00	40.00	290.00	0.00	3.00	35.00	2.00
640	Penne, Spicy, & Ricotta-Smart On	285.6000	10.200	Ounce	12.00	6.00	45.00	280.00	0.00	5.00	5.00	2.00
	Pepper, Stuffed, Single Serving-	283.4930	1.000	Each	10.00	8.00	28.00	220.00	0.00	0.00	0.00	0.00
	Peppers, Stuffed Green-Stouffer'	219.7070	1.000	Each	9.00	8.00	22.00	200.00	0.00	0.00	0.00	0.00
654	Pizza Combo, Deluxe-Smart Ones	184.0000	6.570	Ounce	23.00	11.00	47.00	380.00	0.00	6.00	40.00	3.50
	Pizza, Cheese, 4 - DiGiorno	139.0000	1.000	Slice	16.00	11.00	39.00	320.00	0.00	3.11	25.10	6.10
	Pizza, Cheese, Microwave for One	104.0000	1.000	Each	10.00	11.00	25.00	240.00	0.00	1.00	15.00	3.50
	Pizza, Cheese, Party - Totino's	277.0000	1.000	Slice	15.00	5.00	33.00	320.00	0.00	2.00	20.00	5.00
	Pizza, French Bread, Cheese-Heal	159.4650	1.000	Each	19.00	4.00	46.00	290.00	0.00	0.00	15.00	2.00
	Pizza, French Bread, Cheese-Stou	145.2900	1.000	Each	16.00	14.00	40.00	350.00	0.00	0.00	0.00	0.00
	Pizza, French Bread, Deluxe-Heal	180.7270	1.000	Each	23.00	7.00	41.00	330.00	0.00	0.00	35.00	3.00
	Pizza, French Bread, Deluxe-Stou	173.6390	1.000	Each	21.00	19.00	40.00	420.00	0.00	0.00	0.00	0.00
	Pizza, French Bread, Double Chee	166.5520	1.000	Each	22.00	18.00	43.00	420.00	0.00	0.00	0.00	0.00
	Pizza, French Bread, Hamburger-S	173.6390	1.000	Each	23.00	18.00	39.00	410.00	0.00	0.00	0.00	0.00
	Pizza, French Bread, Pepperoni-H	170.0960	1.000	Each	20.00	7.00	38.00	310.00	0.00	0.00	30.00	3.00
	Pizza, French Bread, Pepperoni-S	159.4650	1.000	Each	19.00	19.00	39.00	400.00	0.00	0.00	0.00	0.00
	Pizza, French Bread, Sausage-Sto	170.0960	1.000	Each	20.00	21.00	40.00	430.00	0.00	0.00	0.00	0.00

Monounsaturated Fat (gm)	Polyunsaturated Fat (gm)	Vitamin D (mg)	Vitamin K (mg)	Vitamin E (mg)	Vitamin A (re)	Vitamin C (mg)	Thiamin (mg)	Riboflavin (mg)	Niacin (mg)	Vitamin B6 (mg)	Folate (mg)	Vitamin B12 (mcg)	Calcium (mg)	Iron (mg)	Magnesium (mg)	Phosphorus (mg)	Potassium (mg)	Sodium (mg)	Zinc (mg)
0.50	2.00	0.00	0.00	0.00	0.00	0.00	1.80	0.10	2.00	0.20	0.00	1.50	0.00	1.80	0.00	0.00	110.00	270.00	0.00
0.50	1.50	0.00	0.00	0.00	60.04	0.00	0.00	0.00	0.00	0.00	0.00	0.00	40.00	0.72	0.00	0.00	180.00	350.00	0.00
2.50	1.50	0.00	0.00	0.00	0.00	0.00	0.00	0.00	0.00	0.00	0.00	0.00	40.00	1.80	0.00	0.00	180.00	420.00	0.00
1.00	1.00	0.00	0.00	0.00	0.00	9.00	0.75	0.34	2.00	0.50	0.00	5.40	60.00	2.70	0.00	0.00	210.00	370.00	0.00
0.00	0.00	0.40	0.00	0.00	225.00	0.00	0.30	0.34	0.00	0.12	0.00	1.80	20.00	1.08	0.00	0.00	60.00	95.00	0.60
1.00	3.00	0.00	0.00	0.00	0.00	0.00	0.75	0.03	0.04	0.08	0.00	0.24	0.00	0.36	0.00	0.00	15.00	220.00	0.00
0.00	0.00	0.00	0.00	0.00	0.00	0.00	0.00	0.00	0.00	0.00	0.00	0.00	0.00	0.72	0.00	0.00	60.00	580.00	0.00
0.00	3.00	0.00	0.00	0.00	0.00	0.00	0.15	0.14	0.76	0.00	0.00	0.00	80.00	1.00	0.00	160.00	250.00	80.00	0.00
0.00	1.00	0.00	0.00	0.00	60.00	3.60	0.45	0.43	2.85	0.00	0.00	0.00	120.00	2.00	0.00	220.00	200.00	510.00	0.00
3.00	2.00	0.00	0.00	0.00	270.00	8.40	0.08	0.12	1.71	0.00	0.00	0.00	32.00	0.70	21.00	0.00	254.00	1009.00	0.75
0.00	0.00	0.00	0.00	0.00	0.00	0.00	0.00	0.01	0.19	0.00	0.00	0.00	1.60	0.20	0.00	0.00	260.39	1992.99	0.00
0.00	0.00	0.00	0.00	0.00	0.00	0.00	0.00	0.00	0.00	0.00	0.00	0.00	0.00	0.00	0.00	0.00	0.00	690.00	0.00
0.00	1.00	0.00	0.00	0.00	60.00	0.00	0.38	0.51	2.85	0.00	0.00	0.00	160.00	2.00	0.00	250.00	590.00	470.00	0.00
0.00	0.00	0.00	0.00	0.00	100.00	3.60	0.45	0.51	1.90	0.00	0.00	0.00	160.00	2.00	0.00	240.00	220.00	480.00	0.00
0.00	0.00	0.00	0.00	0.00	0.00	0.00	0.00	0.00	0.00	0.00	0.00	0.00	0.00	0.00	0.00	0.00	0.00	750.00	0.00
0.00	0.00	0.00	0.00	0.00	0.00	0.00	0.00	0.00	0.00	0.00	0.00	0.00	0.00	0.00	0.00	0.00	0.00	480.00	0.00
0.00	0.00	0.00	0.00	0.00	0.00	0.00	0.00	0.00	0.00	0.00	0.00	0.00	0.00	0.00	0.00	0.00	0.00	700.00	0.00
0.00	0.00	0.00	0.00	0.00	0.00	0.00	0.00	0.00	0.00	0.00	0.00	0.00	0.00	0.00	0.00	0.00	0.00	910.00	0.00
0.00	0.00	0.00	0.00	0.00	0.00	0.00	0.00	0.00	0.00	0.00	0.00	0.00	0.00	0.00	0.00	0.00	0.00	750.00	0.00
0.00	0.00	0.00	0.00	0.00	0.00	0.00	0.00	0.00	0.00	0.00	0.00	0.00	0.00	0.00	0.00	0.00	0.00	640.00	0.00
0.00	0.00	0.00	0.00	0.00	0.00	0.00	0.00	0.00	0.00	0.00	0.00	0.00	0.00	0.00	0.00	0.00	0.00	540.00	0.00
0.00	0.00	0.00	0.00	0.00	0.00	0.00	0.00	0.00	0.00	0.00	0.00	0.00	0.00	0.00	0.00	0.00	0.00	580.00	0.00
0.00	0.00	0.00	0.00	0.00	0.00	0.00	0.00	0.00	0.00	0.00	0.00	0.00	0.00	0.00	0.00	0.00	0.00	530.00	0.00
0.00	0.00	0.00	0.00	0.00	0.00	20.00	0.00	0.00	0.00	0.00	0.00	0.00	160.00	1.20	0.00	0.00	0.00	450.00	0.00
0.00	0.00	0.00	0.00	0.00	0.00	0.00	0.00	0.00	0.00	0.00	0.00	0.00	0.00	0.00	0.00	0.00	0.00	510.00	0.00
0.00	0.00	0.00	0.00	0.00	0.00	0.54	0.00	0.01	0.19	0.00	0.00	0.00	3.45	0.10	0.00	0.00	400.60	891.34	0.00
0.00	0.00	0.00	0.00	0.00	250.00	0.00	0.45	0.26	1.52	0.00	0.00	0.00	32.00	2.50	0.00	0.00	380.00	330.00	0.00
0.00	3.00	0.00	0.00	0.00	60.00	0.00	0.53	0.51	2.85	0.00	0.00	0.00	48.00	2.00	0.00	180.00	540.00	530.00	0.00
0.00	0.00	0.00	0.00	0.00	0.00	6.01	0.11	0.01	0.95	0.00	0.00	0.00	1.04	0.30	0.00	0.00	600.90	781.17	0.00
0.00	0.00	0.00	0.00	0.00	100.00	21.00	0.53	0.43	2.85	0.00	0.00	0.00	320.00	1.50	0.00	240.00	640.00	470.00	0.00
0.00	0.00	0.00	0.00	0.00	150.00	9.00	0.12	0.26	1.90	0.00	0.00	0.00	280.00	1.00	0.00	0.00	480.00	820.00	0.00
0.00	1.00	0.00	0.00	0.00	100.00	6.00	0.45	0.43	6.65	0.00	0.00	0.00	32.00	1.50	0.00	250.00	660.00	430.00	0.00
0.00	2.00	0.00	0.00	0.00	100.00	6.00	0.30	0.34	3.80	0.00	0.00	0.00	48.00	1.50	0.00	200.00	390.00	370.00	0.00
0.00	0.00	0.00	0.00	0.00	0.00	0.00	0.00	0.00	0.00	0.00	0.00	0.00	0.00	0.00	0.00	0.00	0.00	360.00	0.00
0.00	1.00	0.00	0.00	0.00	250.00	6.00	0.30	0.34	2.85	0.00	0.00	0.00	80.00	1.50	0.00	0.00	500.00	410.00	0.00
0.00	0.00	0.00	0.00	0.00	0.00	0.00	0.00	0.00	0.00	0.00	0.00	0.00	0.00	0.00	0.00	0.00	0.00	560.00	0.00
0.00	0.00	0.00	0.00	0.00	0.00	0.00	0.00	0.00	0.00	0.00	0.00	0.00	0.00	0.00	0.00	0.00	0.00	670.00	0.00
0.00	0.00	0.00	0.00	0.00	0.00	0.00	0.00	0.00	0.00	0.00	0.00	0.00	0.00	0.00	0.00	0.00	0.00	560.00	0.00
0.00	0.00	0.00	0.00	0.00	0.00	0.00	0.00	0.00	0.00	0.00	0.00	0.00	0.00	0.00	0.00	0.00	0.00	620.00	0.00
0.00	0.00	0.00	0.00	0.00	0.00	0.00	0.00	0.00	0.00	0.00	0.00	0.00	0.00	0.00	0.00	0.00	0.00	370.00	0.00
0.00	0.00	0.00	0.00	0.00	20.00	6.00	0.23	0.17	2.85	0.00	0.00	0.00	32.00	1.00	0.00	0.00	400.00	1010.00	0.00
0.00	0.00	0.00	0.00	0.00	60.00	6.00	0.12	0.14	2.85	0.00	0.00	0.00	32.00	0.80	0.00	0.00	380.00	650.00	0.00
0.00	0.00	0.00	0.00	0.00	0.00	0.00	0.00	0.00	0.00	0.00	0.00	0.00	0.00	0.00	0.00	0.00	0.00	550.00	0.00
0.00	1.00	0.00	0.00	0.00	138.30	0.00	0.50	0.30	3.00	0.00	0.00	0.00	350.00	0.90	0.00	200.00	330.00	870.00	0.00
0.00	1.00	0.00	0.00	0.00	0.00	0.00	0.00	0.00	0.00	0.00	0.00	0.00	220.00	1.50	0.00	180.00	290.00	530.00	0.00
0.00	1.00	0.00	0.00	0.00	0.00	0.00	0.00	0.00	0.00	0.00	0.00	0.00	300.00	1.50	0.00	200.00	330.00	630.00	0.00
0.00	1.00	0.00	0.00	0.00	20.00	0.00	0.45	0.26	2.85	0.00	0.00	0.00	240.00	2.00	0.00	240.00	310.00	390.00	0.00
0.00	0.00	0.00	0.00	0.00	60.00	3.60	0.45	0.34	2.85	0.00	0.00	0.00	200.00	1.50	0.00	0.00	300.00	630.00	0.00
0.00	1.00	0.00	0.00	0.00	80.00	0.00	0.45	0.34	3.80	0.00	0.00	0.00	200.00	2.50	0.00	280.00	350.00	500.00	0.60
0.00	0.00	0.00	0.00	0.00	100.00	6.00	0.45	0.43	3.80	0.00	0.00	0.00	160.00	1.50	0.00	0.00	350.00	950.00	0.00
0.00	0.00	0.00	0.00	0.00	40.00	6.00	0.45	0.51	3.80	0.00	0.00	0.00	360.00	1.50	0.00	0.00	320.00	850.00	0.00
0.00	0.00	0.00	0.00	0.00	60.00	6.00	0.38	0.34	3.80	0.00	0.00	0.00	160.00	1.50	0.00	0.00	340.00	650.00	0.00
0.00	1.00	0.00	0.00	0.00	150.00	0.00	0.53	0.34	3.80	0.00	0.00	0.00	160.00	2.50	0.00	240.00	350.00	470.00	0.00
0.00	0.00	0.00	0.00	0.00	100.00	6.00	0.53	0.43	3.80	0.00	0.00	0.00	160.00	1.50	0.00	0.00	300.00	880.00	0.00
0.00	0.00	0.00	0.00	0.00	80.00	6.00	0.60	0.43	3.80	0.00	0.00	0.00	160.00	1.50	0.00	0.00	340.00	840.00	0.00

USDA ID Code	Food Name	Weight in Grams*	Quantity of Units	Unit of Measure	Protein (gm)	Fat (gm)	Carbohydrate (gm)	Kcalories	Caffeine (gm)	Fiber (gm)	Cholesterol (mg)	Saturated Fat (gm)
	Pizza, French Bread, Vegetable D	180.7270	1.000	Each	18.00	20.00	41.00	420.00	0.00	0.00	0.00	0.00
	Pizza, Meat, 3 - DiGiorno	154.0000	1.000	Slice	19.00	16.00	40.00	380.00	0.00	3.11	40.00	8.00
	Pizza, Pepperoni	154.0000	1.000	Slice	19.00	24.00	40.00	450.00	0.00	2.00	35.00	9.00
	Pizza, Pepperoni -Weight Watcher	157.6260	1.000	Each	23.00	12.00	46.00	390.00	0.00	4.00	45.00	4.00
	Pizza, Pepperoni, Microwave for	104.0000	1.000	Each	10.00	16.00	25.00	280.00	0.00	1.00	15.00	3.50
	Pizza, Pepperoni, Party - Totino	289.0000	1.000	Slice	14.00	21.00	33.00	380.00	0.00	2.00	20.00	5.00
	Pizza, Sausage & Pepperoni - Tom	132.0000	1.000	Slice	19.00	19.00	25.00	340.00	0.00	2.00	45.00	9.00
	Pizza, Sausage & Pepperoni, Supr	122.0000	1.000	Slice	13.00	20.00	28.00	340.00	0.00	2.00	25.00	7.00
	Pizza, Special Deluxe - Red Baro	129.0000	1.000	Slice	13.00	18.00	32.00	340.00	0.00	2.00	25.00	7.00
	Pizza, Supreme, Party - Totino's	309.0000	1.000	Slice	15.00	20.00	34.00	380.00	0.00	2.00	20.00	4.50
	Pizzas, French Bread, Bacon, Can	163.0080	1.000	Each	18.00	15.00	40.00	370.00	0.00	0.00	0.00	0.00
	Pot Pie, Beef -Swanson	198.4450	1.000	Pie	12.00	19.00	36.00	370.00	0.00	0.00	0.00	0.00
	Pot Pie, Beef-Stouffer's	283.4930	1.000	Each	18.00	27.00	37.00	460.00	0.00	0.00	0.00	0.00
	Pot Pie, Chicken -Swanson	198.4450	1.000	Each	11.00	22.00	35.00	380.00	0.00	0.00	0.00	0.00
	Pot Pie, Chicken-Stouffer's	283.4930	1.000	Each	16.00	27.00	32.00	440.00	0.00	0.00	0.00	0.00
	Pot Pie, Macaroni and Cheese -Sw	198.4450	1.000	Each	7.00	8.00	24.00	200.00	0.00	0.00	0.00	0.00
	Pot Pie, Turkey -Swanson	198.0000	1.000	Each	5.54	10.58	18.14	191.49	0.00	0.00	0.00	0.00
	Pot Pie, Turkey-Stouffer's	283.4930	1.000	Each	16.00	24.00	33.00	410.00	0.00	0.00	0.00	0.00
	Potato Casserole, Garden-Healthy	262.2310	1.000	Each	12.00	4.00	23.00	180.00	0.00	0.00	20.00	2.00
	Potato, Baked, Broccoli and Chee	283.5000	1.000	Each	12.00	7.00	34.00	230.00	0.00	6.00	10.00	2.00
	Potato, Baked, w/ Sour Cream, Le	294.1240	1.000	Each	9.00	5.00	38.00	230.00	0.00	0.00	15.00	2.00
672	Potato, Bkd, Broccoli & Chse -Sm	280.0000	10.000	Ounce	12.00	7.00	35.00	250.00	0.00	6.00	15.00	2.00
	Potatoes Au Gratin-Stouffer's	163.0080	1.000	Each	5.00	9.00	17.00	170.00	0.00	0.00	0.00	0.00
	Potatoes, Scalloped, and Ham, Mi	212.6200	1.000	Each	8.00	16.00	21.00	260.00	0.00	0.00	33.00	6.00
	Potatoes, Scalloped-Stouffer's	163.0080	1.000	Each	4.00	6.00	16.00	130.00	0.00	0.00	0.00	0.00
	Primavera, Chicken-Stouffer's	28.3500	1.000	Ounce	1.60	0.60	1.20	17.00	0.00	0.00	5.00	0.00
689	Ravioli Florentine-Smart Ones	238.0000	8.500	Ounce	9.00	2.00	43.00	220.00	0.00	4.00	5.00	0.50
	Ravioli, Baked Cheese, Lean Cuis	240.9690	1.000	Each	13.00	8.00	30.00	240.00	0.00	0.00	55.00	3.00
	Ravioli, Baked Cheese-Healthy Ch	255.1440	1.000	Each	14.00	2.00	44.00	250.00	0.00	0.00	20.00	1.00
	Ravioli, Beef	243.9350	1.000	Cup	9.00	5.00	35.99	229.94	0.00	4.00	19.99	2.50
	Ravioli, Beef, Micro Cup-Hormel	212.6200	1.000	Each	9.00	11.00	34.00	270.00	0.00	0.00	20.00	4.00
	Ravioli, Cheese	243.9350	1.000	Cup	9.00	3.00	37.99	219.94	0.00	4.00	15.00	1.50
	Ravioli, Cheese-Stouffer's	28.3500	1.000	Ounce	2.80	1.90	6.40	54.00	0.00	0.00	14.00	0.00
	Rice, Confetti-Stouffer's	28.3500	1.000	Ounce	0.50	0.30	4.80	24.00	0.00	0.00	1.00	0.00
692	Rice, Hunan & Vegetables-Smart O	289.5000	10.340	Ounce	7.00	7.00	39.00	250.00	0.00	8.00	5.00	2.00
694	Rice, Sante Fe and Beans-Smart O	280.0000	10.000	Ounce	12.00	9.00	41.00	290.00	0.00	10.00	5.00	4.00
	Rice, Wild - Rice-a-Roni	56.0000	1.000	Cup	5.00	1.00	43.00	240.00	0.00	1.00	0.00	0.00
	Rigatoni Bake, Lean Cuisine-Stou	276.4060	1.000	Each	18.00	8.00	27.00	250.00	0.00	0.00	25.00	3.00
	Rigatoni in Meat Sauce-Healthy C	269.3190	1.000	Each	16.00	6.00	34.00	260.00	0.00	0.00	30.00	2.00
	Rigatoni w/ Meat Sauce-Stouffer'	283.9200	0.500	Cup	16.02	11.02	31.05	290.44	0.00	0.00	30.04	0.00
695	Risotto w/Cheese & Mushrooms-Sma	280.0000	10.000	Ounce	11.00	8.00	44.00	290.00	0.00	4.00	20.00	4.00
	Sauce, Cheddar Cheese-Stouffer's	283.9200	1.000	Cup	26.04	60.09	22.03	731.10	0.00	0.00	130.20	0.00
	Sauce, Marinara-Stouffer's	283.9200	1.000	Cup	3.00	11.02	18.03	180.27	0.00	0.00	0.00	0.00
	Sauce, Newburg, Supreme-Stouffer	283.9200	1.000	Cup	7.01	41.06	20.03	480.72	0.00	0.00	120.18	0.00
	Sauce, Pesto-Stouffer's	283.9200	0.250	Cup	35.05	61.09	21.03	771.16	0.00	0.00	70.11	0.00
	Sauce, Veloute, Supreme-Stouffer	307.5800	1.000	Cup	8.68	49.91	20.61	564.18	0.00	0.00	97.65	0.00
	Shells, Cheese Stuffed-Stouffer'	28.3500	1.000	Ounce	1.50	0.90	3.40	28.00	0.00	0.00	3.00	0.00
	Shrimp Marinara-Healthy Choice	297.6680	1.000	Each	10.00	1.00	51.00	260.00	0.00	0.00	60.00	0.00
697	Shrimp Marinara-Smart Ones	252.0000	9.000	Ounce	9.00	2.00	35.00	190.00	0.00	4.00	40.00	0.50
	Shrimp Marinara-Weight Watchers	255.1500	1.000	Each	9.00	2.00	35.00	190.00	0.00	4.00	40.00	0.50
717	Spaghetti Marinara-Smart Ones	252.0000	9.000	Ounce	9.00	7.00	46.00	280.00	0.00	5.00	5.00	1.50
	Spaghetti w/ Meat Sauce, Lean Cu	326.0170	1.000	Each	15.00	6.00	45.00	290.00	0.00	0.00	20.00	2.00
	Spaghetti w/ Meat Sauce, Top She	283.4930	1.000	Each	14.00	6.00	37.00	260.00	0.00	0.00	20.00	2.00
	Spaghetti w/ Meat Sauce-Healthy	283.4930	1.000	Each	14.00	6.00	42.00	280.00	0.00	0.00	20.00	2.00
718	Spaghetti w/ Meat Sauce-Smart On	280.0000	10.000	Ounce	17.00	6.00	41.00	290.00	0.00	4.00	15.00	2.00

Monounsaturated Fat (gm)	Polyunsaturated Fat (gm)	Vitamin D (mg)	Vitamin K (mg)	Vitamin E (mg)	Vitamin A (re)	Vitamin C (mg)	Thiamin (mg)	Riboflavin (mg)	Niacin (mg)	Vitamin B₆ (mg)	Folate (mg)	Vitamin B₁₂ (mcg)	Calcium (mg)	Iron (mg)	Magnesium (mg)	Phosphorus (mg)	Potassium (mg)	Sodium (mg)	Zinc (mg)
0.00	0.00	0.00	0.00	0.00	250.00	3.60	0.45	0.43	3.80	0.00	0.00	0.00	280.00	1.50	0.00	0.00	230.00	830.00	0.00
0.00	1.00	0.00	0.00	0.00	138.30	0.00	0.50	0.30	3.00	0.00	0.00	0.00	330.00	1.00	0.00	200.00	330.00	1100.00	0.00
0.00	1.00	0.00	0.00	0.00	90.00	0.00	0.00	0.00	0.00	0.00	0.00	0.00	330.00	1.90	0.00	200.00	330.00	920.00	0.00
0.00	0.00	0.00	0.00	0.00	80.00	4.80	0.00	0.00	0.00	0.00	0.00	0.00	540.00	1.00	0.00	0.00	320.00	650.00	0.00
0.00	1.00	0.00	0.00	0.00	0.00	0.00	0.00	0.00	0.00	0.00	0.00	0.00	200.00	1.50	0.00	180.00	290.00	710.00	0.00
0.00	1.00	0.00	0.00	0.00	0.00	0.00	0.00	0.00	0.00	0.00	0.00	0.00	280.00	1.50	0.00	200.00	330.00	920.00	0.00
0.00	1.00	0.00	0.00	0.00	150.00	1.20	0.00	0.00	0.00	0.00	0.00	0.00	350.00	0.90	0.00	200.00	330.00	820.00	0.00
0.00	1.00	0.00	0.00	0.00	40.00	2.40	0.00	0.00	0.00	0.00	0.00	0.00	200.00	1.50	0.00	200.00	330.00	610.00	0.00
0.00	1.00	0.00	0.00	0.00	78.00	0.00	0.00	0.00	0.00	0.00	0.00	0.00	220.00	2.70	0.00	200.00	330.00	690.00	0.00
0.00	1.00	0.00	0.00	0.00	0.00	0.00	0.00	0.00	0.00	0.00	0.00	0.00	280.00	1.50	0.00	200.00	330.00	890.00	0.00
0.00	0.00	0.00	0.00	0.00	80.00	6.00	0.60	0.43	3.80	0.00	0.00	0.00	160.00	1.00	0.00	0.00	300.00	1070.00	0.00
0.00	0.00	0.00	0.00	0.00	250.00	0.00	0.23	0.17	2.85	0.00	0.00	0.00	16.00	1.50	0.00	0.00	0.00	730.00	0.00
0.00	0.00	0.00	0.00	0.00	700.00	2.40	0.30	0.43	3.80	0.00	0.00	0.00	32.00	1.50	0.00	0.00	300.00	1130.00	0.00
0.00	0.00	0.00	0.00	0.00	400.00	0.00	0.23	0.17	2.85	0.00	0.00	0.00	16.00	1.00	0.00	0.00	0.00	760.00	0.00
0.00	0.00	0.00	0.00	0.00	500.00	1.20	0.30	0.43	4.75	0.00	0.00	0.00	80.00	1.00	0.00	0.00	320.00	750.00	0.00
0.00	0.00	0.00	0.00	0.00	80.00	0.00	0.09	0.17	0.76	0.00	0.00	0.00	120.00	0.60	0.00	0.00	0.00	740.00	0.00
0.00	0.00	0.00	0.00	0.00	176.37	0.00	0.11	0.09	1.44	0.00	0.00	0.00	8.06	0.50	0.00	0.00	0.00	362.82	0.00
0.00	0.00	0.00	0.00	0.00	250.00	0.00	0.30	0.43	3.80	0.00	0.00	0.00	80.00	1.00	0.00	0.00	290.00	750.00	0.00
0.00	0.00	0.00	0.00	0.00	0.00	0.00	0.00	0.00	0.00	0.00	0.00	0.00	0.00	0.00	0.00	0.00	600.00	360.00	0.00
0.00	0.00	0.00	0.00	0.00	200.00	9.00	0.00	0.00	0.00	0.00	0.00	0.00	300.00	0.80	0.00	0.00	830.00	510.00	0.00
0.00	0.00	0.00	0.00	0.00	350.00	30.00	0.23	0.26	1.14	0.00	0.00	0.00	160.00	0.60	0.00	0.00	900.00	570.00	0.00
0.00	0.00	0.00	0.00	0.00	0.00	0.00	0.00	0.00	0.00	0.00	0.00	0.00	0.00	0.00	0.00	0.00	0.00	590.00	0.00
0.00	0.00	0.00	0.00	0.00	20.00	3.60	0.00	0.10	0.76	0.00	0.00	0.00	48.00	0.80	0.00	0.00	260.00	670.00	0.00
8.00	2.00	0.00	0.00	0.39	0.00	11.40	0.09	0.10	2.09	0.00	0.00	0.00	32.00	0.40	21.00	0.00	425.00	768.00	0.90
0.00	0.00	0.00	0.00	0.00	0.00	2.40	0.03	0.14	0.76	0.00	0.00	0.00	80.00	0.20	0.00	0.00	375.00	610.00	0.00
0.00	0.00	0.00	0.00	0.00	0.00	1.20	0.00	0.00	0.06	0.00	0.00	0.00	48.00	0.01	0.00	0.00	40.00	119.00	0.00
0.00	0.00	0.00	0.00	0.00	0.00	0.00	0.00	0.00	0.00	0.00	0.00	0.00	0.00	0.00	0.00	0.00	0.00	490.00	0.00
0.00	0.00	0.00	0.00	0.00	60.00	36.00	0.06	0.26	1.14	0.00	0.00	0.00	160.00	0.80	0.00	0.00	380.00	590.00	0.00
0.00	0.00	0.00	0.00	0.00	500.00	4.80	0.30	0.26	1.90	0.00	0.00	0.00	200.00	1.50	0.00	240.00	590.00	420.00	0.00
0.00	0.00	0.00	0.00	0.00	149.96	2.40	0.00	0.00	0.00	0.00	0.00	0.00	0.00	1.50	0.00	0.00	0.00	1149.69	0.00
5.00	1.00	0.00	0.00	0.50	100.00	11.40	0.15	0.27	2.47	0.00	0.00	0.00	48.00	0.90	28.00	0.00	359.00	920.00	1.05
0.00	0.00	0.00	0.00	0.00	59.98	1.20	0.00	0.00	0.00	0.00	0.00	0.00	23.99	1.50	0.00	0.00	0.00	1279.66	0.00
0.00	0.00	0.00	0.00	0.00	0.00	0.00	0.00	0.00	0.02	0.00	0.00	0.00	336.01	0.01	0.00	0.00	16.00	52.00	0.00
0.00	0.00	0.00	0.00	0.00	0.00	0.00	0.00	0.00	0.04	0.00	0.00	0.00	24.00	0.00	0.00	0.00	14.00	136.00	0.00
0.00	0.00	0.00	0.00	0.00	0.00	0.00	0.00	0.00	0.00	0.00	0.00	0.00	0.00	0.00	0.00	0.00	0.00	630.00	0.00
0.00	0.00	0.00	0.00	0.00	80.00	6.00	0.15	0.10	1.52	0.00	0.00	0.00	48.00	0.80	0.00	0.00	0.00	1110.00	0.00
0.00	1.00	0.00	0.00	0.00	200.00	6.00	0.23	0.34	3.80	0.00	0.00	0.00	160.00	1.50	0.00	0.00	620.00	430.00	0.00
0.00	0.00	0.00	0.00	0.00	200.00	2.40	0.30	0.26	2.85	0.00	0.00	0.00	120.00	1.50	0.00	200.00	700.00	540.00	0.00
0.00	0.00	0.00	0.00	0.00	0.00	48.07	0.00	0.01	0.76	0.00	0.00	0.00	2.08	0.30	0.00	0.00	620.93	851.28	0.00
0.00	0.00	0.00	0.00	0.00	0.00	0.00	0.00	0.00	0.00	0.00	0.00	0.00	0.00	0.00	0.00	0.00	0.00	540.00	0.00
0.00	0.00	0.00	0.00	0.00	0.00	0.00	0.00	0.01	0.00	0.00	0.00	0.00	6.33	0.10	0.00	0.00	340.51	1392.09	0.00
0.00	0.00	0.00	0.00	0.00	0.00	66.10	0.00	0.00	0.38	0.00	0.00	0.00	0.00	0.20	0.00	0.00	681.02	1221.83	0.00
0.00	0.00	0.00	0.00	0.00	0.00	0.00	0.00	0.01	0.00	0.00	0.00	0.00	1.84	0.00	0.00	0.00	370.56	1051.58	0.00
0.00	0.00	0.00	0.00	0.00	0.00	12.02	0.00	0.02	0.38	0.00	0.00	0.00	5.69	0.30	0.00	0.00	620.93	1362.04	0.00
0.00	0.00	0.00	0.00	0.00	0.00	0.00	0.00	0.01	0.00	0.00	0.00	0.00	2.26	0.00	0.00	0.00	368.89	1410.45	0.00
0.00	0.00	0.00	0.00	0.00	0.00	0.60	0.00	0.00	0.06	0.00	0.00	0.00	248.01	0.02	0.00	0.00	53.00	59.00	0.00
0.00	0.00	0.00	0.00	0.00	100.00	114.00	0.23	0.14	1.14	0.00	0.00	0.00	48.00	1.50	0.00	130.00	390.00	320.00	0.00
0.00	0.00	0.00	0.00	0.00	0.00	0.00	0.00	0.00	0.00	0.00	0.00	0.00	0.00	0.00	0.00	0.00	0.00	470.00	0.00
0.00	0.00	0.00	0.00	0.00	150.00	6.00	0.00	0.00	0.00	0.00	0.00	0.00	120.00	1.00	0.00	0.00	440.00	400.00	0.00
0.00	0.00	0.00	0.00	0.00	0.00	0.00	0.00	0.00	0.00	0.00	0.00	0.00	0.00	0.00	0.00	0.00	0.00	690.00	0.00
0.00	2.00	0.00	0.00	0.00	100.00	6.00	0.30	0.34	3.80	0.00	0.00	0.00	48.00	2.00	0.00	0.00	500.00	500.00	0.00
2.00	1.00	0.00	0.00	0.11	100.00	2.40	0.23	0.26	3.80	0.00	0.00	0.00	48.00	1.50	45.50	0.00	879.00	980.00	2.40
0.00	2.00	0.00	0.00	0.00	250.00	4.80	0.38	0.26	1.90	0.00	0.00	0.00	48.00	2.00	0.00	160.00	540.00	480.00	0.00
0.00	0.00	0.00	0.00	0.00	0.00	0.00	0.00	0.00	0.00	0.00	0.00	0.00	0.00	0.00	0.00	0.00	0.00	560.00	0.00

USDA ID Code	Food Name	Weight in Grams*	Quantity of Units	Unit of Measure	Protein (gm)	Fat (gm)	Carbohydrate (gm)	Kcalories	Caffeine (gm)	Fiber (gm)	Cholesterol (mg)	Saturated Fat (gm)
	Spaghetti w/ Meat Sauce-Stouffer	364.9980	1.000	Each	16.00	12.00	38.00	320.00	0.00	0.00	0.00	0.00
	Spaghetti w/ Meatballs, Micro Cu	212.6200	1.000	Each	10.00	7.00	27.00	210.00	0.00	0.00	20.00	3.00
	Spaghetti w/ Meatballs-Stouffer'	276.4060	1.000	Each	14.00	9.00	37.00	290.00	0.00	0.00	0.00	0.00
	Spinach Souffle-Stouffer's	170.0960	1.000	Each	9.00	15.00	11.00	220.00	0.00	0.00	0.00	0.00
	Spinach, Creamed-Stouffer's	127.5720	1.000	Each	4.00	16.00	8.00	190.00	0.00	0.00	0.00	0.00
	Steak, Green Pepper, w/ Rice-Sto	297.6680	1.000	Each	20.00	10.00	35.00	310.00	0.00	0.00	0.00	0.00
	Steak, Green Pepper-Stouffer's	28.3500	1.000	Ounce	2.60	1.40	1.30	28.00	0.00	0.00	7.00	0.00
728	Steak, Pepper-Smart Ones	280.0000	10.000	Ounce	18.00	4.50	33.00	240.00	0.00	4.00	35.00	1.50
	Steak, Salisbury, Grilled -Weigh	240.9750	1.000	Each	19.00	9.00	24.00	250.00	0.00	4.00	30.00	3.00
	Steak, Salisbury, Top Shelf-Horm	283.4930	1.000	Each	25.00	15.00	22.00	320.00	0.00	0.00	70.00	7.00
	Steak, Salisbury, w/ Mushroom Gr	311.8430	1.000	Each	21.00	6.00	35.00	280.00	0.00	0.00	55.00	3.00
	Stew, Beef, Dinty Moore -Hormel	253.1620	1.000	Cup	12.28	14.51	17.86	245.58	0.00	0.00	33.49	6.70
	Stew, Chicken, Dinty Moore -Horm	253.1620	1.000	Cup	13.10	21.43	17.86	309.58	0.00	0.00	95.25	4.76
	Stew, Meatball, Dinty Moore -Hor	253.1620	1.000	Cup	12.28	17.86	15.63	267.90	0.00	0.00	33.49	7.81
	Stew, Vegetable, Dinty Moore -Ho	253.1620	1.000	Cup	5.58	6.70	22.33	173.02	0.00	0.00	15.63	2.23
	Stuff'n, Old-Fashion-Stouffer's	283.9200	0.500	Cup	11.02	37.06	61.09	620.93	0.00	0.00	10.02	0.00
	Sweet Potatoes, Whipped-Stouffer	283.9200	0.500	Cup	3.00	18.03	60.09	410.61	0.00	0.00	60.09	0.00
	Taco Shells, Chi-Chi's-Hormel	20.0000	1.000	Each	1.41	4.94	11.99	98.77	0.00	0.00	0.00	0.00
	Tetrazzini, Turkey-Healthy Choic	357.9100	1.000	Each	23.00	6.00	49.00	340.00	0.00	0.00	40.00	3.00
	Tetrazzini, Turkey-Stouffer's	283.4930	1.000	Each	22.00	23.00	26.00	400.00	0.00	0.00	0.00	0.00
	Tortellini w/ Egg Pasta, Cheese-	145.2900	1.000	Each	11.29	8.47	22.22	211.64	0.00	0.00	63.49	0.00
	Tortellini w/ Egg Pasta, Chicken	28.3500	1.000	Ounce	3.10	1.50	6.20	51.00	0.00	0.00	20.00	0.00
	Tortellini w/ Spinach Pasta, Che	28.3500	1.000	Ounce	3.00	2.40	5.70	56.00	0.00	0.00	19.00	0.00
	Tortellini, Beef	257.8940	1.000	Cup	5.00	1.00	45.98	229.91	0.00	9.00	14.99	0.00
	Tortellini, Cheese in Alfredo Sa	251.6000	1.000	Each	26.00	37.00	35.00	580.00	0.00	0.00	0.00	0.00
	Tortellini, Cheese w/ Tomato Sau	262.2310	1.000	Each	18.00	15.00	39.00	360.00	0.00	0.00	0.00	0.00
747	Tuna Noodle Casserole-Smart Ones	266.0000	9.500	Ounce	13.00	7.00	39.00	270.00	0.00	4.00	40.00	3.50
	Tuna Noodle Casserole-Stouffer's	283.4930	1.000	Each	17.00	15.00	33.00	280.00	0.00	0.00	0.00	0.00
	Turkey and Gravy-Stouffer's	255.0000	1.000	Each	11.99	2.47	2.12	77.60	0.00	0.00	23.28	0.00
	Turkey Breast, Sliced, w/ Gravy	283.4930	1.000	Each	27.00	4.00	30.00	270.00	0.00	0.00	50.00	2.00
	Turkey Breast, Sliced, w/ Gravy-	340.1920	1.000	Each	19.00	3.00	46.00	290.00	0.00	0.00	20.00	1.00
748	Turkey Breast, Stuffed-Smart One	280.0000	10.000	Ounce	13.00	7.00	37.00	260.00	0.00	5.00	20.00	2.00
	Turkey Dijon, Lean Cuisine-Stouf	269.3190	1.000	Each	20.00	6.00	20.00	210.00	0.00	0.00	45.00	2.00
	Turkey Dijonnaise-Stouffer's	260.0000	1.000	Each	8.47	5.29	7.05	112.88	0.00	0.00	28.22	0.00
	Turkey Medallions, Roast -Weight	240.9750	1.000	Each	10.00	2.00	34.00	190.00	0.00	4.00	20.00	0.50
750	Turkey Medallions, Rst, /Mush-Sm	238.0000	8.500	Ounce	10.00	2.00	32.00	190.00	0.00	2.00	20.00	0.50
	Turkey, Breast of -Healthy Choic	297.6680	1.000	Each	21.00	5.00	39.00	290.00	0.00	0.00	45.00	2.00
	Turkey, Homestyle w/ Vegetables-	269.3190	1.000	Each	26.00	2.00	34.00	260.00	0.00	0.00	30.00	1.00
	Turkey, Roasted, and Mushrooms i	240.9690	1.000	Each	18.00	3.00	26.00	200.00	0.00	0.00	40.00	1.00
	Turkey, Sliced, w/ Dressing, Lea	223.2510	1.000	Each	16.00	5.00	23.00	200.00	0.00	0.00	25.00	1.00
	Vegetables, Italian Style-Stouff	28.3500	1.000	Ounce	0.30	0.30	1.60	10.00	0.00	0.00	0.00	0.00
	Welsh Rarebit-Stouffer's	141.7460	1.000	Each	13.00	20.00	9.00	270.00	0.00	0.00	0.00	0.00
791	Worthington- Beef, Smoked, Meatl	57.0000	6.000	Slices	11.00	6.00	6.00	120.00	0.00	3.00	0.00	1.00
792	Worthington- Bolono	57.0000	3.000	Slices	10.00	3.50	2.00	80.00	0.00	2.00	0.00	1.00
793	Worthington- Burger, Vegetarian	55.0000	0.250	Cup	9.00	2.00	2.00	60.00	0.00	1.00	0.00	0.00
795	Worthington- Chicken Roll, Meatl	55.0000	1.000	Slice	9.00	4.50	1.00	80.00	0.00	1.00	0.00	1.00
796	Worthington- Chicken Slices, Mea	57.0000	2.000	Slices	9.00	4.50	1.00	80.00	0.00	1.00	0.00	1.00
797	Worthington- Chicken, Diced, Mea	55.0000	0.250	Cup	10.00	0.00	2.00	50.00	0.00	1.00	0.00	0.00
794	Worthington- Chic-Ketts	55.0000	2.000	Slices	13.00	7.00	2.00	120.00	0.00	2.00	0.00	1.00
798	Worthington- Chik Patties, Crisp	71.0000	1.000	Each	8.00	6.00	15.00	150.00	0.00	2.00	0.00	1.00
799	Worthington- Chik Stiks	47.0000	1.000	Each	9.00	7.00	3.00	110.00	0.00	2.00	0.00	1.00
800	Worthington- Chik, Diced	55.0000	0.250	Cup	7.00	0.00	1.00	40.00	0.00	1.00	0.00	0.00
801	Worthington- Chik, Sliced	90.0000	3.000	Slices	14.00	0.50	2.00	70.00	0.00	2.00	0.00	0.00
802	Worthington- Chili	230.0000	1.000	Cup	19.00	15.00	21.00	290.00	0.00	9.00	0.00	2.50
803	Worthington- Chili, Low Fat	230.0000	1.000	Cup	18.00	1.00	21.00	170.00	0.00	11.00	0.00	0.00

Monounsaturated Fat (gm)	Polyunsaturated Fat (gm)	Vitamin D (mg)	Vitamin K (mg)	Vitamin E (mg)	Vitamin A (re)	Vitamin C (mg)	Thiamin (mg)	Riboflavin (mg)	Niacin (mg)	Vitamin B6 (mg)	Folate (mg)	Vitamin B12 (mcg)	Calcium (mg)	Iron (mg)	Magnesium (mg)	Phosphorus (mg)	Potassium (mg)	Sodium (mg)	Zinc (mg)
0.00	12.00	0.00	0.00	0.00	150.00	6.00	0.15	0.17	3.80	0.00	0.00	0.00	80.00	1.50	0.00	0.00	800.00	560.00	0.00
3.00	1.00	0.00	0.00	0.00	140.00	3.60	0.12	0.26	2.28	0.00	0.00	0.00	32.00	1.10	24.50	0.00	341.00	930.00	1.05
0.00	0.00	0.00	0.00	0.00	100.00	6.00	0.30	0.26	3.80	0.00	0.00	0.00	64.00	1.50	0.00	0.00	550.00	790.00	0.00
0.00	0.00	0.00	0.00	0.00	200.00	6.00	0.12	0.34	0.38	0.00	0.00	0.00	120.00	0.40	0.00	0.00	345.00	820.00	0.00
0.00	0.00	0.00	0.00	0.00	400.00	6.00	0.03	0.17	0.00	0.00	0.00	0.00	80.00	0.40	0.00	0.00	400.00	400.00	0.00
0.00	0.00	0.00	0.00	0.00	40.00	6.00	0.15	0.17	3.80	0.00	0.00	0.00	16.00	1.00	0.00	0.00	410.00	700.00	0.00
0.00	0.00	0.00	0.00	0.00	0.00	3.60	0.00	0.00	0.10	0.00	0.00	0.00	48.00	0.02	0.00	0.00	51.00	164.00	0.00
0.00	0.00	0.00	0.00	0.00	0.00	0.00	0.00	0.00	0.00	0.00	0.00	0.00	0.00	0.00	0.00	0.00	0.00	690.00	0.00
0.00	0.00	0.00	0.00	0.00	60.00	0.00	0.00	0.00	0.00	0.00	0.00	0.00	120.00	1.50	0.00	0.00	450.00	590.00	0.00
8.00	1.00	0.00	0.00	0.03	0.00	3.60	0.03	0.26	4.75	8.00	0.00	0.00	16.00	1.50	35.00	0.00	801.00	910.00	5.70
0.00	0.00	0.00	0.00	0.00	0.00	0.00	0.00	0.00	0.00	0.00	0.00	0.00	0.00	0.00	0.00	260.00	630.00	500.00	0.00
5.58	1.12	0.00	0.00	0.00	814.87	2.68	0.03	0.13	2.55	0.00	0.00	0.00	26.79	1.00	23.44	0.00	588.27	971.15	2.85
7.14	8.33	0.00	0.00	0.00	476.27	2.14	0.05	0.28	3.62	0.00	0.00	0.00	38.10	0.71	25.00	0.00	609.63	1012.08	1.25
7.81	1.12	0.00	0.00	2.59	279.06	1.34	0.07	0.15	3.18	0.00	0.00	0.00	26.79	1.23	27.35	0.00	586.04	1093.93	2.68
1.12	2.23	0.00	0.00	0.60	714.41	2.01	0.08	0.09	1.70	0.00	0.00	0.00	35.72	0.67	31.26	0.00	509.01	948.82	0.84
0.00	0.00	0.00	0.00	0.00	0.00	0.84	0.01	0.01	0.74	0.00	0.00	0.00	0.00	0.33	0.00	0.00	200.30	1121.68	0.00
0.00	0.00	0.00	0.00	0.00	0.00	0.00	0.00	0.00	0.19	0.00	0.00	0.00	0.00	0.10	0.00	0.00	400.60	1111.67	0.00
0.00	0.00	0.00	0.00	0.09	0.00	0.00	0.06	0.07	0.54	0.00	0.00	0.00	0.00	0.14	0.00	0.00	0.00	3.53	0.00
0.00	2.00	0.00	0.00	0.00	0.00	72.00	0.23	0.34	3.80	0.00	0.00	0.00	80.00	1.00	0.00	250.00	510.00	490.00	0.00
0.00	0.00	0.00	0.00	0.00	20.00	0.00	0.15	0.43	2.85	0.00	0.00	0.00	80.00	0.80	0.00	0.00	300.00	960.00	0.00
0.00	0.00	0.00	0.00	0.00	0.00	0.00	0.00	0.00	0.20	0.00	0.00	0.00	1.52	0.07	0.00	0.00	70.55	271.61	0.00
0.00	0.00	0.00	0.00	0.00	0.00	0.00	0.00	0.00	0.13	0.00	0.00	0.00	72.00	0.03	0.00	0.00	31.00	57.00	0.00
0.00	0.00	0.00	0.00	0.00	0.00	0.00	0.00	0.00	0.06	0.00	0.00	0.00	0.00	0.02	0.00	0.00	26.00	79.00	0.00
0.00	0.00	0.00	0.00	0.00	149.94	3.60	0.00	0.00	0.00	0.00	0.00	0.00	95.96	1.50	0.00	0.00	0.00	769.68	0.00
0.00	0.00	0.00	0.00	0.00	40.00	3.60	0.30	0.51	1.90	0.00	0.00	0.00	320.00	0.80	0.00	0.00	270.00	830.00	0.00
0.00	0.00	0.00	0.00	0.00	150.00	6.00	0.23	0.34	1.90	0.00	0.00	0.00	240.00	1.00	0.00	0.00	420.00	720.00	0.00
0.00	0.00	0.00	0.00	0.00	0.00	0.00	0.00	0.00	0.00	0.00	0.00	0.00	0.00	0.00	0.00	0.00	0.00	670.00	0.00
0.00	0.00	0.00	0.00	0.00	20.00	0.00	0.15	0.34	3.80	0.00	0.00	0.00	120.00	0.60	0.00	0.00	380.00	1090.00	0.00
0.00	0.00	0.00	0.00	0.00	0.00	0.42	0.00	0.00	0.87	0.00	0.00	0.00	84.66	0.03	0.00	0.00	405.65	296.30	0.00
0.00	1.00	0.00	0.00	0.00	150.00	0.00	0.30	0.34	7.60	0.00	0.00	0.00	48.00	1.00	0.00	310.00	590.00	530.00	0.00
0.00	1.00	0.00	0.00	0.00	150.00	27.00	0.15	0.10	1.52	0.00	0.00	0.00	16.00	0.60	0.00	0.00	360.00	520.00	0.00
0.00	0.00	0.00	0.00	0.00	0.00	0.00	0.00	0.00	0.00	0.00	0.00	0.00	0.00	0.00	0.00	0.00	0.00	680.00	0.00
0.00	0.00	0.00	0.00	0.00	400.00	2.40	0.23	0.34	4.75	0.00	0.00	0.00	120.00	0.40	0.00	0.00	640.00	590.00	0.00
0.00	0.00	0.00	0.00	0.00	0.00	0.63	0.00	0.00	0.27	0.00	0.00	0.00	0.00	0.07	0.00	0.00	176.37	356.27	0.00
0.00	0.00	0.00	0.00	0.00	100.00	4.80	0.00	0.00	0.00	0.00	0.00	0.00	24.00	1.00	0.00	0.00	220.00	530.00	0.00
0.00	0.00	0.00	0.00	0.00	0.00	0.00	0.00	0.00	0.00	0.00	0.00	0.00	0.00	0.00	0.00	0.00	0.00	530.00	0.00
0.00	0.00	0.00	0.00	0.00	40.00	48.00	0.45	0.26	5.70	0.00	0.00	0.00	32.00	1.00	0.00	270.00	540.00	420.00	0.00
0.00	0.00	0.00	0.00	0.00	100.00	4.80	0.03	0.07	0.00	0.00	0.00	0.00	32.00	0.00	0.00	0.00	100.00	550.00	0.00
0.00	1.00	0.00	0.00	0.00	200.00	0.00	0.12	0.14	2.85	0.00	0.00	0.00	16.00	0.80	0.00	150.00	260.00	380.00	0.00
0.00	2.00	0.00	0.00	0.00	500.00	6.00	0.23	0.26	4.75	0.00	0.00	0.00	32.00	0.80	0.00	0.00	400.00	590.00	0.00
0.00	0.00	0.00	0.00	0.00	0.00	1.80	0.00	0.00	0.02	0.00	0.00	0.00	72.00	0.01	0.00	0.00	62.00	147.00	0.00
0.00	0.00	0.00	0.00	0.00	40.00	0.00	0.03	0.34	0.00	0.00	0.00	0.00	280.00	0.20	0.00	0.00	140.00	460.00	0.00
2.50	2.50	0.00	0.00	0.00	0.00	0.00	1.80	0.14	3.00	0.30	0.00	1.80	0.00	1.08	0.00	0.00	150.00	730.00	0.00
1.00	1.50	0.00	0.00	0.00	0.00	0.00	0.60	0.14	0.40	0.40	0.00	0.90	40.00	1.80	0.00	0.00	120.00	720.00	0.00
0.50	1.00	0.00	0.00	0.00	0.00	0.00	0.12	0.07	1.60	0.20	0.00	1.20	0.00	1.80	0.00	0.00	25.00	270.00	0.00
1.00	2.50	0.00	0.00	0.00	0.00	0.00	0.30	0.14	1.20	2.00	0.00	0.90	0.00	1.80	0.00	0.00	270.00	360.00	0.00
1.00	2.50	0.00	0.00	0.00	0.00	0.00	0.30	0.14	1.20	0.20	0.00	0.90	0.00	1.80	0.00	0.00	280.00	370.00	0.00
0.00	0.00	0.00	0.00	0.00	0.00	0.00	0.15	0.14	2.00	0.20	0.00	0.90	0.00	1.44	0.00	0.00	200.00	400.00	0.00
1.50	4.00	0.00	0.00	0.00	0.00	0.00	0.43	0.14	0.80	0.12	0.00	1.20	0.00	1.80	0.00	0.00	30.00	390.00	0.00
1.50	3.50	0.00	0.00	0.00	0.00	0.00	1.20	0.10	0.40	0.20	0.00	0.60	16.00	0.72	0.00	0.00	200.00	600.00	0.00
2.50	3.50	0.00	0.00	0.00	0.00	0.00	0.30	0.03	2.00	0.30	0.00	2.10	0.00	0.72	0.00	0.00	60.00	360.00	0.00
0.00	0.00	0.00	0.00	0.00	0.00	0.00	0.06	0.10	4.00	0.08	0.00	0.24	0.00	1.08	0.00	0.00	100.00	270.00	0.00
0.00	0.00	0.00	0.00	0.00	0.00	0.00	0.12	0.26	7.00	0.12	0.00	0.48	20.00	1.80	0.00	0.00	170.00	430.00	0.00
3.50	9.00	0.00	0.00	0.00	0.00	0.00	0.06	0.07	2.00	0.70	0.00	1.50	40.00	3.60	0.00	0.00	420.00	1130.00	0.00
0.00	0.00	0.00	0.00	0.00	150.00	0.00	0.00	0.00	0.00	0.00	0.00	0.00	40.00	1.80	0.00	0.00	480.00	870.00	0.00

USDA ID Code	Food Name	Weight in Grams*	Quantity of Units	Unit of Measure	Protein (gm)	Fat (gm)	Carbohydrate (gm)	Kcalories	Caffeine (gm)	Fiber (gm)	Cholesterol (mg)	Saturated Fat (gm)
804	Worthington- Choplets	92.0000	2.000	Slices	17.00	1.50	3.00	90.00	0.00	2.00	0.00	1.00
805	Worthington- Choplets, Multigrai	92.0000	2.000	Slices	15.00	2.00	5.00	100.00	0.00	4.00	0.00	0.50
806	Worthington- Corned Beef, Meatle	57.0000	4.000	Slices	10.00	9.00	5.00	140.00	0.00	2.00	0.00	1.00
807	Worthington- Croquettes, Golden	85.0000	4.000	Each	14.00	10.00	14.00	210.00	0.00	3.00	0.00	1.50
808	Worthington- Fillets	85.0000	2.000	Each	16.00	10.00	8.00	180.00	0.00	4.00	0.00	2.00
809	Worthington- FriChik	90.0000	2.000	Each	10.00	8.00	1.00	120.00	0.00	1.00	0.00	1.00
810	Worthington- FriChik, Low Fat	85.0000	2.000	Each	10.00	3.00	2.00	80.00	0.00	1.00	0.00	0.00
811	Worthington- FriPats	64.0000	1.000	Each	14.00	6.00	4.00	130.00	0.00	3.00	0.00	1.00
812	Worthington- Leanies	40.0000	1.000	Each	7.00	7.00	2.00	100.00	0.00	1.00	0.00	1.00
813	Worthington- Links, Super	48.0000	1.000	Each	7.00	8.00	2.00	110.00	0.00	1.00	0.00	1.00
814	Worthington- Links, Veja	31.0000	1.000	Each	5.00	3.00	1.00	50.00	0.00	0.00	0.00	0.50
815	Worthington- Numete	55.0000	1.000	Slice	6.00	10.00	5.00	130.00	0.00	3.00	0.00	2.50
816	Worthington- Prosage Links	45.0000	2.000	Each	8.00	2.50	2.00	60.00	0.00	2.00	0.00	0.50
817	Worthington- Prosage Patties	38.0000	1.000	Each	9.00	3.00	3.00	80.00	0.00	2.00	0.00	0.50
818	Worthington- Prosage Roll, Froze	55.0000	1.000	Slice	10.00	10.00	2.00	140.00	0.00	2.00	0.00	2.00
819	Worthington- Protose	55.0000	1.000	Slice	13.00	7.00	5.00	130.00	0.00	3.00	0.00	1.00
820	Worthington- Roast, Dinner	85.0000	1.000	Slice	12.00	12.00	5.00	180.00	0.00	3.00	0.00	1.50
821	Worthington- Salami, Meatless	57.0000	3.000	Slices	12.00	8.00	2.00	130.00	0.00	2.00	0.00	1.00
822	Worthington- Saucettes	38.0000	1.000	Each	6.00	6.00	1.00	90.00	0.00	1.00	0.00	1.00
823	Worthington- Skallops, Vegetable	85.0000	0.500	Cup	15.00	1.50	3.00	90.00	0.00	3.00	0.00	0.50
824	Worthington- Slices, Savory	84.0000	3.000	Slices	10.00	9.00	6.00	150.00	0.00	3.00	0.00	3.50
825	Worthington- Stakelets	71.0000	1.000	Each	12.00	8.00	6.00	140.00	0.00	2.00	0.00	1.00
826	Worthington- Stakes, Prime	92.0000	1.000	Each	10.00	7.00	4.00	120.00	0.00	4.00	0.00	1.00
827	Worthington- Steaks, Vegetable	72.0000	2.000	Slices	15.00	1.50	3.00	80.00	0.00	3.00	0.00	0.50
828	Worthington- Stew, Country	240.0000	1.000	Cup	13.00	9.00	20.00	210.00	0.00	5.00	0.00	1.00
829	Worthington- Stripples	16.0000	2.000	Each	2.00	4.50	2.00	60.00	0.00	1.00	0.00	0.50
830	Worthington- Tuno	55.0000	0.500	Cup	6.00	6.00	2.00	80.00	0.00	1.00	0.00	1.00
831	Worthington- Turkee Slices	94.0000	3.000	Slices	13.00	12.00	3.00	170.00	0.00	2.00	0.00	1.50
832	Worthington- Turkey, Smoked, Mea	57.0000	3.000	Slices	10.00	0.00	3.00	140.00	0.00	2.00	0.00	2.00
833	Worthington- Wham	45.0000	2.000	Slices	7.00	5.00	1.00	80.00	0.00	0.00	0.00	1.00
948	Ziti Mozzarella-Smart Ones	252.0000	9.000	Ounce	11.00	6.00	45.00	280.00	0.00	4.00	5.00	1.50

Restaurant Chains–Fast Foods

USDA ID Code	Food Name	Weight in Grams*	Quantity of Units	Unit of Measure	Protein (gm)	Fat (gm)	Carbohydrate (gm)	Kcalories	Caffeine (gm)	Fiber (gm)	Cholesterol (mg)	Saturated Fat (gm)
	Arby's-Beef, Roast, Regular	155.9210	1.000	Each	24.68	15.70	38.14	388.12	0.00	1.12	58.33	4.04
	Arby's-Beef, Roast, Super	240.9690	1.000	Each	25.74	22.66	51.49	515.92	0.00	1.65	41.19	8.75
	Arby's-Beef'N Cheddar Sandwich	194.0000	1.000	Each	35.27	19.84	29.76	443.11	0.00	1.21	84.88	9.92
	Arby's-Chicken BBQ, Grilled	201.0000	1.000	Each	23.00	13.00	47.00	388.00	0.00	2.00	43.00	3.00
	Arby's-Chicken Breast Fillet San	204.0000	1.000	Each	25.50	27.72	53.22	546.59	0.00	1.77	100.89	5.65
	Arby's-Chicken Cordon Bleu	240.0000	1.000	Each	38.00	33.00	46.00	623.00	0.00	5.00	77.00	5.65
	Arby's-Chicken Fingers	102.0000	1.000	Each	16.00	16.00	20.00	290.00	0.00	0.50	32.00	2.00
	Arby's-Chicken, Grilled, Delux	230.0000	1.000	Each	23.00	20.00	47.00	430.00	0.00	3.00	61.00	4.00
	Arby's-Chicken, Roast, Delux	195.0000	1.000	Each	20.00	6.00	33.00	276.00	0.00	4.00	33.00	2.00
	Arby's-Chowder, Clam, Boston	226.7950	1.000	Each	10.00	11.00	18.00	207.00	0.00	1.40	28.00	4.00
	Arby's-Fish Fillet Sandwich	221.0000	1.000	Each	23.00	27.00	50.00	526.00	0.00	0.00	43.80	7.00
	Arby's-French Fries	70.8730	1.000	Order	2.10	13.20	29.80	246.00	0.00	0.00	0.00	3.00
	Arby's-French Fries, Curly	99.2230	1.000	Order	4.20	17.70	43.20	337.00	0.00	0.00	0.00	7.40
	Arby's-Ham'N Cheese Sandwich	170.0960	1.000	Each	24.47	18.64	38.45	411.26	0.00	1.17	67.57	7.46
	Arby's-Soup, Broccoli, Cream Of	226.7950	1.000	Each	9.00	8.00	19.00	180.00	0.00	1.80	3.00	5.00
	Arby's-Soup, Cheese, Wisconsin	226.7950	1.000	Each	9.00	19.00	19.00	287.00	0.00	1.80	31.00	8.00
	Arby's-Turkey Sub	277.0000	1.000	Each	32.86	28.17	53.99	598.60	0.00	0.00	82.16	6.22
10	Boston Market-Apples, Cinnamon,	181.0000	0.750	Cup	0.00	4.50	56.00	250.00	0.00	3.00	0.00	0.00
11	Boston Market-Beans, BBQ Baked	201.0000	0.750	Cup	11.00	9.00	53.00	330.00	0.00	9.00	10.00	0.00
12	Boston Market-Brownie	95.0000	1.000	Each	6.00	27.00	47.00	450.00	0.00	3.00	80.00	0.00
13	Boston Market-Caesar, no dressin	225.0000	8.000	Ounce	19.00	13.00	14.00	240.00	0.00	4.00	25.00	0.00
14	Boston Market-Chicken Salad Sand	327.0000	1.000	Each	38.00	33.00	63.00	680.00	0.00	5.00	145.00	0.00
15	Boston Market-Chicken Salad, Chu	158.0000	0.750	Cup	27.00	30.00	3.00	390.00	0.00	1.00	145.00	0.00
16	Boston Market-Chicken Sandwich w	352.0000	1.000	Each	46.00	32.00	71.00	760.00	0.00	12.00	160.00	0.00
17	Boston Market-Chicken Sandwich,	281.0000	1.000	Each	39.00	3.50	61.00	430.00	0.00	11.00	95.00	0.00

Monounsaturated Fat (gm)	Polyunsaturated Fat (gm)	Vitamin D (mg)	Vitamin K (mg)	Vitamin E (mg)	Vitamin A (re)	Vitamin C (mg)	Thiamin (mg)	Riboflavin (mg)	Niacin (mg)	Vitamin B6 (mg)	Folate (mg)	Vitamin B12 (mcg)	Calcium (mg)	Iron (mg)	Magnesium (mg)	Phosphorus (mg)	Potassium (mg)	Sodium (mg)	Zinc (mg)
0.00	0.00	0.00	0.00	0.00	0.00	0.00	0.00	0.00	0.00	0.00	0.00	0.00	0.00	0.36	0.00	0.00	40.00	500.00	0.00
0.50	1.00	0.00	0.00	0.00	0.00	0.00	0.00	0.00	0.00	0.00	0.00	0.00	0.00	0.72	0.00	0.00	30.00	390.00	0.00
2.00	6.00	0.00	0.00	0.00	0.00	0.00	1.80	0.07	1.20	0.30	0.00	1.80	0.00	1.08	0.00	0.00	60.00	520.00	0.00
2.50	6.00	0.00	0.00	0.00	0.00	0.00	0.45	0.07	2.00	0.30	0.00	2.70	40.00	1.44	0.00	0.00	190.00	600.00	0.00
3.50	4.50	0.00	0.00	0.00	0.00	0.00	0.68	0.14	0.80	0.40	0.00	2.70	0.00	1.80	0.00	0.00	130.00	750.00	0.00
2.00	5.00	0.00	0.00	0.00	0.00	0.00	0.09	0.14	0.80	0.16	0.00	2.40	0.00	1.08	0.00	0.00	150.00	430.00	0.00
1.00	2.00	0.00	0.00	0.00	0.00	0.00	0.09	0.14	0.80	0.16	0.00	2.40	0.00	1.08	0.00	0.00	150.00	430.00	0.00
1.50	3.50	0.00	0.00	0.00	0.00	0.00	1.80	0.17	3.00	0.60	0.00	1.20	60.00	1.08	0.00	0.00	125.00	320.00	0.00
1.50	4.50	0.00	0.00	0.00	0.00	0.00	0.23	0.14	0.80	0.20	0.00	0.90	20.00	0.72	0.00	0.00	40.00	430.00	0.00
2.00	4.50	0.00	0.00	0.00	0.00	0.00	0.09	0.10	0.80	0.12	0.00	1.20	0.00	0.00	0.00	0.00	30.00	350.00	0.00
1.50	1.00	0.00	0.00	0.00	0.00	0.00	0.12	0.10	1.60	0.16	0.00	0.48	0.00	0.72	0.00	0.00	20.00	190.00	0.00
4.50	2.50	0.00	0.00	0.00	0.00	0.00	0.09	0.07	0.40	0.20	0.00	0.60	0.00	1.08	0.00	0.00	160.00	270.00	0.00
0.50	1.50	0.00	0.00	0.00	0.00	0.00	1.80	0.14	2.00	0.30	0.00	3.60	0.00	1.44	0.00	0.00	60.00	340.00	0.00
0.50	2.00	0.00	0.00	0.00	0.00	0.00	0.45	0.10	0.40	0.30	0.00	1.50	0.00	1.08	0.00	0.00	100.00	300.00	0.00
3.50	4.50	0.00	0.00	0.00	0.00	0.00	1.05	0.17	1.60	0.20	0.00	0.90	0.00	1.80	0.00	0.00	80.00	390.00	0.00
3.00	2.50	0.00	0.00	0.00	0.00	0.00	0.15	0.14	1.20	0.20	0.00	1.20	0.00	1.80	0.00	0.00	50.00	280.00	0.00
5.00	5.00	0.00	0.00	0.00	0.00	0.00	1.80	0.23	6.00	0.60	0.00	1.50	40.00	0.36	0.00	0.00	55.00	580.00	0.00
1.00	6.00	0.00	0.00	0.00	0.00	0.00	0.75	0.14	1.20	0.20	0.00	0.60	20.00	1.44	0.00	0.00	95.00	930.00	0.00
1.50	3.50	0.00	0.00	0.00	0.00	0.00	0.60	0.07	4.00	0.12	0.00	0.36	0.00	1.08	0.00	0.00	25.00	200.00	0.00
0.50	0.00	0.00	0.00	0.00	0.00	0.00	0.00	0.00	0.00	0.00	0.00	0.00	0.00	0.72	0.00	0.00	10.00	410.00	0.00
4.00	1.50	0.00	0.00	0.00	0.00	0.00	0.23	0.17	1.60	0.30	0.00	1.50	0.00	1.44	0.00	0.00	40.00	540.00	0.00
5.00	2.00	0.00	0.00	0.00	0.00	0.00	1.50	0.14	3.00	0.30	0.00	1.50	40.00	1.08	0.00	0.00	95.00	480.00	0.00
1.50	4.00	0.00	0.00	0.00	0.00	0.00	0.12	0.14	2.00	0.40	0.00	0.90	0.00	0.36	0.00	0.00	80.00	440.00	0.00
0.00	0.00	0.00	0.00	0.00	0.00	0.00	0.53	0.10	4.00	0.20	0.00	3.00	0.00	3.60	0.00	0.00	20.00	300.00	0.00
2.00	5.00	0.00	0.00	0.00	675.45	0.00	1.80	0.23	4.00	0.90	0.00	3.60	60.00	5.40	0.00	0.00	270.00	830.00	0.00
1.00	2.50	0.00	0.00	0.00	0.00	0.00	0.75	0.03	0.40	0.08	0.00	0.24	0.00	0.36	0.00	0.00	15.00	220.00	0.00
1.50	3.00	0.00	0.00	0.00	0.00	0.00	0.15	0.03	1.20	0.30	0.00	2.10	20.00	1.08	0.00	0.00	35.00	290.00	0.00
2.50	8.00	0.00	0.00	0.00	0.00	0.00	1.80	0.14	1.20	0.20	0.00	1.50	0.00	1.44	0.00	0.00	45.00	580.00	0.00
3.50	4.00	0.00	0.00	0.00	0.00	0.00	1.80	0.17	2.00	0.30	0.00	2.10	0.00	1.80	0.00	0.00	70.00	620.00	0.00
1.00	3.00	0.00	0.00	0.00	0.00	0.00	1.80	0.14	1.60	0.20	0.00	1.20	0.00	1.08	0.00	0.00	90.00	430.00	0.00
0.00	0.00	0.00	0.00	0.00	0.00	0.00	0.00	0.00	0.00	0.00	0.00	0.00	0.00	0.00	0.00	0.00	0.00	430.00	0.00
7.63	1.91	0.00	0.00	0.22	70.67	2.24	0.43	0.35	6.62	0.30	44.87	1.37	60.57	4.71	34.77	268.09	354.47	888.41	3.81
8.44	5.56	0.00	0.00	0.41	0.00	0.00	0.65	0.62	9.68	0.49	42.22	4.42	118.42	6.59	59.73	413.97	517.98	821.77	11.02
4.08	3.86	0.00	0.00	0.44	63.93	1.32	0.42	0.51	6.50	0.37	45.19	2.26	201.72	5.62	44.09	442.01	380.28	1801.11	5.95
2.00	1.00	0.00	0.00	0.00	16.63	0.00	0.50	0.43	16.41	0.72	35.48	0.38	123.07	3.88	51.00	321.52	365.87	1002.00	1.88
10.64	11.42	0.00	0.00	2.88	16.63	0.00	0.50	0.43	16.41	0.72	35.48	0.38	123.07	3.88	51.00	321.52	365.87	1129.76	1.88
10.64	11.42	0.00	0.00	2.88	16.63	0.00	0.50	0.43	16.41	0.72	35.48	0.38	123.07	3.88	51.00	321.52	365.87	1594.00	1.88
4.00	4.10	0.00	0.00	1.40	2.60	0.00	0.00	0.00	0.00	0.09	17.00	0.19	92.00	1.90	22.00	140.00	190.00	677.00	0.30
2.00	1.00	0.00	0.00	0.00	16.63	0.00	0.50	0.43	16.41	0.72	35.48	0.38	123.07	3.88	51.00	321.52	365.87	848.00	1.88
2.00	1.00	0.00	0.00	0.00	16.63	0.00	0.50	0.43	16.41	0.72	35.48	0.38	123.07	3.88	51.00	321.52	365.87	777.00	1.88
5.00	2.00	0.00	0.00	0.10	100.00	4.00	0.06	0.22	0.90	0.12	9.00	9.38	170.00	1.40	20.00	143.00	319.00	1157.00	0.70
9.20	10.60	0.00	0.00	0.00	0.00	1.20	0.35	0.31	5.32	0.00	0.00	0.00	72.00	2.10	0.00	0.00	450.00	872.00	0.00
5.50	4.70	0.00	0.00	0.00	0.00	3.60	0.06	0.00	1.90	0.00	0.00	0.00	0.00	0.60	0.00	0.00	240.00	114.00	0.00
7.60	1.50	0.00	0.00	0.00	0.00	0.00	0.06	0.07	1.90	0.00	0.00	0.00	16.00	0.80	0.00	0.00	724.00	167.00	0.00
7.81	1.63	0.00	0.00	1.28	111.84	3.50	0.36	0.57	3.15	0.23	82.72	0.63	151.46	3.84	18.64	177.09	337.86	899.41	1.63
2.00	1.00	0.00	0.00	1.40	50.00	9.00	0.11	0.42	0.80	0.18	46.00	0.59	237.00	0.80	55.00	193.00	455.00	1113.00	0.70
8.00	3.00	0.00	0.00	0.40	90.00	2.00	0.03	0.24	0.70	0.05	7.00	0.00	252.00	1.30	7.00	241.00	441.00	1129.00	1.10
7.04	8.22	0.00	0.00	0.00	0.00	0.00	0.53	0.40	9.39	0.00	0.00	0.00	93.90	3.17	0.00	0.00	0.00	1431.95	0.00
0.00	0.00	0.00	0.00	0.00	0.00	0.00	0.00	0.00	0.00	0.00	0.00	0.00	0.00	0.00	0.00	0.00	0.00	45.00	0.00
0.00	0.00	0.00	0.00	0.00	0.00	0.00	0.00	0.00	0.00	0.00	0.00	0.00	0.00	0.00	0.00	0.00	0.00	630.00	0.00
0.00	0.00	0.00	0.00	0.00	0.00	0.00	0.00	0.00	0.00	0.00	0.00	0.00	0.00	0.00	0.00	0.00	0.00	190.00	0.00
0.00	0.00	0.00	0.00	0.00	0.00	0.00	0.00	0.00	0.00	0.00	0.00	0.00	0.00	0.00	0.00	0.00	0.00	780.00	0.00
0.00	0.00	0.00	0.00	0.00	0.00	0.00	0.00	0.00	0.00	0.00	0.00	0.00	0.00	0.00	0.00	0.00	0.00	1350.00	0.00
0.00	0.00	0.00	0.00	0.00	0.00	0.00	0.00	0.00	0.00	0.00	0.00	0.00	0.00	0.00	0.00	0.00	0.00	790.00	0.00
0.00	0.00	0.00	0.00	0.00	0.00	0.00	0.00	0.00	0.00	0.00	0.00	0.00	0.00	0.00	0.00	0.00	0.00	1810.00	0.00
0.00	0.00	0.00	0.00	0.00	0.00	0.00	0.00	0.00	0.00	0.00	0.00	0.00	0.00	0.00	0.00	0.00	0.00	860.00	0.00

USDA ID Code	Food Name	Weight in Grams*	Quantity of Units	Unit of Measure	Protein (gm)	Fat (gm)	Carbohydrate (gm)	Kcalories	Caffeine (gm)	Fiber (gm)	Cholesterol (mg)	Saturated Fat (gm)
18	Boston Market-Chicken, Dark Meat	125.0000	1.000	Each	31.00	22.00	2.00	330.00	0.00	1.00	180.00	0.00
19	Boston Market-Chicken, Dark Meat	95.0000	1.000	Each	28.00	10.00	1.00	210.00	0.00	1.00	150.00	0.00
22	Boston Market-Chicken, w/ skin,	227.0000	1.000	Each	74.00	37.00	2.00	630.00	0.00	2.00	370.00	0.00
20	Boston Market-Chicken, White Mea	140.0000	1.000	Each	31.00	3.50	0.00	160.00	0.00	0.00	95.00	0.00
21	Boston Market-Chicken, White Mea	152.0000	1.000	Each	43.00	17.00	2.00	330.00	0.00	1.00	175.00	0.00
23	Boston Market-Coleslaw	184.0000	0.750	Cup	2.00	16.00	32.00	280.00	0.00	3.00	25.00	0.00
24	Boston Market-Cookie, Chocolate	79.0000	1.000	Each	4.00	17.00	48.00	340.00	0.00	1.00	25.00	0.00
25	Boston Market-Cookie, Oatmeal Ra	79.0000	1.000	Each	4.00	13.00	48.00	320.00	0.00	1.00	25.00	0.00
26	Boston Market-Corn Bread	68.0000	1.000	Each	3.00	6.00	33.00	200.00	0.00	1.00	25.00	0.00
27	Boston Market-Corn, Buttered	146.0000	0.750	Cup	6.00	4.00	39.00	190.00	0.00	4.00	0.00	0.00
28	Boston Market-Cranberry Relish	225.0000	0.750	Cup	2.00	5.00	84.00	370.00	0.00	5.00	0.00	0.00
29	Boston Market-Fruit Salad	156.0000	0.750	Cup	1.00	0.50	17.00	70.00	0.00	2.00	0.00	0.00
30	Boston Market-Gravy, Chicken	28.0000	1.000	Ounce	0.00	1.00	2.00	15.00	0.00	0.00	0.00	0.00
31	Boston Market-Ham Sandwich w/ Ch	337.0000	1.000	Each	38.00	35.00	71.00	760.00	0.00	5.00	100.00	0.00
32	Boston Market-Ham Sandwich, plai	266.0000	1.000	Each	25.00	9.00	66.00	450.00	0.00	4.00	45.00	0.00
33	Boston Market-Ham, Hearth Honey	142.0000	5.000	Ounce	25.00	9.00	9.00	210.00	0.00	0.00	75.00	0.00
34	Boston Market-Ham/Turkey Club w/	379.0000	1.000	Each	47.00	43.00	79.00	890.00	0.00	4.00	150.00	0.00
35	Boston Market-Ham/Turkey Club, p	266.0000	1.000	Each	29.00	6.00	64.00	430.00	0.00	4.00	55.00	0.00
36	Boston Market-Macaroni & Cheese	192.0000	0.750	Cup	12.00	10.00	36.00	280.00	0.00	1.00	20.00	0.00
37	Boston Market-Meatloaf Sandwich	383.0000	1.000	Each	46.00	33.00	95.00	860.00	0.00	6.00	165.00	0.00
38	Boston Market-Meatloaf w/ Brown	198.0000	7.000	Ounce	30.00	22.00	19.00	390.00	0.00	1.00	120.00	0.00
39	Boston Market-Meatloaf, plain	351.0000	1.000	Each	40.00	21.00	86.00	690.00	0.00	6.00	120.00	0.00
40	Boston Market-Meatloaf/Chunky To	227.0000	8.000	Ounce	30.00	18.00	22.00	370.00	0.00	5.00	120.00	0.00
41	Boston Market-Pot Pie, Chicken,	425.0000	1.000	Each	34.00	34.00	78.00	750.00	0.00	6.00	115.00	0.00
42	Boston Market-Potatoes, Mashed	161.0000	0.660	Cup	3.00	8.00	25.00	180.00	0.00	4.00	25.00	0.00
43	Boston Market-Potatoes, Mashed &	189.0000	0.750	Cup	3.00	9.00	27.00	200.00	0.00	4.00	25.00	0.00
44	Boston Market-Potatoes, New	131.0000	0.750	Cup	3.00	3.00	25.00	140.00	0.00	2.00	0.00	0.00
45	Boston Market-Rice Pilaf	145.0000	0.660	Cup	5.00	5.00	32.00	180.00	0.00	2.00	0.00	0.00
46	Boston Market-Salad, Caesar, Chi	369.0000	13.000	Ounce	45.00	47.00	16.00	670.00	0.00	3.00	120.00	0.00
47	Boston Market-Salad, Caesar, Ent	283.0000	10.000	Ounce	20.00	43.00	16.00	520.00	0.00	3.00	40.00	0.00
48	Boston Market-Salad, Caesar, Sid	113.0000	4.000	Ounce	8.00	17.00	6.00	210.00	0.00	1.00	20.00	0.00
49	Boston Market-Salad, Pasta, Med.	156.0000	0.750	Cup	4.00	10.00	16.00	170.00	0.00	2.00	10.00	0.00
50	Boston Market-Salad, Tortellini	156.0000	0.750	Cup	14.00	24.00	29.00	380.00	0.00	2.00	90.00	0.00
51	Boston Market-Soup, Chicken	257.0000	1.000	Cup	9.00	3.00	4.00	80.00	0.00	2.00	25.00	0.00
52	Boston Market-Soup, Chicken Tort	238.0000	1.000	Cup	10.00	11.00	19.00	220.00	0.00	2.00	35.00	0.00
53	Boston Market-Spinach, Creamed	181.0000	0.750	Cup	10.00	24.00	13.00	300.00	0.00	2.00	75.00	0.00
54	Boston Market-Squash, Butternut	193.0000	0.750	Cup	2.00	6.00	25.00	160.00	0.00	3.00	15.00	0.00
55	Boston Market-Stuffing	174.0000	0.750	Cup	6.00	12.00	44.00	310.00	0.00	3.00	0.00	0.00
56	Boston Market-Turkey Breast, Rot	142.0000	5.000	Ounce	36.00	1.00	1.00	170.00	0.00	0.00	100.00	0.00
57	Boston Market-Turkey Sandwich w/	337.0000	1.000	Each	45.00	28.00	68.00	710.00	0.00	4.00	110.00	0.00
58	Boston Market-Turkey Sandwich, p	266.0000	1.000	Each	32.00	3.50	61.00	400.00	0.00	4.00	60.00	0.00
59	Boston Market-Vegetables, Steame	105.0000	0.660	Cup	2.00	0.50	7.00	35.00	0.00	3.00	0.00	0.00
60	Boston Market-Zucchini Marinara	146.0000	0.750	Cup	2.00	4.00	10.00	80.00	0.00	2.00	0.00	0.00
	Burger King-Biscuit With Bacon,	171.0000	1.000	Each	19.00	31.00	39.00	280.00	0.00	1.00	225.00	10.00
	Burger King-Biscuit with Sausage	151.0000	1.000	Each	16.00	40.00	41.00	360.00	0.00	1.00	45.00	13.00
	Burger King-Cheeseburger	138.0000	1.000	Each	23.00	16.00	28.00	380.00	0.00	1.00	65.00	9.00
	Burger King-Cheeseburger, Bacon	218.0000	1.000	Each	44.00	39.00	28.00	640.00	0.00	1.00	145.00	18.00
	Burger King-Cheeseburger, Double	210.0000	1.000	Each	41.00	36.00	28.00	600.00	0.00	1.00	135.00	17.00
	Burger King-Chicken Salad, Broil	302.0000	1.000	Each	21.00	10.00	7.00	90.00	0.00	3.00	60.00	4.00
	Burger King-Chicken Sandwich	229.0000	1.000	Each	26.00	43.00	54.00	710.00	0.00	2.00	60.00	9.00
	Burger King-Chicken Sandwich- BK	248.0000	1.000	Each	30.00	29.00	41.00	550.00	0.00	2.00	80.00	6.00
	Burger King-Chicken Tenders - 8	117.0000	1.000	Each	21.00	17.00	19.00	310.00	0.00	3.00	50.00	4.00
	Burger King-Coca Cola Classic -	360.0000	1.000	Each	0.00	0.00	70.00	280.00	3.08	0.00	0.00	0.00
	Burger King-Coke, Diet - medium	360.0000	1.000	Each	0.00	0.00	0.00	1.00	3.08	0.00	0.00	0.00
	Burger King-Croissan'Wich, w/ sa	176.0000	1.000	Each	22.00	46.00	25.00	600.00	0.00	1.00	260.00	16.00

Monounsaturated Fat (gm)	Polyunsaturated Fat (gm)	Vitamin D (mg)	Vitamin K (mg)	Vitamin E (mg)	Vitamin A (re)	Vitamin C (mg)	Thiamin (mg)	Riboflavin (mg)	Niacin (mg)	Vitamin B6 (mg)	Folate (mg)	Vitamin B12 (mcg)	Calcium (mg)	Iron (mg)	Magnesium (mg)	Phosphorus (mg)	Potassium (mg)	Sodium (mg)	Zinc (mg)
0.00	0.00	0.00	0.00	0.00	0.00	0.00	0.00	0.00	0.00	0.00	0.00	0.00	0.00	0.00	0.00	0.00	0.00	460.00	0.00
0.00	0.00	0.00	0.00	0.00	0.00	0.00	0.00	0.00	0.00	0.00	0.00	0.00	0.00	0.00	0.00	0.00	0.00	320.00	0.00
0.00	0.00	0.00	0.00	0.00	0.00	0.00	0.00	0.00	0.00	0.00	0.00	0.00	0.00	0.00	0.00	0.00	0.00	960.00	0.00
0.00	0.00	0.00	0.00	0.00	0.00	0.00	0.00	0.00	0.00	0.00	0.00	0.00	0.00	0.00	0.00	0.00	0.00	350.00	0.00
0.00	0.00	0.00	0.00	0.00	0.00	0.00	0.00	0.00	0.00	0.00	0.00	0.00	0.00	0.00	0.00	0.00	0.00	530.00	0.00
0.00	0.00	0.00	0.00	0.00	0.00	0.00	0.00	0.00	0.00	0.00	0.00	0.00	0.00	0.00	0.00	0.00	0.00	520.00	0.00
0.00	0.00	0.00	0.00	0.00	0.00	0.00	0.00	0.00	0.00	0.00	0.00	0.00	0.00	0.00	0.00	0.00	0.00	240.00	0.00
0.00	0.00	0.00	0.00	0.00	0.00	0.00	0.00	0.00	0.00	0.00	0.00	0.00	0.00	0.00	0.00	0.00	0.00	260.00	0.00
0.00	0.00	0.00	0.00	0.00	0.00	0.00	0.00	0.00	0.00	0.00	0.00	0.00	0.00	0.00	0.00	0.00	0.00	390.00	0.00
0.00	0.00	0.00	0.00	0.00	0.00	0.00	0.00	0.00	0.00	0.00	0.00	0.00	0.00	0.00	0.00	0.00	0.00	130.00	0.00
0.00	0.00	0.00	0.00	0.00	0.00	0.00	0.00	0.00	0.00	0.00	0.00	0.00	0.00	0.00	0.00	0.00	0.00	5.00	0.00
0.00	0.00	0.00	0.00	0.00	0.00	0.00	0.00	0.00	0.00	0.00	0.00	0.00	0.00	0.00	0.00	0.00	0.00	10.00	0.00
0.00	0.00	0.00	0.00	0.00	0.00	0.00	0.00	0.00	0.00	0.00	0.00	0.00	0.00	0.00	0.00	0.00	0.00	170.00	0.00
0.00	0.00	0.00	0.00	0.00	0.00	0.00	0.00	0.00	0.00	0.00	0.00	0.00	0.00	0.00	0.00	0.00	0.00	1880.00	0.00
0.00	0.00	0.00	0.00	0.00	0.00	0.00	0.00	0.00	0.00	0.00	0.00	0.00	0.00	0.00	0.00	0.00	0.00	1600.00	0.00
0.00	0.00	0.00	0.00	0.00	0.00	0.00	0.00	0.00	0.00	0.00	0.00	0.00	0.00	0.00	0.00	0.00	0.00	1490.00	0.00
0.00	0.00	0.00	0.00	0.00	0.00	0.00	0.00	0.00	0.00	0.00	0.00	0.00	0.00	0.00	0.00	0.00	0.00	2310.00	0.00
0.00	0.00	0.00	0.00	0.00	0.00	0.00	0.00	0.00	0.00	0.00	0.00	0.00	0.00	0.00	0.00	0.00	0.00	1330.00	0.00
0.00	0.00	0.00	0.00	0.00	0.00	0.00	0.00	0.00	0.00	0.00	0.00	0.00	0.00	0.00	0.00	0.00	0.00	760.00	0.00
0.00	0.00	0.00	0.00	0.00	0.00	0.00	0.00	0.00	0.00	0.00	0.00	0.00	0.00	0.00	0.00	0.00	0.00	2270.00	0.00
0.00	0.00	0.00	0.00	0.00	0.00	0.00	0.00	0.00	0.00	0.00	0.00	0.00	0.00	0.00	0.00	0.00	0.00	1040.00	0.00
0.00	0.00	0.00	0.00	0.00	0.00	0.00	0.00	0.00	0.00	0.00	0.00	0.00	0.00	0.00	0.00	0.00	0.00	1610.00	0.00
0.00	0.00	0.00	0.00	0.00	0.00	0.00	0.00	0.00	0.00	0.00	0.00	0.00	0.00	0.00	0.00	0.00	0.00	1170.00	0.00
0.00	0.00	0.00	0.00	0.00	0.00	0.00	0.00	0.00	0.00	0.00	0.00	0.00	0.00	0.00	0.00	0.00	0.00	2380.00	0.00
0.00	0.00	0.00	0.00	0.00	0.00	0.00	0.00	0.00	0.00	0.00	0.00	0.00	0.00	0.00	0.00	0.00	0.00	390.00	0.00
0.00	0.00	0.00	0.00	0.00	0.00	0.00	0.00	0.00	0.00	0.00	0.00	0.00	0.00	0.00	0.00	0.00	0.00	560.00	0.00
0.00	0.00	0.00	0.00	0.00	0.00	0.00	0.00	0.00	0.00	0.00	0.00	0.00	0.00	0.00	0.00	0.00	0.00	100.00	0.00
0.00	0.00	0.00	0.00	0.00	0.00	0.00	0.00	0.00	0.00	0.00	0.00	0.00	0.00	0.00	0.00	0.00	0.00	600.00	0.00
0.00	0.00	0.00	0.00	0.00	0.00	0.00	0.00	0.00	0.00	0.00	0.00	0.00	0.00	0.00	0.00	0.00	0.00	1860.00	0.00
0.00	0.00	0.00	0.00	0.00	0.00	0.00	0.00	0.00	0.00	0.00	0.00	0.00	0.00	0.00	0.00	0.00	0.00	1420.00	0.00
0.00	0.00	0.00	0.00	0.00	0.00	0.00	0.00	0.00	0.00	0.00	0.00	0.00	0.00	0.00	0.00	0.00	0.00	560.00	0.00
0.00	0.00	0.00	0.00	0.00	0.00	0.00	0.00	0.00	0.00	0.00	0.00	0.00	0.00	0.00	0.00	0.00	0.00	490.00	0.00
0.00	0.00	0.00	0.00	0.00	0.00	0.00	0.00	0.00	0.00	0.00	0.00	0.00	0.00	0.00	0.00	0.00	0.00	530.00	0.00
0.00	0.00	0.00	0.00	0.00	0.00	0.00	0.00	0.00	0.00	0.00	0.00	0.00	0.00	0.00	0.00	0.00	0.00	470.00	0.00
0.00	0.00	0.00	0.00	0.00	0.00	0.00	0.00	0.00	0.00	0.00	0.00	0.00	0.00	0.00	0.00	0.00	0.00	1410.00	0.00
0.00	0.00	0.00	0.00	0.00	0.00	0.00	0.00	0.00	0.00	0.00	0.00	0.00	0.00	0.00	0.00	0.00	0.00	790.00	0.00
0.00	0.00	0.00	0.00	0.00	0.00	0.00	0.00	0.00	0.00	0.00	0.00	0.00	0.00	0.00	0.00	0.00	0.00	580.00	0.00
0.00	0.00	0.00	0.00	0.00	0.00	0.00	0.00	0.00	0.00	0.00	0.00	0.00	0.00	0.00	0.00	0.00	0.00	1140.00	0.00
0.00	0.00	0.00	0.00	0.00	0.00	0.00	0.00	0.00	0.00	0.00	0.00	0.00	0.00	0.00	0.00	0.00	0.00	850.00	0.00
0.00	0.00	0.00	0.00	0.00	0.00	0.00	0.00	0.00	0.00	0.00	0.00	0.00	0.00	0.00	0.00	0.00	0.00	1390.00	0.00
0.00	0.00	0.00	0.00	0.00	0.00	0.00	0.00	0.00	0.00	0.00	0.00	0.00	0.00	0.00	0.00	0.00	0.00	1070.00	0.00
0.00	0.00	0.00	0.00	0.00	0.00	0.00	0.00	0.00	0.00	0.00	0.00	0.00	0.00	0.00	0.00	0.00	0.00	35.00	0.00
0.00	0.00	0.00	0.00	0.00	0.00	0.00	0.00	0.00	0.00	0.00	0.00	0.00	0.00	0.00	0.00	0.00	0.00	470.00	0.00
0.00	0.00	0.00	0.00	0.00	0.00	0.00	0.00	0.00	0.00	0.00	0.00	0.00	0.00	0.00	0.00	0.00	0.00	1530.00	0.00
0.00	0.00	0.00	0.00	0.00	0.00	0.00	0.00	0.00	0.00	0.00	0.00	0.00	0.00	0.00	0.00	0.00	0.00	1390.00	0.00
0.00	0.00	0.00	0.00	0.00	0.00	0.00	0.00	0.00	0.00	0.00	0.00	0.00	0.00	0.00	0.00	0.00	0.00	770.00	0.00
14.50	6.22	0.00	0.00	1.55	73.54	8.29	0.31	0.40	8.39	0.38	32.11	3.36	161.59	4.14	39.36	386.37	479.59	1240.00	6.63
12.24	2.23	0.00	0.00	2.00	111.25	6.68	0.24	0.34	5.45	0.27	34.49	2.01	210.27	3.34	34.49	339.33	382.72	1060.00	4.45
0.00	0.00	0.00	0.00	0.00	0.00	0.00	0.00	0.00	0.00	0.00	0.00	0.00	0.00	0.00	0.00	0.00	0.00	110.00	0.00
0.00	0.00	0.00	0.00	0.00	0.00	0.00	0.00	0.00	0.00	0.00	0.00	0.00	0.00	0.00	0.00	0.00	0.00	1400.00	0.00
0.00	0.00	0.00	0.00	0.00	0.00	0.00	0.00	0.00	0.00	0.00	0.00	0.00	0.00	0.00	0.00	0.00	0.00	4803.00	0.00
0.00	0.00	0.00	0.00	0.00	0.00	0.00	0.00	0.00	0.00	0.00	0.00	0.00	0.00	0.00	0.00	0.00	0.00	710.00	0.00
0.00	0.00	0.00	0.00	0.00	0.00	0.00	0.00	0.00	0.00	0.00	0.00	0.00	0.00	0.00	0.00	0.00	0.00	0.00	0.00
0.00	0.00	0.00	0.00	0.00	0.00	0.00	0.00	0.00	0.00	0.00	0.00	0.00	0.00	0.00	0.00	0.00	0.00	0.00	0.00
0.00	0.00	0.00	0.00	0.00	0.00	0.00	0.00	0.00	0.00	0.00	0.00	0.00	0.00	0.00	0.00	0.00	0.00	1140.00	0.00

USDA ID Code	Food Name	Weight in Grams*	Quantity of Units	Unit of Measure	Protein (gm)	Fat (gm)	Carbohydrate (gm)	Kcalories	Caffeine (gm)	Fiber (gm)	Cholesterol (mg)	Saturated Fat (gm)
	Burger King-Dressing, French	30.0000	1.000	Each	0.00	10.00	11.00	140.00	0.00	0.00	0.00	2.00
	Burger King-Dressing, Italian, R	30.0000	1.000	Each	0.00	0.50	3.00	15.00	0.00	0.00	0.00	0.00
	Burger King-Dressing, Ranch	30.0000	1.000	Each	0.00	19.00	2.00	180.00	0.00	0.00	10.00	4.00
	Burger King-Dressing, Thousand I	30.0000	1.000	Each	0.00	12.00	7.00	140.00	0.00	0.00	15.00	3.00
	Burger King-Fish Sandwich, BK Bi	255.0000	1.000	Each	26.00	41.00	56.00	700.00	0.00	3.00	90.00	6.00
	Burger King-French Fries, Coated	102.0000	1.000	Each	3.00	17.00	43.00	340.00	0.00	3.00	0.00	5.00
	Burger King-French Fries, Medium	116.0000	1.000	Each	5.00	20.00	43.00	180.00	0.00	3.00	0.00	5.00
	Burger King-French Toast Sticks	141.0000	1.000	Each	4.00	27.00	60.00	500.00	0.00	1.00	0.00	27.00
	Burger King-Hamburger	126.0000	1.000	Each	20.00	15.00	28.00	330.00	0.00	1.00	55.00	6.00
	Burger King-Hash Browns	71.0000	1.000	Each	2.00	12.00	25.00	110.00	0.00	2.00	0.00	3.00
	Burger King-Jam, Grape	12.0000	1.000	Each	0.00	0.00	8.00	30.00	0.00	0.00	0.00	0.00
	Burger King-Jam, Strawberry	12.0000	1.000	Each	0.00	0.00	8.00	30.00	0.00	0.00	0.00	0.00
	Burger King-Ketchup	14.0000	1.000	Each	0.00	0.00	4.00	15.00	0.00	0.00	0.00	0.00
	Burger King-Onion Rings	124.0000	1.000	Each	4.00	14.00	41.00	310.00	0.00	6.00	0.00	2.00
	Burger King-Pie, Apple, Dutch	113.0000	1.000	Each	3.00	15.00	39.00	300.00	0.00	2.00	0.00	3.00
	Burger King-Salad w/ 1000 Island	176.0000	1.000	Each	2.00	12.00	9.00	145.00	0.00	0.00	17.00	0.00
	Burger King-Salad w/ Bleu Cheese	176.0000	1.000	Each	3.00	16.00	7.00	184.00	0.00	0.00	22.00	0.00
	Burger King-Salad w/ Dressing, H	176.0000	1.000	Each	3.00	13.00	8.00	159.00	0.00	0.00	11.00	0.00
	Burger King-Salad w/ French	176.0000	1.000	Each	2.00	11.00	13.00	152.00	0.00	0.00	0.00	0.00
	Burger King-Salad w/ Italian, Go	176.0000	1.000	Each	2.00	14.00	7.00	162.00	0.00	0.00	0.00	0.00
	Burger King-Salad w/ Italian, Re	176.0000	1.000	Each	2.00	1.00	7.00	42.00	0.00	0.00	0.00	0.00
	Burger King-Salad, Garden	255.0000	1.000	Each	6.00	5.00	8.00	100.00	0.00	4.00	15.00	3.00
	Burger King-Salad, Side	133.0000	1.000	Each	3.00	3.00	4.00	60.00	0.00	2.00	5.00	2.00
	Burger King-Sauce, Dipping, Barb	28.0000	1.000	Each	0.00	0.00	9.00	35.00	0.00	0.00	0.00	0.00
	Burger King-Sauce, Dipping, Hone	28.0000	1.000	Each	0.00	0.00	21.00	80.00	0.00	0.00	0.00	0.00
	Burger King-Sauce, Dipping, Swee	28.0000	1.000	Each	0.00	0.00	11.00	45.00	0.00	0.00	0.00	0.00
	Burger King-Shake, Chocolate, Me	397.0000	1.000	Each	12.00	10.00	75.00	440.00	0.00	4.00	30.00	6.00
	Burger King-Shake, Vanilla, Medi	397.0000	1.000	Each	13.00	9.00	73.00	430.00	0.00	2.00	30.00	5.00
	Burger King-Whopper	270.0000	1.000	Each	27.00	39.00	45.00	640.00	0.00	3.00	90.00	11.00
	Burger King-Whopper Jr.	164.0000	1.000	Each	21.00	24.00	29.00	420.00	0.00	2.00	60.00	8.00
	Burger King-Whopper Jr. w/ chees	177.0000	1.000	Each	23.00	28.00	29.00	460.00	0.00	2.00	75.00	10.00
	Burger King-Whopper w/ Cheese, D	375.0000	1.000	Each	52.00	63.00	46.00	960.00	0.00	3.00	195.00	24.00
	Burger King-Whopper, Double	351.0000	1.000	Each	33.00	46.00	46.00	730.00	0.00	3.00	115.00	16.00
177	Chick-fil-A-Chicken Club, Chargr	232.0000	1.000	Each	33.00	12.00	38.00	390.00	0.00	2.00	70.00	5.00
178	Chick-fil-A-Chicken Salad Sandwi	167.0000	1.000	Each	25.00	5.00	42.00	320.00	0.00	1.00	10.00	2.00
179	Chick-fil-A-Chicken Sandwich	167.0000	1.000	Each	24.00	9.00	27.00	290.00	0.00	1.00	50.00	2.00
180	Chick-fil-A-Chicken, Chargrilled	150.0000	1.000	Each	27.00	3.00	36.00	280.00	0.00	1.00	40.00	1.00
176	Chick-fil-A-Chick-n-Strips	119.0000	4.000	Each	29.00	8.00	10.00	230.00	0.00	1.00	20.00	2.00
181	Chick-fil-A-Nuggets	110.0000	8.000	Each	28.00	14.00	12.00	290.00	0.00	0.00	60.00	3.00
182	Chick-fil-A-Salad, Ceasar, Chick	241.0000	1.000	Serving	33.00	10.00	5.00	240.00	0.00	2.00	90.00	7.00
184	Chick-fil-A-Salad, Garden w/ Chi	289.0000	1.000	Serving	30.00	8.00	7.00	200.00	0.00	3.00	80.00	3.00
183	Chick-fil-A-Salad, Garden w/ Chi	334.0000	1.000	Serving	32.00	17.00	21.00	370.00	0.00	4.00	113.00	6.00
185	Chick-fil-A-Soup, Chicken Breast	215.0000	1.000	Serving	16.00	1.00	10.00	110.00	0.00	1.00	45.00	0.00
	Fast Food-Beef, Roast Sandwich w	176.0000	1.000	Each	32.23	18.00	45.37	473.44	0.00	0.00	77.44	9.03
	Fast Food-Beef, Roast Sandwich,	139.0000	1.000	Each	21.50	13.76	33.44	346.11	0.00	0.00	51.43	3.60
	Fast Food-Biscuit w/ Egg	136.0000	1.000	Each	11.12	20.20	24.17	315.52	0.00	0.00	232.56	6.17
	Fast Food-Biscuit w/ Egg and Bac	150.0000	1.000	Each	17.00	31.10	28.59	457.50	0.00	0.75	352.50	7.95
	Fast Food-Biscuit w/ Egg and Ham	192.0000	1.000	Each	20.43	27.03	30.32	441.60	0.00	0.77	299.52	5.91
	Fast Food-Biscuit w/ Egg and Sau	180.0000	1.000	Each	19.15	38.70	41.15	581.40	0.00	0.90	302.40	14.98
	Fast Food-Biscuit w/ Egg, Cheese	144.0000	1.000	Each	16.26	31.39	33.42	476.64	0.00	0.00	260.64	11.40
	Fast Food-Biscuit w/ Ham	113.0000	1.000	Each	13.39	18.42	43.79	386.46	0.00	0.79	24.86	11.41
	Fast Food-Biscuit w/ Sausage	124.0000	1.000	Each	12.11	31.78	40.04	484.84	0.00	1.36	34.72	14.22
	Fast Food-Biscuit w/ Steak	141.0000	1.000	Each	13.10	25.99	44.39	455.43	0.00	0.00	25.38	6.94
	Fast Food-Biscuit, Plain	74.0000	1.000	Each	4.31	13.35	34.43	276.02	0.00	0.00	5.18	8.74
	Fast Food-Brownie	60.0000	1.000	Each	2.74	10.10	38.97	243.00	1.20	0.00	9.60	3.13

Monounsaturated Fat (gm)	Polyunsaturated Fat (gm)	Vitamin D (mg)	Vitamin K (mg)	Vitamin E (mg)	Vitamin A (re)	Vitamin C (mg)	Thiamin (mg)	Riboflavin (mg)	Niacin (mg)	Vitamin B_6 (mg)	Folate (mg)	Vitamin B_{12} (mcg)	Calcium (mg)	Iron (mg)	Magnesium (mg)	Phosphorus (mg)	Potassium (mg)	Sodium (mg)	Zinc (mg)
0.00	0.00	0.00	0.00	0.00	0.00	0.00	0.00	0.00	0.00	0.00	0.00	0.00	0.00	0.00	0.00	0.00	0.00	190.00	0.00
0.00	0.00	0.00	0.00	0.00	0.00	0.00	0.00	0.00	0.00	0.00	0.00	0.00	0.00	0.00	0.00	0.00	0.00	50.00	0.00
0.00	0.00	0.00	0.00	0.00	0.00	0.00	0.00	0.00	0.00	0.00	0.00	0.00	0.00	0.00	0.00	0.00	0.00	170.00	0.00
0.00	0.00	0.00	0.00	0.00	0.00	0.00	0.00	0.00	0.00	0.00	0.00	0.00	0.00	0.00	0.00	0.00	0.00	190.40	0.00
0.00	0.00	0.00	0.00	0.00	0.00	0.00	0.00	0.00	0.00	0.00	0.00	0.00	0.00	0.00	0.00	0.00	0.00	980.00	0.00
0.00	0.00	0.00	0.00	0.00	0.00	0.00	0.00	0.00	0.00	0.00	0.00	0.00	0.00	0.00	0.00	0.00	0.00	680.00	0.00
0.00	0.00	0.00	0.00	0.00	0.00	0.00	0.00	0.00	0.00	0.00	0.00	0.00	0.00	0.00	0.00	0.00	0.00	240.00	0.00
0.00	0.00	0.00	0.00	0.00	0.00	0.00	0.00	0.00	0.00	0.00	0.00	0.00	0.00	0.00	0.00	0.00	0.00	490.00	0.00
0.00	0.00	0.00	0.00	0.00	0.00	0.00	0.00	0.00	0.00	0.00	0.00	0.00	0.00	0.00	0.00	0.00	0.00	530.00	0.00
0.00	0.00	0.00	0.00	0.00	0.00	0.00	0.00	0.00	0.00	0.00	0.00	0.00	0.00	0.00	0.00	0.00	0.00	320.00	0.00
0.00	0.00	0.00	0.00	0.00	0.00	0.00	0.00	0.00	0.00	0.00	0.00	0.00	0.00	0.00	0.00	0.00	0.00	0.00	0.00
0.00	0.00	0.00	0.00	0.00	0.00	0.00	0.00	0.00	0.00	0.00	0.00	0.00	0.00	0.00	0.00	0.00	0.00	5.00	0.00
0.00	0.00	0.00	0.00	0.00	0.00	0.00	0.00	0.00	0.00	0.00	0.00	0.00	0.00	0.00	0.00	0.00	0.00	180.00	0.00
0.00	0.00	0.00	0.00	0.00	0.00	0.00	0.00	0.00	0.00	0.00	0.00	0.00	0.00	0.00	0.00	0.00	0.00	810.00	0.00
0.00	0.00	0.00	0.00	0.00	0.00	0.00	0.00	0.00	0.00	0.00	0.00	0.00	0.00	0.00	0.00	0.00	0.00	230.00	0.00
0.00	0.00	0.00	0.00	0.00	0.00	25.80	0.00	0.00	0.19	0.00	0.00	0.00	336.00	0.14	98.00	528.00	405.00	251.00	0.08
0.00	0.00	0.00	0.00	0.00	0.00	25.20	0.00	0.00	0.19	0.00	0.00	0.00	528.00	0.13	101.50	664.00	382.00	333.00	0.09
0.00	0.00	0.00	0.00	0.00	0.00	25.20	0.00	0.00	0.19	0.00	0.00	0.00	352.00	0.13	94.50	592.00	402.00	293.00	0.08
0.00	0.00	0.00	0.00	0.00	0.00	25.80	0.00	0.00	0.19	0.00	0.00	0.00	320.00	0.14	98.00	480.00	410.00	330.00	0.07
0.00	0.00	0.00	0.00	0.00	0.00	5.20	0.00	0.00	0.19	0.00	0.00	0.00	320.00	0.13	98.00	480.00	389.00	292.00	0.06
0.00	0.00	0.00	0.00	0.00	0.00	25.20	0.00	0.00	0.19	0.00	0.00	0.00	320.00	0.14	105.00	472.00	390.00	430.00	0.06
0.00	0.00	0.00	0.00	0.00	0.00	0.00	0.00	0.00	0.00	0.00	0.00	0.00	0.00	0.00	0.00	0.00	0.00	115.00	0.00
0.00	0.00	0.00	0.00	0.00	0.00	0.00	0.00	0.00	0.00	0.00	0.00	0.00	0.00	0.00	0.00	0.00	0.00	55.00	0.00
0.00	0.00	0.00	0.00	0.00	0.00	0.00	0.00	0.00	0.00	0.00	0.00	0.00	0.00	0.00	0.00	0.00	0.00	400.00	0.00
0.00	0.00	0.00	0.00	0.00	0.00	0.00	0.00	0.00	0.00	0.00	0.00	0.00	0.00	0.00	0.00	0.00	0.00	20.00	0.00
0.00	0.00	0.00	0.00	0.00	0.00	0.00	0.00	0.00	0.00	0.00	0.00	0.00	0.00	0.00	0.00	0.00	0.00	50.00	0.00
0.00	0.00	0.00	0.00	0.00	0.00	0.00	0.00	0.00	0.00	0.00	0.00	0.00	0.00	0.00	0.00	0.00	0.00	330.00	0.00
0.00	0.00	0.00	0.00	0.00	0.00	0.00	0.00	0.00	0.00	0.00	0.00	0.00	0.00	0.00	0.00	0.00	0.00	330.00	0.00
14.99	2.39	0.00	0.00	4.24	208.55	14.12	0.02	0.03	5.65	0.34	33.67	3.05	112.96	6.52	54.31	338.89	564.81	870.00	5.76
0.00	0.00	0.00	0.00	0.00	0.00	0.00	0.00	0.00	0.00	0.00	0.00	0.00	0.00	0.00	0.00	0.00	0.00	530.00	0.00
0.00	0.00	0.00	0.00	0.00	0.00	0.00	0.00	0.00	0.00	0.00	0.00	0.00	0.00	0.00	0.00	0.00	0.00	770.00	0.00
0.00	0.00	0.00	0.00	0.00	0.00	0.00	0.00	0.00	0.00	0.00	0.00	0.00	0.00	0.00	0.00	0.00	0.00	1420.00	0.00
0.00	0.00	0.00	0.00	0.00	0.00	0.00	0.00	0.00	0.00	0.00	0.00	0.00	0.00	0.00	0.00	0.00	0.00	1350.00	0.00
0.00	0.00	0.00	0.00	0.00	0.00	0.00	0.00	0.00	0.00	0.00	0.00	0.00	0.00	0.00	0.00	0.00	0.00	980.00	0.00
0.00	0.00	0.00	0.00	0.00	0.00	0.00	0.00	0.00	0.00	0.00	0.00	0.00	0.00	0.00	0.00	0.00	0.00	810.00	0.00
0.00	0.00	0.00	0.00	0.00	0.00	0.00	0.00	0.00	0.00	0.00	0.00	0.00	0.00	0.00	0.00	0.00	0.00	870.00	0.00
0.00	0.00	0.00	0.00	0.00	0.00	0.00	0.00	0.00	0.00	0.00	0.00	0.00	0.00	0.00	0.00	0.00	0.00	640.00	0.00
0.00	0.00	0.00	0.00	0.00	0.00	0.00	0.00	0.00	0.00	0.00	0.00	0.00	0.00	0.00	0.00	0.00	0.00	810.00	0.00
0.00	0.00	0.00	0.00	0.00	0.00	0.00	0.00	0.00	0.00	0.00	0.00	0.00	0.00	0.00	0.00	0.00	0.00	770.00	0.00
0.00	0.00	0.00	0.00	0.00	700.00	6.00	0.00	0.00	0.00	0.00	0.00	0.00	350.00	2.70	0.00	0.00	0.00	990.00	0.00
0.00	0.00	0.00	0.00	0.00	1100.00	18.00	0.00	0.00	0.00	0.00	0.00	0.00	170.00	0.90	0.00	0.00	0.00	790.00	0.00
0.00	0.00	0.00	0.00	0.00	1200.00	15.00	0.00	0.00	0.00	0.00	0.00	0.00	170.00	0.72	0.00	0.00	0.00	725.00	0.00
0.00	0.00	0.00	0.00	0.00	0.00	0.00	0.00	0.00	0.00	0.00	0.00	0.00	0.00	0.00	0.00	0.00	0.00	760.00	0.00
3.66	3.50	0.00	0.00	0.00	45.76	0.00	0.39	0.46	5.90	0.33	63.36	2.06	183.04	5.05	40.48	401.28	344.96	1633.28	5.37
6.81	1.71	0.00	0.00	0.00	20.85	2.09	0.38	0.31	5.87	0.26	56.99	1.22	54.21	4.23	30.58	239.08	315.53	792.30	3.39
8.19	4.22	0.00	0.00	0.00	178.16	0.00	0.34	0.34	0.71	0.08	61.20	0.75	153.68	3.13	20.40	184.96	160.48	654.16	1.10
13.44	7.47	0.00	0.00	2.12	52.50	2.70	0.14	0.23	2.40	0.14	60.00	1.04	189.00	3.74	24.00	238.50	250.50	999.00	1.64
10.96	7.70	0.00	0.00	2.21	240.00	0.00	0.67	0.60	2.00	0.27	65.28	1.19	220.80	4.55	30.72	316.80	318.72	1382.40	2.23
16.40	4.45	0.00	0.00	2.77	163.80	0.00	0.50	0.45	3.60	0.20	64.80	1.37	154.80	3.96	25.20	489.60	320.40	1141.20	2.16
14.23	3.50	0.00	0.00	0.00	165.60	1.58	0.30	0.43	2.30	0.10	53.28	1.05	164.16	2.55	20.16	459.36	230.40	1260.00	1.54
4.84	1.04	0.00	0.00	2.24	33.90	0.11	0.51	0.32	3.48	0.14	38.42	0.03	160.46	2.72	22.60	553.70	196.62	1432.84	1.65
12.82	3.03	0.00	0.00	3.08	13.64	0.12	0.40	0.29	3.27	0.11	45.88	0.51	127.72	2.58	19.84	446.40	198.40	1071.36	1.55
11.08	6.42	0.00	0.00	0.00	15.51	0.14	0.35	0.39	4.16	0.16	63.45	0.94	115.62	4.30	26.79	204.45	234.06	795.24	2.66
3.41	0.52	0.00	0.00	0.00	24.42	0.00	0.27	0.18	1.62	0.03	5.92	0.10	89.54	1.63	8.88	260.48	86.58	583.86	0.29
3.83	2.64	0.00	0.00	0.00	2.40	3.18	0.07	0.13	0.58	0.02	17.40	0.16	25.20	1.29	16.20	87.60	83.40	153.00	0.55

USDA ID Code / Food Name	Weight in Grams*	Quantity of Units	Unit of Measure	Protein (gm)	Fat (gm)	Carbohydrate (gm)	Kcalories	Caffeine (gm)	Fiber (gm)	Cholesterol (mg)	Saturated Fat (gm)
Fast Food-Burrito w/ Beans	217.0000	2.000	Each	14.06	13.50	71.44	447.02	0.00	0.00	4.34	6.88
Fast Food-Burrito w/ Beans and C	186.0000	2.000	Each	15.07	11.70	54.96	377.58	0.00	0.00	27.90	6.84
Fast Food-Burrito w/ Beans and C	204.0000	2.000	Each	16.38	14.67	58.08	412.08	0.00	0.00	32.64	7.61
Fast Food-Burrito w/ Beans and M	231.0000	2.000	Each	22.48	17.81	66.02	508.20	0.00	0.00	48.51	8.32
Fast Food-Burrito w/ Beans, Chee	336.0000	2.000	Each	33.30	22.98	85.18	661.92	0.00	0.00	157.92	11.19
Fast Food-Burrito w/ Beans, Chee	203.0000	2.000	Each	14.58	13.30	39.69	330.89	0.00	0.00	123.83	7.15
Fast Food-Burrito w/ Beef	220.0000	2.000	Each	26.60	20.81	58.52	523.60	0.00	0.00	63.80	10.45
Fast Food-Burrito w/ Beef and Ch	201.0000	2.000	Each	21.51	16.54	49.45	426.12	0.00	0.00	54.27	8.00
Fast Food-Burrito w/ Beef, Chees	304.0000	2.000	Each	40.92	24.78	63.72	632.32	0.00	0.00	170.24	10.40
Fast Food-Burrito w/ Fruit (Appl	74.0000	1.000	Each	2.50	9.52	34.98	230.88	0.00	0.00	3.70	4.57
Fast Food-Cheeseburger, Large, D	258.0000	1.000	Each	37.98	43.65	39.65	704.34	0.00	0.00	141.90	17.67
Fast Food-Cheeseburger, Large, S	185.0000	1.000	Each	30.14	32.99	47.42	608.65	0.00	0.00	96.20	14.84
Fast Food-Cheeseburger, Large, S	195.0000	1.000	Each	32.00	36.76	37.13	608.40	0.00	0.00	111.15	16.24
Fast Food-Cheeseburger, Large, S	219.0000	1.000	Each	28.19	32.94	38.39	562.83	0.00	0.00	87.60	15.05
Fast Food-Cheeseburger, Regular,	228.0000	1.000	Each	29.73	35.27	53.12	649.80	0.00	0.00	93.48	12.77
Fast Food-Cheeseburger, Regular,	102.0000	1.000	Each	14.77	15.15	31.75	319.26	0.00	0.00	49.98	6.47
Fast Food-Cheeseburger, Regular,	154.0000	1.000	Each	17.83	19.79	28.14	358.82	0.00	0.00	52.36	9.19
Fast Food-Cheeseburger, Triple P	304.0000	1.000	Each	56.06	50.95	26.69	796.48	0.00	0.00	161.12	21.71
Fast Food-Chicken Fillet Sandwic	228.0000	1.000	Each	29.41	38.76	41.59	631.56	0.00	0.00	77.52	12.45
Fast Food-Chicken Fillet Sandwic	182.0000	1.000	Each	24.12	29.45	38.69	515.06	0.00	0.00	60.06	8.54
Fast Food-Chicken Nuggets, Plain	17.7000	1.000	Piece	3.01	3.44	2.55	53.28	0.00	0.00	10.27	0.78
Fast Food-Chicken Nuggets, w/ Ba	130.0000	6.000	Each	17.15	17.97	25.03	330.20	0.00	0.00	61.10	5.58
Fast Food-Chicken Nuggets, w/ Ho	115.0000	6.000	Each	16.77	17.54	26.88	328.90	0.00	0.00	60.95	5.50
Fast Food-Chicken Nuggets, w/ Mu	130.0000	6.000	Each	17.42	18.94	20.85	322.40	0.00	0.00	61.10	5.72
Fast Food-Chicken Nuggets, w/ Sw	130.0000	6.000	Each	16.95	17.95	28.95	345.80	0.00	0.00	61.10	5.51
Fast Food-Chili Con Carne	253.0000	1.000	Cup	24.62	8.27	21.94	255.53	0.00	0.00	134.09	3.44
Fast Food-Chimichanga, w/ Beef	174.0000	1.000	Each	19.61	19.68	42.80	424.56	0.00	0.00	8.70	8.51
Fast Food-Chimichanga, w/ Beef a	183.0000	1.000	Each	20.06	23.44	39.33	442.86	0.00	0.00	51.24	11.18
Fast Food-Clams, Breaded and Fri	115.0000	0.750	Cup	12.82	26.40	38.81	450.80	0.00	0.00	87.40	6.60
Fast Food-Cookies, Chocolate Chi	55.0000	1.000	Box	2.89	12.14	36.22	232.65	6.05	0.00	11.55	5.34
Fast Food-Corn On The Cob w/ But	146.0000	1.000	Each	4.47	3.43	31.94	154.76	0.00	0.00	5.84	1.65
Fast Food-Crab, Soft-shell, Frie	125.0000	1.000	Each	10.99	17.86	31.20	333.75	0.00	0.00	45.00	4.40
Fast Food-Croissant w/Egg and Ch	127.0000	1.000	Each	12.79	24.70	24.31	368.30	0.00	0.00	215.90	14.07
Fast Food-Croissant w/Egg, Chees	160.0000	1.000	Each	20.30	38.16	24.72	523.20	0.00	0.00	216.00	18.22
Fast Food-Croissant w/Egg, Chees	129.0000	1.000	Each	16.23	28.35	23.65	412.80	0.00	0.00	215.43	15.43
Fast Food-Croissant w/Egg, Chees	152.0000	1.000	Each	18.92	33.58	24.20	474.24	0.00	0.00	212.80	17.48
Fast Food-Danish Pastry, Cheese	91.0000	1.000	Each	5.83	24.62	28.69	353.08	0.00	0.00	20.02	5.12
Fast Food-Danish Pastry, Cinnamo	88.0000	1.000	Each	4.80	16.72	46.85	349.36	0.00	0.00	27.28	3.48
Fast Food-Danish Pastry, Fruit	94.0000	1.000	Each	4.76	15.93	45.06	334.64	0.00	0.00	18.80	3.32
Fast Food-Egg and Cheese Sandwic	146.0000	1.000	Each	15.61	19.42	25.93	340.18	0.00	0.00	290.54	6.63
Fast Food-Egg, Scrambled	94.0000	2.000	Eggs	13.01	15.21	1.96	199.28	0.00	0.00	400.44	5.78
Fast Food-Enchilada w/ Cheese	163.0000	1.000	Each	9.63	18.84	28.54	319.48	0.00	0.00	44.01	10.60
Fast Food-Enchilada w/ Cheese an	192.0000	1.000	Each	11.92	17.64	30.47	322.56	0.00	0.00	40.32	9.04
Fast Food-Enchirito w/ Cheese, B	193.0000	1.000	Each	17.89	16.08	33.79	343.54	0.00	0.00	50.18	7.95
Fast Food-Fish Fillet, Battered	91.0000	1.000	Each	13.34	11.18	15.44	211.12	0.00	0.46	30.94	2.57
Fast Food-Fish Sandwich w/ Tarta	158.0000	1.000	Each	16.94	22.77	41.02	431.34	0.00	0.00	55.30	5.23
Fast Food-Fish Sandwich w/ Tarta	183.0000	1.000	Each	20.61	28.60	47.63	523.38	0.00	0.00	67.71	8.14
Fast Food-French Toast w/ Butter	135.0000	2.000	Slice	10.34	18.77	36.05	356.40	0.00	0.00	116.10	7.75
Fast Food-Frijoles w/ Cheese	167.0000	1.000	Cup	11.37	7.78	28.71	225.45	0.00	0.00	36.74	4.07
Fast Food-Ham and Cheese Sandwic	146.0000	1.000	Each	20.69	15.48	33.35	351.86	0.00	0.00	58.40	6.44
Fast Food-Ham, Egg, and Cheese S	143.0000	1.000	Each	19.25	16.30	30.95	347.49	0.00	0.00	245.96	7.41
Fast Food-Hamburger, Double Patt	226.0000	1.000	Each	34.28	26.56	40.27	540.14	0.00	0.00	122.04	10.51
Fast Food-Hamburger, Double Patt	215.0000	1.000	Each	31.82	32.47	38.74	576.20	0.00	0.00	103.20	12.00
Fast Food-Hamburger, Double Patt	176.0000	1.000	Each	29.92	27.90	42.93	543.84	0.00	0.00	98.56	10.38
Fast Food-Hamburger, Large, Sing	218.0000	1.000	Each	25.83	27.36	40.00	512.30	0.00	0.00	87.20	10.42

Monounsaturated Fat (gm)	Polyunsaturated Fat (gm)	Vitamin D (mg)	Vitamin K (mg)	Vitamin E (mg)	Vitamin A (re)	Vitamin C (mg)	Thiamin (mg)	Riboflavin (mg)	Niacin (mg)	Vitamin B6 (mg)	Folate (mg)	Vitamin B12 (mcg)	Calcium (mg)	Iron (mg)	Magnesium (mg)	Phosphorus (mg)	Potassium (mg)	Sodium (mg)	Zinc (mg)
4.73	1.19	0.00	0.00	0.00	32.55	1.95	0.63	0.61	4.06	0.30	86.80	1.09	112.84	4.51	86.80	97.65	653.17	985.18	1.52
2.49	1.79	0.00	0.00	0.00	238.08	1.67	0.22	0.71	3.57	0.24	74.40	0.89	213.90	2.27	79.98	180.42	496.62	1166.22	1.64
5.37	0.96	0.00	0.00	0.00	20.40	1.22	0.45	0.71	4.39	0.29	95.88	1.16	99.96	4.55	71.40	114.24	579.36	1044.48	3.41
7.02	1.22	0.00	0.00	0.00	64.68	1.85	0.53	0.83	5.41	0.37	115.50	1.73	106.26	4.90	83.16	140.91	656.04	1335.18	3.83
8.47	1.28	0.00	0.00	0.00	383.04	6.72	0.54	1.21	7.69	0.40	164.64	1.98	288.96	7.69	97.44	285.60	809.76	2059.68	6.08
4.47	1.02	0.00	0.00	0.00	150.22	5.08	0.30	0.71	3.86	0.22	75.11	1.10	129.92	3.74	50.75	140.07	410.06	990.64	2.35
7.41	0.86	0.00	0.00	0.00	28.60	1.10	0.24	0.92	6.45	0.31	129.80	1.96	83.60	6.09	81.40	173.80	739.20	1491.60	4.73
6.07	0.98	0.00	0.00	0.00	46.23	1.61	0.40	0.80	5.09	0.30	96.48	1.29	86.43	4.44	60.30	140.70	498.48	1115.55	4.32
9.94	2.22	0.00	0.00	0.00	112.48	3.65	0.61	1.25	8.33	0.36	139.84	2.07	221.92	7.81	69.92	316.16	665.76	2091.52	7.90
3.42	1.06	0.00	0.00	0.00	37.00	0.74	0.17	0.18	1.86	0.07	24.42	0.51	15.54	1.07	7.40	14.80	104.34	211.64	0.40
17.36	4.70	0.00	0.00	0.00	54.18	1.03	0.36	0.49	7.25	0.41	74.82	3.41	239.94	5.91	51.60	394.74	595.98	1148.10	6.68
12.75	2.44	0.56	0.00	0.00	148.00	0.00	0.48	0.57	11.17	0.28	74.00	2.53	90.65	5.46	38.85	421.80	643.80	1589.15	5.55
14.49	2.71	0.00	0.00	0.00	79.95	2.15	0.31	0.41	6.63	0.31	85.80	2.34	161.85	4.74	44.85	399.75	331.50	1043.25	6.83
12.61	2.04	0.00	0.00	1.18	129.21	7.88	0.39	0.46	7.38	0.28	81.03	2.56	205.86	4.66	43.80	310.98	444.57	1108.14	4.60
12.63	6.36	0.00	0.00	1.98	84.36	2.74	0.57	0.43	8.34	0.27	91.20	2.07	168.72	4.72	36.48	348.84	389.88	921.12	4.13
5.77	1.54	0.31	0.00	0.00	36.72	0.00	0.40	0.40	3.70	0.09	54.06	0.97	140.76	2.44	21.42	195.84	164.22	499.80	2.37
7.16	1.48	0.00	0.00	0.00	70.84	2.31	0.32	0.23	6.38	0.15	64.68	1.23	181.72	2.65	26.18	215.60	229.46	976.36	2.62
21.52	3.16	0.00	0.00	0.00	85.12	2.74	0.61	0.64	11.46	0.61	69.92	5.90	282.72	8.30	60.80	541.12	820.80	1212.96	10.88
13.66	9.94	0.00	0.00	0.00	127.68	2.96	0.41	0.46	9.07	0.41	109.44	0.46	257.64	3.63	43.32	405.84	332.88	1238.04	2.90
10.41	8.39	0.00	0.00	0.00	30.94	8.92	0.33	0.24	6.81	0.20	100.10	0.38	60.06	4.68	34.58	232.96	353.08	957.32	1.87
1.75	0.77	0.00	0.00	0.23	0.00	0.00	0.02	0.03	1.25	0.05	5.13	0.05	2.30	0.16	4.07	48.32	50.98	85.67	0.17
8.76	2.39	0.00	0.00	0.00	46.80	0.78	0.10	0.16	7.02	0.34	29.90	0.30	20.80	1.46	24.70	214.50	318.50	829.40	1.12
8.61	2.22	0.00	0.00	0.00	29.90	0.46	0.09	0.15	6.81	0.31	29.90	0.30	17.25	1.32	19.55	202.50	255.30	537.05	1.08
9.04	2.91	0.00	0.00	0.00	32.50	0.39	0.12	0.16	6.94	0.31	29.90	0.31	24.70	1.48	26.00	218.40	279.50	790.40	1.14
8.65	2.24	0.00	0.00	0.00	72.80	0.78	0.10	0.20	6.86	0.33	29.90	0.36	20.80	1.48	23.40	210.60	276.90	677.30	1.09
3.42	0.53	0.00	0.00	0.00	166.98	1.52	0.13	1.14	2.48	0.33	45.54	1.14	68.31	5.19	45.54	197.34	690.69	1006.94	3.57
8.07	1.13	0.00	0.00	0.00	15.66	4.70	0.49	0.64	5.78	0.28	83.52	1.51	62.64	4.54	62.64	123.54	586.38	910.02	4.96
9.44	0.73	0.00	0.00	0.00	126.27	2.75	0.38	0.86	4.67	0.22	91.50	1.30	237.90	3.84	60.39	186.66	203.13	957.09	3.37
11.44	6.77	0.00	0.00	0.00	36.80	0.00	0.21	0.26	2.86	0.03	42.55	1.10	20.70	3.05	31.05	238.05	265.65	833.75	1.63
5.05	1.03	0.00	0.00	0.37	14.85	0.55	0.09	0.19	1.39	0.03	33.00	0.10	19.80	1.47	16.50	52.25	81.95	188.10	0.34
1.01	0.61	0.00	0.00	0.00	96.36	6.86	0.25	0.10	2.18	0.32	43.80	0.00	4.38	0.88	40.88	108.04	359.16	29.20	0.91
7.69	4.88	0.00	0.00	0.00	3.75	0.75	0.10	0.08	1.75	0.15	20.00	4.48	55.00	1.81	25.00	131.25	162.50	1117.50	1.06
7.54	1.37	0.00	0.00	0.00	255.27	0.13	0.19	0.38	1.51	0.10	46.99	0.77	243.84	2.20	21.59	347.98	173.99	551.18	1.75
14.26	3.01	0.00	0.00	0.00	108.80	0.16	0.99	0.32	4.00	0.11	43.20	0.90	144.00	3.04	24.00	289.60	283.20	1115.20	2.14
9.17	1.75	0.00	0.00	0.00	119.97	2.19	0.35	0.34	2.19	0.12	45.15	0.86	150.93	2.19	22.20	276.06	201.24	888.81	1.90
11.40	2.36	0.00	0.00	0.00	117.04	11.40	0.52	0.30	3.19	0.23	45.60	1.00	144.40	2.13	25.84	335.92	272.08	1080.72	2.17
15.60	2.42	0.00	0.00	0.00	42.77	2.64	0.26	0.21	2.55	0.05	54.60	0.23	70.07	1.85	15.47	80.08	116.48	319.41	0.63
10.60	1.65	0.00	0.00	0.00	5.28	2.55	0.26	0.19	2.20	0.05	54.56	0.22	36.96	1.80	14.08	73.92	95.92	326.48	0.48
10.10	1.57	0.00	0.00	0.00	24.44	1.60	0.29	0.21	1.80	0.06	31.02	0.24	21.62	1.40	14.10	68.62	109.98	332.76	0.48
8.26	2.58	0.00	0.00	0.00	181.04	1.46	0.26	0.57	2.07	0.13	97.82	1.14	224.84	2.98	21.90	302.22	188.34	804.46	1.65
5.54	1.85	1.60	0.00	1.58	251.92	3.10	0.08	0.49	0.20	0.18	52.64	0.95	53.58	2.43	13.16	227.48	138.18	210.56	1.56
6.31	0.81	0.00	0.00	0.00	185.82	0.98	0.08	0.42	1.91	0.39	65.20	0.75	324.37	1.32	50.53	133.66	239.61	784.03	2.51
6.14	1.38	0.00	0.00	0.00	142.08	1.34	0.10	0.40	2.52	0.27	67.20	1.02	228.48	3.07	82.56	167.04	574.08	1319.04	2.69
6.52	0.33	0.00	0.00	0.00	133.17	4.63	0.17	0.69	2.99	0.21	59.83	1.62	218.09	2.39	71.41	223.88	559.70	1250.64	2.76
2.35	5.71	0.00	0.00	0.00	10.92	0.00	0.10	0.10	1.91	0.09	15.47	1.01	16.38	1.92	21.84	155.61	291.20	484.12	0.40
7.69	8.25	0.00	0.00	0.87	30.02	2.84	0.33	0.22	3.40	0.11	85.32	1.07	83.74	2.61	33.18	211.72	339.70	614.62	1.00
8.91	9.42	0.92	0.00	1.83	96.99	2.75	0.46	0.42	4.23	0.11	91.50	1.08	184.83	3.50	36.60	311.10	353.19	938.79	1.17
7.07	2.44	0.00	0.00	0.00	145.80	0.14	0.58	0.50	3.92	0.05	72.90	0.36	72.90	1.89	16.20	145.80	176.85	513.00	0.59
2.62	0.70	0.00	0.00	0.00	70.14	1.50	0.13	0.33	1.49	0.20	111.89	0.68	188.71	2.24	16.20	175.35	604.54	881.76	1.74
6.75	1.37	0.00	0.00	0.29	75.92	2.77	0.31	0.48	2.69	0.20	75.92	0.54	129.94	3.24	16.06	151.84	290.54	770.88	1.37
5.75	1.69	0.00	0.00	0.59	148.72	2.72	0.43	0.56	4.20	0.16	75.79	1.23	211.64	3.10	25.74	346.06	210.21	1005.29	1.99
10.33	2.80	0.00	0.00	0.00	11.30	1.13	0.36	0.38	7.57	0.54	76.84	4.07	101.70	5.85	49.72	314.14	569.52	791.00	5.67
14.13	2.77	0.00	0.00	0.00	4.30	1.08	0.34	0.41	6.73	0.37	83.85	3.33	92.45	5.55	45.15	283.80	526.75	741.75	5.81
12.11	2.34	0.70	0.00	1.32	0.00	0.00	0.33	0.37	8.25	0.32	77.44	2.92	86.24	4.56	36.96	234.08	362.56	554.40	5.72
11.42	2.20	0.00	0.00	0.00	32.70	2.62	0.41	0.37	7.28	0.33	82.84	2.38	95.92	4.93	43.60	233.26	479.60	824.04	4.88

USDA ID Code Food Name	Weight in Grams*	Quantity of Units	Unit of Measure	Protein (gm)	Fat (gm)	Carbohydrate (gm)	Kcalories	Caffeine (gm)	Fiber (gm)	Cholesterol (mg)	Saturated Fat (gm)
Fast Food-Hamburger, Single Patt	106.0000	1.000	Each	12.32	9.77	34.25	272.42	0.00	2.33	29.68	3.56
Fast Food-Hamburger, Single Patt	90.0000	1.000	Each	12.32	11.82	30.51	274.50	0.00	0.00	35.10	4.14
Fast Food-Hamburger, Triple Patt	259.0000	1.000	Each	49.99	41.47	28.59	691.53	0.00	0.00	142.45	15.93
Fast Food-Hot Dog w/ Chili	114.0000	1.000	Each	13.51	13.44	31.29	296.40	0.00	0.00	51.30	4.86
Fast Food-Hot Dog w/ Corn Flour	175.0000	1.000	Each	16.80	18.90	55.79	460.25	0.00	0.00	78.75	5.16
Fast Food-Hot Dog, Plain	98.0000	1.000	Each	10.39	14.54	18.03	242.06	0.00	0.00	44.10	5.11
Fast Food-Ice Milk, Vanilla, Sof	103.0000	1.000	Each	3.89	6.12	24.11	163.77	0.00	0.10	27.81	3.53
Fast Food-Muffin, English w/ But	63.0000	1.000	Each	4.87	5.76	30.36	189.00	0.00	0.00	12.60	2.43
Fast Food-Muffin, English w/ Che	115.0000	1.000	Each	15.34	24.27	29.16	393.30	0.00	1.50	58.65	9.86
Fast Food-Muffin, English w/ Egg	137.0000	1.000	Each	16.69	12.59	26.74	289.07	0.00	1.51	234.27	4.67
Fast Food-Muffin, English w/ Egg	165.0000	1.000	Each	21.66	30.86	30.97	486.75	0.00	0.00	273.90	12.42
Fast Food-Nachos w/ Cheese	113.0000	7.000	Each	9.10	18.95	36.33	345.78	0.00	0.00	18.08	7.79
Fast Food-Nachos w/ Cheese and J	204.0000	7.000	Each	16.81	34.15	60.08	607.92	0.00	0.00	83.64	14.01
Fast Food-Nachos w/ Cheese, Bean	255.0000	7.000	Each	19.79	30.70	55.82	568.65	0.00	0.00	20.40	12.50
Fast Food-Nachos w/ Cinnamon and	109.0000	7.000	Each	7.19	35.98	63.39	591.87	0.00	0.00	39.24	18.21
Fast Food-Onion Rings, Breaded a	83.0000	1.000	Order	3.70	15.51	31.32	275.56	0.00	0.00	14.11	6.96
Fast Food-Oysters, Battered or B	139.0000	6.000	Each	12.54	17.93	39.88	368.35	0.00	0.00	108.42	4.57
Fast Food-Pancakes w/ Butter and	232.0000	2.000	Each	8.26	13.99	90.90	519.68	0.00	0.00	58.00	5.85
Fast Food-Pie, Fried, Fruit (App	85.0000	1.000	Each	2.41	14.37	33.05	266.05	0.00	0.00	12.75	6.51
Fast Food-Pizza w/ Cheese	63.0000	1.000	Slice	7.68	3.21	20.50	140.49	0.00	0.00	9.45	1.54
Fast Food-Pizza w/ Cheese, Sausa	79.0000	1.000	Slice	13.01	5.36	21.29	184.07	0.00	0.00	20.54	1.53
Fast Food-Pizza w/ Pepperoni	71.0000	1.000	Slice	10.12	6.96	19.87	181.05	0.00	0.00	14.20	2.24
Fast Food-Potato, Baked w/ Chees	296.0000	1.000	Piece	14.62	28.74	46.50	473.60	0.00	0.00	17.76	10.57
Fast Food-Potato, Baked w/ Chees	299.0000	1.000	Piece	18.42	25.89	44.43	451.49	0.00	0.00	29.90	10.14
Fast Food-Potato, Baked w/ Chees	339.0000	1.000	Piece	13.66	21.42	46.58	403.41	0.00	0.00	20.34	8.51
Fast Food-Potato, Baked w/ Chees	395.0000	1.000	Piece	23.23	21.84	55.85	481.90	0.00	0.00	31.60	13.04
Fast Food-Potato, Baked w/ Sour	302.0000	1.000	Piece	6.67	22.32	50.01	392.60	0.00	0.00	24.16	10.03
Fast Food-Potato, French Fried I	115.0000	1.000	Large	4.59	18.50	44.36	358.80	0.00	0.00	20.70	8.52
Fast Food-Potato, French Fried I	115.0000	1.000	Large	4.59	18.50	44.36	357.65	0.00	0.00	16.10	7.63
Fast Food-Potato, French Fried I	85.0000	1.000	Small	3.66	15.67	33.84	290.70	0.00	2.98	0.00	3.27
Fast Food-Potato, Mashed	80.0000	0.330	Cup	1.85	0.97	12.90	66.40	0.00	0.00	1.60	0.38
Fast Food-Potatoes, Hashed Brown	72.0000	0.500	Cup	1.94	9.22	16.15	151.20	0.00	0.00	9.36	4.33
Fast Food-Salad, w/o Dressing	104.0000	0.750	Cup	1.30	0.07	3.35	16.64	0.00	0.00	0.00	0.01
Fast Food-Salad, w/o Dressing, w	217.0000	1.500	Cup	8.77	5.79	4.75	101.99	0.00	0.00	97.65	2.97
Fast Food-Salad, w/o Dressing, w	218.0000	1.500	Cup	17.44	2.18	3.73	104.64	0.00	0.00	71.94	0.59
Fast Food-Salad, w/o Dressing, w	417.0000	1.500	Cup	16.43	20.85	31.98	379.47	0.00	0.00	50.04	2.59
Fast Food-Salad, w/o Dressing, w	236.0000	1.500	Cup	14.51	2.48	6.61	106.20	0.00	0.00	179.36	0.66
Fast Food-Scallops, Breaded and	144.0000	6.000	Each	15.75	19.40	38.49	385.92	0.00	0.00	108.00	4.88
Fast Food-Shrimp, Breaded and Fr	164.0000	7.000	Each	18.88	24.90	40.00	454.28	0.00	0.00	200.08	5.38
Fast Food-Steak Sandwich	204.0000	1.000	Each	30.33	14.08	51.96	459.00	0.00	0.00	73.44	3.81
Fast Food-Submarine Sandwich w/	228.0000	1.000	Each	21.84	18.63	51.05	456.00	0.00	0.00	36.48	6.82
Fast Food-Submarine Sandwich w/	216.0000	1.000	Each	28.64	12.96	44.30	410.40	0.00	0.00	73.44	7.08
Fast Food-Submarine Sandwich w/	256.0000	1.000	Each	29.70	27.98	55.37	583.68	0.00	0.00	48.64	5.32
Fast Food-Sundae, Caramel	155.0000	1.000	Each	7.30	9.27	49.31	303.80	0.00	0.00	24.80	4.51
Fast Food-Sundae, Hot Fudge	158.0000	1.000	Each	5.64	8.63	47.67	284.40	1.58	0.00	20.54	5.02
Fast Food-Sundae, Strawberry	153.0000	1.000	Each	6.26	7.85	44.65	267.75	0.00	0.00	21.42	3.73
Fast Food-Taco	171.0000	1.000	Small	20.66	20.55	26.73	369.36	0.00	0.00	56.43	11.37
Fast Food-Taco Salad	198.0000	1.500	Cup	13.23	14.77	23.58	279.18	0.00	0.00	43.56	6.83
Fast Food-Taco Salad w/ Chili Co	261.0000	1.500	Cup	17.41	13.13	26.57	289.71	0.00	0.00	5.22	6.00
Fast Food-Tostada w/ Guacamole	261.0000	2.000	Each	12.48	23.26	32.02	360.18	0.00	0.00	39.15	9.87
Fast Food-Tostada, w/ Beans and	144.0000	1.000	Piece	9.60	9.86	26.52	223.20	0.00	0.00	30.24	5.37
Fast Food-Tostada, w/ Beans, Bee	225.0000	1.000	Piece	16.09	16.94	29.66	333.00	0.00	0.00	74.25	11.48
Fast Food-Tostada, w/ Beef and C	163.0000	1.000	Piece	18.99	16.35	22.77	314.59	0.00	0.00	40.75	10.40
Hardee's-Beef, Roast, Big	163.0080	1.000	Each	21.90	13.38	38.93	364.94	0.00	1.09	54.74	6.08
Hardee's-Beef, Roast, Sandwich	141.7460	1.000	Each	18.65	11.19	38.54	323.28	0.00	0.99	43.52	4.97

Monounsaturated Fat (gm)	Polyunsaturated Fat (gm)	Vitamin D (mg)	Vitamin K (mg)	Vitamin E (mg)	Vitamin A (re)	Vitamin C (mg)	Thiamin (mg)	Riboflavin (mg)	Niacin (mg)	Vitamin B₆ (mg)	Folate (mg)	Vitamin B₁₂ (mcg)	Calcium (mg)	Iron (mg)	Magnesium (mg)	Phosphorus (mg)	Potassium (mg)	Sodium (mg)	Zinc (mg)
3.40	1.01	0.00	0.00	0.01	9.54	2.23	0.29	0.23	3.91	0.12	51.94	1.09	126.14	2.71	23.32	114.48	251.22	534.24	2.25
5.45	0.92	0.27	0.00	0.50	0.00	0.00	0.33	0.27	3.72	0.06	53.10	0.89	63.00	2.40	18.90	102.60	144.90	387.00	2.00
18.23	2.75	0.00	0.00	0.00	15.54	1.30	0.31	0.54	10.96	0.62	75.11	4.92	64.75	8.31	54.39	393.68	784.77	712.25	10.75
6.60	1.19	0.00	0.00	0.00	5.70	2.74	0.22	0.40	3.74	0.05	72.96	0.30	19.38	3.28	10.26	191.52	166.44	479.94	0.78
9.12	3.50	0.00	0.00	0.00	36.75	0.00	0.28	0.70	4.17	0.09	103.25	0.44	101.50	6.18	17.50	166.25	262.50	973.00	1.31
6.85	1.71	0.00	0.00	0.00	0.00	0.10	0.24	0.27	3.65	0.05	48.02	0.51	23.52	2.31	12.74	97.02	143.08	670.32	1.98
1.81	0.36	0.21	0.00	0.38	51.50	1.13	0.05	0.26	0.31	0.06	12.36	0.21	153.47	0.15	15.45	139.05	168.92	91.67	0.57
1.53	1.35	0.00	0.00	0.13	33.39	0.76	0.25	0.32	2.61	0.04	56.70	0.02	102.69	1.59	13.23	85.05	69.30	386.19	0.42
10.09	2.69	0.00	0.00	0.49	86.25	1.27	0.70	0.25	4.14	0.15	66.70	0.68	167.90	2.25	24.15	186.30	215.05	1036.15	1.68
4.67	1.56	1.10	0.00	0.85	156.18	1.78	0.49	0.45	3.33	0.15	43.84	0.67	150.70	2.44	23.29	269.89	198.65	728.84	1.56
12.75	3.32	0.00	0.00	0.00	171.60	1.49	0.84	0.50	4.46	0.20	54.45	1.37	196.35	3.47	29.70	287.10	293.70	1135.20	2.36
7.99	2.24	0.00	0.00	0.00	91.53	1.24	0.19	0.37	1.54	0.20	10.17	0.82	272.33	1.28	55.37	275.72	171.76	815.86	1.79
14.40	4.02	0.00	0.00	0.00	471.24	1.02	0.12	0.49	2.84	0.37	18.36	1.02	620.16	2.45	108.12	393.72	293.76	1736.04	2.90
10.99	5.69	0.00	0.00	0.00	469.20	4.85	0.23	0.69	3.34	0.41	38.25	1.02	385.05	2.78	96.90	387.60	451.35	1800.30	3.65
11.84	4.13	0.00	0.00	0.00	10.90	7.96	0.19	0.45	3.92	0.17	7.63	1.72	85.02	2.89	19.62	32.70	78.48	439.27	0.59
6.65	0.66	0.00	0.00	0.33	0.83	0.58	0.08	0.10	0.92	0.06	54.78	0.12	73.04	0.85	15.77	86.32	129.48	429.94	0.35
6.92	4.64	0.00	0.00	0.00	108.42	4.17	0.31	0.35	4.42	0.03	30.58	1.01	27.80	4.46	23.63	195.99	182.09	676.93	15.64
5.27	1.95	0.00	0.00	1.39	69.60	3.48	0.39	0.56	3.39	0.12	51.04	0.23	127.60	2.62	48.72	475.60	250.56	1104.32	1.02
5.83	1.16	0.00	0.00	0.37	33.15	1.11	0.10	0.08	0.98	0.03	4.25	0.08	12.75	0.88	7.65	37.40	51.00	324.70	0.17
0.99	0.49	0.00	0.00	0.58	73.71	1.26	0.18	0.16	2.48	0.04	34.65	0.33	116.55	0.58	15.75	112.77	109.62	335.79	0.81
2.54	0.92	0.00	0.00	0.00	101.12	1.58	0.21	0.17	1.96	0.09	32.39	0.36	101.12	1.53	18.17	131.14	178.54	382.36	1.11
3.14	1.16	0.00	0.00	0.00	54.67	1.63	0.13	0.23	3.05	0.06	36.92	0.18	64.61	0.94	8.52	75.26	152.65	266.96	0.52
10.72	6.04	0.00	0.00	0.00	227.92	26.05	0.24	0.21	3.34	0.71	26.64	0.18	310.80	3.02	65.12	319.68	1166.24	381.84	1.89
9.72	4.75	0.00	0.00	0.00	173.42	28.70	0.27	0.24	3.98	0.75	29.90	0.33	307.97	3.14	68.77	346.84	1178.06	971.75	2.15
7.70	4.17	0.00	0.00	0.00	277.98	48.48	0.27	0.27	3.59	0.78	61.02	0.34	335.61	3.32	77.97	345.78	1440.75	484.77	2.03
6.83	0.91	0.00	0.00	0.00	173.80	31.60	0.28	0.36	4.19	0.95	47.40	0.24	410.80	6.12	110.60	497.70	1572.10	699.15	3.79
7.88	3.32	0.00	0.00	0.00	277.84	33.82	0.27	0.18	3.71	0.79	33.22	0.21	105.70	3.11	69.46	184.22	1383.16	181.20	0.91
8.03	0.93	0.00	0.00	0.02	3.45	6.10	0.16	0.05	2.60	0.30	37.95	0.14	18.40	1.55	37.95	152.95	818.80	187.45	0.60
8.23	1.99	0.00	0.00	0.00	3.45	6.10	0.16	0.05	2.60	0.30	37.95	0.14	18.40	1.55	37.95	152.95	818.80	187.45	0.60
9.05	2.66	0.00	0.00	1.04	0.00	9.86	0.07	0.03	2.42	0.31	32.30	0.00	11.90	0.66	33.15	109.65	585.65	168.30	0.40
0.28	0.23	0.00	0.00	0.00	8.00	0.32	0.07	0.04	0.96	0.18	6.40	0.04	16.80	0.38	14.40	44.00	235.20	181.60	0.26
3.86	0.47	0.00	0.00	0.12	2.88	5.47	0.08	0.01	1.07	0.17	7.92	0.01	7.20	0.48	15.84	69.12	267.12	290.16	0.22
0.00	0.03	0.00	0.00	0.00	118.56	24.13	0.03	0.05	0.57	0.08	38.48	0.00	13.52	0.66	11.44	40.56	178.88	27.04	0.22
1.76	0.48	0.00	0.00	0.00	115.01	9.77	0.09	0.17	0.98	0.11	84.63	0.30	99.82	0.67	23.87	132.37	371.07	119.35	1.00
0.68	0.57	0.00	0.00	0.00	95.92	17.44	0.11	0.17	5.89	0.44	67.58	0.20	37.06	1.09	32.70	170.04	446.90	209.28	0.89
4.84	9.09	0.00	0.00	0.00	638.01	38.36	0.29	0.21	3.54	0.33	187.65	1.71	70.89	3.17	50.04	204.33	600.48	1572.09	1.67
0.83	0.50	0.00	0.00	0.00	77.88	9.20	0.12	0.17	1.16	0.14	87.32	3.78	59.00	0.90	37.76	160.48	403.56	488.52	1.27
12.56	0.60	0.00	0.00	0.00	41.76	0.00	0.20	0.85	0.00	0.07	53.28	0.43	18.72	2.04	31.68	292.32	293.76	918.72	1.08
17.38	0.64	0.00	0.00	0.00	36.08	0.00	0.21	0.90	0.00	0.07	36.08	0.15	83.64	2.95	39.36	344.40	183.68	1446.48	1.21
5.34	3.35	0.00	0.00	0.00	44.88	5.51	0.41	0.37	7.30	0.37	89.76	1.57	91.80	5.16	48.96	297.84	524.28	797.64	4.53
8.23	2.28	0.00	0.00	0.00	79.80	12.31	1.00	0.80	5.49	0.14	86.64	1.09	189.24	2.51	68.40	287.28	394.44	1650.72	2.58
1.84	2.61	0.00	0.00	0.00	49.68	5.62	0.41	0.41	5.96	0.32	71.28	1.81	41.04	2.81	66.96	192.24	330.48	844.56	4.38
13.41	7.30	0.00	0.00	0.00	40.96	3.58	0.46	0.33	11.34	0.23	102.40	1.61	74.24	2.64	79.36	220.16	335.36	1292.80	1.87
3.04	1.01	0.31	0.00	0.90	68.20	3.41	0.06	0.29	0.95	0.05	12.40	0.60	189.10	0.22	27.90	217.00	317.75	195.30	0.82
2.34	0.81	0.47	0.00	0.66	56.88	2.37	0.06	0.30	1.07	0.13	9.48	0.65	206.98	0.58	33.18	227.52	395.00	181.70	0.95
2.66	1.03	0.46	0.00	0.78	58.14	1.99	0.06	0.28	0.90	0.08	18.36	0.64	160.65	0.32	24.48	154.53	270.81	91.80	0.66
6.58	0.96	0.00	0.00	0.00	147.06	2.22	0.15	0.44	3.21	0.24	68.40	1.04	220.59	2.41	70.11	203.49	473.67	801.99	3.93
5.17	1.74	0.00	0.00	0.00	77.22	3.56	0.10	0.36	2.46	0.22	83.16	0.63	192.06	2.28	51.48	142.56	415.80	762.30	2.69
4.54	1.54	0.00	0.00	0.00	214.02	3.39	0.16	0.50	2.53	0.52	91.35	0.73	245.34	2.66	52.20	153.99	391.50	884.79	3.29
8.48	3.05	0.00	0.00	0.00	216.63	3.65	0.13	0.57	1.98	0.26	114.84	0.99	422.82	1.62	73.08	232.29	649.89	798.66	4.07
3.05	0.75	0.00	0.00	0.00	84.96	1.30	0.10	0.33	1.32	0.16	43.20	0.69	210.24	1.89	59.04	116.64	403.20	542.88	1.90
3.51	0.61	0.00	0.00	0.00	173.25	4.05	0.09	0.50	2.86	0.25	85.50	1.13	189.00	2.45	67.50	173.25	490.50	870.75	3.17
3.34	0.98	0.00	0.00	0.00	96.17	2.61	0.10	0.55	3.15	0.23	74.98	1.17	216.79	2.87	63.57	179.30	572.13	896.50	3.68
6.08	2.43	0.00	0.00	0.24	0.00	0.00	0.36	0.41	6.57	0.34	29.20	2.98	80.29	4.50	40.14	279.79	389.27	1070.50	7.42
4.97	2.49	0.00	0.00	0.25	0.00	0.00	0.32	0.36	5.72	0.30	24.87	2.60	69.63	3.85	34.81	243.70	323.28	907.67	6.47

USDA ID Code	Food Name	Weight in Grams*	Quantity of Units	Unit of Measure	Protein (gm)	Fat (gm)	Carbohydrate (gm)	Kcalories	Caffeine (gm)	Fiber (gm)	Cholesterol (mg)	Saturated Fat (gm)
	Hardee's-Big Cheese	141.7500	1.000	Each	30.00	30.00	28.00	495.00	0.00	0.00	0.00	0.00
	Hardee's-Big Deluxe	248.1000	1.000	Each	31.00	41.00	46.00	675.00	0.00	0.00	0.00	0.00
	Hardee's-Big Twin	141.7460	1.000	Each	18.84	20.48	27.86	368.70	0.00	1.39	45.06	9.01
	Hardee's-Biscuit	77.9610	1.000	Each	5.00	13.00	35.00	275.00	0.00	0.00	0.00	0.00
	Hardee's-Cheeseburger	100.6310	1.000	Each	17.00	17.00	29.00	335.00	0.00	0.00	0.00	0.00
	Hardee's-Chicken Fillet	191.3580	1.000	Each	27.00	26.00	42.00	510.00	0.00	0.00	0.00	0.00
	Hardee's-Fish Sandwich, Big	191.3580	1.000	Each	20.00	26.00	49.00	514.00	0.00	0.00	0.00	0.00
	Hardee's-Ham & Cheese, Hot	141.7460	1.000	Each	23.00	15.00	37.00	376.00	0.00	0.00	0.00	0.00
	Hardee's-Hamburger	100.0630	1.000	Each	17.00	13.00	29.00	305.00	0.00	0.00	0.00	0.00
	Hardee's-Hot Dog	50.0000	1.000	Each	11.00	22.00	26.00	346.00	0.00	0.00	0.00	0.00
	Jack In The Box-Breakfast Jack	126.0000	1.000	Each	18.74	13.54	29.16	313.44	0.00	0.00	189.52	5.31
	Jack In The Box-Cheeseburger, Ba	242.0000	1.000	Each	35.00	45.00	41.00	705.00	0.00	0.00	113.00	14.90
	Jack In The Box-Cheesecake	99.0000	1.000	Each	8.00	18.00	29.00	309.00	0.00	0.00	63.00	9.40
	Jack In The Box-French Fries, Re	109.0000	1.000	Order	4.00	17.00	45.00	351.00	0.00	0.00	0.00	4.00
	Jack In The Box-French Fries, Sm	68.0000	1.000	Order	3.00	11.00	28.00	219.00	0.00	0.00	0.00	2.50
	Jack In The Box-Jumbo Jack	222.0000	1.000	Each	25.27	26.17	40.61	497.24	0.00	0.00	72.20	10.29
	Jack In The Box-Jumbo Jack w/ Ch	242.0000	1.000	Each	28.47	31.14	40.04	558.74	0.00	0.00	97.87	13.35
	K.F.C.-Breast, Center, Original	103.0000	1.000	Each	25.18	15.26	9.16	260.93	0.00	0.08	86.98	3.81
	K.F.C.-Chicken Sandwich, Colonel	166.0000	1.000	Each	20.80	27.00	39.00	482.00	0.00	1.40	47.00	6.00
	K.F.C.-Drumstick, Original Recip	57.0000	1.000	Each	11.57	11.57	4.96	168.52	0.00	0.00	58.65	2.48
	K.F.C.-French Fries	77.0000	1.000	Order	3.20	12.00	31.00	244.00	0.00	0.00	2.00	3.00
	K.F.C.-Potatoes, Mashed, and Gra	98.0000	1.000	Each	2.40	2.00	12.00	71.00	0.00	0.00	0.00	1.00
	K.F.C.-Thigh, Original Recipe	95.0000	1.000	Each	15.97	23.95	11.18	324.12	0.00	0.08	102.98	6.39
	K.F.C.-Wing, Original Recipe	53.0000	1.000	Each	11.80	11.00	5.00	172.00	0.00	0.00	59.00	3.00
	McDonald's-Arch Deluxe	239.0000	1.000	Each	28.00	31.00	39.00	550.00	0.00	4.00	90.00	11.00
	McDonald's-Arch Deluxe w/Bacon	247.0000	1.000	Each	32.00	34.00	39.00	590.00	0.00	4.00	100.00	12.00
	McDonald's-Big Mac	215.0000	1.000	Each	25.00	32.00	43.00	560.00	0.00	0.00	103.00	10.10
	McDonald's-Biscuit w/ Spread	75.0000	1.000	Each	5.00	13.00	32.00	260.00	0.00	1.00	1.00	3.00
	McDonald's-Biscuit, Bacon, Egg a	153.0000	1.000	Each	18.00	28.00	36.00	470.00	0.00	1.00	235.00	8.04
	McDonald's-Biscuit, Sausage	118.0000	1.000	Each	11.00	31.00	35.00	470.00	0.00	0.00	44.00	8.00
	McDonald's-Biscuit, Sausage w/ E	175.0000	1.000	Each	19.00	28.00	27.00	440.00	0.00	0.00	260.00	10.00
	McDonald's-Burrito, Breakfast	117.0000	1.000	Each	13.00	19.00	23.00	320.00	0.00	1.00	195.00	7.00
	McDonald's-Cheeseburger	116.0000	1.000	Each	15.00	13.00	35.00	320.00	0.00	0.00	50.00	5.00
	McDonald's-Chicken McNuggets	18.5000	1.000	Each	3.33	2.50	2.83	45.00	0.00	0.00	9.17	0.58
	McDonald's-Chicken Sld, Grilled,	257.0000	1.000	Each	21.00	1.50	7.00	120.00	0.00	0.00	45.00	0.00
	McDonald's-Chicken, Crispy, Delu	223.0000	1.000	Each	26.00	25.00	43.00	0.00	0.00	3.00	55.00	4.00
	McDonald's-Chicken, Grilled, Del	223.0000	1.000	Each	27.00	20.00	38.00	300.00	0.00	3.00	50.00	1.00
	McDonald's-Cookies, McDonaldland	56.6990	1.000	Each	3.00	5.00	32.00	180.00	0.00	0.00	0.00	1.00
	McDonald's-Danish, Apple	105.0000	1.000	Each	5.00	16.00	51.00	360.00	0.00	1.60	25.00	4.00
	McDonald's-Danish, Cheese, Iced	110.0000	1.000	Each	7.00	22.00	47.00	410.00	0.00	0.00	47.00	6.00
	McDonald's-Eggs, Scrambled	100.0000	1.000	Each	12.00	10.00	1.00	140.00	0.00	0.00	425.00	3.00
	McDonald's-Fish Filet Deluxe	141.0000	1.000	Each	27.00	28.00	54.00	560.00	0.00	1.09	49.65	5.16
	McDonald's-French Fries, Large	122.0000	1.000	Order	6.00	22.00	57.00	450.00	0.00	0.00	0.00	5.00
	McDonald's-French Fries, Small	68.0000	1.000	Order	3.00	12.00	26.00	220.00	0.00	0.00	0.00	2.50
	McDonald's-French Fries, Super S	176.0000	1.000	Each	8.00	26.00	68.00	540.00	0.00	6.00	0.00	4.50
	McDonald's-Hamburger	102.0000	1.000	Each	13.00	9.00	34.00	260.00	0.00	0.00	30.00	3.50
	McDonald's-Hotcakes w/ Margarine	174.0000	1.000	Each	13.00	19.00	100.00	570.00	0.00	0.00	15.00	3.00
	McDonald's-Ice Crm Cone, Vanilla	90.0000	1.000	Each	4.00	4.50	23.00	150.00	0.00	0.00	20.00	3.00
	McDonald's-McMuffin, Egg	135.0000	1.000	Each	17.61	10.76	27.39	283.70	0.00	1.37	221.09	3.72
	McDonald's-McMuffin, Sausage	135.0000	1.000	Each	15.00	20.00	27.00	345.00	0.00	0.00	57.00	7.00
	McDonald's-McMuffin, Sausage w/	159.0000	1.000	Each	21.00	25.00	27.00	430.00	0.00	0.00	270.00	8.00
	McDonald's-Muffin, Apple Bran, L	114.0000	1.000	Each	6.00	3.00	61.00	300.00	0.00	3.00	0.00	0.50
	McDonald's-Muffin, English w/ Sp	58.0000	1.000	Each	5.00	4.00	26.00	170.00	0.00	1.60	9.00	2.40
	McDonald's-Potatoes, Hash Brown	53.0000	1.000	Each	1.00	7.00	15.00	130.00	0.00	0.00	0.00	1.00
	McDonald's-Quarter Pounder	166.0000	1.000	Each	23.00	21.00	37.00	420.00	0.00	0.00	85.00	8.00

Monounsaturated Fat (gm)	Polyunsaturated Fat (gm)	Vitamin D (mg)	Vitamin K (mg)	Vitamin E (mg)	Vitamin A (re)	Vitamin C (mg)	Thiamin (mg)	Riboflavin (mg)	Niacin (mg)	Vitamin B₆ (mg)	Folate (mg)	Vitamin B₁₂ (mcg)	Calcium (mg)	Iron (mg)	Magnesium (mg)	Phosphorus (mg)	Potassium (mg)	Sodium (mg)	Zinc (mg)
0.00	0.00	0.00	0.00	0.00	0.00	0.00	0.00	0.00	0.00	0.00	0.00	0.00	0.00	0.00	0.00	0.00	0.00	1251.00	0.00
0.00	0.00	0.00	0.00	0.00	0.00	0.00	0.00	0.00	0.00	0.00	0.00	0.00	0.00	0.00	0.00	0.00	0.00	1063.00	0.00
7.37	4.10	0.00	0.00	0.74	13.93	2.46	0.23	0.25	5.49	0.22	27.86	1.86	65.55	3.28	28.68	161.41	229.42	475.22	3.77
0.00	0.00	0.00	0.00	0.00	0.00	0.00	0.00	0.00	0.00	0.00	0.00	0.00	0.00	0.00	0.00	0.00	0.00	650.00	0.00
0.00	0.00	0.00	0.00	0.00	0.00	2.00	0.51	0.32	5.50	0.00	0.00	0.00	0.00	0.00	0.00	0.00	0.00	789.00	0.00
0.00	0.00	0.00	0.00	0.00	0.00	0.00	0.00	0.00	0.00	0.00	0.00	0.00	0.00	0.00	0.00	0.00	0.00	360.00	0.00
0.00	0.00	0.00	0.00	0.00	0.00	0.00	0.00	0.00	0.00	0.00	0.00	0.00	0.00	0.00	0.00	0.00	0.00	314.00	0.00
0.00	0.00	0.00	0.00	0.00	0.00	0.00	0.00	0.00	0.00	0.00	0.00	0.00	0.00	0.00	0.00	0.00	0.00	1067.00	0.00
0.00	0.00	0.00	0.00	0.00	0.00	2.00	0.55	0.58	6.40	0.00	0.00	0.00	0.00	0.00	0.00	0.00	0.00	682.00	0.00
0.00	0.00	0.00	0.00	0.00	0.00	0.00	0.00	0.00	0.00	0.00	0.00	0.00	0.00	0.00	0.00	0.00	0.00	744.00	0.00
5.21	2.60	0.00	0.00	0.14	138.50	3.12	0.43	0.49	5.31	0.15	0.00	1.15	184.31	2.60	24.99	322.81	197.85	1079.85	1.87
15.70	8.70	0.00	0.00	0.60	70.00	7.80	0.24	0.48	8.36	0.00	0.00	0.00	200.00	2.80	0.00	0.00	0.00	1240.00	0.00
7.40	1.60	0.00	0.00	0.32	0.00	0.00	0.05	0.24	1.90	0.00	0.00	0.00	88.00	0.30	0.00	0.00	0.00	208.00	0.00
7.00	0.00	0.00	0.00	5.31	0.00	25.80	0.18	0.03	3.61	0.00	0.00	0.00	0.00	0.70	0.00	0.00	0.00	194.00	0.00
7.00	0.00	0.00	0.00	10.36	0.00	16.20	0.11	0.00	2.28	0.00	0.00	0.00	0.00	0.40	0.00	0.00	0.00	121.00	0.00
11.37	2.17	0.00	0.00	0.18	66.78	3.61	0.42	0.31	10.47	0.27	0.00	2.42	120.93	4.06	39.71	235.54	444.00	1023.37	3.79
11.21	1.78	0.00	0.00	0.21	195.74	4.45	0.46	0.34	10.05	0.28	0.00	2.71	242.89	4.09	43.60	365.67	443.96	1482.25	4.27
3.59	1.53	0.00	0.00	0.46	15.26	0.00	0.08	0.13	14.04	0.59	3.81	0.35	16.02	1.22	30.52	238.04	264.75	602.74	1.14
3.90	9.00	0.00	0.00	2.30	14.00	0.00	0.39	0.27	10.64	0.59	29.00	0.31	100.00	3.10	41.00	261.00	297.00	1060.00	1.50
3.06	1.65	0.00	0.00	0.41	14.04	0.00	0.05	0.13	3.39	0.20	4.96	0.18	6.61	0.74	13.22	99.13	129.70	267.65	1.65
7.00	1.00	0.00	0.00	0.00	0.00	15.60	0.15	0.05	1.90	0.00	0.00	0.00	0.00	0.30	0.00	0.00	0.00	139.00	0.00
0.00	0.00	0.00	0.00	0.00	0.00	0.00	0.00	0.03	1.14	0.00	0.00	0.00	16.00	0.20	0.00	0.00	0.00	339.00	0.00
5.59	3.19	0.00	0.00	0.48	27.94	0.00	0.09	0.23	6.55	0.32	7.98	0.29	12.77	1.44	23.15	176.43	223.53	549.24	2.39
6.00	2.00	0.00	0.00	0.00	0.00	0.00	0.03	0.07	2.85	0.00	0.00	0.00	24.00	0.30	0.00	0.00	0.00	383.00	0.00
0.00	0.00	0.00	0.00	0.00	10.00	0.00	0.00	0.00	0.00	0.00	0.00	0.00	6.00	25.00	0.00	0.00	0.00	1010.00	0.00
0.00	0.00	0.00	0.00	0.00	10.00	0.00	0.00	0.00	0.00	0.00	0.00	0.00	6.00	6.00	0.00	0.00	0.00	1150.00	0.00
20.10	1.50	0.00	0.00	0.00	106.00	2.00	0.48	0.41	6.80	0.27	21.00	1.80	256.00	4.00	38.00	314.00	237.00	950.00	4.70
9.00	1.00	0.00	0.00	1.80	0.00	0.00	0.23	0.10	1.52	0.03	6.00	0.10	75.00	1.30	14.00	168.00	100.00	730.00	0.70
15.79	1.96	0.00	0.00	1.47	156.92	0.00	0.35	0.32	2.45	0.17	17.65	0.58	181.44	2.55	30.40	442.33	232.44	1250.00	1.67
17.00	3.00	0.00	0.00	0.00	0.00	0.00	0.45	0.17	3.80	0.00	0.00	0.00	64.00	1.00	0.00	0.00	0.00	1080.00	0.00
20.00	3.00	0.00	0.00	0.00	60.00	0.00	0.45	0.34	3.80	0.00	0.00	0.00	80.00	2.00	0.00	0.00	0.00	1210.00	0.00
0.00	0.00	0.00	0.00	0.00	10.00	15.00	0.00	0.00	0.00	0.00	0.00	0.00	8.00	10.00	0.00	0.00	0.00	600.00	0.00
7.70	1.00	0.00	0.00	0.50	118.00	2.00	0.29	0.21	3.90	0.12	18.00	0.94	199.00	2.30	21.00	177.00	223.00	750.00	2.10
1.67	0.25	0.00	0.00	0.00	0.00	0.00	0.02	0.02	1.27	0.00	0.00	0.00	0.00	0.10	0.00	0.00	0.00	96.67	0.00
0.00	0.00	0.00	0.00	0.00	120.00	40.00	0.00	0.00	0.00	0.00	0.00	0.00	4.00	8.00	0.00	0.00	0.00	240.00	0.00
0.00	0.00	0.00	0.00	0.00	6.00	8.00	0.00	0.00	0.00	0.00	0.00	0.00	6.00	15.00	0.00	0.00	0.00	1060.00	0.00
0.00	0.00	0.00	0.00	0.00	6.00	8.00	0.00	0.00	0.00	0.00	0.00	0.00	6.00	15.00	0.00	0.00	0.00	930.00	0.00
7.00	1.00	0.00	0.00	0.00	0.00	0.00	0.23	0.17	1.90	0.00	0.00	0.00	0.00	1.00	0.00	0.00	0.00	190.00	0.00
11.00	2.00	0.00	0.00	3.80	35.00	15.00	0.30	0.17	2.20	0.03	3.00	0.00	14.00	1.40	8.00	31.00	69.00	290.00	0.20
13.00	2.00	0.00	0.00	0.00	40.00	0.00	0.30	0.26	1.90	0.00	0.00	0.00	32.00	0.80	0.00	0.00	0.00	420.00	0.00
5.00	2.00	0.00	0.00	0.00	100.00	0.00	0.06	0.26	0.00	0.00	0.00	0.00	48.00	1.00	0.00	0.00	0.00	290.00	0.00
10.13	10.72	0.00	0.00	0.00	43.69	0.00	0.30	0.14	2.68	0.10	19.86	0.81	163.84	1.79	26.81	227.39	148.94	1060.00	0.89
15.00	2.00	0.00	0.00	0.00	0.00	15.00	0.23	0.00	2.85	0.00	0.00	0.00	0.00	0.60	0.00	0.00	0.00	290.00	0.00
8.00	1.00	0.00	0.00	0.00	0.00	9.00	0.15	0.00	1.90	0.00	0.00	0.00	0.00	0.20	0.00	0.00	0.00	110.00	0.00
0.00	0.00	0.00	0.00	0.00	0.00	0.00	0.00	0.00	0.00	0.00	0.00	0.00	35.00	8.00	0.00	0.00	0.00	350.00	0.00
5.00	1.00	0.00	0.00	0.00	40.00	4.00	0.30	0.17	3.80	0.00	0.00	0.00	15.00	1.50	0.00	0.00	0.00	580.00	0.00
5.00	5.00	0.00	0.00	0.00	40.00	0.00	0.30	0.34	2.85	0.00	0.00	0.00	80.00	1.00	0.00	0.00	0.00	750.00	0.00
0.00	0.00	0.00	0.00	0.00	6.00	2.00	0.00	0.00	0.00	0.00	0.00	0.00	10.00	2.00	0.00	0.00	0.00	75.00	0.00
5.97	1.27	0.00	0.00	1.76	146.74	0.98	0.46	0.32	3.62	0.16	43.04	0.78	250.43	2.74	32.28	312.07	208.37	723.91	1.76
11.00	2.00	0.00	0.00	0.00	40.00	0.00	0.53	0.26	4.75	0.00	0.00	0.00	160.00	1.50	0.00	0.00	0.00	770.00	0.00
14.00	3.00	0.00	0.00	0.00	100.00	0.00	0.53	0.43	4.75	0.00	0.00	0.00	200.00	2.00	0.00	0.00	0.00	920.00	0.00
0.00	0.00	0.00	0.00	0.00	0.00	0.00	0.00	0.00	0.00	0.00	0.00	0.00	10.00	8.00	0.00	0.00	0.00	380.00	0.00
2.00	1.00	0.00	0.00	0.10	37.00	0.00	0.33	0.14	2.50	0.10	51.00	0.00	151.00	1.60	12.00	60.00	74.00	285.00	0.40
4.00	2.00	0.00	0.00	0.00	0.00	1.20	0.06	0.00	0.76	0.00	0.00	0.00	0.00	0.00	0.00	0.00	0.00	330.00	0.00
11.00	1.00	0.00	0.00	0.00	40.00	3.60	0.38	0.26	6.65	0.00	0.00	0.00	120.00	2.00	0.00	0.00	0.00	645.00	0.00

USDA ID Code	Food Name	Weight in Grams*	Quantity of Units	Unit of Measure	Protein (gm)	Fat (gm)	Carbohydrate (gm)	Kcalories	Caffeine (gm)	Fiber (gm)	Cholesterol (mg)	Saturated Fat (gm)
	McDonald's-Quarter Pounder w/ Ch	200.0000	1.000	Each	28.00	30.00	38.00	530.00	0.00	2.00	95.00	13.00
	McDonald's-Salad, Garden	189.0000	1.000	Each	4.00	2.00	6.00	50.00	0.00	0.00	65.00	0.60
	McDonald's-Shake, Chocolate Lowf	294.1240	1.000	Each	11.04	1.71	66.25	321.23	0.00	0.00	10.04	0.70
	McDonald's-Shake, Strawberry Low	294.1240	1.000	Each	11.00	9.00	60.00	360.00	0.00	0.00	10.00	0.60
	McDonald's-Shake, Vanilla Lowfat	294.1240	1.000	Each	11.00	9.00	60.00	360.00	0.00	0.00	10.00	0.60
	McDonald's-Sweet Roll, Cinnamon	95.0000	1.000	Each	7.00	20.00	47.00	400.00	0.00	2.00	75.00	5.00
	Subway-BLT- 6" white	191.0000	1.000	Each	14.00	10.00	38.00	311.00	0.00	3.00	16.00	3.00
	Subway-BMT- 6" Italian	213.0000	1.000	Each	44.00	55.00	83.00	982.00	0.00	5.00	133.00	20.00
	Subway-BMT- 6" Wheat	253.0000	1.000	Each	21.00	22.00	45.00	460.00	0.00	3.00	56.00	7.00
	Subway-BMT-Classic Italian - 6"	246.0000	1.000	Each	21.00	21.00	39.00	445.00	0.00	3.00	56.00	8.00
	Subway-Bologna - Deli Sandwich	171.0000	1.000	Each	10.00	12.00	38.00	292.00	0.00	2.00	20.00	4.00
	Subway-Chicken Breast, Roasted	246.0000	1.000	Each	26.00	6.00	41.00	332.00	0.00	3.00	48.00	1.00
	Subway-Chicken Taco Sub - 6" whi	286.0000	1.000	Each	24.00	16.00	43.00	421.00	0.00	3.00	52.00	5.00
	Subway-Club - 6" white	246.0000	1.000	Each	21.00	5.00	40.00	297.00	0.00	3.00	26.00	1.00
	Subway-Club Sandwich - 12" Itali	213.0000	1.000	Each	46.00	22.00	83.00	693.00	0.00	5.00	84.00	7.00
	Subway-Club Sandwich - 12" Wheat	220.0000	1.000	Each	47.00	23.00	89.00	722.00	0.00	6.00	84.00	7.00
	Subway-Cold Cut Combo - 12" Ital	184.0000	1.000	Each	46.00	40.00	83.00	853.00	0.00	5.00	166.00	12.00
	Subway-Cold Cut Combo - 12" Whea	184.0000	1.000	Each	48.00	41.00	88.00	853.00	0.00	6.00	166.00	12.00
	Subway-Cold Cut Trio - 6" white	246.0000	1.000	Each	19.00	13.00	39.00	362.00	0.00	3.00	64.00	4.00
	Subway-Ham - 6" white	232.0000	1.000	Each	18.00	5.00	39.00	287.00	0.00	3.00	28.00	1.00
	Subway-Ham - Deli Sandwich	171.0000	1.000	Each	11.00	4.00	37.00	234.00	0.00	2.00	14.00	1.00
	Subway-Ham and Cheese - 12" Ital	184.0000	1.000	Each	38.00	18.00	81.00	643.00	0.00	5.00	73.00	7.00
	Subway-Ham and Cheese Combo - 12	239.0000	1.000	Each	19.00	5.00	45.00	302.00	0.00	3.00	28.00	1.00
	Subway-Italian, Spicy - 12" Ital	213.0000	1.000	Each	42.00	63.00	83.00	1043.00	0.00	5.00	137.00	23.00
	Subway-Italian, Spicy - 6" white	232.0000	1.000	Each	20.00	24.00	38.00	467.00	0.00	3.00	57.00	9.00
	Subway-Meat Ball Sandwich - 12"	215.0000	1.000	Each	42.00	44.00	96.00	918.00	0.00	3.00	88.00	17.00
	Subway-Meat Ball Sandwich - 12"	224.0000	1.000	Each	44.00	45.00	101.00	947.00	0.00	0.00	88.00	17.00
	Subway-Meatballs - 6" white	260.0000	1.000	Each	18.00	16.00	44.00	404.00	0.00	3.00	33.00	6.00
	Subway-Melt - 6" white	251.0000	1.000	Each	22.00	12.00	40.00	366.00	0.00	3.00	42.00	5.00
	Subway-Pizza Sub - 6" white	250.0000	1.000	Each	19.00	22.00	41.00	448.00	0.00	3.00	50.00	9.00
	Subway-Roast Beef - 12" Italian	184.0000	1.000	Each	42.00	23.00	84.00	689.00	0.00	5.00	83.00	8.00
	Subway-Roast Beef - 12" Wheat	189.0000	1.000	Each	41.00	24.00	89.00	717.00	0.00	6.00	75.00	8.00
	Subway-Roast Beef - 6" white	232.0000	1.000	Each	19.00	5.00	39.00	288.00	0.00	3.00	20.00	1.00
	Subway-Roast Beef - Deli Sandwic	180.0000	1.000	Each	13.00	4.00	38.00	245.00	0.00	2.00	13.00	1.00
	Subway-Salad, Club	331.0000	1.000	Each	14.00	3.00	12.00	126.00	0.00	1.00	26.00	1.00
	Subway-Salad, Cold Cut Trio	330.0000	1.000	Each	13.00	11.00	11.00	191.00	0.00	1.00	64.00	3.00
	Subway-Salad, Roast Beef	316.0000	1.000	Each	12.00	3.00	11.00	117.00	0.00	1.00	20.00	1.00
	Subway-Salad, Seafood & Crab	331.0000	1.000	Each	13.00	17.00	10.00	244.00	0.00	2.00	34.00	3.00
	Subway-Salad, Turkey Breast	316.0000	1.000	Each	11.00	2.00	12.00	316.00	0.00	1.00	19.00	1.00
	Subway-Salad, Veggie Delite	260.0000	1.000	Each	2.00	1.00	10.00	51.00	0.00	1.00	0.00	0.00
	Subway-Seafood - 12" Italian	210.0000	1.000	Each	29.00	57.00	94.00	986.00	0.00	0.00	56.00	11.00
	Subway-Seafood - 12" Wheat	219.0000	1.000	Each	31.00	58.00	100.00	1015.00	0.00	2.50	56.00	11.00
	Subway-Seafood & Crab - 6" white	246.0000	1.000	Each	19.00	19.00	38.00	415.00	0.00	3.00	34.00	3.00
	Subway-Steak & Cheese - 6" white	257.0000	1.000	Each	29.00	10.00	41.00	383.00	0.00	3.00	70.00	6.00
	Subway-Steak and Cheese - 12" It	213.0000	1.000	Each	43.00	32.00	83.00	765.00	0.00	6.00	82.00	12.00
	Subway-Tuna - 6" white	246.0000	1.000	Each	18.00	32.00	38.00	527.00	0.00	3.00	36.00	5.00
	Subway-Tuna - Deli Sandwich, lit	178.0000	1.000	Each	11.00	9.00	38.00	279.00	0.00	2.00	16.00	2.00
	Subway-Turkey Breast - 12" Wheat	192.0000	1.000	Each	42.00	20.00	88.00	674.00	0.00	7.00	67.00	6.00
	Subway-Turkey Breast - 6" white	232.0000	1.000	Each	17.00	4.00	40.00	273.00	0.00	3.00	19.00	1.00
	Subway-Turkey Breast - Deli sand	180.0000	1.000	Each	12.00	4.00	38.00	235.00	0.00	2.00	12.00	1.00
	Subway-Turkey Breast & Ham - 6"	232.0000	1.000	Each	18.00	5.00	39.00	280.00	0.00	3.00	24.00	1.00
	Subway-Veggie Delight - 6" white	175.0000	1.000	Each	9.00	3.00	38.00	222.00	0.00	3.00	0.00	0.00
	Subway-Veggie Delite - 6" wheat	182.0000	1.000	Each	9.00	3.00	44.00	237.00	0.00	3.00	0.00	0.00
	Taco Bell-Burrito Supreme	198.0000	1.000	Each	20.00	22.00	55.00	440.00	0.00	3.00	33.00	8.00
	Taco Bell-Burrito Supreme, Light	248.0000	1.000	Each	20.00	8.00	50.00	350.00	0.00	0.00	25.00	0.00

Monounsaturated Fat (gm)	Polyunsaturated Fat (gm)	Vitamin D (mg)	Vitamin K (mg)	Vitamin E (mg)	Vitamin A (re)	Vitamin C (mg)	Thiamin (mg)	Riboflavin (mg)	Niacin (mg)	Vitamin B$_6$ (mg)	Folate (mg)	Vitamin B$_{12}$ (mcg)	Calcium (mg)	Iron (mg)	Magnesium (mg)	Phosphorus (mg)	Potassium (mg)	Sodium (mg)	Zinc (mg)
0.00	0.00	0.00	0.00	0.00	10.00	4.00	0.00	0.00	0.00	0.00	0.00	0.00	15.00	25.00	0.00	0.00	0.00	1290.00	0.00
1.00	0.40	0.00	0.00	0.00	900.00	21.00	0.09	0.10	0.38	0.00	0.00	0.00	32.00	0.80	0.00	0.00	0.00	70.00	0.00
0.90	0.10	0.00	0.00	0.00	92.35	0.00	0.13	0.50	0.40	0.00	0.00	0.00	333.27	0.80	0.00	0.00	0.00	240.92	0.00
0.60	0.10	0.00	0.00	0.00	60.00	0.00	0.12	0.51	0.38	0.00	0.00	0.00	280.00	0.00	0.00	0.00	0.00	170.00	0.00
0.60	0.10	0.00	0.00	0.00	60.00	0.00	0.12	0.51	0.00	0.00	0.00	0.00	280.00	0.00	0.00	0.00	0.00	170.00	0.00
0.00	0.00	0.00	0.00	0.00	10.00	0.00	0.00	0.00	0.00	0.00	0.00	0.00	8.00	8.00	0.00	0.00	0.00	340.00	0.00
0.00	0.00	0.00	0.00	0.00	601.00	15.00	0.00	0.00	0.00	0.00	0.00	0.00	27.00	3.00	0.00	0.00	0.00	945.00	0.00
24.00	7.00	0.00	0.00	5.10	67.00	5.00	0.27	0.34	5.10	0.48	63.00	2.33	64.00	4.30	66.00	308.00	917.00	3139.00	6.10
25.00	7.00	0.00	0.00	0.00	753.00	15.00	0.00	0.00	0.00	0.00	0.00	0.00	44.00	4.00	0.00	0.00	1002.00	3199.00	0.00
0.00	0.00	0.00	0.00	0.00	753.00	15.00	0.00	0.00	0.00	0.00	0.00	0.00	44.00	4.00	0.00	0.00	0.00	1652.00	0.00
0.00	0.00	0.00	0.00	0.00	565.00	14.00	0.00	0.00	0.00	0.00	0.00	0.00	39.00	3.00	0.00	0.00	0.00	744.00	0.00
0.00	0.00	0.00	0.00	0.00	617.00	15.00	0.00	0.00	0.00	0.00	0.00	0.00	35.00	3.00	0.00	0.00	0.00	967.00	0.00
0.00	0.00	0.00	0.00	0.00	1044.00	18.00	0.00	0.00	0.00	0.00	0.00	0.00	118.00	4.00	0.00	0.00	0.00	1264.00	0.00
0.00	0.00	0.00	0.00	0.00	601.00	15.00	0.00	0.00	0.00	0.00	0.00	0.00	29.00	4.00	0.00	0.00	0.00	1341.00	0.00
8.00	4.00	0.00	0.00	1.30	74.00	20.00	0.48	0.33	12.50	0.58	47.00	0.95	58.00	3.10	66.00	384.00	971.00	2717.00	2.50
9.00	4.00	0.00	0.00	4.20	83.00	15.00	0.49	0.35	9.30	0.46	43.00	0.44	96.00	3.20	40.00	247.00	1055.00	2777.00	1.40
15.00	10.00	0.00	0.00	0.90	87.00	17.00	0.36	0.33	3.80	0.20	39.00	1.23	227.00	2.90	28.00	315.00	876.00	2218.00	2.70
15.00	10.00	0.00	0.00	0.90	90.00	18.00	0.37	0.35	3.90	0.21	41.00	1.28	235.00	3.00	29.00	327.00	1010.00	2278.00	2.80
0.00	0.00	0.00	0.00	0.00	649.00	16.00	0.00	0.00	0.00	0.00	0.00	0.00	49.00	4.00	0.00	0.00	0.00	1401.00	0.00
0.00	0.00	0.00	0.00	0.00	601.00	15.00	0.00	0.00	0.00	0.00	0.00	0.00	28.00	3.00	0.00	0.00	0.00	1308.00	0.00
0.00	0.00	0.00	0.00	0.00	565.00	14.00	0.00	0.00	0.00	0.00	0.00	0.00	24.00	3.00	0.00	0.00	0.00	773.00	0.00
8.00	4.00	0.00	0.00	3.80	174.00	17.00	0.53	0.39	3.60	0.34	45.00	0.76	304.00	2.20	50.00	527.00	834.00	1710.00	2.80
8.00	4.00	0.00	0.00	0.00	0.00	0.00	0.00	0.00	0.00	0.00	0.00	0.00	35.00	3.00	0.00	0.00	918.00	1319.00	0.00
28.00	7.00	0.00	0.00	0.00	0.00	0.00	0.00	0.00	0.00	0.00	0.00	0.00	0.00	0.00	0.00	0.00	880.00	2282.00	0.00
0.00	0.00	0.00	0.00	0.00	845.00	15.00	0.00	0.00	0.00	0.00	0.00	0.00	40.00	4.00	0.00	0.00	0.00	1592.00	0.00
17.00	4.00	0.00	0.00	1.00	72.00	19.00	0.33	0.39	9.40	0.40	35.00	3.21	78.00	5.00	47.00	263.00	1210.00	2022.00	6.20
18.00	4.00	0.00	0.00	0.00	0.00	0.00	0.00	0.00	0.00	0.00	0.00	0.00	0.00	0.00	0.00	0.00	1498.00	2082.00	0.00
0.00	0.00	0.00	0.00	0.00	712.00	16.00	0.00	0.00	0.00	0.00	0.00	0.00	32.00	4.00	0.00	0.00	0.00	1035.00	0.00
0.00	0.00	0.00	0.00	0.00	777.00	15.00	0.00	0.00	0.00	0.00	0.00	0.00	93.00	4.00	0.00	0.00	0.00	1735.00	0.00
0.00	0.00	0.00	0.00	0.00	1190.00	16.00	0.00	0.00	0.00	0.00	0.00	0.00	103.00	4.00	0.00	0.00	0.00	1609.00	0.00
9.00	4.00	0.00	0.00	4.40	58.00	5.00	0.23	0.29	4.40	0.42	54.00	2.01	55.00	3.70	57.00	266.00	910.00	2288.00	5.30
9.00	4.00	0.00	0.00	4.50	59.00	5.00	0.24	0.30	4.50	0.43	56.00	2.07	56.00	3.80	59.00	273.00	994.00	2348.00	5.40
0.00	0.00	0.00	0.00	0.00	601.00	15.00	0.00	0.00	0.00	0.00	0.00	0.00	25.00	4.00	0.00	0.00	0.00	928.00	0.00
0.00	0.00	0.00	0.00	0.00	565.00	14.00	0.00	0.00	0.00	0.00	0.00	0.00	23.00	3.00	0.00	0.00	0.00	638.00	0.00
0.00	0.00	0.00	0.00	0.00	1363.00	32.00	0.00	0.00	0.00	0.00	0.00	0.00	26.00	2.00	0.00	0.00	0.00	1067.00	0.00
0.00	0.00	0.00	0.00	0.00	1412.00	33.00	0.00	0.00	0.00	0.00	0.00	0.00	46.00	2.00	0.00	0.00	0.00	1127.00	0.00
0.00	0.00	0.00	0.00	0.00	1363.00	32.00	0.00	0.00	0.00	0.00	0.00	0.00	23.00	2.00	0.00	0.00	0.00	654.00	0.00
0.00	0.00	0.00	0.00	0.00	1366.00	32.00	0.00	0.00	0.00	0.00	0.00	0.00	25.00	2.00	0.00	0.00	0.00	575.00	0.00
0.00	0.00	0.00	0.00	0.00	1363.00	32.00	0.00	0.00	0.00	0.00	0.00	0.00	28.00	2.00	0.00	0.00	0.00	1117.00	0.00
0.00	0.00	0.00	0.00	0.00	1363.00	32.00	0.00	0.00	0.00	0.00	0.00	0.00	23.00	1.00	0.00	0.00	0.00	308.00	0.00
15.00	28.00	0.00	0.00	2.50	107.00	5.00	0.51	0.38	7.00	0.26	91.00	6.54	230.00	4.40	32.00	336.00	641.00	2027.00	5.30
16.00	28.00	0.00	0.00	0.00	0.00	0.00	0.00	0.00	0.00	0.00	0.00	0.00	0.00	0.00	0.00	0.00	557.00	1967.00	0.00
0.00	0.00	0.00	0.00	0.00	604.00	15.00	0.00	0.00	0.00	0.00	0.00	0.00	28.00	3.00	0.00	0.00	0.00	849.00	0.00
0.00	0.00	0.00	0.00	0.00	877.00	18.00	0.00	0.00	0.00	0.00	0.00	0.00	88.00	5.00	0.00	0.00	0.00	1106.00	0.00
12.00	4.00	0.00	0.00	0.80	119.00	6.00	0.33	0.46	5.10	0.38	36.00	2.54	231.00	4.20	43.00	456.00	909.00	1556.00	6.80
0.00	0.00	0.00	0.00	0.00	627.00	15.00	0.00	0.00	0.00	0.00	0.00	0.00	32.00	3.00	0.00	0.00	0.00	875.00	0.00
0.00	0.00	0.00	0.00	0.00	628.00	14.00	0.00	0.00	0.00	0.00	0.00	0.00	26.00	3.00	0.00	0.00	0.00	583.00	0.00
7.00	7.00	0.00	0.00	0.00	0.00	0.00	0.00	0.00	0.00	0.00	0.00	0.00	0.00	0.00	0.00	0.00	605.00	2520.00	0.00
0.00	0.00	0.00	0.00	0.00	601.00	15.00	0.00	0.00	0.00	0.00	0.00	0.00	30.00	4.00	0.00	0.00	0.00	1391.00	0.00
0.00	0.00	0.00	0.00	0.00	565.00	14.00	0.00	0.00	0.00	0.00	0.00	0.00	26.00	3.00	0.00	0.00	0.00	944.00	0.00
0.00	0.00	0.00	0.00	0.00	601.00	15.00	0.00	0.00	0.00	0.00	0.00	0.00	29.00	3.00	0.00	0.00	0.00	1350.00	0.00
0.00	0.00	0.00	0.00	0.00	601.00	15.00	0.00	0.00	0.00	0.00	0.00	0.00	25.00	0.00	0.00	0.00	0.00	3.00	0.00
0.00	0.00	0.00	0.00	0.00	601.00	15.00	0.00	0.00	0.00	0.00	0.00	0.00	32.00	3.00	0.00	0.00	0.00	593.00	0.00
0.00	2.00	0.00	0.00	0.00	0.00	26.00	0.40	2.10	3.60	0.00	0.00	0.00	190.00	4.00	0.00	0.00	501.00	1181.00	0.00
0.00	0.00	0.00	0.00	0.00	600.00	9.00	0.00	0.00	0.00	0.00	0.00	0.00	96.00	1.50	0.00	0.00	0.00	1160.00	0.00

USDA ID Code	Food Name	Weight in Grams*	Quantity of Units	Unit of Measure	Protein (gm)	Fat (gm)	Carbohydrate (gm)	Kcalories	Caffeine (gm)	Fiber (gm)	Cholesterol (mg)	Saturated Fat (gm)
	Taco Bell-Burrito, 7-Layer, Ligh	276.0000	1.000	Each	19.00	9.00	67.00	440.00	0.00	0.00	5.00	0.00
	Taco Bell-Burrito, Bean	206.0000	1.000	Each	15.00	14.00	63.00	387.00	0.00	3.00	9.00	4.00
	Taco Bell-Burrito, Bean, Light	198.0000	1.000	Each	14.00	6.00	55.00	330.00	0.00	0.00	5.00	0.00
	Taco Bell-Burrito, Beef	206.0000	1.000	Each	25.00	21.00	48.00	431.00	0.00	2.00	57.00	8.00
	Taco Bell-Burrito, Chicken, Ligh	170.0000	1.000	Each	12.00	6.00	45.00	290.00	0.00	0.00	30.00	0.00
	Taco Bell-Burrito, Chicken, Supr	248.0000	1.000	Each	18.00	10.00	62.00	410.00	0.00	0.00	65.00	0.00
730	Taco Bell-Cinnamon Twists	28.0000	1.000	Ounce	1.00	6.00	19.00	140.00	0.00	0.00	0.00	0.00
731	Taco Bell-Gordita, Beef, Supreme	154.0000	5.500	Ounce	14.00	13.00	31.00	300.00	0.00	3.00	35.00	6.00
732	Taco Bell-Gordita, Chicken, Gril	154.0000	5.500	Ounce	17.00	14.00	28.00	300.00	0.00	3.00	45.00	5.00
733	Taco Bell-Gordita, Steak, Grille	154.0000	5.500	Ounce	17.00	14.00	27.00	310.00	0.00	3.00	35.00	5.00
734	Taco Bell-MexiMelt, Beef, Big	133.0000	4.750	Ounce	16.00	15.00	23.00	290.00	0.00	4.00	45.00	7.00
	Taco Bell-Nachos	106.0000	1.000	Order	7.00	18.00	37.00	346.00	0.00	1.00	9.00	6.00
	Taco Bell-Nachos Bell Grande	287.0000	1.000	Order	22.00	35.00	61.00	649.00	0.00	4.00	36.00	12.00
735	Taco Bell-Nachos Supreme, Beef ,	98.0000	3.500	Ounce	14.00	24.00	45.00	220.00	0.00	9.00	30.00	8.00
	Taco Bell-Pintos 'N Cheese	128.0000	1.000	Each	9.00	9.00	19.00	190.00	0.00	2.00	16.00	4.00
	Taco Bell-Pizza, Mexican	223.0000	1.000	Each	21.00	37.00	40.00	575.00	0.00	3.00	52.00	11.00
	Taco Bell-Salad, Taco	575.0000	1.000	Each	34.00	61.00	55.00	905.00	0.00	4.00	80.00	19.00
	Taco Bell-Salad, Taco w/o Shell	520.0000	1.000	Each	28.00	31.00	22.00	484.00	0.00	3.00	80.00	14.00
	Taco Bell-Salad, Taco, Light	464.0000	1.000	Each	30.00	9.00	35.00	330.00	0.00	0.00	50.00	0.00
	Taco Bell-Salsa	10.0000	1.000	Each	1.00	0.00	4.00	18.00	0.00	0.40	0.00	0.00
	Taco Bell-Taco	78.0000	1.000	Each	10.00	11.00	11.00	183.00	0.00	1.00	32.00	5.00
736	Taco Bell-Taco, Double Decker	140.0000	5.000	Ounce	14.00	15.00	38.00	340.00	0.00	9.00	25.00	5.00
	Taco Bell-Taco, Light	78.0000	1.000	Each	11.00	5.00	11.00	140.00	0.00	1.00	20.00	4.00
	Taco Bell-Taco, Soft	92.0000	1.000	Each	12.00	12.00	18.00	225.00	0.00	2.00	32.00	5.00
	Taco Bell-Taco, Soft, Chicken, L	120.0000	1.000	Each	9.00	5.00	26.00	180.00	0.00	0.00	30.00	0.00
	Taco Bell-Taco, Soft, Light	99.0000	1.000	Each	13.00	5.00	19.00	180.00	0.00	2.00	25.00	4.00
737	Taco Bell-Taco, Soft, Steak, Gri	126.0000	4.500	Ounce	15.00	10.00	20.00	230.00	0.00	2.00	25.00	2.50
738	Taco Bell-Taco, Soft, Steak, Gri	161.0000	5.750	Ounce	16.00	14.00	24.00	290.00	0.00	3.00	35.00	5.00
	Taco Bell-Taco, Soft, Supreme, L	128.0000	1.000	Each	14.00	5.00	23.00	200.00	0.00	0.00	25.00	0.00
	Taco Bell-Taco, Supreme, Light	106.0000	1.000	Each	14.00	5.00	23.00	160.00	0.00	0.00	20.00	0.00
	Taco Bell-Tostada	156.0000	1.000	Each	9.00	11.00	27.00	243.00	0.00	2.00	16.00	4.00
	Wendy's-Cheeseburger Deluxe, Jr.	180.0000	1.000	Each	18.00	17.00	36.00	360.00	0.00	3.00	50.00	6.00
	Wendy's-Cheeseburger, Bacon, Jr.	166.0000	1.000	Each	20.00	19.00	34.00	380.00	0.00	2.00	60.00	7.00
	Wendy's-Cheeseburger, Jr.	130.0000	1.000	Each	17.00	13.00	34.00	320.00	0.00	2.00	45.00	6.00
	Wendy's-Cheeseburger, Kids' Meal	123.0000	1.000	Each	17.00	13.00	33.00	320.00	0.00	2.00	45.00	6.00
	Wendy's-Chicken Club Sandwich	216.0000	1.000	Each	31.00	20.00	44.00	470.00	0.00	2.00	70.00	4.00
	Wendy's-Chicken, Breaded, Sandwi	208.0000	1.000	Each	28.00	18.00	44.00	440.00	0.00	2.00	60.00	3.50
	Wendy's-Chicken, Grilled, Sandwi	189.0000	1.000	Each	27.00	8.00	35.00	310.00	0.00	2.00	65.00	1.50
	Wendy's-Chicken, Spicy, Sandwich	213.0000	1.000	Each	28.00	15.00	43.00	410.00	0.00	2.00	65.00	2.50
	Wendy's-Chili, Large	340.0000	1.000	Each	28.00	9.00	31.00	290.00	0.00	0.00	60.00	4.00
	Wendy's-Chili, Small	227.0000	1.000	Each	19.00	6.00	21.00	190.00	0.00	0.00	40.00	2.00
	Wendy's-French Fries, Biggie	170.0000	1.000	Order	7.00	23.00	61.00	450.00	0.00	0.00	0.00	5.00
	Wendy's-French Fries, Medium	136.0000	1.000	Order	5.00	17.00	50.00	360.00	0.00	0.00	0.00	4.00
	Wendy's-French Fries, Small	91.0000	1.000	Order	3.00	12.00	33.00	240.00	0.00	0.00	0.00	2.00
	Wendy's-Frosty Dairy Dessert, La	402.2200	1.000	Each	15.00	17.00	91.00	570.00	0.00	0.00	70.00	9.00
	Wendy's-Frosty Dairy Dessert, Me	321.7760	1.000	Each	12.00	13.00	76.00	460.00	0.00	0.00	55.00	7.00
	Wendy's-Frosty Dairy Dessert, Sm	241.3320	1.000	Each	9.00	10.00	57.00	340.00	0.00	0.00	40.00	5.00
	Wendy's-Hamburger, Bacon, Big Cl	285.0000	1.000	Each	34.00	30.00	46.00	580.00	0.00	3.00	100.00	12.00
	Wendy's-Hamburger, Big Classic	251.0000	1.000	Each	27.00	23.00	44.00	480.00	0.00	0.00	75.00	7.00
	Wendy's-Hamburger, Jr.	118.0000	1.000	Each	15.00	10.00	34.00	270.00	0.00	2.00	30.00	3.50
	Wendy's-Hamburger, Kids' Meal	111.0000	1.000	Each	15.00	10.00	33.00	270.00	0.00	2.00	30.00	3.50
	Wendy's-Hamburger, Single w/ eve	219.0000	1.000	Each	25.00	20.00	37.00	420.00	0.00	3.00	70.00	6.00
	Wendy's-Hamburger, Single, Plain	133.0000	1.000	Each	24.00	16.00	31.00	360.00	0.00	2.00	65.00	6.00
	Wendy's-Potato, Bkd w/ Bacon and	380.0000	1.000	Each	17.00	17.00	75.00	510.00	0.00	0.00	15.00	4.00
	Wendy's-Potato, Bkd w/ Broccoli	411.0000	1.000	Each	9.00	14.00	77.00	450.00	0.00	0.00	0.00	2.00

Monounsaturated Fat (gm)	Polyunsaturated Fat (gm)	Vitamin D (mg)	Vitamin K (mg)	Vitamin E (mg)	Vitamin A (re)	Vitamin C (mg)	Thiamin (mg)	Riboflavin (mg)	Niacin (mg)	Vitamin B6 (mg)	Folate (mg)	Vitamin B12 (mcg)	Calcium (mg)	Iron (mg)	Magnesium (mg)	Phosphorus (mg)	Potassium (mg)	Sodium (mg)	Zinc (mg)
0.00	0.00	0.00	0.00	0.00	350.00	4.80	0.00	0.00	0.00	0.00	0.00	0.00	300.00	2.50	0.00	0.00	0.00	1130.00	0.00
0.00	2.00	0.00	0.00	0.00	0.00	53.00	0.40	2.00	2.80	0.00	0.00	0.00	190.00	4.00	0.00	0.00	495.00	1148.00	0.00
0.00	0.00	0.00	0.00	0.00	300.00	2.40	0.00	0.00	0.00	0.00	0.00	0.00	120.00	2.00	0.00	0.00	0.00	1340.00	0.00
0.00	2.00	0.00	0.00	0.00	0.00	2.00	0.40	0.30	3.20	0.00	0.00	0.00	150.00	3.00	0.00	0.00	380.00	1311.00	0.00
0.00	0.00	0.00	0.00	0.00	200.00	3.60	0.00	0.00	0.00	0.00	0.00	0.00	72.00	1.50	0.00	0.00	0.00	900.00	0.00
0.00	0.00	0.00	0.00	0.00	250.00	4.80	0.00	0.00	0.00	0.00	0.00	0.00	72.00	1.50	0.00	0.00	0.00	1190.00	0.00
0.00	0.00	0.00	0.00	0.00	0.00	0.00	0.00	0.00	0.00	0.00	0.00	0.00	0.00	0.00	0.00	0.00	0.00	190.00	0.00
0.00	0.00	0.00	0.00	0.00	0.00	0.00	0.00	0.00	0.00	0.00	0.00	0.00	0.00	0.00	0.00	0.00	0.00	390.00	0.00
0.00	0.00	0.00	0.00	0.00	0.00	0.00	0.00	0.00	0.00	0.00	0.00	0.00	0.00	0.00	0.00	0.00	0.00	540.00	0.00
0.00	0.00	0.00	0.00	0.00	0.00	0.00	0.00	0.00	0.00	0.00	0.00	0.00	0.00	0.00	0.00	0.00	0.00	550.00	0.00
0.00	0.00	0.00	0.00	0.00	0.00	0.00	0.00	0.00	0.00	0.00	0.00	0.00	0.00	0.00	0.00	0.00	0.00	850.00	0.00
0.00	2.00	0.00	0.00	0.00	0.00	2.00	0.00	0.20	0.60	0.00	0.00	0.00	191.00	1.00	0.00	0.00	159.00	399.00	0.00
0.00	3.00	0.00	0.00	0.00	0.00	58.00	0.10	0.30	2.20	0.00	0.00	0.00	297.00	3.00	0.00	0.00	674.00	997.00	0.00
0.00	0.00	0.00	0.00	0.00	0.00	0.00	0.00	0.00	0.00	0.00	0.00	0.00	0.00	0.00	0.00	0.00	0.00	810.00	0.00
0.00	1.00	0.00	0.00	0.00	0.00	52.00	0.10	0.20	0.40	0.00	0.00	0.00	156.00	1.00	0.00	0.00	384.00	642.00	0.00
0.00	10.00	0.00	0.00	0.00	0.00	31.00	0.30	0.30	3.00	0.00	0.00	0.00	257.00	4.00	0.00	0.00	408.00	1031.00	0.00
0.00	12.00	0.00	0.00	0.00	0.00	75.00	0.50	0.60	4.80	0.00	0.00	0.00	320.00	6.00	0.00	0.00	673.00	910.00	0.00
0.00	2.00	0.00	0.00	0.00	0.00	74.00	0.20	0.40	3.20	0.00	0.00	0.00	290.00	4.00	0.00	0.00	612.00	680.00	0.00
0.00	0.00	0.00	0.00	0.00	1200.00	27.00	0.00	0.00	0.00	0.00	0.00	0.00	120.00	1.50	0.00	0.00	0.00	1610.00	0.00
0.00	0.00	0.00	0.00	0.00	0.00	0.00	0.00	0.10	0.00	0.00	0.00	0.00	36.00	1.00	0.00	0.00	376.00	376.00	0.00
0.00	1.00	0.00	0.00	0.00	0.00	1.00	0.10	0.10	1.20	0.00	0.00	0.00	84.00	1.00	0.00	0.00	159.00	276.00	0.00
0.00	0.00	0.00	0.00	0.00	0.00	0.00	0.00	0.00	0.00	0.00	0.00	0.00	0.00	0.00	0.00	0.00	0.00	750.00	0.00
0.00	1.00	0.00	0.00	0.00	40.00	0.00	0.10	0.10	1.20	0.00	0.00	0.00	0.00	0.00	0.00	0.00	159.00	276.00	0.00
0.00	1.00	0.00	0.00	0.00	0.00	1.00	0.40	0.20	2.80	0.00	0.00	0.00	116.00	2.00	0.00	0.00	196.00	554.00	0.00
0.00	0.00	0.00	0.00	0.00	150.00	4.80	0.00	0.00	0.00	0.00	0.00	0.00	48.00	0.80	0.00	0.00	0.00	570.00	0.00
0.00	1.00	0.00	0.00	0.00	40.00	0.00	0.40	0.20	2.80	0.00	0.00	0.00	48.00	0.60	0.00	0.00	196.00	554.00	0.00
0.00	0.00	0.00	0.00	0.00	0.00	0.00	0.00	0.00	0.00	0.00	0.00	0.00	0.00	0.00	0.00	0.00	0.00	1020.00	0.00
0.00	0.00	0.00	0.00	0.00	0.00	0.00	0.00	0.00	0.00	0.00	0.00	0.00	0.00	0.00	0.00	0.00	0.00	1040.00	0.00
0.00	0.00	0.00	0.00	0.00	100.00	2.40	0.00	0.00	0.00	0.00	0.00	0.00	48.00	0.60	0.00	0.00	0.00	610.00	0.00
0.00	0.00	0.00	0.00	0.00	100.00	2.40	0.00	0.00	0.00	0.00	0.00	0.00	0.00	0.00	0.00	0.00	0.00	340.00	0.00
0.00	1.00	0.00	0.00	0.00	0.00	45.00	0.10	0.20	0.60	0.00	0.00	0.00	180.00	2.00	0.00	0.00	401.00	596.00	0.00
0.00	0.00	0.00	0.00	0.00	10.00	10.00	0.00	0.00	0.00	0.00	0.00	0.00	18.00	19.00	0.00	0.00	0.00	890.00	0.00
0.00	0.00	0.00	0.00	0.00	8.00	10.00	0.00	0.00	0.00	0.00	0.00	0.00	17.00	19.00	0.00	0.00	0.00	850.00	0.00
0.00	0.00	0.00	0.00	0.00	6.00	2.00	0.00	0.00	0.00	0.00	0.00	0.00	17.00	18.00	0.00	0.00	0.00	830.00	0.00
0.00	0.00	0.00	0.00	0.00	6.00	0.00	0.00	0.00	0.00	0.00	0.00	0.00	17.00	18.00	0.00	0.00	0.00	830.00	0.00
7.00	9.00	0.00	0.00	0.00	20.00	9.00	0.60	0.43	15.20	0.00	0.00	0.00	80.00	8.00	0.00	0.00	470.00	970.00	0.00
0.00	0.00	0.00	0.00	0.00	4.00	10.00	0.00	0.00	0.00	0.00	0.00	0.00	10.00	16.00	0.00	0.00	0.00	840.00	0.00
0.00	0.00	0.00	0.00	0.00	4.00	10.00	0.00	0.00	0.00	0.00	0.00	0.00	10.00	15.00	0.00	0.00	0.00	790.00	0.00
0.00	0.00	0.00	0.00	0.00	4.00	10.00	0.00	0.00	0.00	0.00	0.00	0.00	11.00	15.00	0.00	0.00	0.00	1280.00	0.00
2.00	1.00	0.00	0.00	0.00	150.00	12.00	0.15	0.17	2.85	0.00	0.00	0.00	80.00	4.50	0.00	0.00	660.00	1000.00	0.00
1.00	1.00	0.00	0.00	0.00	100.00	6.00	0.09	0.14	1.90	0.00	0.00	0.00	64.00	3.00	0.00	0.00	440.00	670.00	0.00
15.00	1.00	0.00	0.00	0.00	0.00	12.00	0.30	0.07	3.80	0.00	0.00	0.00	16.00	0.80	0.00	0.00	950.00	280.00	0.00
12.00	1.00	0.00	0.00	0.00	0.00	9.00	0.23	0.03	2.85	0.00	0.00	0.00	16.00	0.60	0.00	0.00	760.00	220.00	0.00
8.00	1.00	0.00	0.00	0.00	0.00	6.00	0.15	0.03	1.90	0.00	0.00	0.00	0.00	0.40	0.00	0.00	510.00	150.00	0.00
4.00	1.00	0.00	0.00	0.00	100.00	0.00	0.23	1.36	0.76	0.00	0.00	0.00	400.00	1.00	0.00	0.00	1040.00	330.00	0.00
3.00	1.00	0.00	0.00	0.00	100.00	0.00	0.15	1.02	0.76	0.00	0.00	0.00	320.00	0.80	0.00	0.00	830.00	260.00	0.00
3.00	0.00	0.00	0.00	0.00	80.00	0.00	0.12	0.77	0.38	0.00	0.00	0.00	240.00	0.60	0.00	0.00	630.00	200.00	0.00
0.00	0.00	0.00	0.00	0.00	15.00	25.00	0.00	0.00	0.00	0.00	0.00	0.00	25.00	30.00	0.00	0.00	0.00	1460.00	0.00
8.00	7.00	0.00	0.00	0.00	60.00	12.00	0.45	0.26	6.65	0.00	0.00	0.00	120.00	3.50	0.00	0.00	500.00	850.00	0.00
0.00	0.00	0.00	0.00	0.00	2.00	2.00	0.00	0.00	0.00	0.00	0.00	0.00	11.00	17.00	0.00	0.00	0.00	610.00	0.00
0.00	0.00	0.00	0.00	0.00	2.00	0.00	0.00	0.00	0.00	0.00	0.00	0.00	11.00	17.00	0.00	0.00	0.00	610.00	0.00
7.00	7.00	0.00	0.00	0.00	60.00	9.00	0.38	0.17	6.65	0.00	0.00	0.00	80.00	3.00	0.00	0.00	430.00	920.00	0.00
7.00	2.00	0.00	0.00	0.00	0.00	0.00	0.38	0.17	5.70	0.00	0.00	0.00	80.00	3.00	0.00	0.00	280.00	580.00	0.00
3.00	8.00	0.00	0.00	0.00	100.00	36.00	0.45	0.17	6.65	0.00	0.00	0.00	80.00	2.50	0.00	0.00	1370.00	1170.00	0.00
3.00	7.00	0.00	0.00	0.00	200.00	60.00	0.30	0.14	4.75	0.00	0.00	0.00	80.00	2.50	0.00	0.00	1310.00	450.00	0.00

USDA ID Code	Food Name	Weight in Grams*	Quantity of Units	Unit of Measure	Protein (gm)	Fat (gm)	Carbohydrate (gm)	Kcalories	Caffeine (gm)	Fiber (gm)	Cholesterol (mg)	Saturated Fat (gm)
	Wendy's-Potato, Bkd w/ Cheese	383.0000	1.000	Each	14.00	24.00	74.00	550.00	0.00	0.00	30.00	8.00
	White Castle-Cheeseburger Sandwi	64.8000	1.000	Each	7.80	11.20	15.53	199.58	0.00	2.70	0.00	0.00
	White Castle-Chicken Sandwich	63.7860	1.000	Each	7.99	7.45	20.49	185.75	0.00	1.73	0.00	0.00
	White Castle-Fish Sandwich, w/o	59.3330	1.000	Each	5.78	4.98	20.87	155.44	0.00	1.41	0.00	0.00
	White Castle-French Fries	96.8300	1.000	Order	2.49	14.70	37.73	301.14	0.00	4.64	0.00	0.00
	White Castle-Hamburger Sandwich	58.5000	1.000	Each	5.88	7.94	15.38	161.27	0.00	2.13	0.00	0.00
	White Castle-Onion Chips	92.1350	1.000	Each	3.72	16.55	38.83	328.66	0.00	3.52	0.00	0.00
	White Castle-Onion Rings	60.1700	1.000	Each	2.91	13.38	26.62	245.49	0.00	2.61	0.00	0.00
	White Castle-Sausage and Egg San	96.2500	1.000	Each	12.55	22.02	16.05	322.37	0.00	3.03	0.00	0.00
	White Castle-Sausage Sandwich	48.6670	1.000	Each	6.67	12.29	13.30	196.10	0.00	1.95	0.00	0.00

Restaurant Chains—Other

USDA ID Code	Food Name	Weight in Grams*	Quantity of Units	Unit of Measure	Protein (gm)	Fat (gm)	Carbohydrate (gm)	Kcalories	Caffeine (gm)	Fiber (gm)	Cholesterol (mg)	Saturated Fat (gm)
65	Bruegger's Bagels-Bagel, Blueber	101.0000	1.000	Each	10.00	2.00	60.00	300.00	0.00	2.00	0.00	0.00
66	Bruegger's Bagels-Bagel, Cinnamo	101.0000	1.000	Each	10.00	1.50	60.00	290.00	0.00	3.00	0.00	0.00
67	Bruegger's Bagels-Bagel, Egg	101.0000	1.000	Each	10.00	1.00	57.00	280.00	0.00	3.00	25.00	0.50
68	Bruegger's Bagels-Bagel, Everyth	104.0000	1.000	Each	11.00	2.00	58.00	290.00	0.00	2.00	0.00	0.00
69	Bruegger's Bagels-Bagel, Garlic	102.0000	1.000	Each	10.00	1.50	57.00	280.00	0.00	2.00	0.00	0.00
70	Bruegger's Bagels-Bagel, Honey G	103.0000	1.000	Each	11.00	2.50	58.00	300.00	0.00	3.00	0.00	0.50
71	Bruegger's Bagels-Bagel, Onion	102.0000	1.000	Each	10.00	1.50	57.00	280.00	0.00	2.00	0.00	0.00
72	Bruegger's Bagels-Bagel, Plain	101.0000	1.000	Each	10.00	1.50	56.00	280.00	0.00	2.00	0.00	0.00
73	Bruegger's Bagels-Bagel, Poppy S	102.0000	1.000	Each	11.00	1.50	57.00	280.00	0.00	2.00	0.00	0.00
74	Bruegger's Bagels-Bagel, Pumpern	101.0000	1.000	Each	11.00	1.50	56.00	280.00	0.00	4.00	0.00	0.00
75	Bruegger's Bagels-Bagel, Salt	102.0000	1.000	Each	10.00	1.50	55.00	270.00	0.00	2.00	0.00	0.00
76	Bruegger's Bagels-Bagel, Sesame	103.0000	1.000	Each	11.00	2.50	57.00	290.00	0.00	2.00	0.00	0.50
77	Bruegger's Bagels-Bagel, Sun-dri	101.0000	1.000	Each	10.00	1.50	56.00	280.00	0.00	3.00	0.00	0.00
64	Bruegger's Bagels-BLT Sandwich	187.0000	1.000	Each	18.00	18.00	61.00	480.00	0.00	3.00	35.00	7.00
78	Bruegger's Bagels-Brownie	0.0000	1.000	Each	3.00	16.00	27.00	250.00	0.00	1.00	60.00	7.00
79	Bruegger's Bagels-Bruegger Bar	94.0000	1.000	Each	5.00	36.00	39.00	490.00	0.00	2.00	5.00	11.00
80	Bruegger's Bagels-Brueggeroons	71.0000	1.000	Each	4.00	18.00	39.00	320.00	0.00	5.00	0.00	16.00
81	Bruegger's Bagels-Cheese, Veggie	244.0000	8.000	Ounce	5.10	13.00	16.00	200.00	0.00	3.20	15.00	4.50
82	Bruegger's Bagels-Chicken Fajita	250.0000	1.000	Each	28.00	10.00	66.00	460.00	0.00	3.00	80.00	4.50
83	Bruegger's Bagels-Chicken Salad,	116.0000	0.500	Cup	24.00	3.00	4.00	140.00	0.00	1.00	95.00	1.00
84	Bruegger's Bagels-Chicken, Aztec	241.0000	8.000	Ounce	8.00	3.50	14.00	120.00	0.00	2.00	15.00	0.50
85	Bruegger's Bagels-Chile Cilantro	246.0000	8.000	Ounce	8.00	7.00	28.00	200.00	0.00	7.00	0.00	1.00
86	Bruegger's Bagels-Chili, The Big	244.0000	8.000	Ounce	13.00	7.00	26.00	220.00	0.00	6.00	20.00	1.50
87	Bruegger's Bagels-Chowder, Bacon	241.0000	8.000	Ounce	4.00	9.00	25.00	190.00	0.00	1.00	10.00	2.50
88	Bruegger's Bagels-Chowder, Clam	241.0000	8.000	Ounce	8.00	7.00	18.00	170.00	0.00	1.00	10.00	2.00
89	Bruegger's Bagels-Cream Cheese,	27.0000	2.000	Tbsp	1.00	8.00	1.00	90.00	0.00	0.00	20.00	5.00
90	Bruegger's Bagels-Cream Cheese,	30.0000	2.000	Tbsp	2.00	10.00	1.00	100.00	0.00	0.00	30.00	6.00
91	Bruegger's Bagels-Cream Cheese,	26.0000	2.000	Tbsp	2.00	4.50	2.00	60.00	0.00	0.00	15.00	3.00
92	Bruegger's Bagels-Crm Chse, Chiv	26.0000	2.000	Tbsp	2.00	9.00	2.00	100.00	0.00	0.00	25.00	4.50
93	Bruegger's Bagels-Crm Chse, Cucu	28.0000	2.000	Tbsp	2.00	9.00	2.00	100.00	0.00	0.00	25.00	4.50
94	Bruegger's Bagels-Crm Chse, Gard	28.0000	2.000	Tbsp	1.00	8.00	1.00	80.00	0.00	0.00	25.00	5.00
95	Bruegger's Bagels-Crm Chse, Gard	27.0000	2.000	Tbsp	2.00	4.50	2.00	60.00	0.00	0.00	15.00	3.00
96	Bruegger's Bagels-Crm Chse, Herb	27.0000	2.000	Tbsp	2.00	4.50	3.00	60.00	0.00	0.00	15.00	3.00
97	Bruegger's Bagels-Crm Chse, Hone	27.0000	2.000	Tbsp	2.00	9.00	3.00	90.00	0.00	0.00	20.00	5.00
98	Bruegger's Bagels-Crm Chse, Jala	30.0000	2.000	Tbsp	1.00	8.00	1.00	80.00	0.00	0.00	20.00	5.00
99	Bruegger's Bagels-Crm Chse, Salm	29.0000	2.000	Tbsp	2.00	9.00	1.00	90.00	0.00	0.00	20.00	5.00
100	Bruegger's Bagels-Crm Chse, Stra	25.0000	2.000	Tbsp	2.00	4.50	5.00	70.00	0.00	0.00	15.00	3.00
101	Bruegger's Bagels-Crm Chse, Sun	27.0000	2.000	Tbsp	2.00	4.50	2.00	60.00	0.00	0.00	15.00	3.00
102	Bruegger's Bagels-Crm Chse, Wild	30.0000	2.000	Tbsp	1.00	8.00	3.00	90.00	0.00	0.00	20.00	5.00
103	Bruegger's Bagels-Cucumber Dill	236.0000	1.000	Each	18.00	15.00	62.00	450.00	0.00	4.00	40.00	8.00
104	Bruegger's Bagels-Garden Veggie,	227.0000	8.000	Ounce	2.00	1.50	11.00	60.00	0.00	2.00	0.00	0.00
105	Bruegger's Bagels-Gumbo, Cajun	241.0000	8.000	Ounce	3.00	4.50	17.00	120.00	0.00	2.00	0.00	1.00
106	Bruegger's Bagels-Hummus	71.0000	1.000	Scoop	5.00	9.00	13.00	150.00	0.00	4.00	0.00	1.50
107	Bruegger's Bagels-Javahhccino	280.0000	12.000	Fl Oz	9.00	3.00	35.00	210.00	0.00	0.00	10.00	3.00
108	Bruegger's Bagels-Kinnow Bruegge	227.0000	8.000	Fl Oz	1.00	0.00	35.00	140.00	0.00	0.00	0.00	0.00

Monounsaturated Fat (gm)	Polyunsaturated Fat (gm)	Vitamin D (mg)	Vitamin K (mg)	Vitamin E (mg)	Vitamin A (re)	Vitamin C (mg)	Thiamin (mg)	Riboflavin (mg)	Niacin (mg)	Vitamin B$_6$ (mg)	Folate (mg)	Vitamin B$_{12}$ (mcg)	Calcium (mg)	Iron (mg)	Magnesium (mg)	Phosphorus (mg)	Potassium (mg)	Sodium (mg)	Zinc (mg)
6.00	7.00	0.00	0.00	0.00	150.00	36.00	0.30	0.17	3.80	0.00	0.00	0.00	240.00	2.00	0.00	0.00	1210.00	640.00	0.00
0.00	0.00	0.00	0.00	0.00	0.00	0.00	0.00	0.00	0.00	0.00	0.00	0.00	0.00	0.00	0.00	0.00	0.00	361.00	0.00
0.00	0.00	0.00	0.00	0.00	0.00	0.00	0.00	0.00	0.00	0.00	0.00	0.00	0.00	0.00	0.00	0.00	0.00	497.00	0.00
0.00	0.00	0.00	0.00	0.00	0.00	0.00	0.00	0.00	0.00	0.00	0.00	0.00	0.00	0.00	0.00	0.00	0.00	201.00	0.00
0.00	0.00	0.00	0.00	0.00	0.00	0.00	0.00	0.00	0.00	0.00	0.00	0.00	0.00	0.00	0.00	0.00	0.00	193.00	0.00
0.00	0.00	0.00	0.00	0.00	0.00	0.00	0.00	0.00	0.00	0.00	0.00	0.00	0.00	0.00	0.00	0.00	0.00	266.00	0.00
0.00	0.00	0.00	0.00	0.00	0.00	0.00	0.00	0.00	0.00	0.00	0.00	0.00	0.00	0.00	0.00	0.00	0.00	823.00	0.00
0.00	0.00	0.00	0.00	0.00	0.00	0.00	0.00	0.00	0.00	0.00	0.00	0.00	0.00	0.00	0.00	0.00	0.00	566.00	0.00
0.00	0.00	0.00	0.00	0.00	0.00	0.00	0.00	0.00	0.00	0.00	0.00	0.00	0.00	0.00	0.00	0.00	0.00	698.00	0.00
0.00	0.00	0.00	0.00	0.00	0.00	0.00	0.00	0.00	0.00	0.00	0.00	0.00	0.00	0.00	0.00	0.00	0.00	488.00	0.00
0.50	0.50	0.00	0.00	0.00	0.00	0.00	0.00	0.00	0.00	0.00	0.00	0.00	0.00	0.00	0.00	0.00	0.00	480.00	0.00
0.00	0.50	0.00	0.00	0.00	0.00	0.00	0.00	0.00	0.00	0.00	0.00	0.00	0.00	0.00	0.00	0.00	0.00	400.00	0.00
0.50	0.50	0.00	0.00	0.00	0.00	0.00	0.00	0.00	0.00	0.00	0.00	0.00	0.00	0.00	0.00	0.00	0.00	510.00	0.00
0.00	1.00	0.00	0.00	0.00	0.00	0.00	0.00	0.00	0.00	0.00	0.00	0.00	0.00	0.00	0.00	0.00	0.00	700.00	0.00
0.00	0.50	0.00	0.00	0.00	0.00	0.00	0.00	0.00	0.00	0.00	0.00	0.00	0.00	0.00	0.00	0.00	0.00	440.00	0.00
0.50	1.50	0.00	0.00	0.00	0.00	0.00	0.00	0.00	0.00	0.00	0.00	0.00	0.00	0.00	0.00	0.00	0.00	390.00	0.00
0.00	0.50	0.00	0.00	0.00	0.00	0.00	0.00	0.00	0.00	0.00	0.00	0.00	0.00	0.00	0.00	0.00	0.00	430.00	0.00
0.00	1.00	0.00	0.00	0.00	0.00	0.00	0.00	0.00	0.00	0.00	0.00	0.00	0.00	0.00	0.00	0.00	0.00	430.00	0.00
0.00	1.00	0.00	0.00	0.00	0.00	0.00	0.00	0.00	0.00	0.00	0.00	0.00	0.00	0.00	0.00	0.00	0.00	440.00	0.00
0.00	0.50	0.00	0.00	0.00	0.00	0.00	0.00	0.00	0.00	0.00	0.00	0.00	0.00	0.00	0.00	0.00	0.00	390.00	0.00
0.00	0.50	0.00	0.00	0.00	0.00	0.00	0.00	0.00	0.00	0.00	0.00	0.00	0.00	0.00	0.00	0.00	0.00	1670.00	0.00
1.00	1.00	0.00	0.00	0.00	0.00	0.00	0.00	0.00	0.00	0.00	0.00	0.00	0.00	0.00	0.00	0.00	0.00	440.00	0.00
0.00	1.00	0.00	0.00	0.00	0.00	0.00	0.00	0.00	0.00	0.00	0.00	0.00	0.00	0.00	0.00	0.00	0.00	490.00	0.00
0.00	0.00	0.00	0.00	0.00	0.00	0.00	0.00	0.00	0.00	0.00	0.00	0.00	0.00	0.00	0.00	0.00	0.00	820.00	0.00
0.00	0.00	0.00	0.00	0.00	0.00	0.00	0.00	0.00	0.00	0.00	0.00	0.00	0.00	0.00	0.00	0.00	0.00	95.00	0.00
0.00	0.00	0.00	0.00	0.00	150.00	36.00	0.30	0.17	0.00	0.00	0.00	0.00	240.00	0.00	0.00	0.00	0.00	440.00	0.00
0.00	0.00	0.00	0.00	0.00	0.00	0.00	0.00	0.00	0.00	0.00	0.00	0.00	0.00	0.00	0.00	0.00	0.00	140.00	0.00
0.00	0.00	0.00	0.00	0.00	0.00	0.00	0.00	0.00	0.00	0.00	0.00	0.00	0.00	0.00	0.00	0.00	0.00	1010.00	0.00
0.00	0.00	0.00	0.00	0.00	0.00	0.00	0.00	0.00	0.00	0.00	0.00	0.00	0.00	0.00	0.00	0.00	0.00	830.00	0.00
0.00	0.00	0.00	0.00	0.00	0.00	0.00	0.00	0.00	0.00	0.00	0.00	0.00	0.00	0.00	0.00	0.00	0.00	440.00	0.00
0.00	0.00	0.00	0.00	0.00	0.00	0.00	0.00	0.00	0.00	0.00	0.00	0.00	0.00	0.00	0.00	0.00	0.00	570.00	0.00
0.00	0.00	0.00	0.00	0.00	0.00	0.00	0.00	0.00	0.00	0.00	0.00	0.00	0.00	0.00	0.00	0.00	0.00	620.00	0.00
0.00	0.00	0.00	0.00	0.00	0.00	0.00	0.00	0.00	0.00	0.00	0.00	0.00	0.00	0.00	0.00	0.00	0.00	810.00	0.00
0.00	0.00	0.00	0.00	0.00	0.00	0.00	0.00	0.00	0.00	0.00	0.00	0.00	0.00	0.00	0.00	0.00	0.00	700.00	0.00
0.00	0.00	0.00	0.00	0.00	0.00	0.00	0.00	0.00	0.00	0.00	0.00	0.00	0.00	0.00	0.00	0.00	0.00	1230.00	0.00
0.00	0.00	0.00	0.00	0.00	0.00	0.00	0.00	0.00	0.00	0.00	0.00	0.00	0.00	0.00	0.00	0.00	0.00	110.00	0.00
0.00	0.00	0.00	0.00	0.00	0.00	0.00	0.00	0.00	0.00	0.00	0.00	0.00	0.00	0.00	0.00	0.00	0.00	120.00	0.00
0.00	0.00	0.00	0.00	0.00	0.00	0.00	0.00	0.00	0.00	0.00	0.00	0.00	0.00	0.00	0.00	0.00	0.00	130.00	0.00
0.00	0.00	0.00	0.00	0.00	0.00	0.00	0.00	0.00	0.00	0.00	0.00	0.00	0.00	0.00	0.00	0.00	0.00	85.00	0.00
0.00	0.00	0.00	0.00	0.00	0.00	0.00	0.00	0.00	0.00	0.00	0.00	0.00	0.00	0.00	0.00	0.00	0.00	85.00	0.00
0.00	0.00	0.00	0.00	0.00	0.00	0.00	0.00	0.00	0.00	0.00	0.00	0.00	0.00	0.00	0.00	0.00	0.00	120.00	0.00
0.00	0.00	0.00	0.00	0.00	0.00	0.00	0.00	0.00	0.00	0.00	0.00	0.00	0.00	0.00	0.00	0.00	0.00	160.00	0.00
0.00	0.00	0.00	0.00	0.00	0.00	0.00	0.00	0.00	0.00	0.00	0.00	0.00	0.00	0.00	0.00	0.00	0.00	150.00	0.00
0.00	0.00	0.00	0.00	0.00	0.00	0.00	0.00	0.00	0.00	0.00	0.00	0.00	0.00	0.00	0.00	0.00	0.00	90.00	0.00
0.00	0.00	0.00	0.00	0.00	0.00	0.00	0.00	0.00	0.00	0.00	0.00	0.00	0.00	0.00	0.00	0.00	0.00	100.00	0.00
0.00	0.00	0.00	0.00	0.00	0.00	0.00	0.00	0.00	0.00	0.00	0.00	0.00	0.00	0.00	0.00	0.00	0.00	120.00	0.00
0.00	0.00	0.00	0.00	0.00	0.00	0.00	0.00	0.00	0.00	0.00	0.00	0.00	0.00	0.00	0.00	0.00	0.00	60.00	0.00
0.00	0.00	0.00	0.00	0.00	0.00	0.00	0.00	0.00	0.00	0.00	0.00	0.00	0.00	0.00	0.00	0.00	0.00	160.00	0.00
0.00	0.00	0.00	0.00	0.00	0.00	0.00	0.00	0.00	0.00	0.00	0.00	0.00	0.00	0.00	0.00	0.00	0.00	100.00	0.00
0.00	0.00	0.00	0.00	0.00	0.00	0.00	0.00	0.00	0.00	0.00	0.00	0.00	0.00	0.00	0.00	0.00	0.00	630.00	0.00
0.00	0.00	0.00	0.00	0.00	0.00	0.00	0.00	0.00	0.00	0.00	0.00	0.00	0.00	0.00	0.00	0.00	0.00	690.00	0.00
0.00	0.00	0.00	0.00	0.00	0.00	0.00	0.00	0.00	0.00	0.00	0.00	0.00	0.00	0.00	0.00	0.00	0.00	930.00	0.00
0.00	0.00	0.00	0.00	0.00	0.00	0.00	0.00	0.00	0.00	0.00	0.00	0.00	0.00	0.00	0.00	0.00	0.00	140.00	0.00
0.00	0.00	0.00	0.00	0.00	0.00	0.00	0.00	0.00	0.00	0.00	0.00	0.00	0.00	0.00	0.00	0.00	0.00	150.00	0.00
0.00	0.00	0.00	0.00	0.00	0.00	0.00	0.00	0.00	0.00	0.00	0.00	0.00	0.00	0.00	0.00	0.00	0.00	0.00	0.00

USDA ID Code	Food Name	Weight in Grams*	Quantity of Units	Unit of Measure	Protein (gm)	Fat (gm)	Carbohydrate (gm)	Kcalories	Caffeine (gm)	Fiber (gm)	Cholesterol (mg)	Saturated Fat (gm)
109	Bruegger's Bagels-Leonardo da Ve	220.0000	1.000	Each	19.00	11.00	62.00	420.00	0.00	3.00	30.00	6.00
110	Bruegger's Bagels-Mediterranean	231.0000	1.000	Each	20.00	24.00	74.00	610.00	0.00	8.00	30.00	11.00
111	Bruegger's Bagels-Olivia De Hami	239.0000	1.000	Each	29.00	17.00	62.00	520.00	0.00	3.00	75.00	8.00
112	Bruegger's Bagels-Soup, Chicken	241.0000	8.000	Ounce	10.00	3.50	25.00	170.00	0.00	1.00	40.00	1.00
113	Bruegger's Bagels-Soup, Garden S	247.0000	8.000	Ounce	4.00	6.00	19.00	150.00	0.00	3.00	10.00	3.00
114	Bruegger's Bagels-Soup, Marcello	241.0000	8.000	Ounce	4.00	1.00	18.00	90.00	0.00	2.00	0.00	0.00
115	Bruegger's Bagels-Soup, Turkey L	227.0000	8.000	Ounce	14.00	2.50	17.00	150.00	0.00	7.00	20.00	0.50
116	Bruegger's Bagels-Stew, Ratatoui	244.0000	8.000	Ounce	2.00	9.00	12.00	140.00	0.00	3.00	0.00	1.50
117	Bruegger's Bagels-Strawberry Bru	227.0000	8.000	Fl Oz	0.00	0.00	39.00	150.00	0.00	0.00	0.00	0.00
118	Bruegger's Bagels-Tuna Salad	116.0000	0.500	Cup	12.00	19.00	9.00	260.00	0.00	2.00	30.00	3.00
119	Bruegger's Bagels-Turkey Club Sa	258.0000	1.000	Each	27.00	31.00	58.00	620.00	0.00	3.00	55.00	5.00
120	Bruegger's Bagels-Turkey Orzo, T	241.0000	8.000	Ounce	8.00	3.00	13.00	110.00	0.00	1.00	15.00	0.50
121	Bruegger's Bagels-Turkey, Herby	235.0000	1.000	Each	30.00	13.00	67.00	510.00	0.00	3.00	45.00	5.00
122	Bruegger's Bagels-Turkey, Hot Sh	234.0000	1.000	Each	26.00	8.00	68.00	450.00	0.00	3.00	3.00	3.50
123	Bruegger's Bagels-Turkey, Santa	264.0000	1.000	Each	27.00	9.00	63.00	450.00	0.00	3.00	45.00	4.00
220	Denny's-All American Slam	368.5500	1.000	Serving	38.00	62.00	9.00	712.00	0.00	1.00	686.00	20.00
221	Denny's-Bacon, 4 Strips	28.3500	4.000	Each	12.00	18.00	1.00	162.00	0.00	0.00	36.00	5.00
222	Denny's-Bagel, Dry	85.0000	1.000	Each	9.00	1.00	46.00	235.00	0.00	0.00	0.00	0.00
223	Denny's-Big Texas Chicken Fajita	481.0000	1.000	Serving	49.00	70.00	25.00	1217.00	0.00	8.00	518.00	19.00
224	Denny's-Biscuit & Sausage Gravy	198.4500	1.000	Serving	8.00	21.00	45.00	398.00	0.00	0.00	12.00	6.00
225	Denny's-Biscuit, Buttered	85.0000	1.000	Each	5.00	11.00	39.00	272.00	0.00	0.00	0.00	4.00
226	Denny's-Buttermilk Hotcakes (3)	141.7500	3.000	Each	12.00	7.00	95.00	491.00	0.00	3.00	0.00	1.00
227	Denny's-Chicken Fried Steak & Eg	226.8000	1.000	Serving	22.00	36.00	9.00	430.00	0.00	4.00	440.00	12.00
228	Denny's-Chicken Fried Steak Skil	737.0000	1.000	Serving	60.00	104.00	119.00	1745.00	0.00	26.00	607.00	28.00
229	Denny's-Cinnamon Swirl French To	340.0000	1.000	Serving	23.00	49.00	124.00	1030.00	0.00	4.00	280.00	21.00
230	Denny's-Cinnamon Swirl Slam	368.5500	1.000	Serving	38.00	78.00	68.00	1105.00	0.00	2.00	635.00	26.00
231	Denny's-Country Fried Potatoes	170.0000	1.000	Serving	3.00	35.00	23.00	515.00	0.00	9.00	8.00	8.00
232	Denny's-Egg Beaters, Egg Substit	56.7000	1.000	Serving	5.00	5.00	1.00	71.00	0.00	0.00	1.00	1.00
233	Denny's-Eggs Benedict	425.2500	1.000	Serving	34.00	46.00	34.00	695.00	0.00	1.00	515.00	11.00
234	Denny's-English Muffin, Dry, 1mu	113.4000	1.000	Each	5.00	1.00	24.00	125.00	0.00	1.00	0.00	0.00
235	Denny's-Flour Tortillas and Sals	156.0000	1.000	Serving	6.00	8.00	50.50	281.00	0.00	4.00	0.00	1.50
236	Denny's-French Slam	397.0000	1.000	Serving	44.00	71.00	58.00	1029.00	0.00	2.00	777.00	20.00
237	Denny's-French Toast (2)	199.0000	2.000	Each	16.00	24.00	54.00	507.00	0.00	3.00	219.00	6.00
238	Denny's-Grand Slam Slugger	340.0000	1.000	Serving	32.00	46.00	58.00	789.00	0.00	2.00	487.00	14.00
239	Denny's-Grits	113.0000	0.500	Cup	2.00	0.00	18.00	80.00	0.00	0.00	0.00	0.00
241	Denny's-Ham, Grilled, sliced	85.0000	3.000	Ounce	15.00	3.00	2.00	94.00	0.00	0.00	23.00	1.00
240	Denny's-Ham'nCheddar Omelette	283.5000	1.000	Each	37.00	45.00	4.00	581.00	0.00	0.00	672.00	8.00
242	Denny's-Hashed Browns	113.4000	1.000	Serving	2.00	14.00	20.00	218.00	0.00	2.00	0.00	2.00
243	Denny's-Kelloggs Dry Cereal	28.3500	1.000	Serving	2.00	0.00	23.00	100.00	0.00	1.00	0.00	0.00
244	Denny's-Lumberjack Slam	538.6500	1.000	Serving	54.00	70.00	118.00	1259.00	0.00	5.00	481.00	18.00
245	Denny's-Meat Lover's Skillet	425.2500	1.000	Serving	41.00	93.00	24.00	1147.00	0.00	7.00	460.00	26.00
246	Denny's-Oatmeal N' Fixins	538.6500	1.000	Serving	13.00	6.00	95.00	460.00	0.00	7.00	11.00	3.00
247	Denny's-One Egg	56.7000	1.000	Each	6.00	10.00	0.50	120.00	0.00	0.00	210.00	3.00
248	Denny's-Original Grand Slam	283.5000	1.000	Serving	34.00	50.00	65.00	795.00	0.00	2.00	460.00	14.00
249	Denny's-Pork Chop & Eggs	354.3800	1.000	Serving	55.00	47.00	6.00	673.00	0.00	0.00	571.00	13.00
250	Denny's-Quaker Oatmeal	113.4000	0.500	Cup	5.00	2.00	18.00	100.00	0.00	3.00	0.00	0.00
251	Denny's-Sausage Gravy	113.4000	1.000	Serving	3.00	10.00	6.00	126.00	0.00	0.00	12.00	2.00
252	Denny's-Sausage, 4 Links	85.0000	4.000	Each	16.00	32.00	0.00	354.00	0.00	0.00	64.00	12.00
253	Denny's-Sirloin Steak & Eggs	255.0000	1.000	Serving	43.00	49.00	1.00	622.00	0.00	1.00	572.00	18.00
254	Denny's-T-bone Steak & Eggs	397.0000	1.000	Serving	73.00	77.00	1.00	991.00	0.00	1.00	657.00	31.00
255	Denny's-Toast, Dry, 1slice	28.3500	1.000	Slice	3.00	1.00	17.00	90.00	0.00	1.00	0.00	0.00
256	Denny's-Two Egg Breakfast	312.0000	1.000	Serving	31.00	67.00	24.00	825.00	0.00	2.00	538.00	17.00
257	Denny's-Ultimate Omelette	368.5500	1.000	Each	30.00	47.00	9.00	594.00	0.00	2.00	639.00	12.00
258	Denny's-Veggie-Cheese Omelette	340.0000	1.000	Each	26.00	39.00	9.00	480.00	0.00	2.00	644.00	13.00
	Dunkin' Donuts-Apple Filled w/ C	79.0000	1.000	Each	5.00	11.00	33.00	250.00	0.00	1.00	0.00	0.00

Monounsaturated Fat (gm)	Polyunsaturated Fat (gm)	Vitamin D (mg)	Vitamin K (mg)	Vitamin E (mg)	Vitamin A (re)	Vitamin C (mg)	Thiamin (mg)	Riboflavin (mg)	Niacin (mg)	Vitamin B6 (mg)	Folate (mg)	Vitamin B12 (mcg)	Calcium (mg)	Iron (mg)	Magnesium (mg)	Phosphorus (mg)	Potassium (mg)	Sodium (mg)	Zinc (mg)
0.00	0.00	0.00	0.00	0.00	0.00	0.00	0.00	0.00	0.00	0.00	0.00	0.00	0.00	0.00	0.00	0.00	0.00	690.00	0.00
0.00	0.00	0.00	0.00	0.00	0.00	0.00	0.00	0.00	0.00	0.00	0.00	0.00	0.00	0.00	0.00	0.00	0.00	840.00	0.00
0.00	0.00	0.00	0.00	0.00	0.00	0.00	0.00	0.00	0.00	0.00	0.00	0.00	0.00	0.00	0.00	0.00	0.00	1500.00	0.00
0.00	0.00	0.00	0.00	0.00	0.00	0.00	0.00	0.00	0.00	0.00	0.00	0.00	0.00	0.00	0.00	0.00	0.00	1150.00	0.00
0.00	0.00	0.00	0.00	0.00	0.00	0.00	0.00	0.00	0.00	0.00	0.00	0.00	0.00	0.00	0.00	0.00	0.00	1050.00	0.00
0.00	0.00	0.00	0.00	0.00	0.00	0.00	0.00	0.00	0.00	0.00	0.00	0.00	0.00	0.00	0.00	0.00	0.00	890.00	0.00
0.00	0.00	0.00	0.00	0.00	0.00	0.00	0.00	0.00	0.00	0.00	0.00	0.00	0.00	0.00	0.00	0.00	0.00	820.00	0.00
0.00	0.00	0.00	0.00	0.00	0.00	0.00	0.00	0.00	0.00	0.00	0.00	0.00	0.00	0.00	0.00	0.00	0.00	1100.00	0.00
0.00	0.00	0.00	0.00	0.00	0.00	0.00	0.00	0.00	0.00	0.00	0.00	0.00	0.00	0.00	0.00	0.00	0.00	5.00	0.00
0.00	0.00	0.00	0.00	0.00	0.00	0.00	0.00	0.00	0.00	0.00	0.00	0.00	0.00	0.00	0.00	0.00	0.00	580.00	0.00
0.00	0.00	0.00	0.00	0.00	0.00	0.00	0.00	0.00	0.00	0.00	0.00	0.00	0.00	0.00	0.00	0.00	0.00	1420.00	0.00
0.00	0.00	0.00	0.00	0.00	0.00	0.00	0.00	0.00	0.00	0.00	0.00	0.00	0.00	0.00	0.00	0.00	0.00	940.00	0.00
0.00	0.00	0.00	0.00	0.00	0.00	0.00	0.00	0.00	0.00	0.00	0.00	0.00	0.00	0.00	0.00	0.00	0.00	1100.00	0.00
0.00	0.00	0.00	0.00	0.00	0.00	0.00	0.00	0.00	0.00	0.00	0.00	0.00	0.00	0.00	0.00	0.00	0.00	1090.00	0.00
0.00	0.00	0.00	0.00	0.00	0.00	0.00	0.00	0.00	0.00	0.00	0.00	0.00	0.00	0.00	0.00	0.00	0.00	1040.00	0.00
0.00	0.00	0.00	0.00	0.00	390.00	25.80	0.00	0.00	0.00	0.00	0.00	0.00	240.00	3.60	0.00	0.00	0.00	1281.00	0.00
0.00	0.00	0.00	0.00	0.00	0.00	6.00	0.00	0.00	0.00	0.00	0.00	0.00	0.00	0.36	0.00	0.00	0.00	640.00	0.00
0.00	0.00	0.00	0.00	0.00	0.00	0.00	0.00	0.00	0.00	0.00	0.00	0.00	0.00	14.94	0.00	0.00	0.00	495.00	0.00
0.00	0.00	0.00	0.00	0.00	530.00	28.20	0.00	0.00	0.00	0.00	0.00	0.00	220.00	3.06	0.00	0.00	0.00	1817.00	0.00
0.00	0.00	0.00	0.00	0.00	0.00	0.00	0.00	0.00	0.00	0.00	0.00	0.00	0.60	0.18	0.00	0.00	0.00	1267.00	0.00
0.00	0.00	0.00	0.00	0.00	0.00	0.00	0.00	0.00	0.00	0.00	0.00	0.00	0.00	0.00	0.00	0.00	0.00	790.00	0.00
0.00	0.00	0.00	0.00	0.00	0.00	0.00	0.00	0.00	0.00	0.00	0.00	0.00	150.00	1.80	0.00	0.00	0.00	0.00	0.00
0.00	0.00	0.00	0.00	0.00	220.00	0.00	0.00	0.00	0.00	0.00	0.00	0.00	550.00	0.54	0.00	0.00	0.00	861.00	0.00
0.00	0.00	0.00	0.00	0.00	140.00	36.00	0.00	0.00	0.00	0.00	0.00	0.00	130.00	8.10	0.00	0.00	0.00	6184.00	0.00
0.00	0.00	0.00	0.00	0.00	370.00	0.00	0.00	0.00	0.00	0.00	0.00	0.00	180.00	6.48	0.00	0.00	0.00	675.00	0.00
0.00	0.00	0.00	0.00	0.00	540.00	0.00	0.00	0.00	0.00	0.00	0.00	0.00	150.00	5.58	0.00	0.00	0.00	1374.00	0.00
0.00	0.00	0.00	0.00	0.00	0.00	0.00	0.00	0.00	0.00	0.00	0.00	0.00	60.00	1.08	0.00	0.00	0.00	805.00	0.00
0.00	0.00	0.00	0.00	0.00	370.00	0.00	0.00	0.00	0.00	0.00	0.00	0.00	20.00	1.08	0.00	0.00	0.00	138.00	0.00
0.00	0.00	0.00	0.00	0.00	530.00	0.00	0.00	0.00	0.00	0.00	0.00	0.00	190.00	3.96	0.00	0.00	0.00	1718.00	0.00
0.00	0.00	0.00	0.00	0.00	0.00	0.00	0.00	0.00	0.00	0.00	0.00	0.00	80.00	1.80	0.00	0.00	0.00	0.00	0.00
0.00	0.00	0.00	0.00	0.00	150.00	21.00	0.00	0.00	0.00	0.00	0.00	0.00	200.00	2.70	0.00	0.00	0.00	1031.00	0.00
0.00	0.00	0.00	0.00	0.00	530.00	0.00	0.00	0.00	0.00	0.00	0.00	0.00	120.00	5.58	0.00	0.00	0.00	1428.00	0.00
0.00	0.00	0.00	0.00	0.00	130.00	0.00	0.00	0.00	0.00	0.00	0.00	0.00	130.00	3.60	0.00	0.00	0.00	594.00	0.00
0.00	0.00	0.00	0.00	0.00	140.00	0.00	0.00	0.00	0.00	0.00	0.00	0.00	250.00	4.68	0.00	0.00	0.00	1438.00	0.00
0.00	0.00	0.00	0.00	0.00	0.00	0.00	0.00	0.00	0.00	0.00	0.00	0.00	0.00	0.72	0.00	0.00	0.00	520.00	0.00
0.00	0.00	0.00	0.00	0.00	0.00	0.00	0.00	0.00	0.00	0.00	0.00	0.00	0.00	0.72	0.00	0.00	0.00	761.00	0.00
0.00	0.00	0.00	0.00	0.00	390.00	0.00	0.00	0.00	0.00	0.00	0.00	0.00	380.00	2.88	0.00	0.00	0.00	1180.00	0.00
0.00	0.00	0.00	0.00	0.00	30.00	6.60	0.00	0.00	0.00	0.00	0.00	0.00	10.00	0.36	0.00	0.00	0.00	424.00	0.00
0.00	0.00	0.00	0.00	0.00	350.00	9.60	0.00	0.00	0.00	0.00	0.00	0.00	0.00	3.42	0.00	0.00	0.00	276.00	0.00
0.00	0.00	0.00	0.00	0.00	370.00	7.80	0.00	0.00	0.00	0.00	0.00	0.00	230.00	5.22	0.00	0.00	0.00	4028.00	0.00
0.00	0.00	0.00	0.00	0.00	470.00	4.20	0.00	0.00	0.00	0.00	0.00	0.00	220.00	3.42	0.00	0.00	0.00	2507.00	0.00
0.00	0.00	0.00	0.00	0.00	80.00	12.00	0.00	0.00	0.00	0.00	0.00	0.00	250.00	2.70	0.00	0.00	0.00	87.00	0.00
0.00	0.00	0.00	0.00	0.00	20.00	3.60	0.00	0.00	0.00	0.00	0.00	0.00	0.00	0.72	0.00	0.00	0.00	120.00	0.00
0.00	0.00	0.00	0.00	0.00	330.00	0.00	0.00	0.00	0.00	0.00	0.00	0.00	160.00	3.42	0.00	0.00	0.00	2237.00	0.00
0.00	0.00	0.00	0.00	0.00	150.00	0.00	0.00	0.00	0.00	0.00	0.00	0.00	50.00	3.06	0.00	0.00	0.00	1582.00	0.00
0.00	0.00	0.00	0.00	0.00	0.00	0.00	0.00	0.00	0.00	0.00	0.00	0.00	10.00	0.90	0.00	0.00	0.00	175.00	0.00
0.00	0.00	0.00	0.00	0.00	0.00	0.00	0.00	0.00	0.00	0.00	0.00	0.00	10.00	0.18	0.00	0.00	0.00	477.00	0.00
0.00	0.00	0.00	0.00	4.00	0.00	0.00	0.00	0.00	0.00	0.00	0.00	0.00	10.00	1.26	0.00	0.00	0.00	944.00	0.00
0.00	0.00	0.00	0.00	0.00	160.00	1.80	0.00	0.00	0.00	0.00	0.00	0.00	130.00	5.94	0.00	0.00	0.00	632.00	0.00
0.00	0.00	0.00	0.00	0.00	150.00	2.40	0.00	0.00	0.00	0.00	0.00	0.00	200.00	10.80	0.00	0.00	0.00	1003.00	0.00
0.00	0.00	0.00	0.00	0.00	0.00	0.00	0.00	0.00	0.00	0.00	0.00	0.00	30.00	0.72	0.00	0.00	0.00	166.00	0.00
0.00	0.00	0.00	0.00	0.00	170.00	7.80	0.00	0.00	0.00	0.00	0.00	0.00	80.00	3.24	0.00	0.00	0.00	1765.00	0.00
0.00	0.00	0.00	0.00	0.00	320.00	55.20	0.00	0.00	0.00	0.00	0.00	0.00	80.00	3.60	0.00	0.00	0.00	939.00	0.00
0.00	0.00	0.00	0.00	0.00	390.00	16.20	0.00	0.00	0.00	0.00	0.00	0.00	280.00	2.70	0.00	0.00	0.00	535.00	0.00
0.00	0.00	0.00	0.00	0.00	0.00	0.00	0.00	0.00	0.00	0.00	0.00	0.00	0.00	0.00	0.00	0.00	0.00	280.00	0.00

USDA ID Code	Food Name	Weight in Grams*	Quantity of Units	Unit of Measure	Protein (gm)	Fat (gm)	Carbohydrate (gm)	Kcalories	Caffeine (gm)	Fiber (gm)	Cholesterol (mg)	Saturated Fat (gm)
	Dunkin' Donuts-Bavarian Filled w	79.0000	1.000	Each	5.00	11.00	32.00	240.00	0.00	2.00	0.00	0.00
	Dunkin' Donuts-Blueberry Filled	67.0000	1.000	Each	4.00	8.00	29.00	210.00	0.00	2.00	0.00	0.00
	Dunkin' Donuts-Buttermilk Ring,	74.0000	1.000	Each	4.00	14.00	37.00	290.00	0.00	1.00	10.00	0.00
	Dunkin' Donuts-Cake Ring, Plain	62.0000	1.000	Each	4.00	17.00	25.00	270.00	0.00	1.00	0.00	0.00
	Dunkin' Donuts-Chocolate Rings,	71.0000	1.000	Each	3.50	21.00	34.00	324.00	0.00	1.90	0.00	0.00
	Dunkin' Donuts-Coffee Roll, Glaz	81.0000	1.000	Each	5.00	12.00	37.00	280.00	0.00	2.00	0.00	0.00
	Dunkin' Donuts-Cookie, Chocolate	43.0000	1.000	Each	3.00	10.00	25.00	200.00	0.00	1.00	30.00	0.00
	Dunkin' Donuts-Cookie, Chocolate	43.0000	1.000	Each	3.00	11.00	23.00	210.00	0.00	2.00	30.00	0.00
	Dunkin' Donuts-Cookie, Oatmeal P	46.0000	1.000	Each	3.00	9.00	28.00	200.00	0.00	1.00	25.00	0.00
	Dunkin' Donuts-Croissant, Almond	105.0000	1.000	Each	8.00	27.00	38.00	420.00	0.00	3.00	0.00	0.00
	Dunkin' Donuts-Croissant, Chocol	94.0000	1.000	Each	7.00	29.00	38.00	440.00	0.00	3.00	0.00	0.00
	Dunkin' Donuts-Croissant, Plain	72.0000	1.000	Each	7.00	19.00	27.00	310.00	0.00	2.00	0.00	0.00
	Dunkin' Donuts-Cruller, Glazed F	38.0000	1.000	Each	2.00	8.00	16.00	140.00	0.00	0.00	30.00	0.00
	Dunkin' Donuts-Filled, Jelly	67.0000	1.000	Each	4.00	9.00	31.00	220.00	0.00	1.00	0.00	0.00
	Dunkin' Donuts-Filled, Lemon	79.0000	1.000	Each	4.00	12.00	33.00	260.00	0.00	1.00	0.00	0.00
	Dunkin' Donuts-Muffin, Apple 'n	100.0000	1.000	Each	6.00	8.00	52.00	300.00	0.00	2.00	25.00	0.00
	Dunkin' Donuts-Muffin, Banana Nu	103.0000	1.000	Each	7.00	10.00	49.00	310.00	0.00	3.00	30.00	0.00
	Dunkin' Donuts-Muffin, Blueberry	101.0000	1.000	Each	6.00	8.00	46.00	280.00	0.00	2.00	30.00	0.00
	Dunkin' Donuts-Muffin, Bran w/ R	104.0000	1.000	Each	6.00	9.00	51.00	310.00	0.00	4.00	15.00	0.00
	Dunkin' Donuts-Muffin, Corn	96.0000	1.000	Each	7.00	12.00	51.00	340.00	0.00	1.00	40.00	0.00
	Dunkin' Donuts-Muffin, Cranberry	98.0000	1.000	Each	6.00	9.00	44.00	290.00	0.00	2.00	25.00	0.00
	Dunkin' Donuts-Muffin, Oat Bran	100.0000	1.000	Each	7.00	11.00	50.00	330.00	0.00	3.00	0.00	0.00
	Dunkin' Donuts-Yeast Ring, Choco	55.0000	1.000	Each	4.00	10.00	25.00	200.00	0.00	1.00	0.00	0.00
	Dunkin' Donuts-Yeast Ring, Glaze	55.0000	1.000	Each	4.00	9.00	26.00	200.00	0.00	1.00	0.00	0.00
265	Einstein Bros.-Almond Delight	360.0000	12.000	Fl Oz	8.00	4.50	29.00	190.00	0.00	0.00	20.00	3.00
266	Einstein Bros.-Almond Delight, I	480.0000	16.000	Fl Oz	7.00	4.00	28.00	180.00	0.00	0.00	15.00	2.50
267	Einstein Bros.-Almond Delight, N	360.0000	12.000	Fl Oz	8.00	0.00	29.00	150.00	0.00	0.00	5.00	0.00
268	Einstein Bros.-Americano	240.0000	8.000	Fl Oz	0.00	0.00	0.00	0.00	0.00	0.00	0.00	0.00
269	Einstein Bros.-Americano, Iced	360.0000	8.000	Fl Oz	0.00	0.00	0.00	0.00	0.00	0.00	0.00	0.00
270	Einstein Bros.-Bagel Chips, Blue	28.0000	1.000	Each	3.00	1.00	19.00	90.00	0.00	1.00	0.00	0.00
271	Einstein Bros.-Bagel Chips, Cinn	28.0000	1.000	Each	3.00	1.00	19.00	90.00	0.00	1.00	0.00	0.00
272	Einstein Bros.-Bagel Chips, Plai	28.0000	1.000	Each	3.00	0.00	18.00	90.00	0.00	1.00	0.00	0.00
273	Einstein Bros.-Bagel Chips, Sour	28.0000	1.000	Each	3.00	1.00	18.00	90.00	0.00	1.00	0.00	0.00
274	Einstein Bros.-Bagel Chips, Sun-	28.0000	1.000	Each	3.00	1.00	17.00	90.00	0.00	1.00	0.00	0.00
275	Einstein Bros.-Bagel Chips, Sunf	28.0000	1.000	Each	3.00	2.00	18.00	100.00	0.00	1.00	0.00	0.00
276	Einstein Bros.-Bagel, Blueberry,	113.0000	1.000	Each	11.00	1.00	77.00	350.00	0.00	3.00	0.00	0.00
277	Einstein Bros.-Bagel, Choc Chip	113.0000	1.000	Each	11.00	3.00	76.00	370.00	0.00	3.00	0.00	2.00
278	Einstein Bros.-Bagel, Cinnamon R	113.0000	1.000	Each	11.00	1.00	78.00	350.00	0.00	2.00	0.00	0.00
279	Einstein Bros.-Bagel, Cinnamon S	106.0000	1.000	Each	10.00	1.00	74.00	330.00	0.00	2.00	0.00	0.00
280	Einstein Bros.-Bagel, Cranberry	113.0000	1.000	Each	10.00	1.00	78.00	350.00	0.00	3.00	0.00	0.00
281	Einstein Bros.-Bagel, Egg	106.0000	1.000	Each	11.00	3.00	69.00	340.00	0.00	2.00	35.00	1.00
282	Einstein Bros.-Bagel, Everything	111.0000	1.000	Each	13.00	2.00	75.00	340.00	0.00	2.00	0.00	0.00
283	Einstein Bros.-Bagel, Garlic, Ch	119.0000	1.000	Each	13.00	3.00	79.00	380.00	0.00	4.00	0.00	1.00
284	Einstein Bros.-Bagel, Honey 8 Gr	106.0000	1.000	Each	11.00	1.00	69.00	320.00	0.00	4.00	0.00	0.00
285	Einstein Bros.-Bagel, Jalapeno	106.0000	1.000	Each	11.00	1.00	71.00	330.00	0.00	2.00	0.00	0.00
286	Einstein Bros.-Bagel, Nutty Bana	113.0000	1.000	Each	11.00	3.00	74.00	360.00	0.00	2.00	0.00	1.00
287	Einstein Bros.-Bagel, Onion, Chp	106.0000	1.000	Each	11.00	1.00	71.00	330.00	0.00	2.00	0.00	0.00
288	Einstein Bros.-Bagel, Plain	106.0000	1.000	Each	11.00	1.00	71.00	320.00	0.00	2.00	0.00	0.00
289	Einstein Bros.-Bagel, Poppy Dip'	111.0000	1.000	Each	12.00	2.00	74.00	350.00	0.00	2.00	0.00	0.00
290	Einstein Bros.-Bagel, Pumpernick	106.0000	1.000	Each	11.00	1.00	68.00	320.00	0.00	3.00	0.00	0.00
291	Einstein Bros.-Bagel, Rye, Marbl	113.0000	1.000	Each	11.00	2.00	73.00	340.00	0.00	3.00	0.00	0.00
292	Einstein Bros.-Bagel, Salt	111.0000	1.000	Each	11.00	1.00	73.00	330.00	0.00	2.00	0.00	0.00
293	Einstein Bros.-Bagel, Sesame Dip	117.0000	1.000	Each	11.00	5.00	75.00	380.00	0.00	3.00	0.00	1.00
294	Einstein Bros.-Bagel, Spinach He	106.0000	1.000	Each	11.00	1.00	68.00	310.00	0.00	3.00	0.00	0.00
295	Einstein Bros.-Bagel, Sun-dried	106.0000	1.000	Each	11.00	1.00	69.00	320.00	0.00	3.00	0.00	0.00

Monounsaturated Fat (gm)	Polyunsaturated Fat (gm)	Vitamin D (mg)	Vitamin K (mg)	Vitamin E (mg)	Vitamin A (re)	Vitamin C (mg)	Thiamin (mg)	Riboflavin (mg)	Niacin (mg)	Vitamin B_6 (mg)	Folate (mg)	Vitamin B_{12} (mcg)	Calcium (mg)	Iron (mg)	Magnesium (mg)	Phosphorus (mg)	Potassium (mg)	Sodium (mg)	Zinc (mg)
0.00	0.00	0.00	0.00	0.00	0.00	0.00	0.00	0.00	0.00	0.00	0.00	0.00	0.00	0.00	0.00	0.00	0.00	260.00	0.00
0.00	0.00	0.00	0.00	0.00	0.00	0.00	0.00	0.00	0.00	0.00	0.00	0.00	0.00	0.00	0.00	0.00	0.00	240.00	0.00
0.00	0.00	0.00	0.00	0.00	0.00	0.00	0.00	0.00	0.00	0.00	0.00	0.00	0.00	0.00	0.00	0.00	0.00	370.00	0.00
0.00	0.00	0.00	0.00	0.00	0.00	0.00	0.00	0.00	0.00	0.00	0.00	0.00	0.00	0.00	0.00	0.00	0.00	330.00	0.00
0.00	0.00	0.00	0.00	0.00	0.00	0.00	0.00	0.00	0.00	0.00	0.00	0.00	0.00	0.00	0.00	0.00	0.00	383.00	0.00
0.00	0.00	0.00	0.00	0.00	0.00	0.00	0.00	0.00	0.00	0.00	0.00	0.00	0.00	0.00	0.00	0.00	0.00	310.00	0.00
0.00	0.00	0.00	0.00	0.00	0.00	0.00	0.00	0.00	0.00	0.00	0.00	0.00	0.00	0.00	0.00	0.00	0.00	110.00	0.00
0.00	0.00	0.00	0.00	0.00	0.00	0.00	0.00	0.00	0.00	0.00	0.00	0.00	0.00	0.00	0.00	0.00	0.00	100.00	0.00
0.00	0.00	0.00	0.00	0.00	0.00	0.00	0.00	0.00	0.00	0.00	0.00	0.00	0.00	0.00	0.00	0.00	0.00	100.00	0.00
0.00	0.00	0.00	0.00	0.00	0.00	0.00	0.00	0.00	0.00	0.00	0.00	0.00	0.00	0.00	0.00	0.00	0.00	280.00	0.00
0.00	0.00	0.00	0.00	0.00	0.00	0.00	0.00	0.00	0.00	0.00	0.00	0.00	0.00	0.00	0.00	0.00	0.00	220.00	0.00
0.00	0.00	0.00	0.00	0.00	0.00	0.00	0.00	0.00	0.00	0.00	0.00	0.00	0.00	0.00	0.00	0.00	0.00	240.00	0.00
0.00	0.00	0.00	0.00	0.00	0.00	0.00	0.00	0.00	0.00	0.00	0.00	0.00	0.00	0.00	0.00	0.00	0.00	130.00	0.00
0.00	0.00	0.00	0.00	0.00	0.00	0.00	0.00	0.00	0.00	0.00	0.00	0.00	0.00	0.00	0.00	0.00	0.00	230.00	0.00
0.00	0.00	0.00	0.00	0.00	0.00	0.00	0.00	0.00	0.00	0.00	0.00	0.00	0.00	0.00	0.00	0.00	0.00	280.00	0.00
0.00	0.00	0.00	0.00	0.00	0.00	0.00	0.00	0.00	0.00	0.00	0.00	0.00	0.00	0.00	0.00	0.00	0.00	360.00	0.00
0.00	0.00	0.00	0.00	0.00	0.00	0.00	0.00	0.00	0.00	0.00	0.00	0.00	0.00	0.00	0.00	0.00	0.00	410.00	0.00
0.00	0.00	0.00	0.00	0.00	0.00	0.00	0.00	0.00	0.00	0.00	0.00	0.00	0.00	0.00	0.00	0.00	0.00	340.00	0.00
0.00	0.00	0.00	0.00	0.00	0.00	0.00	0.00	0.00	0.00	0.00	0.00	0.00	0.00	0.00	0.00	0.00	0.00	560.00	0.00
0.00	0.00	0.00	0.00	0.00	0.00	0.00	0.00	0.00	0.00	0.00	0.00	0.00	0.00	0.00	0.00	0.00	0.00	560.00	0.00
0.00	0.00	0.00	0.00	0.00	0.00	0.00	0.00	0.00	0.00	0.00	0.00	0.00	0.00	0.00	0.00	0.00	0.00	360.00	0.00
0.00	0.00	0.00	0.00	0.00	0.00	0.00	0.00	0.00	0.00	0.00	0.00	0.00	0.00	0.00	0.00	0.00	0.00	450.00	0.00
0.00	0.00	0.00	0.00	0.00	0.00	0.00	0.00	0.00	0.00	0.00	0.00	0.00	0.00	0.00	0.00	0.00	0.00	190.00	0.00
0.00	0.00	0.00	0.00	0.00	0.00	0.00	0.00	0.00	0.00	0.00	0.00	0.00	0.00	0.00	0.00	0.00	0.00	230.00	0.00
0.00	0.00	0.00	0.00	0.00	0.00	0.00	0.00	0.00	0.00	0.00	0.00	0.00	0.00	0.00	0.00	0.00	0.00	130.00	0.00
0.00	0.00	0.00	0.00	0.00	0.00	0.00	0.00	0.00	0.00	0.00	0.00	0.00	0.00	0.00	0.00	0.00	0.00	120.00	0.00
0.00	0.00	0.00	0.00	0.00	0.00	0.00	0.00	0.00	0.00	0.00	0.00	0.00	0.00	0.00	0.00	0.00	0.00	135.00	0.00
0.00	0.00	0.00	0.00	0.00	0.00	0.00	0.00	0.00	0.00	0.00	0.00	0.00	0.00	0.00	0.00	0.00	0.00	0.00	0.00
0.00	0.00	0.00	0.00	0.00	0.00	0.00	0.00	0.00	0.00	0.00	0.00	0.00	0.00	0.00	0.00	0.00	0.00	0.00	0.00
0.00	0.00	0.00	0.00	0.00	0.00	0.00	0.00	0.00	0.00	0.00	0.00	0.00	0.00	0.00	0.00	0.00	0.00	105.00	0.00
0.00	0.00	0.00	0.00	0.00	0.00	0.00	0.00	0.00	0.00	0.00	0.00	0.00	0.00	0.00	0.00	0.00	0.00	120.00	0.00
0.00	0.00	0.00	0.00	0.00	0.00	0.00	0.00	0.00	0.00	0.00	0.00	0.00	0.00	0.00	0.00	0.00	0.00	140.00	0.00
0.00	0.00	0.00	0.00	0.00	0.00	0.00	0.00	0.00	0.00	0.00	0.00	0.00	0.00	0.00	0.00	0.00	0.00	120.00	0.00
0.00	0.00	0.00	0.00	0.00	0.00	0.00	0.00	0.00	0.00	0.00	0.00	0.00	0.00	0.00	0.00	0.00	0.00	130.00	0.00
0.00	0.00	0.00	0.00	0.00	0.00	0.00	0.00	0.00	0.00	0.00	0.00	0.00	0.00	0.00	0.00	0.00	0.00	190.00	0.00
0.00	0.00	0.00	0.00	0.00	0.00	0.00	0.00	0.00	0.00	0.00	0.00	0.00	0.00	0.00	0.00	0.00	0.00	510.00	0.00
0.00	0.00	0.00	0.00	0.00	0.00	0.00	0.00	0.00	0.00	0.00	0.00	0.00	0.00	0.00	0.00	0.00	0.00	500.00	0.00
0.00	0.00	0.00	0.00	0.00	0.00	0.00	0.00	0.00	0.00	0.00	0.00	0.00	0.00	0.00	0.00	0.00	0.00	490.00	0.00
0.00	0.00	0.00	0.00	0.00	0.00	0.00	0.00	0.00	0.00	0.00	0.00	0.00	0.00	0.00	0.00	0.00	0.00	490.00	0.00
0.00	0.00	0.00	0.00	0.00	0.00	0.00	0.00	0.00	0.00	0.00	0.00	0.00	0.00	0.00	0.00	0.00	0.00	490.00	0.00
0.00	0.00	0.00	0.00	0.00	0.00	0.00	0.00	0.00	0.00	0.00	0.00	0.00	0.00	0.00	0.00	0.00	0.00	510.00	0.00
0.00	0.00	0.00	0.00	0.00	0.00	0.00	0.00	0.00	0.00	0.00	0.00	0.00	0.00	0.00	0.00	0.00	0.00	820.00	0.00
0.00	0.00	0.00	0.00	0.00	0.00	0.00	0.00	0.00	0.00	0.00	0.00	0.00	0.00	0.00	0.00	0.00	0.00	680.00	0.00
0.00	0.00	0.00	0.00	0.00	0.00	0.00	0.00	0.00	0.00	0.00	0.00	0.00	0.00	0.00	0.00	0.00	0.00	510.00	0.00
0.00	0.00	0.00	0.00	0.00	0.00	0.00	0.00	0.00	0.00	0.00	0.00	0.00	0.00	0.00	0.00	0.00	0.00	510.00	0.00
0.00	0.00	0.00	0.00	0.00	0.00	0.00	0.00	0.00	0.00	0.00	0.00	0.00	0.00	0.00	0.00	0.00	0.00	510.00	0.00
0.00	0.00	0.00	0.00	0.00	0.00	0.00	0.00	0.00	0.00	0.00	0.00	0.00	0.00	0.00	0.00	0.00	0.00	500.00	0.00
0.00	0.00	0.00	0.00	0.00	0.00	0.00	0.00	0.00	0.00	0.00	0.00	0.00	0.00	0.00	0.00	0.00	0.00	520.00	0.00
0.00	0.00	0.00	0.00	0.00	0.00	0.00	0.00	0.00	0.00	0.00	0.00	0.00	0.00	0.00	0.00	0.00	0.00	680.00	0.00
0.00	0.00	0.00	0.00	0.00	0.00	0.00	0.00	0.00	0.00	0.00	0.00	0.00	0.00	0.00	0.00	0.00	0.00	730.00	0.00
0.00	0.00	0.00	0.00	0.00	0.00	0.00	0.00	0.00	0.00	0.00	0.00	0.00	0.00	0.00	0.00	0.00	0.00	690.00	0.00
0.00	0.00	0.00	0.00	0.00	0.00	0.00	0.00	0.00	0.00	0.00	0.00	0.00	0.00	0.00	0.00	0.00	0.00	1790.00	0.00
0.00	0.00	0.00	0.00	0.00	0.00	0.00	0.00	0.00	0.00	0.00	0.00	0.00	0.00	0.00	0.00	0.00	0.00	680.00	0.00
0.00	0.00	0.00	0.00	0.00	0.00	0.00	0.00	0.00	0.00	0.00	0.00	0.00	0.00	0.00	0.00	0.00	0.00	520.00	0.00
0.00	0.00	0.00	0.00	0.00	0.00	0.00	0.00	0.00	0.00	0.00	0.00	0.00	0.00	0.00	0.00	0.00	0.00	520.00	0.00

USDA ID Code	Food Name	Weight in Grams*	Quantity of Units	Unit of Measure	Protein (gm)	Fat (gm)	Carbohydrate (gm)	Kcalories	Caffeine (gm)	Fiber (gm)	Cholesterol (mg)	Saturated Fat (gm)
296	Einstein Bros.-Bagel, Sunflower	106.0000	1.000	Each	12.00	5.00	66.00	350.00	0.00	3.00	0.00	1.00
297	Einstein Bros.-Bagel, Veggie Con	106.0000	1.000	Each	11.00	1.00	70.00	320.00	0.00	2.00	0.00	0.00
298	Einstein Bros.-Brownie, Choc Cho	79.5200	2.800	Ounce	3.00	15.00	51.00	346.00	0.00	2.00	18.00	4.00
299	Einstein Bros.-Caf_ Au Lait	360.0000	12.000	Fl Oz	6.00	3.50	9.00	100.00	0.00	0.00	15.00	2.00
300	Einstein Bros.-Caf_ Au Lait, Non	360.0000	12.000	Fl Oz	6.00	0.00	10.00	70.00	0.00	0.00	5.00	0.00
301	Einstein Bros.-Caf_ Latte, Iced	480.0000	16.000	Fl Oz	8.00	4.50	12.00	120.00	0.00	0.00	20.00	3.00
302	Einstein Bros.-Caf_ Latte, Non F	360.0000	12.000	Fl Oz	9.00	0.00	14.00	100.00	0.00	0.00	5.00	0.00
303	Einstein Bros.-Caf_ Latte, Reg	360.0000	12.000	Fl Oz	9.00	5.00	13.00	140.00	0.00	0.00	20.00	3.50
304	Einstein Bros.-Cappuccino	360.0000	12.000	Fl Oz	6.00	3.50	9.00	90.00	0.00	0.00	15.00	2.00
305	Einstein Bros.-Cappuccino, Non F	360.0000	12.000	Fl Oz	6.00	0.00	9.00	60.00	0.00	0.00	5.00	0.00
306	Einstein Bros.-Cheese Melt, Gril	213.0000	1.000	Each	25.00	12.00	74.00	500.00	0.00	3.00	35.00	7.00
307	Einstein Bros.-Chicken Salad, Re	113.6000	4.000	Ounce	16.00	7.00	4.00	150.00	0.00	0.00	45.00	1.50
308	Einstein Bros.-Chili, Turkey, Lo	198.8000	7.000	Ounce	6.00	2.50	9.00	80.00	0.00	3.00	20.00	0.00
309	Einstein Bros.-Chili, Vegetarian	198.8000	7.000	Ounce	3.00	2.00	23.00	120.00	0.00	4.00	0.00	0.00
310	Einstein Bros.-Chix Salad Bagel	324.0000	1.000	Each	28.00	9.00	79.00	510.00	0.00	4.00	45.00	2.00
311	Einstein Bros.-Choc, Hot, Lower	360.0000	12.000	Fl Oz	9.00	7.00	39.00	260.00	0.00	0.00	5.00	6.00
312	Einstein Bros.-Chocolate, Hot, R	360.0000	12.000	Fl Oz	9.00	11.00	39.00	290.00	0.00	0.00	20.00	8.00
313	Einstein Bros.-Chowder, Corn, Am	198.8000	7.000	Ounce	5.00	6.00	25.00	180.00	0.00	2.00	5.00	1.50
314	Einstein Bros.-Chowder, NE Clam	198.8000	7.000	Ounce	9.00	9.00	15.00	170.00	0.00	1.00	25.00	2.50
315	Einstein Bros.-Cinnamon Bun, Ice	142.0000	5.000	Ounce	11.00	16.00	89.00	545.00	0.00	3.00	20.00	5.00
316	Einstein Bros.-Coffee, Reg	360.0000	12.000	Fl Oz	0.00	0.00	0.00	0.00	0.00	0.00	0.00	0.00
317	Einstein Bros.-Coleslaw, Low Fat	113.6000	4.000	Ounce	2.00	3.50	13.00	90.00	0.00	2.00	5.00	0.50
318	Einstein Bros.-Coleslaw, Low Fat	113.6000	4.000	Ounce	1.00	3.50	13.00	90.00	0.00	2.00	5.00	0.50
319	Einstein Bros.-Cookie, Black & W	113.6000	4.000	Ounce	3.00	12.00	68.00	390.00	0.00	1.00	15.00	3.00
320	Einstein Bros.-Cookie, Chocolate	113.6000	4.000	Ounce	6.00	24.00	68.00	510.00	0.00	2.00	35.00	9.00
321	Einstein Bros.-Cookie, Oatmeal R	113.6000	4.000	Ounce	7.00	18.00	70.00	470.00	0.00	3.00	40.00	4.00
322	Einstein Bros.-Cookie, Peanut Bu	113.6000	4.000	Ounce	10.00	31.00	55.00	540.00	0.00	3.00	40.00	6.00
323	Einstein Bros.-Cookie, Sugar	113.6000	4.000	Ounce	6.00	28.00	28.00	530.00	0.00	1.00	45.00	7.00
324	Einstein Bros.-Cream Cheese, Ch	30.0000	2.000	Tbsp	2.00	9.00	2.00	100.00	0.00	0.00	30.00	6.00
325	Einstein Bros.-Cream Cheese, Pl	30.0000	2.000	Tbsp	2.00	5.00	2.00	60.00	0.00	0.00	15.00	3.00
326	Einstein Bros.-Cream Cheese, Cra	30.0000	2.000	Tbsp	2.00	8.00	5.00	100.00	0.00	0.00	25.00	6.00
327	Einstein Bros.-Cream Cheese, Gar	30.0000	2.000	Tbsp	2.00	9.00	2.00	100.00	0.00	0.00	30.00	6.00
328	Einstein Bros.-Cream Cheese, Jal	30.0000	2.000	Tbsp	2.00	8.00	2.00	90.00	0.00	0.00	25.00	6.00
329	Einstein Bros.-Cream Cheese, Map	30.0000	2.000	Tbsp	2.00	9.00	5.00	100.00	0.00	0.00	25.00	6.00
330	Einstein Bros.-Cream Cheese, Pla	30.0000	2.000	Tbsp	2.00	10.00	2.00	100.00	0.00	0.00	30.00	7.00
331	Einstein Bros.-Cream Cheese, Sal	30.0000	2.000	Tbsp	2.00	8.00	2.00	90.00	0.00	0.00	25.00	6.00
332	Einstein Bros.-Cream Cheese, Str	30.0000	2.000	Tbsp	2.00	8.00	5.00	100.00	0.00	0.00	25.00	6.00
333	Einstein Bros.-Cream Cheese, Sun	30.0000	2.000	Tbsp	2.00	9.00	2.00	100.00	0.00	0.00	30.00	6.00
334	Einstein Bros.-Cream Cheese, Veg	30.0000	2.000	Tbsp	2.00	5.00	2.00	60.00	0.00	0.00	16.00	4.00
335	Einstein Bros.-Cream Cheese, Wil	30.0000	2.000	Tbsp	2.00	5.00	6.00	70.00	0.00	0.00	15.00	4.00
336	Einstein Bros.-Cream Cheese-Hone	30.0000	2.000	Tbsp	2.00	9.00	5.00	100.00	0.00	0.00	25.00	6.00
337	Einstein Bros.-Egg, Scr, & Bacon	225.0000	1.000	Each	30.00	23.00	72.00	620.00	0.00	2.00	395.00	10.00
338	Einstein Bros.-Egg, Scr, & Ham B	248.0000	1.000	Each	34.00	18.00	74.00	590.00	0.00	2.00	405.00	8.00
339	Einstein Bros.-Egg, Scr, & Sausa	250.0000	1.000	Each	31.00	30.00	72.00	690.00	0.00	2.00	415.00	12.00
340	Einstein Bros.-Egg, Scr, & Turk	257.0000	1.000	Each	37.00	19.00	72.00	604.00	0.00	2.00	409.00	8.00
341	Einstein Bros.-Egg, Scr, Bagel S	212.0000	1.000	Each	27.00	16.00	72.00	540.00	0.00	2.00	385.00	7.00
342	Einstein Bros.-Espresso	45.0000	1.500	Fl Oz	0.00	0.00	0.00	1.00	0.00	0.00	0.00	0.00
343	Einstein Bros.-Fruit & Yogurt Cu	227.2000	8.000	Ounce	6.00	1.00	32.00	160.00	0.00	4.00	0.00	0.00
344	Einstein Bros.-Fruit Salad	227.2000	8.000	Ounce	1.00	0.50	25.00	110.00	0.00	2.00	0.00	0.00
345	Einstein Bros.-Fruit Salad, Ruby	113.6000	4.000	Ounce	0.00	0.00	23.00	90.00	0.00	1.00	0.00	0.00
346	Einstein Bros.-Fusilli w/ Olives	170.4000	6.000	Ounce	6.00	23.00	33.00	360.00	0.00	3.00	0.00	3.00
347	Einstein Bros.-Ham /Cheese Bagel	275.0000	1.000	Each	32.00	15.00	79.00	580.00	0.00	3.00	70.00	6.00
348	Einstein Bros.-Ham, Deli, Bagel	305.0000	1.000	Each	37.00	17.00	78.00	620.00	0.00	3.00	85.00	10.00
349	Einstein Bros.-Hummus	30.0000	2.000	Tbsp	2.00	3.50	6.00	60.00	0.00	1.00	0.00	0.50
350	Einstein Bros.-Hummus Bagel Sand	248.0000	1.000	Each	15.00	8.00	86.00	480.00	0.00	5.00	0.00	1.00

Monounsaturated Fat (gm)	Polyunsaturated Fat (gm)	Vitamin D (mg)	Vitamin K (mg)	Vitamin E (mg)	Vitamin A (re)	Vitamin C (mg)	Thiamin (mg)	Riboflavin (mg)	Niacin (mg)	Vitamin B6 (mg)	Folate (mg)	Vitamin B12 (mcg)	Calcium (mg)	Iron (mg)	Magnesium (mg)	Phosphorus (mg)	Potassium (mg)	Sodium (mg)	Zinc (mg)
0.00	0.00	0.00	0.00	0.00	0.00	0.00	0.00	0.00	0.00	0.00	0.00	0.00	0.00	0.00	0.00	0.00	0.00	710.00	0.00
0.00	0.00	0.00	0.00	0.00	0.00	0.00	0.00	0.00	0.00	0.00	0.00	0.00	0.00	0.00	0.00	0.00	0.00	490.00	0.00
0.00	0.00	0.00	0.00	0.00	0.00	0.00	0.00	0.00	0.00	0.00	0.00	0.00	0.00	0.00	0.00	0.00	0.00	193.00	0.00
0.00	0.00	0.00	0.00	0.00	0.00	0.00	0.00	0.00	0.00	0.00	0.00	0.00	0.00	0.00	0.00	0.00	0.00	95.00	0.00
0.00	0.00	0.00	0.00	0.00	0.00	0.00	0.00	0.00	0.00	0.00	0.00	0.00	0.00	0.00	0.00	0.00	0.00	100.00	0.00
0.00	0.00	0.00	0.00	0.00	0.00	0.00	0.00	0.00	0.00	0.00	0.00	0.00	0.00	0.00	0.00	0.00	0.00	125.00	0.00
0.00	0.00	0.00	0.00	0.00	0.00	0.00	0.00	0.00	0.00	0.00	0.00	0.00	0.00	0.00	0.00	0.00	0.00	140.00	0.00
0.00	0.00	0.00	0.00	0.00	0.00	0.00	0.00	0.00	0.00	0.00	0.00	0.00	0.00	0.00	0.00	0.00	0.00	140.00	0.00
0.00	0.00	0.00	0.00	0.00	0.00	0.00	0.00	0.00	0.00	0.00	0.00	0.00	0.00	0.00	0.00	0.00	0.00	95.00	0.00
0.00	0.00	0.00	0.00	0.00	0.00	0.00	0.00	0.00	0.00	0.00	0.00	0.00	0.00	0.00	0.00	0.00	0.00	95.00	0.00
0.00	0.00	0.00	0.00	0.00	0.00	0.00	0.00	0.00	0.00	0.00	0.00	0.00	0.00	0.00	0.00	0.00	0.00	970.00	0.00
0.00	0.00	0.00	0.00	0.00	0.00	0.00	0.00	0.00	0.00	0.00	0.00	0.00	0.00	0.00	0.00	0.00	0.00	540.00	0.00
0.00	0.00	0.00	0.00	0.00	0.00	0.00	0.00	0.00	0.00	0.00	0.00	0.00	0.00	0.00	0.00	0.00	0.00	320.00	0.00
0.00	0.00	0.00	0.00	0.00	0.00	0.00	0.00	0.00	0.00	0.00	0.00	0.00	0.00	0.00	0.00	0.00	0.00	730.00	0.00
0.00	0.00	0.00	0.00	0.00	0.00	0.00	0.00	0.00	0.00	0.00	0.00	0.00	0.00	0.00	0.00	0.00	0.00	1060.00	0.00
0.00	0.00	0.00	0.00	0.00	0.00	0.00	0.00	0.00	0.00	0.00	0.00	0.00	0.00	0.00	0.00	0.00	0.00	160.00	0.00
0.00	0.00	0.00	0.00	0.00	0.00	0.00	0.00	0.00	0.00	0.00	0.00	0.00	0.00	0.00	0.00	0.00	0.00	160.00	0.00
0.00	0.00	0.00	0.00	0.00	0.00	0.00	0.00	0.00	0.00	0.00	0.00	0.00	0.00	0.00	0.00	0.00	0.00	670.00	0.00
0.00	0.00	0.00	0.00	0.00	0.00	0.00	0.00	0.00	0.00	0.00	0.00	0.00	0.00	0.00	0.00	0.00	0.00	820.00	0.00
0.00	0.00	0.00	0.00	0.00	0.00	0.00	0.00	0.00	0.00	0.00	0.00	0.00	0.00	0.00	0.00	0.00	0.00	656.00	0.00
0.00	0.00	0.00	0.00	0.00	0.00	0.00	0.00	0.00	0.00	0.00	0.00	0.00	0.00	0.00	0.00	0.00	0.00	0.00	0.00
0.00	0.00	0.00	0.00	0.00	0.00	0.00	0.00	0.00	0.00	0.00	0.00	0.00	0.00	0.00	0.00	0.00	0.00	300.00	0.00
0.00	0.00	0.00	0.00	0.00	0.00	0.00	0.00	0.00	0.00	0.00	0.00	0.00	0.00	0.00	0.00	0.00	0.00	300.00	0.00
0.00	0.00	0.00	0.00	0.00	0.00	0.00	0.00	0.00	0.00	0.00	0.00	0.00	0.00	0.00	0.00	0.00	0.00	260.00	0.00
0.00	0.00	0.00	0.00	0.00	0.00	0.00	0.00	0.00	0.00	0.00	0.00	0.00	0.00	0.00	0.00	0.00	0.00	390.00	0.00
0.00	0.00	0.00	0.00	0.00	0.00	0.00	0.00	0.00	0.00	0.00	0.00	0.00	0.00	0.00	0.00	0.00	0.00	360.00	0.00
0.00	0.00	0.00	0.00	0.00	0.00	0.00	0.00	0.00	0.00	0.00	0.00	0.00	0.00	0.00	0.00	0.00	0.00	620.00	0.00
0.00	0.00	0.00	0.00	0.00	0.00	0.00	0.00	0.00	0.00	0.00	0.00	0.00	0.00	0.00	0.00	0.00	0.00	420.00	0.00
0.00	0.00	0.00	0.00	0.00	0.00	0.00	0.00	0.00	0.00	0.00	0.00	0.00	0.00	0.00	0.00	0.00	0.00	130.00	0.00
0.00	0.00	0.00	0.00	0.00	0.00	0.00	0.00	0.00	0.00	0.00	0.00	0.00	0.00	0.00	0.00	0.00	0.00	110.00	0.00
0.00	0.00	0.00	0.00	0.00	0.00	0.00	0.00	0.00	0.00	0.00	0.00	0.00	0.00	0.00	0.00	0.00	0.00	80.00	0.00
0.00	0.00	0.00	0.00	0.00	0.00	0.00	0.00	0.00	0.00	0.00	0.00	0.00	0.00	0.00	0.00	0.00	0.00	135.00	0.00
0.00	0.00	0.00	0.00	0.00	0.00	0.00	0.00	0.00	0.00	0.00	0.00	0.00	0.00	0.00	0.00	0.00	0.00	140.00	0.00
0.00	0.00	0.00	0.00	0.00	0.00	0.00	0.00	0.00	0.00	0.00	0.00	0.00	0.00	0.00	0.00	0.00	0.00	80.00	0.00
0.00	0.00	0.00	0.00	0.00	0.00	0.00	0.00	0.00	0.00	0.00	0.00	0.00	0.00	0.00	0.00	0.00	0.00	100.00	0.00
0.00	0.00	0.00	0.00	0.00	0.00	0.00	0.00	0.00	0.00	0.00	0.00	0.00	0.00	0.00	0.00	0.00	0.00	210.00	0.00
0.00	0.00	0.00	0.00	0.00	0.00	0.00	0.00	0.00	0.00	0.00	0.00	0.00	0.00	0.00	0.00	0.00	0.00	80.00	0.00
0.00	0.00	0.00	0.00	0.00	0.00	0.00	0.00	0.00	0.00	0.00	0.00	0.00	0.00	0.00	0.00	0.00	0.00	100.00	0.00
0.00	0.00	0.00	0.00	0.00	0.00	0.00	0.00	0.00	0.00	0.00	0.00	0.00	0.00	0.00	0.00	0.00	0.00	150.00	0.00
0.00	0.00	0.00	0.00	0.00	0.00	0.00	0.00	0.00	0.00	0.00	0.00	0.00	0.00	0.00	0.00	0.00	0.00	90.00	0.00
0.00	0.00	0.00	0.00	0.00	0.00	0.00	0.00	0.00	0.00	0.00	0.00	0.00	0.00	0.00	0.00	0.00	0.00	80.00	0.00
0.00	0.00	0.00	0.00	0.00	0.00	0.00	0.00	0.00	0.00	0.00	0.00	0.00	0.00	0.00	0.00	0.00	0.00	950.00	0.00
0.00	0.00	0.00	0.00	0.00	0.00	0.00	0.00	0.00	0.00	0.00	0.00	0.00	0.00	0.00	0.00	0.00	0.00	1120.00	0.00
0.00	0.00	0.00	0.00	0.00	0.00	0.00	0.00	0.00	0.00	0.00	0.00	0.00	0.00	0.00	0.00	0.00	0.00	980.00	0.00
0.00	0.00	0.00	0.00	0.00	0.00	0.00	0.00	0.00	0.00	0.00	0.00	0.00	0.00	0.00	0.00	0.00	0.00	1070.00	0.00
0.00	0.00	0.00	0.00	0.00	0.00	0.00	0.00	0.00	0.00	0.00	0.00	0.00	0.00	0.00	0.00	0.00	0.00	750.00	0.00
0.00	0.00	0.00	0.00	0.00	0.00	0.00	0.00	0.00	0.00	0.00	0.00	0.00	0.00	0.00	0.00	0.00	0.00	0.00	0.00
0.00	0.00	0.00	0.00	0.00	0.00	0.00	0.00	0.00	0.00	0.00	0.00	0.00	0.00	0.00	0.00	0.00	0.00	95.00	0.00
0.00	0.00	0.00	0.00	0.00	0.00	0.00	0.00	0.00	0.00	0.00	0.00	0.00	0.00	0.00	0.00	0.00	0.00	10.00	0.00
0.00	0.00	0.00	0.00	0.00	0.00	0.00	0.00	0.00	0.00	0.00	0.00	0.00	0.00	0.00	0.00	0.00	0.00	20.00	0.00
0.00	0.00	0.00	0.00	0.00	0.00	0.00	0.00	0.00	0.00	0.00	0.00	0.00	0.00	0.00	0.00	0.00	0.00	290.00	0.00
0.00	0.00	0.00	0.00	0.00	0.00	0.00	0.00	0.00	0.00	0.00	0.00	0.00	0.00	0.00	0.00	0.00	0.00	1400.00	0.00
0.00	0.00	0.00	0.00	0.00	0.00	0.00	0.00	0.00	0.00	0.00	0.00	0.00	0.00	0.00	0.00	0.00	0.00	1690.00	0.00
0.00	0.00	0.00	0.00	0.00	0.00	0.00	0.00	0.00	0.00	0.00	0.00	0.00	0.00	0.00	0.00	0.00	0.00	65.00	0.00
0.00	0.00	0.00	0.00	0.00	0.00	0.00	0.00	0.00	0.00	0.00	0.00	0.00	0.00	0.00	0.00	0.00	0.00	640.00	0.00

USDA ID Code	Food Name	Weight in Grams*	Quantity of Units	Unit of Measure	Protein (gm)	Fat (gm)	Carbohydrate (gm)	Kcalories	Caffeine (gm)	Fiber (gm)	Cholesterol (mg)	Saturated Fat (gm)
351	Einstein Bros.-Hummus, Carrot	57.0000	4.000	Tbsp	3.00	2.00	9.00	60.00	0.00	2.00	0.00	0.00
352	Einstein Bros.-Hummus, Carrot, S	248.0000	1.000	Each	15.00	3.00	83.00	420.00	0.00	5.00	0.00	0.00
353	Einstein Bros.-Intellicino, Iced	480.0000	16.000	Fl Oz	6.00	7.00	13.00	140.00	0.00	0.00	15.00	4.00
354	Einstein Bros.-Intellicino, Low	360.0000	12.000	Fl Oz	7.00	3.50	15.00	120.00	0.00	0.00	5.00	2.50
355	Einstein Bros.-Intellicino, Reg	360.0000	12.000	Fl Oz	7.00	7.00	14.00	150.00	0.00	0.00	15.00	4.50
356	Einstein Bros.-Lox & Bagel	318.0000	1.000	Each	26.00	24.00	77.00	630.00	0.00	3.00	75.00	13.00
357	Einstein Bros.-Mocha, Iced	480.0000	16.000	Fl Oz	7.00	6.00	33.00	210.00	0.00	0.00	15.00	4.00
358	Einstein Bros.-Mocha, Low Fat, R	360.0000	12.000	Fl Oz	8.00	2.50	34.00	190.00	0.00	0.00	5.00	2.00
359	Einstein Bros.-Mocha, Reg	360.0000	12.000	Fl Oz	8.00	6.00	34.00	230.00	0.00	0.00	15.00	4.50
360	Einstein Bros.-Muffin, Apple Dat	56.8000	2.000	Ounce	3.00	2.00	35.00	160.00	0.00	2.00	0.00	0.00
361	Einstein Bros.-Muffin, Banana	56.8000	2.000	Ounce	3.00	12.00	25.00	220.00	0.00	0.00	40.00	2.00
362	Einstein Bros.-Muffin, Blueberry	56.8000	2.000	Ounce	3.00	10.00	25.00	200.00	0.00	0.00	40.00	2.00
363	Einstein Bros.-Muffin, Chocolate	56.8000	2.000	Ounce	3.00	13.00	28.00	240.00	0.00	0.00	40.00	3.00
364	Einstein Bros.-Muffin, Cran Oran	56.8000	2.000	Ounce	4.00	0.50	27.00	130.00	0.00	1.00	0.00	0.00
365	Einstein Bros.-Muffin, Lemon Pop	56.8000	2.000	Ounce	3.00	3.00	28.00	150.00	0.00	0.00	0.00	0.00
366	Einstein Bros.-Muffin, Wildberry	56.8000	2.000	Ounce	3.00	0.50	26.00	120.00	0.00	1.00	0.00	0.00
368	Einstein Bros.-Pastrami, Turkey,	305.0000	1.000	Each	37.00	16.00	78.00	600.00	0.00	3.00	85.00	9.00
369	Einstein Bros.-Pastrami, Turkey,	347.0000	1.000	Each	45.00	34.00	77.00	790.00	0.00	3.00	90.00	19.00
367	Einstein Bros.-PB&J Bagel Sandwi	172.0000	1.000	Each	18.00	17.00	99.00	595.00	0.00	4.00	0.00	2.00
370	Einstein Bros.-Peanut Butter, Cr	32.0000	2.000	Tbsp	7.00	16.00	8.00	190.00	0.00	2.00	0.00	2.00
371	Einstein Bros.-Pizza Melt, 3 Che	234.0000	1.000	Each	32.00	18.00	78.00	600.00	0.00	3.00	55.00	10.00
372	Einstein Bros.-Pizza Melt, Peppe	263.0000	1.000	Each	38.00	30.00	79.00	740.00	0.00	3.00	85.00	15.00
373	Einstein Bros.-Pizza Melt, Tomat	277.0000	1.000	Each	32.00	18.00	80.00	610.00	0.00	3.00	55.00	10.00
374	Einstein Bros.-Reuben Bagel Sand	319.0000	1.000	Each	42.00	33.00	82.00	790.00	0.00	5.00	100.00	12.00
375	Einstein Bros.-Salad, Caesar, Ch	269.8000	9.500	Ounce	26.00	37.00	11.00	480.00	0.00	2.00	75.00	8.00
376	Einstein Bros.-Salad, Caesar, La	198.8000	7.000	Ounce	9.00	35.00	10.00	390.00	0.00	2.00	25.00	7.00
377	Einstein Bros.-Salad, Caesar, Re	99.4000	3.500	Ounce	5.00	18.00	7.00	210.00	0.00	1.00	15.00	4.00
378	Einstein Bros.-Salad, Clairemont	113.6000	4.000	Ounce	1.00	4.00	9.00	70.00	0.00	2.00	0.00	0.00
379	Einstein Bros.-Salad, Pasta, Gre	255.6000	9.000	Ounce	12.00	30.00	35.00	270.00	0.00	3.00	45.00	9.00
380	Einstein Bros.-Salad, Pasta, Zit	113.6000	4.000	Ounce	4.00	11.00	20.00	200.00	0.00	2.00	0.00	2.00
381	Einstein Bros.-Salad, Potato & D	113.6000	4.000	Ounce	2.00	0.50	20.00	150.00	0.00	1.00	0.00	0.00
382	Einstein Bros.-Salad, Potato & M	113.6000	4.000	Ounce	2.00	2.50	19.00	110.00	0.00	2.00	0.00	0.00
383	Einstein Bros.-Salad, Potato, Id	113.6000	4.000	Ounce	2.00	7.00	19.00	150.00	0.00	1.00	5.00	1.50
384	Einstein Bros.-Salad, Potato, Ol	113.6000	4.000	Ounce	3.00	8.00	16.00	140.00	0.00	1.00	40.00	1.50
385	Einstein Bros.-Scone, Blueberry	99.4000	3.500	Ounce	8.00	8.50	49.00	295.00	0.00	1.50	20.00	4.50
386	Einstein Bros.-Scone, Cheddar Ch	99.4000	3.500	Ounce	8.00	15.00	37.00	310.00	0.00	2.00	35.00	8.00
387	Einstein Bros.-Scone, Cinnamon	99.4000	3.500	Ounce	8.00	11.00	50.00	325.00	0.00	1.50	20.00	5.50
388	Einstein Bros.-Soup, Bean, Black	198.8000	7.000	Ounce	3.00	1.00	11.00	70.00	0.00	2.00	0.00	0.00
389	Einstein Bros.-Soup, Bean, Monte	198.8000	7.000	Ounce	5.00	2.00	19.00	120.00	0.00	5.00	0.00	0.00
390	Einstein Bros.-Soup, Cheddar & B	198.8000	7.000	Ounce	5.00	10.00	14.00	170.00	0.00	1.00	15.00	3.00
391	Einstein Bros.-Soup, Chicken & R	198.8000	7.000	Ounce	7.00	10.00	15.00	180.00	0.00	0.00	15.00	2.50
392	Einstein Bros.-Soup, Chicken Noo	198.8000	7.000	Ounce	6.00	2.50	13.00	100.00	0.00	1.00	15.00	1.00
393	Einstein Bros.-Soup, Oriental Se	170.4000	6.000	Ounce	7.00	20.00	46.00	390.00	0.00	3.00	0.00	2.50
394	Einstein Bros.-Soup, Pasta Fagio	198.8000	7.000	Ounce	2.00	1.00	11.00	60.00	0.00	1.00	0.00	0.00
395	Einstein Bros.-Soup, Potato, Iri	198.8000	7.000	Ounce	5.00	8.00	19.00	170.00	0.00	1.00	5.00	2.50
396	Einstein Bros.-Soup, Tomato Flor	198.8000	7.000	Ounce	2.00	1.50	14.00	80.00	0.00	2.00	0.00	1.00
397	Einstein Bros.-Soup, Veg, Farmer	198.8000	7.000	Ounce	2.00	0.50	7.00	40.00	0.00	2.00	0.00	0.00
398	Einstein Bros.-Spread, Apricot	28.0000	2.000	Tbsp	0.00	0.00	19.00	75.00	0.00	0.00	0.00	0.00
399	Einstein Bros.-Spread, Butter	14.0000	1.000	Tbsp	0.00	11.00	0.00	100.00	0.00	0.00	30.00	8.00
400	Einstein Bros.-Spread, Butter/Ma	10.0000	1.000	Tbsp	0.00	7.00	0.00	60.00	0.00	0.00	0.00	1.50
401	Einstein Bros.-Spread, Grape Fru	28.0000	2.000	Tbsp	0.00	0.00	19.00	75.00	0.00	0.00	0.00	0.00
402	Einstein Bros.-Spread, Strawberr	28.0000	2.000	Tbsp	0.00	0.00	19.00	75.00	0.00	0.00	0.00	0.00
403	Einstein Bros.-Steamer, Non Fat,	360.0000	12.000	Fl Oz	9.00	0.00	29.00	160.00	0.00	0.00	5.00	0.00
404	Einstein Bros.-Steamer, Reg	360.0000	12.000	Fl Oz	6.00	5.00	30.00	200.00	0.00	0.00	20.00	3.50
405	Einstein Bros.-Syrup, Almond Fla	31.0000	2.000	Tbsp	0.00	0.00	18.00	80.00	0.00	0.00	0.00	0.00

Monounsaturated Fat (gm)	Polyunsaturated Fat (gm)	Vitamin D (mg)	Vitamin K (mg)	Vitamin E (mg)	Vitamin A (re)	Vitamin C (mg)	Thiamin (mg)	Riboflavin (mg)	Niacin (mg)	Vitamin B$_6$ (mg)	Folate (mg)	Vitamin B$_{12}$ (mcg)	Calcium (mg)	Iron (mg)	Magnesium (mg)	Phosphorus (mg)	Potassium (mg)	Sodium (mg)	Zinc (mg)
0.00	0.00	0.00	0.00	0.00	0.00	0.00	0.00	0.00	0.00	0.00	0.00	0.00	0.00	0.00	0.00	0.00	0.00	260.00	0.00
0.00	0.00	0.00	0.00	0.00	0.00	0.00	0.00	0.00	0.00	0.00	0.00	0.00	0.00	0.00	0.00	0.00	0.00	780.00	0.00
0.00	0.00	0.00	0.00	0.00	0.00	0.00	0.00	0.00	0.00	0.00	0.00	0.00	0.00	0.00	0.00	0.00	0.00	140.00	0.00
0.00	0.00	0.00	0.00	0.00	0.00	0.00	0.00	0.00	0.00	0.00	0.00	0.00	0.00	0.00	0.00	0.00	0.00	140.00	0.00
0.00	0.00	0.00	0.00	0.00	0.00	0.00	0.00	0.00	0.00	0.00	0.00	0.00	0.00	0.00	0.00	0.00	0.00	135.00	0.00
0.00	0.00	0.00	0.00	0.00	0.00	0.00	0.00	0.00	0.00	0.00	0.00	0.00	0.00	0.00	0.00	0.00	0.00	1240.00	0.00
0.00	0.00	0.00	0.00	0.00	0.00	0.00	0.00	0.00	0.00	0.00	0.00	0.00	0.00	0.00	0.00	0.00	0.00	120.00	0.00
0.00	0.00	0.00	0.00	0.00	0.00	0.00	0.00	0.00	0.00	0.00	0.00	0.00	0.00	0.00	0.00	0.00	0.00	130.00	0.00
0.00	0.00	0.00	0.00	0.00	0.00	0.00	0.00	0.00	0.00	0.00	0.00	0.00	0.00	0.00	0.00	0.00	0.00	135.00	0.00
0.00	0.00	0.00	0.00	0.00	0.00	0.00	0.00	0.00	0.00	0.00	0.00	0.00	0.00	0.00	0.00	0.00	0.00	210.00	0.00
0.00	0.00	0.00	0.00	0.00	0.00	0.00	0.00	0.00	0.00	0.00	0.00	0.00	0.00	0.00	0.00	0.00	0.00	170.00	0.00
0.00	0.00	0.00	0.00	0.00	0.00	0.00	0.00	0.00	0.00	0.00	0.00	0.00	0.00	0.00	0.00	0.00	0.00	180.00	0.00
0.00	0.00	0.00	0.00	0.00	0.00	0.00	0.00	0.00	0.00	0.00	0.00	0.00	0.00	0.00	0.00	0.00	0.00	180.00	0.00
0.00	0.00	0.00	0.00	0.00	0.00	0.00	0.00	0.00	0.00	0.00	0.00	0.00	0.00	0.00	0.00	0.00	0.00	260.00	0.00
0.00	0.00	0.00	0.00	0.00	0.00	0.00	0.00	0.00	0.00	0.00	0.00	0.00	0.00	0.00	0.00	0.00	0.00	220.00	0.00
0.00	0.00	0.00	0.00	0.00	0.00	0.00	0.00	0.00	0.00	0.00	0.00	0.00	0.00	0.00	0.00	0.00	0.00	260.00	0.00
0.00	0.00	0.00	0.00	0.00	0.00	0.00	0.00	0.00	0.00	0.00	0.00	0.00	0.00	0.00	0.00	0.00	0.00	1590.00	0.00
0.00	0.00	0.00	0.00	0.00	0.00	0.00	0.00	0.00	0.00	0.00	0.00	0.00	0.00	0.00	0.00	0.00	0.00	1780.00	0.00
0.00	0.00	0.00	0.00	0.00	0.00	0.00	0.00	0.00	0.00	0.00	0.00	0.00	0.00	0.00	0.00	0.00	0.00	663.00	0.00
0.00	0.00	0.00	0.00	0.00	0.00	0.00	0.00	0.00	0.00	0.00	0.00	0.00	0.00	0.00	0.00	0.00	0.00	140.00	0.00
0.00	0.00	0.00	0.00	0.00	0.00	0.00	0.00	0.00	0.00	0.00	0.00	0.00	0.00	0.00	0.00	0.00	0.00	1200.00	0.00
0.00	0.00	0.00	0.00	0.00	0.00	0.00	0.00	0.00	0.00	0.00	0.00	0.00	0.00	0.00	0.00	0.00	0.00	1780.00	0.00
0.00	0.00	0.00	0.00	0.00	0.00	0.00	0.00	0.00	0.00	0.00	0.00	0.00	0.00	0.00	0.00	0.00	0.00	1210.00	0.00
0.00	0.00	0.00	0.00	0.00	0.00	0.00	0.00	0.00	0.00	0.00	0.00	0.00	0.00	0.00	0.00	0.00	0.00	1920.00	0.00
0.00	0.00	0.00	0.00	0.00	0.00	0.00	0.00	0.00	0.00	0.00	0.00	0.00	0.00	0.00	0.00	0.00	0.00	1150.00	0.00
0.00	0.00	0.00	0.00	0.00	0.00	0.00	0.00	0.00	0.00	0.00	0.00	0.00	0.00	0.00	0.00	0.00	0.00	900.00	0.00
0.00	0.00	0.00	0.00	0.00	0.00	0.00	0.00	0.00	0.00	0.00	0.00	0.00	0.00	0.00	0.00	0.00	0.00	500.00	0.00
0.00	0.00	0.00	0.00	0.00	0.00	0.00	0.00	0.00	0.00	0.00	0.00	0.00	0.00	0.00	0.00	0.00	0.00	120.00	0.00
0.00	0.00	0.00	0.00	0.00	0.00	0.00	0.00	0.00	0.00	0.00	0.00	0.00	0.00	0.00	0.00	0.00	0.00	960.00	0.00
0.00	0.00	0.00	0.00	0.00	0.00	0.00	0.00	0.00	0.00	0.00	0.00	0.00	0.00	0.00	0.00	0.00	0.00	350.00	0.00
0.00	0.00	0.00	0.00	0.00	0.00	0.00	0.00	0.00	0.00	0.00	0.00	0.00	0.00	0.00	0.00	0.00	0.00	150.00	0.00
0.00	0.00	0.00	0.00	0.00	0.00	0.00	0.00	0.00	0.00	0.00	0.00	0.00	0.00	0.00	0.00	0.00	0.00	340.00	0.00
0.00	0.00	0.00	0.00	0.00	0.00	0.00	0.00	0.00	0.00	0.00	0.00	0.00	0.00	0.00	0.00	0.00	0.00	210.00	0.00
0.00	0.00	0.00	0.00	0.00	0.00	0.00	0.00	0.00	0.00	0.00	0.00	0.00	0.00	0.00	0.00	0.00	0.00	250.00	0.00
0.00	0.00	0.00	0.00	0.00	0.00	0.00	0.00	0.00	0.00	0.00	0.00	0.00	0.00	0.00	0.00	0.00	0.00	560.00	0.00
0.00	0.00	0.00	0.00	0.00	0.00	0.00	0.00	0.00	0.00	0.00	0.00	0.00	0.00	0.00	0.00	0.00	0.00	670.00	0.00
0.00	0.00	0.00	0.00	0.00	0.00	0.00	0.00	0.00	0.00	0.00	0.00	0.00	0.00	0.00	0.00	0.00	0.00	535.00	0.00
0.00	0.00	0.00	0.00	0.00	0.00	0.00	0.00	0.00	0.00	0.00	0.00	0.00	0.00	0.00	0.00	0.00	0.00	460.00	0.00
0.00	0.00	0.00	0.00	0.00	0.00	0.00	0.00	0.00	0.00	0.00	0.00	0.00	0.00	0.00	0.00	0.00	0.00	680.00	0.00
0.00	0.00	0.00	0.00	0.00	0.00	0.00	0.00	0.00	0.00	0.00	0.00	0.00	0.00	0.00	0.00	0.00	0.00	770.00	0.00
0.00	0.00	0.00	0.00	0.00	0.00	0.00	0.00	0.00	0.00	0.00	0.00	0.00	0.00	0.00	0.00	0.00	0.00	1070.00	0.00
0.00	0.00	0.00	0.00	0.00	0.00	0.00	0.00	0.00	0.00	0.00	0.00	0.00	0.00	0.00	0.00	0.00	0.00	910.00	0.00
0.00	0.00	0.00	0.00	0.00	0.00	0.00	0.00	0.00	0.00	0.00	0.00	0.00	0.00	0.00	0.00	0.00	0.00	320.00	0.00
0.00	0.00	0.00	0.00	0.00	0.00	0.00	0.00	0.00	0.00	0.00	0.00	0.00	0.00	0.00	0.00	0.00	0.00	450.00	0.00
0.00	0.00	0.00	0.00	0.00	0.00	0.00	0.00	0.00	0.00	0.00	0.00	0.00	0.00	0.00	0.00	0.00	0.00	650.00	0.00
0.00	0.00	0.00	0.00	0.00	0.00	0.00	0.00	0.00	0.00	0.00	0.00	0.00	0.00	0.00	0.00	0.00	0.00	870.00	0.00
0.00	0.00	0.00	0.00	0.00	0.00	0.00	0.00	0.00	0.00	0.00	0.00	0.00	0.00	0.00	0.00	0.00	0.00	390.00	0.00
0.00	0.00	0.00	0.00	0.00	0.00	0.00	0.00	0.00	0.00	0.00	0.00	0.00	0.00	0.00	0.00	0.00	0.00	8.00	0.00
0.00	0.00	0.00	0.00	0.00	0.00	0.00	0.00	0.00	0.00	0.00	0.00	0.00	0.00	0.00	0.00	0.00	0.00	100.00	0.00
0.00	0.00	0.00	0.00	0.00	0.00	0.00	0.00	0.00	0.00	0.00	0.00	0.00	0.00	0.00	0.00	0.00	0.00	75.00	0.00
0.00	0.00	0.00	0.00	0.00	0.00	0.00	0.00	0.00	0.00	0.00	0.00	0.00	0.00	0.00	0.00	0.00	0.00	3.00	0.00
0.00	0.00	0.00	0.00	0.00	0.00	0.00	0.00	0.00	0.00	0.00	0.00	0.00	0.00	0.00	0.00	0.00	0.00	17.00	0.00
0.00	0.00	0.00	0.00	0.00	0.00	0.00	0.00	0.00	0.00	0.00	0.00	0.00	0.00	0.00	0.00	0.00	0.00	140.00	0.00
0.00	0.00	0.00	0.00	0.00	0.00	0.00	0.00	0.00	0.00	0.00	0.00	0.00	0.00	0.00	0.00	0.00	0.00	150.00	0.00
0.00	0.00	0.00	0.00	0.00	0.00	0.00	0.00	0.00	0.00	0.00	0.00	0.00	0.00	0.00	0.00	0.00	0.00	10.00	0.00

USDA ID Code	Food Name	Weight in Grams*	Quantity of Units	Unit of Measure	Protein (gm)	Fat (gm)	Carbohydrate (gm)	Kcalories	Caffeine (gm)	Fiber (gm)	Cholesterol (mg)	Saturated Fat (gm)
406	Einstein Bros.-Syrup, Caramel Fl	31.0000	2.000	Tbsp	0.00	0.00	18.00	80.00	0.00	0.00	0.00	0.00
407	Einstein Bros.-Syrup, Caramel Fl	31.0000	2.000	Tbsp	0.00	0.00	18.00	80.00	0.00	0.00	0.00	0.00
408	Einstein Bros.-Syrup, Caramel, S	31.0000	2.000	Tbsp	0.00	0.00	0.00	0.00	0.00	0.00	0.00	0.00
409	Einstein Bros.-Syrup, Choc-Hersh	31.0000	2.000	Tbsp	1.00	0.00	24.00	100.00	0.00	0.00	0.00	0.00
410	Einstein Bros.-Syrup, Raspberry	31.0000	2.000	Tbsp	0.00	0.00	18.00	80.00	0.00	0.00	0.00	0.00
411	Einstein Bros.-Syrup, Vanilla, S	31.0000	2.000	Tbsp	0.00	0.00	0.00	0.00	0.00	0.00	0.00	0.00
412	Einstein Bros.-Tabouli, Southwes	284.0000	10.000	Ounce	6.00	1.00	29.00	150.00	0.00	8.00	0.00	0.00
413	Einstein Bros.-Teas, Hot	360.0000	12.000	Fl Oz	0.00	0.00	0.00	1.00	0.00	0.00	0.00	0.00
428	Einstein Bros.-topping, Chocolat	2.5000	0.500	Tsp	0.00	0.00	2.00	10.00	0.00	0.00	0.00	0.00
429	Einstein Bros.-topping, Cinnamon	2.5000	0.500	Tsp	0.00	0.00	2.00	10.00	0.00	0.00	0.00	0.00
414	Einstein Bros.-Topping, Nutmeg	2.5000	0.500	Tsp	0.00	0.00	2.00	10.00	0.00	0.00	0.00	0.00
415	Einstein Bros.-Topping, On Top D	31.0000	2.000	Tbsp	0.00	1.50	2.00	20.00	0.00	0.00	0.00	1.00
416	Einstein Bros.-Topping, Vanilla	2.5000	0.500	Tsp	0.00	0.00	2.00	10.00	0.00	0.00	0.00	0.00
417	Einstein Bros.-Tuna Melt	375.0000	1.000	Each	52.00	36.00	78.00	840.00	0.00	3.00	120.00	19.00
418	Einstein Bros.-Tuna Salad	113.6000	4.000	Ounce	21.00	6.00	3.00	150.00	0.00	0.00	30.00	1.00
419	Einstein Bros.-Tuna Salad Bagel	324.0000	1.000	Each	31.00	8.00	78.00	510.00	0.00	4.00	30.00	1.50
420	Einstein Bros.-Turkey, Deli Smok	305.0000	1.000	Each	35.00	16.00	75.00	590.00	0.00	3.00	65.00	9.00
421	Einstein Bros.-Turkey, Smoked, B	275.0000	1.000	Each	30.00	14.00	75.00	550.00	0.00	3.00	45.00	6.00
422	Einstein Bros.-Turkey, Tasty, Ba	279.0000	1.000	Each	26.00	21.00	77.00	600.00	0.00	3.00	90.00	12.00
423	Einstein Bros.-Veg Out Bagel San	248.0000	1.000	Each	14.00	6.00	78.00	420.00	0.00	3.00	20.00	3.00
424	Einstein Bros.-Veggie Cup	170.4000	6.000	Ounce	1.00	20.00	11.00	230.00	0.00	3.00	5.00	3.00
425	Einstein Bros.-Whipped Cream, Li	31.0000	2.000	Tbsp	0.00	2.00	2.00	30.00	0.00	0.00	10.00	1.50
426	Einstein Bros.-Whitefish Bagel S	245.0000	1.000	Each	23.00	22.00	75.00	590.00	0.00	4.00	45.00	4.00
427	Einstein Bros.-Whitefish Salad	56.8000	2.000	Ounce	8.00	14.00	1.00	160.00	0.00	1.00	30.00	2.00
561	Krispy Kreme-Cinnamon Bun	61.0000	1.000	Each	5.00	11.00	26.00	220.00	0.00	4.00	0.00	3.00
562	Krispy Kreme-Cruller, Fudge Iced	48.0000	1.000	Each	2.00	14.00	26.00	240.00	0.00	0.00	0.00	4.00
563	Krispy Kreme-Cruller, Glazed	43.0000	1.000	Each	2.00	14.00	22.00	220.00	0.00	0.00	0.00	3.00
564	Krispy Kreme-Doughnut, Blueberry	59.0000	1.000	Each	4.00	9.00	26.00	200.00	0.00	2.00	0.00	3.00
565	Krispy Kreme-Doughnut, Cake, Blu	67.0000	1.000	Each	2.00	15.00	37.00	300.00	0.00	1.00	0.00	3.00
566	Krispy Kreme-Doughnut, Cake, Dev	54.0000	1.000	Each	2.00	13.00	29.00	240.00	0.00	3.00	0.00	3.00
567	Krispy Kreme-Doughnut, Cake, Fud	56.0000	1.000	Each	3.00	12.00	28.00	230.00	0.00	0.00	0.00	3.00
568	Krispy Kreme-Doughnut, Cake, Sug	52.0000	1.000	Each	3.00	11.00	26.00	220.00	0.00	0.00	0.00	3.00
569	Krispy Kreme-Doughnut, Cake, Tra	48.0000	1.000	Each	3.00	11.00	22.00	200.00	0.00	0.00	0.00	3.00
570	Krispy Kreme-Doughnut, Cinnamon	66.0000	1.000	Each	4.00	9.00	29.00	210.00	0.00	3.00	0.00	3.00
571	Krispy Kreme-Doughnut, Creme Fil	65.0000	1.000	Each	4.00	14.00	32.00	270.00	0.00	2.00	0.00	3.00
572	Krispy Kreme-Doughnut, Crm Fille	65.0000	1.000	Each	4.00	14.00	32.00	270.00	0.00	2.00	0.00	3.00
573	Krispy Kreme-Doughnut, Custard F	76.0000	1.000	Each	4.00	9.00	38.00	250.00	0.00	3.00	0.00	3.00
574	Krispy Kreme-Doughnut, Fdg Iced	54.0000	1.000	Each	3.00	10.00	31.00	220.00	0.00	0.00	0.00	2.50
575	Krispy Kreme-Doughnut, Fudge Ice	57.0000	1.000	Each	3.00	14.00	30.00	260.00	0.00	1.00	0.00	5.00
576	Krispy Kreme-Doughnut, Lemon Fil	64.0000	1.000	Each	4.00	10.00	28.00	210.00	0.00	0.00	0.00	3.00
577	Krispy Kreme-Doughnut, Maple Ice	51.0000	1.000	Each	3.00	9.00	28.00	200.00	0.00	2.00	0.00	2.50
578	Krispy Kreme-Doughnut, Raspberry	57.0000	1.000	Each	4.00	10.00	28.00	210.00	0.00	0.00	0.00	3.00
579	Krispy Kreme-Doughnut, Yeast, Gl	39.0000	1.000	Each	2.00	10.00	17.00	170.00	0.00	0.00	0.00	2.50
	Pizza Hut-Pizza, Cheese, Hand To	70.0000	1.000	Slice	17.00	10.00	27.50	259.00	0.00	0.00	27.50	6.80
	Pizza Hut-Pizza, Cheese, Pan	70.0000	1.000	Slice	15.00	9.00	28.50	246.00	0.00	0.00	17.00	4.50
	Pizza Hut-Pizza, Cheese, Thin'n	70.0000	1.000	Slice	14.00	8.50	18.50	199.00	0.00	0.00	16.50	5.20
	Pizza Hut-Pizza, Pepperoni, Hand	70.0000	1.000	Slice	14.00	11.50	25.00	250.00	0.00	0.00	25.00	6.45
	Pizza Hut-Pizza, Pepperoni, Pan	70.0000	1.000	Slice	14.50	11.00	31.00	270.00	0.00	0.00	21.00	4.50
	Pizza Hut-Pizza, Pepperoni, Pers	250.0000	1.000	Each	37.00	29.00	76.00	675.00	0.00	0.00	53.00	12.50
	Pizza Hut-Pizza, Pepperoni, Thin	70.0000	1.000	Slice	13.00	10.00	18.00	206.50	0.00	0.00	23.00	5.30
	Pizza Hut-Pizza, Super Sprm, Thi	70.0000	1.000	Slice	14.50	10.50	22.00	231.50	0.00	0.00	28.00	5.15
	Pizza Hut-Pizza, Super Supreme,	70.0000	1.000	Slice	16.50	12.50	27.00	278.00	0.00	0.00	27.00	6.50
	Pizza Hut-Pizza, Super Supreme,	70.0000	1.000	Slice	16.50	13.00	26.50	281.50	0.00	0.00	27.50	6.00
	Pizza Hut-Pizza, Supreme, Hand T	70.0000	1.000	Slice	16.00	13.00	25.00	270.00	0.00	0.00	27.50	6.10
	Pizza Hut-Pizza, Supreme, Pan	70.0000	1.000	Slice	16.00	15.00	26.50	294.50	0.00	0.00	24.00	7.00

Monounsaturated Fat (gm)	Polyunsaturated Fat (gm)	Vitamin D (mg)	Vitamin K (mg)	Vitamin E (mg)	Vitamin A (re)	Vitamin C (mg)	Thiamin (mg)	Riboflavin (mg)	Niacin (mg)	Vitamin B6 (mg)	Folate (mg)	Vitamin B12 (mcg)	Calcium (mg)	Iron (mg)	Magnesium (mg)	Phosphorus (mg)	Potassium (mg)	Sodium (mg)	Zinc (mg)
0.00	0.00	0.00	0.00	0.00	0.00	0.00	0.00	0.00	0.00	0.00	0.00	0.00	0.00	0.00	0.00	0.00	0.00	10.00	0.00
0.00	0.00	0.00	0.00	0.00	0.00	0.00	0.00	0.00	0.00	0.00	0.00	0.00	0.00	0.00	0.00	0.00	0.00	10.00	0.00
0.00	0.00	0.00	0.00	0.00	0.00	0.00	0.00	0.00	0.00	0.00	0.00	0.00	0.00	0.00	0.00	0.00	0.00	20.00	0.00
0.00	0.00	0.00	0.00	0.00	0.00	0.00	0.00	0.00	0.00	0.00	0.00	0.00	0.00	0.00	0.00	0.00	0.00	25.00	0.00
0.00	0.00	0.00	0.00	0.00	0.00	0.00	0.00	0.00	0.00	0.00	0.00	0.00	0.00	0.00	0.00	0.00	0.00	10.00	0.00
0.00	0.00	0.00	0.00	0.00	0.00	0.00	0.00	0.00	0.00	0.00	0.00	0.00	0.00	0.00	0.00	0.00	0.00	20.00	0.00
0.00	0.00	0.00	0.00	0.00	0.00	4.20	0.00	0.00	0.00	0.00	0.00	0.00	0.00	0.00	0.00	0.00	0.00	690.00	0.00
0.00	0.00	0.00	0.00	0.00	0.00	0.00	0.00	0.00	0.00	0.00	0.00	0.00	0.00	0.00	0.00	0.00	0.00	0.00	0.00
0.00	0.00	0.00	0.00	0.00	0.00	0.00	0.00	0.00	0.00	0.00	0.00	0.00	0.00	0.00	0.00	0.00	0.00	0.00	0.00
0.00	0.00	0.00	0.00	0.00	0.00	0.00	0.00	0.00	0.00	0.00	0.00	0.00	0.00	0.00	0.00	0.00	0.00	0.00	0.00
0.00	0.00	0.00	0.00	0.00	0.00	0.00	0.00	0.00	0.00	0.00	0.00	0.00	0.00	0.00	0.00	0.00	0.00	10.00	0.00
0.00	0.00	0.00	0.00	0.00	0.00	0.00	0.00	0.00	0.00	0.00	0.00	0.00	0.00	0.00	0.00	0.00	0.00	5.00	0.00
0.00	0.00	0.00	0.00	0.00	0.00	0.00	0.00	0.00	0.00	0.00	0.00	0.00	0.00	0.00	0.00	0.00	0.00	0.00	0.00
0.00	0.00	0.00	0.00	0.00	0.00	0.00	0.00	0.00	0.00	0.00	0.00	0.00	0.00	0.00	0.00	0.00	0.00	1610.00	0.00
0.00	0.00	0.00	0.00	0.00	0.00	0.00	0.00	0.00	0.00	0.00	0.00	0.00	0.00	0.00	0.00	0.00	0.00	540.00	0.00
0.00	0.00	0.00	0.00	0.00	0.00	0.00	0.00	0.00	0.00	0.00	0.00	0.00	0.00	0.00	0.00	0.00	0.00	1080.00	0.00
0.00	0.00	0.00	0.00	0.00	0.00	0.00	0.00	0.00	0.00	0.00	0.00	0.00	0.00	0.00	0.00	0.00	0.00	1490.00	0.00
0.00	0.00	0.00	0.00	0.00	0.00	0.00	0.00	0.00	0.00	0.00	0.00	0.00	0.00	0.00	0.00	0.00	0.00	1310.00	0.00
0.00	0.00	0.00	0.00	0.00	0.00	0.00	0.00	0.00	0.00	0.00	0.00	0.00	0.00	0.00	0.00	0.00	0.00	1330.00	0.00
0.00	0.00	0.00	0.00	0.00	0.00	0.00	0.00	0.00	0.00	0.00	0.00	0.00	0.00	0.00	0.00	0.00	0.00	690.00	0.00
0.00	0.00	0.00	0.00	0.00	0.00	0.00	0.00	0.00	0.00	0.00	0.00	0.00	0.00	0.00	0.00	0.00	0.00	340.00	0.00
0.00	0.00	0.00	0.00	0.00	0.00	0.00	0.00	0.00	0.00	0.00	0.00	0.00	0.00	0.00	0.00	0.00	0.00	0.00	0.00
0.00	0.00	0.00	0.00	0.00	0.00	0.00	0.00	0.00	0.00	0.00	0.00	0.00	0.00	0.00	0.00	0.00	0.00	1140.00	0.00
0.00	0.00	0.00	0.00	0.00	0.00	0.00	0.00	0.00	0.00	0.00	0.00	0.00	0.00	0.00	0.00	0.00	0.00	410.00	0.00
0.00	0.00	0.00	0.00	0.00	0.00	0.00	0.00	0.00	0.00	0.00	0.00	0.00	0.00	0.00	0.00	0.00	0.00	160.00	0.00
0.00	0.00	0.00	0.00	0.00	0.00	0.00	0.00	0.00	0.00	0.00	0.00	0.00	0.00	0.00	0.00	0.00	0.00	160.00	0.00
0.00	0.00	0.00	0.00	0.00	0.00	0.00	0.00	0.00	0.00	0.00	0.00	0.00	0.00	0.00	0.00	0.00	0.00	150.00	0.00
0.00	0.00	0.00	0.00	0.00	0.00	0.00	0.00	0.00	0.00	0.00	0.00	0.00	0.00	0.00	0.00	0.00	0.00	160.00	0.00
0.00	0.00	0.00	0.00	0.00	0.00	0.00	0.00	0.00	0.00	0.00	0.00	0.00	0.00	0.00	0.00	0.00	0.00	300.00	0.00
0.00	0.00	0.00	0.00	0.00	0.00	0.00	0.00	0.00	0.00	0.00	0.00	0.00	0.00	0.00	0.00	0.00	0.00	180.00	0.00
0.00	0.00	0.00	0.00	0.00	0.00	0.00	0.00	0.00	0.00	0.00	0.00	0.00	0.00	0.00	0.00	0.00	0.00	280.00	0.00
0.00	0.00	0.00	0.00	0.00	0.00	0.00	0.00	0.00	0.00	0.00	0.00	0.00	0.00	0.00	0.00	0.00	0.00	250.00	0.00
0.00	0.00	0.00	0.00	0.00	0.00	0.00	0.00	0.00	0.00	0.00	0.00	0.00	0.00	0.00	0.00	0.00	0.00	280.00	0.00
0.00	0.00	0.00	0.00	0.00	0.00	0.00	0.00	0.00	0.00	0.00	0.00	0.00	0.00	0.00	0.00	0.00	0.00	150.00	0.00
0.00	0.00	0.00	0.00	0.00	0.00	0.00	0.00	0.00	0.00	0.00	0.00	0.00	0.00	0.00	0.00	0.00	0.00	150.00	0.00
0.00	0.00	0.00	0.00	0.00	0.00	0.00	0.00	0.00	0.00	0.00	0.00	0.00	0.00	0.00	0.00	0.00	0.00	150.00	0.00
0.00	0.00	0.00	0.00	0.00	0.00	0.00	0.00	0.00	0.00	0.00	0.00	0.00	0.00	0.00	0.00	0.00	0.00	150.00	0.00
0.00	0.00	0.00	0.00	0.00	0.00	0.00	0.00	0.00	0.00	0.00	0.00	0.00	0.00	0.00	0.00	0.00	0.00	95.00	0.00
0.00	0.00	0.00	0.00	0.00	0.00	0.00	0.00	0.00	0.00	0.00	0.00	0.00	0.00	0.00	0.00	0.00	0.00	105.00	0.00
0.00	0.00	0.00	0.00	0.00	0.00	0.00	0.00	0.00	0.00	0.00	0.00	0.00	0.00	0.00	0.00	0.00	0.00	150.00	0.00
0.00	0.00	0.00	0.00	0.00	0.00	0.00	0.00	0.00	0.00	0.00	0.00	0.00	0.00	0.00	0.00	0.00	0.00	100.00	0.00
0.00	0.00	0.00	0.00	0.00	0.00	0.00	0.00	0.00	0.00	0.00	0.00	0.00	0.00	0.00	0.00	0.00	0.00	160.00	0.00
0.00	0.00	0.00	0.00	0.00	0.00	0.00	0.00	0.00	0.00	0.00	0.00	0.00	0.00	0.00	0.00	0.00	0.00	95.00	0.00
3.20	0.00	0.00	0.00	0.00	50.00	4.80	0.24	0.25	2.57	0.00	0.00	0.30	300.00	1.50	31.50	220.00	198.00	638.00	2.33
4.50	0.00	0.00	0.00	0.00	45.00	3.60	0.28	0.30	2.47	0.00	0.00	0.30	252.00	1.50	26.25	188.00	160.00	470.00	2.03
3.30	0.00	0.00	0.00	0.00	35.00	2.40	0.20	0.20	2.28	0.00	0.00	0.25	264.00	0.90	21.00	188.00	130.50	433.50	1.80
5.05	0.00	0.00	0.00	0.00	50.00	3.60	0.27	0.26	2.66	0.00	0.00	0.33	176.00	1.40	26.25	156.00	207.50	633.50	1.88
6.50	0.00	0.00	0.00	0.00	50.00	4.20	0.32	0.25	2.57	0.00	0.00	0.30	208.00	1.75	24.50	176.00	202.50	563.50	2.10
16.50	0.00	0.00	0.00	0.00	120.00	10.20	0.56	0.66	7.79	0.00	0.00	0.44	584.00	3.20	52.50	360.00	408.00	1335.00	3.75
4.70	0.00	0.00	0.00	0.00	35.00	3.00	0.21	0.21	2.47	0.00	0.00	0.25	180.00	0.90	19.25	148.00	143.50	493.00	1.73
5.35	0.00	0.00	0.00	0.00	50.00	4.20	0.29	0.22	2.57	0.00	0.00	0.35	184.00	1.35	26.25	168.00	231.50	668.00	2.25
6.00	0.00	0.00	0.00	0.00	55.00	6.00	0.35	0.29	3.52	0.00	0.00	0.41	176.00	1.90	33.25	168.00	258.00	824.00	2.40
7.00	0.00	0.00	0.00	0.00	60.00	5.40	0.38	0.33	3.04	0.00	0.00	0.40	216.00	1.85	31.50	188.00	266.00	723.50	2.70
6.90	0.00	0.00	0.00	0.00	55.00	6.00	0.35	0.26	3.42	0.00	0.00	0.40	192.00	2.25	35.00	184.00	289.00	735.00	2.85
8.00	0.00	0.00	0.00	0.00	60.00	4.80	0.41	0.40	2.85	0.00	0.00	0.38	200.00	1.40	33.25	184.00	290.00	831.50	2.78

USDA ID Code	Food Name	Weight in Grams*	Quantity of Units	Unit of Measure	Protein (gm)	Fat (gm)	Carbohydrate (gm)	Kcalories	Caffeine (gm)	Fiber (gm)	Cholesterol (mg)	Saturated Fat (gm)
	Pizza Hut-Pizza, Supreme, Person	250.0000	1.000	Each	33.00	28.00	76.00	647.00	0.00	0.00	49.00	11.20
	Pizza Hut-Pizza, Supreme, Thin'n	70.0000	1.000	Slice	14.00	11.00	20.50	229.50	0.00	0.00	21.00	5.50
	Red Lobster-Calamari, Brded and	141.7460	1.000	Each	13.00	21.00	30.00	360.00	0.00	0.00	140.00	5.60
	Red Lobster-Catfish, Lunch Porti	141.7460	1.000	Each	20.00	10.00	0.00	170.00	0.00	0.00	85.00	2.50
	Red Lobster-Chicken Breast, Skin	113.3970	1.000	Each	26.00	3.00	0.00	140.00	0.00	0.00	70.00	1.00
	Red Lobster-Cod, Atlantic, Lunch	141.7460	1.000	Each	23.00	1.00	0.00	100.00	0.00	0.00	70.00	0.30
	Red Lobster-Crab Legs, King, Lun	453.5900	1.000	Each	32.00	2.00	6.00	170.00	0.00	0.00	100.00	0.50
	Red Lobster-Crab Legs, Snow, Lun	453.5900	1.000	Each	33.00	2.00	1.00	150.00	0.00	0.00	130.00	0.60
	Red Lobster-Flounder, Lunch Port	141.7460	1.000	Each	21.00	1.00	1.00	100.00	0.00	0.00	70.00	0.30
	Red Lobster-Grouper, Lunch Porti	141.7460	1.000	Each	26.00	1.00	1.00	110.00	0.00	0.00	65.00	0.30
	Red Lobster-Haddock, Lunch Porti	141.7460	1.000	Each	24.00	1.00	2.00	110.00	0.00	0.00	85.00	0.30
	Red Lobster-Halibut, Lunch Porti	141.7460	1.000	Each	25.00	1.00	1.00	110.00	0.00	0.00	60.00	0.30
	Red Lobster-Hamburger, Lunch Por	151.1810	1.000	Each	37.00	28.00	0.00	410.00	0.00	0.00	130.00	11.00
	Red Lobster-Langostino, Lunch Po	141.7460	1.000	Each	26.00	1.00	2.00	120.00	0.00	0.00	210.00	0.20
	Red Lobster-Lobster, Live Maine	510.2880	1.000	Each	36.00	8.00	5.00	240.00	0.00	0.00	310.00	1.90
	Red Lobster-Lobster, Rock, Lunch	368.5410	1.000	Each	49.00	3.00	2.00	230.00	0.00	0.00	200.00	0.70
	Red Lobster-Mackerel, Lunch Port	141.7460	1.000	Each	20.00	12.00	1.00	190.00	0.00	0.00	100.00	3.60
	Red Lobster-Monkfish, Lunch Port	141.7460	1.000	Each	24.00	1.00	0.00	110.00	0.00	0.00	80.00	0.20
	Red Lobster-Perch, Atlantic Ocea	141.7460	1.000	Each	24.00	4.00	1.00	130.00	0.00	0.00	75.00	1.10
	Red Lobster-Pollock, Lunch Porti	141.7460	1.000	Each	28.00	1.00	1.00	120.00	0.00	0.00	90.00	0.30
	Red Lobster-Rockfish, Red, Lunch	141.7460	1.000	Each	21.00	1.00	0.00	90.00	0.00	0.00	85.00	0.30
	Red Lobster-Salmon, Norwegian, L	141.7460	1.000	Each	27.00	12.00	3.00	230.00	0.00	0.00	80.00	2.70
	Red Lobster-Salmon, Sockeye, Lun	141.7460	1.000	Each	28.00	4.00	3.00	160.00	0.00	0.00	50.00	1.10
	Red Lobster-Scallops, Deep Sea,	141.7460	1.000	Each	26.00	2.00	2.00	130.00	0.00	0.00	50.00	0.40
	Red Lobster-Shrimp, Lunch Portio	198.4450	1.000	Each	25.00	2.00	0.00	120.00	0.00	0.00	230.00	0.50
	Red Lobster-Snapper, Red, Lunch	141.7460	1.000	Each	25.00	1.00	0.00	110.00	0.00	0.00	70.00	0.40
	Red Lobster-Sole, Lemon, Lunch P	141.7460	1.000	Each	27.00	1.00	1.00	120.00	0.00	0.00	65.00	0.30
	Red Lobster-Steak, Strip, Lunch	255.1440	1.000	Each	47.00	40.00	0.00	560.00	0.00	0.00	150.00	17.00
	Red Lobster-Swordfish, Lunch Por	141.7460	1.000	Each	17.00	4.00	0.00	100.00	0.00	0.00	100.00	1.20
	Red Lobster-Trout, Rainbow, Lunc	141.7460	1.000	Each	23.00	9.00	0.00	170.00	0.00	0.00	90.00	2.50
	Red Lobster-Tuna, Yellow Fin, Lu	141.7460	1.000	Each	32.00	2.00	6.00	180.00	0.00	0.00	70.00	0.50

Seafood and Fish

USDA ID Code	Food Name	Weight in Grams*	Quantity of Units	Unit of Measure	Protein (gm)	Fat (gm)	Carbohydrate (gm)	Kcalories	Caffeine (gm)	Fiber (gm)	Cholesterol (mg)	Saturated Fat (gm)
	Anchovy, European, Cnd In Oil	28.3500	3.000	Ounce	8.19	2.75	0.00	59.54	0.00	0.00	24.10	0.62
	Bass, Freshwater, Ckd, Dry Heat	62.0000	1.000	Each	14.99	2.93	0.00	90.52	0.00	0.00	53.94	0.62
	Bass, Striped, Ckd, Dry Heat	124.0000	1.000	Each	28.19	3.71	0.00	153.76	0.00	0.00	127.72	0.81
	Bluefish, Ckd, Dry Heat	117.0000	1.000	Each	30.06	6.36	0.00	186.03	0.00	0.00	88.92	1.37
	Catfish, Channel, Farmed, Ckd, D	143.0000	1.000	Each	26.77	11.47	0.00	217.36	0.00	0.00	91.52	2.56
	Catfish, Channel, Wild, Ckd, Dry	143.0000	1.000	Each	26.41	4.08	0.00	150.15	0.00	0.00	102.96	1.06
	Catfish, Fried	87.0000	1.000	Each	15.74	11.60	6.99	199.23	0.00	0.65	70.47	2.86
	Caviar, Black and Red, Granular	16.0000	1.000	Tbsp	3.94	2.86	0.64	40.32	0.00	0.00	94.08	0.65
	Clam, Ckd, Breaded and Fried	85.0000	3.000	Ounce	12.10	9.48	8.78	171.70	0.00	0.00	51.85	2.28
	Clam, Ckd, Moist Heat	85.0000	3.000	Ounce	21.72	1.66	4.36	125.80	0.00	0.00	56.95	0.16
	Clam, Cnd, Drained Solids	160.0000	1.000	Cup	40.88	3.12	8.21	236.80	0.00	0.00	107.20	0.30
	Cod, Atlantic, Ckd, Dry Heat	180.0000	1.000	Each	41.09	1.55	0.00	189.00	0.00	0.00	99.00	0.31
	Cod, Atlantic, Cnd	312.0000	1.000	Can	71.01	2.68	0.00	327.60	0.00	0.00	171.60	0.53
	Crab, Alaska King, Ckd, Moist He	134.0000	1.000	Leg	25.93	2.06	0.00	129.98	0.00	0.00	71.02	0.17
	Crab, Alaska King, Imitation	85.0000	3.000	Ounce	10.22	1.11	8.69	86.70	0.00	0.00	17.00	0.22
	Crab, Blue, Ckd, Moist Heat	118.0000	1.000	Cup	23.84	2.09	0.00	120.36	0.00	0.00	118.00	0.27
	Crab, Blue, Cnd	135.0000	1.000	Cup	27.70	1.66	0.00	133.65	0.00	0.00	120.15	0.34
	Crab, Blue, Crab Cakes	60.0000	1.000	Cake	12.13	4.51	0.29	93.00	0.00	0.00	90.00	0.89
	Crab, Dungeness, Ckd, Moist Heat	85.0000	3.000	Ounce	18.97	1.05	0.81	93.50	0.00	0.00	64.60	0.14
	Crab, Queen, Ckd, Moist Heat	85.0000	3.000	Ounce	20.16	1.28	0.00	97.75	0.00	0.00	60.35	0.15
217	Crawfish, Boiled	85.0000	3.000	oz	20.33	1.15	0.00	97.00	0.00	0.00	151.00	0.20
	Crayfish, Farmed, Ckd, Moist Hea	85.0000	3.000	Ounce	14.89	1.11	0.00	73.95	0.00	0.00	116.45	0.19
	Crayfish, Wild, Ckd, Moist Heat	85.0000	3.000	Ounce	14.25	1.02	0.00	69.70	0.00	0.00	113.05	0.15
	Fish Fillets and Sticks, Fried	57.0000	1.000	Piece	8.92	6.97	13.54	155.04	0.00	0.00	63.84	1.80
	Flounder, Ckd, Dry Heat	127.0000	1.000	Each	30.68	1.94	0.00	148.59	0.00	0.00	86.36	0.46

Monounsaturated Fat (gm)	Polyunsaturated Fat (gm)	Vitamin D (mg)	Vitamin K (mg)	Vitamin E (mg)	Vitamin A (re)	Vitamin C (mg)	Thiamin (mg)	Riboflavin (mg)	Niacin (mg)	Vitamin B6 (mg)	Folate (mg)	Vitamin B12 (mcg)	Calcium (mg)	Iron (mg)	Magnesium (mg)	Phosphorus (mg)	Potassium (mg)	Sodium (mg)	Zinc (mg)
16.80	0.00	0.00	0.00	0.00	120.00	10.80	0.59	0.66	7.60	0.00	0.00	0.46	416.00	3.70	52.50	320.00	487.00	1313.00	3.75
5.50	0.00	0.00	0.00	0.00	50.00	4.80	0.30	0.25	2.57	0.00	0.00	0.30	172.00	1.65	29.75	160.00	272.00	664.00	2.33
0.00	1.50	0.00	0.00	0.00	0.00	0.00	0.23	0.14	1.52	0.00	0.00	2.00	0.00	0.60	21.00	360.00	0.00	1150.00	0.90
0.00	1.90	0.00	0.00	0.00	0.00	0.00	0.30	0.14	1.90	0.00	0.00	0.04	0.00	0.00	21.00	160.00	0.00	50.00	0.30
0.00	1.00	0.00	0.00	0.00	0.00	0.00	0.06	0.10	11.40	0.00	0.00	0.08	0.00	0.40	21.00	160.00	0.00	60.00	0.90
0.00	0.60	0.00	0.00	0.00	0.00	0.00	0.03	0.07	0.76	0.00	0.00	0.60	0.00	0.00	28.00	200.00	0.00	200.00	0.30
0.00	1.60	0.00	0.00	0.00	0.00	0.00	0.09	0.17	1.90	0.00	0.00	1.60	48.00	0.00	70.00	320.00	0.00	900.00	6.00
0.00	1.80	0.00	0.00	0.00	0.00	0.00	0.03	0.10	1.90	0.00	0.00	1.60	80.00	0.20	70.00	1630.00	0.00	1630.00	6.00
0.00	0.70	0.00	0.00	0.00	0.00	0.00	0.03	0.00	1.52	0.00	0.00	0.30	16.00	0.00	21.00	48.00	0.00	95.00	0.30
0.00	0.50	0.00	0.00	0.00	0.00	0.00	0.06	0.03	1.52	0.00	0.00	0.08	32.00	0.00	28.00	200.00	0.00	70.00	0.30
0.00	1.10	0.00	0.00	0.00	0.00	0.00	0.03	0.07	2.85	0.00	0.00	0.20	0.00	0.00	21.00	160.00	0.00	180.00	0.30
0.00	0.70	0.00	0.00	0.00	0.00	0.00	0.15	0.00	2.85	0.00	0.00	0.30	0.00	0.00	28.00	240.00	0.00	105.00	0.00
0.00	1.00	0.00	0.00	0.00	0.00	0.00	0.06	0.34	7.60	0.00	0.00	1.20	0.00	1.50	28.00	200.00	0.00	115.00	7.50
0.00	0.60	0.00	0.00	0.00	0.00	0.00	0.12	0.00	1.14	0.00	0.00	2.00	16.00	0.80	35.00	160.00	0.00	410.00	1.50
0.00	4.10	0.00	0.00	0.00	0.00	0.00	0.15	0.17	2.85	0.00	0.00	2.00	320.00	0.80	52.50	320.00	0.00	550.00	6.75
0.00	1.40	0.00	0.00	0.00	0.00	0.00	0.00	0.07	3.80	0.00	0.00	0.50	48.00	0.00	87.50	400.00	0.00	1090.00	6.00
0.00	5.40	0.00	0.00	0.00	0.00	0.00	0.15	0.43	5.70	0.00	0.00	0.80	16.00	0.80	21.00	200.00	0.00	250.00	1.20
0.00	0.70	0.00	0.00	0.00	40.00	0.00	0.06	0.14	0.76	0.00	0.00	0.20	0.00	1.00	14.00	64.00	0.00	95.00	0.30
0.00	1.20	0.00	0.00	0.00	0.00	0.00	0.06	0.10	1.52	0.00	0.00	0.30	0.00	0.00	21.00	160.00	0.00	190.00	0.30
0.00	1.00	0.00	0.00	0.00	0.00	0.00	0.06	0.17	0.38	0.00	0.00	1.00	0.00	0.00	28.00	160.00	0.00	90.00	0.30
0.00	0.50	0.00	0.00	0.00	0.00	0.00	0.09	0.10	0.76	0.00	0.00	0.60	0.00	0.00	21.00	120.00	0.00	95.00	0.30
0.00	4.60	0.00	0.00	0.00	0.00	0.00	0.23	0.07	6.65	0.00	0.00	0.20	16.00	0.00	35.00	240.00	0.00	60.00	0.30
0.00	1.80	0.00	0.00	0.00	0.00	0.00	0.38	0.14	7.60	0.00	0.00	2.00	0.00	0.00	35.00	280.00	0.00	60.00	0.30
0.00	1.50	0.00	0.00	0.00	0.00	0.00	0.00	0.10	1.90	0.00	0.00	0.40	0.00	0.00	52.50	240.00	0.00	260.00	1.50
0.00	1.10	0.00	0.00	0.00	0.00	0.00	0.00	0.03	1.90	0.00	0.00	0.50	32.00	0.00	35.00	120.00	0.00	110.00	1.50
0.00	0.60	0.00	0.00	0.00	0.00	0.00	0.06	0.03	4.75	0.00	0.00	0.30	0.00	0.00	21.00	120.00	0.00	140.00	0.30
0.00	0.40	0.00	0.00	0.00	0.00	0.00	0.06	0.10	0.38	0.00	0.00	0.40	0.00	0.00	21.00	64.00	0.00	90.00	0.30
0.00	2.00	0.00	0.00	0.00	0.00	0.00	0.15	0.34	7.60	0.00	0.00	1.20	0.00	2.00	35.00	280.00	0.00	115.00	9.00
0.00	1.00	0.00	0.00	0.00	20.00	0.00	0.06	0.07	3.80	0.00	0.00	0.30	0.00	0.00	28.00	80.00	0.00	140.00	0.60
0.00	4.00	0.00	0.00	0.00	0.00	0.00	0.12	0.17	2.85	0.00	0.00	1.00	80.00	0.00	21.00	200.00	0.00	90.00	0.90
0.00	1.60	0.00	0.00	0.00	0.00	0.00	0.06	0.03	13.30	0.00	0.00	1.60	0.00	0.60	35.00	240.00	0.00	70.00	0.30
1.07	0.73	0.00	0.00	1.42	5.95	0.00	0.02	0.10	5.64	0.06	3.54	0.25	65.77	1.31	19.56	71.44	154.22	1039.88	0.69
1.14	0.84	0.00	0.00	0.00	21.70	1.30	0.06	0.06	0.94	0.09	10.54	1.43	63.86	1.18	23.56	158.72	282.72	55.80	0.51
1.05	1.25	0.00	0.00	0.00	38.44	0.00	0.15	0.05	3.17	0.43	12.40	5.47	23.56	1.34	63.24	314.96	406.72	109.12	0.63
2.69	1.59	0.00	0.00	0.00	161.46	0.00	0.08	0.12	8.48	0.54	10.53	7.28	12.87	0.73	49.14	340.47	558.09	90.09	1.22
5.95	1.99	0.00	0.00	0.00	21.45	1.14	0.60	0.10	3.59	0.23	10.01	4.00	12.87	1.17	37.18	350.35	459.03	114.40	1.50
1.57	0.92	0.00	0.00	0.00	21.45	1.14	0.33	0.10	3.42	0.16	14.30	4.15	15.73	0.50	40.04	434.72	599.17	71.50	0.87
4.88	2.90	0.00	0.00	0.00	6.96	0.00	0.06	0.11	1.98	0.17	26.10	1.65	38.28	1.24	23.49	187.92	295.80	243.60	0.75
0.74	1.19	0.93	0.00	1.12	89.60	0.00	0.03	0.10	0.02	0.05	8.00	3.20	44.00	1.90	48.00	56.96	28.96	240.00	0.15
3.87	2.44	0.00	0.00	0.00	76.50	8.50	0.09	0.20	1.75	0.05	30.60	34.23	53.55	11.82	11.90	159.80	277.10	309.40	1.24
0.14	0.47	0.00	0.00	0.00	145.35	18.79	0.13	0.37	2.85	0.09	24.48	84.06	78.20	23.77	15.30	287.30	533.80	95.20	2.32
0.27	0.88	0.00	0.00	1.60	273.60	35.36	0.24	0.69	5.36	0.18	46.08	158.22	147.20	44.74	28.80	540.80	1004.80	179.20	4.37
0.22	0.52	0.00	0.00	0.54	25.20	1.80	0.16	0.14	4.52	0.50	14.58	1.89	25.20	0.88	75.60	248.40	439.20	140.40	1.04
0.37	0.90	6.55	0.00	0.62	43.68	3.12	0.28	0.25	7.83	0.87	25.27	3.28	65.52	1.53	127.92	811.20	1647.36	680.16	1.81
0.25	0.72	0.00	0.00	0.00	12.06	10.18	0.07	0.08	1.80	0.24	68.34	15.41	79.06	1.02	84.42	375.20	351.08	1436.48	10.21
0.17	0.57	0.00	0.00	0.09	17.00	0.00	0.03	0.03	0.15	0.03	1.36	1.36	11.05	0.33	36.55	239.70	76.50	714.85	0.28
0.33	0.80	0.00	0.00	1.18	2.36	3.89	0.12	0.06	3.89	0.21	59.94	8.61	122.72	1.07	38.94	243.08	382.32	329.22	4.98
0.30	0.59	0.00	0.00	1.35	2.70	3.65	0.11	0.11	1.85	0.20	57.38	0.62	136.35	1.13	62.65	351.00	504.90	449.55	5.43
1.69	1.36	0.00	0.00	0.00	48.60	1.68	0.05	0.05	1.74	0.10	31.80	3.56	63.00	0.65	19.80	127.80	194.40	198.00	2.45
0.18	0.35	0.00	0.00	0.00	26.35	3.06	0.05	0.17	3.08	0.14	35.70	8.82	50.15	0.37	49.30	148.75	346.80	321.30	4.65
0.28	0.46	0.00	0.00	0.00	44.20	6.12	0.09	0.20	2.46	0.14	35.70	8.82	28.05	2.45	53.55	108.80	170.00	587.35	3.05
0.32	0.28	0.00	0.00	0.00	0.00	2.80	0.00	0.07	2.49	0.00	0.00	2.94	26.00	2.67	27.00	280.00	298.00	58.00	1.42
0.21	0.35	0.00	0.00	0.00	12.75	0.43	0.04	0.07	1.42	0.11	9.35	2.64	43.35	0.94	28.05	204.85	202.30	82.45	1.26
0.20	0.31	0.00	0.00	1.28	12.75	0.77	0.04	0.08	1.94	0.07	37.40	1.83	51.00	0.71	28.05	229.50	251.60	79.90	1.50
2.89	1.81	0.00	0.00	0.78	17.67	0.00	0.07	0.10	1.21	0.03	10.37	1.03	11.40	0.42	14.25	103.17	148.77	331.74	0.38
0.30	0.83	0.00	0.00	2.40	13.97	0.00	0.10	0.14	2.77	0.30	11.68	3.19	22.86	0.43	73.66	367.03	436.88	133.35	0.80

USDA ID Code	Food Name	Weight in Grams*	Quantity of Units	Unit of Measure	Protein (gm)	Fat (gm)	Carbohydrate (gm)	Kcalories	Caffeine (gm)	Fiber (gm)	Cholesterol (mg)	Saturated Fat (gm)
	Grouper, Ckd, Dry Heat	202.0000	1.000	Each	50.18	2.63	0.00	238.36	0.00	0.00	94.94	0.61
	Haddock, Ckd, Dry Heat	150.0000	1.000	Each	36.36	1.40	0.00	168.00	0.00	0.00	111.00	0.26
	Haddock, Smoked	28.3500	1.000	Ounce	7.15	0.27	0.00	32.89	0.00	0.00	21.83	0.05
	Halibut, Ckd, Dry Heat	159.0000	3.000	Ounce	42.44	4.67	0.00	222.60	0.00	0.00	65.19	0.67
	Halibut, Greenland, Ckd, Dry Hea	159.0000	3.000	Ounce	29.29	28.21	0.00	380.01	0.00	0.00	93.81	4.93
	Herring, Ckd, Dry Heat	143.0000	1.000	Each	32.93	16.57	0.00	290.29	0.00	0.00	110.11	3.75
	Herring, Kippered	28.3500	1.000	Ounce	6.97	3.51	0.00	61.52	0.00	0.00	23.25	0.79
	Herring, Pacific, Ckd, Dry Heat	144.0000	1.000	Each	30.25	25.62	0.00	360.00	0.00	0.00	142.56	6.00
	Herring, Pickled	140.0000	1.000	Cup	19.87	25.20	13.50	366.80	0.00	0.00	18.20	3.33
	Lobster, Northern, Ckd, Moist He	145.0000	1.000	Cup	29.73	0.86	1.86	142.10	0.00	0.00	104.40	0.16
	Lobster, Spiny, Ckd, Moist Heat	163.0000	1.000	Lobster	43.05	3.16	5.09	233.09	0.00	0.00	146.70	0.49
	Mackerel, Ckd, Dry Heat	88.0000	1.000	Each	20.99	15.67	0.00	230.56	0.00	0.00	66.00	3.68
	Mullet, Striped, Ckd, Dry Heat	93.0000	1.000	Each	23.07	4.52	0.00	139.50	0.00	0.00	58.59	1.33
	Mussel, Blue, Ckd, Moist Heat	85.0000	3.000	Ounce	20.23	3.81	6.28	146.20	0.00	0.00	47.60	0.72
	Oyster, Eastern, Breaded and Fri	85.0000	3.000	Ounce	7.45	10.69	9.88	167.45	0.00	0.00	68.85	2.72
	Oyster, Eastern, Cnd	162.0000	1.000	Cup	11.44	4.00	6.33	111.78	0.00	0.00	89.10	1.02
	Oysters, Raw	85.0000	3.000	Ounce	4.44	1.32	4.70	50.15	0.00	0.00	21.25	0.37
	Perch, Atlantic, Ckd, Dry Heat	50.0000	1.000	Each	11.94	1.05	0.00	60.50	0.00	0.00	27.00	0.16
	Perch, Ckd, Dry Heat	46.0000	1.000	Each	11.44	0.54	0.00	53.82	0.00	0.00	52.90	0.11
	Pike, Northern, Ckd, Dry Heat	155.0000	3.000	Ounce	38.27	1.36	0.00	175.15	0.00	0.00	77.50	0.23
	Pike, Walleye, Ckd, Dry Heat	124.0000	1.000	Each	30.43	1.93	0.00	147.56	0.00	0.00	136.40	0.40
	Pollock, Atlantic, Ckd, Dry Heat	151.0000	3.000	Ounce	37.63	1.90	0.00	178.18	0.00	0.00	137.41	0.26
655	Pompano, Cooked	85.0000	3.000	Ounce	20.14	10.32	0.00	179.35	0.00	0.00	54.40	3.82
	Pompano, Florida, Ckd, Dry Heat	88.0000	1.000	Each	20.85	10.68	0.00	185.68	0.00	0.00	56.32	3.96
	Rockfish, Pacific, Ckd, Dry Heat	149.0000	1.000	Each	35.82	2.99	0.00	180.29	0.00	0.00	65.56	0.70
	Roughy, Orange, Ckd, Dry Heat	85.0000	3.000	Ounce	16.02	0.77	0.00	75.65	0.00	0.00	22.10	0.02
	Salmon, Atlantic, Wild, Ckd, Dry	154.0000	3.000	Ounce	39.18	12.52	0.00	280.28	0.00	0.00	109.34	1.94
	Salmon, Chinook, Ckd, Dry Heat	154.0000	3.000	Ounce	39.61	20.61	0.00	355.74	0.00	0.00	130.90	4.94
	Salmon, Chum, Ckd, Dry Heat	154.0000	3.000	Ounce	39.76	7.44	0.00	237.16	0.00	0.00	146.30	1.66
	Salmon, Cnd	369.0000	1.000	Can	75.53	26.97	0.00	564.57	0.00	0.00	162.36	6.05
	Salmon, Coho, Farmed, Ckd, Dry H	143.0000	1.000	Each	34.75	11.77	0.00	254.54	0.00	0.00	90.09	2.77
	Salmon, Coho, Wild, Ckd, Dry Hea	178.0000	3.000	Ounce	41.74	7.65	0.00	247.42	0.00	0.00	97.90	1.87
	Salmon, Coho, Wild, Ckd, Moist H	155.0000	3.000	Ounce	42.41	11.63	0.00	285.20	0.00	0.00	88.35	2.48
	Salmon, Pink, Ckd, Dry Heat	124.0000	3.000	Ounce	31.69	5.48	0.00	184.76	0.00	0.00	83.08	0.89
	Sardine, Atlantic, Cnd In Oil	149.0000	1.000	Cup	36.68	17.06	0.00	309.92	0.00	0.00	211.58	2.28
	Scallop, Breaded and Fried	31.0000	2.000	Large	5.60	3.39	3.14	66.65	0.00	0.00	18.91	0.83
	Scallop, Imitation	85.0000	3.000	Ounce	10.85	0.35	9.03	84.15	0.00	0.00	18.70	0.07
	Scallops, Sauteed	28.3500	3.000	Ounce	9.67	0.33	0.67	50.00	0.00	0.00	20.00	0.00
	Sea Bass, Ckd, Dry Heat	101.0000	1.000	Each	23.87	2.59	0.00	125.24	0.00	0.00	53.53	0.67
	Shark, Ckd, Batter-dipped and Fr	85.0000	3.000	Ounce	15.83	11.75	5.43	193.80	0.00	0.00	50.15	2.73
	Shrimp, Ckd, Breaded and Fried	85.0000	3.000	Ounce	18.18	10.44	9.75	205.70	0.00	0.32	150.45	1.78
	Shrimp, Ckd, Moist Heat	85.0000	3.000	Ounce	17.77	0.92	0.00	84.15	0.00	0.00	165.75	0.25
	Shrimp, Cnd	128.0000	1.000	Cup	29.54	2.51	1.32	153.60	0.00	0.00	221.44	0.47
	Shrimp, Fresh	6.0000	1.000	Slice	1.22	0.10	0.05	6.36	0.00	0.00	9.12	0.02
	Shrimp, Imitation	85.0000	3.000	Ounce	10.53	1.25	7.76	85.85	0.00	0.00	30.60	0.25
	Smelt, Rainbow, Ckd, Dry Heat	85.0000	3.000	Ounce	19.21	2.64	0.00	105.40	0.00	0.00	76.50	0.49
	Snapper, Ckd, Dry Heat	170.0000	1.000	Each	44.71	2.92	0.00	217.60	0.00	0.00	79.90	0.63
	Squid, Fried	85.0000	3.000	Ounce	15.25	6.36	6.62	148.75	0.00	0.00	221.00	1.60
	Sunfish, Ckd, Dry Heat	37.0000	1.000	Each	9.20	0.33	0.00	42.18	0.00	0.00	31.82	0.07
	Swordfish, Ckd, Dry Heat	106.0000	1.000	Piece	26.91	5.45	0.00	164.30	0.00	0.00	53.00	1.49
	Trout, Ckd, Dry Heat	62.0000	1.000	Each	16.51	5.25	0.00	117.80	0.00	0.00	45.88	0.91
	Trout, Rainbow, Farmed, Ckd, Dry	71.0000	1.000	Each	17.23	5.11	0.00	119.99	0.00	0.00	48.28	1.50
	Trout, Rainbow, Wild, Ckd, Dry H	143.0000	1.000	Each	32.78	8.32	0.00	214.50	0.00	0.00	98.67	2.32
	Tuna Salad	205.0000	1.000	Cup	32.88	18.98	19.29	383.35	0.00	0.00	26.65	3.16
	Tuna, Light Meat, Cnd In Oil	171.0000	1.000	Can	49.81	14.04	0.00	338.58	0.00	0.00	30.78	2.62

Monounsaturated Fat (gm)	Polyunsaturated Fat (gm)	Vitamin D (mg)	Vitamin K (mg)	Vitamin E (mg)	Vitamin A (re)	Vitamin C (mg)	Thiamin (mg)	Riboflavin (mg)	Niacin (mg)	Vitamin B6 (mg)	Folate (mg)	Vitamin B12 (mcg)	Calcium (mg)	Iron (mg)	Magnesium (mg)	Phosphorus (mg)	Potassium (mg)	Sodium (mg)	Zinc (mg)
0.55	0.81	0.00	0.00	0.00	101.00	0.00	0.16	0.02	0.77	0.71	20.60	1.39	42.42	2.30	74.74	288.86	959.50	107.06	1.03
0.23	0.47	0.00	0.00	0.00	28.50	0.00	0.06	0.08	6.95	0.53	19.95	2.09	63.00	2.03	75.00	361.50	598.50	130.50	0.72
0.05	0.09	0.00	0.00	0.11	6.24	0.00	0.01	0.01	1.44	0.11	4.34	0.45	13.89	0.40	15.31	71.16	117.65	216.31	0.14
1.54	1.49	0.00	0.00	1.73	85.86	0.00	0.11	0.14	11.32	0.64	21.94	2.18	95.40	1.70	170.13	453.15	915.84	109.71	0.84
17.08	2.78	0.00	0.00	0.00	28.62	0.00	0.11	0.16	3.05	0.78	1.59	1.53	6.36	1.35	52.47	333.90	546.96	163.77	0.81
6.85	3.92	0.00	0.00	1.92	44.33	1.00	0.16	0.43	5.89	0.50	16.45	18.79	105.82	2.02	58.63	433.29	599.17	164.45	1.82
1.45	0.83	0.85	0.00	0.28	11.06	0.28	0.04	0.09	1.25	0.12	3.88	5.30	23.81	0.43	13.04	92.14	126.72	260.25	0.39
12.69	4.48	0.00	0.00	0.00	50.40	0.00	0.10	0.37	4.06	0.75	8.64	13.85	152.64	2.07	59.04	420.48	780.48	136.80	0.98
16.73	2.35	23.80	0.00	1.40	361.20	0.00	0.06	0.20	4.62	0.24	3.36	5.98	107.80	1.71	11.20	124.60	96.60	1218.00	0.74
0.23	0.13	0.00	0.00	1.45	37.70	0.00	0.01	0.10	1.55	0.12	16.10	4.51	88.45	0.57	50.75	268.25	510.40	551.00	4.23
0.57	1.24	0.00	0.00	0.00	9.78	3.42	0.02	0.10	7.99	0.28	1.63	6.59	102.69	2.30	83.13	373.27	339.04	370.01	11.85
6.17	3.78	0.00	0.00	0.00	47.52	0.35	0.14	0.36	6.03	0.40	1.32	16.72	13.20	1.38	85.36	244.64	352.88	73.04	0.83
1.28	0.86	0.00	0.00	0.00	39.06	1.12	0.09	0.09	5.86	0.46	9.11	0.23	28.83	1.31	30.69	226.92	425.94	66.03	0.82
0.86	1.03	0.00	0.00	0.00	77.35	11.56	0.26	0.36	2.55	0.09	64.26	20.40	28.05	5.71	31.45	242.25	227.80	313.65	2.27
4.00	2.81	0.00	0.00	0.00	76.50	3.23	0.13	0.17	1.40	0.05	26.35	13.29	52.70	5.91	49.30	135.15	207.40	354.45	74.06
0.41	1.20	0.00	0.00	1.38	145.80	8.10	0.24	0.28	2.01	0.16	14.42	30.99	72.90	10.85	87.48	225.18	370.98	181.44	47.34
0.13	0.50	0.00	0.00	0.00	6.80	4.00	0.09	0.06	1.08	0.05	15.30	13.77	37.40	4.91	28.05	79.05	105.40	151.30	32.23
0.40	0.28	0.00	0.00	0.00	7.00	0.40	0.07	0.07	1.22	0.14	5.20	0.58	68.50	0.59	19.50	138.50	175.00	48.00	0.31
0.09	0.22	0.00	0.00	0.00	4.60	0.78	0.04	0.06	0.87	0.06	2.67	1.01	46.92	0.53	17.48	118.22	158.24	36.34	0.66
0.31	0.40	0.00	0.00	0.00	37.20	5.89	0.11	0.12	4.34	0.22	26.82	3.57	113.15	1.10	62.00	437.10	513.05	75.95	1.33
0.47	0.71	0.00	0.00	0.00	29.76	0.00	0.38	0.25	3.47	0.17	21.08	2.86	174.84	2.07	47.12	333.56	618.76	80.60	0.98
0.21	0.94	0.00	0.00	0.00	18.12	0.00	0.08	0.35	6.01	0.50	4.53	5.56	116.27	0.89	129.86	427.33	688.56	166.10	0.91
2.82	1.24	0.00	0.00	0.00	0.00	0.00	0.58	0.13	3.23	0.20	14.71	1.02	36.55	0.57	26.35	289.85	540.60	64.60	0.59
2.92	1.28	0.00	0.00	0.00	31.68	0.00	0.60	0.13	3.34	0.20	15.22	1.06	37.84	0.59	27.28	300.08	559.68	66.88	0.61
0.67	0.88	0.00	0.00	1.86	98.34	0.00	0.06	0.12	5.84	0.40	15.50	1.79	17.88	0.79	50.66	339.72	774.80	114.73	0.79
0.53	0.02	0.00	0.00	0.00	20.40	0.00	0.10	0.15	3.10	0.30	6.80	1.96	32.30	0.20	32.30	217.60	327.25	68.85	0.82
4.16	5.02	0.00	0.00	0.00	20.02	0.00	0.43	0.75	15.52	1.45	44.66	4.70	23.10	1.59	56.98	394.24	967.12	86.24	1.26
8.84	4.10	0.00	0.00	0.00	229.46	6.31	0.06	0.23	15.48	0.71	53.90	4.42	43.12	1.40	187.88	571.34	777.70	92.40	0.86
3.05	1.77	0.00	0.00	0.00	52.36	0.00	0.14	0.34	13.14	0.71	7.70	5.33	21.56	1.09	43.12	559.02	847.00	98.56	0.92
11.66	6.97	0.00	0.00	5.90	195.57	0.00	0.07	0.70	20.22	1.11	36.16	1.11	881.91	3.91	107.01	1202.94	1391.13	1985.22	3.76
5.18	2.80	0.00	0.00	0.00	84.37	2.15	0.14	0.16	10.57	0.82	20.02	4.53	17.16	0.56	48.62	474.76	657.80	74.36	0.67
2.81	2.26	0.00	0.00	1.44	69.42	2.49	0.14	0.25	14.15	1.01	23.14	8.90	80.10	1.09	58.74	573.16	772.52	103.24	1.00
4.19	3.91	0.00	0.00	0.00	49.60	1.55	0.19	0.25	12.06	0.87	13.95	6.94	71.30	1.10	54.25	461.90	705.25	82.15	0.81
1.49	2.15	0.00	0.00	0.00	50.84	0.00	0.25	0.09	10.58	0.29	6.20	4.29	21.08	1.23	40.92	365.80	513.36	106.64	0.88
5.77	7.67	10.13	0.00	0.45	99.83	0.00	0.12	0.34	7.82	0.25	17.58	13.32	569.01	4.35	58.11	730.10	591.53	752.45	1.95
1.40	0.89	0.00	0.00	0.00	6.82	0.71	0.01	0.03	0.47	0.04	11.47	0.41	13.02	0.25	18.29	73.16	103.23	143.84	0.33
0.05	0.18	0.00	0.00	0.00	17.00	0.00	0.01	0.02	0.26	0.03	1.36	1.36	6.80	0.26	36.55	239.70	87.55	675.75	0.28
0.00	0.00	0.00	0.00	0.00	0.00	0.60	0.00	0.00	0.00	0.00	0.00	0.00	8.00	0.00	0.00	0.00	0.00	91.67	0.00
0.55	0.96	0.00	0.00	0.00	64.64	0.00	0.13	0.15	1.92	0.46	5.86	0.30	13.13	0.37	53.53	250.48	331.28	87.87	0.53
5.05	3.15	0.00	0.00	0.00	45.90	0.00	0.06	0.09	2.36	0.26	12.75	1.03	42.50	0.94	36.55	164.90	131.75	103.70	0.41
3.24	4.33	0.00	0.00	0.00	47.60	1.28	0.11	0.12	2.61	0.09	6.89	1.59	56.95	1.07	34.00	185.30	191.25	292.40	1.17
0.17	0.37	0.00	0.00	0.43	56.10	1.87	0.03	0.03	2.20	0.11	2.98	1.27	33.15	2.63	28.90	116.45	154.70	190.40	1.33
0.37	0.97	0.00	0.00	1.19	23.04	2.94	0.04	0.05	3.53	0.14	2.30	1.43	75.52	3.51	52.48	298.24	268.80	216.32	1.61
0.02	0.04	0.23	0.00	0.05	3.24	0.12	0.00	0.00	0.15	0.01	0.18	0.07	3.12	0.14	2.22	12.30	11.10	8.88	0.07
0.19	0.64	0.00	0.00	0.00	17.00	0.00	0.02	0.03	0.14	0.03	1.36	1.36	16.15	0.51	36.55	239.70	75.65	599.25	0.28
0.70	0.97	0.00	0.00	0.00	14.45	0.00	0.01	0.13	1.50	0.14	3.91	3.37	65.45	0.98	32.30	250.75	316.20	65.45	1.80
0.54	1.00	0.00	0.00	0.00	59.50	2.72	0.09	0.00	0.60	0.78	9.86	5.95	68.00	0.41	62.90	341.70	887.40	96.90	0.75
2.34	1.82	0.00	0.00	0.00	9.35	3.57	0.05	0.39	2.21	0.05	11.90	1.05	33.15	0.86	32.30	213.35	237.15	260.10	1.48
0.06	0.12	0.00	0.00	0.00	6.29	0.37	0.03	0.03	0.54	0.05	6.29	0.85	38.11	0.57	14.06	85.47	166.13	38.11	0.74
2.10	1.25	0.00	0.00	0.00	43.46	1.17	0.04	0.13	12.50	0.40	2.44	2.14	6.36	1.10	36.04	357.22	391.14	121.90	1.56
2.59	1.19	0.00	0.00	0.00	11.78	0.31	0.27	0.26	3.58	0.14	9.30	4.64	34.10	1.19	17.36	194.68	287.06	41.54	0.53
1.49	1.65	0.00	0.00	0.00	61.06	2.34	0.17	0.06	6.24	0.28	17.04	3.53	61.06	0.23	22.72	188.86	313.11	29.82	0.35
2.50	2.62	0.00	0.00	0.00	21.45	2.86	0.21	0.14	8.25	0.50	27.17	9.01	122.98	0.54	44.33	384.67	640.64	80.08	0.73
5.92	8.45	0.00	0.00	0.00	55.35	4.51	0.06	0.14	13.74	0.16	16.40	2.46	34.85	2.05	38.95	364.90	364.90	824.10	1.15
5.04	4.94	0.00	0.00	0.00	39.33	0.00	0.07	0.21	21.20	0.19	9.06	3.76	22.23	2.38	53.01	531.81	353.97	85.50	1.54

USDA ID Code	Food Name	Weight in Grams*	Quantity of Units	Unit of Measure	Protein (gm)	Fat (gm)	Carbohydrate (gm)	Kcalories	Caffeine (gm)	Fiber (gm)	Cholesterol (mg)	Saturated Fat (gm)
	Tuna, Light Meat, Cnd In Water	165.0000	1.000	Can	42.09	1.35	0.00	191.40	0.00	0.00	49.50	0.38
	Tuna, Light, Cnd In Water	154.0000	1.000	Cup	39.29	1.26	0.00	178.64	0.00	0.00	46.20	0.35
	Tuna, Skipjack, Ckd, Dry Heat	154.0000	3.000	Ounce	43.44	1.99	0.00	203.28	0.00	0.00	92.40	0.65
	Tuna, White Meat, Cnd In Oil	178.0000	1.000	Can	47.22	14.38	0.00	331.08	0.00	0.00	55.18	2.94
	Tuna, White Meat, Cnd In Water	172.0000	1.000	Can	40.63	5.11	0.00	220.16	0.00	0.00	72.24	1.36
	Tuna, Yellowfin, Ckd, Dry Heat	85.0000	3.000	Ounce	25.47	1.04	0.00	118.15	0.00	0.00	49.30	0.26
	Whitefish, Ckd, Dry Heat	154.0000	1.000	Each	37.68	11.57	0.00	264.88	0.00	0.00	118.58	1.79
	Whitefish, Smoked	136.0000	1.000	Cup	31.82	1.26	0.00	146.88	0.00	0.00	44.88	0.31
	Yellowtail, Ckd, Dry Heat	146.0000	3.000	Ounce	43.32	9.81	0.00	273.02	0.00	0.00	103.66	0.00
	Yellowtail, Fresh	187.0000	3.000	Ounce	43.27	9.80	0.00	273.02	0.00	0.00	102.85	2.39

Snacks and Sweets

USDA ID Code	Food Name	Weight in Grams*	Quantity of Units	Unit of Measure	Protein (gm)	Fat (gm)	Carbohydrate (gm)	Kcalories	Caffeine (gm)	Fiber (gm)	Cholesterol (mg)	Saturated Fat (gm)
	Brownies	28.3500	1.000	Ounce	1.36	4.62	18.12	114.82	0.57	0.60	4.82	1.20
	Candy Bar, Almond Joy	20.0000	1.000	Small Ba	0.84	5.36	11.66	93.40	0.00	0.96	0.80	3.46
	Candy Bar, Alpine White, w/ Almo	35.0000	1.000	Bar	3.50	12.92	17.64	197.40	0.00	1.89	4.20	6.67
	Candy Bar, Butterfinger Bar	174.0000	1.000	Cup	21.66	32.47	114.07	835.20	6.96	4.18	1.74	18.03
	Candy Bar, Chocolate Bar - Krack	41.0000	1.000	Each	2.71	11.77	25.26	217.71	7.38	0.90	7.79	7.42
	Candy Bar, Chocolate, Milk - Sym	42.0000	1.000	Each	3.02	13.78	24.33	232.26	0.00	0.80	9.24	0.00
	Candy Bar, Chocolate, Special Da	41.0000	1.000	Each	2.01	13.28	24.85	226.32	29.93	2.05	0.41	8.32
	Candy Bar, Chocolate-Mr. Goodbar	49.0000	1.000	Each	5.24	17.10	25.33	267.05	9.80	1.72	3.92	7.30
	Candy Bar, Chunky Bar	35.0000	1.000	Each	3.15	10.22	19.99	173.25	10.15	1.68	3.85	8.13
	Candy Bar, Fifth Avenue Bar	57.0000	1.000	Each	5.13	12.14	37.68	280.44	3.99	1.25	3.42	4.50
	Candy Bar, Milky Way	23.0000	1.000	Each	1.04	3.70	16.49	97.29	1.84	0.39	3.22	1.79
	Candy Bar, Mounds	53.0000	1.000	Each	2.01	13.30	31.22	252.81	9.01	3.13	1.06	10.76
	Candy Bar, Nestle Crunch	40.0000	1.000	Each	2.40	10.52	26.08	208.80	9.60	1.04	5.20	6.08
	Candy Bar, Peanut Bar	28.3500	1.000	Ounce	4.39	9.55	13.44	147.99	0.00	1.62	0.00	1.33
	Candy Bar, Peanut Butter Cups -	7.0000	1.000	Miniatur	0.72	2.19	3.82	37.87	0.70	0.22	0.35	0.78
	Candy Bar, Snickers	57.0000	1.000	Each	4.56	14.01	33.75	273.03	3.99	1.43	7.41	5.12
	Candy Bar, Three Musketeers	23.0000	1.000	Each	0.74	2.97	17.66	95.68	2.53	0.37	2.53	1.50
	Candy Bar, Twix	57.0000	1.000	Each	2.62	13.90	37.38	284.43	1.71	0.63	2.85	5.07
	Candy Bar, Wafer Bar - Kit Kat	42.0000	1.000	Each	2.98	10.71	26.88	215.88	5.04	0.80	2.52	6.85
	Candy, Butterscotch	28.3500	1.000	Ounce	0.03	0.99	27.02	111.98	0.00	0.00	2.55	0.31
	Candy, Caramels	71.0000	1.000	Package	3.27	5.75	54.67	271.22	0.00	0.85	4.97	4.67
	Candy, Goobers	39.0000	1.000	Package	5.34	13.07	18.99	200.07	8.58	2.38	3.51	4.76
	Candy, Gumdrops	182.0000	1.000	Cup	0.00	0.00	180.00	702.52	0.00	0.00	0.00	0.00
	Candy, Jellybeans	11.0000	10.000	Each	0.00	0.06	10.24	40.37	0.00	0.00	0.00	0.02
	Candy, Lollipop	28.3500	1.000	Ounce	0.00	0.06	27.78	111.70	0.00	0.00	0.00	0.00
	Candy, M&M's Almond	42.0000	1.000	Pkg	4.00	13.00	25.00	230.00	0.00	2.00	5.00	4.00
	Candy, M&M's Peanut	170.0000	1.000	Cup	16.10	44.61	102.78	877.20	18.70	5.78	15.30	17.56
	Candy, M&M's Plain	208.0000	1.000	Cup	9.01	43.95	148.12	1023.36	37.44	5.20	29.12	27.21
	Candy, Peanut Brittle	28.3500	1.000	Ounce	2.13	5.41	19.65	128.43	0.00	0.57	3.69	1.42
	Candy, Praline	39.0000	1.000	Piece	1.09	9.48	24.18	177.06	0.00	0.00	0.00	0.73
	Candy, Raisinets	45.0000	1.000	Package	2.12	7.16	32.04	185.40	11.25	2.30	1.80	3.30
	Candy, Reese's Pieces	47.0000	0.250	Cup	6.49	9.92	28.86	230.77	0.00	1.36	0.94	8.51
	Candy, Skittles Bite Size	205.0000	1.000	Cup	0.39	8.96	185.81	830.25	0.00	0.00	0.00	1.78
	Candy, Taffy	15.0000	1.000	Piece	0.02	0.50	13.71	56.40	0.00	0.00	1.35	0.31
	Candy, Toffee	12.0000	1.000	Piece	0.13	3.94	7.72	65.04	0.00	0.00	12.60	2.45
	Candy, Truffles	12.0000	1.000	Piece	0.68	4.12	5.40	58.56	0.00	0.00	6.24	2.58
	Candy, Twizzlers Strawberry	71.0000	1.000	Package	2.41	1.14	54.95	237.14	0.00	0.99	0.00	0.28
	Candy, York Peppermint Pattie (l	42.0000	1.000	Lg Patty	0.92	2.98	33.64	165.06	0.00	0.84	0.42	1.81
	Candy, York Peppermint Pattie (s	14.0000	1.000	Sm Patty	0.31	0.99	11.21	55.02	0.00	0.28	0.14	0.60
	Chips, Bagel	28.3500	1.000	Ounce	4.00	6.00	20.00	150.00	0.00	1.00	0.00	1.00
	Chips, Banana	28.3500	1.000	Ounce	0.65	9.53	16.56	147.14	0.00	2.18	0.00	8.21
	Chips, Corn	2.2310	1.000	Each	0.15	0.85	1.15	12.31	0.00	0.08	0.00	0.12
	Chips, Doritos - Cheese, Nacho	28.0000	1.000	Ounce	2.00	7.00	17.00	140.00	0.00	0.00	0.00	1.00
	Chips, Doritos - Ranch, Cool	28.0000	1.000	Ounce	2.00	7.00	18.00	140.00	0.00	0.00	0.00	1.00
	Chips, Fritos	28.0000	1.000	Ounce	2.00	10.00	15.00	160.00	0.00	0.00	0.00	1.50

Monounsaturated Fat (gm)	Polyunsaturated Fat (gm)	Vitamin D (mg)	Vitamin K (mg)	Vitamin E (mg)	Vitamin A (re)	Vitamin C (mg)	Thiamin (mg)	Riboflavin (mg)	Niacin (mg)	Vitamin B$_6$ (mg)	Folate (mg)	Vitamin B$_{12}$ (mcg)	Calcium (mg)	Iron (mg)	Magnesium (mg)	Phosphorus (mg)	Potassium (mg)	Sodium (mg)	Zinc (mg)
0.26	0.56	0.00	0.00	0.87	28.05	0.00	0.05	0.12	21.91	0.58	6.60	4.93	18.15	2.52	44.55	268.95	391.05	82.50	1.27
0.25	0.52	0.00	0.00	0.82	26.18	0.00	0.05	0.11	20.45	0.54	6.16	4.60	16.94	2.36	41.58	251.02	364.98	520.52	1.19
0.37	0.62	0.00	0.00	0.00	27.72	1.54	0.06	0.18	28.89	1.51	15.40	3.37	56.98	2.46	67.76	438.90	803.88	72.38	1.62
4.41	6.02	0.00	0.00	0.00	42.72	0.00	0.04	0.14	20.83	0.77	8.19	3.92	7.12	1.16	60.52	475.26	592.74	89.00	0.84
1.34	1.91	0.00	0.00	2.73	10.32	0.00	0.02	0.07	9.98	0.38	3.44	2.01	24.08	1.67	56.76	373.24	407.64	86.00	0.83
0.17	0.31	0.00	0.00	0.00	17.00	0.85	0.43	0.05	10.15	0.88	1.70	0.51	17.85	0.80	54.40	208.25	483.65	39.95	0.57
3.94	4.25	0.00	0.00	0.00	60.06	0.00	0.26	0.23	5.93	0.54	26.18	1.48	50.82	0.72	64.68	532.84	625.24	100.10	1.96
0.38	0.39	0.00	0.00	0.27	77.52	0.00	0.04	0.14	3.26	0.53	9.93	4.43	24.48	0.68	31.28	179.52	575.28	1385.84	0.67
0.00	0.00	0.00	0.00	0.00	45.26	4.23	0.26	0.07	12.73	0.28	5.84	1.83	42.34	0.92	55.48	293.46	785.48	73.00	0.98
3.72	2.66	0.00	0.00	0.00	54.23	5.24	0.26	0.07	12.72	0.30	6.92	2.43	43.01	0.92	56.10	293.59	785.40	72.93	0.97
2.54	0.64	0.00	0.00	0.59	1.70	0.00	0.07	0.06	0.49	0.01	5.95	0.02	8.22	0.64	8.79	28.63	42.24	88.45	0.20
1.32	0.30	0.00	0.00	0.00	0.80	0.04	0.01	0.03	0.09	0.01	1.60	0.02	12.20	0.28	13.20	28.00	49.20	29.20	0.16
4.81	0.88	0.00	0.00	0.00	8.75	0.14	0.03	0.15	0.03	0.03	4.55	0.30	80.85	0.20	13.30	81.55	146.30	25.55	0.40
9.67	4.87	0.00	0.00	2.82	0.00	0.00	0.16	0.12	4.35	0.12	46.98	0.02	46.98	1.29	137.46	227.94	662.94	344.52	2.04
3.94	0.37	0.00	0.00	0.00	4.92	0.16	0.02	0.12	0.18	0.01	3.28	0.24	71.75	0.37	22.55	90.61	140.22	56.58	0.50
0.00	0.00	0.00	0.00	0.00	5.46	0.17	0.04	0.16	0.14	0.02	2.94	0.16	90.30	0.50	23.10	105.00	161.70	38.64	0.47
4.59	0.41	0.00	0.00	0.18	1.64	0.00	0.01	0.03	0.16	0.01	0.82	0.00	11.07	0.98	45.51	61.50	122.59	2.87	0.59
5.73	2.35	0.00	0.00	1.34	18.13	0.15	0.08	0.13	1.62	0.04	19.11	0.15	52.92	0.46	42.14	121.52	219.03	73.01	0.89
0.11	1.54	0.00	0.00	0.00	3.85	0.11	0.03	0.14	0.67	0.04	7.70	0.13	50.05	0.44	25.55	72.82	186.90	18.55	0.64
5.70	1.94	0.00	0.00	1.32	8.55	0.11	0.08	0.07	1.97	0.05	21.66	0.07	42.18	0.74	36.48	87.78	169.29	94.05	0.70
1.38	0.14	0.00	0.00	0.15	7.36	0.23	0.01	0.05	0.08	0.01	2.30	0.07	29.90	0.17	7.82	33.12	55.43	55.20	0.16
2.28	0.27	0.00	0.00	0.36	0.53	0.21	0.02	0.03	0.15	0.05	1.59	0.00	7.95	1.11	29.68	48.23	130.91	78.97	0.52
3.44	0.35	0.00	0.00	0.44	8.00	0.12	0.14	0.22	1.58	0.16	31.60	0.15	67.60	0.20	23.20	80.80	137.60	53.20	0.57
4.74	3.02	0.00	0.00	1.30	0.00	0.00	0.03	0.04	2.25	0.05	22.11	0.00	22.11	0.27	32.60	91.29	115.38	44.23	1.17
0.92	0.39	0.00	0.00	0.28	1.33	0.01	0.02	0.01	0.32	0.01	3.85	0.01	5.46	0.08	6.23	14.21	24.64	22.19	0.13
5.96	2.80	0.00	0.00	0.87	22.23	0.34	0.06	0.09	2.39	0.05	22.80	0.09	53.58	0.43	41.04	126.54	184.68	151.62	1.34
0.99	0.10	0.00	0.00	0.15	5.52	0.09	0.01	0.03	0.05	0.00	0.00	0.04	19.32	0.17	6.67	20.93	30.59	44.62	0.13
7.64	0.48	0.00	0.00	0.70	14.25	0.23	0.09	0.13	0.68	0.02	13.68	0.10	51.30	0.46	18.24	68.40	115.14	110.01	0.44
3.11	0.34	0.00	0.00	0.34	20.16	0.29	0.08	0.23	1.07	0.05	59.64	0.07	69.30	0.38	16.38	99.96	122.22	31.50	0.52
0.14	0.02	0.00	0.00	0.02	9.64	0.00	0.00	0.01	0.00	0.00	0.00	0.00	0.85	0.02	0.85	0.85	1.13	104.04	0.01
0.60	0.13	0.00	0.00	0.33	5.68	0.36	0.01	0.13	0.18	0.03	3.55	0.00	97.98	0.10	12.07	80.94	151.94	173.95	0.31
5.75	1.99	0.00	0.00	0.00	0.00	0.00	0.05	0.08	2.03	0.08	3.12	0.11	49.53	0.52	46.41	115.44	195.78	15.99	0.85
0.00	0.00	0.00	0.00	0.00	0.00	0.00	0.00	0.00	0.00	0.00	0.00	0.00	5.46	0.73	1.82	1.82	9.10	80.08	0.00
0.02	0.01	0.00	0.00	0.00	0.00	0.00	0.00	0.00	0.00	0.00	0.00	0.00	0.33	0.12	0.22	0.44	4.07	2.75	0.01
0.00	0.00	0.00	0.00	0.00	0.00	0.00	0.00	0.00	0.00	0.00	0.00	0.00	0.85	0.09	0.85	0.85	1.42	10.77	0.00
0.00	0.00	0.00	0.00	0.00	0.00	0.00	0.00	0.00	0.00	0.00	0.00	0.00	72.00	0.40	0.00	0.00	0.00	20.00	0.00
18.70	7.14	0.00	0.00	4.13	40.80	0.85	0.17	0.29	6.38	0.14	59.50	0.31	171.70	1.96	125.80	387.60	588.20	81.60	3.91
14.31	1.31	0.00	0.00	1.79	110.24	1.04	0.12	0.44	0.46	0.06	12.48	0.56	218.40	2.31	85.28	312.00	553.28	126.88	2.00
2.40	1.33	0.00	0.00	0.46	13.32	0.00	0.05	0.01	0.99	0.03	19.85	0.00	8.51	0.39	14.18	31.47	58.97	128.14	0.27
5.92	2.35	0.00	0.00	0.00	1.95	0.27	0.12	0.02	0.13	0.03	5.46	0.00	12.09	0.46	20.28	42.51	82.29	24.18	0.79
2.67	0.86	0.00	0.00	0.00	4.05	0.09	0.04	0.10	0.18	0.05	2.25	0.09	48.60	0.54	20.25	64.80	231.30	16.20	0.36
0.99	0.47	0.00	0.00	0.98	0.00	0.19	0.05	0.07	1.34	0.03	13.16	0.10	38.54	0.38	20.68	62.04	108.10	69.09	0.36
6.07	0.25	0.00	0.00	0.57	0.00	137.15	0.00	0.04	0.04	0.02	0.00	0.00	0.00	0.02	2.05	4.10	10.25	32.80	0.06
0.14	0.02	0.00	0.00	0.00	4.95	0.00	0.00	0.00	0.00	0.00	0.00	0.00	0.45	0.01	0.15	0.45	0.60	13.35	0.00
1.14	0.15	0.00	0.00	0.00	38.16	0.02	0.00	0.01	0.00	0.00	0.24	0.01	4.08	0.00	0.48	3.96	6.00	22.44	0.02
1.22	0.13	0.00	0.00	0.00	17.16	0.05	0.01	0.03	0.03	0.00	0.12	0.04	18.60	0.12	5.64	21.24	36.60	8.52	0.13
0.00	0.00	0.00	0.00	0.00	0.00	0.00	0.01	0.03	0.07	0.01	0.00	0.00	4.97	0.21	4.26	220.10	45.44	175.37	0.11
1.05	0.08	0.00	0.00	0.00	0.00	0.00	0.00	0.00	0.00	0.00	0.00	0.00	6.30	0.42	0.00	0.00	54.18	10.08	0.00
0.35	0.03	0.00	0.00	0.00	0.14	0.00	0.00	0.01	0.12	0.00	0.56	0.00	2.10	0.14	8.82	13.30	18.06	3.36	0.11
3.00	2.00	0.00	0.00	0.00	0.00	0.00	0.00	0.00	0.00	0.00	0.00	0.00	0.00	0.40	0.00	0.00	0.00	190.00	0.00
0.55	0.18	0.00	0.00	1.53	2.27	1.79	0.03	0.01	0.20	0.07	3.97	0.00	5.10	0.35	21.55	15.88	151.96	1.70	0.21
0.00	0.00	0.00	0.00	0.00	0.00	0.00	0.00	0.00	0.00	0.00	0.00	0.00	5.54	0.02	0.00	0.00	0.00	15.38	0.00
0.00	0.00	0.00	0.00	0.00	0.00	0.00	0.00	0.00	0.00	0.00	0.00	0.00	32.00	0.20	0.00	0.00	0.00	200.00	0.00
0.00	0.00	0.00	0.00	0.00	0.00	0.00	0.00	0.00	0.00	0.00	0.00	0.00	32.00	0.20	0.00	0.00	0.00	170.00	0.00
0.00	0.00	0.00	0.00	0.00	0.00	0.00	0.00	0.00	0.00	0.00	0.00	0.00	0.00	0.00	0.00	0.00	0.00	160.00	0.00

USDA ID Code	Food Name	Weight in Grams*	Quantity of Units	Unit of Measure	Protein (gm)	Fat (gm)	Carbohydrate (gm)	Kcalories	Caffeine (gm)	Fiber (gm)	Cholesterol (mg)	Saturated Fat (gm)
	Chips, Fritos-Barbecue	28.0000	1.000	Ounce	2.00	9.00	16.00	160.00	0.00	0.00	0.00	1.50
	Chips, Pork Skins, Barbecue-flav	28.3500	1.000	Ounce	16.41	9.02	0.45	152.52	0.00	0.00	32.60	3.28
	Chips, Pork Skins, Plain	28.3500	1.000	Ounce	17.38	8.87	0.00	154.51	0.00	0.00	26.93	3.22
	Chips, Potato - Baked Lays	28.0000	1.000	Ounce	2.00	1.50	23.00	110.00	0.00	0.00	0.00	0.00
	Chips, Potato - Barbeque	28.0000	1.000	Ounce	2.00	10.00	15.00	160.00	0.00	0.00	0.00	1.50
	Chips, Potato Sticks	28.3500	1.000	Ounce	1.90	9.75	15.11	147.99	0.00	0.96	0.00	2.52
	Chips, Potato, Barbecue-flavor	28.3500	1.000	Ounce	2.18	9.19	14.97	139.20	0.00	1.25	0.00	2.28
	Chips, Potato, Cheese-flavor	28.3500	1.000	Ounce	2.41	7.71	16.36	140.62	0.00	1.47	1.13	2.44
	Chips, Potato, Cheese-flavor - P	28.3500	1.000	Ounce	1.98	10.49	14.35	156.21	0.00	0.95	1.13	2.71
	Chips, Potato, Light	28.3500	1.000	Ounce	2.01	5.90	18.97	133.53	0.00	1.66	0.00	1.18
	Chips, Potato, Light - Pringles	28.3500	1.000	Ounce	1.59	7.29	18.40	142.03	0.00	1.02	0.00	1.45
	Chips, Potato, Plain - Pringles	28.3500	1.000	Ounce	1.67	10.89	14.46	158.19	0.00	1.02	0.00	2.68
	Chips, Potato, Plain, Salted	28.3500	1.000	Ounce	1.98	9.81	15.00	151.96	0.00	1.28	0.00	3.11
	Chips, Potato, Plain, Unsalted	28.3500	1.000	Ounce	1.98	9.81	15.00	151.96	0.00	1.36	0.00	3.11
	Chips, Potato, Reduced Fat - Ruf	28.0000	1.000	Ounce	2.00	6.70	18.00	140.00	0.00	0.00	0.00	1.00
	Chips, Potato, Sour Cream & Onio	28.3500	1.000	Ounce	1.87	10.49	14.54	155.07	0.00	0.34	0.85	2.68
	Chips, Potato, Sour Cream and On	28.3500	1.000	Ounce	2.30	9.61	14.60	150.54	0.00	1.47	1.98	2.52
	Chips, Potato, w/o Salt Added	28.3500	1.000	Ounce	1.82	10.03	14.70	148.27	0.00	1.36	0.00	2.57
	Chips, Sun, original	28.0000	1.000	Ounce	1.00	6.00	20.00	140.00	0.00	0.00	0.00	1.00
	Chips, Taro	28.3500	1.000	Ounce	0.65	7.06	19.31	141.18	0.00	2.04	0.00	1.82
	Chips, Tortilla, Low-Fat, Baked	2.1810	13.000	Chips	0.23	0.08	1.85	8.46	0.00	0.15	0.00	0.00
	Chips, Tortilla, Nacho Flavor	28.3500	1.000	Ounce	2.21	7.26	17.69	141.18	0.00	1.50	0.85	1.39
	Chips, Tortilla, Nacho-flavor, L	28.3500	1.000	Ounce	2.47	4.31	20.30	126.16	0.00	1.36	0.85	0.82
	Chips, Tortilla, Plain	28.3500	1.000	Ounce	1.98	7.43	17.83	142.03	0.00	1.84	0.00	1.42
	Chips, Tortilla, Ranch Flavor	28.3500	1.000	Ounce	2.15	6.75	18.31	138.92	0.00	1.10	0.28	1.29
	Chips, Tortilla, Taco-flavor	28.3500	1.000	Ounce	2.24	6.86	17.89	136.08	0.00	1.50	1.42	1.32
	Chips, Tostitos, Baked	28.0000	1.000	Ounce	2.00	1.00	24.00	110.00	0.00	0.00	0.00	0.00
	Chips, Tostitos, Baked, Salsa &	28.0000	1.000	Ounce	2.00	3.00	21.00	120.00	0.00	0.00	0.00	0.50
	Chocolate, Milk	168.0000	1.000	Cup	11.59	51.58	99.46	861.84	43.68	5.71	36.96	31.05
	Chocolate, Milk, w/ Almonds	41.0000	1.000	Each	3.69	14.10	21.81	215.66	9.02	2.54	7.79	6.96
191	Cliff Bar, Apple Cherry	68.0000	1.000	Each	4.00	2.00	52.00	250.00	0.00	2.00	0.00	0.50
192	Cliff Bar, Apricot	68.0000	1.000	Each	6.00	0.00	55.00	250.00	0.00	2.00	0.00	0.00
193	Cliff Bar, Berry, Real	68.0000	1.000	Each	4.00	2.00	52.00	250.00	0.00	2.00	0.00	0.50
194	Cliff Bar, Chocolate Chip	68.0000	1.000	Each	4.00	3.00	51.00	250.00	0.00	3.00	0.00	0.50
195	Cliff Bar, Chocolate Chip Peanut	68.0000	1.000	Each	12.00	6.00	40.00	250.00	0.00	5.00	0.00	1.00
196	Cliff Bar, Chocolate Espresso	68.0000	1.000	Each	4.00	2.00	52.00	250.00	0.00	2.00	0.00	0.50
197	Cliff Bar, Peanut Butter, Crunch	68.0000	1.000	Each	10.00	4.00	45.00	250.00	0.00	8.00	0.00	1.00
	Cookie Cakes, Devils Food, Fat F	16.0000	1.000	Each	1.00	0.00	13.00	50.00	0.00	0.50	0.00	0.00
	Cookie Cakes, Double Fudge, Fat	16.0000	1.000	Each	1.00	0.00	12.00	50.00	0.00	0.50	0.00	0.00
	Cookies, Butter	28.3500	1.000	Ounce	1.73	5.33	19.53	132.39	0.00	0.21	33.17	3.13
	Cookies, Chocolate Chip, Reduce	0.4480	2.000	Each	1.00	1.25	10.50	50.00	0.00	0.02	0.00	0.02
	Cookies, Chocolate Chip, Dietary	28.3500	1.000	Ounce	1.11	4.76	20.81	127.58	2.27	0.45	0.00	1.19
	Cookies, Chocolate Chip, Lower F	28.3500	1.000	Ounce	1.64	4.37	20.78	128.43	1.98	1.02	0.00	1.08
	Cookies, Chocolate Chip, Soft-ty	28.3500	1.000	Ounce	0.99	6.89	16.75	129.84	1.98	0.91	0.00	2.10
	Cookies, Chocolate Sandwich, Red	12.5000	2.000	Each	0.50	1.25	10.50	50.00	0.00	0.50	0.00	0.25
	Cookies, Creme Sandwich, Reduced	13.0000	2.000	Each	0.50	1.25	10.50	55.00	0.00	0.50	0.00	0.25
	Cookies, Fig Bars	28.3500	1.000	Ounce	1.05	2.07	20.10	98.66	0.00	1.30	0.00	0.32
	Cookies, Fig Newton, Fat Free	29.0000	2.000	Each	1.00	0.00	22.00	100.00	0.00	0.00	0.00	0.00
	Cookies, Gingersnaps	28.3500	1.000	Ounce	1.59	2.78	21.80	117.94	0.00	0.62	0.00	0.69
	Cookies, Molasses	28.3500	1.000	Ounce	1.59	3.63	20.92	121.91	0.00	0.27	0.00	0.91
	Cookies, Oatmeal Raisin, Reduced	13.5000	2.000	Each	1.00	1.25	10.00	55.00	0.00	0.50	0.00	0.00
	Cookies, Oatmeal, Dietary	28.3500	1.000	Ounce	1.36	5.10	19.82	127.29	0.00	0.81	0.00	0.76
	Cookies, Oatmeal, Regular	28.3500	1.000	Ounce	1.76	5.13	19.48	127.58	0.00	0.79	0.00	1.28
	Cookies, Oatmeal, Soft-type	28.3500	1.000	Ounce	1.73	4.17	18.63	115.95	0.00	0.77	1.42	1.03
	Cookies, Oreos, Dietary	28.3500	1.000	Ounce	1.28	6.27	19.19	130.69	0.85	1.17	0.00	1.09

Monounsaturated Fat (gm)	Polyunsaturated Fat (gm)	Vitamin D (mg)	Vitamin K (mg)	Vitamin E (mg)	Vitamin A (re)	Vitamin C (mg)	Thiamin (mg)	Riboflavin (mg)	Niacin (mg)	Vitamin B6 (mg)	Folate (mg)	Vitamin B12 (mcg)	Calcium (mg)	Iron (mg)	Magnesium (mg)	Phosphorus (mg)	Potassium (mg)	Sodium (mg)	Zinc (mg)
0.00	0.00	0.00	0.00	0.00	0.00	0.00	0.00	0.00	0.00	0.00	0.00	0.00	0.00	0.00	0.00	0.00	0.00	310.00	0.00
4.26	0.98	0.00	0.00	0.00	51.60	0.43	0.02	0.12	0.95	0.05	8.79	0.04	12.19	0.29	0.00	62.37	51.03	756.09	0.20
4.19	1.03	0.00	0.00	0.17	11.06	0.14	0.03	0.08	0.44	0.01	0.00	0.18	8.51	0.25	3.12	24.10	36.00	521.07	0.16
0.00	0.00	0.00	0.00	0.00	0.00	0.00	0.00	0.00	0.00	0.00	0.00	0.00	48.00	0.40	0.00	0.00	0.00	150.00	0.00
0.00	0.00	0.00	0.00	0.00	0.00	6.40	0.00	0.00	0.00	0.00	0.00	0.00	0.00	0.20	0.00	0.00	0.00	300.00	0.00
1.75	5.07	0.00	0.00	1.38	0.00	13.41	0.03	0.03	1.36	0.09	11.34	0.00	5.10	0.64	18.14	48.76	350.69	70.88	0.28
1.85	4.64	0.00	0.00	1.42	6.24	9.61	0.06	0.06	1.33	0.18	23.53	0.00	14.18	0.55	21.26	52.73	357.49	212.63	0.27
2.19	2.71	0.00	0.00	0.00	2.27	15.34	0.05	0.05	1.42	0.10	0.00	0.00	20.41	0.52	21.26	84.77	433.19	224.82	0.26
2.02	5.29	0.00	0.00	0.00	0.00	2.41	0.05	0.03	0.74	0.15	5.10	0.00	31.19	0.45	15.03	46.21	108.01	214.04	0.18
1.36	3.10	0.00	0.00	0.82	0.00	7.29	0.06	0.08	1.98	0.19	7.65	0.00	5.95	0.38	25.23	54.72	494.42	139.48	0.02
1.68	3.82	0.00	0.00	1.42	0.00	3.40	0.05	0.02	1.19	0.22	6.52	0.00	9.64	0.43	17.86	43.66	284.92	121.34	0.17
2.06	5.66	0.00	0.00	1.38	0.00	2.32	0.06	0.03	0.89	0.04	1.98	0.00	6.80	0.43	16.44	44.51	285.77	185.98	0.17
2.79	3.45	0.00	0.00	1.38	0.00	8.82	0.05	0.06	1.09	0.19	12.76	0.00	6.80	0.46	18.99	46.78	361.46	168.40	0.31
2.79	3.45	0.00	0.00	1.38	0.00	8.82	0.05	0.06	1.09	0.19	12.76	0.00	6.80	0.46	18.99	46.78	361.46	2.27	0.31
0.00	0.00	0.00	0.00	0.00	0.00	0.00	0.00	0.00	0.00	0.00	0.00	0.00	0.00	0.20	0.00	0.00	0.00	130.00	0.00
2.02	5.32	0.00	0.00	0.00	27.78	2.69	0.05	0.03	0.71	0.14	6.52	0.00	18.14	0.40	15.59	47.91	140.62	204.12	0.20
1.74	4.94	0.00	0.00	0.00	5.95	10.57	0.05	0.06	1.14	0.19	17.58	0.28	20.41	0.45	20.98	49.90	377.34	177.19	0.28
1.77	5.15	0.00	0.00	2.23	0.00	11.79	0.04	0.01	1.19	0.14	12.81	0.00	6.80	0.34	16.73	43.38	367.98	2.27	0.30
0.00	0.00	0.00	0.00	0.00	0.00	1.20	0.00	0.00	0.00	0.00	0.00	0.00	0.00	0.00	0.00	0.00	0.00	115.00	0.00
1.26	3.65	0.00	0.00	1.39	0.00	1.42	0.05	0.01	0.15	0.12	5.67	0.00	17.01	0.34	23.81	37.14	214.04	96.96	0.11
0.00	0.00	0.00	0.00	0.00	0.00	0.00	0.00	0.00	0.00	0.00	0.00	0.00	3.69	0.00	0.00	0.00	0.00	10.77	0.00
4.28	1.00	0.00	0.00	0.00	11.62	0.51	0.04	0.05	0.41	0.08	3.97	0.01	41.67	0.41	23.25	69.17	61.24	200.72	0.34
2.54	0.60	0.00	0.00	0.00	11.91	0.06	0.06	0.08	0.12	0.07	7.37	0.00	45.08	0.46	27.50	90.15	77.11	284.35	0.00
4.38	1.03	0.00	0.00	0.39	5.67	0.00	0.02	0.05	0.36	0.08	2.84	0.00	43.66	0.43	24.95	58.12	55.85	149.69	0.43
3.98	0.94	0.00	0.00	0.00	7.65	0.26	0.03	0.07	0.41	0.06	4.82	0.00	39.97	0.41	25.23	67.76	69.17	173.50	0.35
4.05	0.95	0.00	0.00	0.00	25.80	0.26	0.07	0.06	0.57	0.09	5.95	0.00	43.94	0.57	24.95	67.76	61.52	223.11	0.36
0.00	0.00	0.00	0.00	0.00	0.00	0.00	0.00	0.00	0.00	0.00	0.00	0.00	32.00	0.20	0.00	0.00	0.00	200.00	0.00
0.00	0.00	0.00	0.00	0.00	0.00	0.00	0.00	0.00	0.00	0.00	0.00	0.00	32.00	0.20	0.00	0.00	0.00	190.00	0.00
16.75	1.78	0.00	0.00	2.08	92.40	0.67	0.13	0.50	0.54	0.07	13.44	0.66	320.88	2.34	100.80	362.88	646.80	137.76	2.32
5.53	0.93	0.00	0.00	0.77	5.74	0.08	0.02	0.18	0.30	0.02	4.92	0.14	91.84	0.67	36.90	108.24	182.04	30.34	0.55
0.00	0.00	0.00	0.00	0.00	0.00	0.00	0.00	0.00	0.00	0.00	0.00	0.00	0.00	0.00	0.00	0.00	270.00	100.00	0.00
0.00	0.00	0.00	0.00	0.00	0.00	0.00	0.00	0.00	0.00	0.00	0.00	0.00	0.00	0.00	0.00	0.00	250.00	55.00	0.00
0.00	0.00	0.00	0.00	0.00	0.00	0.00	0.00	0.00	0.00	0.00	0.00	0.00	0.00	0.00	0.00	0.00	270.00	100.00	0.00
0.00	0.00	0.00	0.00	0.00	0.00	0.00	0.00	0.00	0.00	0.00	0.00	0.00	0.00	0.00	0.00	0.00	330.00	45.00	0.00
0.00	0.00	0.00	0.00	0.00	0.00	0.00	0.00	0.00	0.00	0.00	0.00	0.00	0.00	0.00	0.00	0.00	220.00	110.00	0.00
0.00	0.00	0.00	0.00	0.00	0.00	0.00	0.00	0.00	0.00	0.00	0.00	0.00	0.00	0.00	0.00	0.00	270.00	100.00	0.00
0.00	0.00	0.00	0.00	0.00	0.00	0.00	0.00	0.00	0.00	0.00	0.00	0.00	0.00	0.00	0.00	0.00	330.00	150.00	0.00
0.00	0.00	0.00	0.00	0.00	0.00	0.00	0.00	0.00	0.00	0.00	0.00	0.00	0.00	0.00	0.00	0.00	0.00	25.00	0.00
0.00	0.00	0.00	0.00	0.00	0.00	0.00	0.00	0.00	0.00	0.00	0.00	0.00	0.00	0.20	0.00	0.00	0.00	70.00	0.00
1.56	0.28	0.00	0.00	0.15	47.63	0.00	0.10	0.10	0.90	0.01	11.06	0.10	8.22	0.63	3.40	28.92	31.47	99.51	0.11
0.02	0.00	0.00	0.00	0.00	0.00	0.00	0.00	0.00	0.00	0.00	0.00	0.00	0.00	0.01	0.00	0.00	0.00	2.63	0.00
1.91	1.43	0.00	0.00	0.70	0.00	0.00	0.10	0.05	0.81	0.01	12.76	0.00	13.04	0.99	5.95	30.90	56.42	3.12	0.13
1.73	1.32	0.00	0.00	0.00	0.00	0.00	0.08	0.08	0.79	0.07	19.85	0.00	5.39	0.87	7.94	23.81	34.87	106.88	0.20
3.69	0.99	0.00	0.00	0.00	0.00	0.00	0.03	0.06	0.46	0.05	11.06	0.00	4.25	0.68	9.92	14.18	26.37	92.42	0.13
0.25	0.00	0.00	0.00	0.00	0.00	0.00	0.00	0.00	0.00	0.00	0.00	0.00	0.00	0.20	0.00	0.00	0.00	95.00	0.00
0.50	0.00	0.00	0.00	0.00	0.00	0.00	0.00	0.00	0.00	0.00	0.00	0.04	12.00	0.10	0.00	0.00	0.00	47.50	0.00
0.85	0.79	0.00	0.00	0.35	1.13	0.09	0.05	0.06	0.53	0.02	7.65	0.03	18.14	0.82	7.65	17.58	58.68	99.22	0.11
0.00	0.00	0.00	0.00	0.00	0.00	0.00	0.00	0.00	0.00	0.00	0.00	0.00	0.00	0.00	0.00	0.00	0.00	115.00	0.00
1.52	0.39	0.00	0.00	0.37	0.00	0.00	0.06	0.08	0.92	0.03	20.41	0.00	21.83	1.81	13.89	23.53	98.09	185.41	0.16
2.02	0.49	0.00	0.00	0.48	0.00	0.00	0.10	0.07	0.86	0.03	20.98	0.00	20.98	1.82	14.74	26.93	98.09	130.13	0.13
0.25	0.25	0.00	0.00	0.00	0.00	0.00	0.00	0.00	0.00	0.00	0.00	0.00	12.00	0.20	0.00	0.00	0.00	67.50	0.00
2.14	1.92	0.00	0.00	0.91	0.28	0.09	0.13	0.06	0.92	0.01	14.74	0.00	15.31	1.15	4.82	34.59	49.61	2.55	0.14
2.84	0.72	0.00	0.00	0.71	0.57	0.14	0.08	0.07	0.63	0.02	12.76	0.00	10.49	0.73	9.36	39.12	40.26	108.58	0.22
2.27	0.62	0.00	0.00	0.00	1.42	0.06	0.05	0.07	0.52	0.03	9.64	0.00	25.52	0.79	8.51	59.25	38.27	98.94	0.12
2.62	2.25	0.00	0.00	1.07	0.00	0.00	0.15	0.08	1.13	0.01	17.58	0.01	27.78	1.34	7.37	56.70	83.63	68.89	0.16

USDA ID Code	Food Name	Weight in Grams*	Quantity of Units	Unit of Measure	Protein (gm)	Fat (gm)	Carbohydrate (gm)	Kcalories	Caffeine (gm)	Fiber (gm)	Cholesterol (mg)	Saturated Fat (gm)
	Cookies, Oreos, Regular	28.3500	1.000	Ounce	1.33	5.84	19.93	133.81	3.69	0.91	0.00	1.04
	Cookies, Oreos, w/ Extra Creme F	28.3500	1.000	Ounce	1.02	7.14	19.31	141.75	1.42	0.57	0.00	1.10
	Cookies, Peanut Butter Sandwich,	28.3500	1.000	Ounce	2.84	9.64	14.40	151.67	0.00	0.00	0.00	1.40
	Cookies, Peanut Butter Sandwich,	28.3500	1.000	Ounce	2.49	5.98	18.60	135.51	0.00	0.54	0.00	1.42
	Cookies, Peanut Butter, Regular	28.3500	1.000	Ounce	2.72	6.69	16.70	135.23	0.00	0.51	0.28	1.27
	Cookies, Peanut Butter, Soft-typ	28.3500	1.000	Ounce	1.50	6.92	16.36	129.56	0.00	0.48	0.00	1.74
	Cookies, Raisin, Soft-type	28.3500	1.000	Ounce	1.16	3.86	19.28	113.68	0.00	0.34	0.57	0.98
	Cookies, Shortbread, Pecan	28.3500	1.000	Ounce	1.39	9.21	16.53	153.66	0.00	0.51	9.36	2.32
	Cookies, Shortbread, Plain	28.3500	1.000	Ounce	1.73	6.83	18.29	142.32	0.00	0.51	5.67	1.73
	Cookies, Sugar, Dietary	28.3500	1.000	Ounce	1.16	3.69	21.77	122.19	0.00	0.25	0.00	0.53
	Cookies, Sugar, Regular (include	28.3500	1.000	Ounce	1.45	5.98	19.25	135.51	0.00	0.22	14.46	1.54
	Cookies, Vanilla Sandwich, w/ Cr	28.3500	1.000	Ounce	1.28	5.67	20.44	136.93	0.00	0.43	0.00	0.84
204	Cookies, Wafers, Chocolate	6.0000	1.000	Each	0.40	0.85	4.34	25.98	0.00	0.00	0.12	0.22
	Cookies, Wafers, Vanilla, Higher	28.3500	1.000	Ounce	1.22	5.50	20.16	134.10	0.00	0.57	0.00	1.40
205	Cookies, Wafers, Vanilla, Lower	4.0000	1.000	Each	0.20	0.61	2.94	17.64	0.00	0.00	2.32	0.14
	Cookies,Chocolate Chip, Higher F	28.3500	1.000	Ounce	1.53	6.41	18.94	136.36	3.12	0.71	0.00	2.12
	Cornnuts, Barbecue-flavor	28.3500	1.000	Ounce	2.55	4.05	20.33	123.61	0.00	2.38	0.00	0.73
	Cornnuts, Nacho-flavor	28.3500	1.000	Ounce	2.66	4.03	20.30	124.17	0.00	2.27	0.57	0.73
	Cornnuts, Plain	28.3500	1.000	Ounce	2.41	4.00	20.78	124.46	0.00	1.96	0.00	0.72
	Crackers, Animal	28.3500	1.000	Ounce	1.96	3.91	21.01	126.44	0.00	0.31	0.00	0.98
	Crackers, Classic Golden, Reduce	2.3300	6.000	Each	0.17	0.17	1.83	9.99	0.00	0.00	0.00	0.00
	Crackers, Snack, Cheese, Zesty,	0.9380	32.000	Each	0.09	0.06	0.72	3.75	0.00	0.03	0.16	0.02
	Crackers, Snack, French Onion ,	0.9380	32.000	Each	0.06	0.06	0.72	3.75	0.00	0.03	0.72	0.02
	Crackers, Triscuits	4.4290	7.000	Each	0.43	0.71	3.00	20.00	0.00	0.57	0.00	0.14
	Crackers, Triscuits, Low-Fat	4.0000	8.000	Each	0.38	0.38	3.00	16.25	0.00	0.50	0.00	0.06
	Crackers, Wheat Thins	1.8130	16.000	Each	0.13	0.38	1.19	8.75	0.00	0.13	0.00	0.06
	Crackers, Wheat Thins, Low-Fat	1.6110	18.000	Each	0.11	0.22	1.17	6.67	0.00	0.11	0.00	0.03
	Dip, Bean	15.0000	2.000	Tbsp	0.50	0.00	2.00	10.00	0.00	0.50	0.00	0.00
	Dip, Cheese, Nacho	16.5000	2.000	Tbsp	0.00	1.25	2.00	20.00	0.00	0.00	0.00	0.25
	Dip, French Onion	15.0000	2.000	Tbsp	0.50	2.50	1.00	30.00	0.00	0.00	7.50	1.50
259	Doritos, Corn, Toasted	28.0000	1.000	Ounce	2.00	7.00	18.00	140.00	0.00	1.00	0.00	1.50
260	Doritos, Flamin' Hot	28.0000	1.000	Ounce	2.00	7.00	17.00	140.00	0.00	1.00	0.00	1.50
261	Doritos, Nacho, Spicy	28.0000	1.000	Ounce	2.00	4.00	18.00	140.00	0.00	1.00	0.00	1.50
262	Doritos, Pizza Cravers	28.0000	1.000	Ounce	2.00	6.00	18.00	140.00	0.00	1.00	0.00	1.50
263	Doritos, Taco Bell Taco Supreme	28.0000	1.000	Ounce	2.00	7.00	21.00	150.00	0.00	1.00	0.00	1.50
	Doughnut Holes	15.0000	1.000	Each	0.78	3.44	7.62	63.90	0.00	0.00	4.80	0.80
	Egg Custards	282.0000	1.000	Cup	14.38	13.25	30.17	296.10	0.00	0.00	245.34	6.63
	Frostings, Chocolate, Creamy	462.0000	16.000	Ounce	5.08	81.31	291.98	1834.14	9.24	2.77	0.00	25.55
	Frostings, Cream Cheese-flavor	462.0000	16.000	Ounce	0.46	79.93	308.15	1908.06	0.00	0.00	0.00	23.28
	Frostings, Sour Cream-flavor	462.0000	16.000	Ounce	0.46	79.46	312.31	1903.44	0.00	0.46	0.00	23.15
	Frostings, Vanilla, Creamy	462.0000	16.000	Ounce	0.46	77.62	320.63	1935.78	0.00	0.46	0.00	22.59
	Frozen Bar, Fruit and Juice	77.0000	1.000	Each	0.92	0.08	15.55	63.14	0.00	0.00	0.00	0.00
	Frozen Bar, Pops, Ice	52.0000	1.000	Each	0.00	0.00	9.83	37.44	0.00	0.00	0.00	0.00
	Frozen Bar, Popsicles	56.0000	1.000	Each	0.00	0.00	11.00	40.00	0.00	0.00	0.00	0.00
	Frozen Bar, Pudding Pops, Chocol	47.0000	1.000	Each	1.88	2.21	11.94	71.91	0.00	0.19	0.94	0.00
	Frozen Bar, Pudding Pops, Vanill	47.0000	1.000	Each	1.88	2.07	12.60	74.73	0.00	0.00	0.94	0.00
	Frozen Bars, Pops, Gelatin	44.0000	1.000	Each	0.53	0.04	7.35	30.80	0.00	0.00	0.00	0.00
	Frozen Dessert, Brownie, Fudge-H	132.9690	1.000	Cup	6.00	4.00	54.00	280.00	0.00	0.00	10.00	0.00
	Frozen Dessert, Cherry, Bordeaux	132.9690	1.000	Cup	6.00	4.00	46.00	240.00	0.00	0.00	10.00	0.00
	Frozen Dessert, Chocolate Chip-H	132.9690	1.000	Cup	6.00	4.00	48.00	260.00	0.00	0.00	10.00	0.00
	Frozen Dessert, Coffee Toffee-He	132.9690	1.000	Cup	6.00	4.00	50.00	260.00	0.00	0.00	10.00	0.00
	Frozen Dessert, Cookies 'n Cream	132.9690	1.000	Cup	8.00	4.00	48.00	260.00	0.00	0.00	10.00	0.00
	Frozen Dessert, Fudge Swirl, Dou	132.9690	1.000	Cup	6.00	4.00	48.00	260.00	0.00	0.00	10.00	0.00
	Frozen Dessert, Ice Milk, Vanill	65.0000	3.500	Fl Oz	2.47	2.80	14.76	90.35	0.00	0.00	9.10	1.71
	Frozen Dessert, Ice Milk, Vanill	88.0000	0.500	Cup	4.31	2.29	19.18	110.88	0.00	0.00	10.56	1.43

Monounsaturated Fat (gm)	Polyunsaturated Fat (gm)	Vitamin D (mg)	Vitamin K (mg)	Vitamin E (mg)	Vitamin A (re)	Vitamin C (mg)	Thiamin (mg)	Riboflavin (mg)	Niacin (mg)	Vitamin B6 (mg)	Folate (mg)	Vitamin B12 (mcg)	Calcium (mg)	Iron (mg)	Magnesium (mg)	Phosphorus (mg)	Potassium (mg)	Sodium (mg)	Zinc (mg)
2.43	2.06	0.00	0.00	0.98	0.00	0.00	0.02	0.05	0.59	0.01	12.19	0.01	7.37	1.10	12.76	27.78	49.61	171.23	0.23
3.03	2.66	0.00	0.00	1.27	0.00	0.00	0.02	0.04	0.45	0.01	12.19	0.01	6.80	0.81	9.64	25.80	34.59	139.77	0.18
4.36	3.41	0.00	0.00	1.63	0.00	0.00	0.10	0.04	1.49	0.02	15.31	0.00	12.19	0.72	14.46	43.66	83.35	116.80	0.29
3.17	1.08	0.00	0.00	0.92	0.28	0.03	0.09	0.07	1.06	0.04	12.47	0.07	15.03	0.74	13.89	53.30	54.43	104.33	0.30
3.51	1.56	0.00	0.00	0.96	0.85	0.00	0.05	0.05	1.21	0.03	17.58	0.01	9.92	0.71	12.76	24.38	47.34	117.65	0.15
3.92	0.90	0.00	0.00	0.00	0.00	0.00	0.07	0.05	0.61	0.01	18.99	0.00	3.40	0.25	9.07	24.66	30.33	95.26	0.16
2.17	0.50	0.00	0.00	0.54	0.28	0.11	0.06	0.06	0.56	0.01	12.47	0.01	13.04	0.65	5.95	23.53	39.69	95.82	0.09
5.28	1.17	0.00	0.00	0.00	0.28	0.00	0.08	0.06	0.70	0.01	17.86	0.00	8.51	0.69	5.10	24.10	20.70	79.66	0.16
3.80	0.92	0.00	0.00	0.91	3.40	0.00	0.09	0.09	0.95	0.02	16.73	0.03	9.92	0.78	4.82	30.62	28.35	128.99	0.15
1.49	1.35	0.00	0.00	0.63	0.00	0.00	0.14	0.07	1.04	0.01	16.44	0.00	7.09	1.14	2.55	20.70	29.48	0.85	0.10
3.36	0.75	0.00	0.00	0.80	7.65	0.03	0.07	0.06	0.76	0.02	12.76	0.05	5.95	0.61	3.40	22.68	17.86	101.21	0.12
2.39	2.14	0.00	0.00	1.02	0.00	0.00	0.07	0.07	0.76	0.01	16.73	0.00	7.65	0.63	3.97	21.26	25.80	98.94	0.11
0.45	0.10	0.00	0.00	0.00	0.12	0.00	0.01	0.02	0.17	0.00	0.66	0.00	1.86	0.24	3.18	7.92	12.60	34.80	0.07
3.14	0.69	0.00	0.00	0.00	0.00	0.00	0.10	0.06	0.84	0.01	12.19	0.01	7.09	0.63	3.40	18.14	30.33	86.75	0.09
0.24	0.15	0.00	0.00	0.00	0.72	0.00	0.01	0.01	0.12	0.00	0.36	0.00	1.92	0.10	0.56	4.16	3.88	12.48	0.01
3.31	0.67	0.00	0.00	0.73	0.00	0.00	0.06	0.08	0.77	0.02	11.91	0.00	7.09	0.80	8.79	30.62	38.27	89.30	0.18
2.09	0.91	0.00	0.00	0.00	9.64	0.11	0.10	0.04	0.43	0.05	0.00	0.00	4.82	0.48	30.90	80.23	81.08	276.70	0.53
2.07	0.91	0.00	0.00	0.00	1.13	4.39	0.10	0.02	0.34	0.06	4.25	0.00	9.92	0.48	30.90	87.60	88.17	179.74	0.51
2.06	0.90	0.00	0.00	0.29	0.00	0.00	0.01	0.04	0.48	0.07	0.00	0.00	2.55	0.47	32.04	77.96	78.81	155.64	0.50
2.17	0.53	0.00	0.00	0.52	0.00	0.00	0.10	0.09	0.98	0.01	24.10	0.01	12.19	0.78	5.10	32.32	28.35	111.42	0.18
0.00	0.00	0.00	0.00	0.00	0.00	0.00	0.00	0.00	0.00	0.00	0.00	0.00	3.99	0.07	0.00	0.00	0.00	23.30	0.00
0.02	0.00	0.00	0.00	0.00	0.00	0.00	0.00	0.00	0.00	0.00	0.00	0.00	1.50	0.02	0.00	0.00	0.00	10.94	0.00
0.02	0.00	0.00	0.00	0.00	0.00	0.00	0.00	0.00	0.00	0.00	0.00	0.00	1.50	0.02	0.00	0.00	0.00	9.06	0.00
0.07	0.21	0.00	0.00	0.00	0.00	0.00	0.00	0.00	0.00	0.00	0.00	0.00	0.00	0.11	0.00	11.43	0.00	24.29	0.00
0.00	0.13	0.00	0.00	0.00	0.00	0.00	0.00	0.00	0.00	0.00	0.00	0.00	0.00	0.13	0.00	15.00	0.00	22.50	0.00
0.03	0.16	0.00	0.00	0.00	0.00	0.00	0.00	0.00	0.00	0.00	0.00	0.00	1.50	0.03	0.00	0.00	0.00	10.63	0.00
0.00	0.08	0.00	0.00	0.00	0.00	0.00	0.00	0.00	0.00	0.00	0.00	0.00	1.33	0.02	0.00	4.44	0.00	12.22	0.00
0.00	0.00	0.00	0.00	0.00	0.00	0.00	0.00	0.00	0.00	0.00	0.00	0.00	0.00	0.10	0.00	0.00	0.00	75.00	0.00
0.00	0.00	0.00	0.00	0.00	0.00	0.00	0.00	0.00	0.00	0.00	0.00	0.00	12.00	0.00	0.00	0.00	0.00	100.00	0.00
0.00	0.00	0.00	0.00	0.00	20.00	0.60	0.00	0.00	0.00	0.00	0.00	0.00	12.00	0.00	0.00	0.00	0.00	52.50	0.00
0.00	5.50	0.00	0.00	0.00	0.00	0.00	0.00	0.00	0.00	0.00	0.00	0.00	0.00	0.00	0.00	0.00	0.00	120.00	0.00
0.00	5.50	0.00	0.00	0.00	0.00	0.00	0.00	0.00	0.00	0.00	0.00	0.00	0.00	0.00	0.00	0.00	0.00	210.00	0.00
0.00	4.50	0.00	0.00	0.00	0.00	0.00	0.00	0.00	0.00	0.00	0.00	0.00	0.00	0.00	0.00	0.00	0.00	210.00	0.00
0.00	5.50	0.00	0.00	0.00	0.00	0.00	0.00	0.00	0.00	0.00	0.00	0.00	0.00	0.00	0.00	0.00	0.00	170.00	0.00
0.00	5.50	0.00	0.00	0.00	0.00	0.00	0.00	0.00	0.00	0.00	0.00	0.00	0.00	0.00	0.00	0.00	0.00	170.00	0.00
1.79	0.39	0.00	0.00	0.00	0.45	0.02	0.03	0.03	0.23	0.00	1.80	0.03	9.00	0.16	2.55	17.55	15.30	60.30	0.07
4.26	0.99	0.00	0.00	0.00	169.20	1.41	0.09	0.64	0.24	0.14	28.20	0.87	315.84	0.85	39.48	318.66	431.46	217.14	1.49
41.67	9.84	0.00	0.00	10.95	914.76	0.00	0.05	0.09	0.55	0.05	0.00	0.00	36.96	6.56	97.02	364.98	905.52	845.46	1.34
41.72	10.86	0.00	0.00	0.00	0.00	0.00	0.00	0.05	0.05	0.00	0.00	0.00	13.86	0.74	9.24	13.86	161.70	180.18	0.00
41.53	10.81	0.00	0.00	0.00	563.64	0.00	0.05	0.09	3.10	0.00	4.62	0.05	9.24	0.32	9.24	18.48	896.28	942.48	0.05
40.52	10.53	0.00	0.00	21.81	1044.12	0.00	0.00	0.05	0.05	0.00	0.00	0.00	13.86	0.51	4.62	180.18	170.94	415.80	0.00
0.00	0.02	0.00	0.00	0.00	2.31	7.32	0.01	0.02	0.12	0.02	4.62	0.00	3.85	0.15	3.08	4.62	40.81	3.08	0.04
0.00	0.00	0.00	0.00	0.00	0.00	0.00	0.00	0.00	0.00	0.00	0.00	0.00	0.00	0.00	0.52	0.00	2.08	6.24	0.01
0.00	0.00	0.00	0.00	0.00	0.00	1.20	0.00	0.00	0.00	0.00	0.00	0.00	0.00	0.00	0.00	0.00	0.00	10.00	0.00
0.00	0.00	0.00	0.00	0.01	15.51	0.19	0.02	0.08	0.06	0.01	1.41	0.25	66.27	0.22	9.87	52.64	105.28	77.55	0.17
0.00	0.00	0.00	0.00	0.01	24.44	0.14	0.02	0.09	0.02	0.02	2.35	0.17	60.63	0.03	5.17	47.47	64.86	49.82	0.16
0.00	0.00	0.00	0.00	0.00	0.00	0.00	0.00	0.00	0.00	0.00	0.00	0.00	0.88	0.01	0.44	0.00	0.88	20.24	0.01
0.00	2.00	0.00	0.00	0.00	0.00	0.00	0.06	0.27	0.00	0.00	0.00	0.00	160.00	0.40	0.00	160.00	380.00	140.00	0.00
0.00	2.00	0.00	0.00	0.00	0.00	0.00	0.06	0.34	0.00	0.00	0.00	0.00	160.00	0.00	0.00	200.00	300.00	100.00	0.00
0.00	2.00	0.00	0.00	0.00	0.00	2.40	0.12	0.27	0.00	0.00	0.00	0.00	160.00	0.40	0.00	160.00	320.00	140.00	0.00
0.00	2.00	0.00	0.00	0.00	0.00	2.40	0.12	0.34	0.00	0.00	0.00	0.00	160.00	0.00	0.00	160.00	320.00	160.00	0.00
0.00	2.00	0.00	0.00	0.00	0.00	0.00	0.06	0.34	0.00	0.00	0.00	0.00	240.00	0.00	0.00	200.00	360.00	160.00	0.00
0.00	2.00	0.00	0.00	0.00	0.00	0.00	0.12	0.27	0.00	0.00	0.00	0.00	160.00	0.80	0.00	200.00	420.00	140.00	0.00
0.80	0.10	0.00	0.00	0.00	30.55	0.52	0.04	0.18	0.06	0.05	3.90	0.44	90.35	0.07	9.75	70.85	137.15	55.25	0.29
0.67	0.09	0.00	0.00	0.00	25.52	0.79	0.04	0.18	0.11	0.04	5.28	0.44	138.16	0.05	12.32	106.48	194.48	61.60	0.47

USDA ID Code	Food Name	Weight in Grams*	Quantity of Units	Unit of Measure	Protein (gm)	Fat (gm)	Carbohydrate (gm)	Kcalories	Caffeine (gm)	Fiber (gm)	Cholesterol (mg)	Saturated Fat (gm)
	Frozen Dessert, Mint Chocolate C	132.9690	1.000	Cup	6.00	4.00	50.00	280.00	0.00	0.00	10.00	0.00
	Frozen Dessert, Neapolitan-Healt	132.9690	1.000	Cup	6.00	4.00	44.00	240.00	0.00	0.00	10.00	0.00
	Frozen Dessert, Pecan, Butter, C	132.9690	1.000	Cup	6.00	4.00	52.00	280.00	0.00	0.00	10.00	0.00
	Frozen Dessert, Praline and Cara	132.9690	1.000	Cup	6.00	4.00	52.00	260.00	0.00	0.00	10.00	0.00
	Frozen Dessert, Rocky Road-Healt	132.9690	1.000	Cup	6.00	4.00	64.00	320.00	0.00	0.00	10.00	0.00
	Frozen Dessert, Sherbet, All Fla	74.0000	0.500	Cup	0.81	1.48	22.50	102.12	0.00	0.00	4.44	0.86
	Frozen Dessert, Sorbet, All Flav	180.0530	0.500	Cup	0.00	0.00	50.01	200.06	0.00	2.00	0.00	0.00
	Frozen Dessert, Sorbet-Ben & Jer	110.0000	0.500	Cup	0.00	0.00	32.00	130.00	0.00	0.00	0.00	0.00
	Frozen Dessert, Vanilla-Healthy	132.9690	1.000	Cup	8.00	4.00	42.00	240.00	0.00	0.00	10.00	0.00
	Frozen Desserts, Pops, Ice, w/ A	52.0000	1.000	Each	0.00	0.00	9.83	37.44	0.00	0.00	0.00	0.00
	Fudge, Brown Sugar w/ Nuts	14.0000	1.000	Piece	0.41	1.41	10.86	55.44	0.00	0.00	0.84	0.25
	Fudge, Chocolate	17.0000	1.000	Piece	0.29	1.45	13.52	64.77	2.38	0.14	2.38	0.88
	Fudge, Chocolate w/ Nuts	19.0000	1.000	Piece	0.65	3.06	13.83	80.94	2.66	0.25	2.66	1.07
	Fudge, Peanut Butter	16.0000	1.000	Piece	0.59	1.04	12.53	59.36	0.00	0.00	0.64	0.24
	Fudge, Vanilla	16.0000	1.000	Piece	0.18	0.86	13.17	59.04	0.00	0.00	2.56	0.54
	Fudge, Vanilla w/ Nuts	15.0000	1.000	Piece	0.44	2.00	11.28	62.25	0.00	0.09	2.10	0.56
	Granola Bars, Hard, Almond	28.3500	1.000	Ounce	2.18	7.23	17.58	140.33	0.00	1.36	0.00	3.55
	Granola Bars, Hard, Chocolate Ch	28.3500	1.000	Each	2.07	4.62	20.44	124.17	0.00	1.25	0.00	3.23
	Granola Bars, Hard, Peanut	28.3500	1.000	Ounce	3.12	6.07	18.06	135.80	0.00	1.22	0.00	0.71
	Granola Bars, Hard, Peanut Butte	28.3500	1.000	Ounce	2.78	6.75	17.66	136.93	0.00	0.82	0.00	0.91
	Granola Bars, Hard, Plain	24.5000	1.000	Each	2.47	4.85	15.78	115.40	0.00	1.30	0.00	0.58
	Granola Bars, Low-Fat	28.0000	1.000	Each	2.00	2.00	21.00	110.00	0.00	1.00	0.00	0.00
	Granola Bars, Soft, Chocolate Ch	42.5000	1.000	Each	3.10	7.06	29.37	178.50	0.00	2.04	0.43	4.33
	Granola Bars, Soft, Nut and Rais	28.3500	1.000	Each	2.27	5.78	18.03	128.71	0.00	1.59	0.28	2.70
	Granola Bars, Soft, Peanut Butte	28.3500	1.000	Each	2.98	4.48	18.26	120.77	0.00	1.22	0.28	1.03
	Granola Bars, Soft, Peanut Butte	28.3500	1.000	Each	2.78	5.67	17.63	122.47	0.00	1.19	0.28	1.58
	Granola Bars, Soft, Plain	28.3500	1.000	Each	2.10	4.88	19.08	125.59	0.00	1.30	0.28	2.05
	Granola Bars, Soft, Raisin	42.5000	1.000	Each	3.23	7.57	28.22	190.40	0.00	1.79	0.43	4.07
	Gum, Bubble-Carefree	3.0000	1.000	Each	0.00	0.00	2.00	10.00	0.00	0.00	0.00	0.00
	Gum, Chewing	3.0000	1.000	Stick	0.00	0.01	2.90	10.23	0.00	0.00	0.00	0.00
	Gum, Chewing, Cinnamon	3.0000	1.000	Each	0.00	0.00	2.00	10.00	0.00	0.00	0.00	0.00
	Gum, Chewing, Mint Flavors	3.0000	1.000	Each	0.00	0.00	2.00	10.00	0.00	0.00	0.00	0.00
	Gum,Chewing, Sugar-Free	1.7000	1.000	Stick	0.00	0.00	1.00	5.00	0.00	0.00	0.00	0.00
	Gum-Carefree	3.0000	1.000	Each	0.00	0.00	2.00	8.00	0.00	0.00	0.00	0.00
	Jello, Gelatin	540.0000	3.000	Ounce	6.48	0.00	75.60	318.60	0.00	0.00	0.00	0.00
	Jerky, Beef, Chopped and Formed	28.3500	1.000	Ounce	9.41	7.26	3.12	116.24	0.00	0.51	13.61	3.08
	Jerky, Slim Jims, Smoked	28.3500	1.000	Ounce	6.10	14.06	1.53	155.93	0.00	0.00	37.71	5.90
	Marshmallows	50.0000	1.000	Cup	0.90	0.10	40.65	159.00	0.00	0.05	0.00	0.03
617	Nutri-Grain Bar, Apple Cinnamon-	37.0000	1.000	Each	2.00	2.80	27.00	136.00	0.00	1.00	0.00	0.60
618	Nutri-Grain Bar, Berry, Mixed-Ke	37.0000	1.000	Each	2.00	3.00	27.00	140.00	0.00	1.00	0.00	0.50
619	Nutri-Grain Bar, Blueberry-Kello	37.0000	1.000	Each	2.00	2.80	27.00	136.00	0.00	1.00	0.00	0.60
620	Nutri-Grain Bar, Cherry-Kellogg'	37.0000	1.000	Each	2.00	2.80	27.00	136.00	0.00	1.00	0.00	6.00
621	Nutri-Grain Bar, Peach-Kellogg's	37.0000	1.000	Each	2.00	2.80	27.00	136.00	0.00	1.00	0.00	0.60
622	Nutri-Grain Bar, Raspberry-Kello	37.0000	1.000	Each	2.00	2.80	27.00	136.00	0.00	1.00	0.00	6.00
623	Nutri-Grain Bar, Strawberry-Kell	37.0000	1.000	Each	2.00	2.80	26.00	140.00	0.00	1.00	0.00	0.60
	Pastries, Toaster, Brown-sugar-c	28.3500	1.000	Ounce	1.45	4.03	19.31	116.80	0.00	0.28	0.00	1.03
	Pastries, Toaster, Fruit	28.3500	1.000	Ounce	1.33	2.89	20.16	111.42	0.00	0.59	0.00	0.43
	Peanuts, Chocolate, Milk, Coated	149.0000	1.000	Cup	19.52	49.92	73.61	773.31	32.78	7.00	13.41	21.75
	Pop Tart, Fruit, Frosted	52.0000	1.000	Each	2.00	5.00	38.00	200.00	0.00	1.00	0.00	1.50
	Popcorn, Air-popped	8.0000	1.000	Cup	0.96	0.34	6.23	30.56	0.00	1.21	0.00	0.05
	Popcorn, Air-popped, White Popco	8.0000	1.000	Cup	0.96	0.34	6.23	30.56	0.00	1.21	0.00	0.05
656	Popcorn, Butter, Golden, Fat, Re	14.0000	3.330	Cup	3.00	4.00	21.00	130.00	0.00	4.00	0.00	0.50
660	Popcorn, Butter-Smartfood	14.0000	3.000	Cup	2.00	9.00	15.00	150.00	0.00	1.00	5.00	2.00
	Popcorn, Cakes	10.0000	1.000	Cake	0.97	0.31	8.01	38.40	0.00	0.29	0.00	0.05
	Popcorn, Caramel-coated, w/ Pean	28.3500	0.660	Cup	1.81	2.21	22.88	113.40	0.00	1.08	0.00	0.29

Monounsaturated Fat (gm)	Polyunsaturated Fat (gm)	Vitamin D (mg)	Vitamin K (mg)	Vitamin E (mg)	Vitamin A (re)	Vitamin C (mg)	Thiamin (mg)	Riboflavin (mg)	Niacin (mg)	Vitamin B6 (mg)	Folate (mcg)	Vitamin B12 (mcg)	Calcium (mg)	Iron (mg)	Magnesium (mg)	Phosphorus (mg)	Potassium (mg)	Sodium (mg)	Zinc (mg)
0.00	4.00	0.00	0.00	0.00	0.00	0.00	0.12	0.27	0.00	0.00	0.00	0.00	160.00	0.40	0.00	0.00	340.00	160.00	0.00
0.00	2.00	0.00	0.00	0.00	0.00	0.00	0.06	0.34	0.00	0.00	0.00	0.00	160.00	0.00	0.00	200.00	320.00	120.00	0.00
0.00	2.00	0.00	0.00	0.00	0.00	2.40	0.12	0.34	0.00	0.00	0.00	0.00	160.00	0.00	0.00	160.00	300.00	160.00	0.00
0.00	2.00	0.00	0.00	0.00	0.00	0.00	0.06	0.34	0.00	0.00	0.00	0.00	160.00	0.00	0.00	200.00	320.00	140.00	0.00
0.00	2.00	0.00	0.00	0.00	0.00	0.00	0.06	0.34	0.00	0.00	0.00	0.00	160.00	0.00	0.00	200.00	380.00	140.00	0.00
0.39	0.06	0.00	0.00	0.06	10.36	2.29	0.02	0.06	0.04	0.01	3.70	0.14	39.96	0.10	5.92	29.60	71.04	34.04	0.36
0.00	0.00	0.00	0.00	0.00	0.00	24.01	0.00	0.00	0.00	0.00	0.00	0.00	0.00	0.00	0.00	0.00	0.00	20.01	0.00
0.00	0.00	0.00	0.00	0.00	0.00	0.00	0.00	0.00	0.00	0.00	0.00	0.00	80.00	0.00	0.00	0.00	0.00	10.00	0.00
0.00	2.00	0.00	0.00	0.00	0.00	0.00	0.12	0.51	0.00	0.00	0.00	0.00	240.00	0.00	0.00	200.00	360.00	120.00	0.00
0.00	0.00	0.00	0.00	0.00	0.00	5.56	0.00	0.00	0.00	0.00	0.00	0.00	0.00	0.00	0.52	0.00	2.08	6.24	0.01
0.34	0.76	0.00	0.00	0.00	2.38	0.08	0.01	0.01	0.03	0.01	1.54	0.00	15.54	0.25	6.86	12.04	52.36	13.72	0.09
0.44	0.05	0.00	0.00	0.02	7.82	0.03	0.00	0.01	0.02	0.00	0.34	0.01	7.14	0.08	4.25	9.86	17.51	10.54	0.07
0.82	1.03	0.00	0.00	0.08	8.93	0.11	0.01	0.02	0.04	0.02	1.90	0.01	9.50	0.14	8.55	17.67	30.02	11.40	0.14
0.48	0.27	0.00	0.00	0.00	1.60	0.03	0.00	0.01	0.24	0.01	1.76	0.01	6.72	0.04	3.52	10.40	20.96	11.68	0.07
0.25	0.03	0.00	0.00	0.03	8.00	0.03	0.00	0.01	0.00	0.00	0.16	0.01	6.24	0.01	0.80	5.12	8.00	10.72	0.02
0.50	0.83	0.00	0.00	0.07	6.90	0.09	0.01	0.01	0.03	0.01	1.50	0.01	7.05	0.06	4.05	10.65	16.95	9.15	0.08
2.19	1.07	0.00	0.00	0.00	1.13	0.00	0.08	0.02	0.17	0.01	3.40	0.00	9.07	0.71	22.96	64.64	77.40	72.58	0.45
0.75	0.36	0.00	0.00	0.00	1.13	0.03	0.05	0.03	0.16	0.02	3.69	0.00	21.83	0.86	20.41	57.83	71.16	97.52	0.55
1.63	3.37	0.00	0.00	0.32	0.85	0.00	0.05	0.02	0.41	0.02	6.52	0.00	11.06	0.71	31.19	85.05	86.47	78.81	0.59
1.98	3.42	0.00	0.00	0.00	0.57	0.06	0.06	0.03	0.56	0.03	5.10	0.00	11.62	0.68	15.59	39.41	82.50	80.23	0.35
1.07	2.95	0.00	0.00	0.00	3.68	0.22	0.06	0.03	0.39	0.02	5.64	0.00	14.95	0.72	23.77	67.86	82.32	72.03	0.50
0.00	0.00	0.00	0.00	0.00	0.00	0.00	0.00	0.00	0.00	0.00	0.00	0.00	0.00	0.20	0.00	0.00	0.00	70.00	0.00
1.50	0.84	0.00	0.00	0.00	2.13	0.00	0.10	0.06	0.41	0.04	9.35	0.07	39.53	1.08	33.15	97.75	144.50	115.60	0.64
1.20	1.56	0.00	0.00	0.00	1.13	0.00	0.05	0.05	0.74	0.03	8.51	0.07	23.81	0.62	25.80	68.32	111.13	72.01	0.45
1.87	1.21	0.00	0.00	0.00	0.57	0.00	0.07	0.04	0.89	0.03	9.07	0.06	25.80	0.60	24.38	70.88	82.50	115.95	0.53
2.37	1.31	0.00	0.00	0.00	0.57	0.00	0.03	0.03	0.89	0.03	9.36	0.13	22.68	0.55	24.95	74.28	106.88	92.99	0.48
1.08	1.51	0.00	0.00	0.00	0.00	0.00	0.09	0.05	0.15	0.03	6.80	0.11	29.77	0.73	20.98	65.21	92.14	78.81	0.43
1.21	1.36	0.00	0.00	0.00	0.00	0.00	0.10	0.07	0.47	0.04	8.93	0.08	42.93	1.04	30.60	93.50	153.85	119.85	0.55
0.00	0.00	0.00	0.00	0.00	0.00	0.00	0.00	0.00	0.00	0.00	0.00	0.00	0.00	0.00	0.00	0.00	0.00	0.00	0.00
0.00	0.00	0.00	0.00	0.00	0.00	0.00	0.00	0.00	0.00	0.00	0.00	0.00	0.00	0.00	0.00	0.00	0.00	0.12	0.18
0.00	0.00	0.00	0.00	0.00	0.00	0.00	0.00	0.00	0.00	0.00	0.00	0.00	0.00	0.00	0.00	0.00	0.00	0.00	0.00
0.00	0.00	0.00	0.00	0.00	0.00	0.00	0.00	0.00	0.00	0.00	0.00	0.00	0.00	0.00	0.00	0.00	0.00	0.00	0.00
0.00	0.00	0.00	0.00	0.00	0.00	0.00	0.00	0.00	0.00	0.00	0.00	0.00	0.00	0.00	0.00	0.00	0.00	0.00	0.00
0.00	0.00	0.00	0.00	0.00	0.00	0.00	0.00	0.00	0.00	0.00	0.00	0.00	10.80	0.16	5.40	118.80	5.40	226.80	0.16
3.21	0.29	0.00	0.00	0.14	0.00	0.00	0.04	0.04	0.49	0.05	37.99	0.28	5.67	1.54	14.46	115.38	169.25	627.39	2.30
5.80	1.25	0.00	0.00	0.00	47.91	1.93	0.04	0.12	1.29	0.06	0.00	0.28	19.28	0.96	5.95	51.03	72.86	419.58	0.69
0.04	0.03	0.00	0.00	0.00	0.00	0.00	0.00	0.00	0.04	0.00	0.50	0.00	1.50	0.12	1.00	4.00	2.50	23.50	0.02
1.90	0.30	0.00	0.00	0.00	750.00	0.00	0.38	0.43	5.00	0.50	40.00	0.00	14.00	1.80	8.00	40.00	73.00	110.00	1.50
0.00	0.00	0.00	0.00	0.00	750.00	0.00	0.38	0.43	5.00	0.50	40.00	0.00	0.00	1.80	8.00	40.00	0.00	110.00	1.50
1.90	0.30	0.00	0.00	0.00	750.00	0.00	0.38	0.43	5.00	0.00	40.00	0.00	18.00	1.80	8.00	40.00	73.00	110.00	1.50
1.90	0.30	0.00	0.00	0.00	750.00	0.00	0.38	0.43	5.00	0.00	40.00	0.00	18.00	1.80	8.00	40.00	73.00	110.00	1.50
1.90	0.30	0.00	0.00	0.00	750.00	0.00	0.38	0.43	5.00	0.50	40.00	0.00	18.00	1.80	8.00	40.00	73.00	110.00	1.50
1.90	0.30	0.00	0.00	0.00	750.00	0.00	0.38	0.43	5.00	0.00	4.00	0.00	18.00	1.80	8.00	4.00	73.00	110.00	1.50
1.90	0.30	0.00	0.00	0.00	750.00	0.00	0.38	0.43	5.00	0.50	40.00	0.00	17.00	1.80	0.00	40.00	56.00	110.00	1.50
2.28	0.51	0.00	0.00	0.00	63.50	0.03	0.10	0.16	1.30	0.12	8.22	0.06	9.64	1.14	6.80	37.71	32.32	120.20	0.18
1.17	1.10	0.00	0.00	0.65	0.85	0.17	0.08	0.10	1.12	0.11	18.43	0.00	7.37	0.99	5.10	31.47	31.75	118.79	0.19
19.25	6.45	0.00	0.00	3.80	0.00	0.00	0.18	0.25	6.33	0.31	11.92	0.40	154.96	1.95	140.06	315.88	747.98	61.09	2.89
0.00	0.00	0.00	0.00	0.00	100.00	0.00	0.15	0.17	1.90	0.20	20.00	0.00	0.00	1.00	0.00	16.00	0.00	170.00	1.50
0.09	0.15	0.00	0.00	0.01	1.60	0.00	0.02	0.02	0.16	0.02	1.84	0.00	0.80	0.21	10.48	24.00	24.08	0.32	0.28
0.09	0.15	0.00	0.00	0.00	0.24	0.00	0.02	0.02	0.16	0.02	1.84	0.00	0.80	0.21	10.48	24.00	24.08	0.32	0.28
0.00	0.00	0.00	0.00	0.00	0.00	0.00	0.00	0.00	0.00	0.00	0.00	0.00	0.00	0.00	0.00	0.00	0.00	410.00	0.00
0.00	0.00	0.00	0.00	0.00	0.00	0.00	0.00	0.00	0.00	0.00	0.00	0.00	0.00	0.00	0.00	0.00	0.00	240.00	0.00
0.09	0.14	0.00	0.00	0.01	0.70	0.00	0.01	0.02	0.60	0.02	1.80	0.00	0.90	0.19	15.90	27.70	32.70	28.80	0.40
0.77	0.93	0.00	0.00	0.43	1.70	0.00	0.01	0.04	0.56	0.05	4.54	0.00	18.71	1.11	22.68	36.00	100.64	83.63	0.35

USDA ID Code	Food Name	Weight in Grams*	Quantity of Units	Unit of Measure	Protein (gm)	Fat (gm)	Carbohydrate (gm)	Kcalories	Caffeine (gm)	Fiber (gm)	Cholesterol (mg)	Saturated Fat (gm)
	Popcorn, Caramel-coated, w/o Pea	28.3500	1.000	Ounce	1.08	3.63	22.42	122.19	0.00	1.47	1.42	1.02
657	Popcorn, Cheese, White Cheddar,	14.0000	3.000	Cup	4.00	6.00	19.00	140.00	0.00	4.00	0.00	1.50
658	Popcorn, Cheese, White Cheddar-S	14.0000	2.000	Cup	3.00	12.00	17.00	190.00	0.00	3.00	5.00	2.50
	Popcorn, Cheese-flavor	6.0000	1.000	Cup	1.02	3.65	5.68	57.86	0.00	1.09	1.21	0.71
	Popcorn, Microwave	14.0000	4.000	Cup	0.75	3.00	4.25	42.50	0.00	0.75	0.00	0.75
	Popcorn, Microwave, Low-Fat	14.0000	4.000	Cup	0.67	1.00	3.67	23.33	0.00	0.50	0.00	0.17
659	Popcorn, Microwave, Smart Pop-Re	15.0000	1.000	Cup	3.00	2.00	20.00	105.00	0.00	5.00	0.00	0.00
	Popcorn, Microwave-Pop Secret-94	5.0000	1.000	Serving	1.00	0.00	4.00	20.00	0.00	0.00	0.00	0.00
	Popcorn, Oil-popped	11.0000	1.000	Cup	0.99	3.09	6.29	55.00	0.00	1.10	0.00	0.54
	Popcorn, Oil-popped, White Popco	11.0000	1.000	Cup	0.99	3.09	6.29	55.00	0.00	1.10	0.00	0.54
661	Popcorn, Unpopped, Microwave, Bu	32.0000	2.000	Tbsp	2.70	5.70	19.80	122.00	0.00	4.70	0.00	1.20
662	Popcorn, Unpopped, Microwave, Li	31.0000	2.000	Tbsp	2.60	5.10	18.90	113.00	0.00	4.50	0.00	1.00
663	Popcorn, unpopped, Microwave, No	37.0000	2.000	Tbsp	2.50	12.10	18.70	176.00	0.00	4.50	0.00	2.60
664	Popcorn, Unpopped, Microwave-Sma	30.0000	2.000	Tbsp	2.80	2.10	20.30	92.00	0.00	4.90	0.00	0.40
665	Potato Chips, BBQ, Fat Free-Prin	28.0000	1.000	Ounce	1.00	0.00	15.00	70.00	0.00	1.00	0.00	0.00
666	Potato Chips, Cheezum, Right Cri	51.0000	1.800	Ounce	4.00	24.00	32.00	350.00	0.00	2.00	0.00	6.00
668	Potato Chips, Original, Fat Free	28.0000	1.000	Ounce	1.00	0.00	15.00	70.00	0.00	1.00	0.00	0.00
667	Potato Chips, Original, Right Cr	51.0000	1.800	Ounce	3.00	14.00	36.00	270.00	0.00	2.00	0.00	3.50
	Potato Chips, Pringles, Cheese F	28.3500	1.000	Ounce	1.98	10.49	14.35	156.21	0.00	0.95	1.13	2.71
669	Potato Chips, Ranch, Right Crisp	51.0000	1.800	Ounce	2.00	7.00	18.00	140.00	0.00	1.00	0.00	2.00
670	Potato Chips, S. Cream, Right Cr	51.0000	1.800	Ounce	4.00	23.00	32.00	340.00	0.00	2.00	0.00	6.00
671	Potato Chips, S. Crm/Onion, Fat	28.0000	1.000	Ounce	1.00	0.00	15.00	70.00	0.00	1.00	0.00	0.00
	Power Bar	65.0000	1.000	Each	10.00	2.50	45.00	230.00	0.00	3.00	0.00	0.50
	Pretzels, Cheddar - Combos	28.3500	1.000	Ounce	2.79	4.80	18.85	131.26	0.00	0.00	1.42	0.00
	Pretzels, Hard, Plain, Salted	28.3500	1.000	Ounce	2.58	0.99	22.45	108.01	0.00	0.91	0.00	0.21
	Pretzels, Hard, Plain, Unsalted	28.3500	1.000	Ounce	2.58	0.99	22.45	108.01	0.00	0.79	0.00	0.21
	Pretzels, Hard, Whole-wheat	28.3500	1.000	Ounce	3.15	0.74	23.02	102.63	0.00	2.19	0.00	0.16
	Pudding, Banana	28.3500	1.000	Ounce	0.68	1.02	6.01	36.00	0.00	0.03	0.00	0.16
	Pudding, Bread	252.0000	1.000	Cup	13.10	14.87	61.99	423.36	0.00	0.00	166.32	5.77
	Pudding, Chocolate	28.3500	1.000	Ounce	0.77	1.13	6.46	37.71	1.42	0.28	0.85	0.20
	Pudding, Chocolate, Fat Free	113.0000	0.500	Cup	2.83	0.45	22.71	101.70	0.00	0.90	2.26	0.34
	Pudding, Coconut Cream	140.0000	0.500	Cup	4.34	3.50	24.92	145.60	0.00	0.28	9.80	2.52
	Pudding, Lemon	28.3500	1.000	Ounce	0.03	0.85	7.09	35.44	0.00	0.03	0.00	0.13
	Pudding, Rice	28.3500	1.000	Ounce	0.57	2.13	6.24	46.21	0.00	0.03	0.28	0.33
	Pudding, Tapioca	28.3500	1.000	Ounce	0.57	1.05	5.50	33.74	0.00	0.03	0.28	0.17
	Pudding, Vanilla	28.3500	1.000	Ounce	0.65	1.02	6.21	36.86	0.00	0.03	1.98	0.16
	Pudding, Vanilla, Fat Free	113.0000	0.500	Cup	2.37	0.23	23.17	103.96	0.00	0.11	2.26	0.23
	Raisins, Chocolate, Milk, Coated	180.0000	1.000	Cup	7.38	26.64	122.94	702.00	45.00	7.56	5.40	15.84
	Rice Cakes, Brown Rice, Buckwhea	9.0000	1.000	Cake	0.81	0.32	7.21	34.20	0.00	0.34	0.00	0.06
	Rice Cakes, Brown Rice, Buckwhea	9.0000	1.000	Cake	0.81	0.32	7.21	34.20	0.00	0.00	0.00	0.06
	Rice Cakes, Brown Rice, Corn	9.0000	1.000	Cake	0.76	0.29	7.31	34.65	0.00	0.26	0.00	0.06
	Rice Cakes, Brown Rice, Multigra	9.0000	1.000	Cake	0.77	0.32	7.21	34.83	0.00	0.27	0.00	0.05
	Rice Cakes, Brown Rice, Multigra	9.0000	1.000	Cake	0.77	0.32	7.21	34.83	0.00	0.00	0.00	0.05
	Rice Cakes, Brown Rice, Plain	9.0000	1.000	Cake	0.74	0.25	7.34	34.83	0.00	0.38	0.00	0.05
	Rice Cakes, Brown Rice, Plain, U	9.0000	1.000	Cake	0.74	0.25	7.34	34.83	0.00	0.38	0.00	0.05
	Rice Cakes, Brown Rice, Rye	9.0000	1.000	Cake	0.73	0.34	7.19	34.74	0.00	0.36	0.00	0.05
	Rice Krispie Treats	40.0000	1.000	Cup	1.33	2.00	33.33	160.00	0.00	0.00	0.00	0.00
	Snack Mix, Chex Mix	28.3500	0.660	Cup	3.12	4.90	18.46	120.49	0.00	1.58	0.00	1.57
	Snack Mix, Oriental Mix, Rice-ba	28.3500	1.000	Ounce	4.91	7.25	14.63	155.64	0.00	3.74	0.00	1.07
	Snack Mix, Original Flavor- Doo	56.7000	1.000	Cup	5.84	10.49	36.46	258.55	0.00	3.86	0.57	2.00
	Trail Mix, Regular	150.0000	1.000	Cup	20.70	44.10	67.35	693.00	0.00	0.00	0.00	8.32
	Trail Mix, Regular, Unsalted	150.0000	1.000	Cup	20.70	44.10	67.35	693.00	0.00	0.00	0.00	8.32
	Trail Mix, Regular, w/ Chocolate	146.0000	1.000	Cup	20.73	46.57	65.55	706.64	0.00	0.00	5.84	8.91
	Trail Mix, Tropical	140.0000	1.000	Cup	8.82	23.94	91.84	569.80	0.00	0.00	0.00	11.87

Monounsaturated Fat (gm)	Polyunsaturated Fat (gm)	Vitamin D (mg)	Vitamin K (mg)	Vitamin E (mg)	Vitamin A (re)	Vitamin C (mg)	Thiamin (mg)	Riboflavin (mg)	Niacin (mg)	Vitamin B_6 (mg)	Folate (mcg)	Vitamin B_{12} (mcg)	Calcium (mg)	Iron (mg)	Magnesium (mg)	Phosphorus (mg)	Potassium (mg)	Sodium (mg)	Zinc (mg)
0.82	1.27	0.00	0.00	0.34	2.84	0.00	0.02	0.02	0.62	0.01	0.57	0.00	12.19	0.49	9.92	23.53	30.90	58.40	0.16
0.00	0.00	0.00	0.00	0.00	0.00	0.00	0.00	0.00	0.00	0.00	0.00	0.00	0.00	0.00	0.00	0.00	0.00	280.00	0.00
0.00	0.00	0.00	0.00	0.00	0.00	0.00	0.00	0.00	0.00	0.00	0.00	0.00	0.00	0.00	0.00	0.00	0.00	310.00	0.00
1.07	1.69	0.00	0.00	0.01	4.84	0.06	0.01	0.03	0.16	0.03	1.21	0.06	12.43	0.25	10.01	39.71	28.71	97.79	0.22
0.00	0.00	0.00	0.00	0.00	0.00	0.00	0.00	0.00	0.00	0.00	0.00	0.00	0.00	0.05	0.00	0.00	0.00	72.50	0.00
0.00	0.00	0.00	0.00	0.00	0.00	0.00	0.00	0.00	0.00	0.00	0.00	0.00	0.00	0.07	0.00	0.00	0.00	55.00	0.00
0.00	0.00	0.00	0.00	0.00	0.00	0.00	0.00	0.00	0.00	0.00	0.00	0.00	0.00	0.00	0.00	0.00	0.00	280.00	0.00
0.00	0.00	0.00	0.00	0.00	0.00	0.00	0.00	0.00	0.00	0.00	0.00	0.00	0.00	0.00	0.00	0.00	0.00	40.00	0.00
0.90	1.48	0.00	0.00	0.01	1.65	0.03	0.01	0.02	0.17	0.02	1.87	0.00	1.10	0.31	11.88	27.50	24.75	97.24	0.29
0.90	1.48	0.00	0.00	0.01	0.22	0.03	0.01	0.02	0.17	0.02	1.87	0.00	1.10	0.31	11.88	27.50	24.75	97.24	0.29
0.00	0.00	0.00	0.00	0.00	0.00	0.00	0.00	0.00	0.00	0.00	0.00	0.00	2.00	0.66	0.00	0.00	0.00	357.00	0.00
0.00	0.00	0.00	0.00	0.00	0.00	0.00	0.00	0.00	0.00	0.00	0.00	0.00	2.00	0.63	0.00	0.00	0.00	321.00	0.00
0.00	0.00	0.00	0.00	0.00	0.00	0.00	0.00	0.00	0.00	0.00	0.00	0.00	2.00	0.62	0.00	0.00	0.00	2.00	0.00
0.00	0.00	0.00	0.00	0.00	0.00	0.00	0.00	0.00	0.00	0.00	0.00	0.00	16.00	0.12	0.00	0.00	0.00	307.00	0.00
0.00	0.00	0.00	0.00	0.00	0.00	0.00	0.00	0.00	0.00	0.00	0.00	0.00	0.00	0.00	0.00	0.00	0.00	160.00	0.00
0.00	0.00	0.00	0.00	0.00	0.00	0.00	0.00	0.00	0.00	0.00	0.00	0.00	0.00	0.00	0.00	0.00	0.00	400.00	0.00
0.00	0.00	0.00	0.00	0.00	0.00	0.00	0.00	0.00	0.00	0.00	0.00	0.00	0.00	0.00	0.00	0.00	0.00	160.00	0.00
0.00	0.00	0.00	0.00	0.00	0.00	0.00	0.00	0.00	0.00	0.00	0.00	0.00	0.00	0.00	0.00	0.00	0.00	260.00	0.00
2.02	5.29	0.00	0.00	0.00	0.00	2.41	0.05	0.03	0.74	0.15	5.10	0.00	31.19	0.45	15.03	46.21	108.01	214.04	0.18
0.00	0.00	0.00	0.00	0.00	0.00	0.00	0.00	0.00	0.00	0.00	0.00	0.00	0.00	0.00	0.00	0.00	0.00	160.00	0.00
0.00	0.00	0.00	0.00	0.00	0.00	0.00	0.00	0.00	0.00	0.00	0.00	0.00	0.00	0.00	0.00	0.00	0.00	290.00	0.00
0.00	0.00	0.00	0.00	0.00	0.00	0.00	0.00	0.00	0.00	0.00	0.00	0.00	0.00	0.00	0.00	0.00	0.00	160.00	0.00
1.50	0.50	0.00	0.00	0.00	0.00	0.00	1.50	1.70	19.00	2.00	200.00	2.00	360.00	3.50	122.50	280.00	0.00	90.00	5.25
0.00	0.00	0.00	0.00	0.00	1.98	0.00	0.09	0.16	0.90	0.01	2.27	0.03	55.85	0.26	6.24	40.54	36.86	316.67	0.21
0.39	0.35	0.00	0.00	0.06	0.00	0.00	0.13	0.18	1.49	0.03	48.48	0.00	10.21	1.22	9.92	32.04	41.39	486.20	0.24
0.39	0.35	0.00	0.00	0.06	0.00	0.00	0.13	0.18	1.49	0.03	23.53	0.00	10.21	1.22	9.92	32.04	41.39	81.93	0.24
0.29	0.24	0.00	0.00	0.00	0.00	0.28	0.12	0.08	1.85	0.08	15.31	0.00	7.94	0.76	8.51	35.44	121.91	57.55	0.18
0.43	0.38	0.00	0.00	0.00	8.51	0.14	0.01	0.04	0.05	0.01	0.57	0.05	24.10	0.04	2.27	19.56	31.19	55.57	0.08
5.42	2.39	0.00	0.00	0.00	163.80	2.02	0.23	0.56	1.58	0.19	32.76	0.00	287.28	2.77	47.88	274.68	564.48	582.12	1.31
0.48	0.41	0.00	0.00	0.04	3.12	0.51	0.01	0.05	0.10	0.01	0.85	0.00	25.52	0.14	5.95	22.68	51.03	36.57	0.12
0.00	0.00	0.00	0.00	0.00	0.00	0.34	0.00	0.00	0.00	0.00	0.00	0.00	89.27	0.60	0.00	85.88	235.04	192.10	0.00
0.73	0.10	0.00	0.00	0.10	70.00	0.98	0.04	0.21	0.13	0.21	5.60	0.36	158.20	0.28	22.40	124.60	222.60	228.20	0.52
0.37	0.32	0.00	0.00	0.00	0.00	0.03	0.00	0.00	0.00	0.00	0.00	0.00	0.57	0.02	0.28	1.42	0.28	39.69	0.01
0.91	0.79	0.00	0.00	0.39	9.92	0.14	0.01	0.02	0.05	0.01	0.85	0.06	14.74	0.09	2.27	19.28	17.01	24.10	0.14
0.45	0.39	0.00	0.00	0.03	0.00	0.20	0.01	0.03	0.09	0.01	0.85	0.06	23.81	0.07	2.27	22.40	27.50	45.08	0.08
0.44	0.38	0.00	0.00	0.04	1.70	0.00	0.01	0.04	0.07	0.00	0.00	0.03	24.95	0.04	2.27	19.28	32.04	38.27	0.07
0.00	0.00	0.00	0.00	0.00	0.00	0.34	0.00	0.00	0.00	0.00	0.00	0.00	85.88	0.05	0.00	115.26	123.17	240.69	0.00
8.53	0.92	0.00	0.00	1.75	12.60	0.36	0.14	0.29	0.72	0.14	9.00	0.32	154.80	3.08	81.00	257.40	925.20	64.80	1.46
0.10	0.10	0.00	0.00	0.00	0.00	0.00	0.01	0.01	0.73	0.01	1.89	0.00	0.99	0.10	13.59	34.20	26.91	10.44	0.23
0.10	0.10	0.00	0.00	0.00	0.00	0.00	0.01	0.01	0.73	0.01	1.89	0.00	0.99	0.10	13.59	34.20	26.91	0.36	0.23
0.10	0.10	0.00	0.00	0.00	0.00	0.00	0.01	0.01	0.58	0.01	1.71	0.00	0.81	0.11	10.26	28.80	24.75	26.19	0.20
0.10	0.13	0.00	0.00	0.00	0.00	0.00	0.01	0.02	0.59	0.01	1.80	0.00	1.89	0.18	12.33	33.30	26.46	22.68	0.23
0.10	0.13	0.00	0.00	0.00	0.00	0.00	0.01	0.02	0.59	0.01	1.80	0.00	1.89	0.18	12.33	33.30	26.46	0.36	0.23
0.09	0.09	0.00	0.00	0.06	0.45	0.00	0.01	0.02	0.70	0.01	1.89	0.00	0.99	0.13	11.79	32.40	26.10	29.34	0.27
0.09	0.09	0.00	0.00	0.01	0.45	0.00	0.01	0.02	0.70	0.01	1.89	0.00	0.99	0.13	11.79	32.40	26.10	2.34	0.27
0.12	0.14	0.00	0.00	0.00	0.00	0.00	0.01	0.01	0.63	0.01	0.45	0.00	1.89	0.16	12.96	34.20	27.99	9.90	0.27
1.33	0.00	0.02	0.00	0.00	200.00	20.00	0.50	0.57	6.33	0.67	0.00	0.67	0.00	1.33	0.00	21.33	26.67	226.67	0.00
0.00	0.00	0.00	0.00	0.00	3.97	13.47	0.44	0.14	4.77	0.44	0.00	3.52	9.92	7.00	17.86	53.01	76.26	288.32	0.59
2.80	3.02	0.00	0.00	2.39		0.09	0.09	0.04	0.87	0.02	10.77	0.00	15.31	0.69	33.45	74.28	92.99	117.09	0.75
0.00	0.00	0.00	0.00	0.00	24.38	0.06	0.20	0.15	3.04	0.11	22.68	0.01	41.96	1.42	34.02	167.83	157.06	720.66	1.28
18.80	14.48	0.00	0.00	0.00	3.00	2.10	0.69	0.30	7.07	0.45	106.50	0.00	117.00	4.58	237.00	517.50	1027.50	343.50	4.83
18.80	14.48	0.00	0.00	0.00	3.00	2.10	0.69	0.30	7.07	0.45	106.50	0.00	117.00	4.58	237.00	517.50	1027.50	15.00	4.83
19.77	16.48	0.00	0.00	0.00	7.30	1.90	0.60	0.32	6.44	0.38	94.90	0.00	159.14	4.95	235.06	565.02	946.08	176.66	4.58
3.49	7.22	0.00	0.00	0.00	7.00	10.64	0.63	0.17	2.07	0.46	58.80	0.00	79.80	3.70	134.40	260.40	992.60	14.00	1.64

USDA ID Code	Food Name	Weight in Grams*	Quantity of Units	Unit of Measure	Protein (gm)	Fat (gm)	Carbohydrate (gm)	Kcalories	Caffeine (gm)	Fiber (gm)	Cholesterol (mg)	Saturated Fat (gm)
	Soups											
	Soup, Asparagus, Cream Of	248.0000	1.000	Cup	6.32	8.18	16.39	161.20	0.00	0.74	22.32	3.32
	Soup, Bean and Ham-Healthy Choic	212.6200	1.000	Each	12.00	4.00	35.00	220.00	0.00	0.00	5.00	1.00
	Soup, Bean w/ Bacon	264.9000	1.000	Cup	5.48	2.15	16.37	105.96	0.00	9.01	2.65	0.95
	Soup, Bean w/ Ham	243.0000	1.000	Cup	12.61	8.51	27.12	230.85	0.00	11.18	21.87	3.33
	Soup, Bean w/ Hot Dogs	250.0000	1.000	Cup	9.98	6.98	22.00	187.50	0.00	0.00	12.50	2.13
	Soup, Bean w/ Pork	253.0000	1.000	Cup	7.89	5.95	22.80	172.04	0.00	8.60	2.53	1.52
	Soup, Bean, Black	247.0000	1.000	Cup	5.63	1.51	19.81	116.09	0.00	4.45	0.00	0.40
	Soup, Bean, Navy, w/ Ham-Stouffe	283.9200	1.000	Cup	11.02	8.01	31.05	240.36	0.00	0.00	20.03	0.00
	Soup, Beef and Potato-Healthy Ch	212.6200	1.000	Each	9.00	1.00	17.00	110.00	0.00	0.00	20.00	0.00
	Soup, Beef Mushroom	244.0000	1.000	Cup	5.78	3.00	6.34	73.20	0.00	0.24	7.32	1.49
	Soup, Beef Noodle	244.0000	1.000	Cup	4.83	3.07	8.98	82.96	0.00	0.73	4.88	1.15
	Soup, Beef, Chunky	240.0000	1.000	Cup	11.74	5.14	19.56	170.40	0.00	1.44	14.40	2.54
	Soup, Beef, Hearty-Healthy Choic	212.6200	1.000	Each	9.00	1.00	17.00	120.00	0.00	0.00	20.00	0.00
	Soup, Broccoli, Cream Of,-Stouff	283.9200	1.000	Cup	12.02	21.03	16.02	300.45	0.00	0.00	60.09	0.00
	Soup, Broth or Bouillon, Beef	240.0000	1.000	Cup	2.74	0.53	0.10	16.80	0.00	0.00	0.00	0.26
	Soup, Broth or Bouillon, Chicken	244.0000	1.000	Cup	1.34	1.10	1.44	21.96	0.00	0.00	0.00	0.27
	Soup, Cauliflower	253.0000	1.000	Cup	2.89	1.72	10.73	69.15	0.00	0.00	0.00	0.26
	Soup, Celery, Cream Of	248.0000	1.000	Cup	5.68	9.70	14.53	163.68	0.00	0.74	32.24	3.94
	Soup, Cheddar Cheese, Heat'n Ser	307.5800	1.000	Cup	21.70	35.80	21.70	488.23	0.00	0.00	97.65	0.00
	Soup, Cheddar Cheese-Stouffer's	283.9200	1.000	Cup	21.03	31.05	18.03	440.66	0.00	0.00	70.11	0.00
	Soup, Cheese	247.0000	1.000	Cup	5.41	10.47	10.52	155.61	0.00	0.99	29.64	6.67
	Soup, Chicken Gumbo-Stouffer's	283.9200	1.000	Cup	7.01	5.01	9.01	110.17	0.00	0.00	20.03	0.00
	Soup, Chicken Mushroom	244.0000	1.000	Cup	4.39	9.15	9.27	131.76	0.00	0.24	9.76	2.39
	Soup, Chicken Noodle	241.0000	1.000	Cup	4.05	2.46	9.35	74.71	0.00	0.72	7.23	0.65
	Soup, Chicken Noodle, Chunky	240.0000	1.000	Cup	12.72	6.00	17.04	175.20	0.00	3.84	19.20	1.39
	Soup, Chicken Noodle, Heat'n Ser	283.9200	1.000	Cup	13.02	17.03	28.04	320.48	0.00	0.00	60.09	0.00
	Soup, Chicken Noodle, Old Fashio	212.6200	1.000	Each	5.00	2.00	11.00	90.00	0.00	0.00	20.00	0.00
	Soup, Chicken Noodle-Stouffer's	283.9200	1.000	Cup	7.01	7.01	10.02	130.20	0.00	0.00	20.03	0.00
	Soup, Chicken Pasta-Healthy Choi	212.6200	1.000	Each	7.00	2.00	13.00	100.00	0.00	0.00	15.00	0.00
	Soup, Chicken Rice	240.0000	1.000	Cup	2.33	1.37	8.78	57.60	0.00	0.72	2.40	0.31
	Soup, Chicken Rice, Chunky	240.0000	1.000	Cup	12.26	3.19	12.98	127.20	0.00	0.96	12.00	0.96
	Soup, Chicken w/ Dumplings	241.0000	1.000	Cup	5.62	5.52	6.05	96.40	0.00	0.48	33.74	1.30
	Soup, Chicken w/ Rice	241.0000	1.000	Cup	3.54	1.90	7.16	60.25	0.00	0.72	7.23	0.46
	Soup, Chicken w/ Rice-Healthy Ch	212.6200	1.000	Each	5.00	1.00	14.00	90.00	0.00	0.00	10.00	0.00
	Soup, Chicken, Chunky	240.0000	1.000	Cup	12.14	6.34	16.51	170.40	0.00	1.44	28.80	1.90
	Soup, Chicken, Cream Of	248.0000	1.000	Cup	7.46	11.46	14.98	190.96	0.00	0.25	27.28	4.64
	Soup, Chicken, Creamy-Stouffer's	283.9200	1.000	Cup	17.03	8.01	25.04	240.36	0.00	0.00	20.03	0.00
	Soup, Chicken, Hearty-Healthy Ch	212.6200	1.000	Each	7.00	2.00	17.00	110.00	0.00	0.00	25.00	0.00
	Soup, Chili Beef	250.0000	1.000	Cup	6.70	6.60	21.45	170.00	0.00	9.50	12.50	3.35
	Soup, Clam Chowder, Manhattan St	240.0000	1.000	Cup	7.25	3.38	18.82	134.40	0.00	2.88	14.40	2.11
	Soup, Clam Chowder, New England	248.0000	1.000	Cup	9.47	6.60	16.62	163.68	0.00	1.49	22.32	2.95
	Soup, Clam Chowder, New England-	283.9200	1.000	Cup	14.02	23.03	21.03	340.51	0.00	0.00	40.06	0.00
	Soup, Crab	244.0000	1.000	Cup	5.49	1.51	10.30	75.64	0.00	0.73	9.76	0.39
	Soup, Fiesta Mexicali Heat'n Ser	283.9200	1.000	Cup	3.00	3.00	18.03	110.17	0.00	0.00	10.02	0.00
	Soup, Gazpacho	244.0000	1.000	Cup	7.08	0.24	4.39	46.36	0.00	0.49	0.00	0.02
	Soup, Gumbo, Chicken	244.0000	1.000	Cup	2.64	1.44	8.37	56.12	0.00	1.95	4.88	0.32
	Soup, Hot and Sour	244.0000	1.000	Cup	15.00	8.00	5.00	162.00	0.00	0.50	34.00	3.00
	Soup, Instant	240.0000	1.000	Cup	3.00	1.00	7.00	50.00	0.00	0.70	2.00	0.00
	Soup, Lentil w/ ham	248.0000	1.000	Cup	9.28	2.78	20.24	138.88	0.00	0.00	7.44	1.12
	Soup, Lentil-Healthy Choice	212.6200	1.000	Each	8.00	1.00	23.00	140.00	0.00	0.00	0.00	0.00
	Soup, Minestrone	241.0000	1.000	Cup	4.27	2.51	11.23	81.94	0.00	0.96	2.41	0.55
	Soup, Minestrone Heat'n Serve-St	283.9200	1.000	Cup	5.01	4.01	18.03	130.20	0.00	0.00	0.00	0.00
	Soup, Minestrone, Chunky	240.0000	1.000	Cup	5.11	2.81	20.74	127.20	0.00	5.76	4.80	1.49
	Soup, Minestrone-Healthy Choice	212.6200	1.000	Each	6.00	1.00	30.00	160.00	0.00	0.00	0.00	0.00
	Soup, Minestrone-Stouffer's	283.9200	1.000	Cup	6.01	3.00	20.03	140.21	0.00	0.00	10.02	0.00

Monounsaturated Fat (gm)	Polyunsaturated Fat (gm)	Vitamin D (mg)	Vitamin K (mg)	Vitamin E (mg)	Vitamin A (re)	Vitamin C (mg)	Thiamin (mg)	Riboflavin (mg)	Niacin (mg)	Vitamin B$_6$ (mg)	Folate (mg)	Vitamin B$_{12}$ (mcg)	Calcium (mg)	Iron (mg)	Magnesium (mg)	Phosphorus (mg)	Potassium (mg)	Sodium (mg)	Zinc (mg)
2.08	2.23	0.00	0.00	0.84	84.32	3.97	0.10	0.27	0.89	0.07	29.76	0.50	173.60	0.87	19.84	153.76	359.60	1041.60	0.92
0.00	1.00	0.00	0.00	0.00	60.00	2.40	0.23	0.17	1.14	0.00	0.00	0.00	48.00	1.00	0.00	220.00	630.00	480.00	0.00
0.93	0.16	0.00	0.00	0.26	5.30	1.06	0.05	0.26	0.40	0.03	7.95	0.03	55.63	1.32	29.14	90.07	325.83	927.15	0.69
3.84	0.95	0.00	0.00	0.00	396.09	4.37	0.15	0.15	1.70	0.12	29.16	0.07	77.76	3.23	46.17	143.37	425.25	972.00	1.07
2.73	1.65	0.00	0.00	0.00	87.50	1.00	0.10	0.08	1.03	0.13	30.00	0.08	87.50	2.35	47.50	165.00	477.50	1092.50	1.18
2.18	1.82	0.00	0.00	0.08	88.55	1.52	0.10	0.03	0.56	0.05	31.88	0.05	80.96	2.05	45.54	131.56	402.27	951.28	1.04
0.54	0.47	0.00	0.00	0.07	49.40	0.74	0.07	0.05	0.54	0.10	24.70	0.02	44.46	2.15	41.99	106.21	274.17	1197.95	1.41
0.00	0.00	0.00	0.00	0.00	0.00	0.00	0.00	0.00	0.19	0.00	0.00	0.00	70.11	3.00	0.00	0.00	570.86	1251.88	0.00
0.00	0.00	0.00	0.00	0.00	0.00	2.40	0.03	0.00	0.38	0.00	0.00	0.00	0.00	0.20	0.00	0.00	100.00	550.00	0.00
1.24	0.12	0.00	0.00	0.00		4.64	0.05	0.05	0.95	0.05	9.76	0.20	4.88	0.88	9.76	34.16	153.72	941.84	1.46
1.24	0.49	0.00	0.00	0.00	63.44	0.24	0.07	0.05	1.07	0.05	19.52	0.20	14.64	1.10	4.88	46.36	100.04	951.60	1.54
2.14	0.22	0.00	0.00	0.17	261.60	6.96	0.05	0.14	2.71	0.14	13.44	0.62	31.20	2.33	4.80	120.00	336.00	866.40	2.64
0.00	0.00	0.00	0.00	0.00	150.00	9.00	0.06	0.10	1.90	0.00	0.00	0.00	32.00	0.40	0.00	90.00	280.00	540.00	0.00
0.00	0.00	0.00	0.00	0.00	0.00	0.00	0.00	0.01	0.00	0.00	0.00	0.00	2.48	0.00	0.00	0.00	430.64	791.19	0.00
0.22	0.02	0.00	0.00	0.00	0.00	0.00	0.00	0.05	1.87	0.02	4.80	0.17	14.40	0.41	4.80	31.20	129.60	782.40	0.00
0.41	0.37	0.00	0.00	0.02	12.20	0.00	0.00	0.02	0.20	0.00	2.44	0.02	14.64	0.07	4.88	12.20	24.40	1483.52	0.00
0.74	0.64	0.00	0.00	0.00	0.00	2.56	0.08	0.08	0.51	0.03	2.56	0.18	10.24	0.51	2.56	51.22	105.00	842.57	0.26
2.46	2.65	0.00	0.00	0.97	66.96	1.49	0.07	0.25	0.45	0.07	8.43	0.50	186.00	0.69	22.32	151.28	310.00	1009.36	0.20
0.00	0.00	0.00	0.00	0.00	0.00	0.00	0.00	0.02	0.21	0.00	0.00	0.00	4.95	0.11	0.00	0.00	553.33	770.32	0.00
0.00	0.00	0.00	0.00	0.00	0.00	0.00	0.00	0.01	0.19	0.00	0.00	0.00	4.97	0.00	0.00	0.00	510.77	681.02	0.00
2.96	0.30	0.00	0.00	0.00	108.68	0.00	0.02	0.15	0.40	0.02	4.94	0.00	140.79	0.74	4.94	135.85	153.14	958.36	0.64
0.00	0.00	0.00	0.00	0.00	0.00	0.00	0.00	0.00	0.19	0.00	0.00	0.00	160.24	0.10	0.00	0.00	180.27	1422.13	0.00
4.03	2.32	0.00	0.00	0.00	112.24	0.00	0.02	0.12	1.63	0.05	0.24	0.05	29.28	0.88	9.76	26.84	153.72	941.84	0.98
1.11	0.55	0.00	0.00	0.07	72.30	0.24	0.05	0.07	1.40	0.02	21.69	0.14	16.87	0.77	4.82	36.15	55.43	1106.19	0.39
2.66	1.51	0.00	0.00	0.79	122.40	0.00	0.07	0.17	4.32	0.05	38.40	0.31	24.00	1.44	9.60	72.00	108.00	849.60	0.96
0.00	0.00	0.00	0.00	0.00	0.00	6.01	0.00	0.00	0.57	0.00	0.00	0.00	240.36	0.20	0.00	0.00	310.46	1792.69	0.00
0.00	0.00	0.00	0.00	0.00	80.00	12.00	0.03	0.10	1.90	0.00	0.00	0.00	16.00	0.20	0.00	60.00	130.00	540.00	0.00
0.00	0.00	0.00	0.00	0.00	0.00	0.00	0.00	0.00	0.19	0.00	0.00	0.00	80.12	0.10	0.00	0.00	140.21	1281.92	0.00
0.00	0.00	0.00	0.00	0.00	60.00	0.00	0.03	0.00	0.38	0.00	0.00	0.00	0.00	0.00	0.00	0.00	70.00	560.00	0.00
0.60	0.41	0.00	0.00	0.05	0.00	0.00	0.00	0.00	0.34	0.02	0.48	0.07	7.20	0.00	0.00	9.60	9.60	931.20	0.12
1.44	0.67	0.00	0.00	0.10	585.60	3.84	0.02	0.10	4.10	0.05	3.84	0.31	33.60	1.87	9.60	72.00	108.00	888.00	0.96
2.53	1.30	0.00	0.00	0.14	53.02	0.00	0.02	0.07	1.76	0.05	2.41	0.17	14.46	0.63	4.82	60.25	115.68	860.37	0.36
0.92	0.41	0.00	0.00	0.05	65.07	0.24	0.02	0.02	1.13	0.02	0.96	0.14	16.87	0.75	0.00	21.69	101.22	814.58	0.27
0.00	0.00	0.00	0.00	0.00	80.00	6.00	0.03	0.07	1.90	0.00	0.00	0.00	16.00	0.20	0.00	70.00	140.00	510.00	0.00
2.83	1.32	0.00	0.00	0.17	124.80	1.20	0.07	0.17	4.22	0.05	4.32	0.24	24.00	1.66	7.20	108.00	168.00	849.60	0.96
4.46	1.64	0.00	0.00	0.25	94.24	1.24	0.07	0.25	0.92	0.07	7.69	0.55	181.04	0.67	17.36	151.28	272.80	1046.56	0.67
0.00	0.00	0.00	0.00	0.00	0.00	0.00	0.00	0.02	0.01	0.19	0.00	0.00	2.48	0.00	0.00	0.00	510.77	1281.92	0.00
0.00	0.00	0.00	0.00	0.00	200.00	2.40	0.09	0.17	1.90	0.00	0.00	0.00	32.00	0.40	0.00	90.00	190.00	520.00	0.00
2.80	0.28	0.00	0.00	0.18	150.00	4.00	0.05	0.08	1.08	0.15	17.50	0.33	42.50	2.13	30.00	147.50	525.00	1035.00	1.40
0.98	0.12	0.00	0.00	0.10	328.80	12.24	0.05	0.07	1.85	0.26	9.36	7.92	67.20	2.64	19.20	84.00	384.00	1000.80	1.68
2.26	1.09	0.00	0.00	0.15	39.68	3.47	0.07	0.25	1.04	0.12	9.67	10.24	186.00	1.49	22.32	156.24	300.08	992.00	0.79
0.00	0.00	0.00	0.00	0.00	0.00	0.00	0.00	0.01	0.19	0.00	0.00	0.00	2.48	0.10	0.00	0.00	570.86	961.44	0.00
0.68	0.39	0.00	0.00	0.00	51.24	0.00	0.20	0.07	1.34	0.12	14.64	0.20	65.88	1.22	14.64	87.84	326.96	1234.64	1.46
0.00	0.00	0.00	0.00	0.00	0.00	6.01	0.00	0.00	0.19	0.00	0.00	0.00	2.40	1.00	0.00	0.00	430.64	711.07	0.00
0.02	0.07	0.00	0.00	0.46	261.08	7.08	0.05	0.02	0.93	0.15	9.76	0.00	24.40	0.98	7.32	36.60	224.48	739.32	0.24
0.66	0.34	0.00	0.00	0.05	14.64	4.88	0.02	0.05	0.66	0.07	4.88	0.02	24.40	0.90	4.88	24.40	75.64	954.04	0.37
0.30	0.68	0.00	0.00	0.30	0.03	0.60	0.00	0.00	0.00	0.00	0.00	0.00	32.00	1.65	0.00	0.00	0.00	1011.00	0.00
0.00	0.00	0.00	0.00	0.00	0.03	0.03	0.00	0.00	0.00	0.00	0.00	0.00	27.00	0.45	0.00	0.00	0.00	1222.00	0.00
1.29	0.32	0.00	0.00	0.00	34.72	4.22	0.17	0.12	1.36	0.22	49.60	0.30	42.16	2.65	22.32	183.52	357.12	1319.36	0.74
0.00	0.00	0.00	0.00	0.00	60.00	2.40	0.06	0.03	0.38	0.00	0.00	0.00	0.00	0.00	0.00	0.00	160.00	480.00	0.00
0.70	1.11	0.00	0.00	0.07	233.77	1.21	0.05	0.05	0.94	0.10	36.15	0.00	33.74	0.92	7.23	55.43	313.30	910.98	0.75
0.00	0.00	0.00	0.00	0.00	0.00	0.00	0.00	0.00	0.19	0.00	0.00	0.00	0.00	0.20	0.00	0.00	310.46	1191.79	0.00
0.91	0.26	0.00	0.00	0.72	434.40	4.80	0.05	0.12	1.18	0.24	52.80	0.00	60.00	1.78	14.40	110.40	612.00	864.00	1.44
0.00	0.00	0.00	0.00	0.00	60.00	15.00	0.12	0.14	1.52	0.00	0.00	0.00	32.00	0.60	0.00	130.00	440.00	520.00	0.00
0.00	0.00	0.00	0.00	0.00	0.00	0.00	0.00	0.00	0.19	0.00	0.00	0.00	0.00	0.20	0.00	0.00	370.56	1281.92	0.00

USDA ID Code	Food Name	Weight in Grams*	Quantity of Units	Unit of Measure	Protein (gm)	Fat (gm)	Carbohydrate (gm)	Kcalories	Caffeine (gm)	Fiber (gm)	Cholesterol (mg)	Saturated Fat (gm)
	Soup, Mushroom	253.0000	1.000	Cup	2.23	4.86	11.13	96.14	0.00	0.76	0.00	0.81
	Soup, Mushroom, Cream Of	248.0000	1.000	Cup	6.05	13.59	15.00	203.36	0.00	0.50	19.84	5.13
	Soup, Onion	241.0000	1.000	Cup	3.76	1.74	8.17	57.84	0.00	0.96	0.00	0.27
	Soup, Onion, Cream Of	248.0000	1.000	Cup	6.80	9.37	18.35	186.00	0.00	0.74	32.24	4.04
	Soup, Onion, French-Stouffer's	283.9200	1.000	Cup	4.01	4.01	10.02	100.15	0.00	0.00	0.00	0.00
	Soup, Pea, Green	254.0000	1.000	Cup	12.62	7.04	32.23	238.76	0.00	2.79	17.78	4.01
	Soup, Pea, Split w/ Ham	253.0000	1.000	Cup	10.32	4.40	27.96	189.75	0.00	2.28	7.59	1.77
	Soup, Pea, Split w/ Ham, Chunky	240.0000	1.000	Cup	11.09	3.98	26.81	184.80	0.00	4.08	7.20	1.58
	Soup, Pea, Split, and Ham-Health	212.6200	1.000	Each	10.00	3.00	25.00	170.00	0.00	10.00	10.00	1.00
	Soup, Pea, Split, and Ham-Stouff	283.9200	1.000	Cup	15.02	3.00	35.05	220.33	0.00	0.00	10.02	0.00
	Soup, Potato, Cream Of	248.0000	1.000	Cup	5.78	6.45	17.16	148.80	0.00	0.50	22.32	3.77
	Soup, Potato, Cream Of,-Stouffer	283.9200	1.000	Cup	11.02	13.02	34.05	300.45	0.00	0.00	30.04	0.00
	Soup, Shrimp, Cream Of	248.0000	1.000	Cup	6.82	9.30	13.91	163.68	0.00	0.25	34.72	5.78
	Soup, Sweet & Sour	244.0000	1.000	Cup	3.00	1.00	14.00	72.00	0.00	1.60	5.00	0.00
	Soup, Tomato	248.0000	1.000	Cup	6.10	6.00	22.30	161.20	0.00	2.73	17.36	2.90
	Soup, Tomato Beef w/ noodle	244.0000	1.000	Cup	4.47	4.29	21.15	139.08	0.00	1.46	4.88	1.59
	Soup, Tomato Garden-Healthy Choi	212.6200	1.000	Each	4.00	3.00	22.00	130.00	0.00	0.00	5.00	1.00
	Soup, Tomato Rice	247.0000	1.000	Cup	2.10	2.72	21.93	118.56	0.00	1.48	2.47	0.52
	Soup, Tomato, Garden Heat'n Serv	283.9200	1.000	Cup	4.01	3.00	16.02	110.17	0.00	0.00	10.02	0.00
	Soup, Turkey Noodle	244.0000	1.000	Cup	3.90	2.00	8.64	68.32	0.00	0.73	4.88	0.56
	Soup, Turkey, Chunky	236.0000	1.000	Cup	10.22	4.41	14.07	134.52	0.00	0.00	9.44	1.23
	Soup, Vegetable Beef	253.0000	1.000	Cup	2.93	1.11	8.02	53.13	0.00	0.51	0.00	0.56
	Soup, Vegetable, Beef w/ Barley-	283.9200	1.000	Cup	4.01	13.02	15.02	190.29	0.00	0.00	10.02	0.00
	Soup, Vegetable, Beef-Healthy Ch	212.6200	1.000	Each	8.00	1.00	21.00	130.00	0.00	0.00	15.00	0.00
	Soup, Vegetable, Chicken	241.0000	1.000	Cup	3.62	2.84	8.58	74.71	0.00	0.96	9.64	0.84
	Soup, Vegetable, Chicken, Chunky	240.0000	1.000	Cup	12.31	4.82	18.89	165.60	0.00	0.00	16.80	1.44
	Soup, Vegetable, Chunky	240.0000	1.000	Cup	3.50	3.70	19.01	122.40	0.00	1.20	0.00	0.55
	Soup, Vegetable, Country-Healthy	212.6200	1.000	Each	3.00	1.00	23.00	120.00	0.00	0.00	0.00	0.00
	Soup, Vegetable, Cream Of	260.1000	1.000	Cup	1.90	5.70	12.30	106.64	0.00	0.52	0.00	1.43
	Soup, Vegetable, Garden-Healthy	212.6200	1.000	Each	3.00	1.00	18.00	100.00	0.00	0.00	0.00	0.00
	Soup, Vegetable, Tomato	241.0000	1.000	Cup	1.90	0.82	9.74	53.02	0.00	0.48	0.00	0.36
	Soup, Vegetable, Turkey	241.0000	1.000	Cup	3.08	3.04	8.63	72.30	0.00	0.48	2.41	0.89
	Soup, Vegetable, Turkey-Healthy	212.6200	1.000	Each	4.00	3.00	17.00	110.00	0.00	0.00	15.00	1.00
	Soup, Vegetable, Vegetarian	241.0000	1.000	Cup	2.10	1.93	11.98	72.30	0.00	0.48	0.00	0.29
	Soup, Vegetable, Vegetarian-Stou	283.9200	1.000	Cup	6.01	2.00	20.03	120.18	0.00	0.00	0.00	0.00
	Soup, Won-Ton	241.0000	1.000	Cup	14.00	7.00	14.00	182.00	0.00	0.90	53.00	2.00

Supplements

USDA ID Code	Food Name	Weight in Grams*	Quantity of Units	Unit of Measure	Protein (gm)	Fat (gm)	Carbohydrate (gm)	Kcalories	Caffeine (gm)	Fiber (gm)	Cholesterol (mg)	Saturated Fat (gm)
3	Boost Plus, Chocolate	240.0000	8.000	fl oz	14.00	14.00	45.00	360.00	0.00	0.00	0.00	2.00
4	Boost Plus, Strawberry	240.0000	8.000	fl oz	14.00	14.00	45.00	360.00	0.00	0.00	0.00	2.00
5	Boost Plus, Vanilla	240.0000	8.000	fl oz	14.00	14.00	45.00	360.00	0.00	0.00	0.00	2.00
6	Boost, Chocolate	240.0000	8.000	fl oz	10.00	4.00	40.00	240.00	0.00	0.00	5.00	0.50
7	Boost, Chocolate Mocha	240.0000	8.000	fl oz	10.00	4.00	40.00	240.00	0.00	0.00	5.00	0.50
8	Boost, Strawberry	240.0000	8.000	fl oz	10.00	4.00	40.00	240.00	0.00	0.00	5.00	0.50
9	Boost, Vanilla	240.0000	8.000	fl oz	10.00	4.00	40.00	240.00	0.00	0.00	5.00	0.50
430	Enlive-Ross Labs	243.0000	8.000	Fl Oz	10.00	0.00	65.00	300.00	0.00	0.00	3.00	0.00
431	Ensure Fiber with FOS-Ross Labs	240.0000	8.000	Fl Oz	8.80	6.10	42.00	250.00	0.00	2.80	0.00	0.00
432	Ensure Glucerna OS-Ross Labs	240.0000	8.000	Fl Oz	10.00	11.00	22.00	220.00	0.00	2.00	0.00	1.00
433	Ensure Glucerna Snack Bars-Ross	38.0000	1.000	Bar	6.00	4.00	24.00	140.00	0.00	4.00	3.00	1.00
434	Ensure High Calcium-Ross Labs	240.0000	8.000	Fl Oz	12.00	6.00	31.00	225.00	0.00	0.00	0.00	0.50
435	Ensure High Protein-Ross Labs	240.0000	8.000	Fl Oz	12.00	6.00	30.80	225.00	0.00	0.00	0.00	0.64
436	Ensure Light-Ross Labs	240.0000	8.000	Fl Oz	10.00	3.00	33.30	200.00	0.00	0.00	3.00	0.31
437	Ensure Nutrition Bars-Ross Labs	35.0000	1.000	Bar	6.00	3.00	21.00	130.00	0.00	0.00	3.00	1.00
438	Ensure Plus-Ross Labs	240.0000	8.000	Fl Oz	13.00	11.40	50.10	355.00	0.00	0.00	3.00	0.00
439	Ensure Powder-Ross Labs	240.0000	8.000	Fl Oz	9.00	9.00	34.00	250.00	0.00	0.00	0.00	0.00
440	Ensure Pudding-Ross Labs	120.0000	4.000	Ounce	4.00	5.00	27.00	170.00	0.00	0.00	0.00	0.00
441	Ensure-Ross Labs	240.0000	8.000	Fl Oz	8.80	6.10	40.00	250.00	0.00	0.00	3.00	0.00
677	Power Bar, Apple Cinnamon	65.0000	1.000	Each	10.00	2.50	45.00	230.00	0.00	3.00	0.00	0.50

Monounsaturated Fat (gm)	Polyunsaturated Fat (gm)	Vitamin D (mg)	Vitamin K (mg)	Vitamin E (mg)	Vitamin A (re)	Vitamin C (mg)	Thiamin (mg)	Riboflavin (mg)	Niacin (mg)	Vitamin B6 (mg)	Folate (mg)	Vitamin B12 (mcg)	Calcium (mg)	Iron (mg)	Magnesium (mg)	Phosphorus (mg)	Potassium (mg)	Sodium (mg)	Zinc (mg)
2.25	1.54	0.00	0.00	0.63	0.00	1.01	0.28	0.10	0.51	0.03	5.06	0.25	65.78	0.51	5.06	75.90	199.87	1019.59	0.08
2.98	4.61	0.00	0.00	1.34	37.20	2.23	0.07	0.27	0.92	0.07	9.92	0.50	178.56	0.60	19.84	156.24	270.32	917.60	0.64
0.75	0.65	0.00	0.00	0.29	0.00	1.21	0.02	0.02	0.60	0.05	15.18	0.00	26.51	0.67	2.41	12.05	67.48	1053.17	0.60
3.27	1.59	0.00	0.00	0.07	69.44	2.48	0.10	0.27	0.60	0.07	22.32	0.50	178.56	0.69	22.32	153.76	310.00	1004.40	0.62
0.00	0.00	0.00	0.00	0.00	0.00	0.00	0.02	0.02	0.00	0.00	0.00	0.00	240.36	0.00	0.00	0.00	170.26	2073.11	0.00
2.18	0.53	0.00	0.00	0.18	58.42	2.79	0.15	0.28	1.35	0.10	7.87	0.43	172.72	2.01	55.88	238.76	375.92	970.28	1.75
1.80	0.63	0.00	0.00	0.00	45.54	1.52	0.15	0.08	1.47	0.08	2.53	0.25	22.77	2.28	48.07	212.52	399.74	1006.94	1.32
1.63	0.58	0.00	0.00	0.14	487.20	6.96	0.12	0.10	2.52	0.22	4.56	0.24	33.60	2.14	38.40	177.60	304.80	964.80	3.12
0.00	0.00	0.00	0.00	0.00	100.00	6.00	0.15	0.14	1.90	0.00	0.00	0.00	16.00	0.60	0.00	190.00	450.00	460.00	0.00
0.00	0.00	0.00	0.00	0.00	0.00	0.00	0.01	0.00	0.38	0.00	0.00	0.00	240.36	0.20	0.00	0.00	570.86	1191.79	0.00
1.74	0.57	0.00	0.00	0.10	66.96	1.24	0.07	0.25	0.64	0.10	9.18	0.50	166.16	0.55	17.36	161.20	322.40	1061.44	0.67
0.00	0.00	0.00	0.00	0.00	0.00	0.00	0.00	0.01	0.19	0.00	0.00	0.00	2.08	0.10	0.00	0.00	791.19	1422.13	0.00
2.68	0.35	0.00	0.00	0.87	54.56	1.24	0.07	0.22	0.52	0.45	9.92	1.04	163.68	0.60	22.32	146.32	248.00	1036.64	0.79
0.00	0.00	0.00	0.00	0.00	30.00	16.80	0.00	0.00	0.00	0.00	0.00	0.00	27.00	0.45	0.00	0.00	0.00	1292.00	0.00
1.61	1.12	0.00	0.00	2.60	109.12	67.70	0.12	0.25	1.51	0.17	20.83	0.45	158.72	1.81	22.32	148.80	448.88	744.00	0.30
1.73	0.68	0.00	0.00	0.78	53.68	0.00	0.07	0.10	1.88	0.10	19.52	0.20	17.08	1.12	7.32	56.12	219.60	917.44	0.76
0.00	0.00	0.00	0.00	0.00	100.00	6.00	0.06	0.10	1.14	0.00	0.00	0.00	32.00	0.40	0.00	70.00	440.00	510.00	0.00
0.59	1.36	0.00	0.00	0.79	76.57	14.82	0.07	0.05	1.06	0.07	13.59	0.00	22.23	0.79	4.94	34.58	330.98	815.10	0.52
0.00	0.00	0.00	0.00	0.00	0.00	0.00	0.00	0.00	0.19	0.00	0.00	0.00	240.36	0.30	0.00	0.00	430.64	1051.58	0.00
0.81	0.49	0.00	0.00	0.05	29.28	0.24	0.07	0.07	1.39	0.05	19.52	0.15	12.20	0.95	4.88	48.80	75.64	814.96	0.59
1.77	1.09	0.00	0.00	0.00	715.08	6.37	0.05	0.12	3.59	0.31	11.09	2.12	49.56	1.91	23.60	103.84	361.08	922.76	2.12
0.46	0.05	0.00	0.00	0.03	22.77	1.27	0.03	0.03	0.46	0.05	7.59	0.25	12.65	0.86	22.77	35.42	75.90	1001.88	0.28
0.00	0.00	0.00	0.00	0.00	0.00	0.00	0.00	0.00	0.19	0.00	0.00	0.00	240.36	0.10	0.00	0.00	340.51	1251.88	0.00
0.00	0.00	0.00	0.00	0.00	150.00	15.00	0.09	0.10	1.90	0.00	0.00	0.00	32.00	0.40	0.00	120.00	360.00	530.00	0.00
1.28	0.60	0.00	0.00	0.07	265.10	0.96	0.05	0.05	1.23	0.05	4.82	0.12	16.87	0.87	7.23	40.97	154.24	944.72	0.36
2.16	1.01	0.00	0.00	0.00	600.00	5.52	0.05	0.17	3.29	0.10	12.00	0.24	26.40	1.46	9.60	105.60	367.20	1068.00	2.16
1.58	1.39	0.00	0.00	0.60	588.00	6.00	0.07	0.07	1.20	0.19	16.56	0.00	55.20	1.63	7.20	72.00	396.00	1010.40	3.12
0.00	0.00	0.00	0.00	0.00	200.00	6.00	0.06	0.07	1.52	0.00	0.00	0.00	32.00	0.40	0.00	100.00	380.00	540.00	0.00
2.55	1.48	0.00	0.00	1.25	2.60	3.90	1.22	0.10	0.52	0.03	7.80	0.13	31.21	0.52	10.40	54.62	96.24	1170.45	0.26
0.00	0.00	0.00	0.00	0.00	350.00	9.00	0.09	0.07	0.76	0.00	0.00	0.00	16.00	0.40	0.00	230.00	560.00		0.00
0.29	0.07	0.00	0.00	0.77	19.28	5.78	0.05	0.05	0.75	0.05	9.64	0.00	7.23	0.00	19.28	28.92	98.81	1091.73	0.17
1.33	0.67	0.00	0.00	0.14	243.41	0.00	0.02	0.05	1.01	0.05	4.82	0.17	16.87	0.77	4.82	40.97	175.93	906.16	0.60
0.00	1.00	0.00	0.00	0.00	150.00	4.80	0.03	0.03	0.38	0.00	0.00	0.00	16.00	0.20	0.00	0.00	140.00	540.00	0.00
0.82	0.72	0.00	0.00	0.80	301.25	1.45	0.05	0.05	0.92	0.05	10.60	0.00	21.69	1.08	7.23	33.74	209.67	821.81	0.46
0.00	0.00	0.00	0.00	0.00	0.00	0.00	0.00	0.00	0.19	0.00	0.00	0.00	0.00	0.10	0.00	0.00	400.60	911.37	0.00
0.00	0.00	0.00	0.00	0.00	100.00	3.60	0.00	0.00	0.00	0.00	0.00	0.00	29.00	1.50	0.00	0.00	0.00	543.00	0.00
0.00	0.00	0.00	0.00	0.00	0.00	0.00	0.00	0.00	0.00	0.00	0.00	0.00	0.00	0.00	0.00	0.00	350.00	200.00	0.00
0.00	0.00	0.00	0.00	0.00	0.00	0.00	0.00	0.00	0.00	0.00	0.00	0.00	0.00	0.00	0.00	0.00	350.00	200.00	0.00
0.00	0.00	0.00	0.00	0.00	0.00	0.00	0.00	0.00	0.00	0.00	0.00	0.00	0.00	0.00	0.00	0.00	350.00	200.00	0.00
0.00	0.00	0.00	0.00	0.00	0.00	0.00	0.00	0.00	0.00	0.00	0.00	0.00	0.00	0.00	0.00	0.00	400.00	130.00	0.00
0.00	0.00	0.00	0.00	0.00	0.00	0.00	0.00	0.00	0.00	0.00	0.00	0.00	0.00	0.00	0.00	0.00	400.00	130.00	0.00
0.00	0.00	0.00	0.00	0.00	0.00	0.00	0.00	0.00	0.00	0.00	0.00	0.00	0.00	0.00	0.00	0.00	400.00	130.00	0.00
0.00	0.00	1.50	20.00	3.00	118.12	24.00	0.38	0.34	2.00	0.40	80.00	1.20	60.00	2.70	8.00	20.00	40.00	65.00	3.80
0.00	0.00	2.50	20.00	2.50	118.12	30.00	0.38	0.43	5.00	0.50	100.00	1.50	350.00	4.50	100.00	300.00	370.00	200.00	3.80
0.00	0.00	2.50	20.00	10.00	118.12	60.00	0.38	0.43	5.00	0.50	100.00	1.50	250.00	4.50	100.00	250.00	370.00	210.00	3.80
0.00	0.00	1.50	12.00	10.00	118.12	60.00	0.23	0.26	3.00	0.30	60.00	0.90	250.00	2.70	60.00	150.00	60.00	75.00	2.25
0.00	0.00	3.50	28.00	5.00	118.12	42.00	0.38	0.43	5.00	0.50	120.00	1.80	400.00	4.50	100.00	250.00	500.00	290.00	6.00
0.00	0.00	2.50	20.00	4.00	118.12	30.00	0.38	0.43	5.00	0.50	100.00	1.50	300.00	4.50	100.00	250.00	500.00	290.00	5.70
0.00	0.00	2.50	20.00	2.50	118.12	30.00	0.38	0.43	5.00	0.50	100.00	1.50	250.00	4.50	100.00	250.00	370.00	200.00	3.80
0.00	0.00	1.50	10.00	2.00	67.64	21.00	0.23	0.26	3.00	0.30	60.00	0.90	250.00	2.70	60.00	150.00	200.00	115.00	2.30
0.00	0.00	2.50	20.00	2.50	118.12	30.00	0.38	0.43	5.00	0.50	100.00	1.50	200.00	4.50	100.00	200.00	440.00	240.00	3.80
0.00	0.00	1.25	10.00	1.88	58.62	37.50	0.38	0.43	5.00	0.50	100.00	1.50	125.00	2.25	50.00	125.00	370.00	200.00	2.82
0.00	0.00	1.00	12.00	2.00	45.09	9.00	0.23	0.26	3.00	0.30	60.00	1.20	100.00	2.70	40.00	100.00	180.00	135.00	3.00
0.00	0.00	2.50	20.00	2.50	118.12	30.00	0.38	0.43	5.00	0.50	100.00	1.50	300.00	4.50	100.00	300.00	370.00	200.00	3.80
1.50	0.50	0.00	0.00	0.00	0.00	0.00	0.00	0.00	0.00	0.00	0.00	0.00	0.00	0.00	0.00	0.00	110.00	90.00	0.00

USDA ID Code	Food Name	Weight in Grams*	Quantity of Units	Unit of Measure	Protein (gm)	Fat (gm)	Carbohydrate (gm)	Kcalories	Caffeine (gm)	Fiber (gm)	Cholesterol (mg)	Saturated Fat (gm)
678	Power Bar, Banana	65.0000	1.000	Each	9.00	2.00	45.00	230.00	0.00	3.00	0.00	0.50
679	Power Bar, Berry, Wild	65.0000	1.000	Each	10.00	2.50	45.00	230.00	0.00	3.00	0.00	0.50
680	Power Bar, Chocolate	65.0000	1.000	Each	10.00	2.00	45.00	230.00	0.00	3.00	0.00	0.50
681	Power Bar, Harvest, Apple Crisp	65.0000	1.000	Each	7.00	4.00	45.00	240.00	0.00	4.00	0.00	0.50
682	Power Bar, Harvest, Cherry Crunc	65.0000	1.000	Each	7.00	4.00	45.00	240.00	0.00	4.00	0.00	0.50
683	Power Bar, Harvest, Chocolate	65.0000	1.000	Each	7.00	4.00	45.00	240.00	0.00	4.00	0.00	1.00
684	Power Bar, Harvest, Strawberry	65.0000	1.000	Each	7.00	4.00	45.00	240.00	0.00	4.00	0.00	0.50
685	Power Bar, Malt Nut	65.0000	1.000	Each	10.00	2.50	45.00	230.00	0.00	3.00	0.00	0.50
686	Power Bar, Mocha	65.0000	1.000	Each	10.00	2.50	45.00	230.00	0.00	3.00	0.00	1.00
687	Power Bar, Oatmeal Raisin	65.0000	1.000	Each	10.00	2.50	45.00	230.00	0.00	3.00	0.00	0.50
688	Power Bar, Peanut Butter	65.0000	1.000	Each	10.00	2.50	45.00	230.00	0.00	3.00	0.00	0.50
673	Power Bar, Power Gel, Fruit, Tro	41.0000	1.400	Ounce	0.00	0.00	28.00	110.00	0.00	0.00	0.00	0.00
674	Power Bar, Power Gel, Lemon Lime	41.0000	1.400	Ounce	0.00	0.00	28.00	110.00	0.00	0.00	0.00	0.00
675	Power Bar, Power Gel, Straw-Bana	41.0000	1.400	Ounce	0.00	0.00	28.00	110.00	0.00	0.00	0.00	0.00
676	Power Bar, Power Gel, Vanilla	41.0000	1.400	Ounce	0.00	0.00	28.00	110.00	0.00	0.00	0.00	0.00
698	Slim-Fast Bar, Chocolate, Dutch	34.0000	1.200	Ounce	5.00	5.00	20.00	140.00	0.00	2.00	1250.00	2.00
699	Slim-Fast Bar, Peanut Butter	34.0000	1.200	Ounce	6.00	5.00	19.00	150.00	0.00	2.00	1250.00	3.00
700	Slim-Fast Powder, Chocolate	28.0000	1.000	Ounce	5.00	1.00	20.00	100.00	0.00	2.00	750.00	0.50
701	Slim-Fast Powder, Chocolate Malt	28.0000	1.000	Ounce	5.00	1.00	20.00	100.00	0.00	2.00	750.00	0.50
702	Slim-Fast Powder, Strawberry	28.0000	1.000	Ounce	5.00	0.50	20.00	100.00	0.00	2.00	750.00	0.00
703	Slim-Fast Powder, Vanilla	28.0000	1.000	Ounce	5.00	0.50	20.00	100.00	0.00	2.00	750.00	0.00
740	Tiger Bar, Caf_ Mocha	65.0000	1.000	Each	10.00	2.00	43.00	200.00	0.00	3.00	0.00	0.50
741	Tiger Bar, Chocolate	65.0000	1.000	Each	10.00	2.00	43.00	200.00	0.00	3.00	0.00	0.50
742	Tiger Bar, Vanilla	65.0000	1.000	Each	10.00	2.00	43.00	200.00	0.00	3.00	0.00	0.50
751	Ultra Slim-Fast Bar, Choc Chip C	28.0000	1.000	Ounce	1.00	4.00	16.00	120.00	0.00	2.00	0.00	2.00
752	Ultra Slim-Fast Bar, Peanut Butt	28.0000	1.000	Ounce	2.00	4.00	19.00	120.00	0.00	2.00	0.00	2.00
753	Ultra Slim-Fast Bar, Peanut Cara	28.0000	1.000	Ounce	1.00	4.00	22.00	120.00	0.00	2.00	500.00	2.00
754	Ultra Slim-Fast Powder, Caf_ Moc	33.0000	1.200	Ounce	5.00	1.00	24.00	120.00	0.00	5.00	5.00	0.50
755	Ultra Slim-Fast Powder, Chocolat	33.0000	1.200	Ounce	5.00	2.00	24.00	120.00	0.00	5.00	5.00	1.00
756	Ultra Slim-Fast Powder, Chocolat	33.0000	1.200	Ounce	5.00	1.00	24.00	120.00	0.00	5.00	5.00	0.50
757	Ultra Slim-Fast Powder, Chocolat	33.0000	1.200	Ounce	5.00	1.00	24.00	110.00	0.00	5.00	5.00	0.50
758	Ultra Slim-Fast Powder, Chocolat	33.0000	1.200	Ounce	5.00	1.00	24.00	120.00	0.00	6.00	750.00	0.00
759	Ultra Slim-Fast Powder, Fruit Ju	31.0000	1.100	Ounce	5.00	1.00	24.00	120.00	0.00	5.00	4.00	0.00
760	Ultra Slim-Fast Powder, Strawber	33.0000	1.200	Ounce	5.00	0.50	25.00	120.00	0.00	4.00	5.00	0.00
761	Ultra Slim-Fast Powder, Vanilla	33.0000	1.200	Ounce	5.00	0.50	22.00	110.00	0.00	6.00	5.00	0.00
762	Ultra Slim-Fast, Juice Base, Rtd	350.0000	11.500	Fl Oz	7.00	1.50	46.00	220.00	0.00	5.00	10.00	0.50
763	Ultra Slim-Fast, Juice Base, Rtd	350.0000	11.500	Fl Oz	7.00	1.50	48.00	220.00	0.00	5.00	10.00	0.50
764	Ultra Slim-Fast, Juice Base, Rtd	350.0000	11.500	Fl Oz	7.00	1.50	47.00	220.00	0.00	5.00	10.00	0.50
765	Ultra Slim-Fast, Rtd, Choc Fudge	350.0000	11.000	Fl Oz	10.00	3.00	42.00	220.00	0.00	5.00	5.00	1.00
766	Ultra Slim-Fast, Rtd, Choc Royal	350.0000	11.000	Fl Oz	10.00	3.00	38.00	220.00	0.00	5.00	5.00	1.00
770	Ultra Slim-Fast, Rtd, Chocolate,	350.0000	11.000	Fl Oz	10.00	3.00	42.00	220.00	0.00	5.00	5.00	1.00
767	Ultra Slim-Fast, Rtd, Coffee	350.0000	11.000	Fl Oz	10.00	3.00	38.00	220.00	0.00	5.00	5.00	0.50
768	Ultra Slim-Fast, Rtd, Strawberry	350.0000	11.000	Fl Oz	10.00	3.00	42.00	220.00	0.00	5.00	5.00	1.00
769	Ultra Slim-Fast, Rtd, Vanilla	350.0000	11.000	Fl Oz	10.00	3.00	38.00	220.00	0.00	5.00	5.00	1.00
771	Viactiv-Calcium Chew, Caramel	2.0000	1.000	Each	0.00	0.50	4.00	20.00	0.00	0.00	0.00	0.00
772	Viactiv-Calcium Chew, Chocolate	2.0000	1.000	Each	0.00	0.50	4.00	20.00	0.00	0.00	0.00	0.00
773	Viactiv-Calcium Chew, Mochaccino	2.0000	1.000	Each	0.00	0.50	4.00	20.00	0.00	0.00	0.00	0.00
774	Viactiv-Energy Bar, Fruit Crispy	30.0000	1.000	Each	4.00	2.00	22.00	120.00	0.00	0.00	0.00	0.00
775	Viactiv-Energy Bar, Fruit Crispy	30.0000	1.000	Each	4.00	2.00	20.00	120.00	0.00	0.00	0.00	0.00
776	Viactiv-Energy Bar, Hearty, Appl	45.0000	1.000	Each	6.00	4.50	29.00	180.00	0.00	0.00	0.00	3.50
777	Viactiv-Energy Bar, Hearty, Choc	45.0000	1.000	Each	6.00	4.50	29.00	180.00	0.00	0.00	0.00	3.50
778	Viactiv-Energy Fruit Smoothie, F	240.0000	8.000	Fl Oz	0.00	0.00	37.00	150.00	0.00	0.00	0.00	0.00
779	Viactiv-Energy Fruit Smoothie, S	240.0000	8.000	Fl Oz	0.00	0.00	28.00	110.00	0.00	0.00	0.00	0.00
780	Viactiv-Energy Fruit Spritzer, C	240.0000	8.000	fl oz	0.00	0.00	22.00	90.00	0.00	0.00	0.00	0.00
781	Viactiv-Energy Fruit Spritzer, C	240.0000	8.000	fl oz	0.00	0.00	22.00	90.00	0.00	0.00	0.00	0.00

Monounsaturated Fat (gm)	Polyunsaturated Fat (gm)	Vitamin D (mg)	Vitamin K (mg)	Vitamin E (mg)	Vitamin A (re)	Vitamin C (mg)	Thiamin (mg)	Riboflavin (mg)	Niacin (mg)	Vitamin B$_6$ (mg)	Folate (mg)	Vitamin B$_{12}$ (mcg)	Calcium (mg)	Iron (mg)	Magnesium (mg)	Phosphorus (mg)	Porassium (mg)	Sodium (mg)	Zinc (mg)
1.00	0.50	0.00	0.00	0.00	0.00	0.00	0.00	0.00	0.00	0.00	0.00	0.00	0.00	0.00	0.00	0.00	200.00	90.00	0.00
1.50	0.50	0.00	0.00	0.00	0.00	0.00	0.00	0.00	0.00	0.00	0.00	0.00	0.00	0.00	0.00	0.00	110.00	90.00	0.00
0.50	1.00	0.00	0.00	0.00	0.00	0.00	0.00	0.00	0.00	0.00	0.00	0.00	0.00	0.00	0.00	0.00	145.00	90.00	0.00
0.00	0.00	0.00	0.00	0.00	0.00	0.00	0.00	0.00	0.00	0.00	0.00	0.00	0.00	0.00	0.00	0.00	0.00	80.00	0.00
0.00	0.00	0.00	0.00	0.00	0.00	0.00	0.00	0.00	0.00	0.00	0.00	0.00	0.00	0.00	0.00	0.00	0.00	80.00	0.00
0.00	0.00	0.00	0.00	0.00	0.00	0.00	0.00	0.00	0.00	0.00	0.00	0.00	0.00	0.00	0.00	0.00	0.00	80.00	0.00
1.00	1.00	0.00	0.00	0.00	0.00	0.00	0.00	0.00	0.00	0.00	0.00	0.00	0.00	0.00	0.00	0.00	110.00	90.00	0.00
1.50	0.50	0.00	0.00	0.00	0.00	0.00	0.00	0.00	0.00	0.00	0.00	0.00	0.00	0.00	0.00	0.00	145.00	90.00	0.00
1.00	1.00	0.00	0.00	0.00	0.00	0.00	0.00	0.00	0.00	0.00	0.00	0.00	0.00	0.00	0.00	0.00	180.00	120.00	0.00
1.00	1.00	0.00	0.00	0.00	0.00	0.00	0.00	0.00	0.00	0.00	0.00	0.00	0.00	0.00	0.00	0.00	150.00	110.00	0.00
0.00	0.00	0.00	0.00	0.00	0.00	0.00	0.00	0.00	0.00	0.00	0.00	0.00	0.00	0.00	0.00	0.00	40.00	50.00	0.00
0.00	0.00	0.00	0.00	0.00	0.00	0.00	0.00	0.00	0.00	0.00	0.00	0.00	0.00	0.00	0.00	0.00	40.00	50.00	0.00
0.00	0.00	0.00	0.00	0.00	0.00	0.00	0.00	0.00	0.00	0.00	0.00	0.00	0.00	0.00	0.00	0.00	40.00	50.00	0.00
0.00	0.00	0.00	0.00	0.00	0.00	0.00	0.00	0.00	0.00	0.00	0.00	0.00	0.00	0.00	0.00	0.00	40.00	50.00	0.00
0.00	0.00	0.00	0.00	0.00	0.38	15.00	5.00	0.43	1.50	0.40	40.00	2.50	40.00	0.50	16.00	4.50	40.00	80.00	3.75
0.00	0.00	0.00	0.00	0.00	0.38	15.00	1.50	0.40	1.50	0.40	40.00	2.50	40.00	0.50	16.00	4.50	40.00	80.00	3.75
0.00	0.00	0.00	0.00	0.00	0.45	18.00	7.00	0.26	1.20	0.60	100.00	2.50	150.00	0.40	100.00	6.30	100.00	110.00	4.50
0.00	0.00	0.00	0.00	0.00	0.45	18.00	7.00	0.26	1.20	0.60	100.00	2.50	150.00	0.40	100.00	6.30	100.00	120.00	4.50
0.00	0.00	0.00	0.00	0.00	0.45	18.00	7.00	0.26	1.20	0.60	100.00	2.50	150.00	0.40	100.00	6.30	100.00	130.00	4.50
0.00	0.00	0.00	0.00	0.00	0.45	18.00	7.00	0.26	1.20	0.60	100.00	2.50	150.00	0.40	100.00	6.30	100.00	130.00	4.50
0.00	0.00	0.00	0.00	0.00	0.00	0.00	0.00	0.00	0.00	0.00	0.00	0.00	0.00	0.00	0.00	0.00	0.00	90.00	0.00
0.00	0.00	0.00	0.00	0.00	0.00	0.00	0.00	0.00	0.00	0.00	0.00	0.00	0.00	0.00	0.00	0.00	0.00	90.00	0.00
0.00	0.00	0.00	0.00	0.00	0.00	0.00	0.00	0.00	0.00	0.00	0.00	0.00	0.00	0.00	0.00	0.00	0.00	90.00	0.00
0.00	0.00	0.00	0.00	0.00	750.00	9.00	0.15	0.26	3.00	0.30	60.00	0.90	150.00	2.70	0.00	150.00	110.00	40.00	0.60
0.00	0.00	0.00	0.00	0.00	750.00	9.00	0.23	0.26	3.00	0.30	60.00	0.90	150.00	2.70	16.00	150.00	100.00	45.00	0.60
0.00	0.00	0.00	0.00	0.00	0.23	6.00	3.00	0.26	0.90	0.30	60.00	1.00	150.00	0.00	0.00	2.70	150.00	35.00	0.60
0.00	0.00	0.00	0.00	0.00	750.00	27.00	0.45	0.17	10.00	0.60	100.00	2.10	150.00	6.30	100.00	100.00	210.00	110.00	4.50
0.00	0.00	0.00	0.00	0.00	750.00	27.00	0.45	0.17	10.00	0.60	100.00	2.10	150.00	6.30	100.00	100.00	340.00	100.00	4.50
0.00	0.00	0.00	0.00	0.00	750.00	27.00	0.45	0.17	10.00	0.60	100.00	2.10	150.00	6.30	100.00	100.00	220.00	100.00	4.50
0.00	0.00	0.00	0.00	0.00	750.00	27.00	0.45	0.17	10.00	0.60	100.00	2.10	150.00	6.30	100.00	100.00	280.00	130.00	4.50
0.00	0.00	0.00	0.00	0.00	0.45	27.00	10.00	0.17	2.10	0.60	100.00	4.00	150.00	0.50	100.00	120.00	100.00	120.00	4.50
0.00	0.00	0.00	0.00	0.00	750.00	27.00	0.45	0.17	10.00	0.60	100.00	2.10	150.00	6.30	100.00	200.00	210.00	110.00	4.50
0.00	0.00	0.00	0.00	0.00	750.00	27.00	0.45	0.17	10.00	0.60	100.00	2.10	150.00	6.30	100.00	100.00	170.00	130.00	4.50
0.00	0.00	0.00	0.00	0.00	750.00	27.00	0.45	0.17	10.00	0.60	100.00	2.10	150.00	6.30	100.00	100.00	140.00	130.00	4.50
0.00	0.00	0.00	0.00	0.00	2500.00	60.00	0.38	0.43	5.00	0.50	100.00	1.50	250.00	4.50	100.00	250.00	200.00	240.00	3.75
0.00	0.00	0.00	0.00	0.00	2500.00	60.00	0.38	0.43	5.00	0.50	100.00	1.50	250.00	4.50	100.00	250.00	190.00	260.00	3.75
0.00	0.00	0.00	0.00	0.00	2500.00	60.00	0.38	0.43	5.00	0.50	100.00	1.50	250.00	4.50	100.00	250.00	200.00	240.00	3.75
0.00	0.00	0.00	0.00	0.00	1750.00	21.00	0.53	0.60	7.00	0.70	120.00	2.10	400.00	2.70	140.00	350.00	530.00	300.00	2.25
0.00	0.00	0.00	0.00	0.00	1750.00	21.00	0.53	0.60	7.00	0.70	120.00	2.10	400.00	2.70	140.00	350.00	530.00	220.00	2.25
0.00	0.00	0.00	0.00	0.00	1750.00	21.00	0.53	0.60	7.00	0.70	120.00	2.10	400.00	2.70	140.00	350.00	530.00	220.00	2.25
0.00	0.00	0.00	0.00	0.00	1750.00	21.00	0.53	0.60	7.00	0.70	120.00	2.10	400.00	2.70	140.00	350.00	500.00	300.00	2.25
0.00	0.00	0.00	0.00	0.00	1750.00	21.00	0.53	0.60	7.00	0.70	120.00	2.10	400.00	2.70	140.00	350.00	450.00	460.00	2.25
0.00	0.00	0.00	0.00	0.00	1750.00	21.00	0.53	0.60	7.00	0.70	120.00	2.10	400.00	2.70	140.00	350.00	450.00	460.00	2.25
0.00	0.00	2.50	40.00	0.00	0.00	0.00	0.00	0.00	0.00	0.00	0.00	0.00	500.00	0.00	0.00	0.00	0.00	10.00	0.00
0.00	0.00	2.50	40.00	0.00	0.00	0.00	0.00	0.00	0.00	0.00	0.00	0.00	500.00	0.00	0.00	0.00	0.00	10.00	0.00
0.00	0.00	2.50	40.00	0.00	0.00	0.00	0.00	0.00	0.00	0.00	0.00	0.00	500.00	0.00	0.00	0.00	0.00	10.00	0.00
0.00	0.00	0.00	0.00	33.00	0.00	120.00	0.00	0.00	0.00	2.00	400.00	6.00	0.00	0.00	0.00	0.00	0.00	65.00	0.00
0.00	0.00	0.00	0.00	33.00	0.00	120.00	0.00	0.00	0.00	2.00	400.00	6.00	0.00	0.00	0.00	0.00	0.00	80.00	0.00
0.00	0.00	2.50	40.00	0.00	0.00	0.00	0.00	0.00	0.00	2.00	400.00	6.00	330.00	1.80	0.00	66.66	0.00	90.00	15.00
0.00	0.00	2.50	40.00	0.00	0.00	0.00	0.00	0.00	0.00	2.00	400.00	6.00	330.00	1.80	0.00	66.66	0.00	90.00	15.00
0.00	0.00	0.00	0.00	0.00	0.00	60.00	0.00	0.00	0.00	2.00	400.00	6.00	300.00	0.00	0.00	0.00	0.00	15.00	0.00
0.00	0.00	0.00	0.00	0.00	0.00	60.00	0.00	0.00	0.00	2.00	400.00	6.00	300.00	0.00	0.00	0.00	0.00	5.00	0.00
0.00	0.00	0.00	0.00	0.00	0.00	60.00	0.00	0.00	0.00	2.00	400.00	6.00	0.00	0.00	0.00	0.00	0.00	70.00	0.00
0.00	0.00	0.00	0.00	0.00	0.00	60.00	0.00	0.00	0.00	2.00	400.00	6.00	0.00	0.00	0.00	0.00	0.00	70.00	0.00

USDA ID Code	Food Name	Weight in Grams*	Quantity of Units	Unit of Measure	Protein (gm)	Fat (gm)	Carbohydrate (gm)	Kcalories	Caffeine (gm)	Fiber (gm)	Cholesterol (mg)	Saturated Fat (gm)
	Vitamin Supplement, Centrum	1.0000	1.000	Each	0.00	0.00	0.00	0.00	0.00	0.00	0.00	0.00
782	Vitamin Supplement, Maximum One-	2.0000	1.000	Each	0.00	0.00	0.00	0.00	0.00	0.00	0.00	0.00
	Vitamin Supplement, One-A-Day	1.0000	1.000	Each	0.00	0.00	0.00	0.00	0.00	0.00	0.00	0.00
	Vitamin Supplement, StressTab	1.0000	1.000	Each	0.00	0.00	0.00	0.00	0.00	0.00	0.00	0.00
783	Vitamin Supplement, Theragram	2.0000	1.000	Each	0.00	0.00	0.00	0.00	0.00	0.00	0.00	0.00
784	Vitamite	240.0000	1.000	Cup	3.00	5.00	14.00	110.00	0.00	0.00	0.00	1.50

Toppings and Sauces

USDA ID Code	Food Name	Weight in Grams*	Quantity of Units	Unit of Measure	Protein (gm)	Fat (gm)	Carbohydrate (gm)	Kcalories	Caffeine (gm)	Fiber (gm)	Cholesterol (mg)	Saturated Fat (gm)
	Apple Butter	282.0000	1.000	Cup	1.10	0.00	120.61	487.86	0.00	4.23	0.00	0.00
	Catsup	240.0000	1.000	Cup	3.65	0.86	65.50	249.60	0.00	3.12	0.00	0.12
	Catsup, Low Sodium	240.0000	1.000	Cup	3.65	0.86	65.50	249.60	0.00	3.12	0.00	0.12
	Gravy, Au Jus, Cnd	149.0000	0.250	Cup	2.86	0.48	5.96	38.14	0.00	0.00	0.00	0.24
	Gravy, Beef, Cnd	233.0000	1.000	Cup	8.74	5.50	11.21	123.49	0.00	0.93	6.99	2.68
	Gravy, Chicken, Cnd	238.0000	1.000	Cup	4.59	13.59	12.90	188.02	0.00	0.95	4.76	3.36
	Gravy, Mushroom, Cnd	238.4000	1.000	Cup	3.00	6.46	13.04	119.20	0.00	0.95	0.00	0.95
	Gravy, Turkey, Cnd	298.0000	0.250	Cup	6.20	5.01	12.16	121.58	0.00	0.95	4.77	1.48
	Gravy, Unspecified Type	298.0000	0.250	Cup	3.22	1.99	14.38	86.26	0.00	0.00	0.00	0.71
	Honey	339.0000	1.000	Cup	1.02	0.00	279.34	1030.56	0.00	0.68	0.00	0.00
	Jams and Preserves	20.0000	1.000	Tbsp	0.07	0.01	13.77	55.60	0.00	0.22	0.00	0.00
	Jellies	300.0000	1.000	Cup	0.60	0.09	211.41	849.00	0.00	3.00	0.00	0.06
	Marmalade, Orange	320.0000	1.000	Cup	0.96	0.00	212.16	787.20	0.00	0.64	0.00	0.00
	Mustard	5.0000	1.000	Tbsp	0.00	0.00	0.00	0.00	0.00	0.00	0.00	0.00
	Relish, Pickle, Hamburger	15.0000	1.000	Tbsp	0.09	0.08	5.17	19.35	0.00	0.48	0.00	0.01
	Relish, Pickle, Hot Dog	15.0000	1.000	Tbsp	0.23	0.07	3.50	13.65	0.00	0.23	0.00	0.01
	Relish, Pickle, Sweet	245.0000	1.000	Cup	0.91	1.15	85.87	318.50	0.00	2.70	0.00	0.15
	Salsa	16.5170	2.000	Tbsp	0.00	0.00	2.50	10.01	0.00	0.00	0.00	0.00
	Salt Substitute	4.8000	0.250	Tsp	0.00	0.00	0.00	0.00	0.00	0.00	0.00	0.00
	Salt, Table	292.0000	1.000	Cup	0.00	0.00	0.00	0.00	0.00	0.00	0.00	0.00
	Sauce, A-1 Steak	31.3000	2.000	Tbsp	0.00	0.01	5.00	19.00	0.00	0.50	0.00	0.00
	Sauce, Barbecue	250.0000	1.000	Cup	4.50	4.50	32.00	187.50	0.00	3.00	0.00	0.68
	Sauce, Marinara	250.0000	0.500	Cup	4.00	8.37	25.45	170.00	0.00	0.00	0.00	1.20
	Sauce, Mustard, Chinese	15.0000	1.000	Tbsp	1.00	1.00	1.00	11.00	0.00	0.40	0.00	0.00
	Sauce, Soy (Tamari)	18.0000	1.000	Tbsp	0.93	0.01	1.53	9.54	0.00	0.00	0.00	0.00
	Sauce, Spaghetti	249.0000	0.500	Cup	4.53	11.88	39.67	271.41	0.00	8.47	0.00	1.70
	Sauce, Spaghetti, w/ Garlic & He	113.0000	1.000	Cup	2.00	0.59	9.00	40.00	0.00	0.00	0.00	0.00
	Sauce, Spaghetti-Prego	146.0000	1.000	Cup	3.56	4.15	26.11	154.31	0.00	3.56	0.00	1.19
	Sauce, Spaghetti-Ragu	146.0000	1.000	Cup	3.56	4.75	20.18	130.57	0.00	3.56	0.00	1.78
	Sauce, Teriyaki	288.0000	1.000	Cup	17.08	0.00	45.94	241.92	0.00	0.29	0.00	0.00
	Sauce, White	263.8000	0.500	Cup	10.21	13.45	21.39	240.06	0.00	0.00	34.29	6.41
	Sauce, Worcestershire	34.0000	2.000	Tbsp	0.00	0.00	6.00	23.00	0.00	0.00	0.00	0.00
	Sugar, Brown	220.0000	1.000	Cup	0.00	0.00	214.06	827.20	0.00	0.00	0.00	0.00
	Sugar, Granulated	200.0000	1.000	Cup	0.00	0.00	199.80	774.00	0.00	0.00	0.00	0.00
	Sugar, Powdered	120.0000	1.000	Cup	0.00	0.12	119.40	466.80	0.00	0.00	0.00	0.02
	Syrup, Corn, Dark	328.0000	1.000	Cup	0.00	0.00	251.25	924.96	0.00	0.00	0.00	0.00
	Syrup, Corn, High-fructose	310.0000	1.000	Cup	0.00	0.00	235.60	871.10	0.00	0.00	0.00	0.00
	Syrup, Corn, Light	328.0000	1.000	Cup	0.00	0.00	251.25	924.96	0.00	0.00	0.00	0.00
	Syrup, Malt	384.0000	1.000	Cup	23.81	0.00	273.79	1221.12	0.00	0.00	0.00	0.00
	Syrup, Maple	315.0000	1.000	Cup	0.00	0.63	211.68	825.30	0.00	0.00	0.00	0.13
	Syrup, Pancake, Lo Cal	240.0000	1.000	Cup	0.00	0.00	106.32	393.60	0.00	0.00	0.00	0.00
	Syrup, Pancake, w/ 2% Maple	315.0000	1.000	Cup	0.00	0.32	219.24	834.75	0.00	0.00	0.00	0.06
	Syrup, Pancake, w/ Butter	315.0000	1.000	Cup	0.00	5.04	233.42	932.40	0.00	0.00	12.60	3.18
	Toppings, Butterscotch or Carame	41.0000	2.000	Tbsp	0.62	0.04	27.02	103.32	0.00	0.37	0.41	0.05
	Toppings, Caramel	16.6800	1.000	Tbsp	0.27	0.00	13.01	51.71	0.00	0.00	0.00	0.00
	Toppings, Chocolate	304.0000	1.000	Cup	13.98	27.06	191.22	1064.00	18.24	8.51	6.08	12.10
	Toppings, Fudge, Hot	19.0180	1.000	Tbsp	1.00	2.00	11.01	70.07	0.00	0.00	0.00	0.50
	Toppings, Marshmallow Cream	28.3500	1.000	Ounce	0.23	0.09	22.40	91.29	0.00	0.03	0.00	0.02
	Toppings, Nuts in Syrup	328.0000	1.000	Cup	14.76	72.16	175.15	1338.24	0.00	5.25	0.00	6.43
	Toppings, Pineapple	340.0000	1.000	Cup	0.34	0.34	225.76	860.20	0.00	3.40	0.00	0.07
	Toppings, Strawberry	340.0000	1.000	Cup	0.68	0.34	225.42	863.60	0.00	3.40	0.00	0.03

Monounsaturated Fat (gm)	Polyunsaturated Fat (gm)	Vitamin D (mg)	Vitamin K (mg)	Vitamin E (mg)	Vitamin A (re)	Vitamin C (mg)	Thiamin (mg)	Riboflavin (mg)	Niacin (mg)	Vitamin B6 (mg)	Folate (mg)	Vitamin B12 (mcg)	Calcium (mg)	Iron (mg)	Magnesium (mg)	Phosphorus (mg)	Potassium (mg)	Sodium (mg)	Zinc (mg)
0.00	0.00	5.00	0.00	10.00	1000.00	60.00	1.50	1.70	20.00	2.00	400.00	6.00	162.00	18.00	100.00	109.00	40.00	0.00	15.00
0.00	0.00	0.25	0.00	20.00	1000.00	60.00	1.50	1.70	20.00	2.00	400.00	6.00	130.00	18.00	100.00	0.00	37.50	0.00	15.00
0.00	0.00	5.00	0.00	10.00	1000.00	60.00	1.50	1.70	20.00	2.00	400.00	6.00	0.00	0.00	0.00	0.00	0.00	0.00	0.00
0.00	0.00	0.00	0.00	10.00	0.00	500.00	10.00	0.00	100.00	5.00	400.00	12.00	0.00	18.00	0.00	0.00	0.00	0.00	0.00
0.00	0.00	0.25	0.00	20.00	1100.00	120.00	3.00	3.40	30.00	3.00	400.00	9.00	40.00	27.00	100.00	0.00	7.50	0.00	15.00
0.00	0.00	0.00	0.00	0.00	0.00	0.00	0.00	0.00	0.00	0.00	0.00	0.00	0.00	0.00	0.00	0.00	110.00	120.00	0.00
0.00	0.00	0.00	0.00	0.03	33.84	1.97	0.06	0.06	0.31	0.14	2.82	0.00	39.48	0.87	14.10	28.20	256.62	11.28	0.17
0.14	0.36	0.00	0.00	3.53	244.80	36.24	0.22	0.17	3.29	0.43	36.00	0.00	45.60	1.68	52.80	93.60	1154.40	2846.40	0.55
0.14	0.36	0.00	0.00	3.53	244.80	36.24	0.22	0.17	3.29	0.43	36.00	0.00	45.60	1.68	52.80	93.60	1154.40	48.00	0.55
0.19	0.02	0.00	0.00	0.00	0.00	2.38	0.05	0.14	2.15	0.02	4.77	0.24	9.54	1.43	4.77	71.52	193.10	119.20	2.38
2.24	0.19	0.00	0.00	0.14	0.00	0.00	0.07	0.09	1.54	0.02	4.66	0.23	13.98	1.63	4.66	69.90	188.73	1304.80	2.33
6.07	3.57	0.00	0.00	0.38	264.18	0.00	0.05	0.10	1.05	0.02	4.76	0.24	47.60	1.12	4.76	69.02	259.42	1373.26	1.90
2.79	2.43	0.00	0.00	0.00	0.00	0.00	0.07	0.14	1.60	0.05	28.61	0.00	16.69	1.57	4.77	35.76	252.70	1358.88	1.67
2.15	1.17	0.00	0.00	0.14	0.00	0.00	0.05	0.19	3.10	0.02	4.77	0.24	9.54	1.67	4.77	69.14	259.86	1375.57	1.91
0.78	0.39	0.00	0.00	0.00	0.00	1.83	0.05	0.11	0.78	0.03	3.40	0.18	36.60	0.26	10.46	49.67	65.35	1422.02	0.26
0.00	0.00	0.00	0.00	0.00	0.00	1.70	0.00	0.14	0.41	0.07	6.78	0.00	20.34	1.42	6.78	13.56	176.28	13.56	0.75
0.01	0.00	0.00	0.00	0.00	0.20	1.76	0.00	0.00	0.01	0.00	6.60	0.00	4.00	0.10	0.80	2.20	15.40	6.40	0.01
0.03	0.06	0.00	0.00	0.00	6.00	2.70	0.00	0.09	0.12	0.06	3.00	0.00	24.00	0.60	18.00	15.00	192.00	84.00	0.12
0.00	0.00	0.00	0.00	0.00	16.00	15.36	0.03	0.03	0.16	0.03	115.20	0.00	121.60	0.48	6.40	19.20	118.40	179.20	0.13
0.00	0.00	0.00	0.00	0.00	0.00	0.00	0.00	0.00	0.00	0.00	0.00	0.00	0.00	0.00	0.00	0.00	0.00	75.00	0.00
0.04	0.02	0.00	0.00	0.00	4.05	0.35	0.00	0.01	0.09	0.00	0.15	0.00	0.60	0.17	1.05	2.55	11.40	164.40	0.02
0.03	0.02	0.00	0.00	0.00	2.55	0.15	0.01	0.01	0.08	0.00	0.15	0.00	0.75	0.19	2.85	6.00	11.70	163.65	0.03
0.51	0.29	0.00	0.00	0.10	39.20	2.45	0.00	0.07	0.56	0.05	2.45	0.00	7.35	2.13	12.25	34.30	61.25	1986.95	0.34
0.00	0.00	0.00	0.00	0.00	40.04	1.80	0.00	0.00	0.00	0.00	0.00	0.00	0.00	0.00	0.00	0.00	0.00	120.12	0.00
0.00	0.00	0.00	0.00	0.00	0.00	0.00	0.00	0.00	0.00	0.00	0.00	0.00	0.00	0.00	0.00	0.00	2440.00	0.00	0.00
0.00	0.00	0.00	0.00	0.00	0.00	0.00	0.00	0.00	0.00	0.00	0.00	0.00	70.08	0.96	2.92	0.00	23.36	113173.36	0.29
0.00	0.00	0.00	0.00	0.00	32.00	4.80	0.00	0.00	0.00	0.00	0.00	0.00	12.00	0.30	0.00	0.00	0.00	454.00	0.00
1.93	1.70	0.00	0.00	2.78	217.50	17.50	0.08	0.05	2.25	0.20	10.00	0.00	47.50	2.25	45.00	50.00	435.00	2037.50	0.50
4.28	2.29	0.00	0.00	0.00	240.00	32.00	0.11	0.15	3.97	0.62	33.75	0.00	45.00	2.00	60.00	87.50	1060.00	1572.50	0.67
0.00	0.00	0.00	0.00	0.00	0.00	0.00	0.00	0.00	0.00	0.00	0.00	0.00	12.00	0.30	0.00	0.00	0.00	188.00	0.00
0.00	0.01	0.00	0.00	0.00	0.00	0.00	0.01	0.02	0.60	0.03	2.79	0.00	3.06	0.36	6.12	19.80	32.40	1028.70	0.07
6.07	3.25	0.00	0.00	6.22	306.27	27.89	0.14	0.15	3.75	0.88	53.78	0.00	69.72	1.62	59.76	89.64	956.16	1235.04	0.52
0.00	0.00	0.00	0.00	0.00	56.00	18.00	0.00	0.00	0.00	0.00	0.00	0.00	24.00	0.80	0.00	0.00	0.00	390.00	0.00
0.00	0.00	0.00	0.00	0.00	356.10	21.37	0.00	0.00	0.00	0.00	0.00	0.00	85.46	0.71	0.00	0.00	0.00	724.07	0.00
0.00	0.00	0.00	0.00	0.00	178.05	1.42	0.00	0.00	0.00	0.00	0.00	0.00	56.98	0.71	0.00	0.00	0.00	652.85	0.00
0.00	0.00	0.00	0.00	0.00	0.00	0.00	0.09	0.20	3.66	0.29	57.60	0.00	72.00	4.90	175.68	443.52	648.00	11039.04	0.29
4.70	1.69	0.00	0.00	0.00	92.33	2.64	0.08	0.45	0.53	0.07	15.83	1.06	424.72	0.26	263.80	255.89	443.18	796.68	0.55
0.00	0.00	0.00	0.00	0.00	0.00	4.20	0.00	0.00	0.00	0.00	0.00	0.00	43.00	1.50	0.00	0.00	0.00	333.00	0.00
0.00	0.00	0.00	0.00	0.00	0.00	0.00	0.02	0.02	0.18	0.07	2.20	0.00	187.00	4.20	63.80	48.40	761.20	85.80	0.40
0.00	0.00	0.00	0.00	0.00	0.00	0.00	0.00	0.04	0.00	0.00	0.00	0.00	2.00	0.12	0.00	4.00	4.00	2.00	0.06
0.04	0.06	0.00	0.00	0.00	0.00	0.00	0.00	0.00	0.00	0.00	0.00	0.00	1.20	0.07	0.00	2.40	2.40	1.20	0.04
0.00	0.00	0.00	0.00	0.00	0.00	0.00	0.03	0.03	0.07	0.03	0.00	0.00	59.04	1.21	26.24	36.08	144.32	508.40	0.13
0.00	0.00	5.00	0.00	0.00	0.00	0.00	0.00	0.06	0.00	0.00	0.00	0.00	0.00	0.09	0.00	0.00	0.00	6.20	0.06
0.00	0.00	0.00	0.00	0.00	0.00	0.00	0.03	0.03	0.07	0.03	0.00	0.00	9.84	0.16	6.56	6.56	13.12	396.88	0.07
0.00	0.00	0.00	0.00	0.00	0.00	0.00	0.04	1.50	31.18	1.92	46.08	0.00	234.24	3.69	276.48	906.24	1228.80	134.40	0.54
0.19	0.32	0.00	0.00	0.00	0.00	0.00	0.03	0.03	0.09	0.00	0.00	0.00	211.05	3.78	44.10	0.00	642.60	28.35	13.10
0.00	0.00	0.00	0.00	0.00	0.00	0.00	0.02	0.02	0.05	0.00	0.00	0.00	2.40	0.05	0.00	103.20	7.20	480.00	0.05
0.09	0.16	0.00	0.00	0.00	0.00	0.00	0.03	0.06	0.06	0.00	0.00	0.00	15.75	0.22	6.30	31.50	18.90	192.15	0.72
1.48	0.19	0.00	0.00	0.09	47.25	0.00	0.03	0.03	0.06	0.00	0.00	0.00	6.30	0.28	6.30	31.50	9.45	308.70	0.13
0.01	0.00	0.00	0.00	0.00	11.07	0.12	0.00	0.04	0.02	0.00	0.82	0.04	21.73	0.08	2.87	19.27	34.44	143.09	0.08
0.00	0.00	0.00	0.00	0.00	0.00	0.00	0.00	0.00	0.00	0.00	0.00	0.00	2.34	0.00	0.00	4.67	5.67	11.01	0.03
11.73	0.85	0.00	0.00	8.88	12.16	0.61	0.18	0.67	0.91	0.18	12.16	0.64	246.24	3.95	155.04	410.40	1100.48	1051.84	2.07
0.00	0.00	0.00	0.00	0.00	0.00	0.00	0.00	0.00	0.00	0.00	0.00	0.00	36.03	0.20	0.00	0.00	0.00	35.03	0.00
0.02	0.01	0.00	0.00	0.00	0.00	0.00	0.00	0.00	0.02	0.00	0.28	0.00	0.85	0.06	0.57	2.27	1.42	13.89	0.01
16.30	45.03	0.00	0.00	2.85	13.12	3.61	0.59	0.39	1.34	0.62	68.88	0.00	131.20	3.44	206.64	364.08	685.52	137.76	3.41
0.10	0.17	0.00	0.00	0.00	6.80	199.24	0.10	0.03	0.31	0.07	10.20	0.00	74.80	1.63	6.80	27.20	1077.80	214.20	1.63
0.03	0.17	0.00	0.00	0.48	6.80	84.66	0.03	0.07	0.85	0.07	6.80	0.00	81.60	3.30	13.60	44.20	248.20	71.40	1.67

APPENDIX *B*

Exchange Lists for Meal Planning

Groups/Lists	Carbohydrate (grams)	Protein (grams)	Fat (grams)	Calories
Carbohydrate Group				
Starch	15	3	0-1	80
Fruit	15	—	—	60
Milk				
Fat-free	12	8	0-3	90
Reduced-fat	12	8	5	120
Whole	12	8	8	150
Other carbohydrates	15	varies	varies	varies
Vegetables	5	2	—	25
Meat and Meat Substitute Group				
Very lean	—	7	0-1	35
Lean	—	7	3	55
Medium-fat	—	7	5	75
High-fat	—	7	8	100
Fat Group	—	—	5	45

From American Diabetes Association, American Dietetic Association: Exchange lists for meal planning, rev, Chicago, 1995, ADA/ADA.

STARCH LIST

One starch exchange equals 15 g carbohydrate, 3 g protein, 0-1 g fat, and 80 calories.

Bread

Bagel	½ (1 oz)
Bread, reduced-calorie	2 slices (1½ oz)
Bread, white, whole-wheat, pumpernickel, rye	1 slice (1 oz)
Bread sticks, crisp, 4 in long × ½ in	2 (½ oz)
English muffin	½

Hot dog or hamburger bun	½ (1 oz)
Pita, 6 in across	½
Roll, plain, small	1 (1 oz)
Raisin bread, unfrosted	1 slice (1 oz)
Tortilla, corn, 6 in across	1
Tortilla, flour, 6 in across	1
Waffle, 4½ in square, reduced-fat	1

Cereals and Grains

Bran cereals	½ cup
Bulgur	½ cup
Cereals	½ cup
Cereals, unsweetened, ready-to-eat	¾ cup
Cornmeal (dry)	3 Tbsp
Couscous	⅓ cup
Flour (dry)	3 Tbsp
Granola, low-fat	¼ cup
Grape-Nuts	¼ cup
Grits	½ cup
Kasha	½ cup
Millet	¼ cup
Muesli	¼ cup
Oats	½ cup
Pasta	½ cup
Puffed cereal	1½ cups
Rice milk	½ cup
Rice, white or brown	⅓ cup
Shredded wheat	½ cup
Sugar-frosted cereal	½ cup
Wheat germ	3 Tbsp

Starchy Vegetables

Baked beans	⅓ cup
Corn	½ cup
Corn on cob, medium	1 (5 oz)
Mixed vegetables with corn, peas, or pasta	1 cup
Peas, green	½ cup
Plantain	½ cup
Potato, baked or boiled	1 small (3 oz)
Potato, mashed	½ cup
Squash, winter (acorn, butternut, pumpkin)	1 cup
Yam, sweet potato, plain	½ cup

Crackers and Snacks

Animal crackers	8
Graham crackers, 2½ in square	3
Matzoh	¾ oz
Melba toast	4 slices
Oyster crackers	24
Popcorn (popped, no fat added or low-fat microwave)	3 cups
Pretzels	¾ oz
Rice cakes, 4 in across	2
Saltine-type crackers	6
Snack chips, fat-free (tortilla, potato)	15-20 (¾ oz)
Whole-wheat crackers, no fat added	2-5 (¾ oz)

Beans, Peas, and Lentils

Count as 1 starch exchange, plus 1 very lean meat exchange.

Beans and peas (garbanzo, pinto, kidney, white, split, black-eyed)	½ cup
Lima beans	⅔ cup
Lentils	½ cup
Miso 🖋	3 Tbsp

Starchy Foods Prepared with Fat

Count as 1 starch exchange, plus 1 fat exchange.

Biscuit, 2½ in across	1
Chow mein noodles	½ cup
Corn bread, 2 in-cube	1 (2 oz)
Crackers, round butter type	6
Croutons	1 cup
French-fried potatoes	16-25 (3 oz)
Granola	¼ cup
Muffin, small	1 (1½ oz)
Pancake, 4 in across	2
Popcorn, microwave	3 cups
Sandwich crackers, cheese or peanut butter filling	3
Stuffing, bread (prepared)	⅓ cup
Taco shell, 6 in across	2
Waffle, 4½ in square	1
Whole-wheat crackers, fat added	4-6 (1 oz)

Starches often swell in cooking, so a small amount of uncooked starch will become a much larger amount of cooked food. The following table shows some of the changes.

COMMON MEASUREMENTS

3 tsp = 1 Tbsp
4 oz = ½ cup
4 Tbsp = ¼ cup
8 oz = 1 cup
5⅓ Tbsp = ⅓ cup
1 cup = ½ pint

Food (Starch Group)	Uncooked	Cooked
Oatmeal	3 Tbsp	½ cup
Cream of Wheat	2 Tbsp	½ cup
Grits	3 Tbsp	½ cup
Rice	2 Tbsp	⅓ cup
Spaghetti	¼ cup	½ cup
Noodles	⅓ cup	½ cup
Macaroni	¼ cup	½ cup
Dried beans	¼ cup	½ cup
Dried peas	¼ cup	½ cup
Lentils	3 Tbsp	½ cup

FRUIT LIST

One fruit exchange equals 15 g carbohydrate and 60 calories. The weight includes skin, core, seeds, and rind.

Fruit

Apple, unpeeled, small	1 (4 oz)
Applesauce, unsweetened	½ cup
Apples, dried	4 rings
Apricots, fresh	4 whole (5½ oz)
Apricots, dried	8 halves
Apricots, canned	½ cup
Banana, small	1 (4 oz)

🖋 = 400 mg or more sodium per exchange.

Blackberries	¾ cup
Blueberries	¾ cup
Cantaloupe, small	⅓ melon (11 oz) or 1 cup cubes
Cherries, sweet, fresh	12 (3 oz)
Cherries, sweet, canned	½ cup
Dates	3
Figs, fresh	1½ large or 2 medium (3½ oz)
Figs, dried	1½
Fruit cocktail	½ cup
Grapefruit, large	½ (11 oz)
Grapefruit sections, canned	¾ cup
Grapes, small	17 (3 oz)
Honeydew melon	1 slice (10 oz) or 1 cup cubes
Kiwi	1 (3½ oz)
Mandarin oranges, canned	¾ cup
Mango, small	½ fruit (5½ oz) or ½ cup
Nectarine, small	1 (5 oz)
Orange, small	1 (6½ oz)
Papaya	½ fruit (8 oz) or 1 cup cubes
Peach, medium, fresh	1 (6 oz)
Peaches, canned	½ cup
Pear, large, fresh	½ (4 oz)
Pears, canned	½ cup
Pineapple, fresh	¾ cup
Pineapple, canned	½ cup
Plums, small	2 (5 oz)
Plums, canned	½ cup
Prunes, dried	3
Raisins	2 Tbsp
Raspberries	1 cup
Strawberries	1¼ cup whole berries
Tangerines, small	2 (8 oz)
Watermelon	1 slice (13½ oz) or 1¼ cup cubes

Fruit Juice

Apple juice/cider	½ cup
Cranberry juice cocktail	⅓ cup
Cranberry juice cocktail, reduced-calorie	1 cup
Fruit juice blends, 100% juice	⅓ cup
Grape juice	⅓ cup
Grapefruit juice	½ cup
Orange juice	½ cup
Pineapple juice	½ cup
Prune juice	⅓ cup

MILK LIST

One milk exchange equals 12 g carbohydrate and 8 g protein.

	Carbohydrate (grams)	Protein (grams)	Fat (grams)	Calories
Fat-free/low-fat	12	8	0-3	90
Reduced-fat	12	8	5	120
Whole	12	8	8	150

Fat-Free and Low-Fat Milk

0-3 g fat per serving

Fat-free milk	1 cup
½% milk	1 cup
1% milk	1 cup
Fat-free or low-fat buttermilk	1 cup
Evaporated fat-free milk	½ cup
Fat-free dry milk	⅓ cup dry
Plain nonfat yogurt	¾ cup
Nonfat or low-fat fruit-flavored yogurt sweetened with aspartame or with a nonnutritive sweetener	1 cup

Reduced-Fat

5 g fat per serving

2% milk	1 cup
Plain low-fat yogurt	¾ cup
Sweet acidophilus milk	1 cup

Whole Milk

8 g fat per serving

Whole milk	1 cup
Evaporated whole milk	½ cup
Goat's milk	1 cup
Kefir	1 cup

OTHER CARBOHYDRATES LIST

Substitutes for a starch, fruit, or milk exchange. One exchange equals 15 g carbohydrate, or 1 starch, or 1 fruit, or 1 milk.

Food	Serving Size	Exchanges Per Serving
Angel food cake, unfrosted	¹⁄₁₂th cake	2 carbohydrates
Brownie, small, unfrosted	2 in square	1 carbohydrate, 1 fat
Cake, unfrosted	2 in square	1 carbohydrate, 1 fat
Cake, frosted	2 in square	2 carbohydrates, 1 fat
Cookie, fat-free	2 small	1 carbohydrate
Cookie or sandwich cookie with creme filling	2 small	1 carbohydrate, 1 fat
Cranberry sauce, jellied	¼ cup	1½ carbohydrates
Cupcake, frosted	1 small	2 carbohydrates, 1 fat
Doughnut, plain cake	1 medium (1½ oz)	1½ carbohydrates, 2 fats
Doughnut, glazed	3¾ in across (2 oz)	2 carbohydrates, 2 fats
Fruit juice bars, frozen, 100% juice	1 bar (3 oz)	1 carbohydrate
Fruit snacks, chewy (pureed fruit concentrate)	1 roll (¾ oz)	1 carbohydrate
Fruit spreads, 100% fruit	1 Tbsp	1 carbohydrate
Gelatin, regular	½ cup	1 carbohydrate
Gingersnaps	3	1 carbohydrate
Granola bar	1 bar	1 carbohydrate, 1 fat
Granola bar, fat-free	1 bar	2 carbohydrates
Honey	1 Tbsp	1 carbohydrate
Hummus	⅓ cup	1 carbohydrate, 1 fat

Ice cream	½ cup	1 carbohydrate, 2 fats
Ice cream, light	½ cup	1 carbohydrate, 1 fat
Ice cream, fat-free, no sugar added	½ cup	1 carbohydrate
Jam or jelly, regular	1 Tbsp	1 carbohydrate
Milk, chocolate, whole	1 cup	2 carbohydrates, 1 fat
Pie, fruit, 2 crusts	⅙ pie	3 carbohydrates, 2 fats
Pie, pumpkin or custard	⅛ pie	2 carbohydrates, 2 fats
Potato chips	12-18 (1 oz)	1 carbohydrate, 2 fats
Pudding, regular (made with low-fat milk)	½ cup	2 carbohydrates
Pudding, sugar-free (made with low-fat milk)	½ cup	1 carbohydrate
Salad dressing, fat-free 🖎	¼ cup	1 carbohydrate
Sherbet, sorbet	½ cup	2 carbohydrates
Spaghetti or pasta sauce, canned 🖎	½ cup	1 carbohydrate, 1 fat
Sugar	1 Tbsp	1 carbohydrate
Sweet roll or Danish	1 (2½ oz)	2½ carbohydrates, 2 fats
Syrup, light	2 Tbsp	1 carbohydrate
Syrup, regular	1 Tbsp	1 carbohydrate
Syrup, regular	¼ cup	4 carbohydrates
Tortilla chips	6-12 (1 oz)	1 carbohydrate, 2 fats
Vanilla wafers	5	1 carbohydrate, 1 fat
Yogurt, frozen, low-fat, fat-free	⅓ cup	1 carbohydrate, 0-1 fat
Yogurt, frozen, fat-free, no sugar added	½ cup	1 carbohydrate
Yogurt, low-fat with fruit	1 cup	3 carbohydrates, 0-1 fat

VEGETABLE LIST

One vegetable exchange equals 5 g carbohydrate, 2 g protein, 0 g fat, and 25 calories.

Artichoke
Artichoke hearts
Asparagus
Beans (green, wax, Italian)
Bean sprouts
Beets
Broccoli
Brussels sprouts
Cabbage
Carrots
Cauliflower
Celery
Cucumber
Eggplant
Green onions or scallions
Greens (collard, kale, mustard, turnip)
Kohlrabi
Leeks
Mixed vegetables (without corn, peas, or pasta)

Mushrooms
Okra
Onions
Pea pods
Peppers (all varieties)
Radishes
Salad greens (endive, escarole, lettuce, romaine, spinach)
Sauerkraut 🖎
Spinach
Summer squash
Tomato
Tomatoes, canned
Tomato sauce 🖎
Tomato/vegetable juice 🖎
Turnips
Water chestnuts
Watercress
Zucchini

🖎 = 400 mg or more sodium per exchange.

MEAT AND MEAT SUBSTITUTES LIST

	Carbohydrate (grams)	Protein (grams)	Fat (grams)	Calories
Very lean	0	7	0-1	35
Lean	0	7	3	55
Medium-fat	0	7	5	75
High-fat	0	7	8	100

Very Lean Meat and Substitutes List

One exchange equals 0 g carbohydrate, 7 g protein, 0-1 g fat, and 35 calories.

Poultry: Chicken or turkey (white meat, no skin),
Cornish hen (no skin) .... 1 oz

Fish: Fresh or frozen cod, flounder, haddock,
halibut, trout; tuna, fresh or canned in water .... 1 oz

Shellfish: Clams, crab, lobster, scallops, shrimp,
imitation shellfish .... 1 oz

Game: Duck or pheasant (no skin), venison,
buffalo, ostrich .... 1 oz

Cheese with 1 g or less fat per ounce:
Nonfat or low-fat cottage cheese .... ¼ cup
Fat-free cheese .... 1 oz

Other: Processed sandwich meats with 1 g or less
fat per ounce, such as deli thin, shaved meats,
chipped beef 🔸, turkey ham .... 1 oz
Egg whites 2
Egg substitutes, plain .... ¼ cup
Hot dogs with 1 g or less fat per ounce 🔸 .... 1 oz
Kidney (high in cholesterol) .... 1 oz
Sausage with 1 g or less fat per ounce .... 1 oz
Count as one very lean meat and one starch exchange.
Beans, peas, lentils (cooked) .... ½ cup

Lean Meat and Substitutes List

One exchange equals 0 g carbohydrate, 7 g protein, 3 g fat, and 55 calories.

Beef: USDA Select or Choice grades of lean beef
trimmed of fat, such as round, sirloin, and flank
steak; tenderloin; roast (rib, chuck, rump);
steak (T-bone, porterhouse, cubed), ground round ... 1 oz

Pork: Lean pork, such as fresh ham; canned, cured,
or boiled ham; Canadian bacon 🔸; tenderloin, center
loin chop .... 1 oz

Lamb: Roast, chop, leg .... 1 oz

Veal: Lean chop, roast .... 1 oz

Poultry: Chicken, turkey (dark meat, no skin),
chicken white meat (with skin), domestic
duck or goose (well-drained of fat, no skin) .... 1 oz

🔸 = 400 mg or more sodium per exchange.

Fish:

Herring (uncreamed or smoked)	1 oz
Oysters	6 medium
Salmon (fresh or canned), catfish	1 oz
Sardines (canned)	2 medium
Tuna (canned in oil, drained)	1 oz

Game: Goose (no skin), rabbit — 1 oz

Cheese:

4.5%-fat cottage cheese	¼ cup
Grated Parmesan	2 Tbsp
Cheeses with 3 g or less fat per ounce	1 oz

Other:

Hot dogs with 3 g or less fat per ounce ✒	1½ oz
Processed sandwich meat with 3 g or less fat per ounce, such as turkey pastrami or kielbasa	1 oz
Liver, heart (high in cholesterol)	1 oz

Medium-Fat Meat and Substitutes List

One exchange equals 0 g carbohydrate, 7 g protein, 5 g fat, and 75 calories.

Beef: Most beef products fall into this category (ground beef, meatloaf, corned beef, short ribs, prime grades of meat trimmed of fat, such as prime rib)	1 oz
Pork: Top loin, Boston butt, cutlet	1 oz
Lamb: Rib roast, ground	1 oz
Veal: Cutlet (ground or cubed, unbreaded)	1 oz
Poultry: Chicken (dark meat, with skin), ground turkey or ground chicken, fried chicken (with skin)	1 oz
Fish: Any fried fish product	1 oz

Cheese: With 5 g or less fat per ounce

Feta	1 oz
Mozzarella	1 oz
Ricotta	¼ cup (2 oz)

Other:

Egg (high in cholesterol, limit to 3 per week)	1
Sausage with 5 g or less fat per ounce	1 oz
Soy milk	1 cup
Tempeh	¼ cup
Tofu	4 oz or ½ cup

High-Fat Meat and Substitutes List

One exchange equals 0 g carbohydrate, 7 g protein, 8 g fat, and 100 calories. Remember these items are high in saturated fat, cholesterol, and calories and may raise blood cholesterol levels if eaten on a regular basis.

Pork: Spareribs, ground pork, pork sausage	1 oz
Cheese: All regular cheeses, such as American ✒, cheddar, Monterey Jack, Swiss	1 oz
Other: Processed sandwich meats with 8 g or less fat per ounce, such as bologna, pimento loaf, salami	1 oz
Sausage, such as bratwurst, Italian, knockwurst, Polish, smoked	1 oz

---

✒ = 400 mg or more sodium per exchange.

Hot dog (turkey or chicken) ✎	1 (10/lb)
Bacon	3 slices (20 slices/lb)

Count as one high-fat meat plus one fat exchange.

Hot dog (beef, pork, or combination) ✎	1 (10/lb)

Count as one high-fat meat plus two fat exchanges.

Peanut butter (contains unsaturated fat)	2 Tbsp

FAT LIST

Monounsaturated Fats List

One fat exchange equals 5 g fat and 45 calories.

Avocado, medium	⅛ (1 oz)
Oil (canola, olive, peanut)	1 tsp
Olives: ripe (black)	8 large
green, stuffed ✎	10 large
Nuts	
almonds, cashews	6 nuts
mixed (50% peanuts)	6 nuts
peanuts	10 nuts
pecans	4 halves
Peanut butter, smooth or crunchy	2 tsp
Sesame seeds	1 Tbsp
Tahini paste	2 tsp

Polyunsaturated Fats List

One fat exchange equals 5 g fat and 45 calories.

Margarine: stick, tub, or squeeze	1 tsp
lower-fat (30% to 50% vegetable oil)	1 Tbsp
Mayonnaise: regular	1 tsp
reduced-fat	1 Tbsp
Nuts, walnuts, English	4 halves
Oil (corn, safflower, soybean)	1 tsp
Salad dressing: regular ✎	1 Tbsp
reduced-fat	2 Tbsp
Miracle Whip Salad Dressing®: regular	2 tsp
reduced-fat	1 Tbsp
Seeds: pumpkin, sunflower	1 Tbsp

Saturated Fats List

One fat exchange equals 5 g of fat and 45 calories. Saturated fats can raise blood cholesterol levels.

Bacon, cooked	1 slice (20 slices/lb)
Bacon, grease	1 tsp
Butter: stick	1 tsp
whipped	2 tsp
reduced-fat	1 Tbsp
Chitterlings, boiled	2 Tbsp (½ oz)
Coconut, sweetened, shredded	2 Tbsp
Cream, half and half	2 Tbsp
Cream cheese: regular	1 Tbsp (1/2 oz)
reduced-fat	2 Tbsp (1 oz)

✎ = 400 mg or more sodium per exchange.

Fatback or salt pork, see below*	
Shortening or lard	1 tsp
Sour cream: regular	2 Tbsp
reduced-fat	3 Tbsp

FREE FOODS LIST

>20 calories or >5 g carbohydrates per serving. Foods with a serving size listed should be limited to three servings per day, spread throughout the day.

Fat-Free or Reduced-Fat Foods

Cream cheese, fat-free	1 Tbsp
Creamers, nondairy, liquid	1 Tbsp
Creamers, nondairy, powdered	2 tsp
Mayonnaise, fat-free	1 Tbsp
Mayonnaise, reduced-fat	1 tsp
Margarine, fat-free	4 Tbsp
Margarine, reduced-fat	1 tsp
Miracle Whip®, nonfat	1 Tbsp
Miracle Whip®, reduced-fat	1 tsp
Nonstick cooking spray	
Salad dressing, fat-free	1 Tbsp
Salad dressing, fat-free, Italian	2 Tbsp
Salsa	¼ cup
Sour cream, fat-free, reduced-fat	1 Tbsp
Whipped topping, regular or light	2 Tbsp

Sugar-Free or Low-Sugar Foods

Candy, hard, sugar-free	1 candy
Gelatin dessert, sugar-free	
Gelatin, unflavored	
Gum, sugar-free	
Jam or jelly, low-sugar or light	2 tsp
Sugar substitutes†	
Syrup, sugar-free	2 Tbsp

Drinks

Bouillon, broth, consommé ✐	
Bouillon or broth, low sodium	
Carbonated or mineral water	
Club soda	
Cocoa powder, unsweetened	1 Tbsp
Coffee	
Diet soft drinks, sugar free	
Drink mixes, sugar free	
Tea	
Tonic water, sugar free	

---

*Use a piece 1 inch × 1 inch × ¼ inch if you plan to eat the fatback cooked with vegetables. Use a piece 2 inches × 1 inch × ½ inch when eating only the vegetables with the fatback removed.
†Sugar substitutes, alternatives, or replacements that are approved by the Food and Drug Administration (FDA) are safe to use. Common brand names include: Equal® (aspartame), Sprinkle Sweet® (saccharin), Sweet One® (acesulfame K), Sweet-10® (saccharin), Sugar Twin® (saccharin), and Sweet 'n Low® (saccharin).

✐ = 400 mg or more sodium per exchange.

Condiments

Catsup	1 Tbsp
Horseradish	
Lemon juice	
Lime juice	
Mustard	
Pickles, dill 🖉	1½ large
Soy sauce, regular or light 🖉	
Taco sauce	1 Tbsp
Vinegar	

Seasonings

Be careful with seasonings that contain sodium or are salts, such as garlic or
   celery salt, and lemon pepper.
Flavoring extracts
Garlic
Herbs, fresh or dried
Pimento
Spices
Tabasco® or hot pepper sauce
Wine, used in cooking
Worcestershire sauce

COMBINATION FOODS LIST

Food	Serving Size	Exchanges Per Serving
Entrees		
Tuna noodle casserole, lasagna, spaghetti with meatballs, chili with beans, macaroni and cheese 🖉	1 cup (8 oz)	2 carbohydrates, 2 medium-fat meats
Chow mein (without noodles or rice) 🖉	2 cups (16 oz)	1 carbohydrate, 2 lean meats
Pizza, cheese, thin crust 🖉	¼ of 10 in (5 oz)	2 carbohydrates, 2 medium-fat meats, 1 fat
Pizza, meat topping, thin crust 🖉	¼ of 10 in (5 oz)	2 carbohydrates, 2 medium-fat meats, 2 fats
Pot pie 🖉	1 (7oz)	2 carbohydrates, 1 medium-fat meat, 4 fats
Frozen entrees		
Salisbury steak with gravy, mashed potato 🖉	1 (11 oz)	2 carbohydrates, 3 medium-fat meats, 3-4 fats
Turkey with gravy, mashed potato, dressing 🖉	1 (11 oz)	2 carbohydrates, 2 medium-fat meats, 2 fats
Entree with less than 300 calories 🖉	1 (8 oz)	2 carbohydrates, 3 lean meats
Soups		
Bean 🖉	1 cup	1 carbohydrate, 1 very lean meat
Cream (made with water) 🖉	1 cup (8 oz)	1 carbohydrate, 1 fat
Split pea (made with water) 🖉	½ cup (4 oz)	1 carbohydrate
Tomato (made with water) 🖉	1 cup (8 oz)	1 carbohydrate
Vegetable beef, chicken noodle, or other broth-type 🖉	1 cup (8 oz)	1 carbohydrate

FAST FOODS

Ask at your fast-food restaurant for nutrition information about your favorite fast foods.

Food	Serving Size	Exchanges Per Serving
Burritos with beef ✐	2	4 carbohydrates, 2 medium-fat meats, 2 fats
Chicken nuggets ✐	6	1 carbohydrate, 2 medium-fat meats, 1 fat
Chicken breast and wing, breaded and fried ✐	1 each	1 carbohydrate, 4 medium-fat meats, 2 fats
Fish sandwich/tartar sauce ✐	1	3 carbohydrates, 1 medium-fat meat, 3 fats
French fries, thin ✐	20-25	2 carbohydrates, 2 fats
Hamburger, regular	1	2 carbohydrates, 2 medium-fat meats
Hamburger, large ✐	1	2 carbohydrates, 3 medium-fat meats, 1 fat
Hot dog with bun ✐	1	1 carbohydrate, 1 high-fat meat, 1 fat
Individual pan pizza ✐	1	5 carbohydrates, 3 medium-fat meats, 3 fats
Soft-serve cone	1 medium	2 carbohydrates, 1 fat
Submarine sandwich ✐	1 sub (6 in.)	3 carbohydrates, 1 vegetable, 2 medium-fat meats, 1 fat
Taco, hard shell ✐	1 (6 oz)	2 carbohydrates, 2 medium-fat meats, 2 fats
Taco, soft shell ✐	1 (3 oz)	1 carbohydrate, 1 medium-fat meat, 1 fat

MEAL PLAN

Meal Plan for: _____   Date: _____

Dietitian: _____   Phone: _____

	Grams	Percent
Carbohydrate	_____	_____
Protein	_____	_____
Fat	_____	_____
Calories	_____	_____

Time	Number of Exchanges/Choices	Menu Ideas	Menu Ideas
	_____ Carbohydrate group _____ Starch _____ Fruit _____ Milk _____ _____ Meat group _____ _____ Fat group _____		
	_____ _____ _____ _____ _____ _____		
	_____ Carbohydrate group _____ Starch _____ Fruit _____ Milk _____ ✔ Vegetables _____ Meat group _____ _____ Fat group _____		
	_____ _____ _____ _____ _____ _____		
	_____ Carbohydrate group _____ Starch _____ Fruit _____ Milk _____ ✔ Vegetables _____ Meat group _____ _____ Fat group _____		
	_____ _____ _____ _____ _____ _____		

✐ = 400 mg or more sodium per exchange.

PLANNING INDIVIDUALIZED DIETS USING EXCHANGE LISTS
STEP 1: CONDUCT NUTRITION HISTORY

A 24-hour or 3-day recall can be used to determine usual food intake. Categorize intake into exchanges (or servings) from each list at each meal and snack. Translate into kcalories and grams of carbohydrate, protein, and fat from exchanges. Round off kcalorie level to the nearest 50 or 100 kcalories. Calculations of food intake are not precise enough to allow more accuracy, and patients may consume an extra 50 to 60 kcalories/day from free foods (see Exchange Lists). When in doubt, round up instead of down. Determine percentages of carbohydrate, protein, and fat in current intake.

To determine total kcalories, add up the number of exchanges actually consumed from each Exchange Group. Multiply the number of exchanges by the number of kcalories in each Exchange Group.

Number of exchanges from starch list	= ___ × 80 kcal	= ___
Number of exchanges from fruit list	= ___ × 60 kcal	= ___
Number of exchanges from milk list	= ___ × 80 kcal (skim)	= ___
	= ___ × 120 kcal (low-fat)	= ___
	= ___ × 150 kcal (whole)	= ___
Number of exchanges from vegetable list	= ___ × 25 kcal	= ___
Number of exchanges from meat groups	= ___ × 35 kcal (very lean)	= ___
	= ___ × 55 kcal (lean)	= ___
	= ___ × 75 kcal (medium-fat)	= ___
	= ___ × 100 kcal (high-fat)	= ___
Number of exchanges from fat list	= ___ × 45 kcal	= ___
	TOTAL kcal	___

Using the total number of each Exchange Group, calculate the grams of carbohydrate (CHO), protein (PRO), and fat (FAT).

	Number of Exchanges CHO	Number of Exchanges PRO	Number of Exchanges FAT
Bread list	___ × 15g = ___g	___ × 2g = ___g	___ × 0-3g = ___g
Fruit list	___ × 15g = ___g	___ × 0g = ___g	___ × 0g = ___g
Milk list			
Skim	___ × 12g = ___g	___ × 8g = ___g	___ × 0g = ___g
Low-fat	___ × 12g = ___g	___ × 8g = ___g	___ × 5g = ___g
Whole	___ × 12g = ___g	___ × 8g = ___g	___ × 8g = ___g
Vegetable list	___ × 5g = ___g	___ × 2g = ___g	___ × 0g = ___g
Meat list			
Very lean	___ × 0g = ___g	___ × 7g = ___g	___ × 0-1g = ___g
Lean	___ × 0g = ___g	___ × 7g = ___g	___ × 3g = ___g
Medium-fat	___ × 0g = ___g	___ × 7g = ___g	___ × 5g = ___g
High-fat	___ × 0g = ___g	___ × 7g = ___g	___ × 8g = ___g
Fat group	___ × 0g = ___g	___ × 0g = ___g	___ × 5g = ___g
	TOTAL ___	TOTAL ___	TOTAL ___

Take total kcalories from above and determine the percentage of the diet that is carbohydrate, protein, and fat:

A.
Multiply total grams CHO × 4 kcal = ____kcal
Multiply total grams PRO × 4 kcal = ____kcal
Multiply total grams FAT × 9 kcal = ____kcal
TOTAL   ____kcal

B. Divide each nutrient's total kcalories by the total kcalories for the day, and multiply by 100 to get the percentage of kcalories.

Kcal from CHO × 100 = % kcal from CHO ____ × 100 = ____ Total kcal
Kcal from PRO × 100 = % kcal from PRO ____ × 100 = ____ Total kcal
Kcal from FAT × 100 = % kcal from FAT ____ × 100 = ____ Total kcal

STEP 2: CALCULATE DAILY KILOCALORIE REQUIREMENTS

Kcalorie needs are based on age, weight, and activity level. Use the Harris-Benedict equation to calculate energy needs. Round figure to nearest 100 kcalories. Subtract kcalories if weight loss is desired. Reducing kcaloric intake by 500 kcal/day will theoretically produce a 1 lb weight loss per week. Never reduce kcaloric level to below that required for basal energy needs.

Example: Gail is a 62-year-old woman with type 2 DM. She is 5′5″ tall (medium frame) and weighs 140 lb. Gail walks 10 to 12 miles per week at the mall.

$$655.1 + [9.6 × wt (kg)] + [1.8 × ht (cm)] − [4.7 × age (yrs)]$$
$$655.1 + [9.6 × 63.6 kg] + [1.8 × 165.1 cm] − [4.7 × 62]$$
$$655.1 + 610.6 + 297.2 − 291.4 = 1271.5 kcalories$$
$$1271.5 kcalories × 1.3 (activity factor) = 1652.95 kcalories$$
$$Round off to 1700 kcalories$$

If weight loss is desired, subtract 500 kcalories: 1700 − 500 = 1200 kcalories, which is below her basal energy needs of 1271.5 kcalories. Adjust to 1300 kcalories if weight loss is determined to be a treatment goal.

STEP 3: DETERMINE DISTRIBUTION OF CARBOHYDRATE, PROTEIN, AND FAT KCALORIES

This should be based on the patient's usual intake, blood glucose levels, blood lipid levels, and treatment goals.

Example: Gail's 24-hr recall indicates an intake of approximately 1500 kcalories distributed into 17% protein, 30% fat, and 53% carbohydrate. Her pertinent laboratory values: glycosylated hemoglobin is 6%, cholesterol 210 mg/dl, LDL-cholesterol 179 mg/dl, HDL-cholesterol 55 mg/dl. Although her lipid levels are at the high end of normal or just slightly above normal, her exercise and eating habits appear to be sufficient to control her blood glucose levels. In this case, you would distribute her kcalories in the same pattern as found in her diet recall:

Carbohydrate: 1500 kcal × .53 = 795 kcal ÷ 4 kcal/gm = 199 gm
Protein: 1500 kcal × .17 = 255 kcal ÷ 4 kcal/gm = 64 gm
Fat: 1500 kcal × .30 = 450 kcal ÷ 9 kcal/gm = 50 gm

STEP 4: DETERMINE SERVINGS FROM EACH EXCHANGE LIST

These calculations are based on the amount of carbohydrate, protein, and fat in each exchange list and the patient's preferences for foods within each list or group. The type of milk the patient uses should be calculated into the meal plan. Skim milk and low-fat milks are recommended, but whole milk can be used if the patient will not drink the others. Although lean meats should be encouraged, when calculating fat grams per meat serving, use the fat value that best represents actual intake. People do not need to add or subtract fat exchanges when using different meat categories.

Example: Gail's usual eating pattern indicates she uses the following amounts from the milk, vegetable, and fruit exchange groups:

	Servings	Carbohydrates (gm)	Protein (gm)	Fat (gm)	Kcal
Milk, skim	1	12	8	1	90
Vegetables	4	20	8	0	100
Fruits	4	60	0	0	240
Carbohydrate Subtotal		92	16	1	430

The starch exchange list is the only group remaining that provides carbohydrates. To determine the number of servings to be used from this group, subtract the total grams of carbohydrate (92 gm) from the milk, vegetable, and fruit lists from the total grams of carbohydrate (199 gm) in the meal plan. This amount is divided by 15 gm carbohydrate/serving in the starch list.

	Servings	Carbohydrates (gm)	Protein (gm)	Fat (gm)	Kcal
Carbohydrate Subtotal		92	24	1	460
Starches	7	105	21	7	560
Protein Subtotal		197	45	8	1020

The meat exchange list is the only group remaining that provides protein. To determine the number of servings to be used from this group, subtract the total grams of protein (48 gm) from the milk, vegetable, and starch lists from the total grams of protein (56 gm) in the meal plan. This amount is divided by 7 gm protein/serving in the meat list.

	Servings	Carbohydrates (gm)	Protein (gm)	Fat (gm)	Kcal
Protein Subtotal		197	45	8	1020
Meat/lean	4	0	28	12	220
Fat Subtotal		197	73	20	1240

The fat exchange list is the only group remaining that provides fat. To determine the number of servings to be used from this group, subtract the total grams of fat (20 gm) from the milk, starch, and meat lists from the total grams of fat (50 gm) in the meal plan. This amount is divided by 5 gm fat/serving in the fat list.

	Servings	Carbohydrates (gm)	Protein (gm)	Fat (gm)	Kcal
Fat Subtotal		197	73	20	1240
Fats	6	0	0	30	270
TOTAL		197	73	50	1510

Note: When calculating the number of servings from each exchange list, round to the nearest whole number. It is usually impractical to calculate and plan half servings from the lists.

The daily distribution of servings from the exchange lists is as follows. These servings can now be divided into the appropriate number of meals and snacks per day.

Exchange List Group	Servings	Carbohydrates (gm)	Protein (gm)	Fat (gm)	Kcal
Carbohydrates	12				
Starches	7	105	21	7	560
Fruit	4	60	0	0	240
Milk (skim)	1	0	0	30	270
Vegetables	4	20	8	1	90
Meats/lean	4	0	28	12	220
Fats	6	0	0	30	270

Modified from American Dietetic Association: Exchange lists for meal planning, Alexandria Va, 1995, American Diabetes Association; American Dietetic Association: Handbook of clinical dietetics, ed 2, New Haven, Conn, 1992, Yale University Press; Davis JR, Sherer K: Applied nutrition and diet therapy for nurses, ed 2, Philadelphia, 1994, WB Saunders; American Dietetic Association: Nutrition recommendations and principles for people with diabetes mellitus, J Am Diet Assoc 94:504, 1994; and Tinker LF, Heins JM, Holler HJ: Commentary and translation: 1994 nutrition recommendations for diabetes, J Am Diet Assoc 94:507, 1994.

METRIC-ENGLISH CONVERSIONS

WEIGHT

English (USA) = Metric

grain	= 64.80 mg
ounce	= 28.35 g
pound	= 453.60 g, = 0.45 kg

Metric	English (USA)
milligram	= 0.002 grain (0.000035 oz)
gram	= 0.04 oz
kilogram	= 35.27 oz, 2.20 lb

VOLUME

English (USA) = Metric

ounce	= 0.03 liter (3 ml)*
pint	= 0.47 liter
quart	= 0.95 liter
gallon	= 3.79 liters

Metric	English (USA)
milliliter	= 0.03 oz
liter	= 2.12 pt
liter	= 1.06 qt
liter	= 0.27 gal

1 liter ÷ 1000 = milliliter or cubic centimeter (10^{-3} liter)

1 liter ÷ 1,000,000 = microliter (10^{-6} liter)

*Note: 1 ml = 1 cc

Nutrition and Health Organizations: Sources of Nutrition Information

JOURNALS OF PROFESSIONAL ORGANIZATIONS

This list only includes nutrition journals. A number of nursing and medical journals also feature nutrition-related articles and studies. The asterisked (*) journals are most recommended based on the applicability of their subject content to the nursing setting and/or ease of availability in most libraries.

American Journal of Clinical Nutrition
*American Journal of Public Health**
Annual Review of Nutrition
British Journal of Nutrition
*FDA Consumer**
Human Nutrition: Allied Nutrition
Human Nutrition: Clinical Nutrition
Journal of Food Service
Journal of Food Technology
Journal of Nutrition
*Journal of Nutrition Education**
Journal of Nutrition for the Elderly
Journal of Nutrition Reviews
*Journal of Nutrition Today**
Journal of the American College of Nutrition
*Journal of the American Dietetic Association**
*Journal of the Canadian Dietetic Association**

NEWSLETTERS

Environmental Nutrition
52 Riverside Dr.
New York, NY 10024
(800) 829-5384
www.environmentalnutrition.com

Food and Nutrition News (free)
National Cattlemen's Beef Association
9110 East Nichols Ave., #300
Centennial, CO 80112
(303) 694-0305
www.beef.org

Harvard Medical School Health Letter
Department of Continuing Education
25 Shattuck St.
Boston, MA 02115
(800) 829-9045
www.health.harvard.edu/

Tufts University Health & Nutrition Letter
P.O. Box 10948
Des Moines, IA 50940
(800) 274-7581
www.healthletter.tufts.edu

FEDERAL AGENCIES

Centers for Disease Control and Prevention (CDC)
Public Inquiries
1600 Clifton Rd. NE
Atlanta, GA 30333
(404) 639-3311
www.cdc.gov

Food and Drug Administration
Office of Consumer Affairs
Department of Health and Human Services
U.S. Food and Drug Administration
5600 Fishers Lane
Rockville, MD 20857-0001
888-INFO-FDA (888-463-6332)
www.fda.gov

Food and Nutrition Information Center (FNIC)
National Agricultural Library/USDA
10301 Baltimore Ave.
Beltsville, MD 20705-2351
(301) 504-5719
TTY: (301) 504-6856
www.nal.usda.gov/fnic

Food Safety and Inspection Service
Meat and Poultry Hotline/USDA
Room 1175
1400 Independence Ave., SW
Washington, DC 20250-3700
(800) 535-4555
www.usda.gov/fsis

National Cancer Institute
Cancer Information Center
NCI Public Inquiries Office
Suite 3036A
6116 Executive Blvd., MSC8322
Bethesda, MD 20892-8322
(800) 4-CANCER (800-422-6237)
www.nci.nih.gov

National Diabetes Information Clearinghouse
NIDDK, NIH, Building 31
Room 9A04
31 Center Dr., MSC 2560
Bethesda, MD 20892-2560
(301) 654-3327
www.niddk.nih.gov

National Digestive Diseases Information Clearinghouse
NIDDK, NIH, Building 31
Room 9A04
31 Center Dr., MSC 2560
Bethesda, MD 20892-2560
(301) 654-3810
www.niddk.nih.gov

National Heart, Lung, and Blood Institute (NHLBI)
    Information Center
P.O. Box 30105
Bethesda, MD 20824-0105
(301) 592-8573
TTY: (240) 629-3255
www.nhlbi.nih.gov/index.htm

National Institute on Aging Information Office
Building 31, Room 5C-27
31 Center Dr., MSC 2292
Bethesda, MD 20892
(301) 496-1752
www.nih.gov/nia

Office of Disease Prevention & Health Promotion
Office of Public Health and Science
200 Independence Ave. SW, Room 738G
Washington, DC 20201
(202) 205-8611
www.odphp.osophs.dhhs.gov

Weight-control Information Network
1 Win Way
Bethesda, MD 20892-3665
(877) 946-4627
www.niddk.nih.gov/health/nutrit/win.htm

PROFESSIONAL ASSOCIATIONS AND ORGANIZATIONS

American Academy of Pediatrics
141 Northwest Point Blvd.
Elk Grove Village, IL 60007-1098
(847) 434-4000
www.aap.org

American Association for Health Education
1900 Association Dr.
Reston, VA 20191
(703) 476-3437
www.aahperd.org

American Cancer Society
1599 Clifton Rd. NE
Atlanta, GA 30329
(800) 227-2345
www.cancer.org

American Dental Association Public Information
    and Education
211 E. Chicago Ave.
Chicago, IL 60611
(312) 440-2500
www.ada.org

American Diabetes Association
1660 Duke St.
Alexandria, VA 22314
(800) 342-2383
www.diabetes.org

American Dietetic Association
216 W. Jackson Blvd.
Suite 800
Chicago, IL 60606
(800) 899-0040
www.eatright.org

American Heart Association
National Center
7272 Greenville Ave.
Dallas, TX 75231
(214) 706-1570
www.americanheart.org

American Institute for Cancer Research
1759 R St. NW
Washington, DC 20009
(800) 843-8114
www.aicr.org/index.lasso

American Lung Association
1740 Broadway
New York, NY 10019
(800) 586-4872
www.lungusa.org

American Medical Association
515 N. State St.
Chicago, IL 60610
(800) 621-8335
www.ama-assn.org

American Nurses Association
600 Maryland Ave. SW
Washington, DC 20024
(800) 274-4262
www.nursingworld.org

American Public Health Association
1015 15th St. NW
Suite 300
Washington, DC 20005
(202) 789-5600
www.apha.org

American School Food Service Association
1600 Duke St.
Alexandria, VA 22314
(703) 739-3900
www.asfsa.org

American School Health Association
7263 State, Route 43
P.O. Box 708
Kent, OH 44240
(330) 678-1601
www.ashaweb.org

International Society on Hypertension in Blacks
2045 Manchester St. NE
Atlanta, GA 30324
(404) 875-6263
www.ishib.org

La Leche League International
1400 N. Meacham Rd.
Schaumburg, IL 60173
(847) 519-7730
www.lalecheleague.org

March of Dimes Birth Defects Foundation
1275 Mamaroneck Ave.
White Plains, NY 10605
(914) 428-7100
www.modimes.org

National Osteoporosis Foundation
1150 17th St. NW
Suite 500
Washington, DC 20036
(800) 223-9994
www.nof.org

North American Vegetarian Society
P.O. Box 72
Dolgeville, NY 13329
(518) 568-7970
www.navs-online.org

Penn State Nutrition Information and Resource Center
Pennsylvania State University
5 Henderson Building
University Park, PA 16802
(814) 865-6323 (professionals only)
nirc.cas.psu.edu/index.cfm

Society for Nutrition Education
9202 N. Meridian St.
Suite 200
Indianapolis, IN 46260
(800) 235-6690
www.sne.org

ADVOCACY ORGANIZATIONS

American Association of Retired Persons (AARP)
601 East St. NW
Washington, DC 20049
(800) 424-3410
www.aarp.org

Center for Science in the Public Interest
1875 Connecticut Ave. NW
Suite 300
Washington, DC 20009
(202) 332-9110
www.cspinet.org

The Food Allergy Network
10400 Eaton Pl.
Suite 107
Fairfax, VA 22030
(800) 929-4040
www.foodallergy.org

Food Research and Action Center (FRAC)
1875 Connecticut Ave. NW
Suite 540
Washington, DC 20009
(202) 986-2200
www.frac.org

National Council Against Health Fraud, Inc.
P.O. Box 1276
Loma Linda, CA 92354
(909) 824-4690
www.ncahf.org

Local Resources

- Cooperative extension agents in county extension offices
- Dietitians (contact the state or local Dietetics Association)
- Nutrition faculty affiliated with departments of food and nutrition, home economics, and dietetics
- Registered dietitians (RDs) in city, county, or state agencies

Eating Disorders Resources (For Professionals and the Public)

Anorexia Nervosa and Related Eating Disorders
P.O. Box 5102
Eugene, OR 97405
(541) 344-1144
www.anred.com

International Association of Eating Disorders
 Professionals
123 NW 13th St.
Boca Raton, FL 33432
(800) 800-8126
www.iaedp.com

National Association of Anorexia Nervosa and
 Associated Disorders
P.O. Box 7
Highland Park, IL 60035
(847) 831-3438
www.anad.org

National Eating Disorders Association
603 Stewart St.
Suite 803
Seattle, WA 98101
(206) 382-3587
www.nationaleatingdisorders.org

Overeaters Anonymous, Inc.
6075 Zenith Ct. NE
Rio Rancho, NM 87124
(505) 891-4320
www.overeatersanonymous.org

Remuda Ranch Center
1 E. Apache St.
Wickenburg, AZ 85390
(520) 684-3913
(800) 445-1900
www.remuda-ranch.com

The Renfrew Center
475 Spring Ln.
Philadelphia, PA 19128
(800) 332-8415
www.renfrew.org

Size Acceptance Resources

Council on Size & Weight Discrimination
P.O. Box 305
Mt. Marion, NY 12456
(845) 679-1209
www.cswd.org

National Association to Advance Fat Acceptance
P.O. Box 188620
Sacramento, CA 95818
(916) 558-6880
www.naafa.org

Society for Nutrition Education
Division of Nutrition and Weight Realities
9202 N. Meridian St., Suite 200
Indianapolis, IN 46260
(800) 235-6690
www.sne.org

APPENDIX *D*

Canada's Food Guide to Healthy Eating

These guidelines were developed as the key messages to be communicated to healthy Canadians, older than 2 years of age.

1. Enjoy a VARIETY of foods.
2. Emphasize cereals, breads, other grain products, vegetables, and fruit.
3. Choose lower-fat dairy products, leaner meats, and food prepared with little or no fat.
4. Achieve and maintain a healthy body weight by enjoying regular physical activity and healthy eating.
5. Limit salt, alcohol, and caffeine intake.

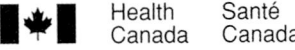
Health   Santé
Canada   Canada

CANADA'S
Food Guide
TO HEALTHY EATING
FOR PEOPLE FOUR YEARS AND OVER

Enjoy a variety
of foods from each
group every day.

Choose lower-
fat foods
more often.

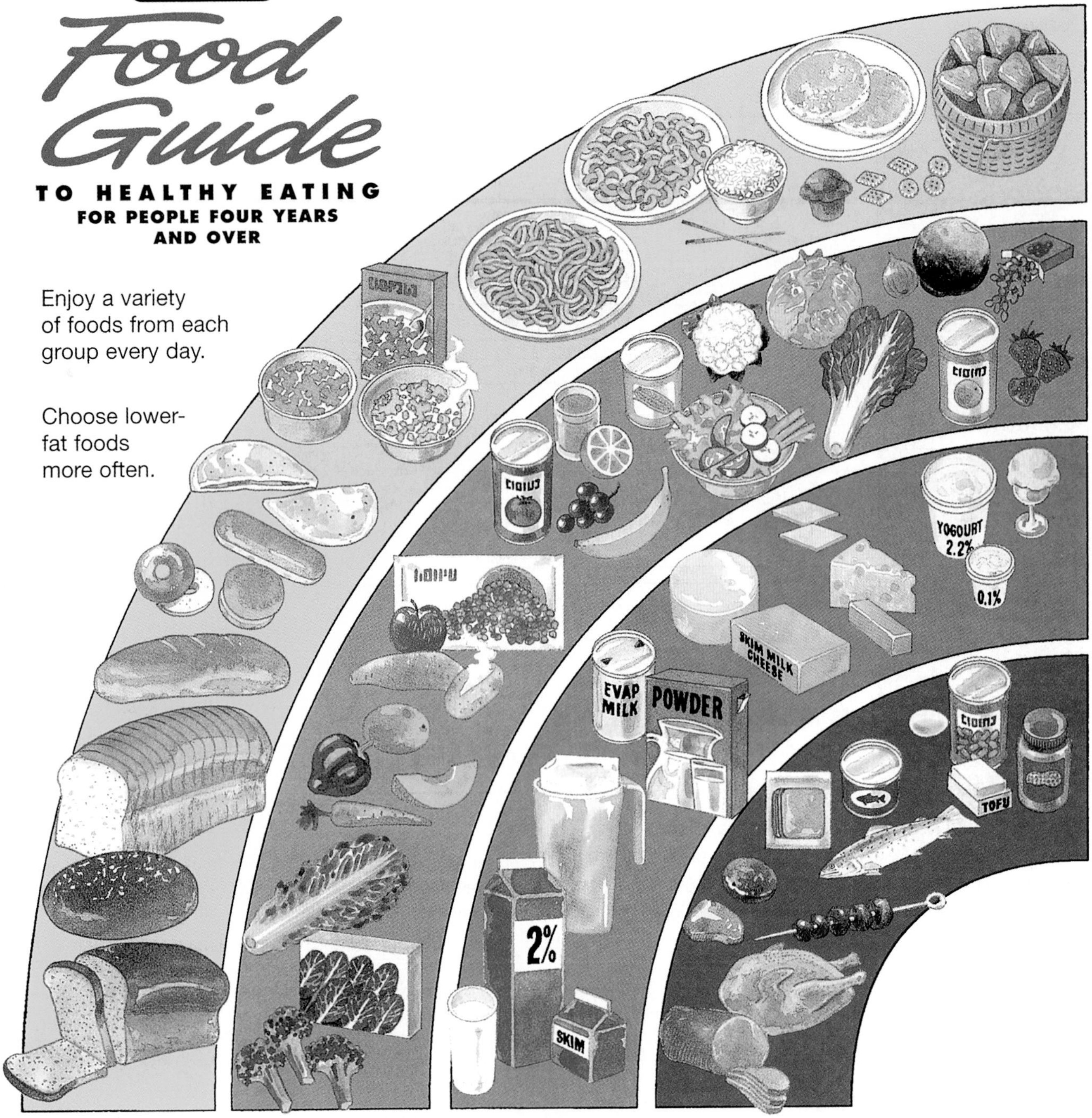

Grain Products
Choose whole grain
and enriched
products more often.

Vegetables and Fruit
Choose dark green and
orange vegetables and
orange fruit more often.

Milk Products
Choose lower-fat milk
products more often.

Meat and Alternatives
Choose leaner meats,
poultry and fish, as well
as dried peas, beans
and lentils more often.

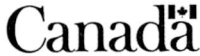
Canada

Grain Products
5–12 SERVINGS PER DAY

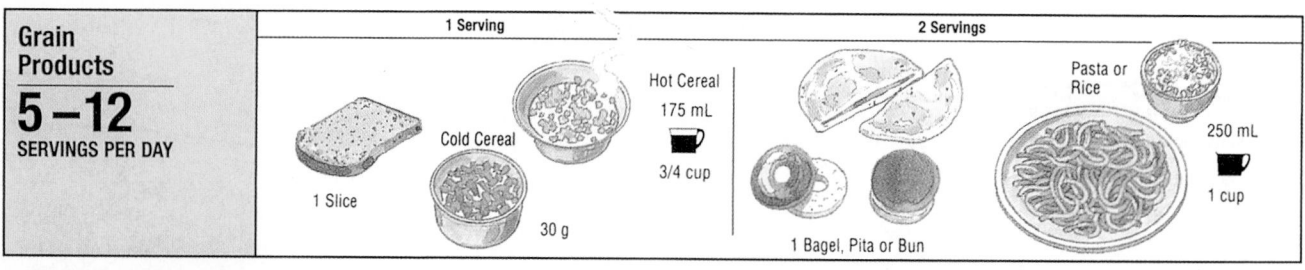

1 Serving — 1 Slice — Cold Cereal 30 g — Hot Cereal 175 mL 3/4 cup

2 Servings — 1 Bagel, Pita or Bun — Pasta or Rice 250 mL 1 cup

Vegetables and Fruit
5–10 SERVINGS PER DAY

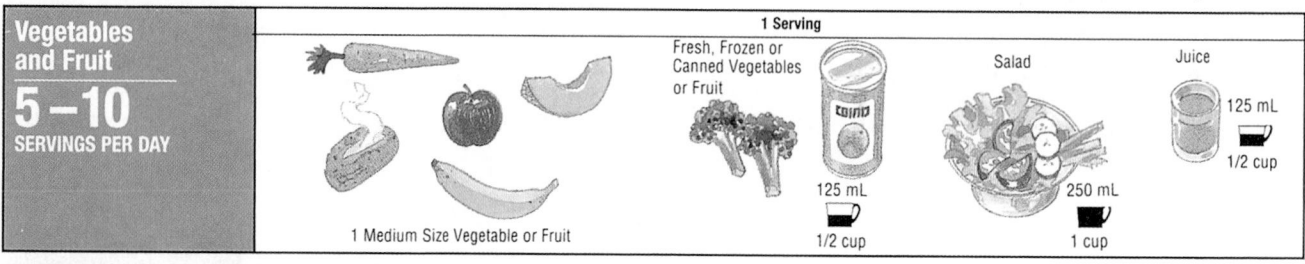

1 Serving — 1 Medium Size Vegetable or Fruit — Fresh, Frozen or Canned Vegetables or Fruit 125 mL 1/2 cup — Salad 250 mL 1 cup — Juice 125 mL 1/2 cup

Milk Products
SERVINGS PER DAY
Children 4–9 years: 2–3
Youth 10–16 years: 3–4
Adults: 2–4
Pregnant and Breast-feeding Women 3–4

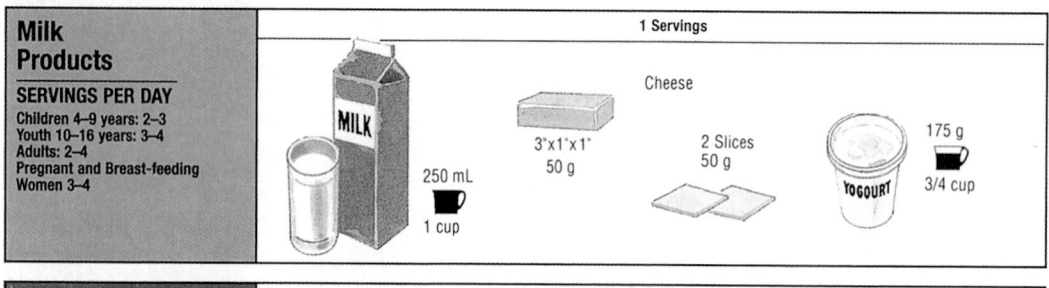

1 Servings — MILK 250 mL 1 cup — Cheese 3"x1"x1" 50 g — 2 Slices 50 g — YOGOURT 175 g 3/4 cup

Other Foods

Taste and enjoyment can also come from other foods and beverages that are not part of the 4 food groups. Some of these foods are higher in fat or Calories, so use these foods in moderation.

Meat and Alternatives
2–3 SERVINGS PER DAY

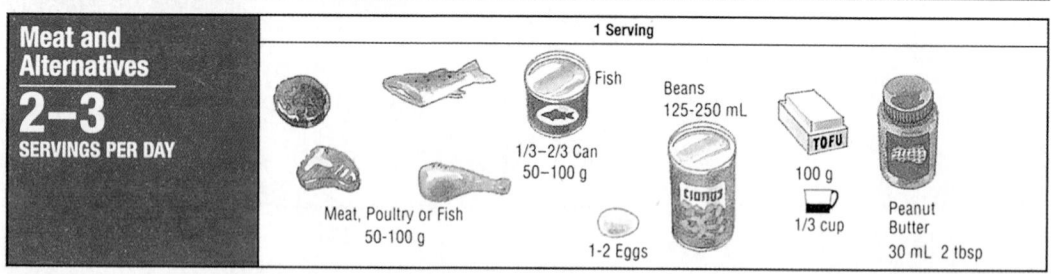

1 Serving — Meat, Poultry or Fish 50-100 g — Fish 1/3–2/3 Can 50–100 g — 1-2 Eggs — Beans 125-250 mL — TOFU 100 g 1/3 cup — Peanut Butter 30 mL 2 tbsp

Different People Need Different Amounts of Food

The amount of food you need every day from the 4 food groups and other foods depends on your age, body size, activity level, whether you are male or female and if you are pregnant or breast-feeding. That's why the Food Guide gives a lower and higher number of servings for each food group. For example, young children can choose the lower number of servings, while male teenagers can go to the higher number. Most other people can choose servings somewhere in between.

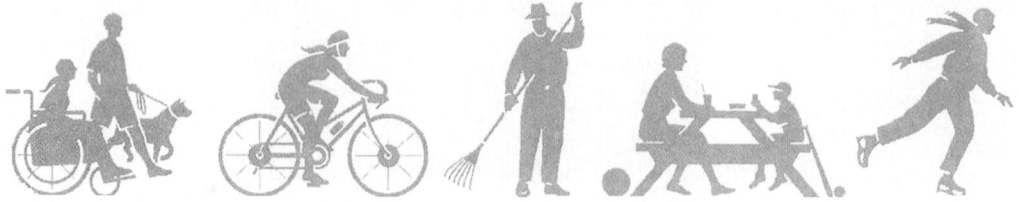

Consult *Canada's Physical Activity Guide to Healthy Active Living* to help you build physical activity into your daily life.

Enjoy eating well, being active and feeling good about yourself. That's VITALITE

APPENDIX E

Body Mass Index Table (Second of Two BMI Tables)

For lower body mass indexes, see Table 10-1 in Chapter 10, "Management of Body Composition."

Body Mass Index Table																		
36	37	38	39	40	41	42	43	44	45	46	47	48	49	50	51	52	53	54
Height (inches)								**Body Weight (pounds)**										
58 172	177	183	186	191	196	201	205	210	215	220	224	229	234	239	244	248	253	258
59 178	183	188	193	198	203	208	212	217	222	227	232	237	242	247	252	257	262	267
60 184	189	194	199	204	209	215	220	225	230	235	240	245	250	255	261	266	271	276
61 190	195	201	206	211	217	222	227	232	238	243	248	254	259	264	269	275	280	285
62 196	202	207	213	218	224	229	235	240	246	251	256	262	267	273	278	284	289	295
63 203	208	214	220	225	231	237	242	248	254	259	265	270	278	282	287	293	299	304
64 209	215	221	227	232	238	244	250	256	262	267	273	279	285	291	296	302	308	314
65 216	222	228	234	240	246	252	258	264	270	276	282	288	294	300	306	312	318	324
66 223	229	235	241	247	253	260	266	272	278	284	291	297	303	309	315	322	328	334
67 230	236	242	249	255	261	268	274	280	287	293	299	306	312	319	325	331	338	344
68 236	243	249	256	262	269	276	282	289	295	302	308	315	322	328	335	341	348	354
69 243	250	257	263	270	277	284	291	297	304	311	318	324	331	338	345	351	358	365
70 250	257	264	271	278	285	292	299	306	313	320	327	334	341	348	355	362	369	376
71 257	265	272	279	286	293	301	308	315	322	329	338	343	351	358	365	372	379	386
72 265	272	279	287	294	302	309	316	324	331	338	346	353	361	368	375	383	390	397
73 272	280	288	295	302	310	318	325	333	340	348	355	363	371	378	386	393	401	408
74 280	287	295	303	311	319	326	334	342	350	358	365	373	381	389	396	404	412	420
75 287	295	303	311	319	327	335	343	351	359	367	375	383	391	399	407	415	423	431
76 295	304	312	320	328	336	344	353	361	369	377	385	394	402	410	418	426	435	443

From NIH/National Heart, Lung, and Blood Institute: Appendix V: Body mass index chart (chart 2), Clinical guidelines on the identification, evaluation, and treatment of overweight and obesity in adults, Bethesda, Md, June 1998, National Institutes of Health.

To use the table, find the appropriate height in the left-hand column. Move across to a given weight. The number at the top of the column is the BMI at that height and weight. Pounds have been rounded off.

APPENDIX F

Kcalorie-Restricted Dietary Patterns

The goal of weight management is weight stabilization through the adoption and maintenance of healthy lifestyle behaviors including consistent eating patterns. Although these changes in behavior may result in minimal weight changes, health status may be improved.

Certain chronic medical conditions are improved by weight loss. Consequently, although physical and psychologic risks of kcalorie-restricted diets may occur, the benefits outweigh the risks. Below are brief reviews of the primary weight loss formats of these diets and a guide for comparison of weight-loss programs. Programs should be contacted directly to determine current fees.

MODERATE RESTRICTION OF KCALORIES

Kcalorie restriction should be at least 500 kcal less than the individual's daily requirement for energy; the amount of daily kcaloric intake should not be lower than about 1200 kcal. Adults, depending on their gender, height, and weight, may lose weight at intakes between 1200 kcal to 1500 kcal. Intake below this level cannot provide sufficient amounts of nutrients unless supplements are prescribed. The diet should still follow general dietary guidelines and provide 45% to 65% kcal from carbohydrates, about 10% to 35% kcal from protein, and 20% to 35% kcal from fat.

The Exchange List for Meal Planning is often used to implement kcalorie-restricted diets. By prescribing the number of each exchange allowed, the individual can then design a dietary pattern based on personal taste preference and scheduling. The following exchanges equal about 1200 kcal: 2 carbohydrates as milk, 3 vegetable, 4 fruit, 5 carbohydrate (either as starch, milk, fruit, or vegetables), 5 lean meat, and 3 fat.

VERY-LOW-CALORIE DIETS (VLCD)

These diets are intended for use by moderately or severely obese individuals (BMI > 30) whose attempts with more traditional methods have been unsuccessful and for individuals with BMI of 27 to 30 or higher whose medical condition depends on weight loss for improvement. Containing only 200 kcal to 800 kcal, a VLCD causes rapid weight loss but increases the risk of gout, gallstones, and other related symptoms, including cardiac complications. Individuals must be under the complete and regular supervision of a physician. The American Dietetic Association (ADA) has developed medical nutrition intervention procedures for the use of VLCD. Maintenance of the weight loss is difficult and depends on nutritional counseling, exercise, and lifestyle changes. Regain of lost weight most often occurs after 5 years even with adjunct support of behavior therapy.

FORMULA DIETS

Developed by pharmaceutical and food manufacturers, these solutions are available in a variety of forms. Designed to replace meals, they may provide a daily total of about 900 kcal and often contain or may be supplemented by vitamins and minerals. Although helpful for quick weight loss, the loss is rarely maintained, as boredom with the solution and the lack of learning new eating approaches soon lead to the weight being regained.

PHARMACOTHERAPY

Criteria for pharmacotherapy are a BMI greater than 30 or clients with comorbidities and BMI of 27. The pharmacotherapy should be accompanied by medical nutri-

From American Dietetic Association: Weight management, *J Am Diet Assoc* 102:1145-1155, 2002; National Institutes of Health/National Heart, Lung, and Blood Institute: *Clinical guidelines on the identification, evaluation, and treatment of overweight and obesity in adults: the evidence report,* June 1998; Standing Committee on the Scientific Evaluation of Dietary Reference Intakes, Institute of Medicine: *Dietary reference intakes for energy, carbohydrate, fiber, fat, fatty acids, cholesterol, protein, and amino acids,* Washington, DC, 2002, National Academy Press; Thomas P, ed.: *Weighing the options: criteria for evaluating weight-management programs,* Washington, DC, 1995, National Academy Press.

tion therapy and exercise. Generally, starting weight loss is only 5% to 15% of original weight. Weight loss is regained when drug therapy is discontinued.

The use of pharmacologic drugs for obesity intervention is controversial among health professionals because of the lack of data on long-term effects of drug usage and the possibility of abuse when prescribed to patients not meeting the criteria for pharmacotherapy.

COMPARISON OF WEIGHT-LOSS PROGRAMS

Do-It-Yourself Programs

Overeaters Anonymous (OA)

Approach/Method. Nonprofit international organization providing volunteer support groups worldwide patterned after the 12-step Alcoholics Anonymous program. Addresses physical, emotional, and spiritual recovery aspects of compulsive overeating. Members encouraged to seek professional help for individualized diet/nutrition plan and for any emotional or physical problems.

Clients. Individuals who define themselves as compulsive eaters.

Staff. Nonprofessional volunteer group members who meet specific criteria lead meetings, sit on the board, and conduct activities.

Expected Weight Loss/Length of Program. Makes no claims for weight loss. Unlimited length.

Healthy Lifestyle Components. Recommends emotional, spiritual, and physical recovery changes. Makes no exercise or food recommendations.

Comments. Inexpensive. Provides group support. No need to follow a specific diet plan to participate. Minimal organization at the group level, so groups vary in approach. No healthcare providers on staff.

Availability. Groups in 47 countries. Headquarters: Rio Rancho, NM; (505) 891-2664; www.oa.org.

Take Off Pounds Sensibly (TOPS)

Approach/Method. Nonprofit support organization whose members meet weekly in groups. Does not prescribe or endorse particular eating or exercise regimen. Mandatory weigh-in at weekly meetings. Provides peer support. Uses award programs for healthy lifestyle changes; special recognition given to best weight losers.

Clients. Members must submit weight goals and diets obtained from a health professional in writing.

Staff. Each group elects a volunteer (nonhealth professional) to direct and organize activities for 1 year. Health professionals, including registered dietitians and psychologists, may be invited to speak at weekly meetings. Organization consults with a medical advisor.

Expected Weight Loss/Length of Program. No claims made for weight loss. Unlimited length.

Healthy Lifestyle Components. No official lifestyle or exercise recommendations, but endorses slow, permanent lifestyle changes. Members encouraged to consult healthcare provider for an exercise regimen to meet their needs.

Comments. Inexpensive form of continuing group support. Used as adjunct to professional care. Nonprofit and noncommercial, so no purchases required. Encourages long-term participation. Lacks professional guidance at chapter level because meetings run by volunteers. Groups vary widely in approach.

Availability. Chapters in 20 countries, mostly the United States and Canada. Headquarters: Milwaukee, Wisc; (800) 932-8677; www.tops.org.

Nonclinical Programs

Diet Center

Approach/Method. Focuses on achieving healthy body composition through diet and personalized exercise recommendations. Diet based on regular supermarket food; Diet Center prepackaged cuisine is optional. Body-fat analysis via electrical impedance taken at start of program and every 4 to 6 weeks thereafter. Clients encouraged to visit center daily for weigh-in. Calorie levels individualized to meet client needs and goals. Minimum level: 1200 kcal/day. Four phases: 2-day conditioning phase prepares dieter for reducing. Reducing phase used until goal achieved. Stabilization, the third phase, has clients adjusting calories and physical activity to maintain weight. Maintenance, the fourth phase, lasts for 1 year. One-on-one counseling. Some group meetings available.

Clients. *Not allowed to join:* pregnant, lactating, anorectic, bulimic, and underweight individuals, and those less than 18 years of age. *Require physician's written approval:* those with more than 50 pounds to lose, kidney or heart disease, diabetes, cancer, or emphysema.

Staff. Clients consult with nonprofessional counselors who typically are program graduates trained by Diet Center. Two staff registered dietitians and scientific advisors, who are made up of a variety of health professionals, design the program at corporate level.

Expected Weight Loss/Length of Program. Not more than 1.5 to 2 lb is lost weekly. Length will vary with individualized client goals, but 1-year maintenance program strongly encouraged.

Healthy Lifestyle Components. Exclusively Me behavior management, as an ongoing part of the program, includes an activity book, audiotapes, and counseling. Used in conjunction with regular one-to-one sessions; counselor helps clients design personal solutions to weight-control problems.

Comments. Emphasizes body composition, not pounds, as a measure of health. Does not require the purchase of Diet Center food for preparation. Professional guidance lacking at the client level. Little group support available. Vitamin supplement required.

Availability. Centers in United States, Canada, Bermuda, Guam, and South America. Headquarters: Pittsburgh, Penn; (800) 333-2581; www.dietcenter.com.

Jenny Craig

Approach/Method. Personal Weight Management menu plans based on Jenny Craig's cuisine with additional store-bought foods. Diet ranges from 1000 to 2600 kcal, depending on client needs. Mandatory weekly one-to-one counseling; group workshops. After clients lose half their goal, they begin planning their own meals using their own foods.

Clients. *Not allowed to join:* individuals who are underweight, pregnant, or younger than age 13; those with celiac disease, diabetes (who inject more than twice daily or who are less than 18 years of age), or allergies to ubiquitous ingredients in company's food products. *Require physician's written permission:* individuals with 18 additional conditions. Regardless of condition, clients encouraged to communicate with personal physician throughout program.

Staff. Program developed by corporate registered dietitians (RDs) and psychologists. Company consults with advisory board of MDs, RDs, and PhDs on program design. Consultants trained by Jenny Craig to implement program and offer support and motivational strategies. Corporate dietitians available for client questions or concerns at no extra charge.

Expected Weight Loss/Length of Program. Clients encouraged to set reasonable weight goals based on personal history and healthy weight standards. Program designed to produce weight loss of 1 to 2 lb/week. A separate, 12-month maintenance program is also offered.

Healthy Lifestyle Components. Clients use program guides to learn cognitive behavioral techniques for relapse prevention and problem management for lifestyle changes. Based on individual priorities, clients address major factors involved with weight management (e.g., exercise, which is addressed through a physical activity module and a walking program). Individual consultations; group workshops provide motivation and peer exchange. The Lifestyle Maintenance program addresses issues such as body image and maintaining motivation to exercise.

Comments. Little food preparation. Vegetarian and kosher meal plans available; also plans for clients who are diabetic, hypoglycemic, and breastfeeding. Recipes provided. Must rely on Jenny Craig cuisine for participation. Lack of professional guidance at client level.

Availability. Centers in five countries; 650 centers in United States. U.S. headquarters: Del Mar, Calif; (800) 815-3669; www.jennycraig.com.

Nutri/System

Approach/Method. Menu plans based on Nutri/System's prepared meals with additional grocery foods. Clients receive individual calorie levels ranging from 1000 to 2200 kcal/day. Multivitamin-mineral supplement available for clients. Personal counseling and group sessions available.

Clients. *Not allowed to join:* individuals who are pregnant, less than 14 years of age, underweight, or anorectic. *Require physician's written permission:* lactating women and those with a variety of conditions including diabetes (if requiring insulin shots), heart disease (that limits normal activity), and kidney disease.

Staff. Staff dietitians, health educators, and PhDs develop program at corporate level. Scientific Advisory Board consisting of MDs and PhDs employed for program design. Counselors with education and experience in psychology, nutrition, counseling, and health-related fields provide weekly guidance to clients. Certified Personal Trainers administer the Personal Trainer Program developed in conjunction with Johnson & Johnson Advanced Behavioral Technologies, Inc. Registered dietitians available through a toll-free number to address client questions.

Expected Weight Loss/Length of Program. Averages 1.5 to 2 lb/week. Clients select weight goal based on a recommended weight range using standard tables. Program length varies with weight-loss goals.

Healthy Lifestyle Components. Wellness and Personal Trainer services developed in conjunction with Johnson & Johnson Health Management have been added to the program.

Comments. Few decisions about what to eat; relatively rigid diet with company foods. Portion-controlled Nutri/System foods allow dieters to focus more on making lifestyle changes than on reducing diet. Program provides both Wellness and Personal Trainer services. Little contact with health professionals.

Availability. 650 centers in the United States and Canada. Headquarters: Horsham, Penn; (800) 315-3577; www.nutrisystem.com.

Weight Watchers

Approach/Method. Emphasis on portion control and healthy lifestyle habits. Dieters choose from regular supermarket food and Weight Watchers foods. Reducing phase: Women average 1250 kcal daily; men 1600 daily. Levels for weight maintenance determined individually. Weekly group meetings with mandatory weigh-in or Internet memberships. Must need to lose at least 5 lb to join.

Clients.   *Not allowed to join:* those not weighing at least 5 lbs above the lowest end of their healthy weight range and those with a medically diagnosed eating disorder. *Require physician's written approval:* pregnant and lactating women and children less than 10 years of age.

Staff.   Group leaders are nonhealth professional graduates of program (Lifetime Members) trained by Weight Watchers. Program developed by corporate registered dietitians. Company consults with medical advisor and advisory board consisting of MDs and PhDs on program design. Health professionals at corporate level, including registered dietitians, direct the program.

Expected Weight Loss/Length of Program.   Up to 2 lb weekly. Unlimited length. Maintenance plan is 6 weeks.

Healthy Lifestyle Components.   Emphasizes making positive lifestyle changes, including regular exercise. Encourages daily minimum physical activity level.

Comments.   Flexible program offering group support and well-balanced diet. Vegetarian plan available, plus healthy eating plans for pregnant and breastfeeding women. Encourages long-term participation for members to attain their weight-loss goals. Lacks professional guidance at client level. No personalized counseling except in select markets.

Availability.   Weekly meetings in 24 countries; Internet access. Headquarters: Jericho, NY; (800) 651-6000; www.weightwatchers.com.

Clinical Programs

Health Management Resources (HMR)

Approach/Method.   Medically supervised very-low-calorie diet (VLCD) of fortified, high-protein liquid meal replacements (520 to 800 kcal daily) or a low-calorie option consisting of liquid supplements and prepackaged HMR entrees (800 to 1300 kcal daily). Dieters receive the HMR Risk Factor Profile that measures and displays an individual's medical and lifestyle health risks. Mandatory weekly 90-minute group meetings. Maintenance meetings are 1 hour per week. One-on-one counseling. Need to have BMI >30 for VLCD.

Clients.   *Not allowed to join:* pregnant or lactating women, acute substance abusers. *Require physician's written approval:* some with acute psychiatric disorders, recent heart disease, cancer, renal or liver disease, type 1 diabetes mellitus, and those who test positive for acquired immunodeficiency syndrome (AIDS).

Staff.   Program developed by physicians, registered dietitians, registered nurses, and psychologists. Each location has at least one physician and health educator on staff. Participants assigned "personal coaches" (i.e., registered dietitians, exercise physiologists, health educators) who help dieters learn and practice weight-

management skills. Dieters on VLCD see a physician or registered nurse weekly.

Expected Weight Loss/Length of Program.   Averages 2 to 5 lb weekly. Reducing phase varies according to weight-loss needs but averages 12 weeks; refeeding phase (after liquids only) lasts about 6 weeks. Maintenance program recommended for up to 18 months.

Healthy Lifestyle Components.   Recommends every client burn a minimum of 2000 kcal in physical activity weekly. Advocates consuming a diet with no more than 30 percent of calories from fat and at least 35 servings of fruits and vegetables per week. Emphasizes lifestyle issues in weekly classes and in personal coaching.

Comments.   Emphasizes exercise as a means for weight loss and control. Few decisions about what to eat. Supervised by a health professional. Requires a strong commitment to physical activity. Side effects of VLCD may include intolerance to cold, constipation, dizziness, dry skin, and headaches. All options include liquid supplement; diet is very high in protein, even at higher calorie levels.

Availability.   Available at 180 hospitals and medical settings nationwide. Headquarters: Boston, Mass; (617) 357-9876; www.hmrprogram.com.

Physicians in a Multidisciplinary Program

Approach/Method.   Multidisciplinary programs may provide a program similar to HMR or Medifast. They may also provide food-based weight-loss programs or modifications of the two approaches. The multidisciplinary aspect implies the coordination of services, availability of individual and/or group counseling, and comprehensive medical supervision.

Staff.   Typically physicians, dietitians, behavior therapists, exercise physiologists, psychologists, and counselors working individually and in group settings. Service providers should be licensed and regulated and should have their activities scrutinized by peers.

Expected Weight Loss/Length of Program.   Variable and adapted to the needs of patient. There should be a maintenance program with continuing patient access to services for sustaining care and reinforcement. Patient use of medications and consequences of surgery will be monitored.

Healthy Lifestyle Components.   Varies. All recognized factors in weight management will be considered.

Comments.   Offers more extensive services than physicians working alone. Professional staff coordinates all aspects of care and long-term management of obesity. Diverse staff adapts care to the needs of patients, including the management of associated medical problems. These are often university-based programs, which have structured peer-review mechanisms and may conduct research. Costs for professional services tend to be high.

Availability. Very limited.

Others

Registered Dietitians (RDs)

Approach/Method. Highly personalized approach to weight loss and maintenance.

Clients. Those acceptable and not acceptable will vary with the RD.

Staff. RDs have, at a minimum, baccalaureate degrees in nutrition or a closely related field and have completed approved or accredited clinical training. Many have advanced degrees. RDs must pass a registration examination given by the Commission on Dietetic Registration of the American Dietetic Association and participate in continuing education.

Expected Weight Loss/Length of Program. Varies according to weight goal. Clients rarely encouraged to lose more than 2 lb weekly.

Healthy Lifestyle Components. Exercise encouraged as part of safe, sensible weight-control program. RDs help clients identify barriers to weight loss and maintenance and provide education about healthy lifestyles.

Comments. Highly adaptable. Personalized approach to clients' health concerns. Trained health professionals who can address medical history and account for it in diet therapy, if necessary. Appropriate for any age group. Can be expensive.

Availability. Located in every state in private practice, outpatient hospital clinics, health maintenance organizations (HMOs), and in physician's practices. For a free referral to a local RD, call (800) 366-1655 or visit www.eatright.org.

Physicians Practicing Alone

Approach/Method. Individualized approach to weight loss and maintenance. Clients able to coordinate the management of their weight with concurrent management of associated medical problems. Services can be adapted to specific needs. Options include medications and surgery to treat obesity.

Staff. Individual physicians possibly working with associates (e.g., nurses and physicians' assistants). Provision of services by licensed professional healthcare providers.

Expected Weight Loss/Length of Program. Varies with client. Program may be of indefinite length and should be coordinated with care of related or unrelated medical issues.

Healthy Lifestyle Components. Varies with the physician and weight-loss approach. Should include exercise and nutrition counseling.

Comments. Professional care. Coordination with other medical problems. Appropriate for clients with complex or serious associated medical problems. Long-term attention in the context of other medical care can be provided. The potential for using medications and/or surgery expands the opportunities for clients at varying stages of their disease. Individual physicians have the ability to vary the client's care and intensity of the effort depending on the client's life circumstances. Physicians often inadequately trained in nutrition and in low-calorie physiology. Cost for services can be high.

Availability. Generally available, but many physicians are reluctant to treat obesity because of their (1) lack of interest or training, (2) recognition that they cannot provide the necessary support services, and (3) concern for the limited usefulness of their intervention.

From American Dietetic Association: Weight management, *J Am Diet Assoc* 102:1145-1155, 2002; National Institutes of Health/National Heart, Lung, and Blood Institute: *Clinical guidelines on the identification, evaluation, and treatment of overweight and obesity in adults: the evidence report,* June 1998; Standing Committee on the Scientific Evaluation of Dietary Reference Intakes, Institute of Medicine: *Dietary reference intakes for energy, carbohydrate, fiber, fat, fatty acids, cholesterol, protein, and amino acids,* Washington, DC, 2002, National Academy Press; Thomas P, ed.: *Weighing the options: criteria for evaluating weight-management programs,* Washington, DC, 1995, National Academy Press.

APPENDIX *G*

Infant and Child Growth Charts: United States, Centers for Disease Control and Prevention (CDC)

CDC Growth Charts: United States

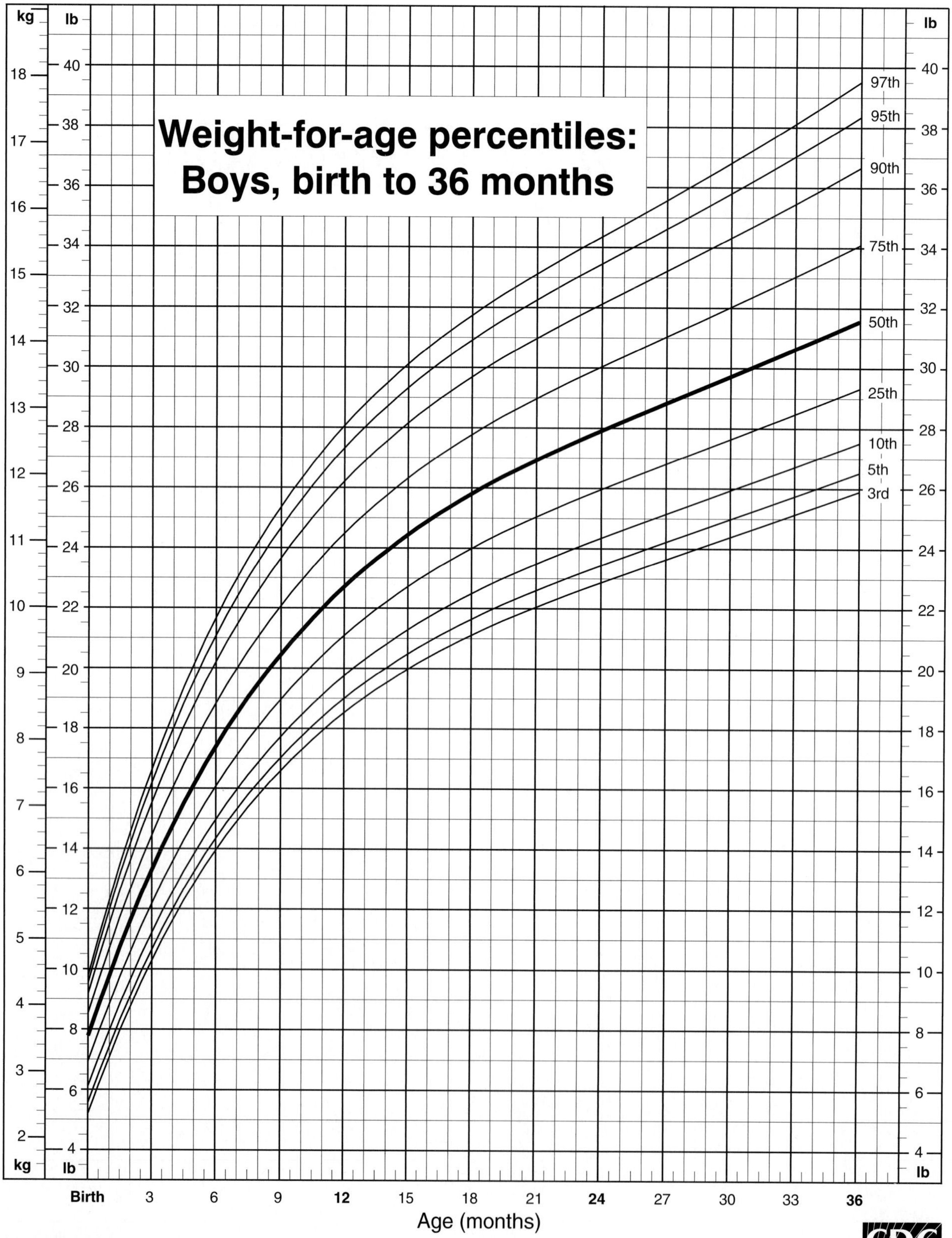
Weight-for-age percentiles:
Boys, birth to 36 months
kg
lb
97th
95th
90th
75th
50th
25th
10th
5th
3rd
Birth
3
6
9
12
15
18
21
24
27
30
33
36
Age (months)

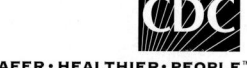

Published May 30, 2000.
SOURCE: Developed by the National Center for Health Statistics in collaboration with the National Center for Chronic Disease Prevention and Health Promotion (2000).

CDC
SAFER • HEALTHIER • PEOPLE™

CDC Growth Charts: United States

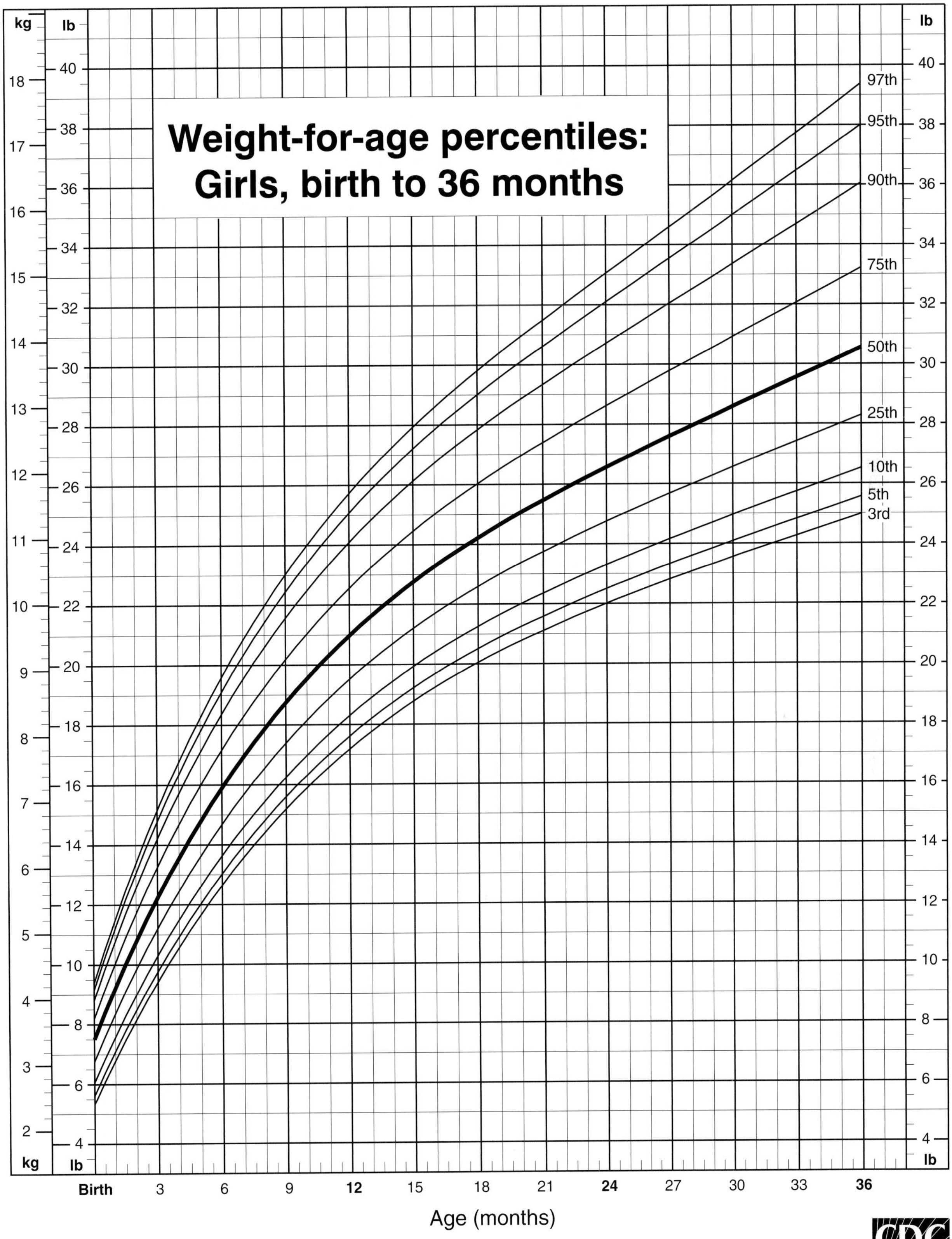
Weight-for-age percentiles:
Girls, birth to 36 months
kg
lb
97th
95th
90th
75th
50th
25th
10th
5th
3rd
18
17
16
15
14
13
12
11
10
9
8
7
6
5
4
3
2
40
38
36
34
32
30
28
26
24
22
20
18
16
14
12
10
8
6
4
Birth
3
6
9
12
15
18
21
24
27
30
33
36
Age (months)

Published May 30, 2000.

SOURCE: Developed by the National Center for Health Statistics in collaboration with the National Center for Chronic Disease Prevention and Health Promotion (2000).

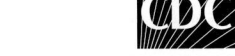

SAFER • HEALTHIER • PEOPLE™

CDC Growth Charts: United States

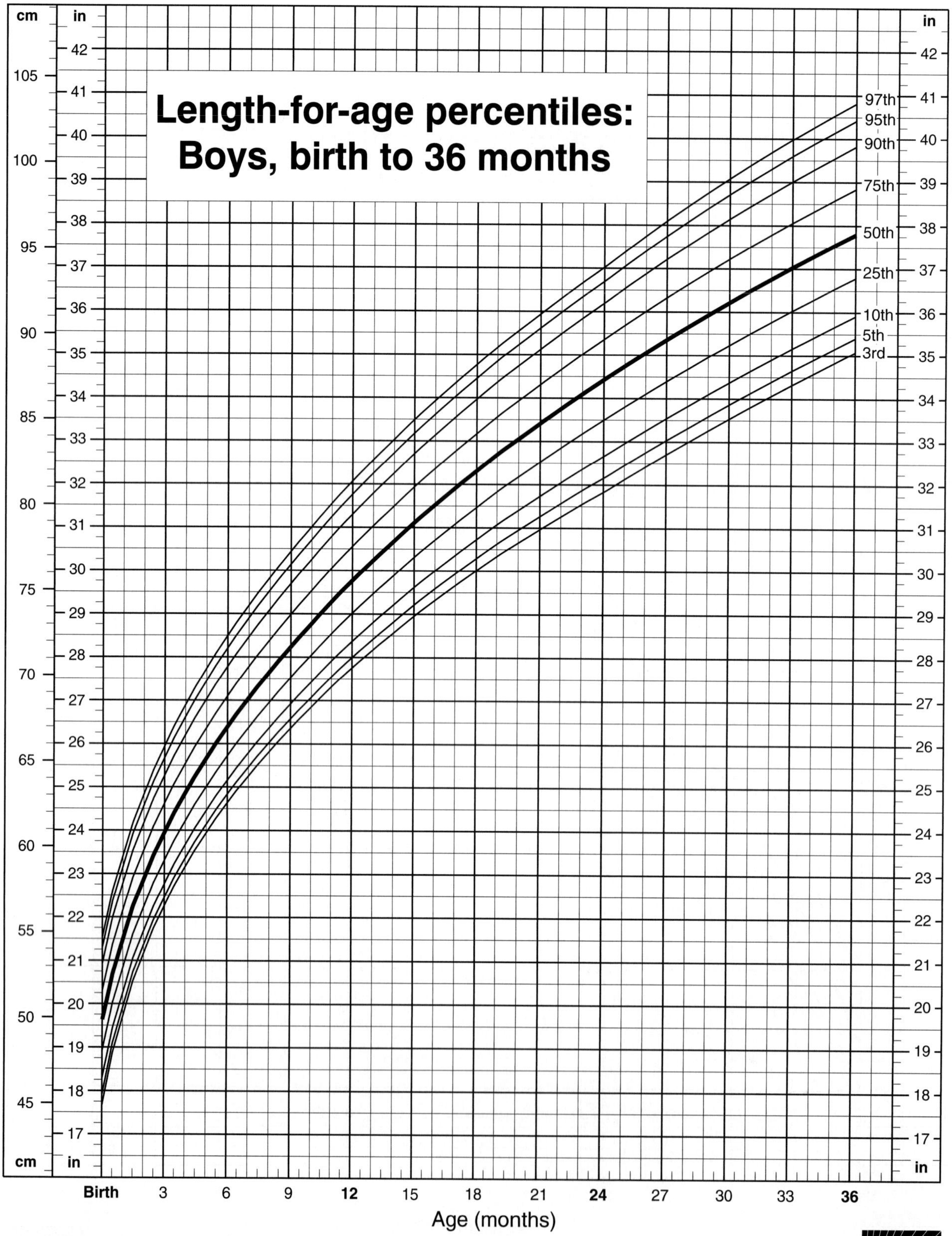
Length-for-age percentiles:
Boys, birth to 36 months
cm
in
97th
95th
90th
75th
50th
25th
10th
5th
3rd
Birth 3 6 9 12 15 18 21 24 27 30 33 36
Age (months)
SAFER • HEALTHIER • PEOPLE™

Published May 30, 2000.

SOURCE: Developed by the National Center for Health Statistics in collaboration with the National Center for Chronic Disease Prevention and Health Promotion (2000).

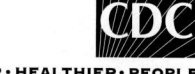

CDC Growth Charts: United States

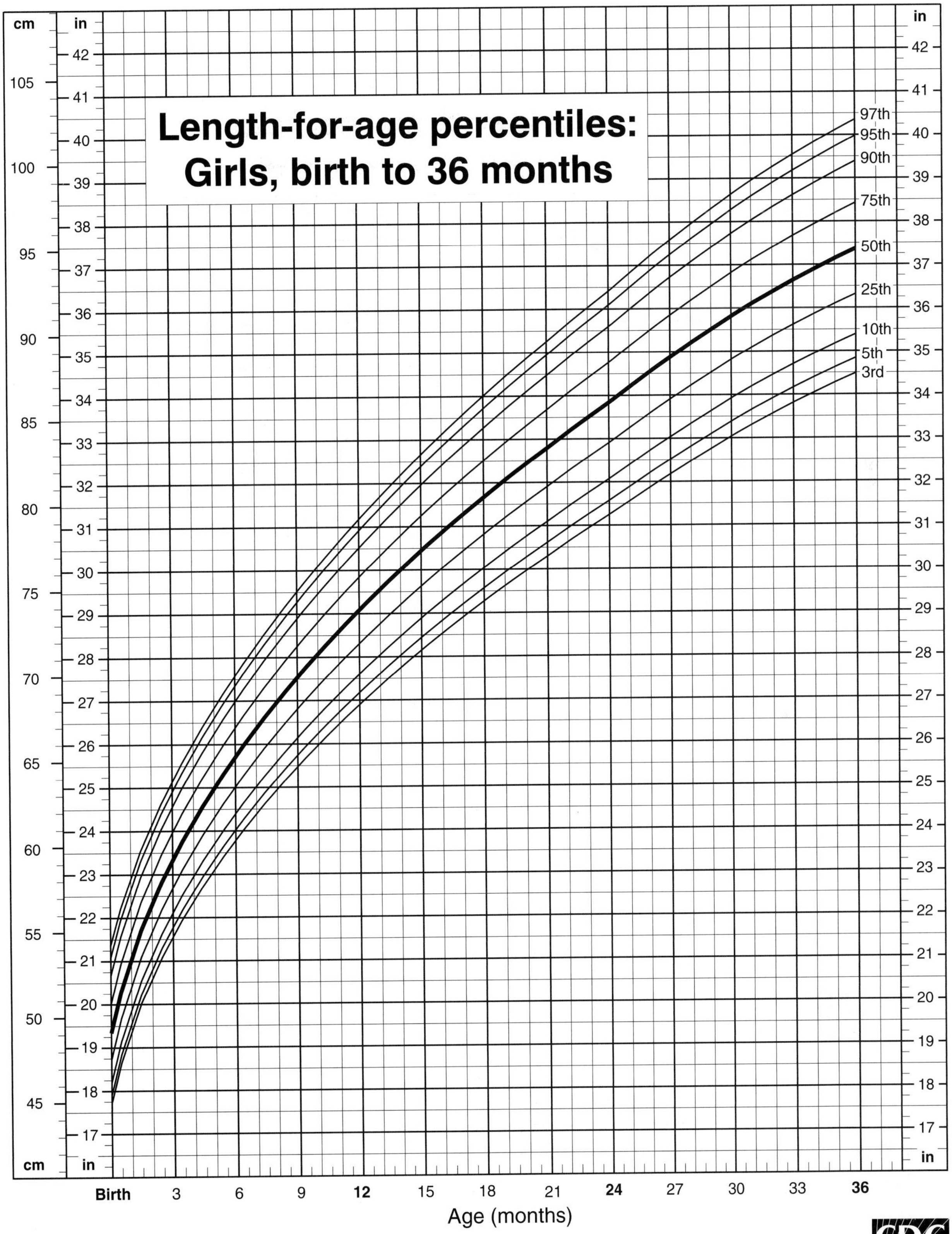

Length-for-age percentiles: Girls, birth to 36 months

97th
95th
90th
75th
50th
25th
10th
5th
3rd

Age (months)

Birth   3   6   9   12   15   18   21   24   27   30   33   36

Published May 30, 2000.
SOURCE: Developed by the National Center for Health Statistics in collaboration with
the National Center for Chronic Disease Prevention and Health Promotion (2000).

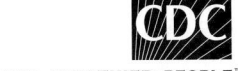

SAFER · HEALTHIER · PEOPLE™

CDC Growth Charts: United States

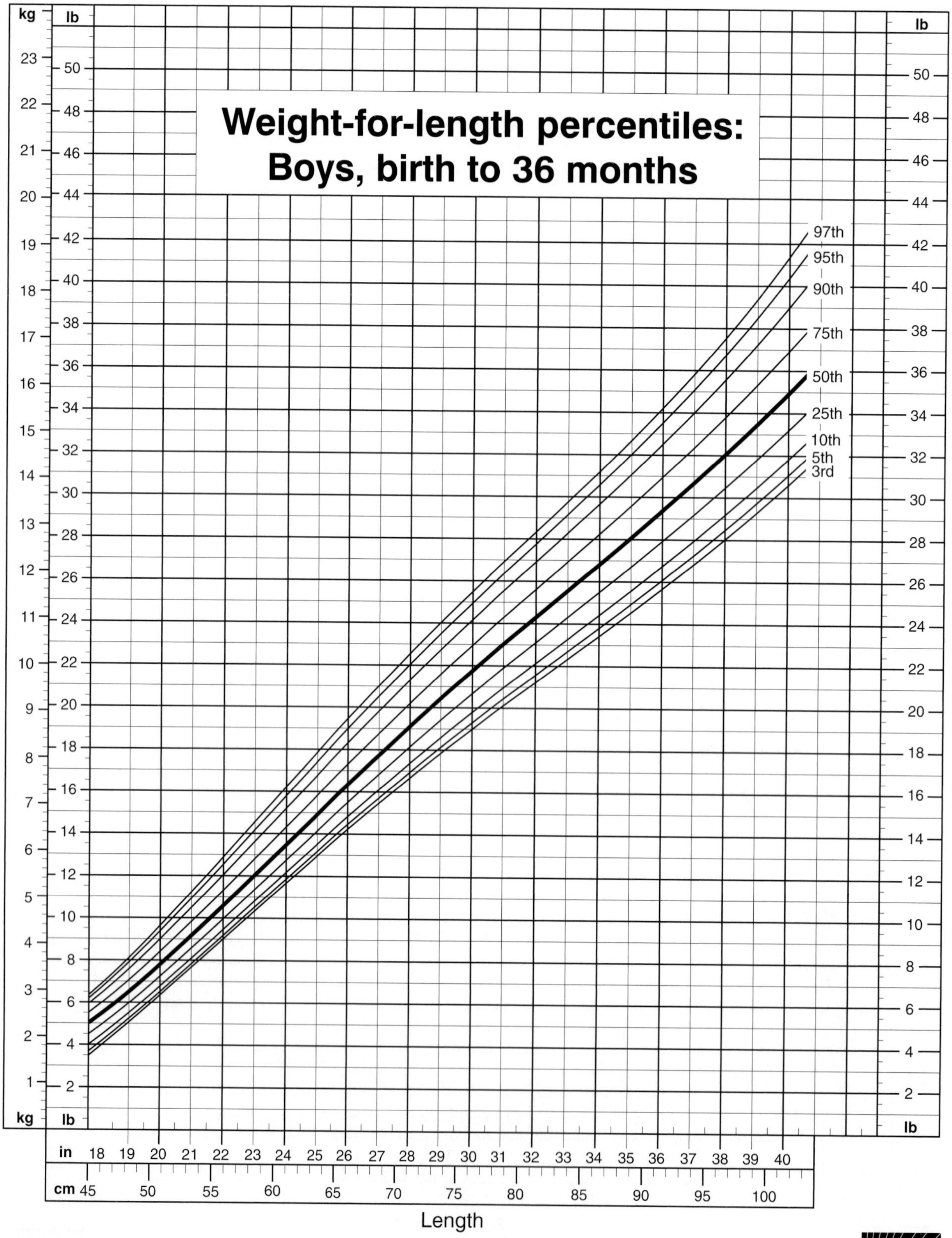
Weight-for-length percentiles:
Boys, birth to 36 months
kg
lb
97th
95th
90th
75th
50th
25th
10th
5th
3rd
in
cm
Length

Published May 30, 2000. (modified 6/8/00).
SOURCE: Developed by the National Center for Health Statistics in collaboration with the National Center for Chronic Disease Prevention and Health Promotion (2000).

CDC
SAFER • HEALTHIER • PEOPLE™

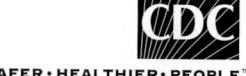

CDC Growth Charts: United States

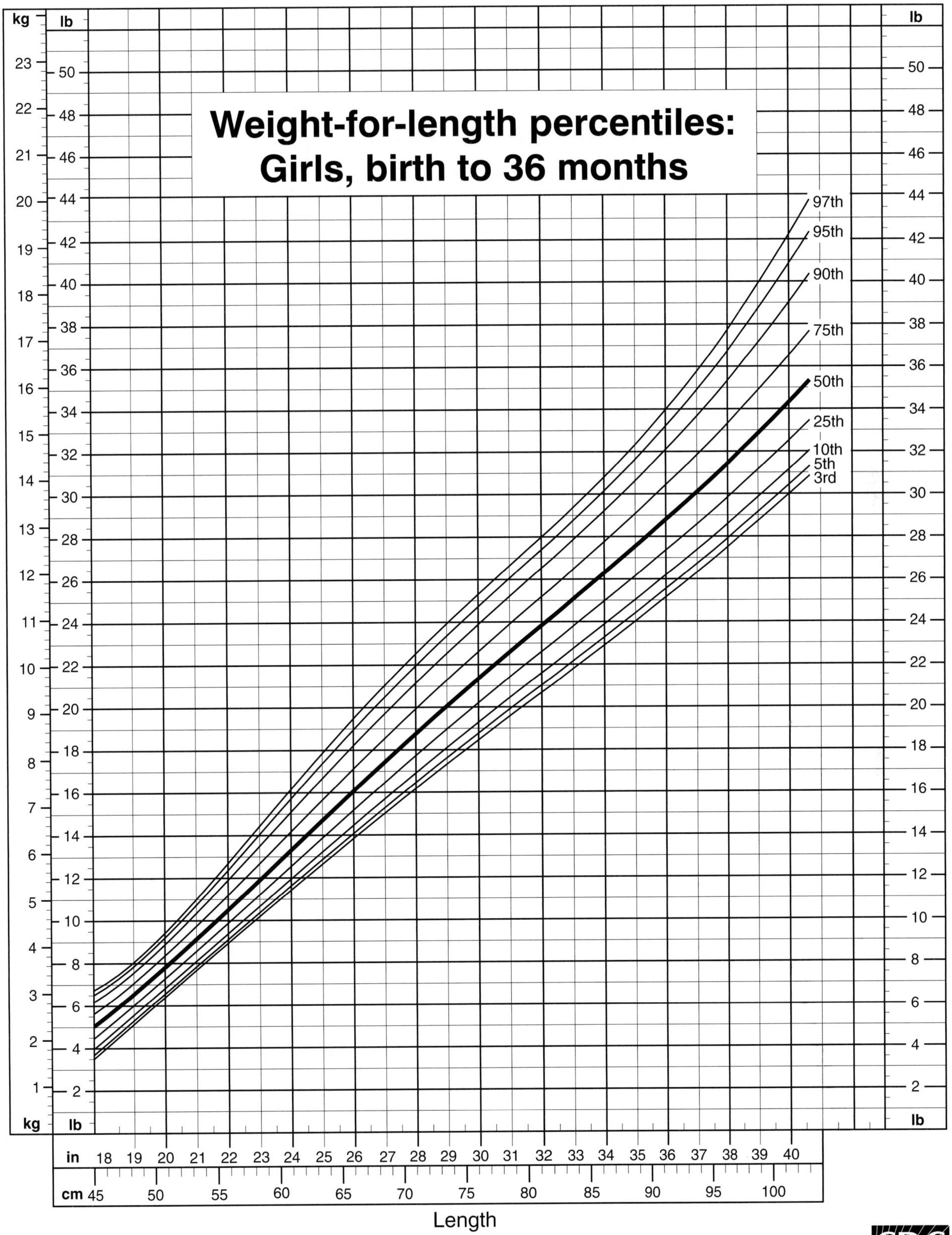
Weight-for-length percentiles:
Girls, birth to 36 months
kg
lb
97th
95th
90th
75th
50th
25th
10th
5th
3rd
in
cm
Length

Published May 30, 2000. (modified 6/8/00).
SOURCE: Developed by the National Center for Health Statistics in collaboration with
the National Center for Chronic Disease Prevention and Health Promotion (2000).

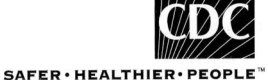

SAFER • HEALTHIER • PEOPLE™

CDC Growth Charts: United States

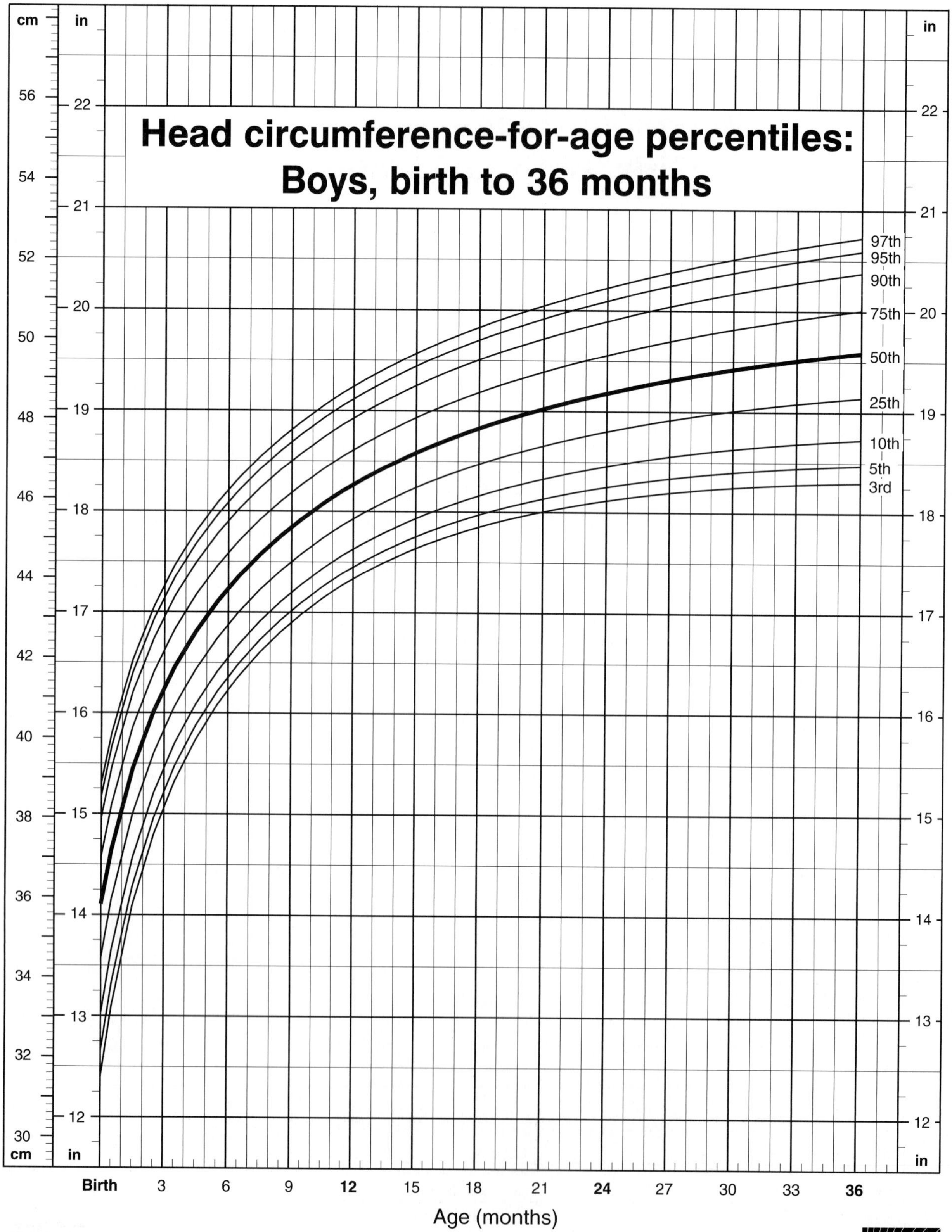
Head circumference-for-age percentiles:
Boys, birth to 36 months
cm
in
97th
95th
90th
75th
50th
25th
10th
5th
3rd
Birth
3
6
9
12
15
18
21
24
27
30
33
36
Age (months)

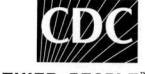

Published May 30, 2000.

SOURCE: Developed by the National Center for Health Statistics in collaboration with the National Center for Chronic Disease Prevention and Health Promotion (2000).

SAFER • HEALTHIER • PEOPLE™

CDC Growth Charts: United States

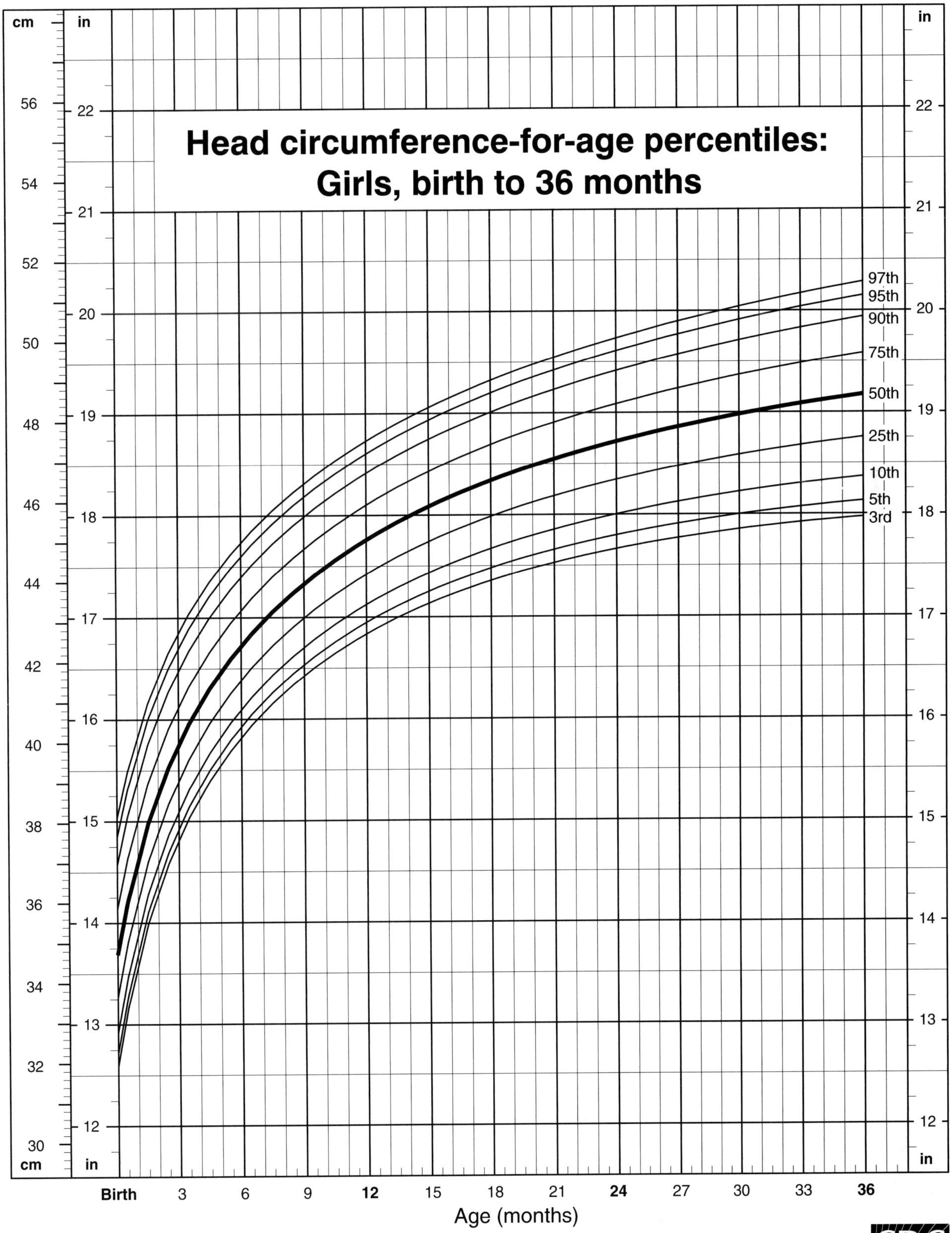

Head circumference-for-age percentiles: Girls, birth to 36 months

97th
95th
90th
75th
50th
25th
10th
5th
3rd

Age (months)

Birth 3 6 9 12 15 18 21 24 27 30 33 36

Published May 30, 2000.
SOURCE: Developed by the National Center for Health Statistics in collaboration with
the National Center for Chronic Disease Prevention and Health Promotion (2000).

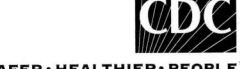

SAFER · HEALTHIER · PEOPLE™

CDC Growth Charts: United States

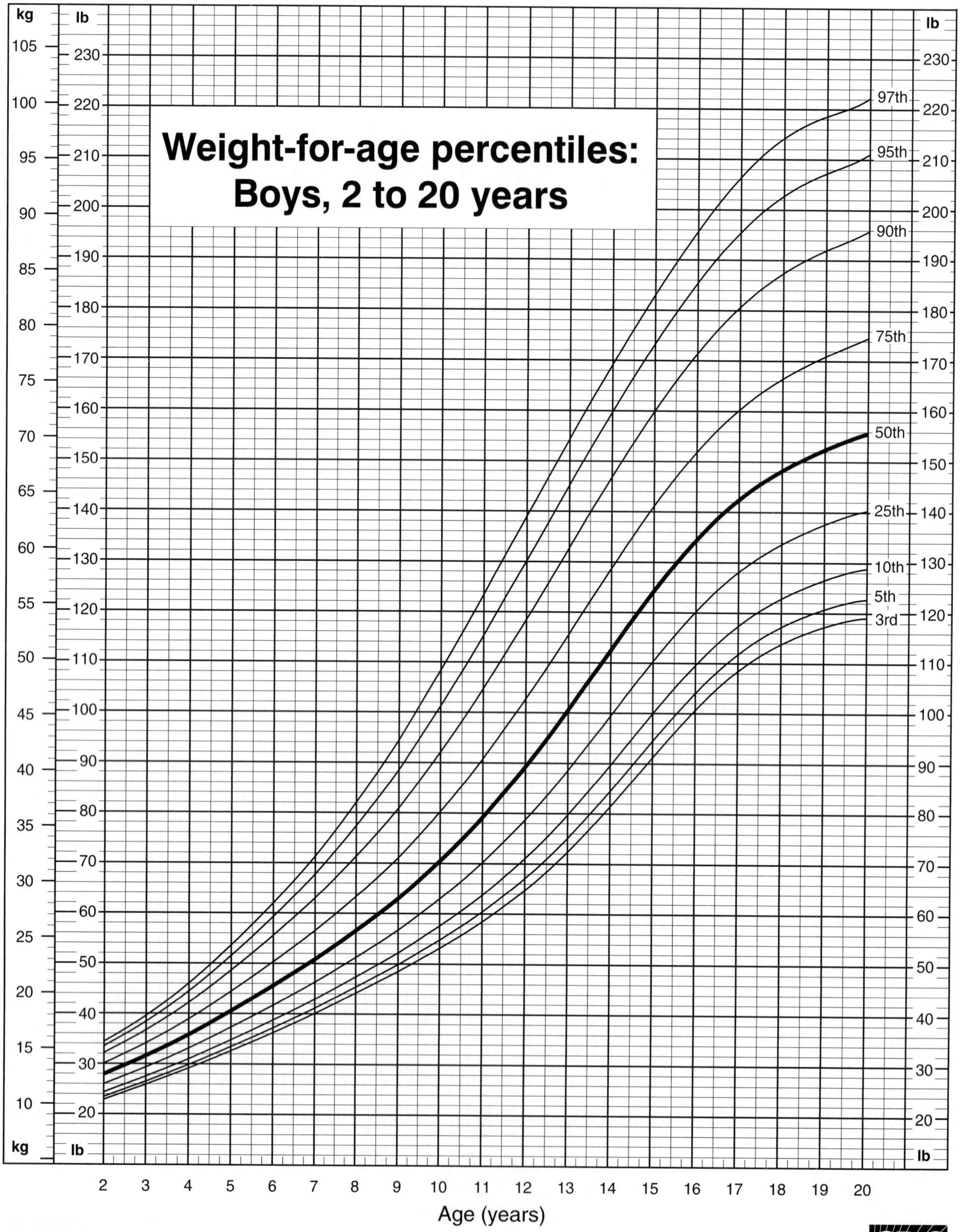

Weight-for-age percentiles: Boys, 2 to 20 years

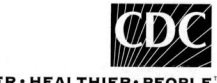

Published May 30, 2000.
SOURCE: Developed by the National Center for Health Statistics in collaboration with
the National Center for Chronic Disease Prevention and Health Promotion (2000).

CDC Growth Charts: United States

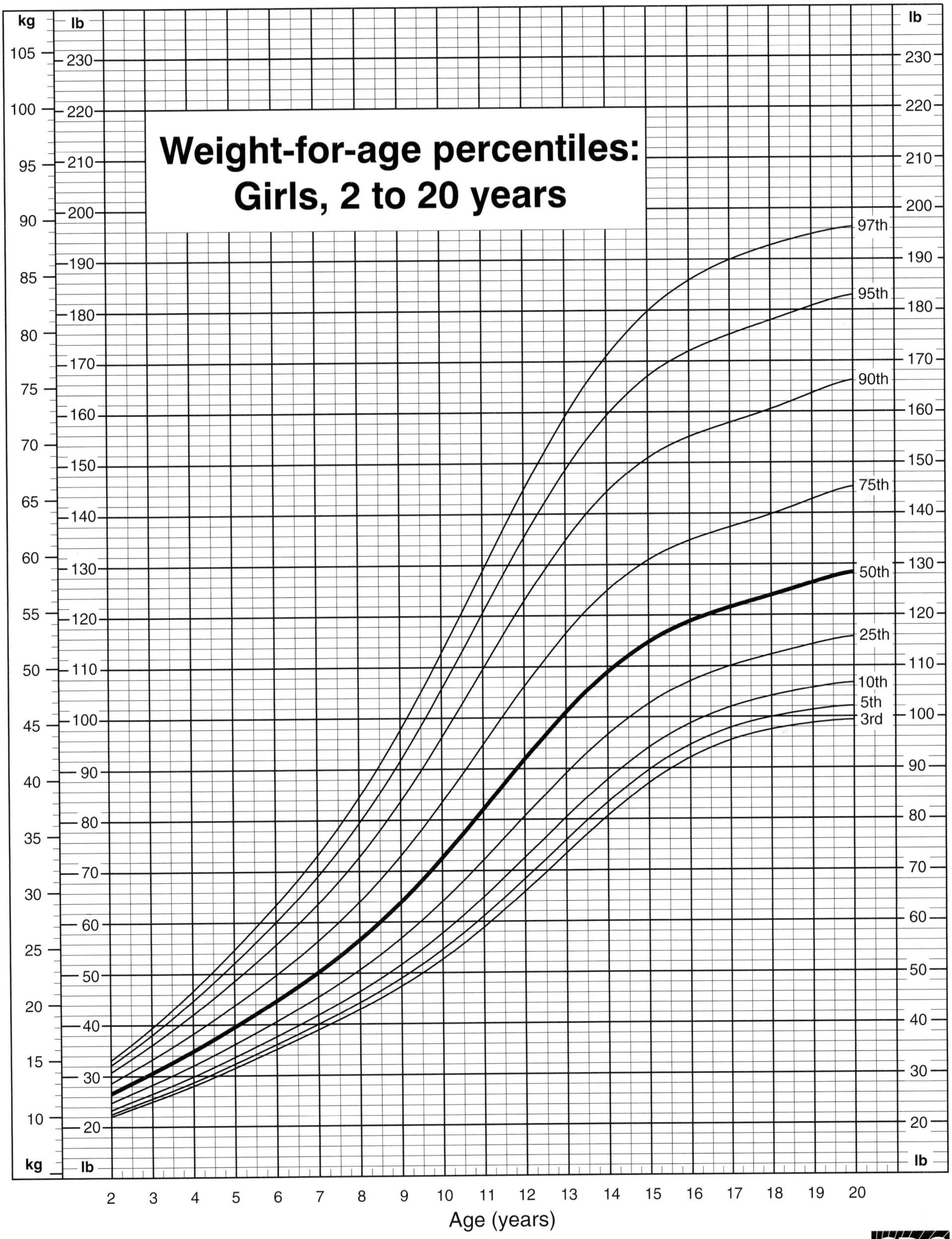

**Weight-for-age percentiles:
Girls, 2 to 20 years**

97th
95th
90th
75th
50th
25th
10th
5th
3rd

Age (years)

Published May 30, 2000.
SOURCE: Developed by the National Center for Health Statistics in collaboration with
the National Center for Chronic Disease Prevention and Health Promotion (2000).

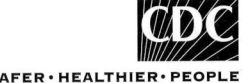

SAFER·HEALTHIER·PEOPLE™

CDC Growth Charts: United States

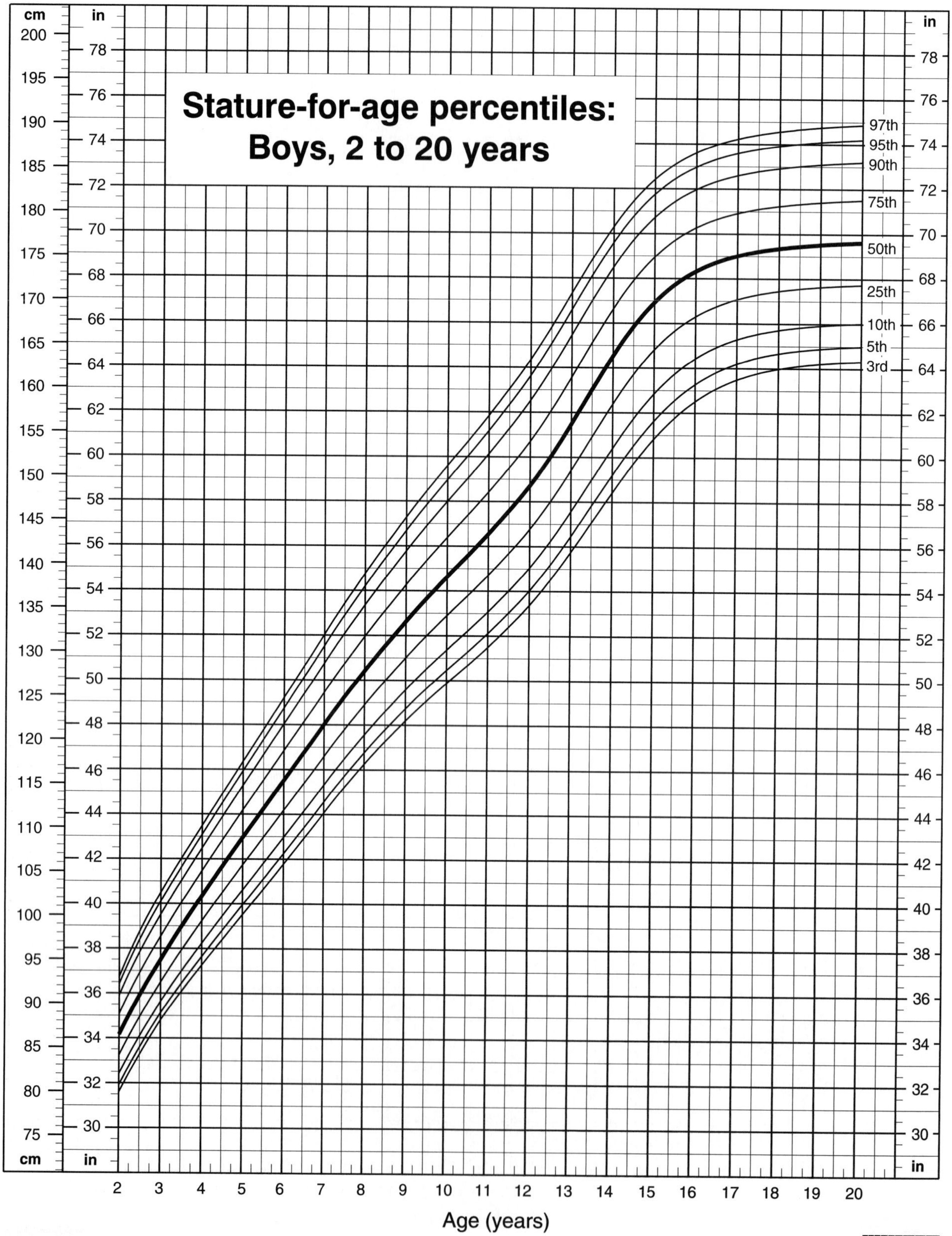

**Stature-for-age percentiles:
Boys, 2 to 20 years**

[Chart with axes: cm (75–200) and in (30–78) on vertical axis; Age (years) 2–20 on horizontal axis. Percentile curves labeled 97th, 95th, 90th, 75th, 50th, 25th, 10th, 5th, 3rd.]

Age (years)

Published May 30, 2000.
SOURCE: Developed by the National Center for Health Statistics in collaboration with
the National Center for Chronic Disease Prevention and Health Promotion (2000).

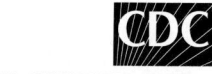

SAFER·HEALTHIER·PEOPLE™

CDC Growth Charts: United States

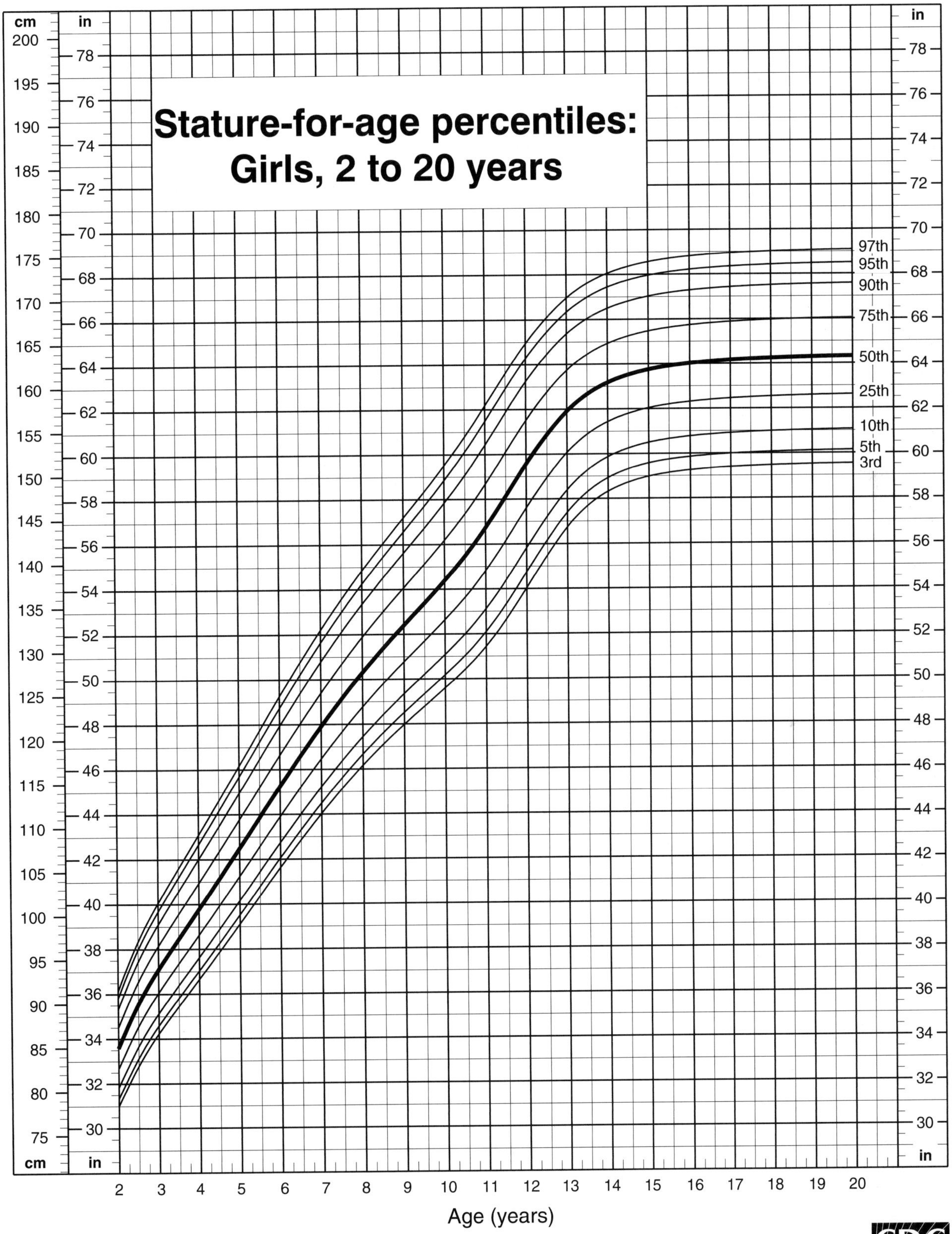

Stature-for-age percentiles: Girls, 2 to 20 years

Age (years)

Published May 30, 2000.
SOURCE: Developed by the National Center for Health Statistics in collaboration with
the National Center for Chronic Disease Prevention and Health Promotion (2000).

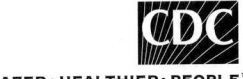

SAFER · HEALTHIER · PEOPLE™

CDC Growth Charts: United States

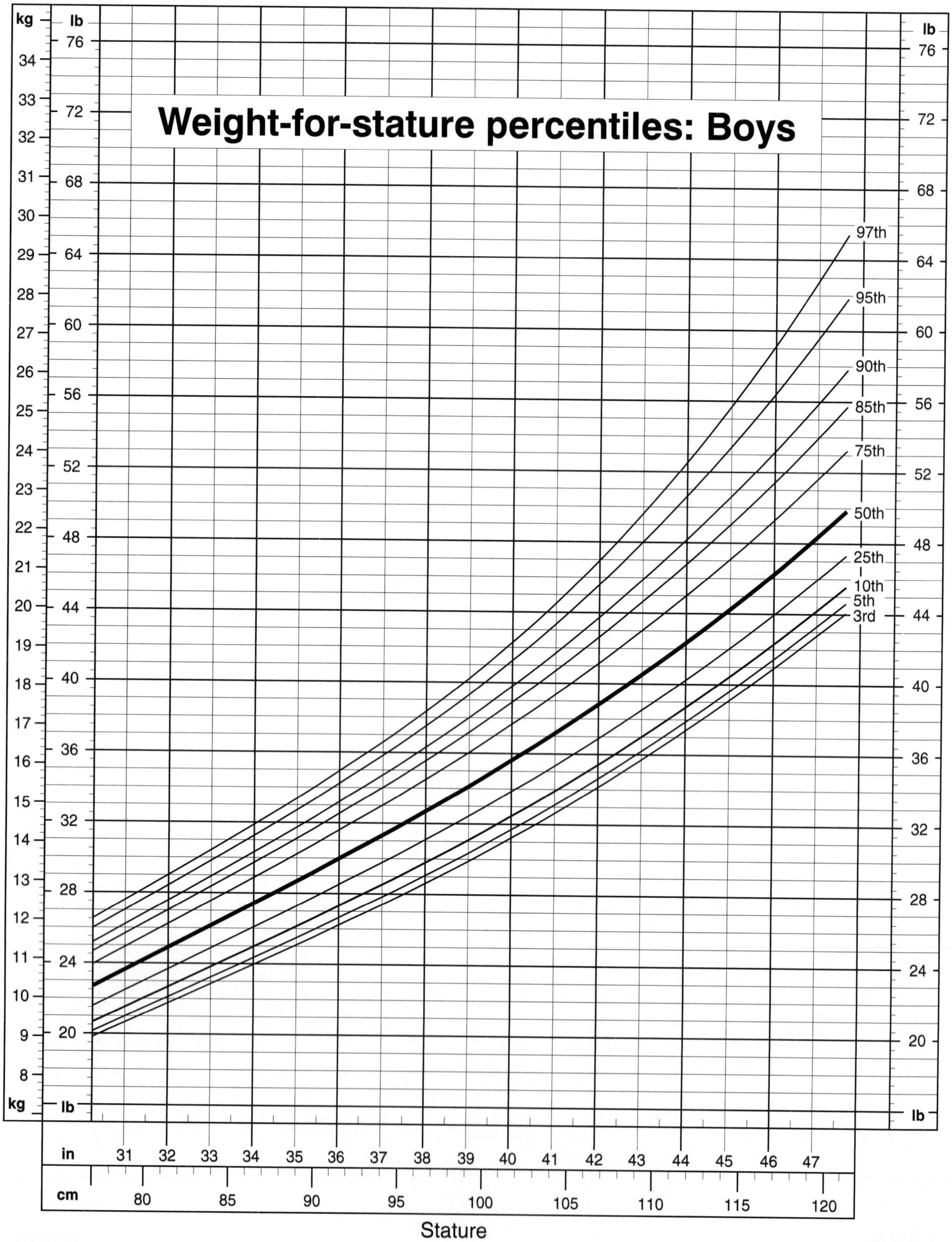

Weight-for-stature percentiles: Boys

Stature

Published May 30, 2000. (modified 11/21/00).
SOURCE: Developed by the National Center for Health Statistics in collaboration with
the National Center for Chronic Disease Prevention and Health Promotion (2000).

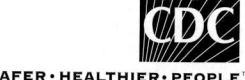

SAFER·HEALTHIER·PEOPLE™

CDC Growth Charts: United States

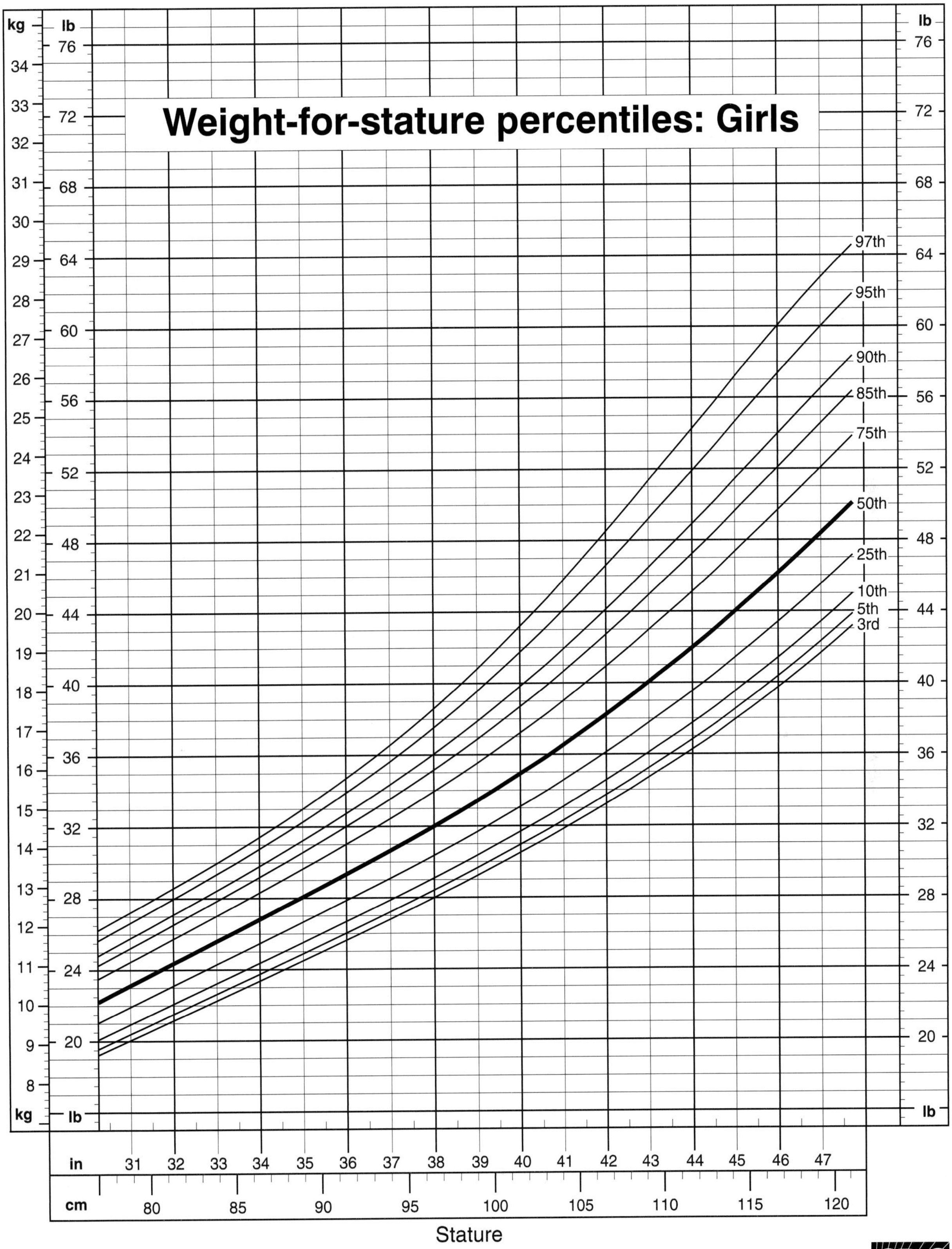
Weight-for-stature percentiles: Girls
kg
lb
97th
95th
90th
85th
75th
50th
25th
10th
5th
3rd
in
cm
Stature

Published May 30, 2000. (modified 11/21/00).
SOURCE: Developed by the National Center for Health Statistics in collaboration with the National Center for Chronic Disease Prevention and Health Promotion (2000).

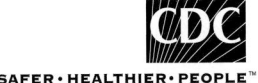

SAFER • HEALTHIER • PEOPLE™

CDC Growth Charts: United States

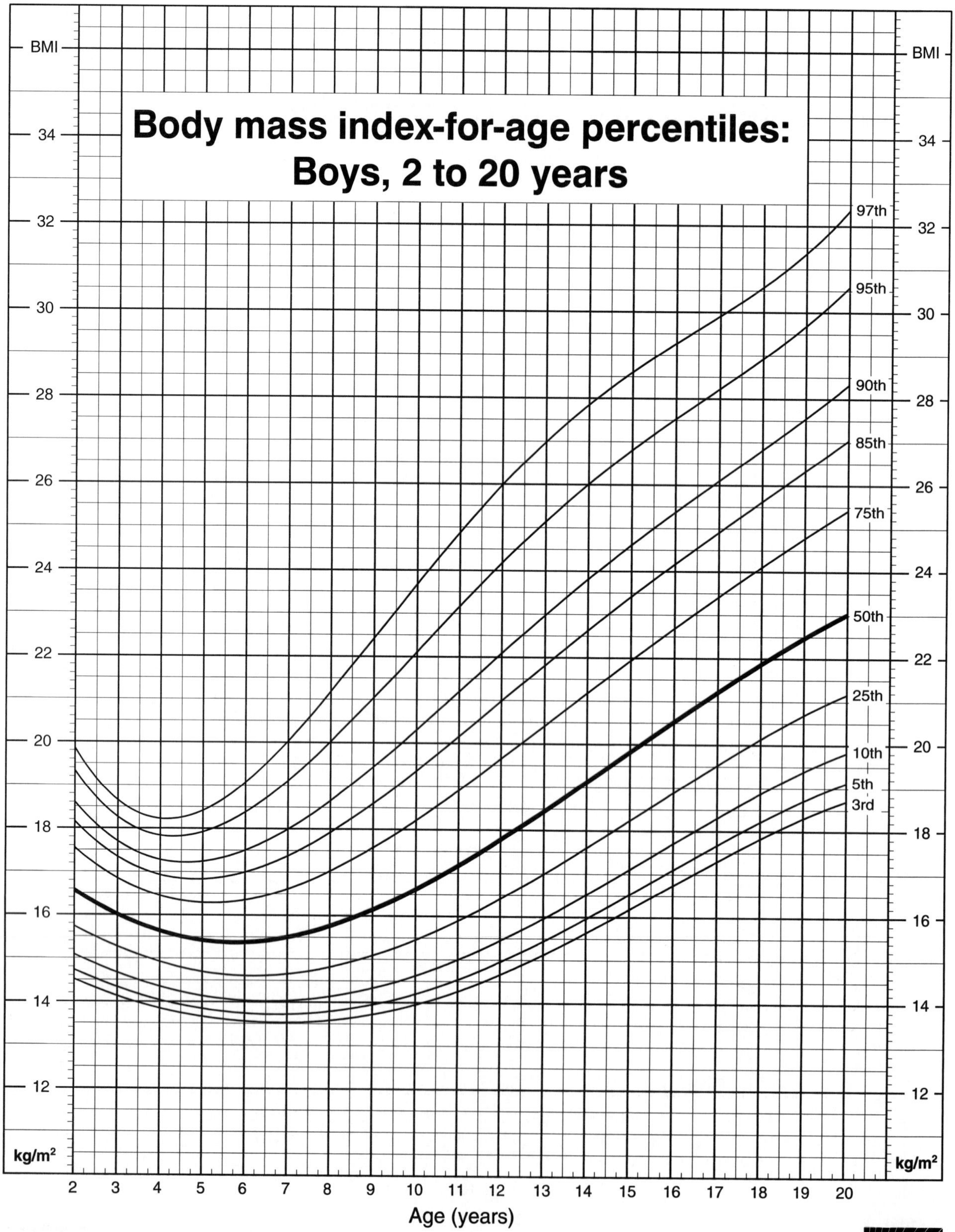

Body mass index-for-age percentiles: Boys, 2 to 20 years

BMI

— 34 —

— 32 —

— 30 —

— 28 —

— 26 —

— 24 —

— 22 —

— 20 —

— 18 —

— 16 —

— 14 —

— 12 —

kg/m²

Age (years)

2 3 4 5 6 7 8 9 10 11 12 13 14 15 16 17 18 19 20

97th
95th
90th
85th
75th
50th
25th
10th
5th
3rd

Published May 30, 2000.
SOURCE: Developed by the National Center for Health Statistics in collaboration with the National Center for Chronic Disease Prevention and Health Promotion (2000).

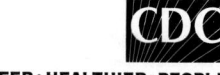

SAFER · HEALTHIER · PEOPLE™

CDC Growth Charts: United States

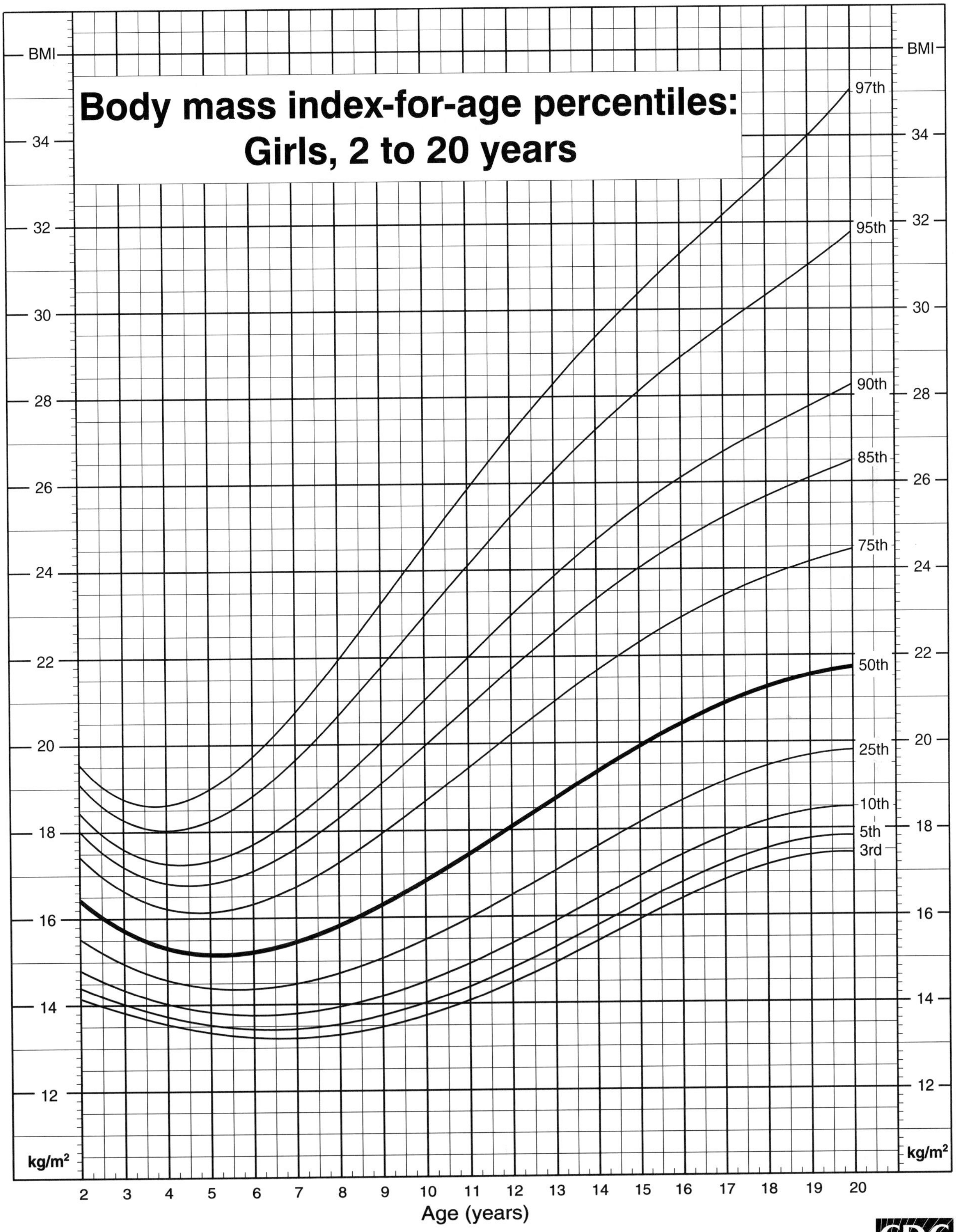
Body mass index-for-age percentiles:
Girls, 2 to 20 years
BMI
kg/m²
34
32
30
28
26
24
22
20
18
16
14
12
97th
95th
90th
85th
75th
50th
25th
10th
5th
3rd
2 3 4 5 6 7 8 9 10 11 12 13 14 15 16 17 18 19 20
Age (years)

Published May 30, 2000.

SOURCE: Developed by the National Center for Health Statistics in collaboration with the National Center for Chronic Disease Prevention and Health Promotion (2000).

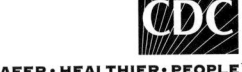

SAFER • HEALTHIER • PEOPLE™

Foods Recommended for Hospital Diet Progressions*

Food Category	Clear Liquid	Full Liquid
Soups	Broth or bouillon	Broth or bouillon; regular or high-protein consomme; strained vegetable, meat, or cream soups containing finely homogenized meat
Beverages	Coffee, tea, decaffeinated coffee, carbonated beverages as tolerated	Coffee, tea, decaffeinated coffee, carbonated beverages as tolerated, eggnogs, instant breakfast beverages, yogurt drinks, fruit-flavored drinks
Meat and meat substitutes	None	Clean, fresh eggs cooked to a liquid consistency or in custards; egg substitutes; pasteurized eggs used in eggnogs or cooking; salmonella-free frozen eggs
Fats	None	Butter, margarine, cream, cream substitute
Milk	None	Milk and milk beverages; plain or flavored yogurt without seeds, nuts, or fruit pieces; cocoa
Starches	None	Refined cooked cereals, strained whole-grain cereals, high-protein cereals; mashed white potato diluted in cream soups
Vegetables	None	Vegetable juice and vegetable purées that are strained and diluted in cream soups

Reference: *American Dietetic Association: Manual of clinical dietetics, ed 6, Chicago, 2000, ADA.*

*Any foods not listed should be excluded from the diet.

Puréed	Mechanical Soft	Soft	Regular
Broth or bouillon, consomme, strained or blenderized cream soup	Soups made with allowed foods	Soups made with allowed foods	All
All	All	All	All
Strained or puréed meat or poultry, cottage cheese, cooked scrambled eggs and egg substitutes puréed as tolerated	Ground or finely diced, moist (gravy or sauces) meats and poultry; flaked fish without bones; eggs; cottage cheese; cheese; creamy peanut butter; soft casseroles	Moist, tender meat, fish, or poultry; eggs; cottage cheese; milk-flavored cheese; creamy peanut butter; soft casseroles	All
Butter, margarine, cream, cream substitute, oil, gravy, white sauce, whipped cream, whipped topping	Butter, margarine, cream, cream substitute, oil, gravy, salad dressing, whipped cream, whipped toppings	Butter, margarine, cream, cream substitute, oil, gravy, salad dressing, whipped cream, whipped toppings, crisp bacon	All
Milk and milk beverages; plain or flavored yogurt without seeds, nuts, or fruit pieces; cocoa	Milk and milk beverages, plain or flavored yogurt without seeds or nuts, cocoa	All	All
Refined cooked cereals; mashed potatoes; puréed rice or noodles thinned with sauce or gravy; soft, crustless bread puréed with milk or other liquid if tolerated; bread crumbs may be added to soups, casseroles, and vegetables	Cooked or refined ready-to-eat cereals; potatoes; rice; pasta; white, refined wheat, or light rye breads or rolls; graham crackers as tolerated; pan-cakes; soft waffles; muffins; plain crackers	Cooked or refined ready-to-eat cereals; potatoes; rice; pasta; white, refined wheat, or light rye breads or rolls; graham crackers as tolerated; pan-cakes; soft waffles; muffins; plain crackers	All
Vegetable juice and strained or puréed vegetables	Soft, cooked vegetables without hulls or tough skin (peas and corn); juices	Soft, cooked vegetables; lettuce and tomatoes; limit gasform-ing vegetables and whole kernel corn	All

Continued

Food Category	Clear Liquid	Full Liquid
Fruits	Clear fruit juices (apple, cranberry, grape) or strained fruit juices	Fruit juices, nectars
Desserts	Flavored gelatin, high-protein gelatin, Popsicles and fruit ices	Flavored gelatin, puddings, high-protein puddings, custard, regular and high-protein gelatin desserts, plain ice cream, frozen yogurt, sherbet, fruit ices, Popsicles
Sweets	Sugar, honey, hard candy, sugar substitute	Sugar, honey, hard candy, sugar substitute, syrup
Miscellaneous	Salt	Salt, pepper, flavorings, chocolate syrup, cinnamon, nutmeg, brewer's yeast
Supplements	High-protein, high-kcalorie, low-residue oral supplements; Polycose	Liquid commercially prepared nutritional supplements, Polycose

Modified from American Dietetic Association: Manual of clinical dietetics, ed 6, Chicago, 2000, ADA.

Puréed	Mechanical Soft	Soft	Regular
Strained or puréed fruit, fruit juice, nectars	Cooked or canned fruit without seeds or skins, banana, fruit juice, nectars, citrus fruit without membrane	Cooked or canned fruit, soft fresh fruit, fruit juice, nectars	All
Flavored gelatin; puddings; custard; plain ice cream without seeds, nuts, or fruit pieces; sherbet; frozen yogurt; fruit ices; Popsicles	Flavored gelatin; puddings; custard; plain ice cream without seeds, nuts, or fruit; sherbet; frozen yogurt; fruit ices; Popsicles	Flavored gelatin, puddings, custard, ice cream without nuts, sherbet, frozen yogurt, fruit ices, Popsicles, cake, cookies without nuts or coconut	All
Sugar, honey, hard candy, sugar substitute, syrup, jelly	Sugar, honey, hard candy, sugar substitute, syrup, jelly	Sugar, honey, candy without nuts or coconut, sugar substitute, syrup, plain chocolate candies, molasses, marshmallows	All
Salt, pepper, flavorings, ground spices, smooth condiments	Salt, pepper, flavorings, ground spices, smooth condiments	Salt, pepper, flavorings, mildly seasoned condiments, herbs, spices, ketchup, mustard, vinegar in moderation	All
Liquid commercially prepared nutritional supplements, Polycose	Liquid commercially prepared nutritional supplements, Polycose	All	All

APPENDIX *I*

Complementary and Alternative Medicine Domains and Therapies

WHAT ARE THE MAJOR TYPES OF COMPLEMENTARY AND ALTERNATIVE MEDICINE?

The National Center for Complementary and Alternative Medicine (NCCAM), a component of the National Institutes of Health, classifies therapies of complementary and alternative medicine (CAM) into five categories, or domains:

1. Alternative Medical Systems

Alternative medical systems are built on complete systems of theory and practice. Often, these systems have evolved apart from and earlier than the conventional medical approach used in the United States. Examples of alternative medical systems that have developed in Western cultures include homeopathic medicine and naturopathic medicine. Examples of systems that have developed in non-Western cultures include traditional Chinese medicine and Ayurveda.

2. Mind-Body Interventions

Mind-body medicine uses a variety of techniques designed to enhance the mind's capacity to affect bodily function and symptoms. Some techniques that were considered CAM in the past have become mainstream (e.g., patient support groups and cognitive-behavioral therapy). Other mind-body techniques are still considered CAM, including meditation, prayer, mental healing, and therapies that use creative outlets such as art, music, or dance.

3. Biologically Based Therapies

Biologically based therapies in CAM use substances found in nature, such as herbs, foods, and vitamins. Some examples include dietary supplements, herbal products, and the use of other so-called "natural" but as yet scientifically unproven therapies (e.g., using shark cartilage to treat cancer).

4. Manipulative and Body-Based Methods

Manipulative and body-based methods in CAM are based on manipulation or movement of one or more parts of the body. Some examples include chiropractic or osteopathic manipulation and massage.

5. Energy Therapies

Energy therapies involve the use of energy fields. They are of two types:

Biofield therapies are intended to affect energy fields that purportedly surround and penetrate the human body. The existence of such fields has not yet been scientifically proven. Some forms of energy therapy ma-

---

NOTES

[1]Conventional medicine is medicine as practiced by holders of M.D. (medical doctor) or D.O. (doctor of osteopathy) degrees and by their allied health professionals, such as physical therapists, psychologists, and registered nurses. Other terms for conventional medicine include allopathy; Western, mainstream, orthodox, and regular medicine; and biomedicine. Some conventional medical practitioners are also practitioners of CAM.

[2]Other terms for CAM include *unconventional, nonconventional, unproven,* and *irregular medicine* or *healthcare.*

[3]Some uses of dietary supplements have been incorporated into conventional medicine. For example, scientists have found that folic acid prevents certain birth defects, and a regimen of vitamins and zinc can slow the progression of an eye disease called *age-related macular degeneration (AMD).*

nipulate biofields by applying pressure or manipulating the body by placing the hands in, or through, these fields. Examples include Qi gong, reiki, and therapeutic touch.

Bioelectromagnetic-based therapies involve the unconventional use of electromagnetic fields, such as pulsed fields, magnetic fields, or alternating current or direct current fields.

Resources

For more information on CAM or NCCAM, contact:
NCCAM Clearinghouse
P.O. Box 7923
Gaithersburg, MD 20898-7923
Toll free: (888) 644-6226
International: (301) 519-3153
TTY (for deaf or hearing-impaired callers):
    (866) 464-3615
FAX: (866) 464-3616
FAX-on-Demand Service: (888) 644-6226
E-mail: info@nccam.nih.gov
Web site: nccam.nih.gov

For more information on dietary supplements, contact:
Office of Dietary Supplements
National Institutes of Health
Web site: ods.od.nih.gov

Center for Food Safety and Nutrition
U.S. Food and Drug Administration
5100 Paint Branch Parkway
College Park, MD 20740-3835
Web site: vm.cfsan.fda.gov

APPENDIX *J*

National Renal Diet

Milk Choices	Per Day
Average per choice: 4 grams protein, 120 kcalories, 80 mg sodium, 100 mg phosphorus	
Milk (fat-free, low-fat, whole)	½ cup
Lo Pro	1 cup
Buttermilk, cultured	½ cup
Chocolate milk	½ cup
Light cream or half and half	½ cup
Ice milk or ice cream	½ cup
Yogurt, plain or fruit-flavored	½ cup
Evaporated milk	¼ cup
Sweetened condensed milk	¼ cup
Cream cheese	3 Tbsp
Sour cream	4 Tbsp
Sherbet	1 cup

Nondairy Milk Substitutes	Per Day
Average per choice: 0.5 gram protein, 140 kcalories, 40 mg sodium, 30 mg phosphorus	
Dessert, nondairy frozen	½ cup
Dessert topping, nondairy frozen	½ cup
Liquid nondairy creamer, polyunsaturated	½ cup

From American Dietetic Association: *National renal diet: professional guide,* Chicago, 1993, American Dietetic Association.

Meat Choices	Per Day
Average per choice: 7 grams protein, 65 kcalories, 25 mg sodium, 65 mg phosphorus	
Prepared without added salt	
Beef	
Round, sirloin, flank, cubed, T-bone, and porterhouse steak; tenderloin, rib, chuck, and rump roast; ground beef or ground chuck	1 oz
Pork	
Fresh ham, tenderloin, chops, loin roast, cutlets	1 oz
Lamb	
Chops, leg, roasts	1 oz
Veal	
Chops, roasts, cutlets	1 oz
Poultry	
Chicken, turkey, Cornish hen, domestic duck and goose	1 oz
Fish	
Fresh and frozen fish	1 oz
Lobster, scallops, shrimp, clams	1 oz
Crab, oysters	1½ oz
Canned tuna, canned salmon (canned without salt)	1 oz
Sardines (canned without salt) ✦	1 oz
Wild game	
Venison, rabbit, squirrel, pheasant, duck, goose	1 oz
Egg	
Whole	1 large
Egg white or yolk	2 large
Low-cholesterol egg product	¼ cup
Chitterlings	2 oz
Organ meats ✦	1 oz
Prepared with added salt	
Beef	
Deli-style roast beef ✏	1 oz
Pork	
Boiled or deli-style ham ✏	1 oz
Poultry	
Deli-style chicken or turkey ✏	1 oz
Fish	
Canned tuna, canned salmon ✏	1 oz
Sardines ✏ ✦	1 oz
Cheese	
Cottage ✏	¼ cup

✏ *High sodium—each serving counts as 1 starch choice and 1 salt choice.*
✦ *High phosphorus.*

The following are high in sodium, phosphorus, and/or saturated fat. They should be used in your diet only as advised by your dietitian.

- Bacon
- Black beans, black-eyed peas, great northern beans, lentils, lima beans, navy beans, pinto beans, red kidney beans, soybeans, split peas, turtle beans
- Frankfurters, bratwurst, Polish sausage
- Luncheon meats, including bologna, braunschweiger, liverwurst, picnic loaf, summer sausage, salami
- Nuts and nut butters
- All cheeses except cottage cheese

Starch Choices	Per Day
Average per choice: 2 grams protein, 90 kcalories, 80 mg sodium, 35 mg phosphorus	
Breads and rolls	
Bagel	½ small
Bread (French, Italian, raisin, light rye, sourdough, white)	1 slice (1 oz)
Bun, hamburger or hot dog type	½
Danish pastry or sweet roll, no nuts	½ small
Dinner roll or hard roll	1 small
Doughnut	1 small
English muffin	½
Muffin, no nuts, bran, or whole wheat	1 small (1 oz)
Pancake 🖊️ 🦴	1 small (1 oz)
Pita or "pocket" bread	½ 6-in diameter
Tortilla, corn	2 6-in diameter
Tortilla, flour	1 6-in diameter
Waffle 🖊️ 🦴	1 small (1 oz)
Cereals and grains prepared without added salt	
Cereals, ready-to-eat, most brands 🖊️	¾ cup
Puffed rice	2 cups
Puffed wheat	1 cup
Cereals, cooked	
Cream of Rice or Wheat, Farina, Malt-O-Meal	½ cup
Oat bran or oatmeal, Ralston	⅓ cup
Cornmeal, cooked	¾ cup
Grits, cooked	½ cup
Flour, all-purpose	2½ Tbsp
Pasta (noodles, macaroni, spaghetti), cooked	½ cup
Pasta made with egg (egg noodles), cooked	⅓ cup
Rice, white or brown, cooked	½ cup

🖊️ *High sodium—each serving counts as 1 starch choice and 1 salt choice.*
🦴 *High phosphorus.*

Starch Choices—cont'd	Per Day
Starchy vegetables **prepared or canned without added salt**	
Corn	⅓ cup or ½ ear
Green peas	¼ cup
Potatoes, baked, white, or sweet	1 small (3 oz)
Potatoes, boiled or mashed	½ cup
Potatoes, French fried	½ cup or 10 small
Potatoes, hashed brown	½ cup
Squash, butternut, mashed	½ cup
Squash, winter, baked (all other varieties), cubed	1 cup
Crackers and snacks	
Crackers: saltines, round butter	4 crackers
Graham crackers	3 squares
Melba toast	3 oblong
Popcorn, plain	1½ cup popped
Potato chips	1 oz, 14 chips
Pretzels, sticks or rings 🖋	¾ oz, 10 sticks
Pretzels, sticks or rings, unsalted	¾ oz, 10 sticks
RyKrisp 🖋	3 crackers
Tortilla chips	¾ oz, 9 chips
Desserts	
Cake	2 × 2-in square or 1½ oz
Cake, angel food	1/20 cake or 1 oz
Sandwich cookie 🖋 🦴	4 cookies
Shortbread cookie	4 cookies
Sugar cookie	4 cookies
Sugar wafer	4 cookies
Vanilla wafer	10 cookies
Fruit pie	⅛ pie
Sweetened gelatin	½ cup

🖋 High sodium—each serving counts as 1 starch choice and 1 salt choice.
🦴 High phosphorus.

The following foods are high in poor-quality protein and/or phosphorus. They should be used only when advised by your dietitian.
- Bran cereal or muffins, Grape-Nuts cereal, granola cereal or bars
- Boxed, frozen, or canned meals, entrees, or side dishes
- Black beans, black-eyed peas, great northern beans, lentils, lima beans, navy beans, pinto beans, red kidney beans, soybeans, split peas, turtle beans
- Pumpernickel, dark rye, whole wheat, or oatmeal bread
- Whole wheat cereals
- Whole wheat crackers

Vegetable Choices

See Starch Choices for other vegetables. Average per choice: 1 gram protein, 25 kcalories, 15 mg sodium, 20 mg phosphorus

Prepared or canned without added salt unless otherwise indicated

1-cup serving

Alfalfa sprouts
Cabbage
Celery
Cucumber (or ½ whole)

Eggplant
Endive

Escarole
Lettuce, all varieties
Pepper, green, sweet
Radishes, sliced
    (or 15 small)
Turnips
Watercress

½-cup serving

Artichoke
Bamboo shoots
Bean sprouts
Beans, green or wax
Beets
Carrots (or 1 small)
Cauliflower
Chard
Chinese cabbage

Collards
Kale
Kohlrabi

Mushrooms, fresh raw
    (or 4 medium)

Onions
Parsnips ✦
Pumpkin
Rutabagas ✦
Sauerkraut ✎ ✎ ✎
Squash, summer
Tomato (or 1 medium)
Tomato juice, unsalted
Tomato juice, canned
    with salt ✎ ✎
Tomato purée
Turnip greens
Vegetable juice
    cocktail, unsalted
Vegetable juice
    cocktail, canned
    with salt ✎ ✎

¼-cup serving

Asparagus (or 2 spears)

Avocado (¼ whole)
Beet greens
Broccoli
Brussels sprouts
Chili pepper

Mushrooms, fresh
    cooked
Mustard greens
Okra
Snow peas
Spinach
Tomato sauce

Prepared or canned with salt

Vegetables canned with salt (use serving size listed below) ✎

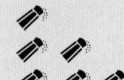 *High sodium—each serving counts as 1 starch choice and 1 salt choice.*
High sodium—each serving counts as 1 vegetable choice and 2 salt choices.
High sodium—each serving counts as 1 vegetable choice and 3 salt choices.
High phosphorus.

Fruit Choices

Average per choice: 0.5 gram protein, 70 kcalories, 15 mg phosphorus

1-cup serving

Apple (1 medium)

Apple juice

Applesauce

Cranberries

Cranberry juice cocktail

Papaya nectar

Peach nectar

Pear nectar

Pear, canned or fresh (1 medium)

Tangerine (1 medium)

½-cup serving

Apricot nectar

Banana (½ small)

Blueberries

Figs, canned

Fruit cocktail

Grapes (15 small)

Grape juice

Grapefruit (½ medium)

Grapefruit juice

Gooseberries

Kiwifruit (½ medium)

Lemon (½ medium)

Lemon juice

Mango (½ medium)

Nectarine (½ medium)

Orange (½ medium)

Peach, canned or fresh (½ medium)

Pineapple

Plums, canned or fresh (1 medium)

Rhubarb

Strawberries

Watermelon

¼-cup serving

Apricots (2 halves)

Apricots, dried (2)

Blackberries

Cantaloupe (⅛ small)

Cherries

Dates (2 Tbsp)

Figs, dried (1 whole)

Honeydew melon (⅛ small)

Orange juice

Papaya (¼ medium)

Prune juice

Prunes, cooked (5)

Raisins (2 Tbsp)

Raspberries

Fat Choices

Average per choice: trace protein, 45 kcalories, 55 mg sodium, 5 mg phosphorus

Unsaturated fats

Margarine	1 tsp
Reduced-calorie margarine	1 Tbsp
Mayonnaise	1 tsp

Continued

Fat Choices-cont'd

Unsaturated fats-cont'd

Low-calorie mayonnaise	1 Tbsp
Oil (safflower, sunflower, corn, soybean, olive, peanut, canola)	1 tsp
Salad dressing (mayonnaise-type)	2 tsp
Salad dressing (oil-type)	1 Tbsp
Low-calorie salad dressing (mayonnaise-type)	2 Tbsp
Low-calorie salad dressing (oil-type) ✏	2 Tbsp
Tartar sauce	1½ tsp

Saturated fats

Butter	1 tsp
Coconut	2 Tbsp
Powdered coffee whitener	1 Tbsp
Solid shortening	1 tsp

✏ *High sodium—each serving counts as 1 starch choice and 1 salt choice.*

High-Calorie Choices

Average per choice: trace protein, 100 kcalories, 15 mg sodium, 5 mg phosphorus

Beverages

Carbonated beverages (fruit flavors, root beer; colas or pepper-type) 🦴	1 cup
Cranberry juice cocktail	1 cup
Fruit-flavored drink	1 cup
Kool-Aid	1 cup
Lemonade	1 cup
Limeade	1 cup
Tang	1 cup
Wine*	½ cup

Frozen desserts

Fruit ice	½ cup
Juice bar (3 oz)	1 bar
Popsicle (3 oz)	1 bar
Sorbet	½ cup

🦴 *High phosphorus.*
*Check with your physician before using alcohol.

High-Calorie Choices—cont'd

Candy and sweets

Butter mints	14
Candy corn	20 or 1 oz
Chewy fruit snacks	1 pouch
Cranberry sauce or relish	¼ cup
Fruit chews	4
Fruit Roll Ups	2
Gumdrops	15 small
Hard candy	4 pieces
Honey	2 Tbsp
Jam or jelly	2 Tbsp
Jelly beans	10
LifeSavers or cough drops	12
Marmalade	2 Tbsp
Marshmallows	5 large
Sugar, brown or white	2 Tbsp
Sugar, powdered	3 Tbsp
Syrup	2 Tbsp

Special low-protein products

Ask your dietitian for information on how to obtain these products.

Low-protein gelled dessert	½ cup
Low-protein bread	1 slice
Low-protein cookies	2
Low-protein pasta	½ cup
Low-protein rusk	2 slices

The following foods are high in poor-quality protein and/or phosphorus. They should be used only when advised by your dietitian.

- Beer*
- Chocolate
- Nuts and nut butters

Salt Choices

Average per choice: 25 mg sodium

Salt	⅛ tsp
Seasoned salts (onion, garlic, etc)	⅛ tsp
Accent	¼ tsp
Barbecue sauce	2 Tbsp
Bouillon	⅓ cup
Chili sauce	1½ Tbsp
Dill pickle	⅙ large or ½ oz

Continued

*Check with your physician before using alcohol.

Salt Choices—cont'd

Ketchup	1½ Tbsp
Mustard	4 tsp
Olives, black	3 large or 1 oz
Olives, green	2 medium or ⅓ oz
Soy sauce	¾ tsp
Light soy sauce	1 tsp
Steak sauce	2½ tsp
Sweet pickle relish	2½ Tbsp
Taco sauce	2 Tbsp
Tamari sauce	¾ tsp
Teriyaki sauce	1¼ tsp
Worcestershire sauce	1 Tbsp

A Healthy Food Guide: Kidney Disease

Name: _____   _____ grams protein
Date:_____   _____ calories
Your dietitian is: _____   _____ milligrams phosphorus
Telephone number: _____   _____ milligrams sodium

Your Daily Meal Plan

Breakfast   Sample Menu   **Snack**   Sample Menu
Milk   ____ choices _____   ____ choices _____
Nondairy Milk Substitute   ____ choices _____   ____ choices _____
Meat   ____ choices _____
Starch   ____ choices _____   **Dinner**
Fruit   ____ choices _____   Milk   ____ choices _____
Fat   ____ choices _____   Nondairy Milk Substitute   ____ choices _____
High-Calorie   ____ choices _____   Meat   ____ choices _____
Salt   ____ choices _____   Starch   ____ choices _____
                                                                Vegetable   ____ choices _____
Snack   Fruit   ____ choices _____
                                                                Fat   ____ choices _____
                              ____ choices _____   High-Calorie   ____ choices _____
                              ____ choices _____   Salt   ____ choices _____

Lunch   **Snack**
Milk   ____ choices _____
Nondairy Milk Substitute   ____ choices _____   ____ choices _____
Meat   ____ choices _____   ____ choices _____
Starch   ____ choices _____
Vegetable   ____ choices _____
Fruit   ____ choices _____
Fat   ____ choices _____
High-Calorie   ____ choices _____
Salt   ____ choices _____

Foods High in Lactose, Purines, and Oxalates

LACTOSE CONTENT OF FOODS

Lactose contents are approximate, depending on portion size and product preparation. Foods not listed do not usually contain lactose. Most individuals can experiment with different lactose-containing foods to determine their level of tolerance. Although dairy products all contain lactose, processing reduces the lactose in some products.

High-Lactose Foods

Buttermilk
Cheesecake, cream pies
Cold cuts and hot dogs (some may contain varying amounts of lactose)
Cottage cheese (nonfat, low fat, regular)
Cream
Cream cheese
Cream or milk soups
Creamy sauces (white sauce, Alfredo sauce, vegetables au gratin)
Evaporated milk
Half and half
Ice cream (regular and low fat), ice milk, frozen yogurt
Milk (nonfat, skim, low fat, whole)
Milk-related products
Powdered milk
Pudding, custard
Ricotta cheese
Salad dressings with milk
Sour cream
Yogurt

Low-Lactose Foods

Aged cheese (cheddar, Swiss)
Butter/margarine
Commercial bread or cake products (bread, muffins, pancakes, waffles, biscuits)
Drug preparations (tablets) (may contain lactose as filler, but usually tolerated)
Lactose-reduced milk (nonfat, skim, low fat, whole)
Processed cheese (depending on milk solids added)
Processed foods containing dry milk solids or whey
Ready-to-eat cereals containing milk/lactose
Sherbet
Yogurt (may be tolerated)

From Nelson JK et al: *Mayo Clinic diet manual*, ed 7, St Louis, 1994, Mosby; and Dietary Department, University of Iowa Hospital and Clinics, Iowa City: *Recent advances in therapeutic diets*, ed 5, Ames, Iowa, 1996, Iowa State University Press.

PURINE CONTENT OF FOODS

High-Purine Foods: Content 150-825 mg/100 g

Fish/Seafood

Anchovies
Herring
Mackerel
Sardines
Scallops

Meats

Brains
Goose
Gravies
Kidney
Liver
Meat extracts
Sweetbreads
Wild game

Moderate-Purine Foods: Content 50-150 mg/100 g

Vegetables

Asparagus
Cauliflower
Green peas
Mushrooms
Spinach

Grains and Legumes

Legumes (split peas, beans, lentils)
Oatmeal
Wheat bran and germ
Whole grain breads and cereals

Fish/Seafood

Crabs
Eel
Fish (all kinds)
Lobsters
Oysters

Meats and Related Products

Beef
Lamb
Pork
Veal

Poultry

Chicken
Duck
Turkey

Low-Purine Foods: Content 0-50 mg/100 g

Beverages

Carbonated beverages
Coffee
Tea

Grains

Breads and cereals (refined white flour)

Dairy

Cheese
Milk (all fat levels)

Miscellaneous

Eggs
Fats
Fish roe
Fruits, fruit juices
Gelatin
Nuts
Sugars (all types) and sweet foods
Vegetables

OXALATE CONTENT OF FOODS

High-Oxalate Foods: >10 mg/Serving

Vegetables

Beans (wax, green, dried)
Beets
Cassava
Celery
Chives
Collards
Cucumbers
Dandelion greens
Green peppers
Okra
Parsley
Rutabagas
Spinach
Summer squash
Sweet potatoes
Swiss chard

Fruits and Juices

Blackberries
Blueberries
Citrus peel (lemon, lime, orange)
Fruit cocktail
Gooseberries
Grapes (purple/Concord)
Plums
Raspberries (black, red)
Red currants
Rhubarb
Strawberries
Tangerines

Starches/Breads

Amaranth
Bran
Breads
Fruit cake
Grits
Pasta
Soybean crackers
Wheat germ

Meat and Protein Sources

Baked beans (tomato sauce)
Tofu

Fats

Almonds
Cashews
Nut butters
Peanuts
Pecans
Sesame seeds
Tahini
Walnuts

Beverages

Beer
Chocolate milk
Cocoa
Coffee (instant)
Colas
Ovaltine
Tea

Others

Chocolate
Cocoa powder
Tomato soup
Vegetable soup

Appendix *L*

Cultural Dietary Patterns

CULTURAL FOODS

Foods specifically associated with these cultural groups are noted. Individuals may consume typical American foods as well; assumptions of dietary patterns cannot be made, but knowledge of these unique foods provides a common understanding of the range of possible food choices.

Native American

Each tribe may have specific foods; listed here are commonly consumed foods.

1. Bread, Cereal, Rice, and Pasta Group

Blue corn flour (ground dried blue corn kernels) used to make cornbread, mush dumplings; fruit dumplings (walakshi); fry bread (biscuit dough deep fried); ground sweet acorn; tortillas; wheat or rye used to make cornmeal and flours.

2. Vegetable Group

Cabbage, carrots, cassava, dandelion greens, eggplant, milkweed, onions, pumpkin, squash (all varieties), sweet and white potatoes, turnips, wild tullies (a tuber), yellow corn.

3. Fruit Group

Dried wild cherries and grapes; wild banana, berries, and yucca.

4. Milk, Yogurt, and Cheese Group

None.

5. Meat, Poultry, Fish, Dry Beans, Eggs, and Nuts Group

Duck, eggs, fish eggs (roe), geese, groundhog, kidney beans, lentils, nuts (all), peanuts, pine nuts, pinto beans, all nuts, venison, wild rabbit.

6. Fats, Oils, and Sweets

None.

African-American

1. Bread, Cereal, Rice, and Pasta Group

Biscuits, cornbread as spoon bread, cornpone or hush puppies, grits.

2. Vegetable Group

Leafy greens including dandelion greens, kale, mustard greens, collard greens, turnips.

3. Fruit Group

None.

4. Milk, Yogurt, and Cheese Group

Buttermilk.

5. Meat, Poultry, Fish, Dry Beans, Eggs, and Nuts Group

Pork and pork products, scrapple (cornmeal and pork), chitterlings (pork intestines), bacon, pig's feet, pig ears, souse, pork neck bones, fried meats and poultry, organ meats (kidney, liver, tongue, tripe), venison, rabbit, catfish, buffalo fish, mackerel, legumes (black-eyed peas, kidney, navy, chickpeas).

6. Fats, Oils, and Sweets

Lard.

Japanese

1. Bread, Cereal, Rice, and Pasta Group

Rice and rice products, rice flour (mochiko), noodles (comen/soba), seaweed around rice with or without fish (sushi).

2. Vegetable Group

Bamboo shoots (takenoko), burdock (gobo), cabbage (nappa), dried mushrooms (shiitake), eggplant, horseradish (wasabi), Japanese parsley (seri), lotus root (renkon), mustard greens, pickled cabbage (kimchee), pickled vegetables, seaweed (laver, nori, wakame, kombu), vegetable soup (mizutaki), white radish (daikon).

3. Fruit Group

Pear-like apple (nasi), persimimmons.

4. Milk, Yogurt, and Cheese Group

None.

5. Meat, Poultry, Fish, Dry Beans, Eggs, and Nuts Group

Fish and shellfish including dried fish with bones, raw fish (sashimi), and fish cake (kamaboko); soybeans as soybean curd (tofu), fermented soy bean paste (miso), and sprouts; red beans (azuki).

6. Fats, Oils, and Sweets

Soy and rice oil.

Chinese

1. Bread, Cereal, Rice, and Pasta Group

Rice and related products (flour, cakes, and noodles); noodles made from barley, corn, and millet; wheat and related products (breads, noodles, spaghetti, stuffed noodles [won ton] and filled buns [bow]).

2. Vegetable Group

Bamboo shoots; cabbage (napa); Chinese celery; Chinese parsley (coriander); Chinese turnips (lo bok); dried day lilies; dry fungus (Black Juda's ear); leafy green vegetables including kale, Chinese cress, Chinese mustard greens (gai choy), Chinese chard (bok choy), amaranth greens (yin choy), wolfberry leaves (gou gay), and Chinese broccoli (gai lan); lotus tubers; okra; snow peas; stir-fried vegetables (chow yuk); taro roots, white radish (daikon).

3. Fruit Group

Kumquat.

4. Milk, Yogurt, and Cheese Group

None.

5. Meat, Poultry, Fish, Dry Beans, Eggs, and Nuts Group

Fish and seafood (all kinds, dried and fresh), hen, legumes, nuts, organ meats, pigeon eggs, pork and pork products, soybean curd (tofu), steamed stuffed dumplings (dim sum).

6. Fats, Oils, and Sweets

Peanut, soy, sesame and rice oil; lard.

Filipino

1. Bread, Cereal, Rice, and Pasta Group

Noodles, rice, rice flour (mochiko), stuffed noodles (won ton), white bread (pan de sal).

2. Vegetable Group

Bamboo shoots, dark green leafy vegetables (malunggay and salvyot), eggplant, sweet potatoes (camotes), okra, palm, peppers, turnips, root crop (gabi).

3. Fruit Group

Avocado, bitter melon (ampalaya), guavas, jackfruit, limes, mangoes, papaya, pod fruit (tamarind), pomelos, tangelo (naranghita).

4. Milk, Yogurt, and Cheese Group

Custards.

5. Meat, Poultry, Fish, Dry Beans, Eggs, and Nuts Group

Fish in all forms; dried fish (dilis); egg roll (lumpia); fish sauce (alamang and bagoong); legumes such as mung beans, bean sprouts, chickpeas, organ meats (liver, heart, intestines); pork with chicken in soy sauce (adobo); pork sausage; soybean curd (tofu).

6. Fats, Oils, and Sweets

None.

Southeastern Asians: (Laos, Cambodia, Thailand, Vietnam, the Hmong, and the Mien)

1. Bread, Cereal, Rice, and Pasta Group

Rice (long and short grain) and related products such as noodles; Hmong cornbread or cake.

2. Vegetable Group

Bamboo shoots, broccoli, Chinese parsley (coriander), mustard greens, pickled vegetables, water chestnuts, Thai chili peppers.

3. Fruit Group

Apple pear (Asian pear), bitter melon, coconut cream and milk, guava, jackfruit, mango.

4. Milk, Yogurt, and Cheese Group

Sweetened condensed milk.

5. Meat, Poultry, Fish, Dry Beans, Eggs, and Nuts Group

Beef; chicken; deer; eggs; fish and shellfish (all kinds of freshwater and saltwater); legumes including black-eyed peas, peanuts, kidney beans, and soybeans; organ meats (liver, stomach); pork; rabbit; soybean curd (tofu).

6. Fats, Oils, and Sweets

Lard, peanut oil.

Mexican

1. Bread, Cereal, Rice, and Pasta Group

Corn and related products; taco shells (fried corn tortillas); tortillas (corn and flour); white bread.

2. Vegetable Group

Cactus (nopoles), chili peppers, salsa, tomatoes, yam-bean root (jicama), yucca root (cassava or manioc).

3. Fruit Group

Avocado, guacamole (mashed avocado, onion, cilantro [coriander], and chilies), papaya.

4. Milk, Yogurt, and Cheese Group

Cheese, flan, sour cream.

5. Meat, Poultry, Fish, Dry Beans, Eggs, and Nuts Group

Black or pinto beans (reijoles); refried beans (frijoles refritos); flour tortilla stuffed with beef, chicken, eggs, or beans (burrito); corn tortilla stuffed with chicken, cheese, or beef topped with chili sauce (enchilada); Mexican sausage (chorizo).

6. Fats, Oils, and Sweets

Bacon fat, lard (manteca), salt pork.

Puerto Rican and Cuban

1. Bread, Cereal, Rice, and Pasta Group

Rice; starchy green bananas, usually fried (plantain).

2. Vegetable Group

Beets, eggplant, tubers (yucca), white yams (boniato).

3. Fruit Group

Coconuts, guava, mango, oranges (sweet and sour), prune and mango paste.

4. Milk, Yogurt, and Cheese Group

Flan, hard cheese (queso de mano).

5. Meat, Poultry, Fish, Dry Beans, Eggs, and Nuts Group

Chicken, fish (all kinds and preparations including smoked, salted, canned, and fresh), legumes (all kinds especially black beans), pork (fried), sausage (chorizo).

6. Fats, Oils, and Sweets

Olive and peanut oil, lard.

Jewish

The foods below reflect both religious and cultural customs of Jewish people. Adherence to religious dietary patterns by followers of the different forms of Judaism (Orthodox, Conservative, Reform, and Reconstructionist) vary. Generally, Orthodox Jews and many Conservative Jews follow kosher dietary rules both when eating at home and when dining out. Others may only observe these rules when in their own homes. These rules of "keeping kosher" are reviewed in the next section on religious dietary patterns.

1. Bread, Cereal, Rice, and Pasta Group

Bagel, buckwheat groats (kasha), dumplings made with matzoh meal (matzoh balls or knaidelach), egg bread (challah), noodle or potato pudding (kugel), crepe filled with farmer cheese and/or fruit (blintz), unleavened bread or large cracker made with wheat flour and water (matzoh).

2. Vegetable Group

Potato pancakes (latkes); a vegetable stew made with sweet potatoes, carrots, prunes, and sometimes brisket (tzimmes); beet soup (borscht).

3. Fruit Group

None.

4. Milk, Yogurt, and Cheese Group

None.

5. Meat, Poultry, Fish, Dry Beans, Eggs, and Nuts Group

A mixture of fish formed into balls and poached (gefilte fish); smoked salmon (lox).

6. Fats, Oils, and Sweets

Chicken fat.

RELIGIOUS DIETARY PATTERNS

Beliefs of several major religions include practices that affect or prescribe specific dietary patterns or prohibit consumption of certain foods. Individuals practicing these religions may or may not adhere to all of the prescribed customs. A brief review of some of these practices follows.

Muslim

Pork and pork-related products are not eaten. Meats that are consumed must be slaughtered by prescribed rituals; these procedures are similar to the Judaic kosher slaughtering of animals, so Muslims may eat kosher meats. Coffee, tea, and alcohol are not consumed. During the month of Ramadan, Muslims fast during the day from dawn to sunset.

Christianity

Some sects may not eat meat on holy days; others prohibit alcohol consumption.

Hinduism

Animal foods of beef, pork, lamb, and poultry are not eaten. Followers are lacto-vegetarians or vegans.

Judaism

Food consumption is guided by religious doctrines; no pork or pork-related products nor seafood or fish without scales and fins are eaten. Dairy foods are not consumed with meat or animal-related foods (excludes fish). If meat or dairy is eaten, 6 hours must pass for the other to be acceptable for consumption. Animals are slaughtered according to a ritual in which blood is drained and the carcass is salted and rinsed; meat prepared in this manner is "kosher." The preparation of all processed foods eaten must also adhere to these guidelines. Because meat and dairy must not mix, two sets of dishes and utensils are used at home and in kosher restaurants. Foods that are neither meat nor dairy are called *parve* and are often so labeled by food manufacturers. Additional customs affect food consumption on Saturday, the Sabbath, during which no cooking occurs. Special foods are associated with each religious holiday. Fasting (no water or food) for 24 hours occurs during Yom Kippur (Day of Atonement). During Passover, an 8-day holiday, no leavened bread is consumed—only matzoh (made from flour and water) and products made from matzoh flour. Other symbolic food restrictions may also be observed.

Seventh Day Adventist

General restrictions of pork and pork-related products, shellfish, alcohol, coffee, and tea are followed. Some followers are ovo-lacto vegetarians, whereas others are vegans.

APPENDIX *M*

Activities Expenditure Table

Total Kcalories Burned for Each 1 Hour of Expenditure Item Using Body Weight Shown

Expenditure Description	Body Weight (lb)						
	100	125	150	175	200	225	250
Aerobics, easy	269	336	403	470	538	605	672
Aerobics, medium	278	348	418	487	557	626	696
Aerobics, hard	360	450	540	630	720	810	900
Archery	216	270	324	378	432	486	540
Assembly work, standing	132	164	197	230	263	296	329
Badminton, competition	389	486	583	680	778	875	972
Badminton, recreation	230	288	346	403	461	518	576
Bartending, standing	115	144	173	201	230	259	288
Baseball, pitcher	240	300	360	420	480	540	600
Baseball, player	187	234	281	328	374	421	468
Basketball, competition	394	492	591	689	787	886	984
Basketball, half-court	197	246	295	344	394	443	492
Basketball, moderate	283	354	425	496	566	637	708
Bathing, in tub	96	120	144	168	192	216	240
Bicycling (level) 13 mph	427	534	641	748	855	962	1068
Bicycling (level) 5.5 mph	202	252	302	353	403	454	504
Bowling, nonstop	269	336	403	470	538	605	672
Boxing, sparring	202	252	302	353	403	454	504
Calisthenics	202	252	302	353	403	454	504
Canoeing, 2.5 mph	110	138	166	193	221	248	276
Canoeing, 4.0 mph	283	354	425	496	566	637	708
Chambermaid	110	137	164	192	219	247	274
Childcare, general	138	173	207	242	276	311	345
Computer work, e-mailing, etc.	77	96	115	134	154	173	192
Construction, brick layer	359	449	539	628	718	808	898
Construction, carpentry	155	194	233	272	311	349	388
Construction, electrical/plumbing	150	187	224	262	299	336	374
Construction, painting, papering, etc.	169	212	254	297	339	381	424
Construction, remodeling, etc.	243	304	364	425	486	546	607
Construction, road building, laborers	276	345	415	484	553	622	691
Construction, shoveling, digging ditches	379	473	568	663	758	852	947
Cooking	86	108	130	151	173	194	216
Dance, fox-trot	178	222	266	311	355	400	444
Dance, modern, moderate	168	210	252	294	336	378	420

Developed by SureQuest Systems, Inc. Includes all of the activities listed in *Mosby's NutriTrac Nutrition Analysis CD-ROM, Version III,* which accompanies every copy of this text.

Total Kcalories Burned for Each 1 Hour of Expenditure Item Using Body Weight Shown—cont'd

Expenditure Description	Body Weight (lb)						
	100	125	150	175	200	225	250
Dance, modern, vigorous	226	282	338	395	451	508	564
Dance, rumba	278	348	418	487	557	626	696
Dance, square	274	342	410	479	547	616	684
Dance, waltz	206	258	310	361	413	464	516
Driving	62	78	94	109	125	140	156
Eating	62	78	94	109	125	140	156
Elliptical machine, moderate	303	379	455	531	607	683	758
Fencing, moderate	202	252	302	353	403	454	504
Fencing, vigorous	413	516	619	723	826	929	1032
Firefighter, fighting fires	517	646	775	904	1034	1163	1292
Fishing, general	157	196	235	274	313	352	391
Football, moderate	202	252	302	353	403	454	504
Football, vigorous	331	414	497	579	662	745	828
Frisbee	264	330	396	462	528	594	660
Golf, 2-some	216	270	324	378	432	486	540
Golf, 4-some	163	204	245	286	326	367	408
Hacky sack	158	197	237	276	316	355	395
Handball	389	486	583	680	778	875	972
Hiking, 40 lb pack, 3.0 mph	274	342	410	479	547	616	684
Hockey, field	360	450	540	630	720	810	900
Hockey, ice	380	475	570	665	760	855	950
Home gym equipment, general	267	334	401	468	535	602	669
Horseback riding, trot	269	336	403	470	538	605	672
Horseback riding, walk	134	168	202	235	269	302	336
Horseshoe pitching	144	180	216	252	288	324	360
Housecleaning	144	180	216	252	288	324	360
Hunting, general	201	251	301	351	402	452	502
Ironing, standing	103	128	154	180	205	231	256
Jai alai	544	680	816	952	1088	1224	1360
Jazzercise	283	353	424	495	566	636	707
Jet skiing	199	249	299	349	399	449	499
Jogging, 4.0-5.0 mph	302	377	453	528	604	679	755
Judo, karate	514	642	771	899	1027	1156	1284
Lacrosse	398	498	598	697	797	896	996
Lying at ease	58	72	86	101	115	130	144
Machine operator, standing	110	137	164	192	219	247	274
Marching, general	210	262	314	367	419	472	524
Marching band, drum major	164	205	245	286	327	368	409
Marching band, playing instrument	188	234	281	328	375	422	469
Masseuse	161	202	242	282	323	363	403
Meditation	62	78	94	109	125	140	156
Mountain climbing	403	504	605	706	806	907	1008
Movers, furniture, boxes, etc.	331	414	497	579	662	745	828
Mowing lawn, riding mower	115	144	173	202	231	260	288
Mowing lawn, walking, power mower	199	249	299	349	399	449	499
Office work, at desk	77	96	115	134	154	173	192
Paddle ball, racquetball	389	486	583	680	778	875	972
Playing instrument, drums	158	197	237	276	316	355	395
Playing instrument, general	113	141	170	198	226	255	283
Playing instrument, guitar	113	141	170	198	226	255	283
Playing instrument, piano	113	141	170	198	226	255	283
Police work, driving squad car	101	127	152	178	203	228	254
Pool, billiards	72	90	108	126	144	162	180
Racquetball	480	600	720	840	960	1080	1200
Raking leaves	170	213	255	298	341	383	426
Reading, sitting	70	87	105	122	140	157	175

Continued

Total Kcalories Burned for Each 1 Hour of Expenditure Item Using Body Weight Shown—cont'd

Expenditure Description	Body Weight (lb)						
	100	125	150	175	200	225	250
Rollerblading	312	390	468	546	624	702	780
Rope jumping, 110 rpm	389	486	583	680	778	875	972
Rope jumping, 120 rpm	370	462	555	647	739	832	924
Rope jumping, 130 rpm	346	432	518	605	691	778	864
Rowing, machine	547	684	821	958	1095	1232	1369
Rowing, recreation	202	252	302	353	403	454	504
Rugby	355	444	533	622	710	799	888
Running, 5-min mile, 12 mph	787	984	1181	1378	1575	1772	1969
Running, 7-min mile, 9 mph	629	786	943	1101	1258	1415	1572
Running, 8.5-min mile, 7 mph	562	702	843	983	1124	1264	1404
Running, 11-min mile, 5.5 mph	432	540	648	756	864	972	1080
Sailing	115	144	173	202	230	259	288
SCUBA diving	320	400	479	559	639	719	799
Shopping, grocery w/cart	153	192	230	268	306	345	383
Shopping, walking, nongrocery	108	136	163	190	217	244	271
Showering, towel drying	135	169	203	237	271	305	338
Sitting quietly	62	78	94	109	125	140	156
Skateboarding/scooter	202	252	302	353	403	454	504
Skating, ice	230	288	346	403	461	518	576
Skating, roller	413	516	619	723	826	929	1032
Skiing, downhill	389	486	583	680	778	875	972
Skiing, level, 5 mph	470	588	705	823	940	1058	1176
Skiing, racing downhill	658	822	987	1151	1316	1480	1645
Sleeping	48	60	72	84	96	108	120
Snorkeling	224	280	336	392	448	504	560
Snow shoeing, 2.3 mph	250	312	374	437	499	562	624
Snow shoeing, 2.5 mph	360	450	540	630	720	810	900
Snowboarding	261	326	391	457	522	587	652
Soccer	360	450	540	630	720	810	900
Softball	187	234	281	328	374	421	468
Sprinting	922	1152	1382	1613	1843	2074	2304
Squash	418	522	626	731	835	939	1044
Stair climbing and descending	384	480	576	672	768	864	960
Standing	72	90	108	126	144	162	180
Stationary running, 140 counts/min	979	1223	1468	1713	1958	2202	2447
Stretching, hatha yoga	158	197	237	276	316	355	395
Surfing	288	360	432	504	576	648	720
Swimming, back 20 yds/min	154	192	230	269	307	346	384
Swimming, back 30 yds/min	211	264	317	370	422	475	528

Total Kcalories Burned for Each 1 Hour of Expenditure Item Using Body Weight Shown—cont'd

Expenditure Description	Body Weight (lb)						
	100	125	150	175	200	225	250
Swimming, back 40 yds/min	336	420	504	588	672	756	840
Swimming, breast 20 yds/min	192	240	288	336	384	432	480
Swimming, breast 30 yds/min	288	360	432	504	576	648	720
Swimming, breast 40 yds/min	384	480	576	672	768	864	960
Swimming, butterfly 50 yds/min	470	588	705	823	940	1058	1176
Swimming, crawl 20 yds/min	192	240	288	336	384	432	480
Swimming, crawl 45 yds/min	350	438	526	613	701	789	876
Swimming, crawl 50 yds/min	427	534	641	748	855	962	1068
Swimming, pleasure 25 yds/min	240	300	360	420	480	540	600
Synchronized swimming	378	473	567	662	756	851	945
Table tennis, ping-pong	154	192	230	269	307	346	384
Talking, sitting	70	87	105	122	140	157	175
Tennis, competition	389	486	583	680	778	875	972
Tennis, recreation	278	348	418	487	557	626	696
Timed calisthenics	585	732	878	1024	1171	1317	1463
Volleyball, beach	389	486	583	680	778	875	972
Volleyball, casual, 6-9 team members	152	190	228	265	303	341	379
Volleyball, competitive, in gym	230	288	346	403	461	518	576
Walking, 110-120 steps/min	206	258	310	361	413	464	516
Walking, 2.0 mph	139	174	209	244	278	313	348
Walking, 4.5 mph	264	330	396	462	528	594	660
Walking, to work or class	158	197	237	276	316	355	395
Walking, with stroller	109	136	164	191	218	245	273
Washing car	199	249	299	349	399	449	499
Washing dishes, standing	103	128	154	180	205	231	256
Water aerobics	158	197	237	276	316	355	395
Water polo	454	567	681	794	908	1021	1135
Water skiing	312	390	468	546	624	702	780
Weight training	322	402	482	563	643	723	804
Wrestling	514	642	771	899	1027	1156	1284
Writing, sitting	77	96	115	134	154	173	192

Developed by SureQuest Systems, Inc. Includes all of the activities listed in *Mosby's NutriTrac Nutrition Analysis CD-ROM, Version III,* which accompanies every copy of this text.

NOTE: To determine kcalories used for more or less than 1 hour use the following formula:

Actual min/60 × Total kcalories used (from table above) = Actual kcalories burned

Example: Using "Aerobics, easy" for 150 lb body weight from table above

Actual minutes = 45

(45/60) × 403 = Total kcalories burned

.75 × 403 = 302 Total kcalories burned

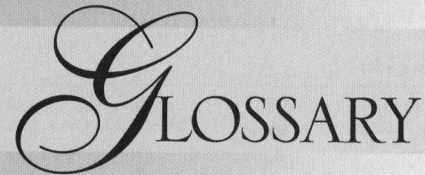

GLOSSARY

A

absorption the process by which substances pass through the intestinal mucosa into the blood or lymph

acanthosis nigricans hyperpigmentation and thickening of the skin into velvety irregular folds in the neck and flexural areas

acesulfame K a nonnutritive sweetener

acetyl coenzyme A (acetyl CoA) important intermediate by product in metabolism formed from the breakdown of glucose, fatty acids, and certain amino acids

acupuncture use of fine needles to open blockages of the flow of Qi, or life force, and restore balance

acute respiratory failure (ARF) sudden absence of respirations with confusion or unresponsiveness caused by obstructed air flow or failure of the pulmonary gas exchange mechanism

acute tubular necrosis (ATN) acute death of cells in the small tubules of the kidneys as a result of disease or injury

adaptive thermogenesis energy (or heat released) used by the body to adjust to changing physical and biologic environments

adenosine triphosphate (ATP) an energy-rich compound used for all energy-requiring processes in the body

Adequate Intake (AI) the approximate level of an average nutrient intake determined by observation of or experimentation with a particular group or population that appears to maintain good health

adipocytes cells specifically used for fat storage

adrenocorticotropic hormone (ACTH) an adrenal cortex hormone that stimulates secretion of more hormones

aerobic glycolysis the conversion of glucose to adenosine triphosphate (ATP) for energy when oxygen is available

aerobic pathway a form of energy production that depends on oxygen and increases the use of fat

aerophagia swallowing of air, usually the result of eating with the mouth open, followed by belching, gastric distress, or flatulence

alcoholic cirrhosis associated with chronic alcohol abuse; accounts for 50% of all cases; also called *Laënnec's cirrhosis*

aldosterone a hormone secreted by the adrenal gland in response to sodium levels in kidneys; helps kidneys balance fluid levels as needed

alternative medicine healing practices that replace conventional medical treatment

alternative sweeteners nonnutritive sweeteners (or artificial sweeteners) synthetically produced to be sweet-tasting but that provide no nutrients and few, if any, kcalories; examples are aspartame, saccharin, acesulfame K, and sucralose

amino acid pool the assortment of amino acids available to cells

amino acid score a simple measure of an amino acid composition of a food as compared with a reference protein; based on the limiting amino acid

amino acids organic compounds that contain carbon, hydrogen, oxygen, and nitrogen

aminopeptidase an intestinal peptidase that releases free amino acids from the amino end of short-chain peptides

amyloidosis a disorder characterized by accumulation of waxy starchlike glycoprotein (amyloid) in organs and tissues that affects function

anaerobic glycolysis the conversion of glucose to pyruvate to provide energy in the absence of oxygen

anaerobic pathway a form of energy production that does not require oxygen

anaphylaxis a severe immune system response to an allergen

anencephaly a congenital defect in which the brain does not develop; death occurs shortly after birth

angina pectoris chest pain that often radiates down the left arm and is frequently accompanied by a feeling of suffocation and impending death

anorexia nervosa a mental disorder characterized by self-imposed starvation; may include binge eating episodes associated with bulimic behaviors

antidiuretic hormone (ADH) a hormone secreted by the pituitary gland in response to low fluid levels; helps kidneys decrease excretion of water; also called *vasopressin*

antineoplastic therapy substance, procedure, or measure that prevents the proliferation of malignant cells; usually chemotherapy, radiation therapy, surgery, biologic response modifiers, or bone marrow transplantation

antioxidant a compound that guards other compounds from damaging oxidation

anuria excretion of less than 250 ml of urine every 24 hours

appetite desire for food

ariboflavinosis a group of symptoms associated with riboflavin deficiency

aromatherapy use of extracts or essences of herbs, flowers, and trees in the form of essential oils to support health and well-being

arteriosclerosis thickening, loss of elasticity, and calcification of arterial walls, which results in decreased blood supply

ascites abnormal intraperitoneal accumulation of fluid that contains large amounts of protein and electrolytes; usually results in swollen abdomen, hemodilution, edema, or decreased urinary output

aspartame a nonnutritive sweetener formed by bonding the amino acids of phenylalanine and aspartic acid

asthma a chronic respiratory disorder characterized by airway obstruction caused by excessive mucus production and respiratory mucosa edema; may be triggered by infection, cold air, vigorous exercise, stress, or inhalation of environmental allergens or pollutants

ataxia muscle weakness and loss of coordination

atherosclerosis development of lesions (also called *fatty streaks*) in the intima of arteries; during aging, the lesions develop into fibrous plaques that project into the vessel lumen and begin to disturb blood flow by blocking the arteries

athetoid purposeless weaving motions of the body or extremities

atonic lacking normal muscle tone

Ayurveda a system of healing focusing on diet and herbal remedies that emphasizes the use of body, mind, and spirit to prevent and treat disorders

azotemia retention of excessive amounts of nitrogenous compounds in the blood caused by the kidney's failure to remove urea from the blood; characterized by uremia

B

barium enema rectal infusion of a radiopaque contrast medium to diagnose obstruction, tumors, or other abnormalities (e.g., ulcerative colitis)

basal metabolism the amount of energy required to maintain life-sustaining activities for a specific period

beikost (pronounced BYE-cost) supplemental or weaning foods

beriberi a severe chronic deficiency of thiamine characterized by muscle weakness and pain, anorexia, mental disorientation, and tachycardia

beta cells insulin-producing cells situated in the islets of Langerhans of the pancreas

bezoars physical obstacles created by tangles of fibrous material in the gastrointestinal tract that may cause dangerous gastrointestinal obstructions

bile a substance that emulsifies fats to aid the digestion of lipids; produced by the liver and stored in the gallbladder

biliary atresia a congenital condition in which the major bile duct is blocked, limiting the availability of bile for fat digestion

biliary cirrhosis associated with obstruction of biliary drainage or biliary disorders; accounts for 15% of all cases

binge eating disorder (BED) a mental disorder characterized by frequent binge eating behaviors, not accompanied by purging or compensatory behaviors; commonly called *compulsive overeating*

bingeing feeling out of control when eating, which results in the consumption of excessive amounts of food

bioelectric impedance analysis (BIA) a method using a mild electric charge to estimate lean body mass to determine body fat composition

biofeedback use of special devices to convey physiologic information to enable a person to learn how to consciously control these medically important functions

biologic value a method to determine the quality of food protein by measuring the amount of nitrogen kept in the body after digestion and absorption

body mass index (BMI) a measure that describes relative weight for height and is significantly correlated with total body fat content

bolus a masticated lump or ball of food ready to be swallowed

branched-chain amino acids (BCAA) leucine, isoleucine, and valine

bulimia nervosa a mental disorder characterized as the binge and purge syndrome; includes experiencing repetitive food binges accompanied by purging or compensatory behaviors

C

cachexia general ill health and malnutrition, marked by weakness and emaciation

calcitonin a hormone that reacts in response to high blood levels of calcium; released by the special C cells of the thyroid gland

calcitriol active vitamin D hormone that raises blood calcium levels

calcium rigor a condition of hardness or stiffness of muscles when blood calcium levels get too high

calcium tetany a condition of spasms and nerve excitability when blood calcium levels get too low

cancer uncontrolled growth of cells that tend to invade surrounding tissue and metastasize to distant body sites

carbohydrates organic compounds composed of carbon, hydrogen, and oxygen

carboxypeptidase   a pancreatic protease that hydrolyzes polypeptides and dipeptides into amino acids

carcinogenesis   the process of cancer production

cardiac decompensation   impaired cardiac output (reasons not entirely understood)

cardiovascular endurance   the ability of the body to take in, deliver, and obtain oxygen for physical work

cheilosis   inflammation of the mucous membrane of the mouth and lips (angular stomatitis) caused by riboflavin and other B vitamin deficiencies

chemical digestion   the chemical altering effects of digestive secretions, gastric juices, and enzymes on food substance composition

chiropractic manipulation   a manipulation modality addressing the ties between body structure (particularly of the spine) and function and how those ties impact the maintenance and return to health

cholecystectomy   surgical removal of the gallbladder, performed to treat cholelithiasis and cholecystitis

cholecystitis   acute inflammation of the gallbladder associated with pain, tenderness, and fever

cholecystokinin-pancreozymin (CCK)   a hormone that initiates pancreatic exocrine secretions, acts against gastrin, and activates the gallbladder to release bile; secreted by the small intestine

choledocholithiasis   gallstones in the common bile duct

cholelithiasis   presence of stones in the gallbladder

chronic dieting syndrome   a lifestyle inhibited or controlled by a constant concern about food intake, body shape, or weight that affects an individual's physical and mental health status

chronic hunger   a continual experience of undernutrition

chronic obstructive pulmonary disease (COPD)   a progressive and irreversible condition identified by obstruction of air flow; chronic bronchitis, asthma, and emphysema (also called *chronic obstructive lung disease*)

chronic ulcerative colitis (CUC)   an inflammatory process confined to the mucosa of any or all of the large intestine

chylomicrons   the first lipoproteins formed after absorption of lipids from food

chyme   a semiliquid mixture of food mass

chymotrypsin   a pancreatic protease that hydrolyzes polypeptides into dipeptides

cis fatty acids   *cis* indicates the configuration of the double bond of fatty acids in a natural oil

coenzyme   a substance that activates an enzyme

colic   sharp visceral pain

colonoscopic examination   examination of the mucosal lining of the colon using a colonoscope (an elongated endoscope)

colostomy   a surgical creation of an artificial anus on the abdominal wall by incising the colon and bringing it out to the surface; may be single-barreled (one opening) or double-barreled (distal and proximal loops open onto the abdomen)

colostrum   the fluid secreted from the breast during late pregnancy and first few days postpartum; contains immunologic active substances (maternal antibodies) and essential nutrients

complementary and alternative medicine (CAM)   a cluster of medical and healthcare approaches, methods, and items not associated with conventional medicine

complementary medicine   non-Western healing approaches used at the same time as conventional medicine

complete protein   proteins containing all nine essential amino acids

complex carbohydrates   polysaccharides of starch and fiber

component puréeing   each food item is puréed separately (food thickeners may be added to help maintain consistency), then presented in a manner that resembles the original product (e.g., a pork chop can be puréed, then molded into a pork-chop shape and served)

computed tomography (CT)   an imaging technique for determining body fat composition

congestive heart failure (CHF)   circulatory congestion resulting in the heart's inability to maintain adequate blood supply to meet oxygen demands

constipation   straining to pass hard, dry stools; slow movement of feces through colon

cor pulmonale   an abnormal cardiac condition characterized by hypertrophy of the right ventricle as a result of hypertension of the pulmonary circulation

coronary artery disease (CAD)   a term used for several abnormal conditions that affect the arteries of the heart and produce various pathologic effects, especially reduced flow of oxygen and nutrients to the cardiac tissue

Crohn's disease   an inflammatory disorder that involves all layers of the intestinal wall and may involve small or large intestine or both; associated with stricture formation, fistulous tracts, and abscesses

cystic fibrosis (CF)   a genetic disorder in which excessive mucus is produced, primarily affecting respiratory airways; also limits fat absorption in the digestive system; most common among Caucasian populations

D

Daily Reference Values   a set of daily nutrient and food constituent values for which there are no Recommended Dietary Allowances (RDAs), including fat, fiber, cholesterol, and sodium (for food labeling only)

Daily Values (DVs)   a system for food labeling composed of two sets of reference values: Reference Daily Intakes and Daily Reference Values

deamination a process through which an amino group breaks off from an amino acid molecule, resulting in molecules of ammonia and keto acid

denatured a change in the shape of protein structures caused by heat, light, acids, alcohol, or mechanical actions

densitometry underwater weighing

diabetes mellitus (DM) a disorder of carbohydrate metabolism characterized by hyperglycemia caused by insulin that is either defective or deficient

diagnostic related groups (DRGs) classifications used to determine Medicare payments for inpatient care, based on primary and secondary diagnosis, primary and secondary procedures, age, and length of hospitalization

dialysate dialysis solution

dialysis a procedure that involves diffusion of particles from an area of high to lower concentration, osmosis of fluid across the membrane from an area of lesser to greater concentration of particles, and the ultrafiltration or movement of fluid across the membrane as a result of an artificially created pressure differential

diarrhea frequent passing of loose, watery bowel movements

diet manual the reference book (usually in a three-ring binder or on computer) used by nurses and dietitians that describes the rationale and indications for using a specific diet, lists the allowed and restricted foods, and provides sample menus

dietary fiber polysaccharides in plant foods that cannot be digested by humans

Dietary Reference Intakes (DRIs) dietary standards including Estimated Average Requirement (EAR), Recommended Dietary Allowance (RDA), Adequate Intake (AI), and Tolerable Upper Intake Level (UL)

dietary standards a guide to adequate nutrient intake levels against which to compare the nutrient values of foods consumed

dietary supplements substances consumed orally as an addition to dietary intake

digestion the process through which foods are broken down into smaller and smaller units to prepare nutrients for absorption

digestive system a series of organs that functions to prepare ingested nutrients for digestion and absorption

dipeptidase an intestinal peptidase that completes the hydrolysis of proteins to amino acids

disaccharides a sugar formed by two single carbohydrate units bound together; sucrose, maltose, and lactose are disaccharides

disease prevention the recognition of a danger to health that could be reduced or alleviated through specific actions or through changes in lifestyle behaviors

diverticula pouchlike herniations protruding from the muscular layer of the colon

diverticulitis inflammation of one or more diverticula

diverticulosis the presence of diverticula

dry beriberi thiamin deficiency affecting the nervous system, producing paralysis and extreme muscle wasting

dumping syndrome contents from the stomach empty too rapidly into the duodenum, causing symptoms of profuse sweating, nausea, dizziness, and weakness

durable power of attorney a legal document in which a competent adult authorizes another competent adult to make decisions for him or her in the event of incapacitation

dysphagia the inability to swallow normally or freely or to transfer liquid or solid foods from the oral cavity to the stomach; may be caused by an underlying central neurologic or isolated mechanical dysfunction

E

eating disorders a group of behaviors fueled by unresolved emotional conflicts, resulting in altered food consumption

edema excess accumulation of fluid in interstitial spaces caused by seepage from the circulatory system

edentulous toothless

eicosapentaenoic acid (EPA) the main omega-3 fatty acid in fish

elemental formula a solution that provides ready-to-absorb basic nutrients that require minimal digestion

emetic a substance that causes vomiting

emulsifier a substance that works by being soluble in water and fat at the same time

endogenous originating from within the body or produced internally

endometrium mucous membrane of the uterus

enrichment returning nutrients that were lost because of processing to their original levels

enteral nutrition administration of nourishment via the gastrointestinal tract

enteritis infection of the small intestine caused by a virus, bacteria, or protozoa

ergogenic aids drugs and dietary regimens believed by some (but not proven) to increase strength, power, and endurance

esophageal varices large and swollen veins at the lower end of the esophagus that are especially vulnerable to ulceration and hemorrhage, usually the result of portal hypertension

esophagitis inflammation of the lower esophagus

essential amino acids amino acids that cannot be manufactured by the human body

essential fat certain components of body fat that are essential for life

essential fatty acids (EFAs)   polyunsaturated fatty acids that cannot be made in the body and thus must be consumed in the diet

Estimated Average Requirement (EAR)   the amount of a nutrient needed to meet the basic requirements of half the individuals in a specific group; the basis for setting the Recommended Dietary Allowances (RDAs)

exocrine glands   glands that secrete chemicals into ducts that release into a cavity or to the surface of the body, such as the salivary glands (mouth) and the liver (gallbladder)

exogenous   originating outside the body or produced from external sources

extracellular fluid   all fluids outside cells including interstitial fluid, plasma, and watery components of body organs and substances

F

faith healing   healing by invoking divine intervention without the use of conventional or surgical therapy

fasting blood glucose   level of glucose circulating in blood serum after an 8-hour fast; also called *fasting blood sugar*

fatty infiltration   accumulation of fat (triglycerides) in the liver

feeding relationship   the interactions or patterns of behaviors surrounding food preparation and consumption within a family

fetal alcohol syndrome (FAS) or fetal alcohol spectrum disorders (FASD)   a disorder caused by alcohol consumption during pregnancy that produces a range of specific anatomic and central nervous system defects

flatus   intestinal gas

flexibility   the ability to move muscles to their full extent without injury

fluid volume deficit (FVD)   the state in which a person experiences vascular, cellular, or intracellular dehydration

fluid volume excess   the state in which a person experiences increased fluid retention and edema

fluorosis   a condition of mottling or brown spotting of the tooth enamel caused by excessive intake of fluoride

food allergy   the overreaction to a food protein or other large molecule producing an immune response

food choice   the specific foods that are convenient to choose when we are actually ready to eat

food intolerance   an adverse reaction to a food not involving the immune system

food liking   foods we really like to eat

food preferences   the foods we choose to eat when all foods are available at the same time and in the same quantity

fractionation   administration of radiation in smaller doses over time rather than in a single large dose; minimizes tissue damage

G

galactosemia   an autosomal recessive disorder resulting in an inability to metabolize galactose and lactose milk products

gastrin   a hormone that increases the release of gastric juices; secreted by stomach mucosa

gastroesophageal reflux disease (GERD)   return of gastric contents into the esophagus that results in a severe burning sensation under the sternum, commonly called heartburn; may be referred to as gastroesophageal reflux (GER) during early onset

gastrointestinal (GI) tract   the main organs of the digestive system that form a tube that runs from the mouth to the anus

gerontology   the study of aging

gestational diabetes mellitus (GDM)   a form of diabetes occurring during pregnancy, most commonly after the 20th week of gestation

glomerulonephritis   inflammation of the glomerulus of the kidney, characterized by proteinuria, hematuria, decreased urine production, and edema

glossitis   inflammation of the tongue

glucagon   a pancreatic hormone that releases glycogen from the liver

glucocorticoid   an adrenal cortex hormone that affects food metabolism

gluconeogenesis   the process that produces glucose from fat and protein

glycogen   carbohydrate energy stored in the liver and in muscles

glycogenesis   the process by which glucose is converted to glycogen

glycogenolysis   the process by which glycogen is converted back to glucose

glycolysis   the conversion of glucose to carbon compound

glycosylated hemoglobin (HgbA$_{1c}$)   a substance— glycohemoglobin—formed when hemoglobin combines with some of the glucose in the bloodstream

goiter   enlargement of the thyroid gland caused by iodine deficiency

H

hard water   water that contains high amounts of minerals such as calcium and magnesium

health   the merging and balancing of five physical and psychologic dimensions of health: physical, mental, emotional, social, and spiritual

health promotion strategies to increase the level of health of individuals, families, and communities

heme iron dietary iron found in animal foods (i.e., meat, fish, and poultry)

hemochromatosis a genetic disorder causing excessive dietary iron absorption characterized by excess iron deposits throughout the body

hemodialysis a procedure to remove impurities or wastes from the blood in treating renal insufficiency by shunting the blood from the body through a machine for diffusion and ultrafiltration and then returning it to the patient's circulation

hemodilution dilution of the blood

hemoglobin oxygen-transporting protein in red blood cells

hemosiderosis a condition in which too much iron is stored in the body

heparinized use of an antithrombin factor to prevent intravascular clotting

hepatic coma neuropsychiatric symptom of extensive liver damage caused by chronic or acute liver disease

hepatic encephalopathy a type of brain damage caused by liver disease and consequent ammonia intoxication

hepatotoxic potentially destructive to liver cells

hiatal hernia herniation of a portion of the stomach into the chest through the esophageal hiatus of the diaphragm

high-density lipoproteins (HDLs) lipoproteins that carry fats and cholesterol from body cells to the liver and are made of large proportions of proteins

high-quality protein a food containing the best balance and assortment of essential and nonessential amino acids for protein synthesis

homeopathic medicine an alternative medical system through which a small amount of a diluted substance is prescribed to relieve symptoms for which the same substance, given in larger amounts, will cause the same symptoms

homeostasis a state of physiologic equilibrium produced by a balance of functions and of chemical composition within an organism

hormones substances that act as messengers between organs to cause the release of needed secretions

hunger a physiologic need for food

hydrogenation breaking a double bond on a fatty acid carbon chain and saturating it with hydrogen

hydroxyapatite a natural mineral structure of bones and teeth

hyperbilirubinemia a neonatal condition of excessively high levels of bilirubin (red bile pigment) leading to jaundice, in which bile is deposited in tissues throughout the body

hypercaloric more than 1 kcalorie per ml

hypercholesterolemia total blood cholesterol levels greater than 200 mg/dl; greater than normal amounts of cholesterol in the blood; may be reduced or prevented by avoiding saturated fats

hyperemesis gravidarum severe and unrelenting vomiting in the second trimester of pregnancy that severely interferes with the mother's life; a serious condition usually requiring intravenous replacement of nutrients and fluids

hyperglycemia elevated blood glucose levels (>120 mg/dl)

hyperlipidemic excess lipids in the blood

hyperosmolar abnormally increased osmolarity

hyperplasia an increase in the number of cells occurring during the growth spurts that accompany normal development

hypertension an average systolic blood pressure greater than 140 mmHg and/or a diastolic pressure greater than 90 mmHg (or both)

hypertonic having greater concentration of solute than another solution

hypertrophy an increase in the size of cells

hypoglycemia blood glucose levels that are below normal values

hypogonadism a deficiency in the secretory activity of the ovary or testis

hypophosphatemia low serum phosphorus levels

hyporeflexia a neurologic condition characterized by weakened reflex reactions

hypoxia lack of oxygen to the cells

I

iatrogenic inadvertently caused by treatment or diagnostic procedure

idiopathic steatorrhea fat malabsorption as a result of unknown causes

ileostomy removal of entire colon and rectum; surgical formation of an opening of the ileum onto the surface of the abdomen, through which fecal matter is emptied

incidental additives substances that inadvertently contaminate processed foods

incomplete protein proteins lacking one or more of the essential amino acids

insensible perspiration water lost invisibly through evaporation from the lungs and skin

insoluble dietary fibers dietary fibers that do not dissolve in fluids

insulin   a hormone produced by the pancreas that regulates blood glucose levels

integrative medicine   merging of conventional medical therapies with complementary and alternative medicine (CAM) modalities for which safety and efficacy, based on scientific data, have been demonstrated

intentional food additives   substances purposely added to food products during manufacturing

interstitial fluid   fluid between the cells containing concentrations of sodium and chloride

intracellular fluid   fluid within the cells composed of water plus concentrations of potassium and phosphates

intrinsic factor   a substance produced by stomach mucosa that is required for vitamin B_{12} absorption

irradiation   a procedure by which food is exposed to radiation that destroys microorganisms, insect growth, and parasites that could spoil food or cause illness

ischemia   decreased or completely blocked blood supply to a body organ

isotonic   having the same concentration of solute as another solution; therefore, exerting the same amount of osmotic pressure as that solution

K

keratomalacia   a condition caused by vitamin A deficiency in which the cornea becomes dry and thickens from the formation of hard protein tissue

ketone bodies   a breakdown product of fatty acid catabolism

ketosis   a condition in which the absence of plasma glucose results in partial oxidation of fatty acids and the formation of excessive amounts of ketones

Kt/V   a measurement of adequacy and protein nutritional status

kwashiorkor   malnutrition caused by a lack of protein although adequate energy is consumed

L

lactation   the production of breast milk

lacto-vegetarian dietary pattern   a food plan consisting of only plant foods plus dairy products

lifestyle   a pattern of behaviors

limiting amino acid   the essential amino acid or amino acids that incomplete proteins lack

linoleic acid   an essential polyunsaturated fatty acid with the first double bond located at the sixth carbon atom from the omega end

lipogenesis   anabolism (synthesis) of lipids

lithotripsy   extracorporeal shock wave lithotripsy (ESWL), a noninvasive technique whereby high intensity shock waves cause fragmentation of kidney stones from a device outside the body

locus of control   the perception of one's ability to control life events and experiences

low birth weight   weighing less than 5.5 lbs (2500g) at birth

low-density lipoproteins (LDLs)   lipoproteins that carry fats and cholesterol to body cells and are made of large proportions of cholesterol

lupus erythematosus   a chronic inflammatory disease of unknown cause that affects many systems of the body; pathophysiology includes severe vasculitis, renal involvement, and lesions of the skin and nervous system

M

macrophages   cells that are able to surround, engulf, and digest microorganisms and cellular debris; big scavenger cells

macrosomia   larger body size

major minerals   essential nutrient minerals required daily in amounts of 100 mg or higher

malnutrition   an imbalanced nutrient or energy intake

marasmus   malnutrition caused by a lack of energy (kcalorie) intake

MCT fat (oil)   specialized modular formulas made of medium-chain triglycerides that do not require pancreatic lipase or bile for digestion and absorption; absorbed directly into the portal vein (like amino acids and monosaccharides) rather than the lymphatic system like other lipids

mechanical digestion   the crushing and twisting effects of teeth and peristalsis that divide foods into smaller pieces

medical nutrition therapy   (1) definition may be dictated by state laws licensing registered dietitians, but typically involves provision of nutrient, dietary, and nutrition education needs by a registered dietitian based on a comprehensive nutritional assessment; (2) the use of specific nutrition services to treat an illness, injury, or condition

meditation   a self-directed technique of relaxing the body and calming the mind

megacolon   massive, abnormal dilation of the colon that may be congenital, toxic, or acquired in nature

menopause   the end of menstruation because of the cessation of ovarian, follicular function

metabolism   a set of processes through which absorbed nutrients are used by the body for energy and to form and maintain body structures and functions

metastasis   the spread of malignant cells from the original tumor location to other sites

monosaccharides   a sugar composed of a single carbohydrate unit; glucose, fructose, and galactose are monosaccharides

monounsaturated fatty acid a fatty acid containing a carbon chain with one double bond

mucosa the inside gastrointestinal muscle tissue layer composed of mucous membrane

mucositis inflammation of mucous membranes

multifactorial phenotype a characteristic that is the product of numerous genetic and environmental factors

multiple organ dysfunction syndrome (MODS) the progressive failure of two or more organ systems at the same time (e.g., the renal, hepatic, cardiac, or respiratory systems)

muscular strength and endurance the ability of the muscles to perform hard work or prolonged work

muscularis a thick layer of muscle tissue surrounding the submucosa

myocardial infarction occlusion of a coronary artery; sometimes called *heart attack*

myoglobin oxygen-transporting protein in muscle

N

naturopathic medicine use of the body's natural healing forces to recover from disease and to achieve wellness; incorporates techniques from Eastern and Western traditions

nephrosclerosis necrosis of the renal arterioles, associated with hypertension

nephrotoxic toxic or destructive injury to a kidney

night blindness the inability of the eyes to readjust vision from bright to dim light as a result of vitamin A deficiency

nitrogen-balance studies measurement of the amount of nitrogen entering the body compared with the amount excreted

nocturia excessive urination at night

nonessential amino acids (NEAA) amino acids manufactured by the human body

nonheme iron dietary iron found in plant foods

nutrients substances in foods required by the body for energy, growth, maintenance, or repair

nutrition the study of essential nutrients and the processes by which nutrients are used by the body

nutritional risk the potential to become malnourished because of primary (inadequate intake of nutrients) or secondary (caused by disease or iatrogenic effects) factors

nutritional support although commonly used in reference to enteral and parenteral nutrition delivery systems, it can refer to any nutrition intervention used to minimize patient morbidity, mortality, and complications

nutritionist a professional who has completed graduate degrees of MS, EdD, or PhD in foods and nutrition

O

oliguria excretion of less than 400 ml urine every 24 hours

osmolality concentration of electrically charged particles per kilogram of solution

osmotic diarrhea diarrhea associated water retention in the large intestine resulting from an accumulation of non-absorbable water-soluble solutes

osteomalacia an adult disorder caused by vitamin D or calcium deficiency characterized by soft, demineralized bones

osteopathic medicine an approach based on the assumption that the systems of the body function together with disease stemming from the musculoskeletal system

osteoporosis a multifactorial disorder in which bone density is reduced and remaining bone is brittle and breaks easily

overnutrition consumption of too many nutrients and too much energy compared with Dietary Reference Intake (DRI) levels

ovo-lacto vegetarian dietary pattern a food plan consisting of only plant foods plus dairy products and eggs

oxygen debt the amount of oxygen required to clear lactic acid buildup from the body

oxytocin a hormone that initiates uterine contractions of labor and has a role in the ejection of milk during lactation

P

pancreatitis inflammation of the pancreas; may be acute or chronic

paralytic ileus decrease in or absence of intestinal peristalsis

parathormone a hormone that raises blood calcium levels; secreted by the parathyroid gland in response to low blood calcium levels

parenteral nutrition administration of nutrients by a route other than the gastrointestinal tract, usually intravenously

pellagra the deficiency disorder of niacin characterized by diarrhea, dermatitis, and dementia

pepsin the gastric protease

pepsinogen the inactive form of pepsin

percutaneous endoscopic placement placement of feeding tube into stomach via the esophagus and then drawing it through the abdominal skin using a stab incision

perimenopause the time before menopause during which hormonal, biologic, and clinical changes begin to occur

peristalsis the rhythmic contractions of muscles causing wavelike motions that move food down the gastrointestinal tract

peritoneal dialysis   a dialysis procedure performed to correct an imbalance of fluid or electrolytes in the blood or other wastes by using the peritoneum as the diffusible membrane

pernicious anemia   inadequate red blood cell formation caused by a lack of intrinsic factor in the stomach with which to absorb vitamin B_{12}

phenylketonuria (PKU)   a genetic disorder in which the body cannot break down excess phenylalanine

phospholipids   lipid compounds that form part of cell walls and act as a fat emulsifier

physical activity   any body movement produced by skeletal muscles that results in energy expenditure

physical fitness   the limits on the actions that the body is capable of making

phytochemicals   nonnutritive substances in plant-based foods that appear to have disease-fighting properties

pica   a condition characterized by a hunger and appetite for nonfood substances

plaque   deposits of fatty substances, including cholesterol, that attach to arterial walls

polydipsia   excessive thirst

polymeric formula   a solution that provides intact nutrients (e.g., whole proteins and long-chain triglycerides), which require a normally functioning gastrointestinal tract

polyphagia   excessive hunger and eating

polysaccharide   a carbohydrate consisting of many units of monosaccharides joined together; starch and fiber are food sources and glycogen is a storage form in the liver and muscles

polyunsaturated fatty acid (PUFA)   a fatty acid containing one or more double bonds on the carbon chain

polyuria   excessive urination

portal hypertension   increased blood pressure in the portal circulation caused by compression or occlusion in the portal or hepatic vascular system

postischemic   injury after decreased blood supply to a body organ or part

postnecrotic cirrhosis   associated with history of viral hepatitis, improperly treated hepatitis, or hepatic damage from toxic chemicals; accounts for about 20% of all cases

postprandial   occurring after a meal

pregnancy-induced hypertension (PIH)   a sudden rise in arterial blood pressure accompanied by rapid weight gain and marked edema during pregnancy; formerly known as *toxemia of pregnancy*

primary or essential hypertension   elevated blood pressure for which the cause is unknown

prolactin   a hormone responsible for milk synthesis

proteases   protein enzymes

protein efficiency ratio (PER)   a method to determine the quality of food protein by comparing weight gain with protein intake

protein-energy malnutrition (PEM)   malnutrition caused by the lack of protein, energy, or both

proteins   organic compounds formed from chains of amino acids

Q

Qi gong   a modality of Traditional Chinese Medicine that merges breathing regulation, movement, and meditation to increase the flow of Qi or life force in the body

R

reactant   a substance that enters into and is altered during a chemical reaction

recombinant erythropoietin (EPO)   recombinant human erythropoietin; drug used to treat anemia by replacing erythropoietin for patients with chronic renal failure who do not produce this hormone in adequate amounts

Recommended Dietary Allowance (RDA)   the level of nutrient intake sufficient to meet the needs of almost all healthy individuals of a life-stage and gender group

recumbent measures   measurements taken while the subject is lying down or reclining

refeeding syndrome   physiologic and metabolic complications associated with reintroducing nutrition (refeeding) too rapidly to a person with protein-energy malnutrition (PEM); these complications can include malabsorption, cardiac insufficiency, congestive heart failure, respiratory distress, convulsions, coma, and perhaps death

Reference Daily Intakes   a set of daily nutrient values for protein, vitamins, and minerals based on allowances of the 1968 Recommended Dietary Allowances (RDAs)

refined grains   grains that contain only some of the edible kernel

regional enteritis   Crohn's disease

registered dietitian (RD)   a professional trained in foods and the management of diets (dietetics) who is credentialed by the Commission on Dietetic Registration of the American Dietetic Association; credentialing is based on completing a bachelor's degree from an approved program, receiving clinical and administrative training, and passing a registration examination

reiki   an energy therapy based on the belief that by healing the patient's spirit, the physical body will also heal

renal transplantation   the transfer of a kidney from one person to another

respiratory distress syndrome (RDS)   a respiratory disorder identified by insufficient respiration and abnormally low levels of circulating oxygen in the blood

respiratory quotient (RQ)   ratio of CO_2 exhaled to O_2 inhaled; depending on the net metabolic needs of the body, the ratio ranges from 0.7 to 1.0 and averages around 0.8; carbohydrate metabolism produces an RQ = 1; protein metabolism RQ = 0.8; and fat metabolism RQ = 0.7

retrovirus   a ribonucleic acid (RNA) virus that becomes integrated into the deoxyribonucleic acid (DNA) of a host cell during replication; human immunodeficiency virus (HIV) is a retrovirus

rickets   a childhood disorder caused by vitamin D calcium deficiency leading to insufficient mineralization of bone and tooth matrix

S

saccharin   a nonnutritive sweetener

saliva   the secretions of the salivary glands of the mouth

saturated fatty acid   a fatty acid with carbon chains completely saturated or filled with hydrogen

scurvy   extreme vitamin C deficiency disorder characterized by inflammation of connective tissues, gingivitis, muscle degeneration, bruising, and hemorrhaging as the vascular system weakens

secondary hypertension   elevated blood pressure for which the cause can be identified

secretin   a hormone secreted by the small intestine that causes the pancreas to release bicarbonate to the small intestine

segmentation   the forward and backward muscular action that assists in controlling the mass movement of food through the gastrointestinal tract

senescence   older adulthood

sepsis   systemic infection

serosa   the outermost layer of the gastrointestinal wall, made of serous membrane

set point   a natural level (of some characteristic) that the body regulates or defends

simple carbohydrates   monosaccharides and disaccharides

small for gestational age (SGA)   having a lower birth weight than expected for the length of gestation

soft water   water that has been filtered to replace some of the minerals with sodium

soluble dietary fibers   dietary fibers that dissolve in fluids

solute   a substance dissolved in another substance

solvent   the liquid in which another substance (the solute) is dissolved to form a solution

somatic proteins   skeletal muscle proteins

somatostatin   a hormone produced by the pancreas and hypothalamus that inhibits insulin and glucagons

spina bifida   a congenital defect of the spinal column causing the spinal cord to be unprotected, resulting in a range of disabilities including paralysis and incontinence

steodystrophy   defective bone development associated with disturbances in calcium and phosphorus metabolism and renal insufficiency

sterols   fatlike class of lipids that serve vital functions in the body

stomatitis   inflammation of mucous membranes of the mouth

storage fat   layers and cushions of fat providing stored energy and protection from extremes of environmental temperatures; also protects internal organs against physical trauma

submucosa   a layer of connective muscle tissue under the mucosa

sucralose   a nonnutritive sweetener

sugar alcohols   nutritive sweeteners related to carbohydrates that provide 4 kcalories per gram; sorbitol, mannitol, and xylitol are sugar alcohols

T

tachycardia   rapid beating of the heart

TCA cycle   cellular reactions that liberate energy from fragments of carbohydrates, fats, and protein; also called the *tricarboxylic acid cycle* or *Krebs cycle*

teratogen   an agent capable of producing a malformation or a defect in the unborn fetus

therapeutic touch   an energy system based on the blockage of energy flow in and around the body

thermic effect of food (TEF) or diet-induced thermogenesis   an increase of cellular activity when food is eaten

third space (or third spacing)   refers to a condition in which fluid shifts from the blood into a body cavity or tissue where it is no longer available as circulating fluid

thrombosis   an abnormal vascular condition in which a blood clot (thrombus) develops within a blood vessel

thrombus   blood clot

thyrotoxicosis   iodine-induced goiter

Tolerable Upper Intake Level (UL)   the level of nutrient intake that should not be exceeded to prevent adverse health risks

trace minerals   essential nutrient minerals required daily in amounts less than or equal to 20 mg

trans fatty acids   fatty acids with unusual double-bond structures caused by hydrogenated unsaturated oils

triglycerides   the largest class of lipids found in food and body fat; composed of three fatty acids and one glycerol molecule

trypsin   the primary pancreatic protease

type 1 diabetes mellitus (DM)   a form of diabetes mellitus in which the pancreas produces no insulin at all

type 2 diabetes mellitus (DM)   a form of diabetes mellitus in which the pancreas produces some insulin that is defective and unable to serve the complete needs of the body

U

undernutrition   the underconsumption of energy or nutrients based on Recommended Dietary Allowance (RDA)/Dietary Reference Intake (DRI) values

unrefined grains   grains prepared for consumption that contain all edible portions of kernels

urea   product of ammonia conversion produced during deamination

uremia   excessive amounts of urea and other nitrogenous waste products in the blood

uremic toxicity   buildup of toxic waste products (urea and other nitrogenous waste products) in the blood; symptoms include anorexia, nausea, metallic taste in the mouth, irritability, confusion, lethargy, restlessness, and pruritus (itching)

V

vegan dietary pattern   a food plan consisting of only plant foods

very low-calorie diets (VLCDs)   usually defined as diets containing 800 kcalories a day or less

very low-density lipoproteins (VLDLs)   lipoproteins that carry fats and cholesterol to body cells and that are made of the largest proportions of cholesterol

villi   fingerlike projections on the walls of the small intestine

visceral fat   fat that is within the abdominal cavity

visceral protein stores   proteins contained in the internal organs

visceral proteins   proteins other than muscle tissue (e.g., internal organs and blood)

vitamin   essential organic molecules needed in very small amounts for cellular metabolism

vomiting   reverse peristalsis

W

wasting syndrome   an involuntary weight loss of more than 10% in 1 month with the presence of either chronic diarrhea, weakness, or fever for more than 30 days in the absence of a concurrent illness or condition

wellness   a lifestyle enhancing our level of health

Wernicke-Korsakoff syndrome   cerebral form of beriberi affecting the central nervous system

wet beriberi   thiamine deficiency with edema that affects cardiac function by weakening the heart muscle and vascular system

whole grain products   food items made using unrefined grains

Wilson's disease   a rare, inherited disorder of copper metabolism in which copper accumulates slowly in the liver and is then released and taken up in other parts of the body; as copper accumulates in red blood cells, hemolysis and hemolytic anemia occur

X

xerophthalmia   a condition caused by vitamin A deficiency ranging from night blindness to keratomalacia; may result in complete blindness

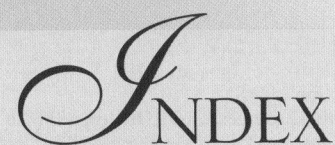

INDEX

Page numbers followed by "b" indicate boxes. Page
numbers followed by "f" indicate figures. Page numbers followed by "t" indicate tables.

Median Heights and Weights and Recommended Energy Intake, 10th Edition RDA

Category	Age (years) or Condition	Weight (kg)	Weight (lb)	Height (cm)	Height (in)	REE[a] (kcal/day)	Average Energy Allowance (kcal) Multiples of REE	Per kg	Per Day[b]
Infants	0.0-0.5	6	13	60	24	320		108	650
	0.5-1.0	9	20	71	28	500		98	850
Children	1-3	13	29	90	56	740		102	1300
	4-6	20	44	112	44	950		90	1800
	7-10	28	62	132	52	1130		70	2000
Males	11-14	45	99	157	62	1440	1.70	55	2500
	15-18	66	145	176	69	1760	1.67	45	3000
	19-24	72	160	177	70	1780	1.67	40	2900
	25-50	79	174	176	70	1800	1.60	37	2900
	51+	77	170	173	68	1530	1.50	30	2300
Females	11-14	46	101	157	62	1310	1.67	47	2200
	15-18	55	120	163	64	1370	1.60	40	2200
	19-24	58	128	164	65	1350	1.60	38	2200
	25-50	63	138	163	64	1380	1.55	36	2200
	51+	65	143	160	63	1280	1.50	30	1900
Pregnant	1st Trimester								+0
	2nd Trimester								+300
	3rd Trimester								+300
Lactating	1st 6 months								+500
	2nd 6 months								+500

From Recommended Dietary Allowances, 10th ed., © 1989 by the National Academies of Sciences. Published by the National Academies Press.

[a]Resting energy expenditure (REE); calculation based on FAQ equations, then rounded. This is the same as RMR.

[b]Figure is rounded.

Body Mass Index Chart*

Height (inches)	19	20	21	22	23	24	25	26	27	28	29	30	31	32	33	34	35
							Body Weight (pounds)										
58	91	96	100	105	110	115	119	124	129	134	138	143	148	153	158	162	167
59	94	99	104	109	114	119	124	128	133	138	143	148	153	158	163	168	173
60	97	102	107	112	118	123	128	133	138	143	148	153	158	163	168	174	179
61	100	106	111	116	122	127	132	137	143	148	153	158	164	169	174	180	185
62	104	109	115	120	126	131	136	142	147	153	158	164	169	175	180	186	191
63	107	113	118	124	130	135	141	146	152	158	163	169	175	180	186	191	197
64	110	116	122	128	134	140	145	151	157	163	169	174	180	186	192	197	204
65	114	120	126	132	138	144	150	156	162	168	174	180	186	192	198	204	210
66	118	124	130	136	142	148	155	161	167	173	179	186	192	198	204	210	216
67	121	127	134	140	146	153	159	166	172	178	185	191	198	204	211	217	223
68	125	131	138	144	151	158	164	171	177	184	190	197	203	210	216	223	230
69	128	135	142	149	155	162	169	176	182	189	196	203	209	216	223	230	236
70	132	139	146	153	160	167	174	181	188	195	202	209	216	222	229	236	243
71	136	143	150	157	165	172	179	186	193	200	208	215	222	229	236	243	250
72	140	147	154	162	169	177	184	191	199	206	213	221	228	235	242	250	258
73	144	151	159	166	174	182	189	197	204	212	219	227	235	242	250	257	265
74	148	155	163	171	179	186	194	202	210	218	225	233	241	249	256	264	272
75	152	160	168	176	184	192	200	208	216	224	232	240	248	256	264	272	279
76	156	164	172	180	189	197	205	213	221	230	238	246	254	263	271	279	287

*To use the table, find the appropriate height in the left-hand column. Move across to a given weight. The number at the top of the column is the BMI at that height and weight. Pounds have been rounded off. Additional BMI listed in Appendix E.

Modified from National Institutes of Health/National Heart, Lung, and Blood Institute: Clinical guidelines on the identification, evaluation, and treatment of overweight and obesity in adults: the evidence report, June 1998.

Key: Underweight = <19, Healthy Weight = 19-25, Overweight = 25-30, Obese = ≥30.